Noninvasive diagnostic techniques in vascular disease

Edited by

EUGENE F. BERNSTEIN, M.D., Ph.D.

Division of Vascular and Thoracic Surgery,
Scripps Clinic and Research Foundation,
La Jolla; Adjunct Professor of Surgery,
University of California, San Diego Medical Center,
San Diego, California

THIRD EDITION

With 688 illustrations,

including 2 color plates

The C. V. Mosby Company

ST. LOUIS • TORONTO • PRINCETON   1985

MOSBY

A TRADITION OF PUBLISHING EXCELLENCE

Editor: Carol Trumbold
Assistant editor: Anne Gunter
Editing supervisor: Elaine Steinborn
Manuscript editors: Barry Thornell, Carol Sullivan Wiseman
Book design: Jeanne Genz
Cover design: Suzanne Oberholtzer
Production: Carol O'Leary, Barbara Merritt, Ginny Douglas

THIRD EDITION

The C.V. Mosby Company
11830 Westline Industrial Drive, St. Louis, Missouri 63146

Library of Congress Cataloging in Publication Data

Main entry under title:

Noninvasive diagnostic techniques in vascular disease.

   Includes bibliographies and index.
   1. Blood-vessels—Diseases—Diagnosis.   2.   Diagnosis, Noninvasive.   I.   Bernstein, Eugene F., 1930-
[DNLM: 1. Vascular Diseases—diagnosis.   WG 500   N813]
RC691.6.N65N66   1985   616.1′3075   85-2974
ISBN 0-8016-0596-2

GW/MV/MV 9 8 7 6 5 4   01/B/083

To the conviction that
precise and quantitative diagnostic methods
have enriched our knowledge and helped the study of vascular disease
emerge as a scientific medical discipline

CONTRIBUTORS

ROBERT H. ACKERMAN, M.D.

Director, Carotid Evaluation Laboratory and Cerebral Blood Flow and Metabolism Laboratory, Massachusetts General Hospital, Boston, Massachusetts

NATHANIEL M. ALPERT, Ph.D.

Associate Applied Physicist, Division of Nuclear Medicine, Massachusetts General Hospital, Boston, Massachusetts

FREDERICK A. ANDERSON, Jr., Ph.D.

Assistant Professor, Department of Surgery, University of Massachusetts Medical Center, Worcester, Massachusetts

NICOS A. ANGELIDES, M.D., Ph.D.

Senior Consultant Vascular Surgeon; Director of Vascular Unit and Vascular Laboratory, Nicosia General Hospital, Nicosia, Cyprus

ROBERT W. BARNES, M.D.

Professor and Chairman, Department of Surgery, University of Arkansas for Medical Sciences; Surgical Service, McClellan Memorial Veterans Administration Medical Center, Little Rock, Arkansas

KIRK W. BEACH, Ph.D., M.D.

Research Associate Professor, Department of Surgery, University of Washington School of Medicine, Seattle, Washington

HENRY D. BERKOWITZ, M.D.

Associate Professor of Surgery, Department of Surgery, University of Pennsylvania; Director, Peripheral Vascular Laboratory, University of Pennsylvania Hospital, Philadelphia, Pennsylvania

EUGENE F. BERNSTEIN, M.D., Ph.D.

Division of Vascular and Thoracic Surgery, Scripps Clinic and Research Foundation, La Jolla; Adjunct Professor of Surgery, University of California, San Diego Medical Center, San Diego, California

EDWIN C. BROCKENBROUGH, M.D.

Clinical Professor of Surgery, University of Washington School of Medicine; Institute of Applied Physiology and Medicine, Seattle, Washington

NORMAN LESLIE BROWSE, M.D., F.R.C.S.

Professor of Surgery, Department of Surgery, St. Thomas' Hospital and Medical School, University of London, London, England

STEFAN A. CARTER, M.D., M.Sc.

Professor of Physiology and Medicine, Departments of Physiology and Medicine, University of Manitoba; Director, Vascular Laboratory, St. Boniface General Hospital, Winnipeg, Manitoba, Canada

ANTHONY J. COMEROTA, M.D.

Chief, Section of Vascular Surgery; Director, Vascular Laboratory; Assistant Professor, Department of Surgery, Temple University Hospital, Philadelphia, Pennsylvania

JOHN A. CORREIA, Ph.D.

Associate Professor of Radiology, Department of Radiology, Harvard Medical School and Massachusetts General Hospital, Boston, Massachusetts

JOHN J. CRANLEY, M.D.

Director of Medical Education; Director of Surgery; Director of Kachelmacher Memorial Laboratory for Venous Disease, Good Samaritan Hospital, Cincinnati, Ohio

RALPH B. DILLEY, M.D.

Head, Division of Vascular and Thoracic Surgery, Scripps Clinic and Research Foundation, La Jolla, California

BERT C. EIKELBOOM, M.D., Ph.D.

Consultant Surgeon; Director, Noninvasive Vascular Laboratory, St. Antonius Hospital, Utrecht, The Netherlands

ARNOST FRONEK, M.D., Ph.D.

Professor of Surgery and Bioengineering, University of California, San Diego Medical Center, San Diego, California

DON P. GIDDENS, Ph.D.

Regents' Professor, School of Aerospace Engineering, Georgia Institute of Technology, Atlanta, Georgia

DAVID GUR, Sc.D.

Professor of Radiology and Radiation Health, Department of Radiology, School of Medicine, Department of Radiation Health, Graduate School of Public Health, The University of Pittsburgh, Pittsburgh, Pennsylvania

RONALD D. HARRIS, M.D.

Head, Department of Radiology, Geisinger Clinic, Danville, Pennsylvania; Head, Tomography and Ultrasound, Scripps Clinic and Medical Institutions, La Jolla, California

WILLIAM G. HAYDEN, M.D.

Clinical Assistant Professor of Radiology (Cardiovascular), Stanford University School of Medicine, Stanford; Director, Noninvasive Vascular Laboratory, Sequoia Hospital, Redwood City, California

JACK HIRSH, M.D.

Professor and Chairman, Department of Medicine, McMaster University Medical Center, Hamilton, Ontario, Canada

RUSSELL D. HULL, M.B.B.S., M.Sc.

Associate Professor, Department of Medicine, McMaster University Medical Center, Hamilton, Ontario, Canada

KURT A. JÄGER, M.D.

Department of Internal Medicine/Angiology, University Hospital, Zurich, Switzerland

GARY R. JOHNSON, M.D.

Instructor in Medicine, Harvard Medical School; Member, Division of Peripheral Vascular Disease, New England Deaconess Hospital, Boston, Massachusetts

K. WAYNE JOHNSTON, M.D., F.R.C.S.(C), F.A.C.S.

Professor of Surgery and Biomedical Engineering, University of Toronto and the Toronto General Hospital, Toronto, Ontario, Canada

DARRELL N. JONES, Ph.D.

Department of Surgery, University of Colorado Health Sciences Center, Denver, Colorado

MARK M. KARTCHNER, M.D.

Medical Director, Vascular Laboratory, Tucson Medical Center, Tucson, Arizona

MAHMOOD S. KASSAM, M.A.Sc.

Research Associate, Institute of Biomedical Engineering, University of Toronto, Toronto, Ontario, Canada

J. PHILIP KISTLER, M.D.

Associate Professor of Neurology, Harvard Medical School; Assistant Neurologist, Massachusetts General Hospital, Boston, Massachusetts

RICHARD I. KITNEY, Ph.D.

Lecturer, Department of Electrical Engineering, Imperial College of Science and Technology, London, England

CYNTHIA A. KUPPER, B.S.N., R.V.T.

Clinical Assistant Professor, Department of Surgery, University of North Carolina; Supervisor, Peripheral Vascular Laboratory, North Carolina Memorial Hospital, Chapel Hill, North Carolina

YVES F. LANGLOIS, M.D., F.R.C.S.(C)

Fellow, Department of Surgery, University of Washington School of Medicine, Seattle, Washington

BO M.T. LANTZ, M.D.

Professor of Radiology; Chief, Section of Vascular and Interventional Radiology, Division of Diagnostic Radiology, School of Medicine, University of California, Davis Medical Center, Sacramento, California

NIELS A. LASSEN, M.D., Ph.D.

Chief, Department of Clinical Physiology, Bispebjerg Hospital, Copenhagen, Denmark

ROBERT S. LEES, M.D.

Professor of Cardiovascular Disease, Department of Applied Biological Sciences, Massachusetts Institute of Technology; Director of Medical Research and Head, Division of Peripheral Vascular Disease, New England Deaconess Hospital, Boston, Massachusetts

GEORGE R. LEOPOLD, M.D.

Professor of Radiology and Head, Division of Diagnostic Ultrasound, University of California, San Diego Medical Center, San Diego, California

JAMES M. MALONE, M.D.

Associate Professor Surgery, University of Arizona Health Sciences Center; Chief, Vascular Surgery, Tucson Veterans Administration, Tucson, Arizona

LORIN P. McRAE, Ph.D.

Technical Director, Vascular Laboratory, Tucson Medical Center, Tucson, Arizona

RICHARD D. MILES, Ph.D.

Biomedical Engineer; Assistant Professor, Department of Surgery, Southern Illinois University School of Medicine, Springfield, Illinois

ARNOLD MILLER, M.B., Ch.B., F.R.C.S.

Surgeon, Tel Hashomer Hospital, Tel Aviv, Israel

DERMOT J. MOORE, M.D., F.R.C.S.I.

Research Fellow in Vascular Surgery, Department of Peripheral Vascular Surgery, Southern Illinois University School of Medicine, Springfield, Illinois

WESLEY S. MOORE, M.D.

Professor and Chief, Section of Vascular Surgery, University of California at Los Angeles, Los Angeles, California

ANDREW N. NICOLAIDES, M.D., F.R.C.S.

Professor of Vascular Surgery, University of London; Academic Surgical Unit, Cardiovascular Unit and Irvine Laboratory for Cardiovascular Investigation, St. Mary's Hospital Medical School, London, England

STEEN L. NIELSEN, M.D., Ph.D.

Chief, Department of Clinical Physiology, Herlev Hospital, University of Copenhagen, Copenhagen, Denmark

M. LEE NIX, B.S.N., R.V.T.

Clinical Instructor, Department of Surgery; Director, Vascular Laboratory, University of Arkansas School for Medical Science, Little Rock, Arkansas

C. SCOTT NORRIS, M.D.

Resident in Surgery, University of Massachusetts Medical Center, Worcester, Massachusetts

CARL-GUSTAV OLSSON, M.D.

Physicist, Department of Clinical Physiology, University of Lund, Lund, Sweden

THERON W. OVITT, M.D.

Professor, Department of Radiology; Chief, Section of Cardiovascular Radiology, The University of Arizona Health Sciences Center, Tucson, Arizona

BILL C. PENNEY, Ph.D.

Research Associate, Department of Surgery, University of Massachusetts Medical School, Worcester, Massachusetts

DAVID J. PHILLIPS, Ph.D.

Research Assistant Professor, Departments of Surgery and Nuclear Medicine, University of Washington School of Medicine, Seattle, Washington

GERALD M. POHOST, M.D.

Professor, Department of Medicine, Division of Cardiovascular Disease, University of Alabama School of Medicine, Birmingham, Alabama

LUIS A. QUERAL, M.D.

Associate Professor of Surgery, University of Maryland Medical School, Baltimore, Maryland

JEFFREY K. RAINES, Ph.D., F.A.C.C.

Adjunct Professor of Surgery, University of Miami; Director, Vascular Laboratory, Miami Heart Institute, Miami, Florida

GARY E. RASKOB, B.Sc.

Research Associate, Department of Medicine, McMaster University, Hamilton, Ontario, Canada

RUSSELL C. REEVES, M.D.

Assistant Professor, Department of Medicine, Division of Cardiovascular Disease, University of Alabama School of Medicine, Birmingham, Alabama

H. J. RICKETTS, M.D.

Associate Professor of Radiology, Department of Radiology, University of Washington School of Medicine, Seattle, Washington

GHISLAINE O. ROEDERER, M.D.

Research Fellow, Department of Surgery, University of Washington School of Medicine, Seattle, Washington

JAMES B. RUSSELL, B.S.

Southern Illinois University School of Medicine, Springfield, Illinois

ROBERT B. RUTHERFORD, M.D.

Professor, Department of Surgery, University of Colorado Health Sciences Center, Denver, Colorado

MERRILL P. SPENCER, M.D.

Director, Institute of Applied Physiology and Medicine, Seattle, Washington

D. EUGENE STRANDNESS, Jr., M.D.

Professor of Surgery; Head, Section of Vascular Surgery, University of Washington School of Medicine, Seattle, Washington

DAVID S. SUMNER, M.D.

Professor of Surgery and Chief, Section of Peripheral Vascular Surgery, Department of Surgery, Southern Illinois University School of Medicine, Springfield, Illinois

THORALF M. SUNDT, Jr., M.D.

Professor and Chairman, Department of Neurosurgery, Mayo Clinic and Medical School, Rochester, Minnesota

BRIAN L. THIELE, M.D.

Professor of Surgery, Department of Surgery, The Pennsylvania State University College of Medicine, The Milton S. Hershey Medical Center, Hershey, Pennsylvania

MARTIN H. THOMAS, M.D.

Consultant Surgeon, St. Peter's Hospital, Chertsey, Surrey, United Kingdom

OLAV THULESIUS, M.D., Ph.D.

Professor, Medical Faculty, Kuwait University, Kuwait

H. BROWNELL WHEELER, M.D.

Professor and Chairman, Department of Surgery, University of Massachusetts Medical School, Worcester, Massachusetts

DENIS N. WHITE, M.D.

Professor Emeritus, Queens University at Kingston, Kingston, Ontario, Canada

KATHRYN F. WITZTUM, M.D.

Assistant Professor, Department of Radiology, Nuclear Medicine Division, University of California, San Diego School of Medicine; Chief, Nuclear Medicine Service, Veterans Administration Medical Center, La Jolla, California

SIDNEY K. WOLFSON, Jr., M.D.

Professor of Neurological Surgery, Department of Neurological Surgery, University of Pittsburgh School of Medicine, Pittsburgh, Pennsylvania

JAMES S.T. YAO, M.D., Ph.D.

Professor of Surgery, Director, Blood Flow Laboratory, Northwestern University Medical School, Chicago, Illinois

HOWARD YONAS, M.D.

Associate Professor of Neurological Surgery, Department of Neurological Surgery, University of Pittsburgh School of Medicine, Pittsburgh, Pennsylvania

R. EUGENE ZIERLER, M.D.

Assistant Professor of Surgery, University of Washington School of Medicine; Chief, Vascular Surgery Section, Seattle Veterans Administration Medical Center, Seattle, Washington

P. ZUECH, M.A. Sc.

Research Associate, Institute of Biomedical Engineering, University of Toronto, Toronto, Ontario, Canada

PREFACE

This book was originally conceived in 1976 at a meeting in Marseilles, France, when it became clear that a new and exciting field of noninvasive vascular diagnosis had been created by the almost simultaneous development of several applications of ultrasound and plethysmography. The first edition, published in 1978, attempted to survey the emerging field by asking the principal authors of each new approach to describe their methods, with editorial comments focusing on controversial issues.

The rapid expansion of the field during the next several years, in terms of both new modalities and new applications, appeared to justify the second edition, published in 1982. By that time interest in noninvasive vascular technology had spread from the few early pioneers, mostly vascular surgeons, to a much broader group of physicians, including neurologists, radiologists, cardiologists, and internists. In addition, an entire corps of vascular technologists had evolved, a number of whom participated in the subsequent development of new and important applications of diagnostic equipment. Most significant at this time was the development of vascular imaging techniques, including the Duplex scanner. Also, investigators who were not involved in the original development of noninvasive technology were able to provide thoughtful and objective evaluations of some of the earlier methods.

Now another level of maturity and technologic advancement has been reached. As a result, approximately 50 chapters of the current edition are new or radically revised. Not only the development of better methods, but also the changing indications for earlier techniques must be placed into proper perspective for the volume to remain a state-of-the-art resource for both the practicing clinician and the research investigator. Thus many modalities are now described by new authors, selected because of their experience with and comparative knowledge of alternative or supplementary approaches. In addition, a growing body of information that has been learned from the careful application of noninvasive methodology has been included in this volume.

Fortunately, the original editors, including Drs. Robert W. Barnes, Ralph B. Dilley, George R. Leopold, D. Eugene Strandness, and James S.T. Yao, who contributed so much to the first edition and were joined by Dr. Arnost Fronek in helping prepare the second edition, have continued their active roles in the planning, writing, and editing of this edition. If we have succeeded in presenting a comprehensive and balanced view of the topic, it is because of the willingness of these editors to contribute so generously of their time and knowledge. In addition, the number of contributors and their increasingly diverse backgrounds have added immeasurably to the breadth of the volume. To these contributors and their staffs the editors wish to express their most sincere appreciation. We also would like to acknowledge our pleasure in being able to work with the very capable staff of The C.V. Mosby Company, and in particular with our editors, Carol Trumbold, Anne Gunter, and Elaine Steinborn.

Eugene F. Bernstein

CONTENTS

COLOR PLATES

Noninvasive diagnostic techniques
in vascular disease

CHAPTER 1

Introduction

EUGENE F. BERNSTEIN

Within the past decade noninvasive vascular technology has emerged from the research laboratory and become an accepted method of assessing vascular disease throughout the world. Before 1970 a few pioneers were using specialized devices or methods that they had developed in their own laboratories for isolated measurements of vascular functions. The strain gauge and other plethysmographs were available to evaluate pulsation and the filling and emptying of vessels in the extremities. Rarely, physicians measured blood pressure in the legs. However, the true impetus for the expansion of the field was associated with the development of ultrasound, because both the imaging and the Doppler effect modalities provided significant new insight into vascular conditions.

In the early 1960s the Doppler effect, which detects the velocity of moving particles, was being studied using only the audio output. Scanning with the Doppler systems involved learning to listen to signals from normal and diseased vessels, both arterial and venous, and assessing changes in velocity caused by stenosis or turbulence. Although this information was indeed useful and the technique was picked up in several centers, the method was too subjective and too difficult to learn to attract the busy physician interested in vascular disease.

A- and then B-mode ultrasound for the evaluation of abdominal aortic aneurysms was a significant noninvasive vascular imaging modality used to obtain pertinent clinical information as early as 1970. At that time ultrasound was the only accurate means of studying the external size of aneurysms, which offered invaluable insight into the clinical management of the condition.

The development of two oculoplethysmographic instruments, by Kartchner and Gee, further stimulated the mid-1970s explosion of noninvasive

technology. These systems provided simple means of noninvasive detection of carotid artery stenosis. They were based on the detection of diminished pulsations, or blood pressure, in the orbit of the eye, could be applied by a technician, and justified the development of new laboratory facilities dedicated to vascular screening. In addition the introduction of impedance plethysmography and the pulse volume recorder demonstrated the usefulness of volumetric techniques in the evaluation of peripheral venous and arterial disease. As it became clear that the information obtained from the vascular laboratory was unique and clinically significant and new instruments and methods were introduced, the technology mushroomed and the number of vascular laboratories grew to the present estimate of 1500 in the United States alone.

CURRENT ROLE OF VASCULAR LABORATORY

By the early 1980s the vascular laboratory had achieved a firm role in the management of vascular disease in most major medical institutions. It is a facility akin to the pulmonary function laboratory or the cardiac catheterization suite, where special expertise can be brought to bear on various aspects of vascular disease and can provide functional and hemodynamic information as well as the anatomic location of most vascular problems. The specific role of the laboratory in each of the major clinical conditions is detailed in subsequent chapters of this volume, but it is fair to say that the major functions of the laboratory include detection and documentation of vascular disease, characterization of obstruction and its functional significance, localization of its anatomic site, confirmation of appropriate indications for angiography in questionable cases, and evaluation of the results of treatment. In addition, the surgeon has developed a special reliance on vascular laboratory data for evaluating asymptomatic carotid disease, multilevel peripheral arterial disease, intraoperative monitoring, and postoperative screening. Finally, laboratory data can be the basis for objective epidemiologic studies. In each of these areas the vascular laboratory provides information not otherwise readily available by noninvasive methods.

NEW TECHNOLOGY

Since publication of the second edition of this book in 1982 the field of vascular technology has continued to grow rapidly. Thus the justification for this third edition is sufficient new material to fill approximately 50 chapters. The new technology includes more information on the fundamentals of blood flow disturbances, Doppler signal processing and waveform analysis, and particularly spectral analysis. In addition, information regarding the proper selection of Doppler instrumentation and pitfalls regarding the use of such devices is available. The older techniques of ocular plethysmography and ocular pneumoplethysmography are still useful for certain applications but have been superseded by the entirely new technology of direct carotid evaluation. Additional radioisotopic methods, for use in both the brain and the extremities, are also increasing our ability to measure blood flow semiinvasively.

Perhaps the greatest advance in vascular laboratory technology in the mid-1980s, however, is in the area of vascular imaging. Data regarding the place of digital subtraction angiography, which at one point was considered a competitor but now is appreciated as a supplement to the vascular laboratory examination, are well detailed in two new chapters, as are the relative values of quantitative angiographic techniques and the exciting new fields of positron emission tomography and nuclear magnetic resonance, both of which offer the promise of new, wonderfully sensitive, and physiologically relevant imaging techniques that will have a significant place in the study of vascular disease both for research and clinical purposes. In addition, the intraoperative ultrasonic assessment of vascular surgery is rapidly becoming an important adjunct in assuring a technically acceptable procedure, which is the first prerequisite in minimizing postoperative problems.

More sophisticated vascular laboratory functions and the increasing volume of patient examinations have also mandated the use of the computer for both analytic and bookkeeping purposes. In addition, computer programs offer an opportunity for standardization of testing, classifying, and reporting data, which may permit the development of more generalized agreement and therefore universal usefulness of vascular laboratory measurements. An entirely new data base derived from the vascular laboratory now permits discussion of the evolution of carotid arterial disease in asymptomatic patients, the risks of asymptomatic carotid disease with various surgical procedures, and the natural outcome of such disease on the side not operated on in association with a carotid endarterectomy.

In peripheral arterial disease, too, new technology and new information have dictated the inclusion of information regarding isotope technology, the prediction of amputation level healing, and monitoring the results of reconstructive arterial surgery. Applications of the duplex scanner to peripheral arterial disease promise to resolve some of the persisting problems in evaluation of multilevel disease above and below the common femoral artery. The value of postoperative screening of peripheral arterial disease is clearly documented, as is its usefulness as an indication for subsequent angioplasty or reoperation in the still asymptomatic patient with clinically silent recurrent stenosis. In addition, entirely new areas of testing have emerged in the important areas of renal arterial stenosis and impotence.

The noninvasive evaluation of peripheral venous disease was initially confined to the detection and evaluation of acute deep venous thrombosis. More recently, additional techniques, including thermography and newer isotope methods, have been applied to this problem. In addition, adequate data are now available to permit firm conclusions regarding the cost-benefit value of screening asymptomatic patients for deep venous thrombosis as well as the accepted indications for studying symptomatic patients. Information regarding tests that can be used to study chronic venous insufficiency promises help in assessment of this difficult disorder, particularly with respect to the newer surgical techniques now available for the repair of chronic venous valve insufficiency and venous obstruction.

The technology is growing, not only in the availability of new instrumentation and techniques but also in the accumulation of useful information based on reproducible and objective data. This expanded body of knowledge regarding vascular disease has been obtained from and is centralized in the files of the noninvasive vascular laboratories.

MEDICAL AND TECHNICAL SPECIALITIES

In the development of any new technical area of expertise, a core of specialists who are skilled in the application and interpretation of the methods emerges. With the exception of central Europe, where angiology has long been a well-recognized medical specialty, vascular disease has not been a recognized area of medical specialization. Except in a few large institutions, in the United States internists interested primarily in vascular disease have been rare. However, the development of the vascular laboratory and the knowledge necessary for its proper application have stimulated a new generation of physicians to become seriously involved in the study of vascular disease. This group was originally recruited from the ranks of vascular surgery, where most clinical knowledge regarding these conditions existed. However, as the laboratories began to have a greater impact in other areas of medicine and to consume more of the supervising physician's time and energy, physicians were recruited from neurology, radiology, ultrasound, cardiology, and internal medicine. In many institutions these laboratories still serve a secondary function and the physicians continue to perform their primary roles; in others, however, the vascular laboratory is becoming so important and busy that a full-time commitment to its operation is essential. Thus because of the emergence of the laboratory as an important and valuable resource, a new specialty of vascular medicine is developing centered about the clinical and quantitative evaluation of vascular disease. It seems only logical that this evolution will soon result in the development of a bona fide, well-rounded medical specialty for the evaluation of patients with vascular disease and their treatment by nonsurgical modalities. The development of such a group of physicians is also important and desirable for the vascular surgical fraternity, because the availability of such medical colleagues with clinical expertise and sophistication will ease the referral of many patients for study and treatment by physicians who are now reluctant to refer directly to surgeons. In addition, such full-time devotion to the study of vascular disease can

only increase the quality of information and expertise that can be applied to patient care.

The new technology of noninvasive vascular instrumentation also necessitates special training for those responsible for the operation and application of the machines: the technician or technologist. Thus the Society for Noninvasive Vascular Technologists was born at a symposium in San Diego in 1976, which was the first major meeting in the United States devoted to this area. This group of technicians and technologists rapidly matured and developed standards of training and certification, means for the dissemination of information, programs for continuing education, and all of the other activities relevant to a separate profession. The important role of the technologists in the vascular laboratory is well defined and is critical to its proper operation. Clearly, technologists have progressed more rapidly than physicians in developing a separate discipline that formally defines their area of expertise.

PROBLEMS

Perhaps the most important problem facing existing vascular laboratories is the lack of standard methods of investigation, data evaluation, and reporting. The measurement of a serum sodium level or pulmonary artery wedge pressure is so universal in its reliability, the units used, and the reproducibility of the data that studies performed in any quality laboratory can be fully accepted by physicians in another practice setting. This is not true for vascular laboratories, where local routines have evolved based on selection of instrumentation, evaluation procedures, and data analysis systems, with a great variety in quality and completeness. Thus data transfer from laboratory to laboratory, as well as from time to time, remains difficult, imprecise, and unreliable.

A second problem facing the continuing development of vascular technology is the need for objective study of new devices, which continue to be introduced. Methodical study by interested but unbiased observers occupies a large fraction of the investigative energy in this field and is most appropriate. As a result, this volume is able to place in proper perspective a number of noninvasive techniques that have progressed from early enthusiasm to a documented level of usefulness and reliability.

Many additional problems face us in new and

as yet unexplored areas, including evaluation of the regional cerebral arterial circulation, noninvasive studies of the interior of the thoracic and abdominal aorta and visceral arterial branches for functionally and anatomically important lesions, differentiation between the relative importance of venous obstruction and valvular insufficiency, and myriad other clinically important subjects. The field is still young, with great promise for the future and much room for evolution and development. Yet its scientific basis is firm, it has rapidly become an accepted methodology, and it is clear that the vascular laboratory has become the central core of a new and rapidly evolving medical specialty devoted to the study and care of vascular disease.

CHAPTER 2

Validation and classification

D. EUGENE STRANDNESS, Jr.

The noninvasive laboratory has now entered into the practice of medicine in a significant way. One only need visit the commercial exhibits at national and regional meetings to sense the economic impact this relatively new discipline has in terms of our approach to vascular disease. In addition, the organization of the Society of Noninvasive Technologists is clear proof of the growth of the field. However, rapid growth, much like adolescence, introduces new problems, some of which can be anticipated but others of which can catch us entirely by surprise.

VALIDATION

The introduction of a new testing procedure requires validation by the best available standard diagnostic procedure. In the field of noninvasive testing this has traditionally been arteriography. With this approach, anatomic findings are used to verify the results of testing procedures designed to detect physiologic abnormalities. Enough experience has accumulated to review this approach for a variety of testing procedures and draw some conclusions concerning results. Before reviewing examples, it is important to restate a few essential principles for validation of a new test. The new procedure and that used as the standard should be interpreted independently of each other *without* prior knowledge of the other test result. In addition, the tests used for validation must be interpreted by an individual not concerned with the development or application of the noninvasive test. These are the only ways that bias can be avoided. If these approaches had been routinely followed in the evaluation of new procedures, some of the confusion that currently exists could have been avoided or at least minimized.

Another, almost universal occurrence when new tests are introduced is the considerable variability in accuracy reported by different authors. Why? Those scientists who develop new methods are usually enthusiastic and often report the results at an early stage before all the pitfalls of the procedure are appreciated. In addition, they often understand the method very well and often do not present all the nuances required for best performance and interpretation of the test. Thus the early, often glowing results tempt the uninitiated to use the technique before its application is completely understood. This sets the stage for confusion and may delay the implementation of a worthwhile test. On the other hand, even if the test is worthless, this does not mean it will not be used. Unfortunately, there are many examples of this.

To put the problems associated with validation in proper perspective, I would like to review a few situations in which it has worked successfully and the dilemmas we face in other areas that remain controversial even at the present time.

Acute venous thrombosis

Acute venous thrombosis has been recognized since antiquity, but it was not until 1940 that we began to appreciate how this disease could be documented by phlebography.[3] The classic work by Gunnar Bauer described in rather exquisite detail the diagnostic findings associated with this prevalent disorder. It is unfortunate, however, that Bauer himself did not appreciate the importance of this diagnostic technique. In fact, as late as 1957 he stated that the bedside diagnosis of venous thrombosis was sufficiently accurate and that phlebography was not necessary.[4] With the passage of time the medical community slowly began to realize that the clinical findings were so nonspecific that the diagnosis often had to be verified by some independent test, the best being phlebography.[11]

As with most invasive procedures, there are occasional serious complications. In the case of phlebography the patients quickly informed us of associated discomfort, and physicians became aware of the danger of contrast medium–induced "phlebitis." These problems, combined with the poor accuracy of the bedside diagnosis, set the stage for noninvasive testing. The use of noninvasive testing began when Dahn and Eiriksson introduced the use of plethysmography as another diagnostic method for this disorder.[9] In 1972 we reported the initial use of Doppler ultrasound for the diagnosis of acute venous thromboses.[17]

From this time forward, progress was rapid as more investigators became involved, and the end result tells an excellent success story. As the newer approaches such as impedance plethysmography[22] and phleborheography were introduced,[8] the validity of the methods were clearly documented and have come to occupy an important place in our diagnostic armamentarium. At the present time it is accepted that it is not only safe but proper and cost-effective to evaluate patients suspected of having deep vein thrombosis by noninvasive means. Thus most patients can be spared a painful procedure that may result in serious complications.

Peripheral arterial disease

The progress in diagnosis of peripheral arterial disease has been equally rapid, but some areas still remain controversial. Here the problem has not been so much a matter of validation as one of acceptance. Although everyone agrees that the diagnosis of arterial occlusion can be established by noninvasive means, skeptics have claimed that the data obtained provide little additional information of value in planning therapy. This criticism remains but has been blunted by the realization that the results of therapy, that is, surgery and transluminal angioplasty, are best documented by noninvasive testing. For example, it is now generally accepted that a change in the ankle/arm index of greater than 0.15 during follow-up is associated with the development of either new disease or worsening of the narrowing associated with an area of stenosis.

From a clinical standpoint, a critically important problem is the assessment of the aortoiliac segment, particularly in patients with multilevel disease. For me this became clearly evident when I examined the results of aortoiliac reconstruction in

patients with associated femoropopliteal disease. In this group of patients, 19% failed to show improvement after the proximal reconstruction.[20] This was not satisfactory and emphasized the need for a better standard than arteriography in trying to evaluate the hemodynamic significance of a diseased segment.

Other investigators have also appreciated this problem and attempted to solve it by using a variety of noninvasive tests ranging from segmental limb blood pressure determinations to analysis of the velocity patterns from the common femoral artery. These have not been uniformly successful, possibly for a reason that has escaped the notice of many workers in the field. The standard used was the arteriogram, a diagnostic test with its own inadequacies. This problem is finally being overcome with the realization that a better standard for validation is direct pressure measurement across the aortoiliac-femoral segments.[21]

Carotid artery disease

Carotid artery disease poses unique challenges and problems. Because transient ischemic attacks and strokes can occur secondary to disease in the carotid bulb, the importance of this area is beyond question. Major problems revolve about how best to evaluate both symptomatic and asymptomatic patients.

Before considering the available diagnostic approaches it is important to review a few basic considerations. The carotid bulb is a unique region in that this segment is normally larger than the common carotid artery and its connection, the internal carotid artery. Selective injection of the common carotid artery, with multiplanar views, is the standard approach used to evaluate the location and extent of other sclerotic involvement. From a physiologic standpoint, the factors controlling the hemodynamics of the external and internal carotid arteries are entirely different. The external carotid artery is similar to other peripheral arteries in terms of its flow patterns, whereas the internal carotid artery feeds a vascular bed of very low resistance. Thus, from a diagnostic standpoint, unusual anatomic and physiologic complexities of the carotid bulb make the use of any diagnostic procedure more difficult.

The initial efforts in this field were physiologic tests (periorbital Doppler, oculoplethysmography) to detect changes in blood flow at a point distal to the bifurcation.[6,10,12] In practice it was found that these tests could be used for the detection of very high grade stenoses and occlusions. But even here, problems with regard to reported accuracy were encountered. This may in large part be the result of our inability to predict from a selective arteriogram the hemodynamic consequences of a stenosis or even, in some cases, a total occlusion. We lack a standard for this anatomic segment that permits certain documentation of the hemodynamic consequences of stenosis, and often we are forced to presume that if the indirect tests are positive the lesion must be hemodynamically significant.

When the direct tests such as ultrasonic arteriography[13] and Duplex scanning[2] became available the validation process became even more difficult, because these tests could, in theory at least, detect carotid bifurcation disease in all stages of development. Chikos et al.[7] systematically examined the variability associated with reading selective arteriograms. The variability obviously differed for different degrees of involvement, but in general it appears unrealistic to attempt to predict the degree of stenosis to within $\pm 20\%$ even with multiple views of the carotid bulb.

Because the standard is not perfect, our difficulties in attempting to validate noninvasive testing are further compounded. For this reason it is prudent to classify stenosis of the carotid bulb into rather broad categories: normal, 1% to 15% occlusion, 16% to 49%, 50% to 70%, 81% to 99%, and total occlusion.[5] We have found this categorization to be useful for both initial evaluation and follow-up. Some uncertainty will always exist but once the criteria for the noninvasive tests have been established they should be usable from one laboratory to another as long as the equipment and test procedure provide the same data. However, when there is a change in the instrumentation or technique, it is necessary to revalidate the diagnostic technique. Inasmuch as this can be very tedious and time consuming, this task is often best done in laboratories experienced with the procedure.

The recent introduction of intravenous digital subtraction arteriography (DSA) has created new and unexpected problems.[16] Initially heralded as the immediate answer for screening, it was predicted that DSA would replace noninvasive testing. Experience has now demonstrated that this is not the case, and even if DSA were to become the standard diagnostic test for clinical purposes, it would not be an acceptable standard to use in the evaluation of noninvasive testing. The resolution is not as good as with selective arterial injections. Furthermore, limited views are frequently obtained, often making interpretation and estimation of the degree of involvement difficult.

An interesting trend has begun that may affect the future of both the digital method and noninvasive testing procedures such as ultrasonic duplex scanning. It is our practice to insist, whenever possible, that the noninvasive test be done first because the findings can be a great help in planning the arteriographic procedure to be used. For example, if a high-grade stenosis is found, it may be appropriate to use a venous injection site. On the other hand, when lesser degrees of involvement are found it is appropriate to insist on the use of the standard selective approach that provides the best possible visualization and resolution of the entire bifurcation.

CLASSIFICATION

The need to arrange according to a systematic division is an essential feature of the biologic sciences. To classify any disease or state correctly, it is necessary to identify and use the proper criteria. Failure to pay attention to this fundamental approach usually leads to confusion and uncertainty. In the field of noninvasive testing there are numerous examples of the problem. For example, different investigators have over the years used different sites of measurement to define the degree of stenosis in the carotid bulb. Some have used the bulb itself, whereas others have related the degree of narrowing in the bulb to the uninvolved internal carotid artery. If a physiologic parameter such as a change in the Doppler spectrum is used to categorize the degree of stenosis, it is likely that two investigators using different sites of measurement will arrive at differing conclusions. This may also explain why one investigator finds test results positive for one degree of stenosis and another arrives at an entirely different outcome. Unfortunately, it is not likely that this problem will be resolved, because there is very little movement in this direction. However, each of us must examine all of the criteria used in reported studies, perhaps to explain some of the discrepancies between investigators.

An equally important and frustrating problem is seen in the classification of clinical problems that the vascular laboratory is frequently asked to evaluate, for example, cold sensitivity and the thoracic outlet syndrome.

With regard to cold sensitivity, there is not even agreement as to how the two broad categories of the disorder should be classified. For example, I consider Raynaud's disease to be idiopathic, benign, and not associated with the development of digital artery occlusive disease or fingertip ulcerations.[1] The other and much more serious category includes cold sensitivity with an underlying cause such as scleroderma that is commonly associated with digital artery occlusive disease[16] and the frequent development of fingertip ulceration and, on some occasions, gangrene. If this classification scheme is correct, then the vascular laboratory could be helpful in separating patients into these two broad categories by simply determining whether there is occlusive disease in the arteries of the hand and fingers. Although this has been my practice, it is not an approach that is universally accepted by the medical community.

Thoracic outlet compression syndrome is another example of confusion in classification.[15] Although there is no doubt that vascular complications can occur, particularly when a cervical rib is present, it is now quite clear that most symptoms attributable to this syndrome are caused by compression of the lower roots of the brachial plexus. Yet the most commonly used test, even today, is the Adson maneuver or some variation thereof. This might be acceptable if the demonstration of arterial compression was uniformly associated with simultaneous compression of the brachial plexus, but this is obviously not the case. Yet we continue to get referrals to the vascular laboratory to determine whether there is vascular compression when the results, positive or negative, have little bearing on either the clinical diagnosis or subsequent treatment.

Another common area of confusion is differentiating between acute and chronic venous disease. The most frequently used term to describe acute venous thrombosis is *thrombophlebitis*. Yet it is now well established that acute occlusion of the deep venous system is not caused by or associated with inflammation. On the other hand, thrombosis of the superficial veins is frequently associated with fever, marked erythema, and local tenderness, all of which fulfill the criteria for an inflammatory process. "Thrombophlebitis" should be used to describe this superficial venous process that appears to be a separate and distinct entity from the acute involvement of the deep venous system. Deep vein thrombosis should be described simply as such and not as phlebitis, a term that is neither appropriate nor descriptive of the underlying disease.

The issue with regard to chronic venous disease is equally frustrating from a classification standpoint. Primary varicose veins rarely lead to ulceration, yet ulcers in the region of the medial malleolus are referred to as "varicose ulcers." This is incorrect, and more appropriate descriptive terminology that reflects the etiology should be used. "Stasis ulcer" would appear to be more appropriate, but even here there is no firm evidence that stasis exists under these circumstances. Perhaps, the best term would be "postthrombotic syndrome with ulceration."[19] This at least suggests that the initiating event was in all likelihood an episode of venous thrombosis that led over time to the development of valvular incompetence, which appears to be essential in the development of this late complication.

Finally, there is confusion related to the vascular disorders associated with diabetes mellitus. It is now clear that diabetes cannot be presented as a single disorder, because both morbidity and mortality vary according to the specific type. Thus diabetes mellitus must be qualified as to type and form of therapy used.[14] At present it is preferable to describe the disease in relationship to insulin dependence (type 1) and to further qualify by treatment the non-insulin-dependent form (type 2, NIDDM). Thus for non-insulin-dependent diabetes there are three forms of therapy: diet, sulfonylurea, and insulin (NIDDM-D, NIDDM-S, NIDDM-I). These are important because it appears that prevalence of disease, location, and associated risk factors may differ for each category of treatment. It is also clear that the prevalence of vascular disease in insulin-dependent diabetes (IDDM) is entirely different from that in NIDDM.

As you read the subsequent chapters, it is essential to ask the following questions: (1) Is the clinical classification of disease accepted and standard? (2) Has the diagnostic test been properly validated with safeguards to prevent bias? (3) Can the test be used in the clinical situation for which it was designed? (4) Will the test provide information that is useful for both diagnostic purposes and long-term follow-up?

REFERENCES

1. Allen, E.V., and Brown, G.E.: Raynaud's disease: a critical review of minimal requisites for diagnosis, Am. J. Med. Sci. 183:187, 1932.
2. Barber, F.E., et al.: Ultrasonic duplex echo-Doppler scanner, IEEE Trans. Biomed. Eng. 21:109, 1974.
3. Bauer, G.: A venographic study of thromboembolic problems, Acta Chir. Scand. 84(suppl. 6):1, 1940.
4. Bauer, G.: Diagnosis and management of peripheral venous diseases, Am. J. Med. 23:713, 1957.

5. Breslau, P.J.: Ultrasonic duplex scanning in the evaluation of carotid artery disease, medical thesis, Maastricht, Holland, 1982, University of Limburg.

6. Brockenbrough, E.J.: Screening for the prevention of stroke: use of a Doppler flowmeter, Seattle, 1970, Information and Education Resource Support Unit of Washington/Alaska Regional Medical Program.

7. Chikos, P.M., et al.: Observer variability in evaluating extracranial artery stenosis, Stroke 14:885, 1983.

8. Cranley, J.J., et al.: A plethysmographic technique for the diagnosis of deep venous thrombosis of the lower extremities, Surg. Gynecol. Obstet. 136:385, 1973.

9. Dahn, I., and Eiriksson, E.: Plethysmographic diagnosis of deep venous thrombosis of the leg, Acta. Chir. Scand. 398(Suppl.):33, 1968.

10. Gee, W., Oller, D.W., and Wylie, E.J.: Noninvasive diagnosis of carotid occlusion by ocular pneumoplethysmography, Stroke 7:18, 1976.

11. Haeger, K.: Problems of acute venous thrombosis. I. The interpretation of signs and symptoms, Angiology 20:219, 1969.

12. Kartchner, M.M., McRae, L.P., and Morrison, F.D.: Noninvasive detection and evaluation of carotid occlusive disease, Arch. Surg. 106:528, 1973.

13. Mozersky, D.J., et al.: Ultrasonic visualization of the arterial lumen, Surgery 72:253, 1972.

14. Pecoraro, R.E., and Porte, D., Jr.: What is diabetes mellitus? Vasc. Diagn. Ther. 3:9, 1982.

15. Porter, J.M., et al.: Thoracic outlet syndrome: a conservative approach, Vasc. Diagn. Ther. 3:35, 1982.

16. Strandness, D.E., Jr.: Carotid-vertebral digital subtraction angiography: a surgeon's view, Cardiovasc. Intervent. Radiol. 6:203, 1983.

17. Strandness, D.E., Jr., and Sumner, D.S.: Ultrasonic velocity detector in the diagnosis of thrombophlebitis, Arch. Surg. 104:180, 1972.

18. Strandness, D.E., Jr., and Sumner, D.S.: Raynaud's disease and Raynaud's phenomenon. In Strandness, D.E., Jr., and Sumner, D.S., editors: Hemodynamics for surgeons, New York, 1975, Grune & Stratton, Inc.

19. Strandness, D.E., Jr., and Thiele, B.L.: Postthrombotic venous insufficiency. In Strandness, D.E., Jr., and Thiele, B.L., editors: Selected topics in venous disorders: pathophysiology, diagnosis and treatment, Mt. Kisco, N.Y., 1981, Futura Publishing Co.

20. Sumner, D.S., and Strandness, D.E., Jr.: Aortoiliac reconstruction in patients with combined iliac and superficial femoral arterial occlusion, Surgery 84:348, 1978.

21. Thiele, B.L., et al.: A systematic approach to the assessment of aortoiliac disease, Arch. Surg. 118:477, 1983.

22. Wheeler, H.B., and Mullick, S.C.: Detection of venous obstruction in the leg by measurement of electrical impedance, Ann. NY Acad. Sci. 170:804, 1970.

PART ONE

FUNDAMENTALS OF MEASUREMENT AND CURRENT INSTRUMENTATION

CHAPTER 3

Doppler ultrasonic techniques in vascular disease

D. EUGENE STRANDNESS, Jr.

Since publication of the last edition of this book, remarkable progress has been made in both the development and the application of Doppler techniques. The instruments available range from pencil-sized units to highly sophisticated duplex systems that combined both Doppler and B-mode ultrasound. In addition, considerable progress has been made in the area of Doppler signal processing, permitting a more quantitative analysis of the important data in the Doppler spectrum. Finally, and most gratifying, has been the application of these methods to gain a broader understanding of vascular disease and its natural history with and without treatment.

PHYSICAL PRINCIPLES[1,4]

Three areas are of immediate concern to those who use ultrasound: (1) the Doppler effect, (2) the relationship between the ultrasonic frequency and attenuation, and (3) the velocity of transmission of ultrasound.

Doppler ultrasound is based on the fact that any moving object in the path of the sound beam will shift the frequency of the transmitted signal. This is expressed by the following formula:

$$f = 2f_e v \, (\cos \theta)/c$$

where:

f = Frequency shift
f_e = Frequency of transmitted signal
v = Velocity of the objects
θ = Angle of the incidence beam with the object path
c = Velocity of sound in the medium being studied

Each of these factors should be understood to appreciate the application of the current systems. It should be obvious that doubling the frequency of the transmitted signal will result in doubling of the frequency shift. The angle (θ) at which the

sound beam encounters the moving object is important to know whenever possible, particularly if the velocity of the object is to be quantitated. For example, in theory, a sound beam at right angles to the moving object gives a zero frequency shift because the cosine of 90 degrees is zero. The greatest frequency shift is encountered when the angle is 0 degrees, which has a cosine value of 1.0. This is rarely attainable with transcutaneous probes but is always the case when the crystals are mounted in the end of an intravascular probe. Although the angle to be used can vary by user preference, we have found an angle of 60 degrees to be relatively easy to obtain, particularly when the position of the vessel being studied is known from the use of a B-mode image. In practice, the transmitting frequency used will depend on intended application. It is important to remember that there is a relationship between the transmitting frequency and the attenutation (power) observed. For a 10 MHz system the attenuation is twice as great as with a 5 MHz system. Thus, for interrogation of deeper vessels, such as in the abdomen, a lower frequency is required than for the more superficial vessels of the arm and leg. In general, for most vascular applications a frequency in the 5 MHz range is most suitable.

There is another fact that tends to compensate for the loss of power when higher transmitting frequencies are used. The red blood cells, which are the principal reflectors, tend to scatter the higher frequencies better than the lower frequencies. This effect acts to minimize the increased attenuation of the higher ultrasound frequencies (Chapter 4).

The velocity of ultrasound determines the travel time between the transducer and the moving reflectors of interest. With the use of a continuous-wave system, everything in the path of the beam

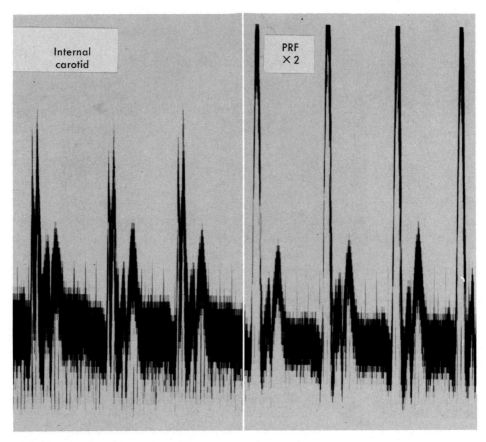

Fig. 3-1. Illustration of problem of sharing pulse repetition frequency *(PRF)* of pulsed Doppler and B-mode system. On left is velocity spectrum recorded from normal internal carotid artery when PRF is shared. Fold over (aliasing) occurs, which is eliminated when B-mode portion of Duplex system is shut off and PRF doubled.

is insonated, and it is impossible to estimate the site from which flow is detected. With a pulsed system, when a short burst is generated the receiver is activated to obtain a short sample of the return signal. To ensure that the sample originates from only one depth in tissue the echo from each transmission must be received before the next sample is transmitted. This limits the rate at which the pulses can be transmitted and obeys the following relationship:

$$PRF \ (maximum) \ = \ C/2d$$

where C is the velocity of sound in tissue (1540 m/sec), d is the distance of the reflector, and PRF is the pulse repetition frequency.

When the expected peak Doppler shift is higher than twice PRF the frequency generated by the instrument will be lower than expected. The highest Doppler shift that can be generated is called the

Nyquist frequency. For example, if the maximum PRF is 10 kHz, the highest Doppler shift that can be recorded is 5 kHz. Frequencies above this limit will not be displayed as expected and will appear as an aliased signal. This can often be recognized audibly but is best demonstrated by examining the spectral display of an analyzed signal. Those higher frequencies (above the Nyquist limit) are anomalously displayed as reverse flow (Fig. 3-1). The PRF will have to be lower when deeper vessels are being examined because of the increased travel times to reach these depths (Chapter 5).

AVAILABLE METHODS
Peripheral arterial disease[3]

Doppler techniques are currently being used to measure limb blood pressures and to survey the arterial and venous velocity patterns from nearly every region of the body. Limb blood pressures are

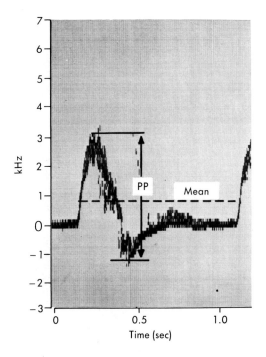

Fig. 3-2. Waveform typical of normal velocity pattern recorded from peripheral artery. Triphasic nature of waveform is readily seen. Values used to calculate pulsatility index *(PI)* are shown: (1) peak to peak *(PP)* and (2) mean value, derived by integrating area under curve.

easily measured with the simple and inexpensive pocket devices that are most commonly used with a stethoscope headset. Very little expertise is required other than a knowledge of the location of the posterior tibial, anterior tibial, and peroneal arteries at the ankle and foot. The transmitting frequency for most of these systems is 5 MHz. These devices are also commonly used in the recovery room and intensive care unit to monitor limb blood pressures after direct arterial surgery.

When the physician or technician attempts to survey the velocity patterns from specific sites along the course of the major arteries, the problem becomes more difficult, because the velocity patterns themselves are complex and influenced in a variety of ways by disease. Normally, in the resting state the velocity patterns of the peripheral arteries are triphasic, with two periods of forward flow and one of reverse flow (Fig. 3-2). They occur in forward-reverse-forward sequence and are quite distinct and recognizable by simply listening to the audio output of the Doppler device. When the transducer is placed over an area of stenosis the peak velocity increases in proportion to the degree of narrowing. Beyond the region of a stenosis or oc-

clusion there is damping of the velocity patterns with loss of the triphasic character. These waveforms are best described as monophasic and are usually quite distinct.

It is becoming more common to record the velocity patterns as an analog display that permits an immediate, visual inspection of the shape of the waveform. This has the additional advantage in that a permanent record is available for comparison with updated studies at some later time. It is also possible to derive quantitative information from a waveform even if the angle of the sound beam is unknown. Gosling and King[2] have described the use of the pulsatility index, expressed by the following formula:

$$PI = \text{Peak to peak/mean}$$

While there is some disagreement as to its application, it has been useful in the evaluation of aortoiliac disease. (See Chapters 7 and 53 for studies on quantitative measurements of velocity signals.)

Peripheral venous disease[7]

Doppler techniques are used to answer two simple questions: Is a major vein patent or occluded? Are the valves competent or incompetent? These questions can be answered with the continuous-wave pocket devices, but these require considerable experience and expertise for proper application. Just as the velocity patterns in peripheral arteries have a typical sequence in relationship to each cardiac cycle, the flow in the venous system of the supine subject is dominated by respiratory events. Acute venous occlusion alters the venous flow patterns in the patent veins distal to the site of involvement in predictable but often subtle ways. Flow tends to lose its phasic quality and become continuous.

Valvular incompetence is recognized by reversal of flow during periods of transient venous hypertension proximal to the segment being examined. This can be elicited by either limb compression or by performance of a Valsalva maneuver monitored from the common femoral vein. Although this phenomenon of venous reflux can be documented by an analog recording, this is usually not required in clinical practice.

Preliminary work suggests that ultrasonic duplex scanning may be of value in the study of venous disease. In theory, the ability to image major veins as well as evaluate flow should make this a powerful method.

Extracranial arterial disease[5,8]

Perhaps the greatest variation in applicable Doppler devices is found in evaluation of extracranial arterial disease. The price alone is indicative of the broad spectrum of instruments that can be used: from $400.00 to $100,000.00. The simplest instruments are of course used for periorbital studies and for direct scanning across the bifurcation. With the more expensive systems it is now possible to examine the plaque directly and estimate the functional effects of varying degrees of stenosis on the velocity patterns. The applicaton of these powerful methods is covered in considerable detail in this volume. Although it might appear that imaging and Doppler techniques are competitive, this is really not the case. As the two approaches become more sophisticated and combined in a single instrument, they will become the standard method for evaluating the extracranial circulation.

Signal processing[1]

Of all the areas related to the use of Doppler ultrasound, signal processing is perhaps the most confusing, yet the most promising for the future of the field. When I first started applying Doppler techniques, the audible interpretation of the detected velocity changes seemed adequate. Why? When new methods are applied to the study of disease, they are initially applied to obviously healthy individuals and patients with advanced disease. The normal person was noted to have triphasic arterial signals, whereas in the patient with total arterial occlusion the velocity signals distal to sites of involvement were of low frequency and monophasic. This distinction seemed so obvious that little further signal processing appeared to be needed.

However, as investigators began examining the velocity patterns in more detail it became clear that some method of analog display was desirable. The most obvious, cheapest, and simplest approach was the zero-crossing detector. This method, which generates a voltage proportional to the number of zero crossings of the received Doppler signal, appeared to be ideal, but very quickly problems became apparent.[6]

The disadvantages of the zero-crossing detector included the following: (1) it worked poorly, with a poor signal-to-noise ratio; (2) the output is dependent on signal amplitude; (3) with very high velocities the low-amplitude high-frequency com-

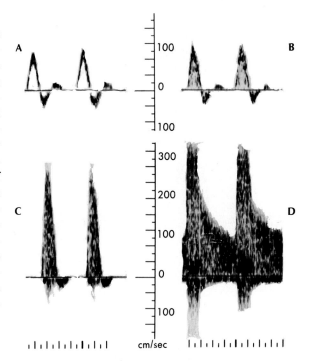

Fig. 3-3. Spectra illustrated can be used to classify degree of stenosis present in peripheral arteries. *A,* Normal spectrum with narrow band of frequencies throughout entire pulse cycle. *B,* Spectrum found with 1% to 19% stenosis, showing some increase in spectral width. *C,* Spectrum found with 16% to 49% stenosis. There is both an increase in peak velocity and marked spectral broadening. *D,* Spectrum in 50% to 99% stenosis. There is marked increase in peak frequency, spectral broadening, and simultaneous forward and reverse flow during systole. (From Jager, K.A., et al.: Noninvasive assessment of lower extremity ischemia. In Bergan, J.J., and Yao, J.S.T., editors: Evaluation and treatment of upper and lower extremity circulatory disorders, New York, 1983, Grune & Stratton, Inc.)

ponents may be lost entirely; and (4) unless there is complete resolution of directional changes, the forward-reverse flow relationships may not be accurately depicted.

Because the problems of the zero-crossing detector appeared insurmountable, it was only natural that more sophisticated techniques would appear and be applied. The Doppler spectrum proved to be extremely complex, not only with regard to frequency (as a reflection of velocity) but also as related to those changes in the spectrum that reflected complex alterations in the velocity patterns in areas of disturbed and turbulent flow. Thus it became apparent that for any signal processing technique to be useful, it had to be operable in a wide variety of flow states. For example, it was found important to be able to describe the flow patterns where laminar flow is altered either at bifurcations or in areas of disease that produce both directional and amplitude changes in the Doppler spectra.

The most popular method of digital frequency analysis is the fast Fourier transform, a method of analyzing periodic signals to assess their frequency content. This method is a true transform in that the method converts the function from time to frequency domain. The result may then be subjected to an inverse conversion to restore the original function. The magnitude of the function in the frequency domain is the spectrum. The display itself is in terms of time and frequency coordinates with magnitude displayed as gray-scale density (Fig. 3-3).

The spectral waveforms not only display the velocity versus time relationships for each cardiac cycle, but they can be used to provide data on flow disturbances, which are displayed in terms of spectral broadening. One problem that is not critical for visual interpretation of the spectra but can be for quantitative application is the poor statistical sampling of the data. This is noted by the variability between adjacent spectra, which results in the ragged appearance of the waveform. This may be overcome in large part by ensemble averaging over several cardiac cycles. This is particularly important in deriving quantitative data from the spectrum.

In attempting to obtain quantitative data from the Doppler signal it is possible to work with the entire spectrum or with a single derived value that corresponds to a frequency event at some point in time. The information can be used to generate absolute values of frequency events for calculations of flow or as dimensionless indices such as the pulsatility index (Fig. 3-2), which does not require knowledge of the Doppler angle. To make measurements of absolute velocity the Doppler angle must be known. Until the development of duplex scanners this information was rarely known with any precision. However, at the present time, not only is it feasible to measure the angle of the sound beam, but it is also a simple matter to measure arterial dimensions at the site of the velocity measurement at any level of the arterial system (Chapter 60). Thus it is now also possible to measure volume flow, a variable rarely available in the past.

The exact single feature in the spectrum to use for quantitative measurements remains somewhat uncertain. For example, it is possible to measure the mean, mode, or median frequency. The mean,

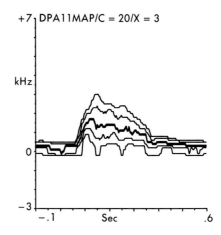

Fig. 3-4. Ensemble averaged waveform from 20 heartbeats. Dark line is mode (frequency of greatest amplitude). Other contours are 3 and 9 dB levels above and below the mode. This is a computer-generated waveform from output of fast Fourier transform spectrum analyzer.

or average, frequency is the most commonly discussed and is the most sensitive to the presence of noise. The mode frequency is that of greatest magnitude within the spectrum. It, too, is subject to some of the problems of the mean but appears to provide a better waveform (Fig. 3-4). In the median frequency one half of the power lies above the median and one half below.

Quantification of flow variables

Since the introduction of Doppler techniques for the study of vascular disease, data have usually been expressed in terms of frequency shift (Δf) of backscattered signal with the realization that it was not possible to calculate velocity because the necessary angle information for the incident sound beam ($\cos \theta$) was never available. For this reason investigators used ratios such as the pulsatility index (Fig. 3-2), where values were independent of Doppler angle. In addition, it has never been clear whether quantitative expression of the velocity information has any clinical value. For example, it has long been known that volume flow to the limbs, because of wide range for normal individuals, was not a useful diagnostic variable. Some authors have used variables such as deceleration and decay time in clinical studies (Chapter 56).

The development of ultrasonic duplex systems in conjunction with fast Fourier spectral analysis has made it possible to quantitate many variables that previously were unobtainable. It is now possible to obtain the following information from the arterial system: (1) dimensions, (2) movement of the arterial wall, (3) absolute measurements of flow velocity (peak and mean), (4) volume flow, (5) timing of events that make up the pulse cycle, and (6) a beginning examination of the flow events that occur in regions of disturbed and turbulent flow.

The possibility of using these variables to quantitate certain aspects of vascular function is particularly attractive in the limb arteries, where the vessels are relatively straight and there is not the complex geometry seen in the carotid bulb. For example, it is possible to examine in detail these variables from precise sites within the arterial system of the limbs. Although it is not yet clear how this information will be clinically helpful, it may be useful for the early detection of atherosclerosis and, in particular, in following its progress over time.

REFERENCES

1. Beach, K.W., and Phillips, D.J.: Doppler instrumentation for the evaluation of arterial and venous disease. (In press.)
2. Gosling, R.G., and King, D.H.: Processing arterial Doppler signals for clinical data. In de Vlieger, M., editor: Handbook of clinical ultrasound, New York, 1978, John Wiley & Sons, Inc.
3. Jager, K.A., et al.: Noninvasive assessment of lower extremity ischemia. In Bergan J.J., and Yao, J.S.T., editors: Evaluation and treatment of upper and lower extremity circulatory disorders, New York, 1983, Grune & Stratton, Inc.
4. Nippa, J.H., et al.: Phase rotation for separating forward and reverse blood velocity signals, IEEE Trans. Sonics Ultrasonics 22:340, 1975.
5. Phillips, D.J., et al.: Detection of peripheral vascular disease using the duplex scanner. III, Ultrasound Med. Biol. 6:205, 1980.
6. Reneman, R.S., et al.: In vivo comparison of electromagnetic and Doppler flowmeters with special attention to the processing of the analogue Doppler signal, Cardiovasc. Res. 7:557, 1973.
7. Strandness, D.E., Jr., and Thiele, B.L.: Methods of studying venous anatomy and function. In Strandness, D.E., Jr., and Thiele, B.L., editors: Selected topics in venous disorders: pathophysiology, diagnosis and treatment, Mt. Kisco, N.Y., 1981, Futura Publishing Co., Inc.
8. Zierler, R.E., et al.: The use of frequency spectral analysis in carotid artery surgery. In Bergan, J.J., and Yao, J.S.T., editors: Cerebrovascular insufficiency, New York, 1982, Grune & Stratton, Inc.

CHAPTER 4

Continuous-wave Doppler ultrasound

ROBERT W. BARNES

Continuous-wave (CW) Doppler ultrasound is the most commonly used noninvasive diagnostic technique to evaluate cardiovascular disorders. The instrument detects blood flow velocity from the Doppler effect by means of continuous-wave transmission of ultrasound into the tissues.[1] Backscattered ultrasound is detected and amplified by the instrument as an audible signal, or the signal may be processed for graphic recording by analog or sound spectrum analysis techniques. CW Doppler permits simple, inexpensive, and rapid evaluation of peripheral arterial, cerebrovascular, and venous disorders. The technique lacks range resolution and will detect flow from any vessel insonated by the Doppler probe. Despite these limitations, CW Doppler is the most widely used technique to evaluate peripheral vascular disease. The physical principles, instrument design, methods of signal processing and display, and brief clinical applications are outlined in this chapter; more specific clinical applications are described in other chapters.

PHYSICAL PRINCIPLES

Fig. 4-1 depicts the block diagram of the essential components of a CW Doppler instrument. An oscillator causes a sinusoidal electrical waveform to drive a transmitting piezoelectric crystal at its resonant frequency to emit a continuous beam of ultrasound into the tissues through acoustic gel coupling with the skin. The transmitted ultrasound is reflected from varying acoustic interfaces within the body. Moving structures such as red blood cells provide a reflective interface, which causes backscattered ultrasound to be shifted in frequency by an amount proportional to the velocity of blood flow, according to the following Doppler formula:

$$\Delta f = \frac{2 f_t \, v \, \text{Cos} \, \theta}{C}$$

where

Δf = Doppler frequency shift
f_t = Transmitter frequency
v = Velocity of blood cells
θ = Angle between the transmitted sound beam and the direction of blood flow
c = Velocity of sound in the tissues (1540 m/sec for soft tissue)

The backscattered signal is received by a second piezoelectric crystal in the Doppler probe. This received signal is referenced to the transmission frequency, and the frequency difference is detected and amplified as an audible signal; it may be recorded as an analog waveform or be analyzed by sound spectrum analysis techniques. For ultrasonic transmission frequencies in the range of 3 to 10 MHz and a normal range of blood flow velocity, the frequency shift will be in the range of 0 to 10 kHz. This means that the signals from moving blood can be made audible with appropriate electronic processing.

The Doppler signal constitutes a variety or spectrum of frequencies. The frequency distribution depends on such factors as differences in red blood cell velocity distribution across the cross-section of the vessel, variations in blood cell interspace, nonuniformity, and divergence of sound beams with resultant variations in the incident angle θ when the red blood cells pass through the ultrasonic beam. The power of the ultrasonic signal received at the crystal is determined by the amount of backscattering of the insonant energy received from the red blood cell–plasma interface and the quantity of sound absorbed by the tissues. The amount of

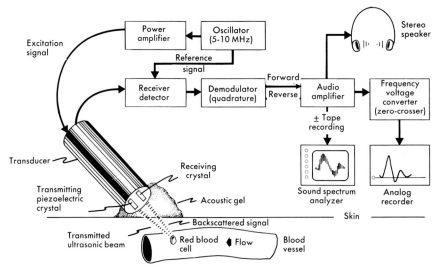

Fig. 4-1. Block diagram of components of CW Doppler ultrasonic velocity detector.

both backscatter and absorption of ultrasound increases at higher transmitter frequencies. The higher the number of red blood cells moving through the ultrasonic beam, the higher the power of the received Doppler signal. Backscattered ultrasound is received not only from moving red blood cells but also from the motion of the blood vessel wall. The wall motion signals are low in frequency but high in amplitude because of the better reflection of the flat blood–vessel wall interface compared with the blood–red cell interface.

INSTRUMENT DESIGN
Detector

The CW Doppler circuitry is relatively simple and may be housed in small portable units. Such units often contain not only the transmission and receiving circuitry but also the piezoelectric crystals and loudspeaker for audible signal analysis. Units as small as a penlight are available, permitting the use of stethoscope earpieces for audible signal analysis. Other units are portable tabletop models that permit additional features such as direction-sensing capability, velocity meters, multiple selection of transmission frequencies, and built-in graphic strip chart recorders. CW Doppler instruments may be an integral part of ultrasonic imaging devices, particularly for noninvasive screening of extracranial carotid occlusive disease. CW Doppler instruments vary in cost from $250 to $3000, with imaging devices costing up to $30,000.

Transducer

The CW Doppler transducer contains transmitting and receiving crystals, usually mounted at angles to focus the ultrasonic beam at the appropriate level of selected use in specific clinical circumstances. A focusing lens of plastic or epoxy is often used to protect the transducer. The Doppler probe may be a pencil-shaped device that is detachable from the detector itself, or the transmitting and receiving crystals may be housed in the self-contained portable device. Separate Doppler probes are particularly useful when used under sterile conditions for intraoperative monitoring purposes. Some Doppler probes are attached to the appropriate oscillator so that different transmission frequencies may be used by exchanging the probe and oscillator units with the main Doppler housing. The Doppler probe requires cold gas sterilization and should be handled with care to avoid damage to the connecting wires, the crystals, and the protective material over the crystal surfaces. The acoustic coupling of the Doppler probe with the skin should be achieved with a gel or other coupling agent of high acoustic transmissivity. Intraoperatively, physiologic saline solution or blood may be used as the acoustic coupling medium.

Direction sensor

The simplest CW Doppler instrument is incapable of determining the direction of blood flow relative to the Doppler probe. Direction-sensing instruments use special demodulation techniques.

Using the phase-shift detection technique of McLeod,[2] the identification and separation of positive and negative Doppler frequency shifts is possible. The phase-shift technique permits flow direction sensing by means of stereo earphones or by frequency-to-voltage conversion, which permits analog recordings of separate forward and reverse flow velocity or differentially as mean velocity recording. The refinement in CW Doppler direction-sensing capability by Nippa et al.[3] permits phase rotation for separation of forward and reverse flow without ambiguity, so that audible assessment of forward or reverse flow may be possible with a monaural speaker. Such circuitry permits more complete flow velocity separation with a sound spectrum analyzer.

Frequency selection

Simple CW Doppler devices have one inherent transmission frequency, designed for specific applications depending on the anticipated range of blood flow from the Doppler transducer. The most common devices used for clinical evaluation of peripheral vascular disease range between 5 and 10 MHz. Some devices permit selection of multiple transmission frequencies either with a selector switch or by means of exchange of Doppler probes with separate oscillators attached to each probe. The oscillator frequency must be matched to the resonant frequency of the piezoelectric crystals in the Doppler probe. Instruments with higher transmission frequencies usually have smaller transmission and receiving crystals, permitting greater lateral resolution. However, because of the increased absorption and backscattering of ultrasound at higher transmission frequencies, the range or depth penetration of such devices is limited. Doppler units operating at lower transmission frequencies usually have larger transmission and receiving crystals, a wider ultrasonic beam, and reduced lateral resolution, although such devices are more suitable for interrogating blood flow at greater tissue depths.

Portability

CW Doppler devices used for rapid qualitative screening of peripheral vascular disease should be readily portable and simple in operation. However, for more precise recording of Doppler frequency spectra, more sophisticated tabletop devices that have optimum frequency and spectral characteristics should be used. Most vascular laboratories will find the need for several types of Doppler instruments for both portable and laboratory-based studies.

SIGNAL PROCESSING AND DISPLAY

CW Doppler ultrasound may be analyzed by one of four principal techniques: (1) audible interpretation of the Doppler waveform, (2) analog recording of the average velocity signal, (3) sound spectrum analysis, and (4) vascular imaging.

Audible interpretation

The CW Doppler signal may be interpreted through the use of stethoscope-type earpieces, earphones, or a loudspeaker. An experienced observer learns to distinguish the audible Doppler signal characteristics that detect not only differences in arterial and venous signals but also the presence or absence of disease through disturbances in blood flow velocity. The characteristics of the normal and abnormal arterial velocity signals are reviewed in Chapter 53, and the use of CW Doppler for evaluation of venous disease is discussed in Chapter 71. With experience a technician or physician can learn to audibly recognize the flow perturbations that permit an accurate diagnosis of the presence or absence of arterial or venous disease with an accuracy exceeding 90%. However, the audible interpretation of CW Doppler signals requires considerable experience for maximal accuracy. The extent of this commitment is similar to that necessary to achieve maximal accuracy in the use of a stethoscope for diagnosing heart disease from abnormalities of heart sounds and murmurs. It is for this reason that other more objective graphic display techniques of the Doppler signal have been devised.

Analog recording

The most common device to translate Doppler frequency shifts into voltage changes for analog recording is the zero-crossing meter.[6] With this device the average frequency shift is determined and converted to a proportional electric signal for recording on a strip chart recorder. The zero-crossing circuitry does not measure the true mean frequency shift (and thus the velocity) but a close approximation to the root mean square, which is slightly greater than the mean. Although such analog recordings are relatively inexpensive, several limitations of the technique must be recognized. The recordings may be significantly altered by changes in probe-vessel angle; misalignment of the probe and vessel; presence of a broad frequency spectrum, which is particularly common with disturbed or turbulent blood flow; mixture of arterial and venous signals; vessel wall motion; and varying velocity profiles. In addition, the zero-crossing circuit may lead to inaccurate readings at the high flow velocities often seen in arteries with stenotic lesions. Although other modifications of frequency analysis, such as the maximum frequency follower,[9] have been developed, most investigators currently use real-time sound spectrum analysis for the most accurate recording and display of Doppler frequency shifts.[7]

Sound spectrum analysis

Graphic display of the entire range of frequencies and amplitudes of the Doppler spectrum may be carried out with a sound spectrum analyzer. Such analysis can be carried out with off-line[5] or real-time techniques.[7] Most investigators use real-time sound spectrum analyzers, which portray varying frequencies and amplitudes of the Doppler spectrum with respect to time. A more thorough discussion of this technology is the subject of Chapter 7.

CW Doppler signals may be sound spectrum analyzed for the evaluation of peripheral arterial or cerebral vascular disease. The Doppler frequency spectrum from a CW Doppler system is broader than that of a pulsed Doppler system because of the sample volume that encompasses the cross-section of the interrogated vessel. Thus the backscattered CW Doppler spectrum will include the high frequency associated with centerline blood flow velocity as well as the lower frequencies associated with slower moving blood cells near the vessel wall. In addition, the frequency shifts associated with vessel wall motion may also be included in the Doppler spectrum unless such unwanted signals are specifically rejected by appropriate band-pass filter techniques. Although CW Doppler spectra are broader, diagnostic information is still available within the displayed spectrum. The normal Doppler arterial spectra reveal pulsatile waveforms with most of the Doppler signal amplitude along the upper border of the velocity waveform. The resultant clear area beneath peak systole is relatively smaller than the corresponding window beneath the peak systolic waveform of a pulsed Doppler spectrum from the same vessel. Nevertheless, qualitative or quantitative analysis[8] of spectral broadening in the detection of peripheral arterial or cerebral vascular disease is possible with CW Doppler ultrasound. In addition, arterial occlusive disease is detectable not only by Doppler spectral broadening but also by the resulting increased peak velocity at an arterial stenosis. The diagnostic accuracy of Doppler spectrum analysis using either CW or pulsed Doppler techniques is relatively similar in the reported results from independent investigators.

Vascular imaging

The CW Doppler system is used in several commercially available Doppler ultrasonic arteriographs.[4,10] These devices use a CW Doppler transducer joined to a position-sensing arm. The loci of detected blood flow are translated by means of the position-sensing arm to appropriate positions on a storage oscilloscope, where spots are created when blood flow velocity exceeds a certain threshold value. By moving the CW Doppler probe along the course of the underlying artery or vein a vascular image may be developed on the screen of the storage oscilloscope. At selected sites along the course of the imaged vessel the CW Doppler signal may be sampled and recorded by analog or sound spectrum analysis techniques. Electronic processing of the frequency shifts associated with the Doppler signal may be color coded on the display screen of a color monitor to permit depiction of different blood cell velocities associated with vascular stenoses (Echoflow). The technique and clinical application of these CW Doppler ultrasonic arteriographs are described in Chapters 20 and 36.

CLINICAL APPLICATIONS

CW Doppler ultrasound forms the basis of many of the noninvasive techniques described in this textbook. Some applications of these commonly used versatile instruments are summarized.

Peripheral arterial disease

An audible assessment of peripheral arterial blood velocity signals permit qualitative screening of peripheral arterial disease. An experienced technician or physician may use the Doppler instrument as a sensitive electronic stethoscope to detect and localize arterial stenoses or occlusions.

CW Doppler ultrasound is often used to measure systolic blood pressures at various segmental levels along the limb. Such segmental blood pressures permit quantification and localization of peripheral arterial occlusive disease.

Recent use of analog or sound spectrum recordings of Doppler velocity signals from the common femoral artery permits rapid assessment of aorto-iliac stenosis in patients who may have normal segmental limb blood pressures. The absence of the normal reversed blood flow velocity in early diastole in the common femoral artery signal is a useful guide to the presence of significant aortoiliac stenosis.

The Doppler detector permits assessment of acute and chronic arterial occlusive disease, vasospastic or occlusive digital artery occlusive disease, and in selected cases the presence of visceral artery obstructions. In addition, Doppler probes may be sterilized and used for intraoperative monitoring and for evaluating arterial reconstructions. After treatment, the efficacy of medical or surgical therapy may be evaluated by defining the incidence of disease progression or the development of complications in reconstructed arterial segments.

Cerebral vascular disease

CW Doppler ultrasound is one of the most versatile methods of evaluating extracranial cerebral vascular occlusive disease. The technique may be used not only to assess the direction of blood flow in branches of the ophthalmic artery but also to detect abnormal flow velocity signals in the carotid artery and its branches in the neck. Although audible signal analysis has formed the basis of many previous studies, current investigators are improving the diagnostic accuracy of Doppler ultrasonic evaluation of cerebral vascular disease through use of real-time sound spectrum analysis techniques. With such indirect and direct carotid screening techniques, CW Doppler ultrasound permits identification of arterial stenosis or occlusion of the extracranial carotid arteries with an accuracy exceeding 90%. The applications are discussed in greater detail in Chapters 34 and 39. In addition to interpretation of CW Doppler signals, CW Doppler ultrasonic arteriographs permit visualization of the extracranial carotid arteries for more precise signal sampling and sound spectrum analysis.

Venous disease

CW Doppler ultrasound has proved to be the most rapid and versatile method to evaluate the venous system, as indicated in Chapter 71. Although the Doppler technique is sensitive to deep vein thrombosis in more than 95% of cases, this accuracy can only be achieved with long-term experience with the technique. The advantages of Doppler ultrasound include its ability to distinguish deep from superficial venous disease and to evaluate patients in plaster casts or traction devices. The technique can also be applied to the upper extremity. Despite its accuracy and versatility in experienced hands, the subjective nature of this technique has limited its widespread application.

ADVANTAGES AND LIMITATIONS

CW Doppler velocity detectors are electronically simpler and less expensive than pulsed Doppler devices. These devices are rapid, and for most clinical purposes the diagnostic information is as accurate as that provided by pulsed Doppler instruments. CW Doppler devices have a greater Doppler band width than that of pulsed units. This characteristic increases the maximum blood velocity detectable with the instrument. Because of the larger sample volume, a CW Doppler device is capable of rapid localization of blood flow, facilitating the examination.

The disadvantages of CW Doppler ultrasound include the following: All blood flow within the range of the Doppler probe is detected by the instrument, leading to confusion of arterial and venous flow signals. The diameter of the vessel cannot be ascertained, and thus quantification of blood flow is generally not feasible with CW Doppler devices. Vessel wall motion artifacts are sometimes difficult to eliminate without losing information from low blood flow velocities. Flow velocity profiles within the vessel lumen cannot be detected with CW Doppler ultrasound.

CONCLUSIONS

Despite the limitations of CW Doppler ultrasound, its simplicity, low cost, and versatility make it a most valuable instrument for evaluating peripheral vascular disease. With the use of more sophisticated sound spectrum analysis and imaging techniques, CW Doppler velocity detectors have assumed an important role in the evaluation of peripheral arterial, cerebral vascular, and venous disease.

REFERENCES

1. Franklin, D.L., Schlegel, W., and Rushmer, R.F.: Blood flow measured by Doppler frequency shift of backscattered ultrasound, Science 134:564, 1961.
2. McLeod, F.D.: A directional Doppler flowmeter, Dig. Int. Conf. Med. Biol. Eng. 7:213, 1967.
3. Nippa, J.H., et al.: Phase rotation for separating forward and reverse blood velocity signals, IEEE Trans. Sonics Ultrasonics 22:340, 1975.

4. Reid, J.M., and Spencer, M.P.: Ultrasonic Doppler technique for imaging blood vessels, Science 176:1235, 1972.

5. Reneman, R.S., and Spencer, M.P.: Local Doppler audio spectra in normal and stenosed carotid arteries in man, Ultrasound Med. Biol. 5:1, 1979.

6. Reneman, R.S., et al.: In vivo comparison of electromagnetic and Doppler flowmeters, with special attention to the processing of the analogue Doppler flow signal, Cardiovasc. Res. 7:557, 1973.

7. Rittgers, S.E., Putney, W.W., and Barnes, R.W.: Real-time spectrum analysis and display of directional Doppler ultrasound blood velocity signals, IEEE Trans. Biomed. Eng. BME-27:723, 1980.

8. Rittgers, S.E., Thornhill, B.M., and Barnes, R.W.: Quantitative analysis of carotid artery Doppler spectral waveforms: diagnostic value of parameters, Ultrasound Med. Biol. 9:255, 1983.

9. Skidmore, R., and Follett, D.H.: Maximum frequency follower for the processing of ultrasonic Doppler shift signals, Ultrasound Med. Biol. 4:145, 1978.

10. White, D., and Lyons, E.A.: A comparison of 424 carotid bifurcations examined by angiography and the Doppler Echoflow, Ultrasound Med. Biol. 4:363, 1978.

CHAPTER 5

Pulsed Doppler ultrasound for blood velocity measurements

KIRK W. BEACH and D. EUGENE STRANDNESS, Jr.

The earliest ultrasonic Doppler instruments were nondirectional continuous-wave devices that transmitted at an ultrasonic frequency of about 5 MHz. The choice of that frequency was fortunate because it produces the strongest reflected signal from blood at a depth of 2 cm when viewed (with ultrasound) through muscle. Suppose that the blood velocity is 15.4 cm/sec and the blood is insonated with a 5 MHz ultrasound beam colinear with the blood velocity (a Doppler angle of zero). Because the velocity of sound in tissue is 154,000 cm/sec, ultrasound reflecting off the moving erythrocytes would experience a 1/10,000 shift in frequency on reaching the erythrocytes and another 1/10,000 shift on reflecting from them, for a total shift of 2/10,000. A 2/10,000 shift in the frequency of 5,000,000 Hz is equal to 1000 Hz, a frequency that, by chance, is well within the normal human hearing range. It is only by chance that over the normal range of blood flow velocities, 3 to 150 cm/sec, the Doppler shift produces Doppler signals of 200 Hz to 10,000 kHz with a Doppler angle of zero degrees, or 100 Hz to 5000 kHz with a Doppler angle of 60 degrees (cos 60 = 0.5).

Those relationships, in combination with a simple set of electronics capable of extracting the "beat" (difference) frequency between the transmitted and the received frequencies,[3] made the first Doppler instruments possible. These instruments extended the acoustic examination of patients beyond the stage of the passive stethoscope, but they had limitations. The two major limitations, the inability to separate mixed signals and the need to quantify velocities, could be overcome using technology already developed for radio and radar.

The first limitation appears when two blood vessels are insonated simultaneously by the instrument; the signals appear superimposed in the output. The two signals are hard to separate. Although both vessels might be arteries, usually one is an artery and the other a vein. Two strategies were available to separate these signals, one based on the difference in flow direction in arteries and veins, and the other on the fact that the two vessels are spatially separated. Flow direction can be identified by using methods developed by radio engineers working with single sideband receivers. It was only necessary to recognize the similarity in the two systems and apply the method to Doppler systems. Because flow toward the probe shifts ultrasound to slightly higher frequencies, and flow away from the probe shifts ultrasound to slightly lower frequencies, flows in two directions appear as two "sidebands" of the transmitted frequency and can be separated using sideband technology. The bidirectional ultrasonic Doppler system is based on this technology.[5,6] Spatial separation is achieved by focusing the ultrasonic beam to allow the ultrasound to be directed toward one vessel while avoiding the other, and by an electronic method of selecting the Doppler-shifted signal from a single depth in tissue while rejecting signals from all other depths. The pulsed Doppler system was devised to accomplish this.

The second limitation is that there is a direct proportional relationship between blood velocity and frequency. The relationship is expressed as the Doppler equation:

$$\Delta f = \frac{2f_0 \cdot v \cdot \cos(\theta)}{C}$$

where

Δf = Audio output frequency
2 = Round trip of the ultrasound
C/f_0 = Wavelength of ultrasound
$v \cos(\theta)$ = Closing speed between the erythrocytes and the Doppler probe

Examiners, aware of this relationship, wanted to quantify blood velocity. Two things were needed: a method of measuring the Doppler angle and a quantitative frequency display. Fortunately, imaging systems are now capable of displaying the Doppler angle, and frequency analyzers are capable of displaying the quantitative spectral waveform.

Of all the advances in ultrasonic Doppler technology, the pulsed Doppler system is the most intriguing. It provides the ability to monitor blood velocity at different depths in tissue, pulsed Doppler systems combine the spatial ability on which ultrasonic imaging is based with the ultrasound phase detection on which Doppler measurement is based.

PHYSICAL BASIS OF PULSED DOPPLER SYSTEM

When a pulse of ultrasound is transmitted into tissue the echo returned by the tissue consists of a series of radio frequency oscillations. The duration of the echo is dependent on the power of the ultrasound pulse and on the attenuation of the tissue. The attenuation in turn is dependent on the ultrasonic frequency and the tissue type. There is a direct relationship between the duration of a segment of the echo and the depth of tissue involved in that time segment. The relationship is based on the velocity of ultrasound in tissue (154,000 cm/sec) as the pulse travels to and from the reflectors. Each centimeter in tissue depth is displayed as 13 μsec in echo duration. Thus to receive an echo from a depth of 3 cm, you must wait about 40 μsec after the transmission. To accept the signal from a 1 mm slice of tissue at that depth, you would have to accept the signal for 1.3 μsec after waiting 40 μsec for the desired echo.

If the ultrasound frequency is 6 MHz and the sound is passing through muscle, the attenuation rate is 10 dB/cm tissue depth. Inasmuch as the ultrasound must pass through each centimeter

twice, once going down, the other coming back, echoes are attenuated 20 dB, or a factor of 100 in power for each centimeter of tissue depth represented (each 13 μsec on the display). Most ultrasonic pulsed echo instruments (imaging and Doppler) are equipped with *time-gain controls* (TGC; sometimes called depth gain compensation [DGC]) to compensate for the attenuation. Such a control will amplify echoes from the first 13 μsec after pulse transmission by a factor of 100 (representing the first centimeter), echoes from the next 13 μsec (second centimeter) by a factor of 10,000, those from the next 13 μsec (another centimeter) by 1,000,000, and each successive 13 μsec (representing successive centimeters) by successive factors of 100. Thus the intensity of the echoes varies over a wide range, strong from shallow reflectors and weak from deep reflectors. Undesired echoes from beyond the desired depth are ignored because the amplification is inadequate to make these signals visible.

In continuous-wave (CW) Doppler systems two transducers are used, one for transmitting and the other for receiving. In pulsed Doppler systems a single crystal is used for both transmitting and receiving. Voltages required for ultrasound transmission range from 20 to 100 V. Echoes, returning from tissue, generate voltages in the range of 1 to 10 mV. It is therefore very important to electrically isolate the receiver from the transmitter. In CW Doppler systems the separation is accomplished by having separate transducers. In pulsed Doppler systems the separation is achieved by switching the same transducer from transmitting to receiving. The beam patterns from the two transducers used in CW Doppler systems do not overlap near the skin. Thus the strong echoes from shallow depths are avoided. CW Doppler systems are therefore able to operate without electronic depth gain compensation; instead the limited overlap of the beam patterns provides automatic depth gain compensation. In pulsed Doppler systems the transmitter beam pattern and the receiver beam pattern are identical, so that all of the depth gain compensation must be done by timing. With CW Doppler systems it is not possible to perform depth gain compensation with timing from the transmitted pulse, because ultrasound is transmitted continuously and echoes are received from all depths at all times.

An ultrasonic pulsed Doppler instrument consists of a radio frequency oscillator operating in the range of 1 to 20 MHz, a gate (or switch) to

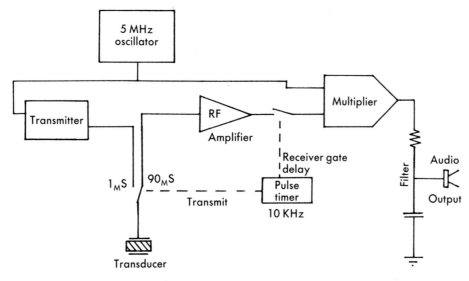

Fig. 5-1. Pulsed Doppler circuit. The 5 MHz oscillator is source of radio frequency signal. A 5-cycle burst of this signal is transmitted into tissue every 0.1 msec. Echoes from burst are amplified and directed into receiver gate. Pulse timing circuit selects time interval between transmission pulse and echo from selected depth and directs echo into multiplier. If phase and amplitude of gated echo are constant with respect to oscillator signal, constant peak-to-peak voltage appears at output of multiplier at PRF. Shifting of phase reflecting blood flow will appear as oscillation in voltage superimposed on PRF. Filter removes PRF, leaving audio Doppler signal from selected depth.

determine the transmission timing and the pulse length, a timing circuit that opens the receiver for the desired echo, an amplifier, a mixer-detector to compare the phase and amplitude of the echo to the reference oscillator, and an audio amplifier to amplify the resultant Doppler signal (Fig. 5-1). The ultrasonic pulse generated by an ultrasonic pulsed Doppler instrument differs from the pulse generated by an ultrasonic pulsed echo imaging instrument. The pulsed echo instrument transmits the shortest possible burst into tissue (Fig. 5-2, *A*). This is to assure the best possible depth resolution of the image. The Doppler pulse consists of a series of cycles at the ultrasonic carrier frequency (Fig. 5-2, *B*). The returned echo contains variations in both amplitude and phase (Fig. 5-2, *C*). As the echo is received the portion of the echo from the desired depth is accepted by the receiver gate. That portion, the gated echo, is usually equal in length to the transmitted pulse. The gated echo is multiplied times a reference wave within the instrument. The reference wave is the Doppler carrier frequency. The output voltage of the multiplier is dependent on the phase relationship between the echo and the reference. If that phase relationship is constant, as with a stationary reflector, the output will be a constant voltage containing no audio signal.

If the phase relationship is changing, as with a moving reflector, the output voltage will vary up and down, generating the audio output, a sound with frequency proportional to blood velocity. Superimposed on that signal is the pulse repetition frequency (PRF), which is suppressed by a low pass filter set to reject the PRF while preserving the lower frequency audio Doppler signal.

The audio signal generated by the pulsed Doppler unit is similar to the CW Doppler signal. The nondirectional or directional output signals from the pulsed Doppler system can be handled and analyzed just like the CW signals. Pulsed Doppler signals differ from CW Doppler signals in two ways. First, usually pulsed Doppler signals represent velocities in smaller sample volumes than do CW Doppler signals. While CW Doppler units display velocities from the entire vessel cross-section, a pulsed Doppler system can obtain Doppler data from a sample volume as small as 3 mm.[3] The small sample volume allows data gathering from many adjacent regions in a single artery. This enables the operator to examine in detail the complex nature of the blood flow. Second, because the pulsed Doppler system samples the data rather than gathering data continuously, an artifact of the sampling rate occurs. There is a limit to the Doppler

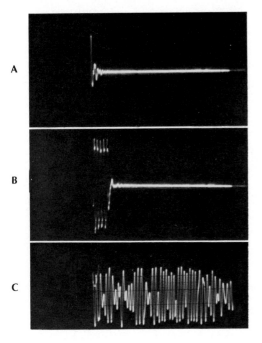

Fig. 5-2. Transmitted and received ultrasonic signals. **A,** Ultrasonic pulsed echo transmission burst. Note few weak oscillations (ringing) following single cycle transmitted. In most systems ringing is suppressed to improve depth resolution of system. **B,** Ultrasonic pulsed Doppler transmission pulse. Five cycles of 5 MHz ultrasound are transmitted in pulse 1 μsec long. **C,** Radio frequency A-mode echo. This is echo received at transducer over first 8 μsec after completion of Doppler pulse transmission. This represents first 6 mm of tissue depth. Appropriate time gain amplification has been applied to prevent attentuation of trace from left (skin) to right (deep).

shift frequency that can be displayed by a pulsed Doppler unit.

ALIASING

The output of the pulsed Doppler system is generated by displaying the phase of successive pulse echoes as sound. To faithfully create an audible sound of a particular frequency, at least one point must be available for each peak and one for each valley of the output frequency (Fig. 5-3). This means that the audio Doppler output signal will have a frequency that is lower than half of the PRF of the pulsed Doppler. The limiting audio frequency (PRF/2) is called the Nyquist frequency. If the PRF is less than half of the expected Doppler frequency, a sound will be generated based on the phase samples available, but the audio output generated is the lowest frequency that satisfies the phase shift. If the PRF is 10 kHz, the highest magnitude Doppler shift frequencies that can be correctly displayed on the audio channel or the spectral waveform output are ±5 kHz. A tabulation of the effect is helpful for a PRF of 10 kHz (Table 5-1).

Aliasing can be easily recognized on a velocity waveform tracing (Fig. 5-4). Frequencies that should appear in the forward direction at frequencies higher than the Nyquist frequency are plotted in the reverse direction. The same effect will appear on the audio output channels. Because CW Doppler

Table 5-1. Aliasing frequencies for a pulse repetition frequency of 10 kHz

Expected Doppler shift (kHz)	Observed nondirectional Doppler shift (kHz)	Observed directional Doppler shift (kHz)
3	3	+3
4	4	+4
5	5*	±5*
6	4†	−4†
7	3†	−3†
8	2†	−2†
9	1†	−1†
10	0†	0†
11	1†	+1†
12	2†	+2†

*Half of PRF equals aliasing frequency.
†$F(observed) = F(expected) - n \cdot (PRF)/2$, where n is an integer chosen to locate the result between $-(PRF)/2$ and $+(PRF)/2$; the nondirectional result displays only the magnitudes of the aliased frequencies.

systems do not sample the phase of the ultrasonic echoes but monitor the phase continuously, they do not exhibit aliasing. Digital spectra derived from CW Dopplers may alias because the spectrum analyzer samples the audio output of the Doppler at a frequency equal to twice the maximum frequency of the spectrum analyzer display, and thus if the Doppler frequency is higher than the maximum of

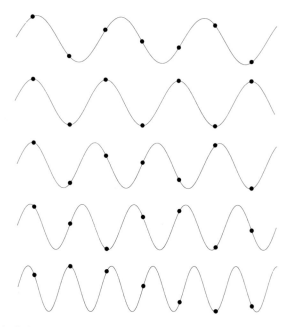

Fig. 5-3. Aliasing of high-frequency Doppler shift signal. Dots represent ultrasound pulses that sample phase of echo from a particular depth. Horizontal dimension represents timing of pulses; vertical distance represents phase alignment measurement from each ultrasonic echo. As frequency exceeds Nyquist frequency (equal to half of PRF), line connecting samples would produce erroneously low output frequency rather than expected frequency drawn. Upper two tracings show correctly represented frequencies; lower three tracings represent signals that would be aliased if signals were reconstructed from dot samples. In lowest tracing, effect is shown with greatest clarity. There Doppler shift frequency is nearly equal to sample frequency.

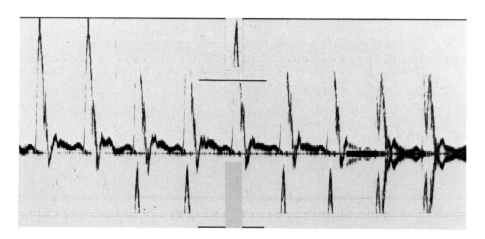

Fig. 5-4. Pulsed Doppler signal with aliasing. First two cardiac cycles were obtained with PRF of 19.6 kHz. Range of kHz spectral tracing is +7 to −3 kHz. Next five cardiac cycles were obtained with directional pulsed Doppler system with PRF of 7.6 kHz. Aliasing begins at 3.8 kHz. Lines drawn at +3.8 kHz and −3.8 kHz allow aliased signal to be moved to correct location on waveform by aligning −3.8 kHz mark with +3.8 kHz mark. Last two cardiac cycles were gathered with nondirectional pulsed Doppler system at PRF of 7.6 kHz. Note that nondirectional aliased signal produces **M**-shaped waveform.

the display (half of the spectrum analyzer sample rate), aliasing will result on the display but not on the audio channels.

PULSED DOPPLER SIGNALS

Pulsed Doppler and CW Doppler systems are both subject to the Doppler equation, but the signals obtained from the two instruments are different. Because the pulsed Doppler systems can measure flow velocity in the midstream of a vessel while rejecting signals from near the vessel walls, the width of the frequency spectrum generated by the pulsed Doppler unit is narrower than those from a CW Doppler unit (Fig. 5-5). This difference in

spectral width can be heard. The sound from a pulsed Doppler system is a purer tone than that from a CW Doppler system.

A flow profile across the vessel can be generated by stepping the angle of the probe laterally across the vessel or by stepping the Doppler sample volume across the vessel[4] by incrementally increasing the depth (Fig. 5-6). If the steps occur in 1 mm increments, the vessel dimensions can be determined by observing the points where velocity goes to zero. This is not an ideal way to measure arterial dimensions because the vessel walls move during the cardiac cycle. The motion of the arterial wall will introduce an intense, low-frequency Doppler

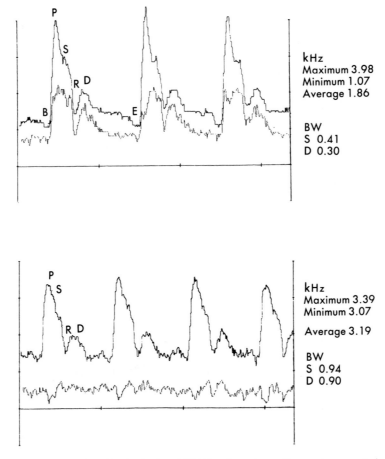

Fig. 5-5. Comparing spectral width of pulsed and CW Doppler systems. Figures show spectral waveform and spectral width by plotting 12th and 88th percentile contour lines. Upper curve is from pulsed Doppler system, and lower trace is from CW Doppler system. Both signals were taken at angle of 45 degrees to skin. While wave shapes are similar, spectral width of pulsed Doppler signal is narrower than CW tracing. Note that peak frequency appears lower on CW tracing even though upper envelopes of signals as viewed on a spectrum analyzer are similar. *S,* Systole; *D,* diastole; *BW,* spectral bandwidth; *B,* automatically selected systolic upslope; *P,* automatically selected peak systole; *B* to *S,* automatically selected systolic period; *R,* automatically selected first zero slope after systole; *S* to *D,* automatically selected diastolic interval; *E,* end diastolic frequency.

signal that will make the vessel appear wider. If low-frequency filters are used to suppress these signals, the vessel width will appear incorrectly small and the width measurement will be velocity dependent.

MULTIGATE PULSED DOPPLER SYSTEMS

The pulsed Doppler system is more difficult to operate than the CW Doppler system. To receive a signal from a CW Doppler unit the Doppler probe must be coupled with the skin and directed at a blood vessel. This requires that the operator have knowledge of the vascular system as projected in the skin. To obtain a signal with a pulsed Doppler unit, in addition to pointing the probe at the vessel of interest, the operator must adjust the range (depth setting) of the machine so that the Doppler signal will be obtained from within the vessel. This requires that the operator have knowledge of the depth of the blood vessels in addition to their projection on the skin. Recognizing this difficulty, investigators have attempted to develop a convenient pulsed Doppler system that could interrogate multiple depths simultaneously.[2]

As the pulsed Doppler system operates, the echoes from tissue include data from a broad range of depths. The data from all depths of tissue except the depth of the sample gate are discarded. Like the echo from the depth of interest, the data from all other depths can be processed by additional sample gates without degrading the data from the first. Such a system allows the velocity profile across the vessel to be displayed. The operation of such a system requires that the phase of the ultrasound signal from various depths be stored separately. The phase from each depth during successive pulse echoes can be compared with the phase from the preceding pulse to establish the Doppler phase shift. This storage can be accomplished in digital memory devices[1] or in analog delay lines.[7] In either case, flow profiles across a vessel diameter can be obtained.

Additional insight to the multigate pulsed Doppler system and its nature can be obtained by playing with the operation of a B-mode imaging system. When a B-mode image is viewed, a speckle pattern is apparent in the image. The size of the

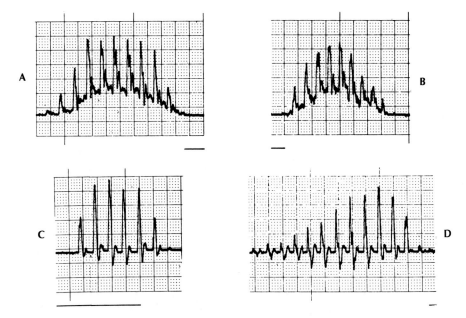

Fig. 5-6. Stepping pulsed Doppler sample volume across common carotid artery and external iliac artery. **A,** Stepping sample volume laterally across common carotid artery indicates blunt flow in systole and rounded flow in diastole. Probe was held by hand without guidance. **B,** Stepping sample volume in depth at same point in common carotid artery indicates more parabolic flow along that diameter of common carotid artery. **C,** Stepping sample volume laterally across external iliac artery shows profile of both forward and reverse flow. **D,** Stepping sample volume in depth in same external iliac artery. Probe is looking into curve; velocities on left are on inside of arterial bend. Peak velocities show asymmetry, whereas reverse velocities have rounded symmetry.

speckles in the depth direction is dependent on the length of the transmission pulse and the response time of the receiver. The speckle does not represent density fluctuations in the tissue but constructive and destructive interference between the reflections coming from slightly different depths. This is superimposed on the image intensity fluctuations caused by changes in tissue density.

In normal B-mode imaging the transmission pulse is so short that the speckles may be too small to be apparent. If, however, the B-mode image is generated from a long Doppler transmission pulse the speckle will be prominent. The speckle associated with stationary regions of tissue will be stationary, but the speckle pattern representing moving tissues such as blood will fluctuate. This "sparkling" of the image is the visual manifestation of the Doppler effect. If attention is focused on a single spot of the speckle pattern the fluctuation frequency of the spot is exactly equal to the expected Doppler frequency. Of course, in Doppler signals, the Doppler frequency may vary from a few hundred to thousands of cycles per second (Hertz). It is not possible to follow such frequencies by eye because the flicker fusion rate of the eye is about 20 Hz. By chance, aliasing makes the effect visible.

In a two-dimensional, real-time B-mode imaging system the frame rate is about 30 Hz. This means that the PRF for each B-mode line comprising the image is about 30 Hz. The PRF is much higher, because the pulser also is used to obtain data from many other lines in the image. A pulsed Doppler system operating at 30 Hz will alias at 15 Hz, below the flicker fusion rate of the eye. Suppose that the velocity in a blood vessel is such that it would create a Doppler shift of 1000 Hz. The pulsed Doppler system operates at a PRF of 30 Hz, so that aliasing will occur at 15 Hz. Doppler frequencies that are multiples of 30 Hz will appear stationary because they exhibit an exact integral number of phase shifts between pulses. Thus an expected Doppler shift frequency of 990 Hz would produce a zero Doppler shift in this pulsed system and a stationary speckle pattern. A 1000 Hz shift, 10 Hz higher than 990 Hz, will produce a periodic cycle in the brightness of the speckle pattern at a frequency of 10 Hz. For other frequencies the fluctuation of the speckle pattern will range in frequency between zero and 15 Hz, well within the range of visibility.

The pattern does not show velocity in an easily understandable manner, but it does show those regions where blood flow is present as a sparkling area of the image and those where it is absent. We first observed the pattern on a wide-aperture B-mode imaging system. The engineers were installing a new transmitter so that the instrument could be used with pulsed Doppler system. Creating the B-mode image with the Doppler transmitter produced the effect of "worms crawling" within the arteries and veins. The observation was never exploited by the manufacturer.

CONCLUSION

Pulsed Doppler systems are now most popular when used with two-dimensional B-mode imaging systems in the form of duplex scanners. Such systems allow the visualization of a blood vessel in longitudinal section and the location of the Doppler sample volume within the vessel under visual control. The angle between the vessel axis and the Doppler ultrasound can be measured directly, and the location of the measurement with respect to curves and bifurcations can be positively established. In addition, periodic vessel motion with respect to the Doppler sample volume can be observed. Pulsed Doppler signals are usually analyzed with real-time spectrum analyzers that allow the details of the frequencies generated to be displayed. In this context the pulsed Doppler system can be used to display the details of the flow within the vascular system.

Even though many advances have been made using CW and pulsed Doppler systems for the diagnosis of arterial, venous, and cardiac disease, there are still many opportunities to expand the usefulness of the information available from pulsed Doppler systems.

REFERENCES

1. Hoeks, A.P.G., Reneman, R.S., and Peronneau, P.A.: A multigate Doppler system with serial data processing, IEEE Trans. Sonics Ultrasonics SU-28:4 1981.
2. Hokanson, D.E., Mozersky, D.J., and Sumner, D.S.: Ultrasonic arteriography, Biomed. Eng. 6:420, 1971.
3. Jaffe, J.: Listen to your heart with Doppler ultrasound, Popular Electronics, August 1975, pp. 60-63.
4. Ku, D.N., Phillips, D.J., Giddens, D.P., Strandness, D.E. Jr.: Hemodynamics of the normal human carotid bifurcation: in vitro and in vivo studies. (Submitted for publication.)
5. McLeod, F.D.: A directional Doppler flowmeter, Dig. Int. Conf. Med. Biol. Eng. 7:196-217, 1967.
6. McLeod, F.D.: A Doppler ultrasonic physiologic flowmeter, Proceedings of the 17th Annual Conference for Engineering in Medicine and Biology, 1968.
7. Nowicki, A., and Reid, J.M.: An infinite gate pulsed Doppler, Ultrasound Med. Biol. 7:41-50, 1981.

CHAPTER 6

Criteria for selection of Doppler instrumentation

K. WAYNE JOHNSTON, P. ZUECH, and MAHMOOD S. KASSAM

Doppler ultrasound equipment is widely used in the noninvasive vascular laboratory for the diagnosis of peripheral arterial, carotid arterial, and venous disease. A typical continuous-wave (CW) system or pulsed Doppler system includes the following components: (1) the Doppler probe, (2) a CW or pulsed Doppler velocity meter, (3) a frequency analyzer or alternative method for processing the Doppler signals, (4) a display system, (5) a technique for quantifying the Doppler spectral waveforms, and (6) a method for obtaining hard copy recordings. A flow-map imaging system will include not only the components listed but also an x-y arm and a display of the flow map. The Doppler components of a duplex scanning system are similar to those mentioned and will not be considered separately. There are a relatively large number of possible components in a Doppler system, and the exact configuration will be determined by the requirements of the laboratory, including the types of studies to be carried out (peripheral arterial, carotid, or venous), the severity of arterial stenoses that must be detected (minor stenoses or severe hemodynamically significant stenoses), and the money available for the purchase of the equipment.

The purpose of this chapter is to describe the criteria for selecting each component in a Doppler system.

DOPPLER PROBE

The Doppler probe forms a critical link between the hemodynamic changes in the artery and the recorded frequency spectrum. Consequently, the accuracy of the Doppler information obtained depends on the characteristics of the Doppler probe.

☐ Supported by a grant from the Ontario Heart Foundation.

The important features of Doppler probes are discussed in the following sections.

Probe frequency

The selection of the optimum probe frequency is based on a compromise between frequency resolution and depth of penetration. With a high probe frequency (8 to 10 MHz), the frequency range of the transduced spectral information is increased, but because of the properties of ultrasonic transmission through tissue, the effective penetration depth is reduced. Generally, for carotid arterial examinations a 4 to 5 MHz probe frequency is recommended. For peripheral arterial studies an 8 to 10 MHz probe is adequate for examination of the pedal arteries but a 4 to 5 MHz probe will achieve better penetration for the femoral and popliteal arteries.

Probe beam field pattern

The uniformity of a CW Doppler ultrasound beam determines the accuracy with which the Doppler information can be obtained from the artery under examination. Ideally the beam should be as wide as the vessel and should have uniform intensity over the entire cross section of the artery. The factors that determine the overall beam field pattern of CW Doppler probes include the frequency of operation, the geometric configurations of both the transmitter and the receiver crystals, the angle and position of the two crystals with respect to each other, and the care and accuracy with which the probe is manufactured.

To determine which commercially available probes had beam characteristics potentially suitable for quantitative assessment of arterial disease, an in vitro model was used to map the beam patterns of ultrasound probes from different manufacturers.[8] Certain probes had beam characteristics that were not uniform, some had shallow depths of penetration, and others showed insufficient beam widths. Previous reports[9,30,31] also noted significant differences in the beam field patterns between probes of different design and different nominal frequencies. When designing probes for quantitative Doppler studies, manufacturers must give more attention to the probe field response characteristics, since any deviation from the ideal beam characteristics can alter the spectral information sufficiently to mask subtle changes that may be of diagnostic value.

Power

Most commercial Doppler probes are within what is generally considered a safe upper limit of acoustic power output (100 mW/cm^2). Probes with a low power output (<50 mW/cm^2) have problems picking up flow signals from vessels where the Doppler signal is attenuated by obesity, scar tissue, or an atherosclerotic plaque.

Pulsed Doppler sample volume

The characteristics of the pulsed Doppler sample volume are of great importance. The recorded Doppler waveform will not be representative and consistent from one recording to another or from one instrument to another if the sample size or shape varies or if the sample is positioned at different sites across the artery.

DOPPLER VELOCITY METER

Over the years, considerable improvement has been made in the design of both CW[21,22,26] and pulsed Doppler velocity meters. Demodulation techniques have been refined so that now, with current instruments, the quality of the raw Doppler signal is quite good. Most Doppler velocity meters provide bidirectional flow outputs as separate forward and reverse flow channels; however, to maintain compatibility with various types of commercial frequency analyzers, additional dual-channel phase quadrature outputs should be available. Cross-talk rejection between the two flow channels of greater than 40 dB is not uncommon but must be specified.

Since different probe frequencies may be used, depending on the depth of the artery being studied, many Doppler velocity meters accept two or three different frequencies. Battery-operated equipment

has the advantages of increased patient safety, portability, and resistance to interference.

Some CW and pulsed Doppler velocity meters have inadequate shielding and an isolated receiver. A poorly designed receiver often will pick up interference noise, from hospital pagers for example, and as a consequence the spectral information is unsatisfactory. Usually a Doppler velocity meter will operate with minimal interference when it is used on its own; however, as soon as it is connected to other instruments, such as a frequency analyzer, display, or recorder, the interference increases dramatically. Proper shielding of the receiver and isolation of signal grounds within the Doppler velocity meter are essential to minimize these problems. In general, users are advised to test a manufacturer's Doppler velocity meter by connecting it to the equipment with which it will be used.

An important specification of a pulsed Doppler system that is often ignored by the user is the pulse repetition frequency (PRF). The maximum detectable Doppler shift frequency is limited to PRF/2. For example, a PRF of 11 kHz will limit the maximum frequency to 5.5 kHz. This is inadequate for carotid examination, since Doppler frequencies above 5.5 kHz will be recorded at the site of a stenosis and will "fold over" and contaminate the spectral information.

Relative advantages of CW vs. pulsed Doppler systems

There is no clear evidence supporting the preferential use of either CW or pulsed Doppler systems in the clinical vascular laboratory. A CW Doppler system insonates the entire vessel, is less expensive, and is generally easier for the technologist to operate. With a pulsed Doppler system, velocity signals can be recorded from any point across the vessel. Although some workers have argued that the early flow disturbances produced by minor arterial stenoses can be detected with a pulsed Doppler system by recording the signals from the center line of flow,[2,3] current evidence suggests that the early disturbances of flow beyond a stenosis occur near the vessel wall. With a pulsed Doppler system, the sample volume may be positioned incorrectly even if a duplex scanning system is used. Also, throughout the cardiac cycle the vessel may move in relation to the fixed position of the sample volume. In these situations the recordings may not be representative.

FREQUENCY ANALYZER

Frequency analysis is generally accepted as the optimum method for processing the Doppler signals.* The following sections describe the important features to consider in evaluating a frequency analyzer.

General features

Simplicity of operation, with careful attention to the human factor, is very important in the design of the analysis system and should efficiently increase patient throughput. Remote control of analyzer and display from the bedside is of great value. Clinical vascular studies are usually carried out by a technician, who must record spectral data as completely as possible so that the supervising physician can interpret the results of the study at a later time. A clinically cost-effective system must be sturdy and reliable, with modular components designed so that service can be carried out quickly by the local distributor, who can simply replace a defective component when a breakdown occurs. It is important that the analyzer system be flexible enough to adapt to rapidly advancing technology, to allow quantitative analysis of Doppler spectral information in the future.

Real time. In some research applications, off-line frequency analysis may be optimum; however, frequency analyzers for use in the clinical vascular laboratory must process the Doppler signals in real time. This feature is of fundamental importance, since real-time analysis provides visual feedback and permits the technician to alter the probe position if necessary to obtain representative recordings. Moreover, quantification of the spectral data can be made available in real time.

Two channels. Bidirectional display is important for both peripheral and carotid arterial studies. In studies of the peripheral arterial system, where the waveform normally contains both forward and reverse flow components, display of both the forward and reverse flow signals is necessary. Bidirectional frequency analysis is also important for carotid studies to allow the examiner to accurately recognize a coexisting venous flow signal and accurately detect the reverse flow signals produced by the eddies and vortices that occur distal to a stenosis. Ideally the frequency analyzer should process the two channels of information separately.

*References 5, 11, 12, 20, 24, 25, 32.

Some analyzers are actually single-channel systems that are adapted to bidirectional analysis using a constant off-set frequency modulator; however, with this approach there may be cross talk between the forward and reverse flow channels.

Time and frequency resolution. The Doppler frequency spectra recorded from pulsatile blood flow may span a wide frequency range and change quite rapidly over time. Current analyzers produce a new spectrum approximately every 10 msec. If a much shorter time segment is analyzed, the resulting spectrum will have significant variability and little meaning. If a longer time sample is used, the dynamic properties of the spectra may be lost. Since normal carotid Doppler signals span a frequency range from 0 to 5 kHz and peripheral arterial signals from 3 kHz in the reverse flow channel to 8 kHz in the forward flow channel, the 100 Hz frequency resolution offered by most analyzers is optimum. With all frequency analyzers it is important to note that there are limitations to the frequency and time resolution which can be achieved, since the frequency bandwidth and the sample time required to produce a complete spectrum are inversely related. For example, if a complete spectrum is produced every 10 msec with most analyzers, the best frequency resolution that can be achieved is approximately 100 Hz; 50 Hz resolution can be achieved if the sampling time is increased to 20 msec. In some systems, a sliding method of analysis is used to improve the frequency resolution. For example, 50 Hz resolution may be obtained and spectra displayed every 5 msec by doing a running average of the most recent 20 msec time sample. With this technique there may be a loss of time resolution because of the averaging effect.

Compatability. The frequency analyzer is an integral part of the Doppler system and must be compatible with currently available CW or pulsed Doppler receivers and with Doppler imaging systems in terms of input signal level, frequency range and resolution, and configuration. Since both components are often made by the same manufacturer, the input signal level, frequency range and resolution, and configuration are not usually a problem.

DISPLAY

The optimum characteristics of a display for carotid Doppler spectral waveforms are somewhat different from those for peripheral arterial waveforms and are described in this section. The important features of a peripheral arterial display are summarized at the end of the section.

Display screen

The technician must view the display screen from a distance. Consequently, it must be large enough and it must have good resolution. A selective frequency range is of benefit, since this will display the waveforms with maximum detail.

Display scan time

Current displays move from right to left so that the operator has a long period of time to evaluate the waveforms and freeze representative waveforms on the screen. The optimum sweep time depends on the size of the screen, but a 2-second sweep is usually too short to allow the technician to accurately evaluate the waveform. A 4- or 5-second sweep time is preferred, but unfortunately with some low-resolution video monitors this sweep speed reduces the time resolution to one spectrum every 25 to 30 msec.

Gray scale or color

In carotid studies, the proportion of spectral energy at every frequency is of interest and consequently must be included in the spectral display. Information concerning spectral content is typically presented to the user through gray-scale modulation of the display intensity or color content. The optimum number of gray-scale levels is difficult to determine. The technician cannot assimilate numerous gray-scale levels in real time, but with the use of only one or two gray-scale levels, only the coarse features of the waveform can be evaluated. In our experience, the display of approximately 10 gray-scale levels has proven to be adequate.

Schemes have been devised using various colors and color intensities to display the spectral intensity. Some technicians find the color display easier to interpret, but this is largely a matter of personal preference. There is a trend toward color display, and it would be advantageous if the choice of a color scheme could be standardized among the manufacturers so that results can be compared and subjectively interpreted.

Linear or decibel

As with the choice between gray scale or color, personal experience plays an important role in the choice of linear or decibel intensity modulation. Basically, a linear scale preserves a direct linear relationship between the spectral strength and display intensity (or color), whereas a decibel scale compresses the information into a logarithmic scale. With a decibel scale it is possible to display a wider range of spectral intensities, but in some cases the visual detection of certain features is hampered. For example, the clear window under the systolic peak of a normal carotid waveform is harder to see. Some manufacturers transform the spectral information in a nonlinear fashion to highlight some of the features of the waveform. However, with this approach quantitative measurements may be in error.

Gain control

The strength of the Doppler signal can vary greatly between recording sites. Since most analysis schemes operate best over a certain range of signal strengths, a gain control is needed in the analyzer to adjust signal levels to within the dynamic range of the analyzer and thereby optimize processing. Both manual and automatic gain controls have advantages and limitations. The manual gain control is more versatile, but the choice of setting is subjective. With an automatic gain control, the signals are adjusted to a relatively constant average power level, but after the operator locates the artery there is a time delay before the automatic gain control adjusts the gain to the predefined level. Also, the effective range of the automatic gain control is sometimes limited and a coarse manual range setting is necessary. Further difficulties may occur when signals are recorded just beyond a stenosis, where low frequency high amplitude signals from eddies and vortices are present along with high frequency low amplitude signals from the jet of blood passing through the stenosis. Automatic adjustment of gain to accommodate both signal components is difficult, and the high frequency peak may not be recorded satisfactorily.

Other criteria

The following features are also helpful: clear frequency and time-scale markings; display of recording site and patient identification; cursors for marking distinct time and frequency points of interest; and gray-scale or color calibration markers. Also there should be provision for display of quantification indices, so they can be recorded on hard copy along with the spectral waveforms.

Peripheral arterial display

For peripheral arterial studies, a bi-level display (black and white) is quite adequate for the following reasons. Because of the complex nature of the peripheral arterial waveform, the gray-scale information has no known diagnostic value. The shapes of the waveforms at the proximal and distal sites of a particular limb segment are used to quantify the severity of the arterial occlusive disease. The bi-level display is usually satisfactory for detecting waveforms with artifacts resulting from noise, co-existing arterial or venous flow, or atypical flow patterns that may occur at a bifurcation or a stenosis. Since the maximum velocity waveform is used for quantitative analysis (Chapter 7), a bi-level display is appropriate. A bi-level display will cut down on the amount of information presented to the operator and present a sharper and more clearly defined waveform for analysis.

QUANTIFICATION

The analog zero-crossing detector waveform has been shown to be artifactual in certain situations[14,15] and should not be used for quantitative analysis. The instantaneous mean waveform derived by analog methods[1,10,22] or preferably from the digital output of a frequency analyzer, and the instantaneous maximum velocity waveform[17] from the outline of the Doppler spectral waveform are commonly used in the quantitative assessment of carotid and peripheral arterial Doppler recordings. Quantitative indices should only be used if they have been validated in careful clinical studies. This section lists some of the indices that have proven to be of value and refers the reader to other chapters in this book where they are reviewed in greater detail.

Quantification of carotid waveforms

Chapter 39 describes in detail the quantitative methods for analyzing carotid Doppler waveforms. At the site of a stenosis the peak frequency is increased, and beyond the stenosis, where there is a disturbed flow, spectral broadening is recorded. Clinical studies have documented that the measurement of peak frequency can accurately detect moderate and severe stenoses.[4,19,29] Several alternatative methods for quantifying the instantaneous Doppler spectrum and thus measuring the severity of spectral broadening are currently being investigated.[7,22,23,28]

Quantification of peripheral arterial waveforms

Chapter 53 describes the alternative methods for quantifying peripheral arterial Doppler waveforms. The methods are based on the subjective obser-

vation that distal to a stenosis, the normal triphasic waveform is dampened, that is, the peak is delayed and reduced and the reverse flow component is reduced or absent. Pulsatility index[11,12,16,18] is the most popular method for quantitative analysis, but other indices are of equivalent value.[18]

HARD COPY

As mentioned previously in this chapter, the data from Doppler studies must be recorded as completely as possible for interpretation at a later time. Videotape recordings preserve all of the Doppler spectral information and have relatively low initial expense but are quite time-consuming for the physician to review. The ideal hard-copy display method should produce a record of the waveforms frozen on the frequency analysis display screen. Polaroid photographs of the display screen have the advantage of a low initial cost, but unfortunately they are time-consuming, and each photograph is quite expensive. A video printer has a high capital cost but a relatively low operating expense and can produce a hard copy of the display in less than 10 seconds. In the future, analysis systems will store displays and data on computer disk, and a small microcomputer will be used to review and print the recordings and produce a report.

For peripheral arterial studies, simple recordings of the maximum frequency waveform have proven to be ideal, thus alleviating the need for a hard copy of the entire spectral display. The technologist uses the frequency analyzer and display to obtain optimum and representative recordings that are free of artifacts and then records only the maximum waveform for documentation. As described in Chapter 7, this can be done automatically by a small microprocessor board in the frequency analyzer.

FLOW-MAP IMAGE

A map of the carotid bifurcation or peripheral arteries can be produced by detecting the presence or absence of a Doppler signal within an x-y plane.[13,27] A Doppler probe attached to an x-y arm is scanned back and forth across the artery, and a display is produced based on the presence or absence of flow at each x-y coordinate. Instead of merely detecting flow and recording it as present or absent, the imaging systems can code the received flow spectral information into various colors or gray-scale levels depending on predetermined frequency bands.[6] With this method, at each arterial site a particular color or gray-scale level represents the dominant velocity band and stenoses can be diagnosed by noting increased frequencies. With most current systems, in addition to the flow map coded with the peak frequency, spectral waveforms are displayed and analyzed as described earlier.[29]

With a flow-map system, the Doppler beam should be as narrow as possible so that adequate spatial resolution is achieved to clearly separate the internal and external carotid arteries and the bifurcation. When a narrow beam is used, more points must be analyzed to construct the image than if a wider beam is employed. In contrast, with a CW Doppler system, if the Doppler spectra are to be analyzed quantitatively, the beam should insonate the entire vessel uniformly. This requires a relatively wide beam. Consequently, to obtain both good spatial resolution and complete insonation of the vessel, a probe with an adjustable beam field pattern may be ideal, but this feature is not yet available in commercial systems.

In any flow-map imaging system, the x-y arm must have good spatial resolution. The computer logic must determine the presence or absence of flow within a few cardiac cycles and discriminate between Doppler signals resulting from probe movement artifacts and line Doppler signals. Well-defined criteria are necessary for color coding areas of peak frequency if errors are to be avoided.

SUMMARY AND CONCLUSIONS

The ideal ultrasound system should have the following characteristics: simplicity of operation; versatility (because the same equipment is often used for various types of examinations); reliability; accuracy for detecting the hemodynamic changes that result from a stenosis; and cost-effectiveness.

In this chapter we have described the criteria for selecting the different components of a continuous-wave or pulsed Doppler system and flow-map imaging system. The components may be configured in several different ways depending on the requirements of the noninvasive laboratory.

ACKNOWLEDGMENTS

The authors wish to acknowledge the secretarial assistance of Mrs. C. Czarnowski.

REFERENCES

1. Arts, M.J.G., and Roevros, J.M.J.G.: On the instantaneous measurement of bloodflow by ultrasonic means, Med. Biol. Eng. 10:23, 1972.
2. Blackshear, W.M., et al.: Detection of carotid occlusive disease by ultrasonic imaging and pulsed Doppler spectrum analysis, Surgery 86:698, 1979.
3. Blackshear, W.M., et al.: Carotid artery velocity patterns in normal and stenotic vessels, Stroke 11:67, 1980.
4. Brown, P.M., et al.: A critical study of ultrasound Doppler spectral analysis for detecting carotid disease, Ultrasound Med. Biol. 8:515, 1982.
5. Coghlan, B.A., Taylor, M.G., and King, D.H.: On-line display of Doppler-shift spectra by a new time compression analyser. In Reneman, R.S., editor: Cardiovascular applications of ultrasound, Amsterdam, 1974, North Holland Publishing Co.
6. Curry, G.R., and White, D.N.: Color-coded ultrasonic differential velocity arterial scanner (Echoflow), Ultrasound Med. Biol. 4:27, 1978.
7. Douville, Y., et al.: An in vitro study of carotid Doppler spectral broadening, Ultrasound Med. Biol. 9:347, 1983.
8. Douville, Y., et al.: Critical evaluation of continuous-wave Doppler probes for carotid studies, J. Clin. Ultrasound 11:83, 1983.
9. Evans, D.H., and Parton, L.: The directional characteristics of some ultrasonic Doppler blood-flow probes, Ultrasound Med. Biol. 7:51, 1981.
10. Gerzberg, L., and Meindl, J.D.: Mean frequency estimator with applications in ultrasonic Doppler flowmeters. In White, D.N., and Brown, R., editors: Ultrasound in medicine; Engineering aspects, New York, 1977, Plenum Publishing Corp.
11. Gosling, R.G., King, D., and Woodcock, J.: Blood-velocity waveforms in the valuation of atheromatous changes. In Roberts, V.C., editor: Blood flow measurement, London, 1972, Sector Publishing.
12. Harris, P.L.: The role of ultrasound in the assessment of peripheral arterial disease, doctoral dissertation, Manchester, England, 1975, University of Manchester.
13. Hokanson, D.E., et al.: Ultrasonic arteriography: a noninvasive method of arterial visualization, Radiology 102:435, 1972.
14. Johnston, K.W., Maruzzo, B.C., and Cobbold, R.S.C.: Errors and artifacts of Doppler flowmeters and their solution, Arch. Surg. 112:1335, 1977.
15. Johnston, K.W., Maruzzo, B.C., and Cobbold, R.S.C.: Inaccuracies of a zero-crossing detector for recording Doppler signals, Surg. Forum 28:201, 1977.
16. Johnston, K.W., Maruzzo, B.C., and Cobbold, R.S.C.: Doppler methods for quantitative measurement and localization of peripheral arterial disease of analysis of the blood flow velocity waveform, Ultrasound Med. Biol. 4:209, 1978.
17. Johnston, K.W., et al.: Methods of obtaining, processing and quantifying Doppler blood flow velocity waveforms. In Nicolaides, A.N., and Yao, J.S.T., editors: Investigation of vascular disorders, Edinburgh, 1980, Churchill Livingstone.
18. Johnston, K.W., et al.: Comparative study of four methods for quantifying Doppler ultrasound waveforms from the femoral artery, Ultrasound Med. Biol. 10:1, 1984.
19. Johnston, K.W., et al: Accuracy of carotid Doppler peak frequency analysis: Results determined by receiver operating characteristic curves and likelihood ratios, Stroke. (In Press).
20. Kaneko, J., et al.: Analysis of ultrasonic blood rheogram by the sound spectrograph, Jpn. Circ. J. 34:1035, English edition, 1970.
21. Kassam, M.S., Johnston, K.W., and Cobbold, R.S.C.: A critical assessment of heterodyne demodulation techniques for directional Doppler ultrasound, Digest of XII International Conference on Medical and Biological Engineering, part II, session 28, paper 3, Jerusalem, 1979.

22. Kassam, M.S., et al.: Method for estimating the Doppler mean velocity waveform, Ultrasound Med. Biol. 8:537, 1982.
23. Kassam, M.S., et al.: Quantification of carotid arterial disease by Doppler ultrasound, IEEE Ultrasonics Symp., pp. 675, 1982.
24. Light, L.H.: A recording spectrograph for analysing Doppler blood velocity signals (particularly from aortic flow) in real time, J. Physiol. (Lond.) 207:42, 1971.
25. Maruzzo, B.C., Johnston, K.W., and Cobbold, R.S.C.: Real-time spectral analysis of directional Doppler flow signals, Digest of XI International Conference on Medical and Biological Engineering, pp. 158, Ottawa, 1976.
26. Nippa, J.H., et al.: Phase rotation for separating forward and reverse blood velocity signals, IEEE Trans. Sonics and Ultrasonics, SU-22:340, 1975.
27. Reid, J.M., and Spencer, M.P.: Ultrasonic Doppler technique for imaging blood vessels, Science 176:1235, 1972.
28. Rittgers, S.E., Thornhill, B.M., and Barnes, R.W.: Quantitative analysis of carotid artery Doppler spectral waveforms—Diagnostic value of parameters, Ultrasound Med. Biol. 9:255, 1983.
29. Spencer, M.P., and Reid, J.M.: Quantitation of carotid stenosis with continuous-wave (CW) Doppler ultrasound, Stroke 10:326, 1979.
30. Wells, P.N.T.: The directivities of some ultrasonic Doppler probes, Med. Biol. Eng. 8:241, 1970.
31. Wells, P.N.T.: Ultrasonic Doppler probes. In Reneman, R.S., editor: Cardiovascular application of ultrasound, Amsterdam, 1974, North Holland Publishing Co.
32. Zuech, P., et al.: The application of CCD transversal filters for real-time spectral analysis of Doppler ultrasound signals, Ultrasound Med. Biol. 8:57, 1982.

CHAPTER 7

Processing Doppler signals and analysis of peripheral arterial waveforms: problems and solutions

K. WAYNE JOHNSTON and MAHMOOD S. KASSAM

In the assessment of patients with occlusive arterial disease, continuous-wave (CW) Doppler velocity meters are most commonly used in combination with a blood pressure cuff to measure limb systolic blood pressures. In addition, many vascular laboratories also use them to record blood flow velocity waveforms from peripheral arteries, extracranial cerebral arteries, or the aortic arch.

The purpose of this chapter is to describe the principles and problems of Doppler signal processing and wave-form analysis of peripheral arterial signals and to outline how these limitations can be overcome. To present these data in a format that is easily understood, we have confined our remarks to the problems encountered in the diagnosis of occlusive peripheral arterial disease. Similar problems may occur in processing and analyzing signals from the carotid arteries or the aortic arch.

To obtain valid and useful clinical data by processing CW Doppler signals and analyzing the Doppler waveform, it is essential that representative Doppler signals be transduced from the artery, that the Doppler equipment process the signals accurately and display a waveform that is free of artifacts, and that the waveforms be quantified accurately. As shown diagrammatically in Fig. 7-1, problems in Doppler signal processing and waveform analysis may be the result of errors introduced by (1) the Doppler equipment, (2) the vascular laboratory technician, or (3) the patient's patho-

☐ Supported by grants from The Medical Research Council of Canada and NSERC.

physiologic state. In the following sections these errors will be outlined and solutions to the problems described.

ERRORS INTRODUCED BY THE DOPPLER EQUIPMENT

The waveform recorded noninvasively from a peripheral artery by using Doppler ultrasound has little or no value unless one can be certain that it is proportional to the true blood flow velocity waveform in the artery. Probably the most common cause of an artifactual waveform is the use of a Doppler system that does not accurately transduce, process, display, or quantify the Doppler waveform. The following subsections will describe the errors that may result from the use of an inappropriate Doppler probe, Doppler demodulation technique, Doppler signal analyzer, display system, or quantitative method for assessment of waveforms. The solutions to these problems will be described.

The Doppler probe

Clinicians have noted that superficial arteries (for example, dorsalis pedis, posterior tibial) are optimally studied with a 9 or 10 MHz Doppler probe, whereas a lower frequency is preferable for deep vessels (for example, femoral, popliteal). As illustrated in Fig. 7-2, for a vessel of d cm depth, the optimum probe frequency (f_{opt}) in MHz is given by[45]

$$f_{opt} \approx \frac{9}{d} \qquad (1)$$

If an inappropriate probe frequency is used, the signal-to-noise ratio may be poor; as a result, it

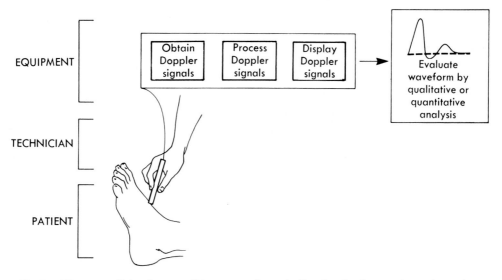

Fig. 7-1. Diagram outlining three possible sources of error in Doppler signal processing and waveform analysis.

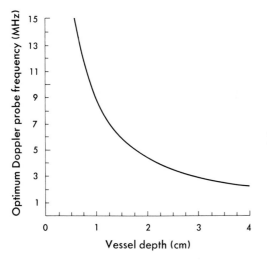

Fig. 7-2. Relationship between optimum Doppler probe frequency and vessel depth.[45]

may be impossible to obtain a useful Doppler signal. Moreover, the waveform may appear to be abnormally dampened in the normal subject. When both superficial and deep vessels are to be studied, this problem can be overcome by choosing a two-probe system (for example, 5 and 10 MHz).

Doppler demodulation techniques

In humans the normal peripheral arterial blood flow velocity waveform contains forward and reverse flow information. The early work with CW Doppler systems used *nondirectional* Doppler techniques and thus it was necessary to determine sub-jectively which portions of the recorded trace corresponded to forward flow and which to reverse flow.[33,54,55] It is apparent that this technique is associated with considerable potential for error or ambiguity and that quantitative assessment of Doppler signals requires that the Doppler demodulating technique clearly separate the forward and reverse flow signals even if they coexist.

The methods available for obtaining the Doppler frequency spectrum with *directional information* have been reviewed by Coghlan and Taylor[9] and Johnston et al.[31,33] Most commercially available systems make use of one of the new phase quadrature demodulation schemes[40,41,44] or other improved techniques.[37] These schemes are all limited in their ability to achieve perfect separation between the forward and reverse flow channels and as a result cross talk may be present (that is, some of the reverse flow signal may appear in the forward channel and vice versa). Since the cross talk arises from a cancellation effect, long-term drift of the circuit and aging of the components, as well as production tolerances, can result in inadequate performance. Over the past several years, awareness of the potential inaccuracies that may result from cross talk has led the manufacturers of Doppler velocity meters to specify cross-talk rejections of more than 40 dB. Such high rejection values are now possible through improved designs and stringent quality control.

Doppler signal analyzer (real-time frequency analyzer)

Having obtained undistorted Doppler signals, it is necessary to process and display them in a clinically useful way. In a previous publication we have described the alternatives for processing the Doppler frequencies and have reviewed the errors and limitations associated with the use of a zero-crossing detector, first moment processor, or frequency follower.[34] In particular, it is important to realize that the zero-crossing detector is associated with certain inherent errors and is less satisfactory for producing a waveform that is suitable for quantitative analysis.[30] In a clinical vascular laboratory study we found that a zero-crossing detector system accurately recorded the velocity wave in only 15% of the femoral, 31% of the popliteal, 67% of the dorsalis pedis, and 62% of the posterior tibial artery recordings.[30]

Arts and Roevros[5] and Gerzberg and Meindl[16] have described circuits that calculate the true analog mean velocity waveform, that is, the first moment of the Doppler spectrum. However, these circuits have many of the problems encountered with the zero-crossing detector, especially if the signal-to-noise ratio is poor or there is coexisting arterial or venous flow. Also, the recorded mean will be correct only if the entire vessel is uniformly insonated with ultrasound and there is no attenuation of the ultrasound beam across the vessel.

Full spectral analysis is the method of choice for processing the Doppler signals from peripheral arteries, since it retains all the Doppler information and allows the examiner to determine if the wave-

form contains an artifact. The artifacts that can be detected may be the result of significant background noise, high-amplitude low-frequency signals arising from arterial wall or probe movement, or signals recorded simultaneously from two arteries or an artery and vein.

In early studies,[12] frequency analysis was accomplished by an off-line method. The Kay sonograph was a reliable method for processing Doppler signals, but unfortunately only 2.5 seconds of the Doppler trace could be recorded. It was extremely time-consuming, and directional Doppler information could not be displayed easily.

Real-time frequency analysis is preferable and can be performed by the time compression technique,[10,54] fast Fourier analysis (FFT), or by multiple band-pass filter analysis.[38,41]

If the Doppler signals are processed by a frequency analyzer, the operator can be certain that there are no artifacts and can use the following methods to display the Doppler information.

Display of Doppler waveform

Having obtained directional Doppler signals and processed them by a real-time frequency analyzer, it is necessary to display and analyze the resulting spectral information. In this subsection we will discuss the methods for displaying and recording (1) the Doppler frequency waveform and (2) the instantaneous maximum velocity waveform.

Doppler frequency waveform. The Doppler frequency waveform obtained from the frequency analyzer can be displayed on an oscilloscope or a video display in real time. The waveforms move across the screen from right to left and when representative waveforms are present on the screen, the examiner uses a remote control button to freeze the display.

For peripheral arterial studies, the gray-scale information within the waveform has little meaning and is difficult to quantify. Consequently, only the shape of the spectral waveform is used to assess the severity of arterial disease. The maximum velocity waveform is used for quantitative analysis, and for this reason, in peripheral arterial studies, it is preferable to use a bi-level spectral display. This format provides optimum quality control of the waveform and establishes a one-to-one correspondence between what the technician views and what is quantified. Fig. 7-3 illustrates that a bi-level display records the shape of the waveform without the complex gray-scale levels. Fig. 7-4

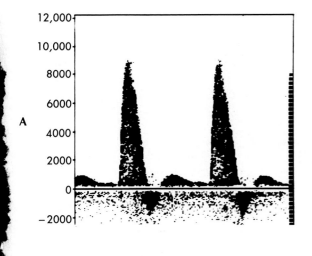

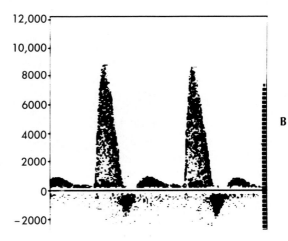

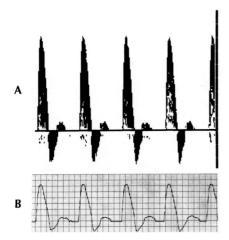

Fig. 7-3. Normal femoral artery waveform. *A,* Ten levels of gray scale (note several levels of gray scale are lost in photographic reproduction). *B,* Four levels of gray scale. *C,* Bi-level display.

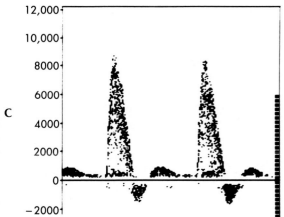

Fig. 7-4. *A,* Doppler spectral waveform. *B,* Corresponding instantaneous maximum velocity waveform.

illustrates the correspondence between the Doppler spectral waveform and the instantaneous maximum velocity waveform derived from the outline of the spectral waveform.

Permanent recordings of the spectral waveform can be obtained by photographing the display, by using an oscillographic recorder, or by using a video printer.

Instantaneous maximum velocity waveform. The instantaneous maximum velocity waveform represents the velocity of the fastest moving red cells. As illustrated in Fig. 7-4, *B,* this waveform is the envelope of the Doppler frequency waveform. We have used this waveform for quantitative analysis, since it is the easiest to obtain clinically. It is only necessary to adjust the probe position so that the maximum amplitude and frequency are obtained.

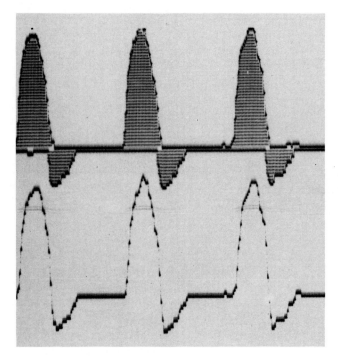

Fig. 7-5. Instantaneous maximum velocity waveform is envelope of Doppler frequency waveform. Circuit that detects envelope also is able to reject artifacts arising from cross talk.

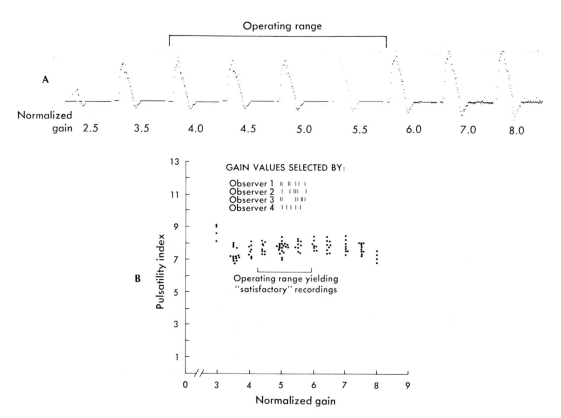

Fig. 7-6. A, As Doppler gain is increased, amplitude of instantaneous maximum velocity waveform increases, although shape remains unchanged. ***B,*** Within normal operating region, pulsatility index (peak-to-peak height divided by mean height) is independent of Doppler gain.

We have developed an electronic circuit that detects the envelope and displays the maximum velocity waveform on a standard analog recorder. An additional and very valuable feature of this circuit is its ability to reject artifacts arising from cross talk (Fig. 7-5).

Since the amplitude of the Doppler signal depends on the probe-to-vessel angle, vessel depth, tissue depth, tissue attenuation, and other factors, the operator either must adjust the gain control to achieve a satisfactory recording or use an automatic gain control (AGC) feature. Although the amplitude of the wave increases with increasing gain, the shape of the wave does not change. As illustrated in Fig. 7-6, *A,* with increasing gain the peak-to-peak height of the wave increases and the mean height increases, but within the normal operating region, the normalized peak-to-peak height (that is, peak-to-peak height divided by mean height, or pulsatility index) is independent of gain (Fig. 7-6, *B*). In other words, within the normal operating region the gain setting is not critical in obtaining quantitative information.

Summary. Display of the Doppler frequency waveform in realtime allows the examiner to position the Doppler probe and obtain representative waveforms that are free of artifacts. This waveform may be photographed from the oscilloscope display or recorded by an oscillographic recorder or video printer. However, we have found that it is easier to obtain a permanent record by recording the instantaneous maximum velocity waveform by using one of the methods already described. The use of an analog signal simplifies on-line quantitative analysis.

Assessment of waveforms

Subjective analysis. Subjective evaluation of Doppler velocity recordings from peripheral arteries is widely used in vascular laboratories for the diagnosis and localization of occlusive peripheral arterial disease. As illustrated in Fig. 7-7, the normal Doppler blood flow velocity waveform is triphasic, consisting of forward flow, reverse flow, and a second forward flow component, whereas distal to an arterial stenosis or occlusion, the waveform is dampened, that is, the amplitude of the velocity wave is decreased, the peak is delayed, and the reverse *flow component* is attenuated or absent.* Fig. 7-8 illustrates the progressive dampening of the waveform shape that occurs beyond stenoses. In the usual vascular laboratory study, waveforms are recorded from the femoral, popliteal, dorsalis pedis, and posterior tibial arteries (Fig. 7-9), and by subjective analysis vascular disease is detected and regionally localized. Subjective analysis may be of value in many situations, but unfortunately, it requires experience and the results cannot be used to compare patients or to provide objective quantitative follow-up.

Quantification. Quantitative analysis of Doppler waveforms is the ideal goal. As described earlier, quantification is possible only if directional Doppler signals are obtained by a reliable method and the Doppler signals are processed and displayed accurately.

The most direct way to quantify the Doppler waveform is to calibrate the waveform as velocity.

*References 12,15,20,30,31,33,55,58.

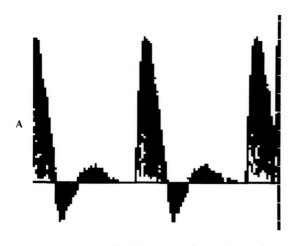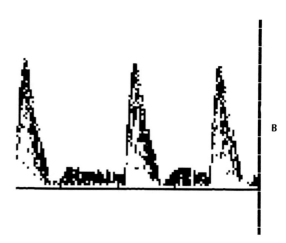

Fig. 7-7. A, Normal spectral waveform from bi-level display. *B,* Abnormal waveform.

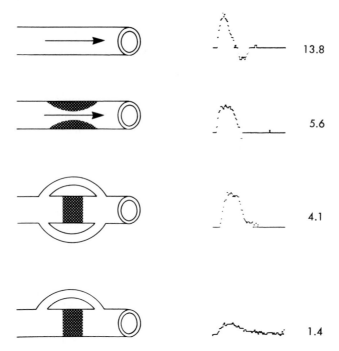

Fig. 7-8. Doppler blood flow velocity waveform is dampened by proximal arterial stenosis. Numbers refer to pulsatility index.

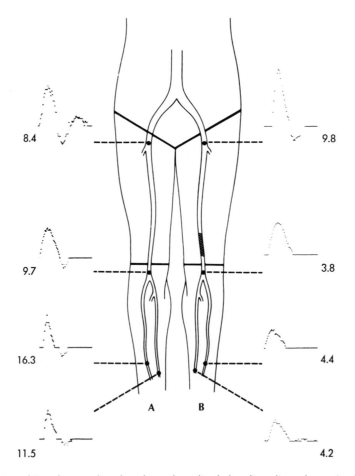

Fig. 7-9. A, Normal Doppler recordings from femoral, popliteal, dorsalis pedis, and posterior tibial arteries. **B,** Doppler recordings from patient with superficial femoral artery occlusion.

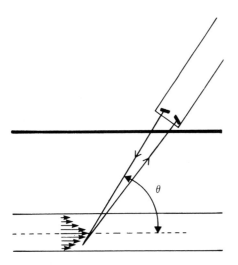

Fig. 7-10. Doppler output can be converted to velocity only if angle between ultrasound probe and axis of blood flow is known.

However, the Doppler output can be converted to velocity only if the angle between the ultrasound probe and the axis of blood flow is known or the angle yielding the maximum velocity signal is employed both in calibration and in clinical use (Fig. 7-10). Fish and Walters[11] have reviewed the proposed techniques for accurately measuring the probe-to-vessel angle, and they have implemented a technique in their pulsed Doppler system.

Although a CW Doppler velocity meter can only be used to measure velocity or flow if previously calibrated (Chapter 53), quantitative data still can be obtained. For any measurement from the Doppler waveform to be of value, it is necessary to show that the measurement is independent of probe-to-vessel angle and that it is clinically useful.

Distal to an arterial stenosis, the waveform is dampened and the following changes are characteristic: reduced peak amplitude, delayed peak, broadened systolic wave, and reduction or elimination of the reverse flow component. Any index that incorporates one or more of these changes may be useful.

Of the possible indices described in this discussion, we have found that peak-to-peak pulsatility index is of practical value and can be computed quite simply in real time.

Fourier pulsatility index. Gosling et al.[17,19] and Woodcock et al.[57] were the first to recognize that Fourier analysis could be used to quantify the Doppler waveform. Any periodic wave, including the

Doppler blood flow velocity waveform, can be expressed as a series of sine waves (harmonics) that oscillate about a mean velocity. The frequencies of these sine waves are integral multiples of the fundamental frequency (that is, heart rate). Each sine wave has a characteristic frequency, amplitude (that is, velocity) and phase angle. In the same way that the amplutude of blood flow velocity waveform depends on the probe-to-vessel angle, the amplitudes of each of the Fourier harmonics and of the mean value of the wave also depend on this angle; but since the same constant of proportionality applies to all the amplitudes, the ratio from the amplitudes of each harmonic (A_n) to the mean amplitude of the wave (A_0) is independent of the probe-to-vessel angle. The Fourier pulsatility index was defined by

$$\text{PI}_f = \sum_{n=1}^{\infty} \frac{A_n^2}{A_0^2} \qquad (2)$$

Since both the numerator and the denominator depend on the velocity squared, the unknown constant of proportionality, which relates the maximum instantaneous frequency waveform to the maximum instantaneous velocity waveform, disappears in the calculation. Theoretically this index is independent of probe-to-vessel angle, and indeed this has been confirmed by Kaneko et al.[36]

Since energy is proportional to velocity squared, the Fourier pulsatility index is related to the maximum oscillatory energy of the wave divided by the energy of the mean forward flow. Distal to an arterial stenosis, the oscillatory energy of the wave is reduced, and thus it was predicted that the Fourier pulsatility index would be reduced and would be useful for detecting occlusive arterial disease. The diagnostic value of the Fourier pulsatility index has been confirmed in clinical studies by Gosling et al.[19] and Johnston and Taraschuk.[33]

Peak-to-peak pulsatility index. It is apparent that the calculation of the Fourier pulsatility index is quite cumbersome and time consuming, so it is impractical for routine clinical use. Gosling and King[17] have suggested an alternative definition of the pulsatility index with roughly the same diagnostic sensitivity. As illustrated in Fig. 7-11, they defined peak-to-peak pulsatility index by

$$\text{PI}_{p/p} = \frac{\text{Peak-to-peak velocity}}{\text{Mean velocity}} \qquad (3)$$

It should be noted that the peak-to-peak pulsatility index is also independent of the probe-to-vessel

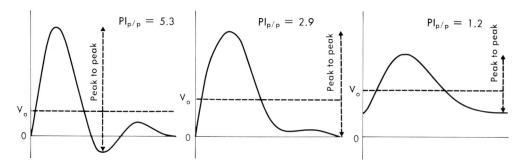

Fig. 7-11. Calculation of peak-to-peak pusatility index.

angle, since the unknown constant of proportionality is present in both the numerator and the denominator and disappears in the calculation. We have found that peak-to-peak pulsatility index and Fourier pulsatility index are related by[31]

$$PI_{pp} = 1.9(PI_f)^{0.57} \qquad (4)$$

As illustrated in Fig. 4-9, *A*, the pulsatility index will usually increase if one progresses distally from the aorta to the pedal arteries. To quantify these changes and permit regional localization of occlusive arterial disease, it is convenient to define a second index, namely, the damping factor (DF)[19] given by

$$DF = \frac{\text{Proximal pulsatility index}}{\text{Distal pulsatility index}} \qquad (5)$$

Because most clinical measurement indices decrease with increasing severity of disease, to conform to this convention, we feel it is preferable to use inverse damping factor DF^{-1}.

Clinical studies by Woodcock et al.,[57] Gosling et al.,[17,19] Harris,[20] and Johnston et al.* have shown that the pulsatility index is of diagnostic value. In a typical study (Fig. 7-9) recordings are made from the femoral, popliteal, dorsalis pedis, and posterior tibial arteries. Femoral pulsatility index and femoral, popliteal, and tibial inverse damping factors are calculated.

Recordings were made from 224 limbs and compared to arteriographic grades to obtain the data presented in Figs. 7-12 to 7-14.

In other arteriographic studies, investigators have confirmed that the measurement of peak-to-peak pulsatility index could detect and regionally localize significant peripheral arterial occlusive disease.[1,20,21] Because of the uncertainties of arterio-

*References 24,25,29,31,32,34.

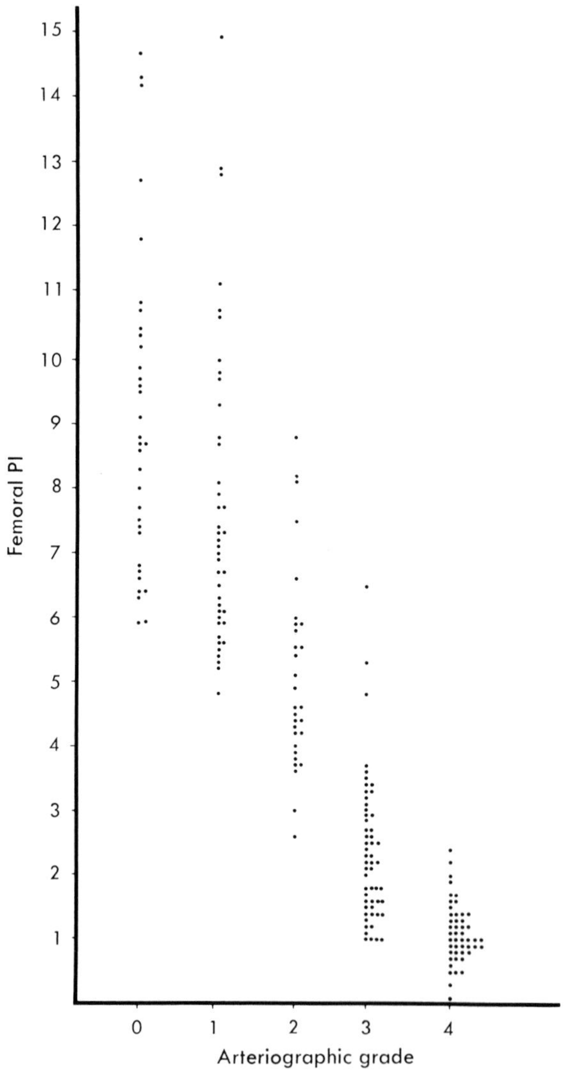

Fig. 7-12. Femoral artery pulsatility index plotted against corresponding aortoiliac arteriographic grade. Grade 0, normal; Grade 1, intimal disease; Grade 2, less than 50% stenosis; Grade 3, greater than 50% stenosis; Grade 4, complete arterial occlusion. (Reproduced courtesy PSG Publishing Co., Inc., Littleton, Mass.)

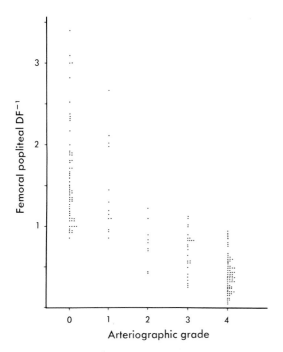

Fig. 7-13. Inverse femoral popliteal damping factor plotted against femoral artery arteriographic grades. (Reproduced courtesy PSG Publishing Co., Inc., Littleton, Mass.)

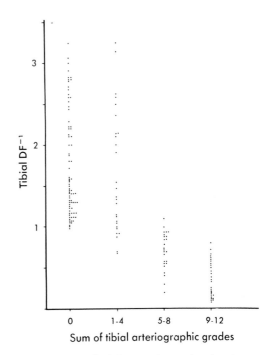

Fig. 7-14. Inverse tibial damping factor plotted against sum of tibial artery arteriographic grades. (Reproduced courtesy PSG Publishing Co., Inc., Littleton, Mass.)

graphic grading, we studied 175 aortofemoral segments and determined the accuracy of peak-to-peak pulsatility index by comparison to the systolic pressure difference between the aorta and common femoral artery as measured at the time of arteriography.[27] In Fig. 7-15, *A,* the receiver operating characteristic (ROC) curve[42,43] is shown for all pulsatility index measurements. An aortofemoral systolic pressure difference equal to or greater than 10 mm Hg was considered a positive test. The highest pulsatility index recorded from the femoral artery at the level of the inguinal ligament or 2 to 3 cm distally was used. In the ROC curve, the sensitivities and specificities are plotted in increments of 0.1 for threshold values of pulsatility index between 4.5 and 6.0. The maximum overall accuracy is approximately 95%.

The effect of distal peripheral arterial occlusive disease on the accuracy of femoral pulsatility index measurements is illustrated in the ROC curve plotted in Fig. 7-15, *B.* The diagnostic accuracy of the pulsatility index in patients without significant distal occlusive disease is slightly higher than for those patients with significant distal disease, that is, patients with greater than 50% stenosis or occlusion of the femoral popliteal segment or occlusion of two or three tibial arteries.

Although some research[2,3,4] has indicated that the pulsatility index is of value in diagnosing hemodynamically significant aortoiliac disease even if the patient has distal occlusive disease, other investigators[6,7,56] have suggested that pulsatility index is strongly influenced by the severity of distal disease and that femoral pulsatility index is less accurate when distal disease is present. We have demonstrated that accurate reproducible measurements can be obtained only if attention is given to certain important technical details. These factors probably explain why pulsatility index measurements have been less accurate in some studies.

Pulsatility index compared to other indices. Although a number of indices, including transit time,[13,17,23] rise time, and rise time ratio,[23] have been suggested for quantifying Doppler ultrasound recordings, in a recent study[28] we have compared the accuracy of the following indices in the diagnosis of peripheral arterial occlusive disease: peak-to-peak pulsatility index, height-width index, path length index, and a transfer function index.

Peak-to-peak pulsatility index (PI) is defined by equation 3 in this chapter.

Height-width index (HWI) is based on the observation that waveforms recorded distal to an ar-

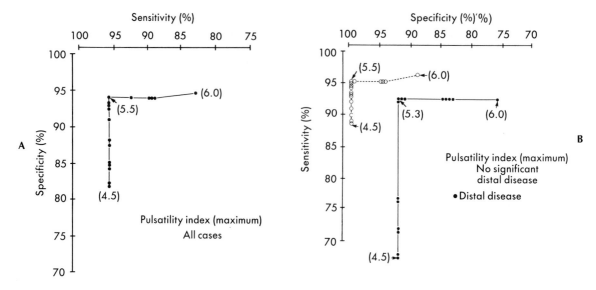

Fig. 7-15. Receiver operating characteristic (ROC) curves. Aortofemoral systolic pressure difference greater than or equal to 10 mm Hg was considered positive test. Sensitivities and specificities are plotted for different values of pulsatility index in increments of 0.1. **A,** All cases. **B,** Effect of distal arterial occlusive disease. (From Johnson, K.W., Kassam, M., and Cobbold, R.S.C.: Ultrasound Med. Biol. 9:271, 1983.)

terial stenosis have smaller peak forward and smaller peak reverse flow frequencies relative to the mean value, and the duration of the systolic peak is greater than that of a normal waveform. This dimensionless index is given by the following formula

$$\text{(6)}$$

$$\text{HWI} = \frac{\text{Peak-to-peak frequency/Mean frequency}}{\text{(Duration of systolic peak/Duration of cardiac cycle)}}$$

where the systolic peak duration is measured between the half-amplitude points.

Path length index (PLI). The effect of increased damping on the instantaneous frequency waveform is to decrease the total path traced out over one cardiac cycle. Consequently, the path length, normalized by mean amplitude (to remove the angle dependence) and normalized by the cardiac period (to reduce the dependence on heart rate), should be reasonably well correlated with the disease grade. We define the path length index by

$$\text{PLI} = \sum_{i=0}^{n-1} [(f_{i+1} - f_i)^2/\bar{f}^2 - (t_{i+1} - t_i)^2/T]^{1/2} \qquad \text{(7)}$$

where the time axis has been divided into n segments, the maximum instantaneous frequency at the time t_i is f_i, $\bar{f}$ is the mean frequency, and T is the total waveform duration.

Transfer-function index. Brown et al.,[8] Skidmore and Woodcock,[48,49] and Skidmore et al.[52] have suggested that arterial occlusive disease can be diagnosed by determining the poles of the transfer function that relate the flow velocity waveform measured at two locations. Subsequently, Skidmore and Woodcock[50,51,53] proposed that the velocity waveform could fit in the frequency domain to the third-order Laplace transform

$$H(s) = 1/(s^2 + 2\delta\omega_o s + \omega_o^2)(s + \gamma) \qquad \text{(8)}$$

where $s = j\omega$. It is evident that the same set of parameters could also be obtained by fitting the waveform in the time domain to the inverse Laplace transform of equation 5, that is to

$$\text{(9)}$$

$$f(t) = \frac{\gamma(\alpha^2 + \beta^2)}{(\gamma - \alpha)^2 + \beta^2} [e^{-\gamma t} + e^{-\alpha t}(\frac{\gamma - \alpha}{\beta} \sin\beta t - \cos\beta t)]$$

where $\alpha = \omega_o\delta$ and $\beta^2 = \omega_o^2 - \alpha^2$.

Skidmore and Woodcock presented experimental evidence to support the hypothesis that parameter δ is related to the degree of proximal disease, that ω_o is related to the arterial elasticity, and that γ is related to the distal impedance. Skidmore et al. calculated δ from the femoral Doppler recordings and investigated the sensitivity to aortoiliac disease and concluded that δ is a sensitive index for de-

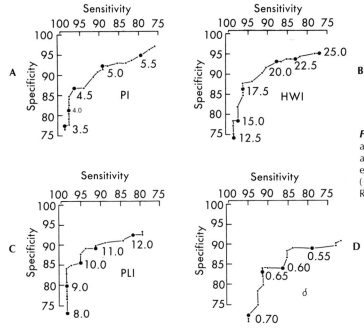

Fig. 7-16. ROC curves for *A,* PI; *B,* HWI; *C,* PLI; and *D,* δ. Iliac disease was defined as present if arteriogram showed less than 50% stenosis, greater than 50% stenosis, or complete occlusion. (From Johnson, K.W., Kassam, M., and Cobbold, R.S.C.: Ultrasound Med. Biol. 9:271, 1983.)

termining the presence of aortoiliac stenoses. In addition, they also investigated the pulsatility index but found that, unlike δ, it did not seem to differentiate between stenoses of less than 50% and greater than 50%.

To determine the optimum index, recordings of the Doppler spectral waveforms from the common femoral artery of 234 limbs were digitized to obtain the maximum velocity waveforms.[28] The data were analyzed on a computer, and the various indices were computed and compared with the arteriographic grades as defined in Fig. 7-12. The calculations of peak-to-peak pulsatility index, height-width index, and path length index were straightforward, but the transfer function parameters were more complicated. Although we used the method described by Skidmore[48] and confirmed the accuracy of our methods, there were significant problems with the frequency domain fitting technique.[28] Specifically, we found that a significant number of waveforms did not yield complex poles, we noted significant discrepancies in the reconstructed waveform of certain recordings, and we observed discrepancies in many of the natural frequencies. Because of these problems, we carried out our curve-fitting procedure in the time domain and specifically calculated δ, which is reported to be related to the severity of proximal disease.

The accuracy of each index for detecting aortoiliac disease was determined by calculating the ROC curves.[22] Two definitions of a positive test were used. In the first, an iliac arteriographic lesion of less than 50% or greater than 50% or a complete occlusion was used; this resulted in the ROC curves in Fig. 7-16. For the second, iliac disease was defined to be present if the stenosis was either greater than 50% or a complete occlusion. For this definition, the curves in Fig. 7-17 resulted. In both sets of curves, the sensitivities and specificities are plotted for different cut off values of each index.

The presence of coexisting femoral popliteal occlusive disease reduced the accuracy of all indices when the definition of iliac disease is a stenosis of less than 50%, greater than 50%, or complete occlusion. On the other hand, for the other definition (that is, greater than 50% stenosis or a complete occlusion) the effect of femoral popliteal disease on the accuracy is less marked, particularly for peak-to-peak pulsatility index and height-width index.

Although arteriography may not be the ideal standard for evaluating noninvasive Doppler data, its shortcomings are not particularly important, since all four indices in this study were calculated from the same waveforms. We have concluded that all the indices had very similar diagnostic accu-

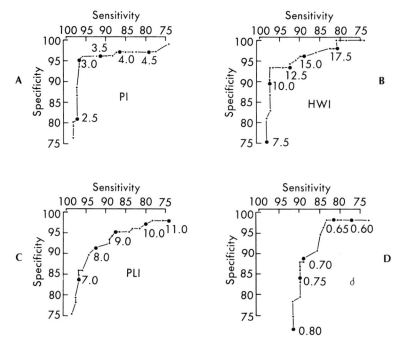

Fig. 7-17. ROC curves for ***A,*** PI; ***B,*** HWI; ***C,*** PLI; and ***D,*** δ. Iliac disease was defined as present if arteriograms showed greater than 50% stenosis or complete occlusion. (From Johnson, K.W., Kassam, M., and Cobbold, R.S.C.: Ultrasound Med. Biol. 9:271, 1983.)

racies. In contrast to the previous report by Skidmore et al.,[53] the index δ did not prove to be superior to pulsatility index. In view of the approximately equivalent diagnostic accuracy of the four indices studied, we feel that pulsatility index has the advantages of simplicity and ease of real-time calculation.

ERRORS INTRODUCED BY THE TECHNICIAN

As with most diagnostic techniques, the operator must acquire experience and appreciate the technical and physiologic limitations of Doppler signal processing and quantitative waveform analysis before representative blood flow velocity recordings can be obtained and reproducible results achieved. For example, errors in recording the femoral artery waveform may be made (1) if only part of the artery is insonated with ultrasound or recordings are inadvertently made from a side branch, (2) if two arteries or an artery and a vein are recorded simultaneously, or (3) if the technician fails to realize that the Doppler signal may be attenuated if the vessel is covered with scar tissue, hematoma, or excessive fat or if it has an atherosclerotic plaque on the anterior wall. The technician must alter the probe position and/or frequency to obtain a representative waveform recording.

If Doppler recordings are to be of quantitative diagnostic value, the technician must be adequately trained and must have a reasonable technical facility. We have found that the use of frequency analysis with a real-time bi-level moving display allows the technician to position the probe optimally, avoid artifacts, and record representative waveforms.

ERRORS INTRODUCED BY THE PATIENT (PATHOPHYSIOLOGIC ERRORS)

Quantitative analysis of Doppler waveforms has been shown to be of diagnostic value; however, problems may be introduced by certain uncontrollable physiologic or pathologic variables.

Attenuation of the Doppler signal

Ultrasound is attenuated as it passes through tissue; hence when the distance between the probe and the vessel is increased by obesity, by hematoma from an arteriogram or operation, or by scar tissue, the Doppler blood flow signals are significantly attenuated. As a result, the Doppler signals may not be distinguishable from background noise, or the waveform may appear abnormal. This problem can usually be overcome if the technician uses the optimum Doppler probe frequency and position. Similarly an atherosclerotic plaque on the anterior wall of the femoral artery may attenuate the ultrasound signal and give the false impression that the waveform is dampened. However, with the help of a real-time display, the operator can in most cases position the probe and obtain a representative waveform.

As the Doppler ultrasound passes across the vessel, those signals arising from blood cells close to the distant wall are attenuated more than those from the blood cells close to the near wall. Thus in large vessels the spectral density may be distorted. The instantaneous maximum velocity waveform will usually be recorded correctly, but if the power spectrum is distorted, the instantaneous mean velocity waveform may not be accurately recorded.

Variations with respiration, heart rate, and peripheral resistance

Peripheral blood flow fluctuates with respiration, so it is not surprising that the peripheral arterial blood flow velocity waveform and thus the pulsatility index also change with respiration. However, we have found that the effect of normal respiration on pulsatility index is insignificant in most patients.

Pulsatility index is calculated by dividing the peak-to-peak height of the wave by the mean height. The mean height is the net area under the wave (forward minus reverse) divided by the pulse length. In other words, it is to be expected that pulsatility index will vary linearly with heart rate. We have confirmed this observation by studying patients with cardiac arrhythmias[35] but have not found this to be a common limitation.

Quantitative analysis of the Doppler waveform, like the determination of many other physiologic parameters, assumes that the patient is in a basal state. If vasodilation occurs, limb blood flow and therefore mean velocity increase and consequently pulsatility index falls, even though the wave may remain very oscillatory. This problem may be minimized by examining subjects at rest, in a quiet room, and at a temperature of $21° \pm 2°$ C. No exercise should be permitted for at least 20 minutes before the examination, and subjects should be asked to refrain from smoking for 1 hour before examination.

Minor arterial stenoses

Minor and usually asymptomatic and hemodynamically insignificant arterial stenoses are not consistently detected by calculation of the pulsatility index from Doppler velocity waveforms.

Major stenoses and occlusions

Major arterial stenoses and arterial occlusions cannot always be distinguished by waveform analysis. Although Gosling and King[17] suggested that the addition of transit time measurement to those of pulsatility index and inverse damping factor may improve this separation, we have not found this measurement to be of additional value. Moreover, it is rarely of clinical significance to be able to distinguish severe stenosis from complete occlusion in the peripheral arteries, and indeed, hemodynamically, a complete occlusion with good collateralization may be similar to a major stenosis.

Multisegmental severe disease

Using pulsatility index and inverse damping factor, it is usually possible to detect and localize occlusive peripheral arterial disease even if more than one arterial segment is involved; however, if severe occlusive disease is present in a proximal segment and the waveforms are very dampened, it may be impossible to make meaningful quantitative measurements from the more distal segments.

Tibial artery assessment

Collateral flow between the three tibial arteries is usually quite satisfactory, so it is not surprising that atherosclerotic occlusion of one tibial vessel cannot be detected or always distinguished from the common normal variation where one tibial artery is congenitally small. Nonetheless, as illustrated in Fig. 7-14, significant occlusive tibial arterial disease (that is, disease in two or three vessels) can usually be detected by the calculation of the tibial inverse damping factor.

Summary of recommendations for reliable and reproducible quantification using pulsatility index

It is now accepted that Doppler systems can be used to quantify the severity of peripheral arterial occlusive disease and that this leads to more precise diagnosis. However, quantitative analysis of Doppler waveforms can be achieved only if the following recommendations are followed.

Appropriate Doppler probe. Accurate recordings

can be obtained only if a Doppler probe with the proper field pattern, operating close to the optimum frequency, is used. The importance of the frequency of the Doppler probe has often been overlooked. Some investigators[6,56] have used 8 to 10 MHz probes to record Doppler signals from the femoral artery. In our experience, with an 8 MHz probe it may be difficult to obtain a Doppler signal much above the noise level, especially if the common femoral artery is deep, is surrounded by hematoma or scar tissue, or has a significant atherosclerotic plaque on the anterior wall. Although femoral recordings can be made with this high frequency, 4 to 5 MHz probes generally are preferable, since they reduce the attenuation and result in a better signal-to-noise ratio.

Optimum Doppler velocity meter. The transmitter-receiver must have an adequate power output, good signal-to-noise ratio, and clear separation between forward and reverse flow channels. Often a high-pass filter is used to reject wall thump artifacts. For peripheral arterial studies, this filter cutoff should not exceed 100 Hz (when using 8 MHz probe) so that important reverse flow information is not lost. The presence or absence of reverse flow is a very sensitive indicator of the disease state and is reflected in the pulsatility index value. In many commercial instruments that allow both carotid and peripheral arterial studies, the wall thump filter may be set at 400 Hz to reject the wall thump artifacts experienced in the carotid artery.

Frequency analyzer. To obtain representative waveforms free of electronic and physiologic artifacts, we feel that it is important to use a frequency analyzer to process the Doppler signals. Through the use of a real-time frequency analyzer, the technician obtains both visual and audio feedback and thus can position the Doppler probe to achieve better ''quality control'' of the waveforms selected for analysis. Thus waveforms that contain artifacts caused by a poor signal-to-noise ratio, coexisting arterial or venous flow, or atypical flow patterns like those that may occur directly over a stenosis or at an arterial bifurcation can be excluded. For peripheral arterial studies, a bi-level spectral display is simpler than a multilevel gray-scale display.

Analyze maximum velocity waveform. As previously described, the maximum velocity waveform is preferable for the following reasons[26,27]: The operator does not need to be sure that the vessel is completely and uniformly insonated but rather, with the probe/vessel angle constant, simply searches for the largest spectral waveform. Whereas noise or coexisting arterial or venous signals may seriously affect the mean velocity waveform,* the maximum waveform is less susceptible to these artifacts. Complete insonation of the vessel is required to obtain the true mean waveform but not the maximum waveform.

We use the maximum velocity waveform derived directly from the envelope of the spectral waveform.[26] The baseline reference is always fixed, and cross talk is rejected by a special circuit. To avoid tracking the instantaneous maximum frequency outline of the minor images of the spectral waveform caused by cross talk, the tracking decision should be made based on the relative instantaneous powers in the forward and reverse flow channels. In other words, the channel with the higher instantaneous power should be used to determine the instantaneous maximum frequency. In this way, the cross-talk image is not tracked, since the spectral power of the cross-talk signal is lower.

The zero flow baseline reference must be stable at all times. Slight changes in the baseline may cause significant errors in the calculated values of pulsatility index from certain waveforms. Baseline variation resulting from electronic drift should be detected and compensated before quantification.

Once the envelope of the maximum spectral waveform is obtained, we recommend prefiltering before quantification. A digital or an analog low-pass filter with a cutoff at approximately 30 Hz should be used to smooth out any spikes that may arise as a result of background noise or physiologic artifacts. Although this situation does not occur often, it will cause significant errors in the calculation of pulsatility index.

Calculate pulsatility index online. As illustrated in Fig. 7-18, on-line calculation of pulsatility index is performed by a small dedicated microprocessor, which is an integral part of the Doppler system. The values of pulsatility index are printed above the corresponding maximum velocity waveforms. The algorithm for identifying the waves without the use of an electrocardiogram (ECG) trigger and for calculation of pulsatility index have been described in a previous publication.[26] Not only is on-line quantification convenient but, more important,

*References 5, 14, 17, 29, 39, 46, 47.

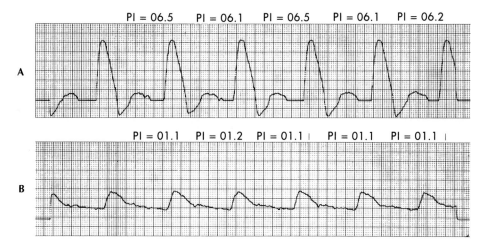

PI = 06.5   PI = 06.1   PI = 06.5   PI = 06.1   PI = 06.2

A

PI = 01.1   PI = 01.2   PI = 01.1 | PI = 01.1   PI = 01.1 |

B

Fig. 7-18. A, Normal maximum instantaneous Doppler velocity waveforms recorded from common femoral artery. Pulsatility indices have been calculated by small microprocessor integrated into Doppler system, and values are printed above corresponding waveforms. ***B,*** Abnormal Doppler waveforms and pulsatility indices.

by quantifying each waveform it minimizes the subjectivity in selecting appropriate waveforms for quantification and eliminates the errors in the calculation of pulsatility index.

Technician must be experienced. The technician who performs waveform analysis must be well trained, must acquire experience in Doppler technique, and must recognize the problems associated with waveform analysis. The use of a real-time frequency analyzer and visual display of the bidirectional Doppler information permits optimum interaction between the operator and the Doppler system and allows the technologist to obtain representative and reproducible blood flow velocity recordings.

Ideal test conditions. Limb blood flow and consequently Doppler blood flow velocity waveforms are affected significantly by the factors that change peripheral arterial resistance. To minimize the physiologic variations in pulsatility index, patients should be examined in a room with a temperature between 21° and 22° C and after a minimum of 15 minutes' rest.

CONCLUSION

Doppler recordings from peripheral arteries can be quantified if attention is directed to the details of Doppler signal processing methods, if the technician is well trained and experienced, and if certain physiologic and pathologic limitations are recognized.

ACKNOWLEDGMENTS

The technical assistance of Mrs. B. Hanson, R.N., and Mrs. S. Ungaro, R.N., and the secretarial assistance of Mrs. J. Behrens are acknowledged.

REFERENCES

1. Altstaedt, F., Storz, L.W., and Ruckert, U.: Erste erfahrungen mit einer semiquantitativen analyse von Doppler-fluss-kurven in der gefasschirurgie. In Kriessman, A., and Bollinger, A., editors: Ultrashall-Doppler-Diagnostik in der Angiologie, Stuttgart, 1979, Thieme.
2. Archie, J.P.: Nondimensional normalized femoral Doppler wave-form indices to predict the hemodynamic significance of iliac artery stenosis. Surg. Forum 30:191, 1979.
3. Archie, J.P., and Feldtman, R.W.: Intraoperative assessment of the hemodynamic significance of iliac and profunda femoris artery stenosis, Surgery 90:876, 1981.
4. Archie, J.P., and Feldtman, R.W.: Determination of the hemodynamic significance of iliac artery stenosis by noninvasive Doppler ultrasonography, Surgery 91:419, 1982.
5. Arts, M.G., and Roevros, J.M.: On the instantaneous measurement of bloodflow by ultrasonic means, Med. Biol. Eng. 10:23, 1972.
6. Baird, R.N., et al.: Upstream stenosis—its diagnosis by Doppler signals from the femoral artery, Arch. Surg. 115:1316, 1980.
7. Barrie, W.E., Evans, D.H., and Bell, P.R.F. The relationship between ultrasonic pulsatility index and proximal arterial stenosis, Br. J. Surg. 66:366, 1979.
8. Brown, J.M., et al.: Transfer-function modelling of arteries, Med. Biol. Eng. Comput. 16:161, 1978.
9. Coghlan, B.A., and Taylor, M.G.: Directional Doppler techniques for detection of blood velocities, Ultrasound Med. Biol. 2:181, 1976.
10. Coghlan, B.A., Taylor, M.G., and King, D.H.: On-line display of Doppler-shift spectra by a new time compression analyser. In Reneman, R.S., editor: Cardiovascular applications of ultrasound, Amsterdam, 1974, North Holland Publishing Co.

11. Fish, P., and Walters, D.: Beam/vessel angle problem in Doppler flow measurement. In Taylor, D.E.M., and Whamond, D., editors: Non-invasive clinical measurement, Tunbridge Wells, England, 1977, Pitman Medical Publishing.
12. Fitzgerald, D.E., and Carr, J.: Doppler ultrasound diagnosis and classification as an alternative to arteriography, Angiology 26:183, 1975.
13. Fitzgerald, D.E., Gosling, R.G., and Woodcock, J.P.: Grading dynamic capability of arterial collateral circulation, Lancet 1:66, 1971.
14. Flax, S.W., Webster, J.G., and Updike, S.J.: Pitfalls using Doppler ultrasound to transduce blood flow, IEEE Trans. Biomed. Eng. 20:306, 1973.
15. Fronek, A., Coel, M., and Bernstein, E.F.: Quantitative ultrasonographic studies of lower extremity flow velocities in health and in disease, Circulation 53:953, 1976.
16. Gerzberg, L., and Meindl, J.D.: Mean frequency estimator with applications in ultrasonic Doppler flowmeters. In White, D.N., and Brown, R., editors: Ultrasound in medicine; engineering aspects, vol. 3B, New York, 1977, Plenum Publishing Corp.
17. Gosling, R.G., and King, D.H.: Continuous wave ultrasound as an alternative and complement to X-rays in vascular examinations. In Reneman, R.S., editor: Cardiovascular applications of ultrasound, Amsterdam, 1974, North Holland Publishing Co.
18. Gosling, R.G., King, D., and Woodcock, J.: Blood-velocity waveforms in the evaluation of atheromatous changes. In Roberts, V.C., editor: Blood flow measurement, London, 1972, Sector Publishing.
19. Gosling, R.G., et al.: The quantitative analysis of occlusive peripheral arterial disease by a non-intrusive technique, Angiology 22:52, 1971.
20. Harris, P.L.: The role of ultrasound in the assessment of peripheral arterial disease, doctoral dissertation, Manchester, England, 1975, University of Manchester.
21. Harris, P.L., et al.: The relationship between Doppler ultrasound assessment and angiography in occlusive arterial disease of the lower limbs, Surg. Gynecol. Obstet. 138:911, 1974.
22. Haynes, B.L.: How to read clinical journals. II. To learn about a diagnostic test, Can. Med. Assoc. J. 124:703, 1981.
23. Humphries, K.N., et al.: Quantitative assessment of the common femoral to popliteal arterial segment using continuous wave Doppler ultrasound, Ultrasound Med. Biol. 6:99, 1980.
24. Johnston, K.W.: Role of Doppler ultrasonography in determining the hemodynamic significance of aortoiliac disease, Can. J. Surg. 21:319, 1978.
25. Johnston, K.W., Demorais, D., and Colopinto, R.F.: Difficulty in assessing the severity of aorto-iliac disease by clinical and arteriographic methods, Angiology 32:609, 1982.
26. Johnston, K.W., Kassam, M., and Cobbold, R.S.C.: On-line identification and quantification of Doppler ultrasound waveforms, Med. Biol. Eng. Comput. 20:336, 1982.
27. Johnston, K.W., Kassam, M., and Cobbold, R.S.C.: Relationship between Doppler pulsatility index and direct femoral pressure measurements in the diagnosis of aroto-iliac occlusive disease, Ultrasound Med. Biol. 9:271, 1983.
28. Johnston, K.W., et al.: Comparative study of four methods for quantifying Doppler ultrasound waveforms from the femoral artery, Ultrasound Med. Biol. 10:1, 1984.
29. Johnston, K.W., Maruzzo, B.C., and Cobbold, R.S.C.: Errors and artifacts of Doppler flowmeters and their solution, Arch. Surg. 112:1335, 1977.
30. Johnston, K.W., Maruzzo, B.C., and Cobbold, R.S.C.: Inaccuracies of a zero-crossing detector for recording Doppler signals, Surg. Forum 28:201, 1977.
31. Johnston, K.W., Maruzzo, B.C., and Cobbold, R.S.C.: Doppler methods for quantitative measurement and localization of peripheral arterial disease by analysis of the blood flow velocity waveform, Ultrasound Med. Biol. 4:209, 1978.
32. Johnston, K.W., Maruzzo, B.C., and Taraschuk, I.C.: Fourier and peak-to-peak pulsatility indices—quantitation of arterial occlusive disease. In Taylor, D.E.M. and Whamond, D., editors: Non-invasive clinical measurement, Tunbridge Wells, England, 1977, Pitman Medical Publishing.
33. Johnston, K.W., and Taraschuk, I.: Validation of the role of pulsatility index in quantitation of the severity of peripheral arterial occlusive disease, Am. J. Surg. 131:295, 1976.
34. Johnston, K.W., et al.: Methods for obtaining, processing and quantifying Doppler blood flow velocity waveforms. In Nicolaides, A.N., and Yao, J.S.T., editors: Investigation of vascular disorders, Edinburgh, 1981, Churchill Livingstone. (In press.)
35. Johnston, K.W., et al.: Quantitative analysis of Doppler blood flow velocity recordings using pulsatility index. In Nicolaides, A.N., and Yao, J.S.T., editors: Investigation of vascular disorders, Edinburgh, 1980, Churchill Livingstone.
36. Kaneko, J., et al.: Analysis of ultrasonic blood rheogram by the sound spectrograph, Jpn. Circ. J. 34:1035, English edition, 1970.
37. Kassam, M., Johnston, K.W., and Cobbold, R.S.C.: A critical assessment of heterodyne demodulation techniques for directional Doppler ultrasound, Digest of XII International Conference on Medical and Biological Engineering, part II, session 28, paper 3, Jerusalem, 1979.
38. Light, L.H.: A recording spectrograph for analysing Doppler blood velocity signals (particularly from aortic flow) in real time, J. Physiol. (Lond.) 207:42P, 1971.
39. Lunt, M.J.: Accuracy and limitations of the ultrasonic Doppler blood velocimeter and zero-crossing detector, Ultrasound Med. Biol. 2:1, 1975.
40. Mackay, R.S.: Non-invasive cardiac output measurement, Microvasc. Res. 4:438, 1972.
41. Maruzzo, B.C., Johnston, K.W., and Cobbold, R.S.C.: Real-time spectral analysis of directional Doppler flow signals, Digest of XI International Conference on Medical and Biological Engineering, pp. 158, Ottawa, 1976.
42. McNeil, B.J., Keller, E., and Adelstein, S.J.: Primer on certain elements of medical decision making, N. Engl. J. Med. 293:211, 1975.
43. Metz, C.E.: Basic principles of ROC analysis, Semin. Nucl. Med. 8:283, 1978.
44. Nippa, J.H., et al.: Phase rotation for separating forward and reverse blood velocity signals, IEEE Trans. Sonics Ultrasonics, SU-22:340, 1975.
45. Reid, J.M., and Baker, D.W.: Physics and electronics of the ultrasonic Doppler method. In Bock, J., and Ossoinig, K., editors: Ultrasonographia medica, vol. I, pp. 109, Vienna, 1971, Verlag Wien Medizinisch Akademie.
46. Reneman, R.S., and Spencer, M.P.: Difficulties in processing of an analogue Doppler flow signal; with special reference to zero-crossing meters and quantification. In Reneman, R.S., editor: Cardiovascular Applications of Ultrasound, Amsterdam, 1974, North Holland Publishing Co.
47. Roberts, C.: Ultrasound in the assessment of vascular function, Med. Prog. Technol. 4:3, 1976.

48. Skidmore, R.: The use of the transcutaneous ultrasonic flowmeter in the dynamic analysis of blood flow, doctoral dissertation, Bristol, England, 1979, University of Bristol.
49. Skidmore, R., and Woodcock, J.P.: Physiological significance of arterial models derived using transcutaneous ultrasonic flowmeters, J. Physiol. (Lond.) 277:29, 1978.
50. Skidmore, R., and Woodcock, J.P.: Physiological interpretation of Doppler-shift waveforms. I. Theoretical considerations, Ultrasound Med. Biol. 6:7, 1980.
51. Skidmore, R., and Woodcock, J.P.: Physiological interpretation of Doppler-shift waveforms. II. Validation of the Laplace transform method for characterisation of the common femoral blood-velocity/time waveform, Ultrasound Med. Biol. 6:219, 1980.
52. Skidmore, R., et al.: Transfer function analysis of common femoral artery Doppler waveforms, Br. J. Surg. 66:883, 1979.
53. Skidmore, R., et al.: Physiological interpretation of Doppler-shift waveforms. III. Clinical results. Ultrasound Med. Biol. 6:227, 1980.
54. Stevens, A., and Roberts, V.C.: On-line signal processing of CW Doppler shifted ultrasound, Digest of XI International Conference on Medical and Biological Engineering, pp. 160, Ottawa, 1976.
55. Strandness, D.E., Jr.: Peripheral arterial disease, a physiologic approach, Boston, 1967, Little, Brown & Co.
56. Ward, A.S., and Martin, T.P.: Some aspects of ultrasound in the diagnosis and assessment of aortoiliac disease, Am. J. Surg. 140:260, 1980.
57. Woodcock, J.P., Gosling, R.G., and Fitzgerald, D.E.: A new noninvasive technique for assessment of superficial femoral arterial obstruction, Br. J. Surg. 59:226, 1972.
58. Yao, S.T.: Haemodynamic studies in peripheral arterial disease, Br. J. Surg. 57:761, 1970.

CHAPTER 8

Blood flow disturbances and spectral analysis

DON P. GIDDENS and RICHARD I. KITNEY

The ideal noninvasive method for detecting and quantifying atherosclerosis should be capable of describing the level of disease over its entire spectrum, including configuration, function, composition, and complication. While a single test cannot as yet accomplish these goals, duplex scanning—the combination of high-resolution β-mode imaging with pulsed Doppler ultrasound—has allowed significant progress in disease identification by virtue of its ability to provide both anatomic information and functional data on blood flow and its behavior near plaques. It is now possible, for example, to grade stenoses in rather broad categories based on peak Doppler frequency and spectral broadening.[15] On the other hand, a major weakness is the difficulty in distinguishing flow patterns induced by minimal disease from those inherent in normal vessels; this differentiation is not significantly enhanced by current imaging capability.

Despite present limitations, however, there is optimism that further advances in disease description are possible through a greater knowledge of arterial fluid dynamics, particularly as related to branching and poststenotic flows, and of signal analysis methods capable of extracting relevant information from Doppler-derived measurements. In this chapter we shall discuss recent advances in the understanding of arterial flow disturbances along with examples of modern signal analysis techniques, which appear to offer promise for improvements in data processing of velocity measurements. These will first be treated using data obtained from laboratory and animal models to exhibit fundamental phenomena. Next, problems associated with transferring this knowledge to noninvasive measurements with Doppler ultrasound will be discussed before finally speculating on future work, which has potential for improving clinical diagnoses.

FLUID MECHANICS

The vast majority of fluid dynamics knowledge is based on flow velocity, whereas noninvasive Doppler ultrasound measurements present data whose frequency content is related to but not necessarily the same as flow velocity. Therefore the interpretation of Doppler-derived data requires a knowledge of the relationship between Doppler frequency and fluid velocity and also of the complex flow fields that can occur in branching and stenotic vessels. In this section we concentrate on the nature of poststenotic flow disturbances using a simple configuration—that of an axisymmetric constriction in an unbranched tube or vessel. The data examined will be velocity results obtained either with a laser Doppler velocity meter in vitro or a hot-film anemometer in vivo. Relationships with Doppler ultrasound will be discussed subsequently.

In earlier work it was shown that rather mild stenoses in the descending canine thoracic aorta produced notable velocity disturbances.[14] An example of this is shown in Fig. 8-1, which displays the velocity measured at the centerline of a dog aorta by a hot-film anemometer probe located 2 cm distal to a 40% stenosis (by area reduction).[13] Disturbances in the velocity waveform are clearly seen during the deceleration phase of systole, although it is difficult to determine by visual inspection whether these fluctuations are indeed turbulent. As the degree of stenosis increases, the intensity of the disturbances also increases, as well as their duration,[14,17] until flow becomes extremely turbulent throughout the cycle.

Because of the ability to control flow conditions carefully, in vitro model studies are useful for examining the nature and evolution of poststenotic flow disturbances. An ideal instrument for such studies is the laser Doppler velocity meter (LDV),

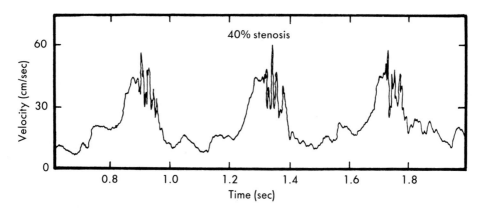

Fig. 8-1. Velocity waveforms measured distal to 40% stenosis (by area reduction) in dog aorta. Data were obtained by hot-film anemometry. (From Giddens, D.P., and Kitney, R.I.: Autoregressive spectral estimation of poststenotic blood flow disturbances, J. Biomech. Eng. 105:401, 1983. By permission of the American Society of Mechanical Engineers.)

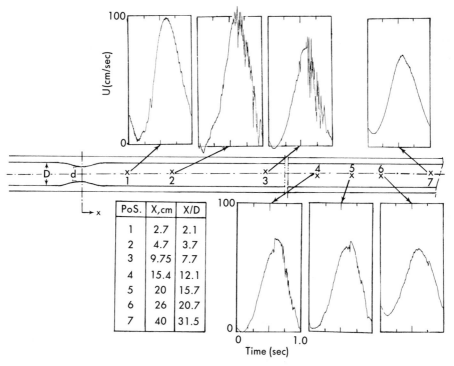

Fig. 8-2. Centerline velocity waveforms measured at seven axial positions downstream of 50% axisymmetric stenosis. Measurements were performed with laser Doppler anemometer. *U*, Measured fluid velocity; *D*, diameter of unoccluded portion of vessel; *X*, distance downstream from constriction; *Pos.*, position of measurement site. (From Khalifa, A.M.A., and Giddens, D.P.: J. Biomech. 14:279, 1981.)

which is noninvasive and possesses far superior resolution and accuracy than Doppler ultrasound instruments. The major drawback of the LDV is its requirement of a good optical path between instrument and sample volume. Khalifa and Giddens[18] performed a series of LDV velocity measurements in Plexiglas tubes containing varying de-

grees of constriction using pulsatile flow that was representative of conditions in the dog aorta. Fig. 8-2 presents examples of velocity waveforms measured at the centerline of the tube for several axial locations distal to a 50% (by area) stenosis. By carefully examining data such as these and employing time series signal analysis methods, some of which will be discussed in the next section, it was shown that three distinct types of flow disturbances exist:

1. A coherent structure associated with the start-up process of each cycle (termed a *starting structure*)
2. Oscillations of discrete frequency originating in the shear layer formed in the diverging section of the stenosis (termed a *shear layer oscillation*)
3. Turbulent structures, characterized by some degree of random velocity behavior

Of further interest is the fact that these disturbances are listed in the order of their occurrence as the degree of stenosis increases. For example, depending on the Reynolds number, frequency parameter, and contour, a mild stenosis may result in only a starting structure with no evidence of shear layer oscillation or turbulence. Furthermore, studies currently in progress in our laboratories indicate that the turbulence seen distal to mild and moderate stenoses contains ordered structures that are only pseudorandom; that is, structures that are essentially reproducible from beat-to-beat, but somewhat random in their phase and amplitude.

It must be noted that the studies that model the dog aorta are typically at mean Reynolds numbers of about 1000, whereas the corresponding mean in the human common carotid artery is approximately 400. Therefore production of truly turbulent poststenotic flow is more difficult than in the dog aorta experiments and requires a greater degree of stenosis to produce the same effect. An extensive series of steady and pulsatile flow experiments for more moderate Reynolds number values has been recently completed by Ahmed[1] (see also Ahmed and Giddens[2,3]).

Finally, the discussion of flow disturbances would be incomplete without consideration of a more realistic geometry. In view of the interest and importance of the carotid arteries with regard to atherosclerosis, we developed a model bifurcation based on extensive and quantitative studies of angiograms[4] and examined steady[4,5] and pulsatile[21,22] flow through this model using flow visualization techniques and LDV instrumentation. These studies were directed toward defining normal hemodynamic behavior in the bifurcation and toward relating hemodynamic factors with localization of atherosclerotic lesions in humans. An important finding was that plaques localize in regions of low mean shear in the carotid bulb and not in

regions of high flow velocity or shear.[26] Furthermore, when employing physiologic flow waveforms at appropriate Reynolds numbers, no turbulence was observed for the normal bifurcation.[5,21] There were, however, very strong secondary or helical flow patterns in the bifurcation, which cannot be considered flow disturbances in the true sense because they occur for normal hemodynamic conditions. Fig. 8-3 gives a sche-

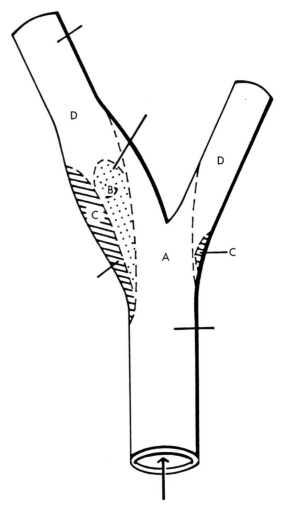

Fig. 8-3. Schematic presentation of general flow conditions at four regions in carotid bifurcation. Region *A* is one of basically axial flow. Region *B* contains evolving secondary helical structures that change direction through pulsatile cycle. Transient separation with oscillatory velocity directions characterize region *C*, while region *D* has steep near-wall velocity gradients and blunt, entrance-type velocity profiles. (From Ku, D.N.: Hemodynamics and atherogenesis at the human carotid bifurcation, doctoral dissertation, Atlanta, 1983, Georgia Institute of Technology.)

matic of the carotid bifurcation and the location and nature of unsteady flow phenomena that exist under pulsatile conditions.[21] Using the LDV to measure velocity at various locations allows a quantitative assessment of velocity as a function of position and time. Fig. 8-4 presents an example, shown in a three-dimensional perspective, of the axial velocity component measured midway of the carotid bulb and in the plane of the bifurcation.[21] The two parts of the figure are simply two different projections of the same data, and the region of reverse flow over a large part of the bulb during systole is viewed particularly well in Fig. 8-4, *B*. Such reverse velocity behavior has now been documented in human subjects using duplex scanning instrumentation, and the similarity between model and human measurements is striking.[23] Studies are under way to examine the effects of lesions in the models, and these data will be related to similar work in humans using Doppler ultrasound.

In summary, then, it is now possible to make the following statements regarding the fluid dynamics of flow disturbances:

1. There are at least three distinct types of post-stenotic flow disturbances, which occur as the degree of stenosis increases: starting structures, shear layer oscillations, and turbulence.
2. Because disturbances evolve during each cycle, they are of a nonstationary nature, and care must be exercised when employing standard methods of time series analysis.
3. While the normal human carotid bifurcation does not exhibit turbulence, complex secondary laminar flow patterns that may give the appearance of flow disturbances are created transiently with each beat.
4. Lowering the threshold of recognition of localized arterial disease using flow disturbance analysis will best be achieved by understanding the role of coherent disturbance features, not by measurement of turbulence.

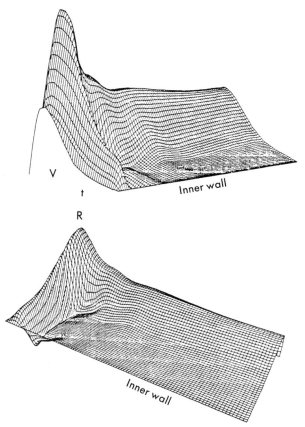

Fig. 8-4. Axial velocity vs. radial position and phase within cycle as measured midway of the carotid sinus in plane of bifurcation with laser Doppler anemometer. (From Ku, D.N.: Hemodynamics and atherogenesis at the human carotid bifurcation, doctoral dissertation, Atlanta, 1983, Georgia Institute of Technology.)

SIGNAL ANALYSIS

Because flow characteristics of interest contain recurring features on a beat-to-beat basis, most analyses of velocity data assume that an underlying waveform exists that can be determined by appropriate ensemble averaging over a number of beats.[14,19] Hence a single beat in the ensemble is assumed to be of the form

$$u(t) = U(t) + u'(t) \qquad (1)$$

where U(t) is the underlying ensemble average and u'(t) is a random velocity component. The ensemble average of N beats is determined by

$$U(t) = \frac{1}{N} \sum_{n=0}^{N-1} u(t + nP) \qquad (2)$$

where P is the period of the waveform and t = 0 is the time that is referenced to the ECG signal. Note also that $0 \leq t \leq P$. Any waveform features that are repeatable and in phase from cycle to cycle will appear in U(t). The accuracy of this form of velocity decomposition is affected by several aspects of physiologic variability, including respiration, heart rate changes, and stroke consistency. It is possible to reduce physiologic variability somewhat by the technique of phase-shift averaging as described by Kitney and Giddens,[20] a method in which cross correlation between U(t) and u(t) is employed to minimize phase errors.

Using equations 1 and 2 along with the phase-shift averaging to construct the ensemble average, a series of 25 waveforms of the 40% occlusion data were employed to form U(t) as shown in Fig. 8-5. It is interesting to note that, after averaging, several disturbance structures remain in the waveform. These are flow characteristics that are not random in nature and in themselves would not be classified as turbulent—although they may be orderly structures which are precursors of, or imbedded phasically within, turbulence. Fig. 8-6 gives the square root of the corresponding ensemble average of $u'^2(t)$, that is, $\langle u'^2(t) \rangle^{1/2}$, where $\langle \rangle$ indicates ensemble average. It is seen that the disturbance level is fairly low during the acceleration and peak velocity phases of systole and increases abruptly at the same time that U(t) shows obvious disturbance activity. This type of behavior in U(t) and u'(t) is seen consistently in both animal and in vitro poststenotic flow studies and emphasizes the fact that flow disturbances related to localized plaques are clearly nonstationary phenomena.

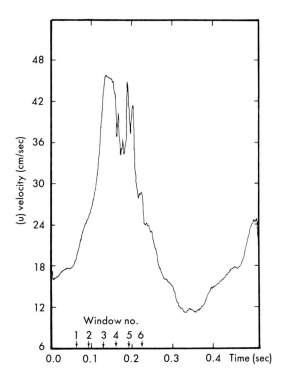

Fig. 8-5. Phase-shifted ensemble average waveform for 25 beats taken from 40% stenosis data illustrated in Fig. 8-1. Ensemble averaged velocity is denoted by *u,* and windows are used for subsequent spectral analysis. (From Giddens, D.P., and Kitney, R.I.: Autoregressive spectral estimation of poststenotic blood flow disturbances, J. Biomech. Eng. 105:401, 1983. By permission of the American Society of Mechanical Engineers.)

While the methods of equations 1 and 2, as exemplified in Figs. 8-5 and 8-6, provide a form of signal decomposition, further analysis is required to characterize the nature of the flow disturbances. One such technique is spectral analysis, in which the frequency content of a signal is determined with the objective of ultimately relating that content to physical phenomena. We emphasize that the present discussion of spectral analysis deals with analyzing the *velocity* signal, not a Doppler frequency signal.

First, we are reminded that spectrum estimates require data to be gathered over an interval of time that must be at least as long as the period of the lowest frequency present. Actually, for good accuracy the traditional methods of Fourier analysis require on the order of five cycles of the lowest frequency present. Consequently, for flow disturbances in pulsatile flows we face a dilemma: To obtain good spectrum estimates, data must be gathered over a sufficiently long time interval within

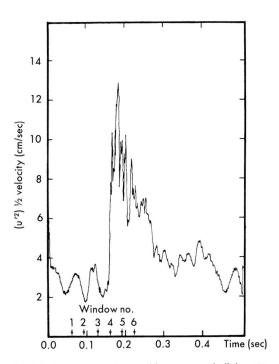

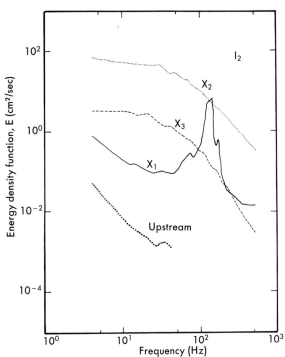

Fig. 8-6. Square root of ensemble average of u'^2 for 40% stenosis data of Fig. 8-1, taken over 25 beats. (From Giddens, D.P., and Kitney, R.I.: Autoregressive spectral estimation of poststenotic blood flow disturbances, J. Biomech. Eng. 105:401, 1983. By permission of the American Society of Mechanical Engineers.)

Fig. 8-7. Energy spectra of disturbance velocity u' measured at several axial positions distal to 75% (by area) axisymmetric stenosis under pulsatile flow conditions. Spectra are calculated over 0.25-second period taken near peak systolic velocity in each cycle. Velocity was measured at tube axis using laser Doppler anemometer. (From Khalifa, A.M.A., and Giddens, D.P.: J. Biomech. 14:279, 1981.)

the cycle, yet the characteristics of the disturbance are changing during this interval. If the latter changes are not large during the observation time, it is possible to treat the signal as quasi-stationary—and this is the approach usually taken.

An example of the information afforded by spectral analysis of the velocity component $u'(t)$ is given in Fig. 8-7.[18] This figure presents spectra of the energy in $u'(t)$ as measured distal to a 75% stenosis with an LDV at several axial positions along the centerline. The interval over which the spectra are calculated is a 0.25-second period taken near the peak systolic velocity in each cycle. It can be seen that at position X_1, which is two tube diameters distal to the stenosis, there is a sharp peak in the spectrum. This corresponds to an oscillation of discrete frequency arising in the poststenotic shear layer as discussed earlier. On the other hand, spectra further downstream at X_2 and X_3 show characteristically broadband turbulent shapes. The frequency content of the underlying waveform, $U(t)$,

may also be of value, a point to which we shall return shortly.

Because of the transient behavior of flow disturbances during each cycle, the problem may be looked on as one of analyzing data records of short duration. For such cases, Fourier methods may lack accuracy, and linear estimation techniques[6] developed recently for such applications may prove of value. We have examined the potential of a class of these techniques—autoregressive methods—when applied to both underlying $[U(t)]$[20] and random $[u'(t)]$[13] velocities. The theory behind these methods can be found in other literature[6,16,20,25] and will not be repeated here.

An example of applying fast Fourier transform (FFT) and autoregressive (AR) methods of spectrum estimation is shown in Figs. 8-8 and 8-9. Fig. 8-8 presents an ensemble average $U(t)$ waveform determined from hot-film anemometer measurements of velocity taken distal to an 88% (by area) stenosis in the dog aorta.[13] Flow was so turbulent

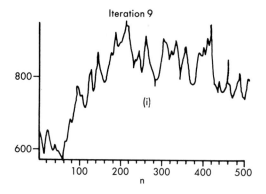

Fig. 8-8. Phase-shifted ensemble average of 100 very turbulent velocity waveforms measured distal to 88% stenosis in dog aorta with hot-film anemometer. Final ensemble average shows disturbances occurring at discrete frequency in each cycle that survive the averaging process. Value of *n* is related to time in seconds such that time = n/2560. (From Kitney, R.I., and Giddens, D.P.: Analysis of blood velocity waveforms by phase shift averaging and autoregressive spectral estimation, J. Biomech. Eng. 105:398, 1983. By permission of the American Society of Mechanical Engineers.)

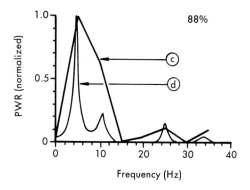

Fig. 8-9. Spectral content of curve in Fig. 8-8 as estimated by FFT and autoregressive methods. (From Kitney, R.I., and Giddens, D.P.: Analysis of blood velocity waveforms by phase shift averaging and autoregressive spectral estimation, J. Biomech. Eng. 105:398, 1983. By permission of the American Society of Mechanical Engineers.)

that it was difficult to detect any of the individual beats in the raw data. However, by phase-shift averaging 100 beats, a well-defined U(t) waveform emerged that apparently contains distinct frequency components. Fig. 8-9 gives the spectral estimations obtained by FFT and AR methods. The fundamental peak at about 5 Hz arises from the data window employed (that is, 0.20 sec). Both FFT and AR methods give higher frequency peaks at about 25 and 35 Hz; however, the peak at 10 Hz is not resolved by the FFT approach. Additionally, the FFT resolution is basically 5 Hz and will give no peaks other than in multiples of this value. On the other hand, the AR method provides a continuous estimate of the spectrum, resulting in better resolution.

As a final example to illustrate application of the AR method to u′(t) data, as well as to show the evolution of spectra during a cycle, we return to the 40% occlusion data shown in Fig. 8-5 and 8-6. Referring to these figures, it will be noted that six "windows" are identified along the time axis. The numbers shown correspond to the locations of the centers of six windows of 0.064-second dura-

tion; each successive window is shifted by 0.032 second, resulting in a 50% overlap. The AR method was applied to the u′(t) data during each of these data windows, and the results are graphed in Fig. 8-10.[13] It is seen that windows 1 and 2 give very little high-frequency activity, indicating that flow is essentially laminar and cyclically repeatable during these times, in agreement with the curve of Fig. 8-6. Window 3 begins to show an increase in high-frequency disturbances, but this is still a relatively low level. On the other hand, windows 4 to 6 display a greater amplitude of disturbance and much greater high-frequency activity than the first three windows. These latter three spectra are characteristically turbulent and correspond to the high levels of disturbance seen in Figs. 8-5 and 8-6.

In summary, we may make the following statements regarding analysis of blood velocity signals:

1. Certain aspects of data interpretation are facilitated by decomposition of the velocity into an underlying waveform, U(t), determined by ensemble averaging and a random velocity component, u′(t).

2. Although not shown by example here, it is impossible to obtain accurate underlying waveforms by low pass filtering,[19] as has been suggested by others.
3. Phase-shift averaging to obtain U(t) reduces physiologic variability.
4. Because data records are relatively short as a result of the evolving nature of flow disturbances, AR spectral estimation techniques offer an improvement over FFT estimates in many cases.

NONINVASIVE MEASUREMENTS

Presently, the primary means of obtaining blood velocity information is with Doppler ultrasound, most notably with pulsed Doppler ultrasound, which is guided by real-time imaging—that is, duplex scanning. However, a dilemma exists as we have stated earlier. The vast majority of fluid dynamics knowledge is based on the velocity field, while the output of Doppler ultrasound instruments is an amplitude and frequency modulated signal whose frequency content is derived from scattering by moving particles. Although the relationship between Doppler frequency and flow velocity seems straightforward, such is not the case. Unfortunately, Doppler systems suffer from Doppler ambiguity, which results from factors such as mean velocity gradient (spatial resolution), rapid variations in velocity (temporal resolution), transit time and geometric broadening, instrument bandwidth, and noise. George and Lumley[11] provide an excellent discussion of Doppler ambiguity and focus attention on laser Doppler systems, whereas Garbini et al.[9,10] discuss similar considerations for ultrasonic Doppler devices. Because of the much longer wavelength of ultrasound systems, Doppler ambiguity is a central problem; perhaps as a consequence of this, most commercial Doppler ultrasound devices have tended to display Doppler spectra. Extensive clinical experience with such systems has led to diagnostic improvements, and descriptions of flow disturbances have been given in terms of "filling in the window" and "spectral broadening." However, these descriptions have not yet been properly connected to physical phenomema occurring in arterial flows, so we suggest it is perhaps more appropriate to call the output of these devices *spectral displays* rather than spectral analyses.

It is important, therefore, to recognize that (1) extraction of velocity information from Doppler

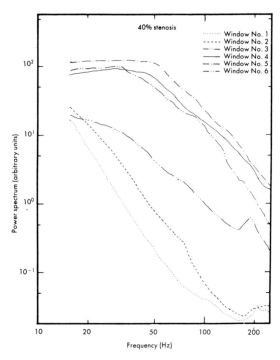

Fig. 8-10. Power spectra for disturbance velocity u' as calculated by autoregressive spectral estimation for six data windows during cycle. Results are for 40% stenosis and give evolving spectral content of u'. Refer to Fig. 8-6 for location of 0.064-second windows. (From Giddens, D.P., and Kitney, R.I.: Autoregressive spectral estimation of poststenotic blood flow disturbances, J. Biomech. Eng. 105:401, 1983. By permission of the American Society of Mechanical Engineers.)

signals arising from disturbed flows or from complex, but normal, flow patterns is not simple, and that (2) spectral broadening results from many sources that are strictly instrument related, such as sample volume size, transmission frequency and bandwidth, and the resolution and accuracy of the spectrum estimator.

While spectral broadening descriptions may be useful as an interim stage, it is our opinion that converting to velocity information holds more promise for diagnosis of mild to moderate lesions. This opinion is based on the fact that the vast body of fluid dynamics knowledge deals with the velocity field, not with descriptions of Doppler spectra. Thus converting the Doppler signal to fluid velocity data allows one to bring to bear the full power of fluid dynamics on the interpretation of blood flow disturbances induced by arterial disease. One approach that appears promising is to use phase lock loop (PLL) frequency tracking of the Doppler sig-

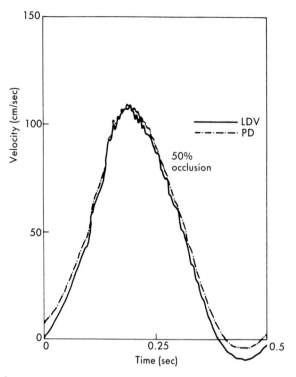

Fig. 8-11. Ensemble average axial velocity waveforms measured by pulsed Doppler (PD) ultrasound and laser Doppler velocity meters (LDV) distal to 50% stenosis in pulsatile flow. Ultrasound data were processed by frequency tracker. (From Giddens, D.P., and Khalifa, A.M.A.: Ultrasound Med. Biol. 8:427, 1982.)

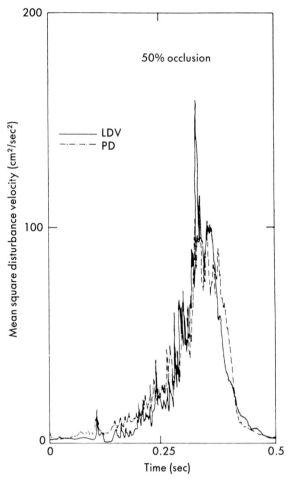

Fig. 8-12. Ensemble averages of axial mean square disturbance velocity measured by pulsed Doppler (PD) ultrasound and laser Doppler velocity meters (LDV) distal to 50% contoured stenosis in pulsatile flow. Ultrasound data were processed by frequency tracker. (From Giddens, D.P., and Khalifa, A.M.A.: Ultrasound Med. Biol. 8:427, 1982.)

nal in which the output of a variable frequency oscillator is caused to lock in phase with the Doppler signal and follow its frequency through a feedback system. In a series of in vitro experiments, measurements of flow disturbances were performed in pulsatile flow distal to stenoses of 50% and 75% area reduction.[12] Pulsed Doppler ultrasound (PDU) with PLL tracking was compared with data obtained from the LDV, an instrument whose ambiguity is substantially less than that for ultrasound because of its much shorter wavelength.[11] Figs. 8-11 and 8-12 give results obtained downstream of a 50% stenosis. For both U(t) and u'(t) the PDU-PLL system gave good agreement with the LDV. However, when the stenosis increased to 75% area reduction, the PDU-PLL system suffered from excessive loss in tracking, resulting in disturbance velocity measurements that were approximately 50% too large. In view of the ambiguity problems discussed earlier this result is not surprising.

The PLL method may be applied to human subjects, although in such cases there is no indepen-

dent method of evaluating its accuracy. Casty and Giddens[7] studied several subjects using a multichannel pulsed Doppler system in which one of the channels was located at the centerline and employed to measure disturbances. Fig. 8-13 shows the results obtained from the left common carotid artery of a 65-year-old patient with failure of the aortic valve and a systolic bruit transmitted to the carotids. The presence of coherent flow disturbances during the peak phase of systole and an increase in disturbance level during the peak and deceleration phases can be seen clearly in the figures.

Another approach of converting Doppler data to velocity is that of rapid calculation of the mean

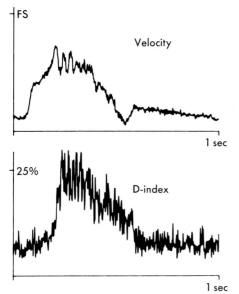

Fig. 8-13. Ensemble average waveform and disturbance velocity obtained via pulsed Doppler ultrasound from patient with failure of aortic valve and transmitted systolic bruit. Doppler data were processed with frequency tracker. D-index is *disturbance index* defined by relation

$$D(t) = \frac{\sqrt{<u'(t)^2>}}{\overline{U}}$$

where $\overline{U}$ is mean velocity averaged over heart cycle and $<u'(t)^2>$ is ensemble average (see equation 2) of square of disturbance velocity. (From Casty, M., and Giddens, D.P.: Ultrasound Med. Biol. 10(2):161, 1984.)

value of the frequency from frequency spectra. This procedure assumes that the mean frequency may be determined from

$$f_m(t) = \frac{\int fP(f)df}{\int P(f)df} \qquad (3)$$

where P(f) is the Doppler power spectrum and is assumed to represent a probability distribution function for Doppler frequency. Because equation 3 is the first moment of P(f) and because the process was implemented digitally, we called this procedure a digital first moment (DFM) method.[8] If appropriate windows are used, equation 3 gives excellent results when employed with simulated Doppler signals.[8,24] However, again because of Doppler ambiguity, the accuracy is degraded when the method is applied to real Doppler signals. The net effects are that rapid variations in velocity cannot be followed and the output of the estimator is somewhat noisy. However, the approach may be useful when applied for detecting coherent, low-frequency velocity disturbances and has not yet been fully explored.

Finally, it is our opinion that

1. Spectral analysis of the Doppler signal, as presently practiced, is no more than a spectral display of the audio signal whose relationship to hemodynamic phenomena is poorly understood.

2. For low to moderate levels of velocity fluctuation, frequency tracking by PLL provides reasonably accurate conversion of the Doppler signal to fluid velocity.

3. Improved methods of spectral estimation that will account for ambiguity phenomena are needed.

FUTURE DIRECTIONS

The hemodynamic behavior of normal and mildly diseased vessels is just beginning to be understood properly. Additional work is necessary in this area, particularly with regard to the three-dimensional geometries of relevant vessels. Model studies have been shown to be very important in elucidating flow behavior under controlled conditions with accurate instrumentation. These results can then be employed to aid in the interpretation of data obtained under clinical conditions with noninvasive methods. Also, research should be focused on better modeling of the Doppler signal at its fundamental level and on accurate conversion to fluid velocity information so that a broader knowledge of fluid dynamics can be brought to bear on clinical measurements.

REFERENCES

1. Ahmed, S.A.: An experimental investigation of steady and pulsatile flow through a constricted tube, doctoral dissertation, Atlanta, 1981, Georgia Institute of Technology.

2. Ahmed, S.A., and Giddens, D.P.: Velocity measurements in steady flow through axisymmetric stenoses at moderate Reynolds numbers, J. Biomech. 16:505, 1983.

3. Ahmed, S.A., and Giddens, D.P.: Flow disturbance measurements through a constricted tube at moderate Reynolds numbers, J. Biomech. 16:955, 1983.

4. Bharadvaj, B.K., Mabon, R.F., and Giddens, D.P.: Steady flow in a model of the carotid bifurcation. Part I—Flow visualization, J. Biomech. 15:349, 1982.

5. Bharadvaj, B.K., Mabon, R.F., and Giddens, D.P.: Steady flow in a model of the carotid bifurcation. Part II—Laser-Doppler anemometer measurements, J. Biomech. 15:363, 1982.

6. Box, G.E., and Jenkins, G.H.: Time series analysis: Forecasting and control, San Francisco, 1976, Holden-Day, Inc.

7. Casty, M., and Giddens, D.P.: 25 + 1 channel pulsed ultrasound Doppler velocity meter for quantitative flow measurements and turbulence analysis, Ultrasound Med. Biol. 10(2):161, 1984.

8. Craig, J.I., Saxena, V., and Giddens, D.P.: A minicomputer-based scheme for turbulence measurements with pulsed Doppler ultrasound, IEEE Proceedings of the third annual symposium on Computer Applications in Medical Care, p. 638, Washington, D.C., 1979.

9. Garbini, J.L., Forster, F.K., and Jorgensen, J.E.: Measurement of fluid turbulence based on pulsed ultrasound techniques. Part 1. Analysis, J. Fluid Mech. 118:445, 1982.

10. Garbini, J.L., Forster, F.K., and Jorgensen, J.E.: Measurement of fluid turbulence based on pulsed ultrasound techniques. Part 2. Experimental investigation, J. Fluid Mech. 118:471, 1982.

11. George, W.F., and Lumley, J.L.: The laser-Doppler velocimeter and its application to the measurement of turbulence, J. Fluid Mech. 60:321, 1973.

12. Giddens, D.P., and Khalifa, A.M.A.: Turbulence measurements with pulsed Doppler ultrasound employing a frequency tracking method, Ultrasound Med. Biol. 8:427, 1982.

13. Giddens, D.P., and Kitney, R.I.: Autoregressive spectral estimation of poststenotic blood flow disturbances, J. Biomech. Eng. 105:401, 1983.

14. Giddens, D.P., Mabon, R.F., and Cassanova, R.A.: Measurements of disordered flows distal to subtotal vascular stenoses in the thoracic aortas of dogs, Circ. Res. 39:112, 1976.

15. Greene, F.M., Jr., et al.: Computer-based pattern recognition of carotid arterial disease using pulsed Doppler ultrasound, Ultrasound Med. Biol. 8:161, 1982.

16. Kay, S.M.: The effects of noise on the autoregressive spectral estimator, IEEE Trans. Acoustics Speech Signal Processing 5:478, 1979.

17. Khalifa, A.M.A., and Giddens, D.P.: Analysis of disorder in pulsatile flows with application to poststenotic blood velocity measurement in dogs, J. Biomech. 11:129, 1978.

18. Khalifa, A.M.A., and Giddens, D.P.: Characterization and evolution of poststenotic flow disturbances, J. Biomech. 14:279, 1981.

19. Kitney, R.I., and Giddens, D.P.: Extraction and characterisation of underlying velocity waveforms in poststenotic flow, IEE Proceedings 129(A):651, 1982.

20. Kitney, R.I., and Giddens, D.P.: Analysis of blood velocity waveforms by phase shift averaging and autoregressive spectral estimation, J. Biomech. Eng. 105:398, 1983.

21. Ku, D.N.: Hemodynamics and atherogenesis at the human carotid bifurcation, doctoral dissertation, Atlanta, 1983, Georgia Institute of Technology.

22. Ku, D.N., and Giddens, D.P.: Pulsatile flow in a model carotid bifurcation, Arteriosclerosis 3:31, 1983.

23. Ku, D.N., et al.: Hemodynamics of the normal human bifurcation: in vitro and in vivo studies, Manuscript submitted for publication, 1984.

24. Saxena, V.: Turbulence measurements using pulsed Doppler ultrasound, doctoral dissertation, Atlanta, 1978, Georgia Institute of Technology.

25. Ulrych, T.F., and Bishop, T.N.: Maximum entropy spectral analysis and autoregressive decomposition, Rev. Geophysics Space Physics 13:198, 1975.

26. Zarins, C.K., et al.: Carotid bifurcation atherosclerosis: quantitative correlation of plaque localization with flow velocity profiles and wall shear stress, Circ. Res. 53:502, 1983.

CHAPTER 9

Accuracy and potential pitfalls of carotid Doppler frequency analysis

K. WAYNE JOHNSTON, P. ZUECH, and MAHMOOD S. KASSAM

Frequency analysis of Doppler signals is a widely used method for diagnosing extracranial carotid arterial disease because it can reliably detect moderately severe and severe stenoses.[6,7,8,22] Although various methods for Doppler frequency analysis have been used for almost a decade,[18] clinically practical systems have become widely available only in the last few years. The advantages of carotid frequency analysis are generally accepted. Specifically, the technologist can separate the true Doppler signals from other artifactual signals. Also, recordings of the spectral waveforms provide additional diagnostic information; namely, at the site of a stenosis the peak frequency is increased,[8,11,15,22] and beyond the stenosis the spectrum of Doppler frequencies is broadened because of the presence of disturbed or turbulent flow.[2,8,11,21]

The purposes of this chapter are (1) to review the changes in the Doppler spectral waveform produced by a stenosis, (2) to describe the carotid Doppler technique, and (3) to identify problems that limit the accuracy of the method.

CHANGES IN THE DOPPLER SPECTRAL WAVEFORM PRODUCED BY A STENOSIS

In Fig. 9-1 frequency analysis recordings from our in vitro model illustrate the two abnormalities that are of value in diagnosing carotid stenoses. First, the Doppler frequency increases at the site of the stenosis, and second, the Doppler spectrum is broadened beyond the stenosis where the flow is disturbed.

Peak frequency. The relationship between the peak Doppler frequency and the severity of the stenosis has been studied in vitro and clinically. As

□ Supported by the Ontario Heart Foundation.

illustrated in Fig. 9-2, from the results obtained with our pulsatile flow in vitro model[11] with a nominal flow rate of 225 ml/min and a 4 MHz probe kept at a constant angle of 60 degrees, it can be seen that the peak frequency is directly related to the percentage area of stenosis. The comparable clinical results are shown in Fig. 9-3 where the peak Doppler frequency is plotted against the percentage of internal carotid diameter stenosis measured from arteriograms in 397 cases.

The reason for the increased Doppler frequency at the site of a stenosis is quite well understood.[8,11] In a nonbranched artery, the volumetric flow is the same at all points along the artery, and since the cross-sectional area is reduced at the stenosis, the mean velocity increases. Clinical recordings such as those illustrated in Fig. 9-4 clearly show that the maximum peak frequency is detected directly over the stenosis.

Spectral broadening. While the basis for the increased peak frequency over a stenosis is well understood, the significance of spectral broadening has not been critically evaluated. In a normal carotid Doppler recording, there is a clear window beneath the systolic peak because at this point the flow velocity profile is nearly flat. Beyond a stenosis where the flow is disturbed, the clear window is obliterated (that is, the spectrum is broadened) because the directions of the vectors of flow change with respect to the orientation of the Doppler probe.

CAROTID DOPPLER TECHNIQUE AND RESULTS

Over the last 4 years more than 2800 patients have been studied in our clinical vascular laboratory at the Toronto General Hospital.

Technique. These studies were performed by one nurse technologist using a 4 MHz continuous-wave

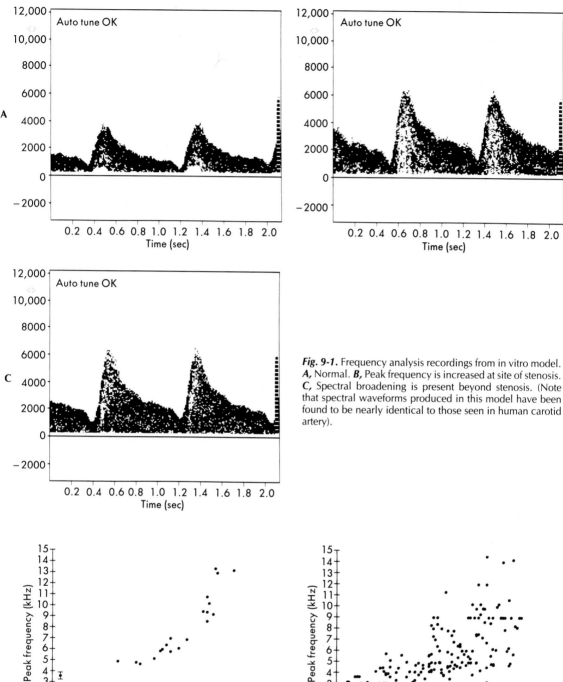

Fig. 9-1. Frequency analysis recordings from in vitro model. *A,* Normal. *B,* Peak frequency is increased at site of stenosis. *C,* Spectral broadening is present beyond stenosis. (Note that spectral waveforms produced in this model have been found to be nearly identical to those seen in human carotid artery).

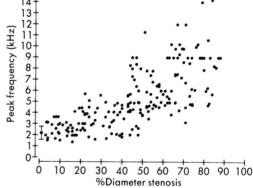

Fig. 9-2. In vitro results showing relationship between percentage *area* of stenosis and peak Doppler frequency.

Fig. 9-3. Clinical results showing relationship between peak Doppler frequency and percentage of internal carotid *diameter* stenosis (that is, minimum residual lumen diameter divided by diameter of distal internal carotid). Normal peak frequency ± 1 standard deviation is shown (2.2 ± 0.6 kHz, N = 149).

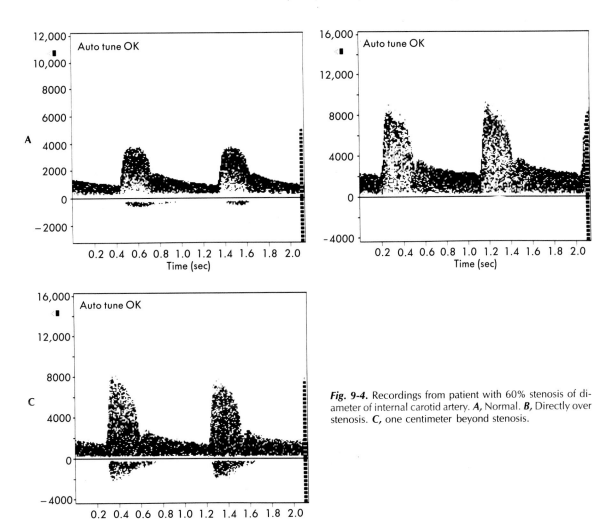

Fig. 9-4. Recordings from patient with 60% stenosis of diameter of internal carotid artery. **A,** Normal. **B,** Directly over stenosis. **C,** one centimeter beyond stenosis.

(CW) Doppler velocity meter,* a frequency analyzer of our own design[23] with 16.6 msec time resolution and 100 Hz frequency resolution from −1.6 to 8 kHz or 200 Hz resolution from −3.2 kHz to 16.0 kHz, a real-time, high-resolution video display with 16 levels of gray scale, and a video image recorder. The technologist held the Doppler probe and maintained a probe-to-skin angle that was as constant as possible, usually betweeen 45 and 60 degrees. Representative recordings were made at 0.5 to 1.0 cm increments along the common carotid/internal carotid axis. At each site the probe was positioned to obtain waveforms that were free of artifacts and showed the least amount of spectral broadening under the peak.

*Medasonics, Mountainview, Calif.

Clinical studies. The accuracy of the carotid Doppler frequency analysis technique has been determined by comparison to arteriography in 397 arteries. The minimum residual lumen diameter at the stenosis[5] was measured with calipers from carotid arteriograms by an independent observer who was unaware of the Doppler results. The percentage of internal carotid diameter stenosis was calculated from this measurement and the diameter of the distal internal carotid. The maximum peak Doppler frequency over the stenosis was measured and the severity of spectral broadening was graded subjectively as grade 0 if the width of the Doppler spectrum at peak systole was less than 50% of the peak frequency, grade 1 if the width was 50% to 99%, grade 2 if the width was 100%, and grade 3 if reverse flow was also present.[1]

Clinical results. Fig. 9-5 is the receiver operating characteristic curve[12,19,20] obtained when a stenosis greater than 40% diameter was considered a positive test (prevalence of disease = 45.4%). The sensitivity and specificity are plotted for different peak frequency threshold values. The maximum accuracy was achieved when the peak frequency threshold value was 4.1 kHz: accuracy = 90.3%, sensitivity = 90.2%, specificity = 90.4%, positive predictive value = 88.7%, and negative predictive value = 91.7%.

The accuracy of subjectively grading the severity of spectral broadening in detecting carotid stenosis

greater than 40% is quite similar. If spectral-broadening grades 3 and 4 are considered a positive test, then the overall accuracy is 86.2%, the specificity 90.3%, the sensitivity 83.5%, the positive predictive value 78.6% and the negative predictive value 92.8%.

These data confirm our initial observations[6,7,8] and those of Spencer and Reid[22] and show that frequency analysis of CW Doppler recordings can accurately diagnose moderately severe and severe stenoses or occlusions but not minor stenoses.

POTENTIAL PITFALLS OF THE CAROTID DOPPLER TECHNIQUE

Fig. 9-6 shows the components of a typical carotid Doppler system.[13] Errors can occur at any point in the system, from the probe to the method of quantification. The pitfalls of the Doppler technique have been identified through experiments using in vitro models with steady and pulsatile flow and through studies in our clinical vascular laboratory and will be discussed in the following subsections.

Technician errors

The use of frequency analysis provides visual feedback to the technician, augmenting the audio interpretation of the signals and thereby aiding the collection of representative waveforms that are free of artifacts. Despite these advantages, the accuracy of the carotid Doppler technique depends on the skill of the technician. For example, the common, internal, and external carotid arteries are usually distinguished by the morphological differences in the shape of their waves, and failure to correctly identify the arteries can lead to serious errors in diagnosis. Also, as our in vitro and clinical studies

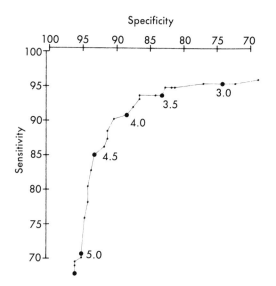

Fig. 9-5. Receiver operating characteristic curve. Carotid arteriographic stenosis of greater than 40% diameter was considered positive test. Sensitivities and specificities are plotted for different peak frequency threshold values in increments of 0.1 kHz.

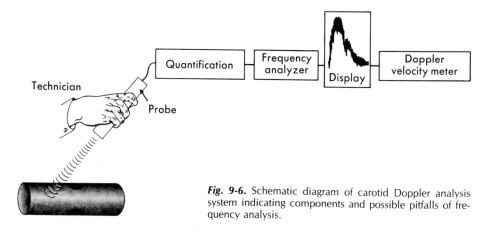

Fig. 9-6. Schematic diagram of carotid Doppler analysis system indicating components and possible pitfalls of frequency analysis.

have demonstrated, measurements of peak frequency will be variable unless the technician holds the Doppler probe at a relatively constant angle and carefully locates the site of the maximum stenosis.[17] Since the maximum peak frequency occurs directly over the stenosis, if the technician does not carefully identify the site of the maximum stenosis, errors in the clinical estimation of the severity of stenosis will occur.

Doppler probe

The Doppler probe is central in any system to evaluate blood flow velocity patterns.

Frequency. In the study of carotid arteries, the best quality Doppler recordings can be made with a 5 MHz probe. With an 8 to 10 MHz probe we have noted that the Doppler signal may be weak and there may be a large amount of background noise. This is a result of signal attenuation in patients having a deep vessel, scar tissue in the neck, or a significant plaque present on the anterior wall of the vessel.

Beam characteristics. Ideally the ultrasonic beam produced by the Doppler probe should uniformly insonate the vessel cross section. We have mapped the beam pattern of commercially available probes and have shown that some have beam patterns that are very wide or do not uniformly insonate the vessel.[10] In our clinical vascular laboratory studies we noted that the clear window under the systolic peak of a normal recording could not be identified

if certain probes were used. In contrast, other probes allowed us to evaluate the severity of spectral broadening quite accurately. Thus if the probe beam pattern is not ideal and distorts the spectral waveform, the subtle changes produced by minor flow disturbances may be masked.

Incomplete insonation of the vessel. The CW Doppler probe can be positioned over the carotid artery so that the vessel is not completely insonated with ultrasound, and consequently the Doppler spectral waveform may be distorted. The effect of incomplete vessel insonation has been studied in vitro with a steady-flow model. As shown in Fig. 9-7, *A*, when the tube is completely insonated, the Doppler spectrum is quite flat, closely matching the spectrum theoretically expected for a parabolic velocity profile. In contrast, Fig. 9-7, *B*, shows the spectrum recorded when the beam center is located near the edge of the tube. Thus partial insonation may distort the spectrum, and the measured mean and maximum frequencies may be in error. We have calculated that the mean frequency could be in error up to 7% if the probe beam was centered at the edge of the vessel,[9] but the error in the maximum frequency is less. In all cases the degree of distortion will be highest when the profile is parabolic and lowest when it is flat. In some clinical applications these errors are not likely to be important; however, they may introduce inaccuracies in quantitative measurements from the instantaneous Doppler spectra of carotid arteries.

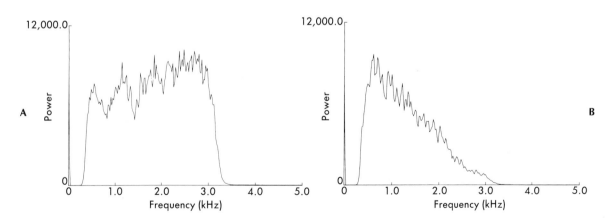

Fig. 9-7. Effect of incomplete insonation studied in vitro with steady parabolic flow. Instantaneous spectrum recorded *(A)* when vessel is completely insonated with probe directed at center of tube and *(B)* when vessel is incompletely insonated with center of beam at edge of tube. (Note the lower part of each recorded spectrum is removed by wall thump filter on Doppler demodulator.)

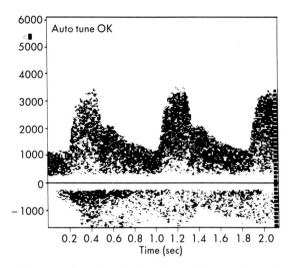

Fig. 9-8. With good quality Doppler velocity meter, forward and reverse flow signals are clearly separated. This example shows normal carotid arterial signal in upper channel and coexisting venous signal in lower channel.

Doppler velocity meter

As illustrated in Fig. 9-8, a high-quality Doppler receiver clearly separates the forward and reverse flow signals. The carotid arterial waveform is shown in the upper or forward channel; a coexisting venous flow signal is shown in the reverse channel. With an inferior Doppler velocity meter the forward and reverse flow signals may not be adequately separated. In this case some of the venous flow signal will appear along with the arterial signal, and as a consequence, accurate evaluation of the spectral waveform is impossible. Fortunately, over the last several years, commercially available Doppler velocity meters have been improved considerably, and as a result, the quality of the Doppler signal is generally quite good.

There is no agreement as to whether a CW or pulsed Doppler system is preferable. The CW Doppler system insonates the entire vessel with ultrasound, is less expensive, is technically simpler, and is easier to operate. Some workers[3,4] have argued that the pulsed Doppler system has the advantage of being more accurate, since it can record the velocity changes in the center line of flow of the vessel. However, there is no clear evidence supporting the use of pulsed over CW Doppler systems. In fact, some of the early disturbances of flow beyond the stenosis occur near the vessel wall and not in the center line of flow.[16] Furthermore, with the pulsed Doppler system, if the sample vol-

ume is positioned incorrectly, or if the vessel itself moves significantly throughout the cardiac cycle, inconsistent recordings can be obtained. We prefer the CW Doppler technique; other workers prefer the pulsed method. A direct comparison of the accuracy and the limitations of both methods is now being carried out in our laboratory.

Frequency analyzer

Gain control. Frequency analyzers require some type of gain control to modify the strength of the incoming Doppler signal. If not properly adjusted, an automatic gain control (AGC) may result in a saturated spectral waveform or an unsaturated waveform that is lost in background noise. Although an AGC is convenient, the use of only two or three preset gain levels will not accommodate all normal and abnormal input signals. A manual gain control is versatile, but the gain setting is subjective and additional training is required. The optimum system would incorporate an AGC but would also give the operator the option to intervene and use a manual gain control in selected cases.

Resolution. The resolution in both the frequency and the time axes is important, but unfortunately they are not independent. In our experience, the optimum frequency resolution is 50 to 100 Hz for carotid studies, but if the peak frequency is very high, 200 Hz may be satisfactory. In the time axis, 10 msec resolution is optimum and will allow the observer to evaluate the rapid acceleration phases of the Doppler waveform. With most systems, 50 Hz resolution is obtained only if the maximum sampling time is increased to 20 msec. To alleviate this problem and maintain good time resolution, some manufacturers use a sliding method, in which the last 20 msec sample is analyzed every 5 msec. In other words, 50 Hz resolution is achieved, but still there may be a significant loss in the time resolution because of the integrating effect of the sampling process.

Spectral variability. One of the fundamental problems of frequency analysis is the variability of the instantaneous spectrum from the one spectrum to another. The spectra in Fig. 9-9 were recorded from an in vitro model with steady parabolic flow. In Fig. 9-9, *A*, 256 spectra were averaged to obtain the smooth waveform. In Fig. 9-9, *B* and *C*, the significant variations between the various spectra are apparent.

This variability may be a result of the inherent random nature of the Doppler signal itself or the sampling and processing errors introduced by the

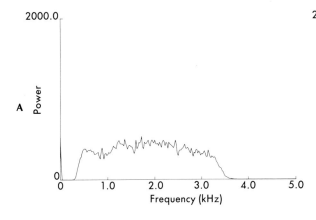

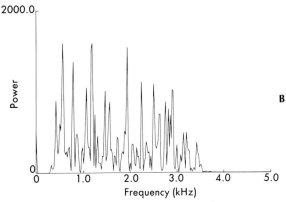

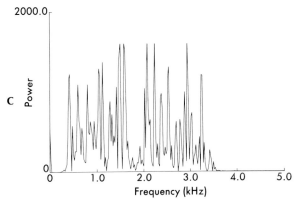

Fig. 9-9. Variability of instantaneous Doppler spectrum recorded from steady parabolic flow. *A,* Signal averaged over 256 samples. *B,* Individual Doppler power spectrum. *C,* Individual Doppler power spectrum.

frequency analyzer. By averaging spectra from the same point in consecutive pulsatile waveforms, it is possible to obtain a more representative spectrum, but this is difficult to do under clinical conditions. In the future, with improved methods of spectral estimation, the accuracy of individual spectral recordings may be improved; however, at this time, because of the variability of individual spectra, a clinician should be cautious about deriving quantitative data from displays of individual spectra.

DISPLAY OF THE SPECTRAL WAVEFORM

The spectral analysis display presents a vast amount of information to the technologist in real time, and this can be overwhelming and confusing even to the experienced observer. Based on our experience, we have concluded that the technician can assimilate only the gross characteristics of the spectral waveform in real time.

Most commercial frequency analyzers have a gray-scale or color display with 16 or more levels, but there are advantages in reducing the number of gray-scale levels so that the technician can eval-

uate the waveforms more easily. With a higher number of gray-scale levels the display is more complex and potentially more confusing, especially if the technician is only interested in recording the peak frequency and determining the presence or absence of a window under the systolic peak. By reducing the complexity of the display it may be easier for the technician to evaluate the peak frequency and the window in real time.

QUANTIFYING THE SPECTRAL WAVEFORM

Although there is general agreement that peak frequency measurements are of diagnostic value and that the extent of spectral broadening can be graded subjectively, the optimum method for quantifying the Doppler spectral waveform remains a problem. As described previously, the measurement of the peak frequency is quite accurate, but errors may occur if the technician fails to identify the internal and external carotid arteries correctly or record the maximum frequency that occurs directly over the stenosis. Since the peak frequency depends on the probe/vessel angle and since this angle is usually unknown (unless a duplex scanner is used), the clinical measurements of peak frequency cannot be related to an exact cross-sectional area stenosis but can only be proportionally related, in an approximate way, to the severity of the stenosis (Fig. 9-3).[17]

The potential accuracy and the value of quantitative measurements of spectral broadening remain uncertain, but this is an area of active research at this time.[4,8,11,14,21] By using a pulsatile flow in vitro model, we have found that the extent of spectral broadening depends on several factors, including the recording site in relation to the stenosis, the severity of the stenosis, and the shape of the stenosis, but is not strongly influenced by the flow rate or the phase of the cardiac cycle.[11] After further clarification of these complex relationships, it should be possible to quantify the severity of spectral broadening and relate it to the severity of carotid stenosis, as suggested by several workers.[4,8,11,21]

CONCLUSION

Frequency analysis presently is the logical method for processing the Doppler signals. In this chapter we have reviewed our current clinical results and presented various potential problems associated with frequency analysis. Through our clinical experience and experiments using in vitro flow models, we have identified certain problems with the frequency analysis technique that are related to errors introduced by the technician, our fundamental lack of knowledge of the underlying hemodynamic events, the Doppler probe, the Doppler velocity meter, the frequency analyzer, the display system, and the methods used for analysis or quantification of the waveforms. Future research and further developments will solve many of these problems.

ACKNOWLEDGMENTS

The authors wish to acknowledge the technical assistance of Mrs. S. Ungaro and Mrs. M. Bleach and the secretarial help of Mrs. D. Reynolds and Mrs. C. Czarnowski.

REFERENCES

1. Barnes, R.W., Rittgers, S.E., and Putney, W.: Screening for carotid artery disease: Comparison of plethysmographic and Doppler techniques. In Courbier, R. editor: Arteriopathies cerebrales extracraniennes asymptomatiques, Paris, 1980, Medical Oberval.
2. Barnes, R.W., et al.: Non-invasive ultrasonic carotid angiography: perspective validation by contrast arteriography, Surgery 80:328, 1976.
3. Blackshear, W.M., et al.: Detection of carotid occlusive disease by ultrasonic imaging and pulsed Doppler spectrum analysis, Surgery 86:698, 1979.
4. Blackshear, W.M., et al.: Carotid Artery velocity patterns in normal and stenotic vessels, Stroke 11:67, 1980.
5. Brown, P.M., and Johnston, K.W.: The difficulty of quantifying the severity of carotid stenosis, Surgery 92:468, 1982.
6. Brown, P.M., Johnston, K.W., and Douville, Y.: Detection of occlusive disease of the carotid artery with continuous wave Doppler spectral analysis, Surg. Gynecol. Obstet. 155:183, 1982.
7. Brown, P.M., Johnston, K.W., and Kassam, M.: Real-time Doppler spectral analysis for the measurement of carotid stenosis. In Diethrich, E.B., editor: Non-invasive cardiovascular diagnosis, ed. 3, Littletown, Mass., 1982, PSG Publishing Co., Inc.
8. Brown, P.M., et al.: A critical study of ultrasound Doppler spectral analysis for detecting carotid disease, Ultrasound Med. Biol. 8:515, 1982.
9. Cobbold, R.S.C., Veltink, P., and Johnston, K.W.: Influence of beam profile and degree of insonation on the CW Doppler ultrasound spectrum and mean velocity, IEEE Trans. Sonics Ultrasonics 30:364, 1983.
10. Douville, Y., et al.: Critical evaluation of continuous wave Doppler probes for carotid studies, J. Clin. Ultrasound 11:83, 1983.
11. Douville, Y., et al.: An in vitro study of carotid Doppler spectral broadening, Ultrasound Med. Biol. 9:347, 1983.
12. Haynes, B.L.: How to read clinical journals. II. To learn about a diagnostic test, Can. Med. Assoc. J. 124:703, 1981.
13. Johnston, K.W., et al.: Methods for obtaining, processing and quantifying Doppler blood flow velocity waveforms. In Nicolaides, A.N., and Yao, J.S.T., editors: Investigation of vascular disorders, Edinburgh, 1980, Churchill Livingstone.
14. Kassam, M., et al.: Quantification of carotid arterial disease by Doppler ultrasound, IEEE Ultrasonics Symp., p. 675, 1982.
15. Keagy, B.A., et al.: Evaluation of the peak frequency ratio (PFR) measurement in the detection of internal carotid artery stenosis, J. Clin. Ultrasound 10:109, 1982.
16. Khalifa, A.M.A., and Giddens, D.P.: Characterization and evolution of post stenotic flow disturbances, J. Biomech. 14:279, 1981.
17. Lally, M., Johnston, K.W., and Cobbold, R.S.C.: Limitations in the accuracy of peak frequency measurements in the diagnosis of carotid disease, J. Clin. Ultrasound 12:403, 1984.
18. Maruzzo, B.C., Johnston, K.W., and Cobbold, R.S.C.: Real-time spectral analysis of directional Doppler flow signals, Digest of XI International Conference on Medical and Biological Engineering, Ottawa, p. 158, 1976.
19. McNeil, B.J., Keller, E., and Adelstein, S.J.: Primer on certain elements of medical decision making, N. Engl. J. Med. 293:211, 1975.
20. Metz, C.E.: Basic principles of ROC analysis, Semin. Nucl. Med. 8:283, 1978.
21. Rittgers, S.E., Thornhill, B.M., and Barnes, R.W.: Quantitative analysis of carotid artery Doppler spectral waveforms—diagnostic value of parameters, Ultrasound Med. Biol. 9:255, 1983.
22. Spencer, M.P., and Reid, J.M.: Quantitation of carotid stenosis with continuous wave (CW) Doppler ultrasound, Stroke 10:326, 1979.
23. Zuech, P., et al.: The application of CCD transversal filters for real-time spectral analysis of Doppler ultrasound signals, Ultrasound Med. Biol. 8:57, 1982.

CHAPTER 10

Principles of pressure measurement

OLAV THULESIUS

The principles of pressure measurement in the detection of occlusive arterial disease are based on the pressure-flow relationships in the peripheral vascular bed. A decrease in the effective perfusion pressure (the arteriovenous pressure gradient) is roughly proportional to the severity of occlusive disease. The reduction in effective blood flow, however, is dependent on the degree of autoregulation in the peripheral vascular bed. In the case of the cutaneous circulation, autoregulation, that is, a higher blood flow in proportion to pressure reduction, is not present; on the contrary, a situation of stopped flow caused by a critical vascular closing or yield pressure related to rheologic factors may be expected. In the muscular circulation, on the other hand, autoregulation is usually present. However, the clinically most important situation is encountered in the cutaneous acral regions with a risk of the development of gangrene.

DETECTION OF ARTERIAL STENOSES AND OCCLUSIONS

Experimental studies have shown that a severe arterial stenosis is required before there is a significant change in mean pressure or flow. Beyond the so-called *critical stenosis* there is a rapid fall in both distal pressure and flow. The most important factors determining the "critical" value for a stenosis are the flow rate in the unstenosed vessel and the ratio of areas between the stenosed and unstenosed segments. Therefore a stenosis may first become apparent with increased flow rates, such as after exercise (Fig. 10-1). A pressure gradient will develop as a result of energy loss through conversion of lateral pressure energy into kinetic energy and the subsequent development of turbulence and vortex shedding in the poststenotic segment. The pressure gradient across a stenosis is

equal to the sum of the frictional pressure loss through the body of the stenosis and the pressure loss created by turbulence at the exit from the stenosis. Turbulence will develop at Reynolds numbers well below the critical value for an unobstructed tube.[13] Turbulence is also responsible for audible murmurs, which may be the earliest indication of an arterial stenosis. A bruit is more likely to become audible when narrowing in the artery reaches 50% of the cross-sectional area, but the sound may disappear when the narrowing exceeds 85% to 90%.[2] Changes in pressure and flow profiles with pulsatile flow, with periods of acceleration and retrograde flow, are more complex than with steady flow, and disturbances can be observed with as little as 25% stenosis during the deceleration phase.[1]

Multiple stenoses do not result in flow changes in proportion to the simple addition of individual stenoses. Each additional stenosis causes less effect than the preceding one. This is partly a result of the fact that each stenosis brings about larger reductions in *peak* flow and *peak* pressure than in mean flow and mean pressure. Therefore pressure and flow waves distal to the previously placed stenoses are characterized by reduced peaks. Acceleration- and deceleration-induced energy losses because of turbulence are successively reduced.[3] The *length* of the stenosis has much less effect on pressure drop and flow reduction than the *percentage stenosis* (area ratio). The length factor is directly proportional to the pressure drop, whereas the pressure loss as a result of the degree of stenosis is proportional to the second power of the area ratio of the obstructed to unobstructed artery.[14]

Pressure analysis is further complicated by the presence of reflected pressure waves traveling from the peripheral reflecting site to the point of mea-

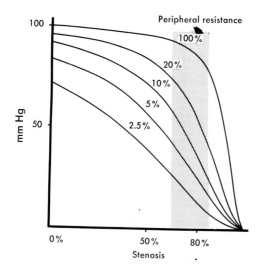

Fig. 10-1. Relationship of percentage of stenosis to distal arterial pressure at various levels of peripheral resistance (gradual increase inflow). Stippled area indicates region of "critical stenosis" during resting conditions.

Table 10-1. Systolic blood pressure (mm Hg) in healthy individuals (0) and in patients with obliterative arterial disease (I and II)

	Leg	Arm	L/A	L—A	N
At rest					
0	158.9 ± 17.5	141.5 ± 14.5	1.12 ± 0.09	17.4 ± 12.3	27
I	152.1 ± 30.9	150.3 ± 29.3	1.02 ± 0.07	3.6 ± 10.3	59
II	102.5 ± 22.9	154.1 ± 23.9	0.67 ± 0.13	−51.5 ± 25.3	14
After exercise					
0	179.3 ± 22.6	163.5 ± 22.0	1.10 ± 0.09	16.1 ± 15.3	27
I	131.4 ± 28.1	166.4 ± 28.3	0.79 ± 0.15	−35.0 ± 25.5	14
II	62.5 ± 30.2	184.4 ± 27.9	0.34 ± 0.19	−121.1 ± 44.5	58

I, no symptoms, slight stenosis; II, intermittent claudication, occlusions.
Mean values ± 1 standard deviation (mm Hg);
L = leg, A = arm, N = number of extremities.

surement. The presence of a stenosis leads to the production of a partial standing wave with an antinode of pressure immediately proximal to the stenosis. Therefore the best chance to detect a stenosis is to record the whole flow profile or to determine the pressure gradient with measuring sites immediately proximal and distal to the stenosis, preferably by direct pressure measurement. Newman et al.[7] have shown that changes in oscillatory flow and pressure begin to occur at 60% stenosis, whereas changes in mean pressure or flow do not become apparent unless there is an 80% stenosis.

The most frequently encountered symptomatic lesion is not presence of stenosis but *complete occlusion* with collateral flow. In this situation the effect of distal blood flow and pressure is dependent on the input impedance of the collateral vascular bed. With multiple total occlusions the resultant pressure drop is not additive, but is 22% of the expected pressure drop in femoroiliac occlusions and 9% in femorotibial occlusions.[6]

DETECTION OF STENOSES AND OCCLUSIONS

From the preceding theoretical discussion it is apparent that methods that detect peak oscillatory flow or pressure (that is, systolic pressure) must be more sensitive than those measuring mean flow or pressure. Moreover, mild stenosis must be more easily detected under conditions of increased flow (for example, active or reactive hyperemia). This has been shown frequently in cases in which pressure measurement after treadmill exercise can be performed.[11] Normal values for healthy individuals and for patients with arterial insufficiency before and after exercise are given in Table 10-1. As can be seen, leg systolic pressure is about 17 mm higher at the ankle than in the brachial artery, an example of systolic pressure amplification because of re-

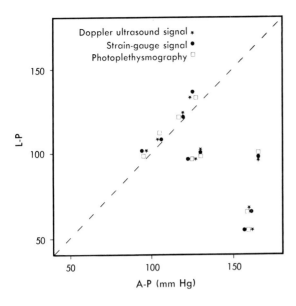

Fig. 10-2. Simultaneous determination of arm systolic pressure (A-P) and leg systolic pressure (L-P) determined with three different detectors in healthy individuals and in patients with arterial insufficiency.

flected waves. These values are in accordance with directly measured pressure levels.[8] Asymptomatic individuals with normal arm-leg pressures and stenotic lesions may demonstrate significant gradients after exercise, since the increased flow rate produces an enhanced pressure gradient, and at the same time systemic arterial pressure rises.

Absolute values of distal arterial pressure are a valuable guide for assessing the prognosis of skin lesions. Previous experience gathered from the Copenhagen group[4] and our own material indicates that an ankle pressure below 50 mm Hg and a toe pressure below 20 mm Hg are limits below which gangrene may be expected.

Noninvasive pressure measurements are usually performed with proximal arterial occluding cuffs and distal detection of flow signals, for example, in the posterior tibial or dorsalis pedis artery. The "on-signal" indicating start of flow is taken as coincident with the simultaneously measured systolic pressure level. Several pulse-sensing devices have been used, including the following:

1. Doppler ultrasound signal
2. Photoelectric plethysmography
3. Strain-gauge signal
4. Clearance of radioactive tracers

We have performed a parallel investigation of simultaneous measurements with Doppler signals, photoelectric plethysmographs, and strain-gauge signals in healthy individuals and in patients with obliterative arterial disease. Essentially all of these methods give reliable signals down to a pressure

level of 50 mm Hg (Fig. 10-2). Doppler signals were the most easily discernible indication of blood flow. Another advantage of Doppler detection is the possibility of transforming it to an audible sound that facilitates measurements and makes expensive recording instruments unnecessary. Strain-gauge recordings from the great toe are recommended particularly with advanced arterial disease, since blood flow may be nonpulsatile in these circumstances. Signals from clearance curves of radioactive tracers have been used in conjunction with occluding cuffs covering the measuring site. These values are slightly lower than strain-gauge signals, since they presumably reflect arteriolar pressure.[5]

PRESSURE GRADIENTS

For assessment of arterial insufficiency in the lower extremities, the brachial artery systolic pressure generally serves as a reference for the determination of a pressure gradient or the ankle-to-arm pressure ratio. To get a reliable frame of reference, it should be mandatory to record brachial and ankle pressures simultaneously, since fluctuations of the basal blood pressure occur frequently, especially if painful arterial occlusions with tourniquets are being performed. We have therefore made a series of consecutive and simultaneous measurements in 100 extremities of healthy individuals and patients with arterial stenoses and total occlusions, both at rest and after exercise (Fig. 10-3). In this study a much better distinction between healthy individuals

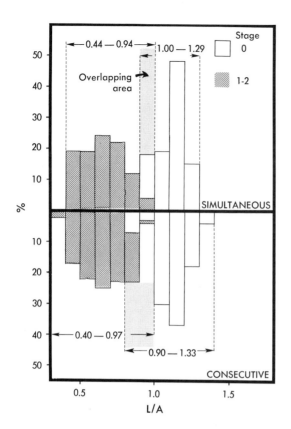

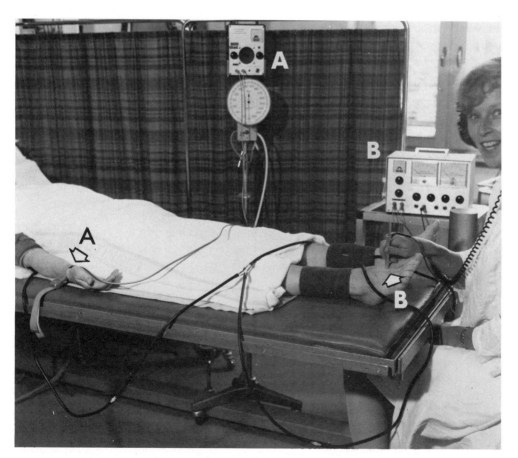

Fig. 10-3. Result of simultaneous and consecutive leg and arm systolic pressure measurements in healthy individuals (stage 0) and in patients with arterial insufficiency (stages 1 and 2). Stages are identical with those in Table 10-1. Percent indicates frequency distribution of cases, and L/A represents leg/arm pressure ratio.

Fig. 10-4. Procedure for simultaneous determination of arm (A with arrow) and leg (B with arrow) systolic pressure using two Doppler detectors, one (A) with a flashing light and the other (B) with an audio signal.

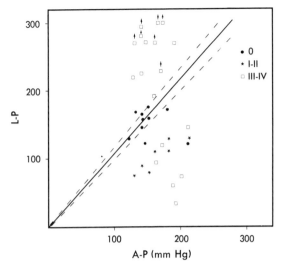

Fig. 10-5. Simultaneous arm systolic pressure (A-P) and leg systolic pressure (L-P) levels in 36 patients with diabetes—10 patients without evidence of arterial lesions and 26 patients with various degrees of arterial insufficiency. I-II, Stenoses and occlusions; III-IV, occlusions with rest pain or gangrene.

and those with various degrees of arterial insufficiency was observed when simultaneous rather than consecutive measurements of arm and ankle pressure were obtained.[10] The technique we are presently using is shown in Fig. 10-4. Two Doppler detectors are used, one (a flat probe) attached to the radial artery and the other held over a foot artery. To distinguish between the two flow signals, we use a photo-diode for the pulsating flow from the radial artery and an audible signal from the foot. Both the arm and leg tourniquets are inflated and deflated simultaneously from the same line.

ARTIFACTS

The main source of error is associated with incomplete occlusion of the artery, which may be a result of the following:
1. Rigid arteries
2. Extravascular structures
3. Tourniquet that is too small

In the presence of rigid arteries, indirect measurement of blood pressure with tourniquets often involves a delayed closure that gives rise to an overestimation of intravascular pressure. In this situation it is more reliable to record systolic blood pressure only during deflation. A delayed opening is characteristic of the vasospasm seen in digital arteries of patients with Raynaud's phenomenon (Chapter 62). Therefore it is important to standardize the rate of cuff deflation and read systolic blood pressure only during deflation.[12]

Rigid arteries as a result of medial sclerosis are most frequently seen in patients with diabetes and yield erroneously high pressure levels in the leg, even in cases with proximal occlusion (Fig. 10-5). Hence it is essential to use additional methods to determine the actual flow condition. We therefore combine our evaluation with an analysis of the Doppler flow profile, oscillometric indices, and an assessment of toe pressure and toe plethysmography. There is some evidence that medial sclerosis is less prominent in digital arteries.

Extravascular components such as obesity and edema may interfere with proper arterial cuff occlusion. It is always essential to use tourniquets of proper dimensions, totally encircling the extremity and with a width of at least 120% of the extremity diameter. Bladder diameters in excess of 120% do not yield falsely low values.[9]

Segmental distal pressure measurements at the thigh, calf, and ankle have been used to disclose multiple-level occlusions. Yet because of an obvious perturbation of the system during measurement, the more proximal pressures cannot be relied on to reflect the actual intraarterial pressure. When inflating the cuff above the local systolic pressure, all circulation in the tissue mass distal to the cuff ceases; the closer the cuff is to the occlusion, the larger is the fraction of the tissue mass supplied by the collaterals that will be excluded. In this situation a measurable rise in local arterial pressure will occur because the flow rate through the collaterals decreases.[4]

REFERENCES

1. Cassanova, R.A., and Giddens, D.P.: Disorder distal to modeled stenoses in steady and pulsatile flow, J. Bio-mech. 11:441, 1978.
2. Fields, W.S.: Management of asymptomatic carotid bruit, Am. Heart J. 98:1, 1979.
3. Flanigan, D.P., et al.: Multiple subcritical stenoses, Ann. Surg. 186:663, 1977.
4. Lassen, N.A., Tönnesen, K.H., and Holstein, P.: Distal blood pressure, Scand. J. Clin. Lab. Invest. 36:705, 1976.
5. Lassen, N.A., et al.: Distal blood pressure measurement in occlusive arterial disease, strain gauge compared to Xenon-133, Angiology 23:211, 1972.
6. Martin, M., and Müller-Scholtes, G.: Die systolische Blutdruckmessung über der A. tibialis posterior mit Hilfe der Ultraschall-Doppler-Technik. In Hild, R., and Spaan, G., editors: Therapiekontrolle in der angiologie, Baden-Baden, West Germany, 1979, Gerhard Witzstrock.
7. Newman, D.L., Walesby, R.K., and Bowden, N.L.R.: Hemodynamic effects of acute experimental aortic coarctation in the dog, Circ. Res. 36:165, 1975.
8. Nielsen, P.E., Barras, J.P., and Holstein, P.: Systolic pressure amplification in the arteries of normal subjects, Scand. J. Clin. Lab. Invest. 33:371, 1974.
9. Thulesius, O.: Några synpunkter på indirekt blodtrycksmätning, Opusc. Med. 17:52, 1972.
10. Thulesius, O.: Simultane Doppler-Sonographic von Arm- und Bein-gefässen bei arteriellen Occlusionen. In Kreissmann, A., and Bollinger, A., editors: Ultraschall-Doppler Diagnostik in der Angiologie, Stuttgart, 1978, Georg Thième.
11. Thulesius, O.: Systemic and ankle blood pressure before and after exercise in patients with arterial insufficiency, Angiologia 29:374, 1978.
12. Thulesius, O., and Lanne, T.: The importance of arterial compliance and tone for the determination of ankle systolic pressure, Presented at the thirteenth World Congress of the International Union of Angiology, Rochester, Minn., 1983.
13. Yougchareon, W., and Young, D.: Initiation of turbulence in models of arterial stenoses, J. Biomech. 12:185, 1979.
14. Young, D.F., Cholvin, N.R., and Roth, A.: Pressure drop across artificially induced stenoses in the femoral artery of dogs, Circ. Res. 36:735, 1975.

CHAPTER 11

Noninvasive techniques of measuring lower limb arterial pressures

JAMES S. T. YAO

Ever since Hales[14] successfully measured mean blood pressure from the carotid artery in an unanesthetized horse in 1733, investigators have sought better and more convenient ways of measuring the same phenomenon. It was not until more than a century later that von Basch first developed an arterial occluding device to measure blood pressure in humans.[30] The use of the air-inflated arm-occluding cuff, introduced by Riva-Rocci[25] and further modified by Von Recklinghausen,[31] revolutionized the method of recording blood pressure. By means of palpation of the radial pulse distal to the cuff or by the oscillometric technique, systolic blood pressure may be measured indirectly. In 1905 Korotkoff[19] proposed his auscultatory method and successfully established the basic sphygmomanometric technique for measuring brachial systolic and diastolic blood pressure.

At present the measurement of blood pressure may be classified into direct and indirect methods. The former requires placement of a needle or catheter in an artery, and the latter is generally determined by placing a cuff around the part of the limb to be measured. This is done by inflating the cuff to a pressure sufficient to stop blood flow and then slowly deflating the cuff with some method to detect the pressure at which distal blood flow is resumed. Because of the noninvasive nature of the indirect technique, measurement of brachial blood pressure is now routine medical practice.

Measurement of upper extremity pressure with a conventional stethoscope seldom presents problems, except under shock conditions and in a noisy environment. The use of the stethoscope to measure lower limb pressure, however, is often difficult. Even in normal subjects, the inability to detect Korotkoff sounds in pedal arteries or even in popliteal arteries has made measurement of lower limb pressures by the conventional stethoscope a difficult procedure.[16] In the presence of arterial occlusion, the decrease of systolic pressure further limits the use of the conventional technique. Because of this limitation, various techniques are now available to aid in recording blood pressure of a lower limb noninvasively.

CURRENT INSTRUMENTATION FOR PULSE REGISTRATION

Many time-honored techniques such as the flush method, oscillometry, and volume (air or water) plethysmography are too cumbersome for clinical use. Therefore these techniques will not be discussed here. Only those methods that are currently in use will be reviewed.

Mercury-in-Silastic strain-gauge plethysmography

The Silastic gauge filled with mercury is used to detect the change of circumference of a digit or a part of the limb to be measured. When the gauge is placed around the terminal digit (toe) or the foot, the volume changes that occur with each heartbeat produce a change in the circumference of the gauge. By balancing the gauge on a Wheatstone bridge together with an amplifier, it is possible to detect the pulse of a digit in a lower extremity.[23,28] Measurement of the systolic pressure is performed by placing a cuff proximal to the gauge. After rapid inflation of the cuff to about 20 mm Hg above the systolic pressure, the pulse signals disappear. During deflation of the cuff, the systolic pressure is

☐ Supported in part by the Northwestern University Vascular Research Fund.

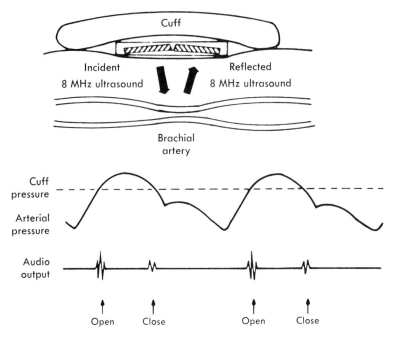

Fig. 11-1. Using ultrasound to measure vessel wall movement during deflation of pneumatic cuff. (From Stegall, H.F., Kardon, H.B., and Kemmerer, W.T.: J. Appl. Physiol. 25:793, 1968.)

recorded at the time of reappearance of the pulse. In the low flow state or in vasoconstriction, pulse registration from the toe may not be apparent. Under this circumstance, a DC mode may be used. The sudden increase in volume during deflation of the inflated cuff causes a shift of the baseline. This shift may be used as the endpoint for systolic pressure.

Isotope clearance

Xenon-133(^{133}Xe) injected into tissue may be used to calculate muscle flow by recording the wash-out curve of the isotope.[8] Using a cuff proximal to the site of the depot of ^{133}Xe, systolic pressure is recorded at the level during slow inflation when the washout stops. Such a pressure level represents perfusion pressure in the muscle. Similarly Lassen and Holstein[20] have found that the flow cessation pressure measured by inflating a blood pressure cuff placed over a radioactive depot injected into the skin was nearly equal to the diastolic pressure in normal subjects. This pressure level represents skin pressure, or it may merely represent systolic pressure in small arteries, as suggested by Carter.[6]

Transcutaneous ultrasound techniques

Wall-motion technique. Wall-motion technique is based on the use of a specially constructed trans-ducer to detect changes in Doppler-shifted ultrasound generated by arterial wall motion. The technique was first described by Ware.[24] When cuff pressure is above systolic arterial pressure, the artery remains closed throughout the cardiac cycle and no signal is heard. As cuff pressure falls below systolic, a short thump is heard, which splits into distinct "opening" and "closing" phases (Fig. 11-1). As cuff pressure falls further, separation between the opening and closing signals widens until a closing signal begins to encroach on the subsequent opening signal. When these two merge, cuff pressure is equivalent to diastolic pressure. Because the technique measures wall motion, it is also termed Doppler ultrasound kinetoarteriography.

Flow velocity detector. Arterial flow signals are now readily detected by various types of Doppler instruments using the Doppler-shift flow detection principle. These Doppler instruments range from pocket-size portable devices to the directional flow detector equipped with analog output. Through the use of the flow probe in a manner similar to the stethoscope, the Doppler flow velocity detector has greatly facilitated measurement of systolic pressure of lower limbs.

A sphygmomanometer cuff is applied just above the ankle, and a flow probe is placed over the posterior tibial artery or the dorsal artery of the

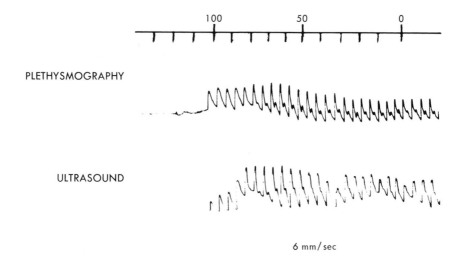

Fig. 11-2. Comparison of systolic pressure (in millimeters of mercury) measured by strain-gauge plethysmography and Doppler ultrasound. Systolic pressure of 100 mm Hg was recorded by both methods.

foot. Flow signals cease as the cuff is inflated to 20 mm Hg or more above the brachial systolic pressure. During deflation of the cuff, a return of flow signals indicates the level of the systolic pressure at the ankle (Fig. 11-2). The flow velocity detector, however, is useful in the detection of systolic pressure only.

Photosensor technique

Measurement of skin blood pressure using photoelectric plethysmography has been recently reported.[24] A probe into which a lamp and a photoelectric resistance are built is placed under a cuff in direct contact with the skin, and the reflected light is recorded on a potentiometer writer. When the cuff is inflated to above systolic level, blanching of the skin occurs and pulsation disappears. During slow deflation of the cuff, a DC-register curve shift or baseline shift indicates the return of blood inflow, and hence the level of skin systolic pressure. Recently an infrared photoplethysmograph has been introduced. This technique is particularly useful for toe pressure measurements. A DC mode is also available, if pulse registration of the first toe is not feasible. Again, a shift in baseline of the DC-register curve indicates the endpoint of systolic pressure.

EQUIPMENT

Proper blood pressure cuffs, manometers, and control valves are prerequisites for accurate blood pressure recording.

Cuff size for recording blood pressure

Regardless of the type of instrument used, the cuff size applied to the limb is of paramount importance in achieving accurate readings. An inflatable bladder is surrounded by an unyielding cover, called the cuff. The width of the bladder is critical. If it is too narrow (undercuffing), the blood pressure reading will be erroneously high, and if it is too wide (overcuffing), the reading may be too low. In a recent study by Manning et al.[21], miscuffing was found to distort the blood pressure reading in the arm by an average of 8.5 mm Hg.

For the accurate indirect measurement of blood pressure, the American Heart Association (AHA) now recommends that the cuff size be based on limb circumference.[18] It is recommended that the width of the inflatable bladder be 40% of the circumference of the midpoint of the limb, or 20% wider than the diameter. The circumference of the limb, not the age of the patient, is the factor that determines cuff size. The length of the bladder should be twice its width (bladder length equal to 80% of the arm circumference). Table 11-1 illustrates the recommendations for blood pressure cuff bladder dimensions made by the AHA in 1980.[18] Since the recording of ankle pressure closely parallels the recording of brachial pressure, the bladder dimension and ankle circumference must be taken into consideration for accurate measurement. For measurement of ankle blood pressure the conventional arm cuff is sufficient, although some investigators prefer a wider cuff.[29] In a study com-

Table 11-1. Recommended bladder dimensions for blood pressure cuff

Arm circumference at midpoint* (cm)	Cuff name	Bladder width (cm)	Bladder length (cm)
5-7.5	Newborn	3	5
7.5-13	Infant	5	8
13-20	Child	8	13
17-26	Small adult	11	17
24-32	Adult	13	24
32-42	Large adult	17	32
42-50†	Thigh	20	42

From Kirkendall, W.M., et al.: Recommendations for human blood pressure determination by sphygmomanometers. Subcommittee of the AHA Postgraduate Education Committee, Circulation 62:1146A, 1980. By permission of the American Heart Association, Inc.
*Midpoint of arm is defined as half the distance from the acromion to the olecranon.
†In persons with very large limbs, the indirect blood pressure should be measured in the leg or forearm.

Table 11-2. Recommended cuff size for lower limb pressure measurement

Cuff location	Cuff size
Adult upper thigh	11 cm
Adult lower thigh	19 cm
Adult thigh (contour-type cuff)	22 cm
Adult ankle	12 cm
Adult finger	2 to 2.5 cm
Adult toe	2.5 to 3 cm

paring different sized cuffs, Gundersen[13] recommended that the ankle cuff be 7 to 8 cm, the calf cuff 11 to 14 cm, and the thigh cuff 16 to 23 cm wide. Standard adult arm cuffs used in clinical medicine at the present time contain an air-inflatable rubber bladder that is 23 cm long and 12 to 12.5 cm wide, which should be sufficient for use at the ankle level. Measurements using cuffs of this size yield values that agree with intraarterial measurements.[4,23,26]

The size of the thigh cuff is important. It should be 18 to 20 cm wide. Because of the shape of the thigh, Hokanson[17] has devised a contoured thigh cuff. The bladder in this cuff is 22 cm wide and 71 cm long and is shaped to conform to the taper of the thigh. Although no study has been done to prove the superiority of the contour cuff as compared with the ordinary thigh cuff, the idea of con-

tour cuffs is a good one and merits further application. For recording pressure of the lower thigh, we have found that a 19 cm cuff is useful. Barnes[2] has suggested a narrow cuff (11 cm) for upper thigh pressure measurement. In obese patients a wider cuff may be more appropriate because of the large size of the thigh.

Digital cuffs for recording finger or toe pressures may be constructed of a bladder made of Penrose drain on a backing of nylon Velcro strip[13] (Fig. 11-3). Digital cuff width varies from finger to toe, and the proper size for a finger is 2 to 2.5 cm and for a toe, 2.5 to 3 cm. According to Gundersen,[13] a 2.4 cm wide cuff was found to be the most suitable for finger pressure recording on a medium-sized man. Table 11-2 summarizes the different sizes of cuffs that should be used for recording lower limb pressure.

Obviously, for extremely obese patients or patients with odd-shaped ankles, the size of the cuff should be adjusted accordingly to avoid unusually high readings. Steinfeld et al.[27] have proposed that, for the conically shaped obese leg, a bladder of trapezoidal design should be used so that, when applied to the limb, it would conform more closely to its natural contours. Recently the same group of investigators[1] have constructed a new cuff with the bladder completely encircling the limb, thus avoiding the narrow cuff effect. In general, a large cuff probably should be used in obese patients. Error in blood pressure measurement resulting from incorrect cuff size in such patients has been reported.[22]

Control valves and tubings

Defects in the control valve or air leaks may cause false or inaccurate readings. Such defects have been claimed to be a major source of error in blood pressure recording.[7] Conceicao et al.[7] have recommended the following maneuvers to test for air leaks and the function of the control valve as well as the connecting tubes:

1. The pump should have a competent nonreturn valve and no leaks.

2. The control valve should allow the free passage of air without excessive muscular effort when the filter is clean. When closed, it should hold the mercury at a constant level. When released, it should allow a controlled fall of the mercury column.

To test the valve, roll the cuff in its own ''tail,'' pump to 200 mm Hg, and wait 10 seconds, during

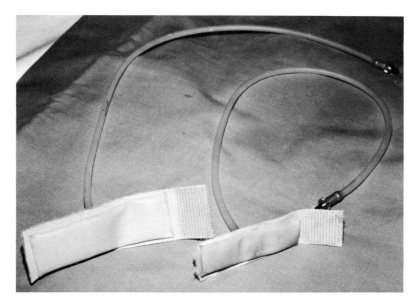

Fig. 11-3. Digital cuffs for measuring toe and finger pressures.

which time the level should not fall more than 2 mm Hg. If a leak is detected, the circuit is clamped in sections to find the site; in fact, most such leaks can be traced to control valves. Slowly release the valve on four occasions. During at least two of these attempts, it should be possible to control the rate of fall readily to not more than 1 mm/sec and to change to and from a faster rate at will. Ideally, this should be possible at every attempt, but a more demanding test would result in condemning nearly all sphygmomanometers, including many new ones, with the present design of control valves.

3. The connections should fit without an air leak and should come apart easily.

4. The tube should be airtight and of appropriate length.

5. The mercury tube should not be cracked. There should be a patent air vent at the top of the column.

6. The cuff should fit comfortably around the arm and stay in place when inflated. The rubber bag should be long enough to encircle the arm.

Manometers

Two types of pressure-registering systems are in general use: the mercury gravity manometer and the aneroid. Both give accurate and reproducible results when working properly. The aneroid manometer is probably more versatile for bedside or laboratory use. If an aneroid manometer is used, efforts should be made to calibrate the instrument yearly. Such calibration can be made by interposing a Y connector in the tube from the cuff to a mercury manometer and attaching the sphygmomanometer to be tested to the free end of the connector.

MEASURING TECHNIQUES

Brachial pressure is recorded with a Doppler or a conventional stethoscope before lower limb pressure measurement. All measurements are made with the patient in the supine position after a 10- to 15-minute period of rest.

Ankle systolic pressure

The arm pressure cuff is applied snugly above the malleolus (Fig. 11-4). The cuff is then inflated above the brachial systolic pressure (about 20 to 30 mm Hg). The endpoint of systolic pressure is determined by the reappearance of the pulse (an audible sound by Doppler method or pulse waveform by plethysmography). Two or three measurements should be made on each limb.

Upper thigh pressure

A narrow cuff (11 cm) is placed just below the inguinal ligament, and the Doppler probe is placed over the popliteal artery for endpoint determination.

Lower thigh pressure

The thigh cuff is applied just above the knee. If the Doppler ultrasound method is used, the sound

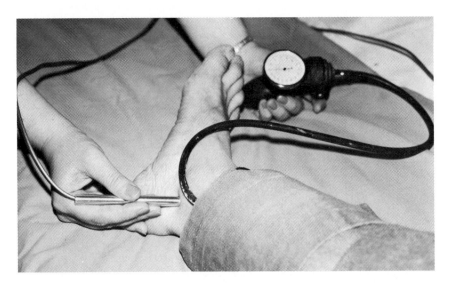

Fig. 11-4. Method of recording ankle systolic pressure.

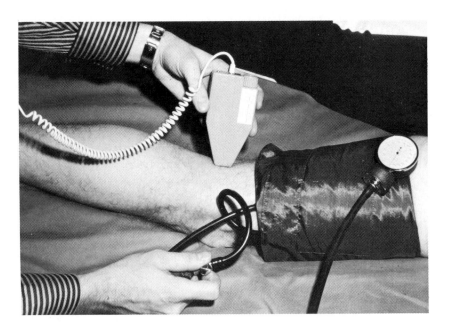

Fig. 11-5. Method of recording thigh pressure.

probe is placed over the popliteal artery to detect sound signals (Fig. 11-5). It has been shown that placing the sensor close to the pressure cuff is critical to obtaining accurate thigh pressure measurement, especially in patients with multiple-level occlusions.[11] For the plethysmographic method, the pulse registration is normally done on the big toe. The endpoint of the systolic pressure is determined by the same maneuver used to obtain the ankle pressure.

Toe pressure

A strain gauge or photosensor is placed on the big toe to record pulse or volume changes with the cuff placed at the base of the toe.

Postexercise measurements

Ankle pressure can be measured after exercise in a similar manner. Standard treadmill walking is used. Immediately after termination of the treadmill exercise, the patient resumes the supine position, and ankle pressure is recorded at 1-minute intervals until the pressure reaches the preexercise level.

Postischemic measurement (reactive hyperemia)

To simulate the reactive hyperemia induced by exercise, the pressure cuff applied to the thigh may be used to induce distal ischemia. The cuff is inflated to a level of 50 mm Hg above the systolic pressure for a period of 3 to 5 minutes and then abruptly deflated. Reactive hyperemia will follow immediately. Ankle systolic pressure is then recorded at 1-minute intervals until it returns to the resting pressure level.

Comparative study with intraarterial technique

Noninvasive measurement of ankle pressure using Doppler ultrasound has been compared with the intraarterial technique in normal subjects by Bollinger et al.[3] Continuous monitoring of pressure in the posterior tibial or dorsalis pedis artery was used, and there was good correlation ($\sqrt{} = 0.87$) between the systolic pressure values measured by the two techniques. Recently the use of upper thigh pressure has been compared with intraarterial pressure measurements in the femoral artery.[9,10] From this analysis it was found that the upper thigh pressure does not differentiate between aortoiliac and superficial femoral artery disease.

SUMMARY

Recording of blood pressure is one of the fundamental measurements in understanding the hemodynamics of occlusive arterial disease. Proper equipment, especially the size of the cuff, the dimension of the bladder, and proper measuring technique are important to achieve accurate readings. The choice of instrumentation depends on the resources of the institution. At present the Doppler ultrasound technique is probably the least expensive and the most versatile. Unlike pulse registration techniques such as plethysmography, which requires cumbersome equipment, the pocket or portable Doppler instruments allow systolic pressure recording at the bedside, in the office, in the operating room, or in the intensive care area. The technique is simple and requires little training. It can be performed readily by a nurse or competent technician. For toe pressure measurement, however, the photoplethysmograph appears to be more useful because of difficulty in recording the toe pulse.

As with all measuring techniques, indirect pressure recording has its limitations. In the lower limb an important limitation is the inability of the pressure cuff to compress a heavily calcified artery. Such a condition is commonly seen in patients with diabetes mellitus or those with chronic renal failure and calcified arteries.[12,15] Because of such arterial calcification, a falsely high ankle systolic pressure may be recorded in some patients with diabetes mellitus or with chronic renal failure. In addition, when two parallel vessels of comparable size are compressed by the cuff, the measurement will reflect the pressure in the artery with the highest pressure and may not detect a significant stenotic or occlusive lesion in the other vessel.

Of pressures recorded at different levels of the lower limb, the ankle systolic pressure is probably the most reliable in detection of abnormalities. Both upper and lower thigh pressures are subject to more variation and are less sensitive in detection of arterial occlusion or stenosis.[3,9,10] Difficulties with thigh pressure measurement are caused by inability of the cuff to compress the artery completely, obesity, and inherent problems with the size and dimension of the bladder of the pressure cuff.

REFERENCES

1. Alexander, M., Cohen, M.L., and Steinfeld, L.: Criteria in the choice of an occluding cuff for indirect measurement of blood pressure, Med. Biol. Eng. Comput. 15:2, 1977.
2. Barnes, R.W., and Wilson, M.R.: Doppler ultrasound evaluation of peripheral arterial disease. A programmed audiovisual instruction, Iowa City, 1976, University of Iowa.
3. Bernstein, E.F., et al.: Thigh pressure artifacts with noninvasive techniques in an experimental model, Surgery 89:391, 1981.
4. Bollinger, A., Barras, J.P., and Mahler, F.: Measurement of foot artery blood pressure by micromanometry in normal subjects and in patients with arterial occlusive disease, Circulation 53:506, 1976.
5. Bone, G.E., and Pomajzl, M.J.: Toe blood pressure by photoplethysmography: an index of healing in forefoot amputation, Surgery 89:569, 1981.
6. Carter, S.A.: Peripheral blood flow, blood pressure and metabolism in occlusive arterial disease. Application to control of surgical and medical therapy, Scand. J. Clin. Lab. Invest. 31(suppl. 128):147, 1973.
7. Conceicao, S., Ward, M.K., and Kerr, D.N.S.: Defects in sphygmomanometers: an important source of error in blood pressure recordings, Br. Med. J. 1:886, 1976.
8. Dahn, I., Lassen, N.A., and Westling, H.: Blood flow in human muscles during external pressure or venous stasis, Clin. Sci. 32:467, 1967.
9. Flanigan, D.P. et al.: Correlation of Doppler-derived high thigh pressure and intra-arterial pressure in the assessment of aorto-iliac occlusive disease, Br. J. Surg. 68:423, 1981.
10. Flanigan, D.P., et al.: Utility of wide and narrow blood pressure cuffs in the hemodynamic assessment of aortoiliac occlusive disease, Surgery 92:16, 1982.

11. Franzeck, U.K., Bernstein, E.F., and Fronek, A.: The effect of sensing site on the limb segmental blood pressure determination, Arch. Surg. 116:912, 1981.

12. Gipstein, R.M., Coburn, J.W., Adams, D.A., et al.: Calciphylaxis in man. A syndrome of tissue necrosis and vascular calcification in 11 patients with chronic renal failure, Arch. Intern. Med. 136:1273, 1976.

13. Gundersen, J.: Segmental measurements of systolic blood pressure in the extremities including the thumb and the great toe, Acta Chir. Scand. (suppl.) 426:1, 1972.

14. Hales, S.: Statistical essays: containing haemastaticks, vol. 2, London, 1733, W. Innys & R. Manby.

15. Hobbs, J.T., et al.: A limitation of the Doppler ultrasound method of measuring ankle systolic pressure, Vasa 3:160, 1974.

16. Hocken, A.G.: Measurement of blood pressure in the leg, Lancet 1:466, 1967.

17. Hokanson, G.: Personal communication, 1976.

18. Kirkendall, W.M., et al.: Recommendations for human blood pressure determination by sphygmomanometers. Subcommittee of the AHA Postgraduate Education Committee, Circulation 62(5):1146A, 1980.

19. Korotkoff, N.S.: On the subject of methods of measuring blood pressure, Bull. Imperial Military Med. Acad. 11:365, 1905.

20. Lassen, N.A., and Holstein, P.: Use of radioisotopes in assessment of distal blood flow and distal blood pressure in arterial insufficiency, Surg. Clin. North Am. 54:39, 1974.

21. Manning, D.M., Kuchirka, C., and Kaminski, J.: Miscuffing: inappropriate blood pressure cuff application, Circulation 68:763, 1983.

22. Maxwell, M.H., et al.: Error in blood-pressure measurement due to incorrect cuff size in obese patients, Lancet 2:33, 1982.

23. Nielsen, P.E., Bell, G., and Lassen, N.A.: The measurement of digital systolic blood pressure by strain-gauge technique, Scand. J. Clin. Lab. Invest. 29:371, 1972.

24. Nielsen, P.E., Poulsen, N.L., and Gyntelberg, F.: Arterial blood pressure in the skin measured by a photoelectric probe and external counter pressure, Vasa 2:65, 1973.

25. Riva-Rocci, S.: Un nuovo sfigmomanometro, Gaz. Med. Torino 47:981, 1896.

26. Stegall, H.F., Kardon, M.B., and Kemmerer, W.T.: Indirect measurement of arterial blood pressure by Doppler ultrasonic sphygmomanometry, J. Appl. Physiol. 25:793, 1968.

27. Steinfeld, L., Alexander, H., and Cohen, M.L.: Updating sphygmomanometry (editorial), Am. J. Cardiol. 33:107, 1974.

28. Strandness, D.E., Jr., and Bell, J.W.: Peripheral vascular disease. Diagnosis and objective evaluation using a mercury strain-gauge, Ann. Surg. 161(suppl. 4):3, 1965.

29. Thulesius, O., and Gjores, J.E.: Use of Doppler-shift detection for determining peripheral arterial blood pressure, Angiology 22:594, 1971.

30. von Basch, S.: Ueber die Messung des Blutdrucks am Menschen, Z. Klin. Med. 2:79, 1881.

31. Von Recklinghausen, H.: Ueber Blutdruckmessung beim Menschen, Arch. Exper. Pathol. Pharmakol. 46:78, 1901.

CHAPTER 12

Physiologic principles of ocular pneumoplethysmography

BERT C. EIKELBOOM

Soon after the introduction of the ophthalmoscope, Donders[2], among others, studied the pulsation of the vessels at the optic disk during compression of the ocular globe with the finger. In principle the possibility of measuring blood pressure in the eye originated. It was not recognized until the beginning of this century that ophthalmic artery pressure reflects distal internal carotid artery pressure and can be used in the diagnosis of carotid stenosis.

In 1917 clinical ophthalmodynamometry originated from the springdynamometer developed by Baillart[1] in which external pressure is put on the eye during simultaneous fundoscopy. The ophthalmic artery pressure was calculated from the pressure needed to stop the pulsations in the fundus arteries. Galin[4] modified this technique by the application of a suction cup to the sclera to increase ocular pressure and obliterate ocular pulsations. Gee[5-7] combined Galin's technique with ocular plethysmography and obtained a graphic reproduction of the pulsations of both eyes simultaneously at different degrees of vacuum, thus making it possible to calculate both ophthalmic artery pressures in a more objective manner. His technique, known as OPG-Gee, has been used since 1973. Ever since, OPG-Gee has remained a valuable technique in the evaluation of carotid disease, even though many more sophisticated techniques have been developed in recent years. This is a result of the sound physiologic principle of pressure measurement that has proved to be valuable in assessing arterial and venous disease.

DEVELOPMENT OF INSTRUMENTATION

Gee distinguishes four phases in the development of OPG-Gee. From 1967 to 1971 two experimental machines were tested that proved to be of no clinical use. In the second phase (1971 to 1973) tests were performed with a monocular unit that produced a variable vacuum that increased stepwise until pulsations disappeared. However, a few seconds after reaching that level, pulsations reappeared. This was explained by the fact that an elevated eye pressure brings along a faster outflow of ocular fluid via the Schlemm system, resulting in a decrease of ocular pressure and the reappearance of ocular pulsations. Gee also recognized that since the systemic blood pressure fluctuates, both ophthalmic artery pressures should be measured simultaneously for an accurate comparison of the left side and right side and for an accurate determination of the ophthalmic/systemic pressure ratio.

The instrument was redesigned to produce binocular registration and rapid accumulation of vacuum up to 300 mm Hg, followed by automatic gradual release over 30 seconds. This machine became commercially available in 1973 and was produced until 1978. The maximum ophthalmic artery pressure that could be measured was 110 mm Hg, and it was soon recognized that this caused a problem in hypertensive patients. This led to the development of the OPG-500, which could create a vacuum of 500 mm Hg, allowing determination of systolic ophthalmic arterial pressures up to 143 mm Hg. The original three-channel recorder was replaced by a four-channel recorder that made simultaneous electrocardiogram (ECG) registration possible.

VALIDATION STUDIES

The correlation between the amount of vacuum applied to the eye, the resulting intraocular pressure, and the ophthalmic artery pressure was par-

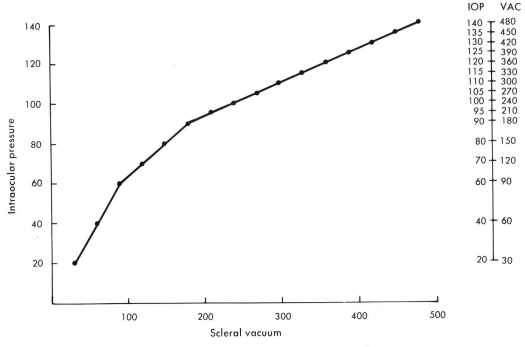

Fig. 12-1. Correlation of intraocular pressure induced by application of scleral vacuum. All figures are in millimeters of mercury. (From Gee, W., et al.: Arch. Surg. 115:183, 1980. Copyright 1975, 1978, 1980, American Medical Association.)

tially determined in animal and human experimental work by Gee[5-7] and was partially copied from Galin[4] (Fig. 12-1). Galin tonometrically determined the relation between intraocular pressure and vacuum applied to the eye cup in increments of 25 mm Hg. Gee performed multiple animal experiments in which simultaneous intraoperative direct stump pressure measurements were made with OPG recordings. The level of the eye cup vacuum at which a pulse wave was first detected was noted and related to the internal carotid artery back pressure with the common and external carotid arteries clamped.

Three independent researchers proved that the ophthalmic artery pressure, as measured with OPG, truly reflects the distal internal carotid artery pressure. Johnston[9] investigated artificial carotid stenosis in dogs and demonstrated a good correlation between OPG pressures and direct intraarterial pressures. Eikelboom[3] compared stump pressures measured in 13 carotid endarterectomies with simultaneously determined OPG pressures. The mean difference was only 4.6%. Finally, Ricotta[10] measured arterial pressure proximal and distal to a carotid stenosis in 49 patients who had a carotid

endarterectomy. He defined a drop of 5 mm Hg or more as hemodynamically significant. OPG pressures were accurate in 96% of the cases.

Ophthalmic artery pressure and carotid artery stenosis

OPG is based on pressure measurements and will detect only those obstructions that cause a reduction in arterial pressure. There is general agreement that pressure and flow are almost equally affected by a stenosis, but there is disagreement about the percentage of diameter reduction that results in a hemodynamically significant pressure reduction. Various definitions of diameter reduction between 50% and 75% have been used. In experimental situations there is a fixed percentage of stenosis that serves as a threshold between pressure-reducing lesions and non-pressure reducing-lesions. This is also valid when pressure gradients across a stenosis are measured intraoperatively. However, it is not valid when ophthalmic artery pressures are compared to stenoses on angiograms primarily because accurate classification of an angiogram is hard to obtain. Ophthalmic artery pressures measured with OPG might be a better standard for hemodynamic significance of a carotid stenosis than the angiographically determined percentage of stenosis. There is no fixed angiographic threshold, but there is a border zone in which a stenosis can be pressure reducing or not (Fig. 12-2). In our early experience with the OPG-300 this zone was between 60% and 70% of diameter reduction.

The length of a stenosis does not influence its hemodynamic significance. The effect of two separate stenoses in the same vessel is only determined by the most severe stenosis when there is no collateral bed between the two stenoses. It does not matter which stenosis is proximal and which is distal, although this may be important in the presence of combined carotid bifurcation and siphon disease. The branching of the ophthalmic artery generally takes place from the distal point of the siphon, so the OPG can be used to determine the hemodynamic significance of most siphon lesions. Siphon lesions distal to the branching of the ophthalmic artery may cause an increase in ophthalmic artery pressure, but these lesions are rarely encountered. Lesions of the ophthalmic artery itself, which will cause a reduction in ophthalmic artery pressure, are also rarely seen.

Central retinal artery occlusion will be associated with normal ophthalmic artery pressures when determined with the OPG, whereas the pressures measured with ophthalmodynamometry will be abnormal. A rare case of a reduced ophthalmic artery pressure has been described with a carotid-cavernous sinus fistula.[8] These fistulas are characterized by an increased ocular blood flow.

Similar to internal carotid stenosis, lesions in the common carotid and innominate arteries may cause a reduction in ophthalmic artery pressure, although these large vessels may have larger critical diameters. However, the hemodynamic significance of a carotid lesion does not depend only on the degree of stenosis, but it also depends on cardiac output, peripheral resistance, flow velocity, blood viscosity, and pulse rate.

Theoretically the intrinsic eye pressure might influence the ophthalmic artery pressure as measured with the OPG. We studied the OPG measurements of 88 patients in whom the intrinsic eye pressure was known, since tonometry had been performed by an ophthalmologist. We were able to prove that the absolute value of the intrinsic eye pressure does not influence the ophthalmic artery pressure. Even differences in intrinsic pressure between both eyes of up to 10 mm Hg did not cause unequal ophthal-

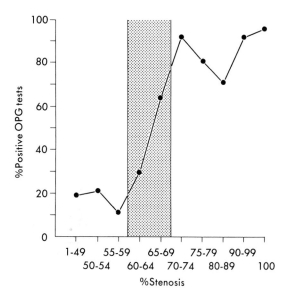

Fig. 12-2. Percentage of positive OPG tests for different degrees of carotid obstructions. Highest percentage of left and right carotid stenosis is taken.

Table 12-1. Right-left differences in intrinsic eye pressure and ophthalmic artery pressure (OAP) in patients without significant lesions on angiography[3]

1 − r intrinsic eye pressure difference	no. of patients	1 − r equal	OAPs unequal
1	3	2	1 (3 mm Hg)
2	3	2	1 (4 mm Hg)
3	6	4	2 (3 mm Hg)
4	4	4	—
10	1	1	—
TOTAL	17	13	4

mic artery pressures (Table 12-1). Another factor that might influence the ophthalmic artery pressure is the position of the body, but there are no data available on OPG performed in another position than supine. However, postural tests have been done with ophthalmodynamometry and may have some diagnostic value.[3]

A question often asked is whether the size of reduction in ophthalmic artery pressure has any value in predicting the severity of a pressure-reducing obstruction. The ability to differentiate between a severe stenosis or an occlusion is important. A group of 95 patients who had undergone angiography was selected. They had unequal left

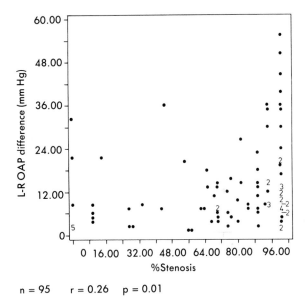

n = 95   r = 0.26   p = 0.01

Fig. 12-3. Correlation between difference in left and right ophthalmic artery pressures and severity of carotid stenosis.

location of the obstruction becomes more proximal. This is the main reason why occlusions of proximal branches of the aorta arch vessels are usually asymptomatic. Distal obstructions have fewer collateral pathways and tend to be more symptomatic. This is mainly determined by the patency of the circle of Willis, which is abnormal in about 50% of the cases. Anterior and posterior communicating arteries may be stringlike or even completely absent. Several autopsy studies have shown a higher incidence of cerebral softening in patients with an abnormal circle of Willis compared to those with a normal circle.

The adequacy of collateral circulation can be assessed using OPG with common carotid compression,[3,6] which provides a preoperative prediction of the internal carotid artery back pressure or stump pressure. This test may be useful in assessing the risk of a carotid stenosis when there is doubt about whether to operate, for example, in a patient with an asymptomatic stenosis and a prior myocardial infarction. In patients scheduled for carotid endarterectomy, OPG with carotid compression helps predict the necessity of a shunt. Whenever carotid ligation is considered, preoperative knowledge on the collateral potential is essential to determine the safety of the operation.

The residual ophthalmic artery pressure on the side of carotid compression is called the collateral ophthalmic artery pressure (COAP) and varies greatly among different patients. There may also be a considerable difference in the COAPs of both sides in an individual patient. Compression of the carotid bifurcation, if performed inappropriately over the bifurcation area, may stimulate the baroreceptors and may therefore decrease the systemic blood pressure. Our experience with 5000 patients showed no such effect when carotid compression was performed low in the neck. Simultaneous automatic brachial artery pressure monitoring taught us that the systemic blood pressure tends to be higher during compression than before. In 6.3% of the cases it was necessary to discontinue compression because of ischemic neurologic symptoms. Carotid occlusion should be avoided in these patients. If 60 mm Hg is taken as a threshold between good and poor collateral potential, half of the COAPs can be classified as poor and half as good.

Since the progression of carotid stenosis might coincide with an increase in COAP, whether a correlation existed between the COAP and the severity

and right pressures and did not have more than 50% stenosis on the side of the higher pressure, which excluded pressure-reducing lesions on that side. Fig. 12-3 shows the correlation between the pressure difference and the degree of carotid stenosis. Although a statistically significant correlation was found (r = 0.26), it is clear that the correlation in a given patient is very low, and that differentiation between stenosis and occlusion cannot be made.

Ophthalmic artery pressure and collateral circulation

The risk of cerebral damage from occlusion of the carotid artery is extremely variable and depends primarily on the availability of a collateral circulation. This does not only apply to the progression of a carotid stenosis into occlusion, but also to carotid ligation, which may be necessary in embolization from surgically inaccessible carotid lesions, distal cervical aneurysms, tumor surgery, or carotid trauma. Occlusion may cause no symptoms whatsoever or may result in transitory symptoms, frank stroke, or death. These differences in clinical outcome are caused by differences in the anatomy of the many potential collateral channels, including the circle of Willis. Collateral circulation can be established at several different levels of the extracranial and intracranial blood supply. The number of potential collateral pathways increases as the

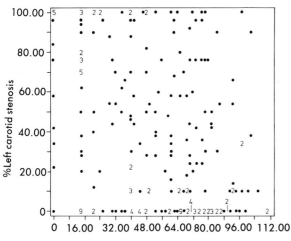

Fig. 12-4. Correlation between right COAP and left carotid obstruction.

n = 241   r = 0.30   p = <0.01

Table 12-2. COAP with various intracranial circulatory situations[3]

| | | COAP | | | |
| | | ≤60 mm Hg | | >60 mm Hg | |
Condition	Total no.	No.	%	No.	%
Anterior communicating artery present	153	73	48	80	52
Posterior communicating artery present	45	18	40	27	60
Embryonic circle of Willis	20	14	70	6	30
Absent first part of anterior cerebral artery	18	16	89	2	11

of carotid obstruction on the same side was investigated in 241 patients who underwent angiography. This was not the case (r = 0.03, p = .623). Since the collateral supply of a carotid territory comes mainly from the contralateral carotid artery, we also investigated whether a correlation existed between the COAP and the severity of contralateral carotid disease. Fig. 12-4 shows the results for the same 241 patients. A statistically significant negative correlation was found (r = −0.30, p = <.01), which implies that significant carotid disease diminishes the collateral circulation to the contralateral side. However, a statistically significant correlation does not imply that a prediction can be made in an individual patient, as is clearly shown by the scattergram. We also investigated whether some of the intracranial arterial distribution patterns as shown by selective carotid and semiselective vertebral injections correlated with differences in COAPs. Even if the anterior or posterior

communicating arteries are seen angiographically, there is no guarantee of a good collateral circulation as measured with OPG (Table 12-2).

An embryonic type of circle of Willis is accompanied by a poor collateral circulation in 70% of the cases. Absence of the first part of an anterior cerebral artery may be seen by filling the middle cerebral artery on that side only and two anterior cerebral arteries on the other side. The COAP on the side with the two anterior cerebral arteries (the dominant side) was poor in 16 of the 18 cases (89%).

We also investigated whether differences in COAPs existed for different groups of patients according to their symptoms. There were no differences between a control group of patients without bruits or symptoms and patients with asymptomatic bruits or nonhemispheric symptoms of transient ischemic attack (TIA). However, 84 stroke patients had statistically significant poorer COAPs than 134

TIA patients (t = 2.64, p < .05). This difference is especially striking, since the stroke group consisted of a selection of patients who survived the stroke and whose condition was good enough to undergo angiography. Therefore the stroke patients with the poorest COAPs may not be included in the study. This retrospective study supports the hypothesis that a poor COAP may be a risk factor for stroke and that OPG may noninvasively identify stroke-prone patients.

REFERENCES

1. Baillart, J.P.: La pression artérielle dans les branches de l'artère centrale de la rétine, nouvelle technique pour la déterminer, Ann. Ocul. 154:648, 1917.
2. Donders, F.C.: Ueber die sichtbaren Erscheinungen der Blutbewegung im Auge, Graefes Arch. Opht. 1:75, 1855.
3. Eikelboom, B.C.: Evaluation of carotid artery disease and potential collateral circulation by ocular pneumoplethysmography, thesis, Leiden, The Netherlands, 1981, University of Leiden.
4. Galin, M.A., et al.: Methods of suction ophthalmodynamometry, Ann. Ophthalmol. 1:439, 1970.
5. Gee W., et al.: Ocular pneumoplethysmography in carotid artery disease, Med. Instrum. 8:244, 1974.
6. Gee, W., Mehigan J.T., and Wylie E.J.: Measurement of collateral cerebral hemispheric blood pressure by ocular pneumoplethysmography, Am. J. Surg. 110:1516, 1975.
7. Gee, W., et al.: Simultaneous bilateral determination of the systolic pressure of the ophthalmic arteries by ocular pneumoplethysmography, Invest. Ophthalmol. Vis. Sci. 16:86, 1977.
8. Gee, W., et al.: Ocular pneumoplethysmography in carotid-cavernous sinus fistulas, J. Neurosurg. 59:40, 1983.
9. Johnston, C.G., and Bernstein, E.F.: Quantitation of internal carotid artery stenosis by ocular plethysmography, Surg. Forum 26:290, 1975.
10. Ricotta, J.J.: Definition of extracranial carotid disease: comparison of oculo pneumoplethysmography continuous wave Doppler angiography and measurement at operation, In Greenhalgh, R.M., and Clifford, R.F., editors: Progress in stroke research 2, London, 1983, Pitman Publishing, Ltd.

CHAPTER 13

Volume plethysmography in vascular disease: an overview

DAVID S. SUMNER

Although plethysmography was among the earliest methods devised for measuring blood flow in the extremities, it remains one of the most useful and most accurate. Much of our basic knowledge of vascular physiology and the pathophysiology of human arterial and venous disease has been derived from information obtained plethysmographically. More recently the technique has been applied to the diagnostic evaluation of peripheral vascular disease and now enjoys widespread use in many clinics throughout the world.

Plethysmography was first employed in 1622 by Glisson[22] and in 1737 by Swammerdam[61] to study contractions of isolated muscle, but it was not until the latter half of the nineteenth century that it was applied to blood flow measurements. The first recorded attempt to determine limb blood flow with venous occlusion techniques was by François-Franck in 1876.[21] However, credit for the basic concept is usually given to Brodie and Russell,[10] who studied renal blood flow by enclosing the kidney in a chamber and then recording the increase in volume produced by clamping the renal vein. Four years later Hewlett and van Zwaluwenburg[27] applied the same principle to the measurement of blood flow in human limbs, thus ushering in the era of venous occlusion plethysmography. Since that time methodology has improved, new instruments have been invented, and old instruments have been perfected.[35]

BASIC PRINCIPLES

The term *plethysmograph* is derived from the Greek word for increase, *plethysmos,* and the word to write, *graphein.* Thus the origin of the word encompasses the fundamental principle of the technique, which is simply the recording of changes in volume of portions of the body. Although these parts can be the entire body, the chest cavity, the heart, kidney, liver, or any other organ, in vascular physiology plethysmography is usually applied to the limbs or portions thereof. Since transient changes in the volume of most parts of the body (except the lungs) are related to their content of blood, plethysmography serves to measure changes in the volume of blood in the part being examined. At this point it must be emphasized that all varieties of plethysmographs do just this—measure changes in volume. Much confusion has arisen from the idea that some plethysmographs do more or less than others. The basic differences between instruments are in the method by which they record increases or decreases in volume, the ease with which they are used, and their stability and sensitivity.

Pulse plethysmography refers to the transient changes in volume related to the beat-by-beat activity of the left ventricle, the part expanding when arterial inflow exceeds venous outflow and contracting when the opposite occurs. More gradual changes in volume of the part are a result of dilation or contraction of the encompassed arteries and veins, as well as expansion of the interstitial fluid space. Pulsatile information is superimposed on these gradual and sometimes periodic fluctuations in volume.

Mean blood flow can be measured by recording the rate of increase in volume that occurs when the venous outflow to a part is suddenly, but temporarily, interrupted (venous occlusion plethysmography). It is only in this way that plethysmography can be used to determine blood flow. There is no way of deriving flow information from pulsatile waveforms, despite occasional claims to the contrary. The venous occlusion method has also been adapted to measure the rate of venous outflow under standardized conditions of elevated venous pressure. Here again the rate of blood flow under resting conditions is not measured, but relative venous resistance can be estimated.

INSTRUMENTATION

Although many instruments have been devised for recording plethysmographic information, they all fall into one of several distinct categories. Some measure volume change directly by fluid displacement (water-filled). Others depend on the compression of air in a closed system to produce comparable changes in pressure (air-filled), on changes in the circumference of the limb (strain gauge), or on changes in electrical resistance (impedance), or on the reflection of light from blood cells (photoelectric).

In the following discussion the basic principles of these methods will be described. Subsequent chapters will provide further details.

Water-filled plethysmographs

The earliest plethysmographs were water filled. In essence they consist of a water-filled watertight container in which the body part is immersed.[2,24,71] Any change in volume of the enclosed part will displace an equivalent quantity of water, and this displacement can be measured by a variety of means. Thus this technique provides the most direct measurement of volume change.

Although many types of instruments have been constructed, their basic idea is embodied in the diagrams in Figs. 13-1 and 13-2. The part to be studied is enclosed in a rigid container filled with water. Leakage is prevented by either sealing the part with cement to a rubber diaphragm at the point where it enters or leaves the container (Fig. 13-2) or by enclosing the part in a thin latex rubber sleeve or glove (Fig. 13-1). Because of hydrostatic pressure exerted by the surrounding fluid, the rubber sleeve or glove is kept in close contact with the skin. Bulging of the rubber diaphragm or sleeve at the entrance and exit points of the rigid container is avoided by means of a metal iris diaphragm.

When the enclosed part expands, water is displaced into a glass chimney where it compresses a column of air that activates a spirometer. This in turn writes a record on a kymograph. Various types of spirometers have been used, including the so-called Brodie bellows; but better results are obtained by miniature Krogh spirometers, which are counterbalanced to avoid the effect of gravity.[2] Because of the cushion of air within the bellows and chimney, the frequency response of this assembly is necessarily reduced. Optical methods for recording the fluid level in the chimney are quite accurate but have the disadvantages of requiring photosensitive paper and of not being available for immediate inspection.[38] Variations in the height of the fluid in the chimney may also be recorded by measuring the change in resistance between conductors that dip into the fluid.[13] Another method that can be used is to record changes in inductance of a coil, the core of which is floated on the fluid. Pressure changes in the enclosed air above the fluid-filled chimney may be used to activate a pressure transducer. The simplest method is to measure hydrostatic pressure changes in the fluid column by means of a sensitive pressure transducer.[36]

Calibration is achieved by adding or subtracting a known quantity of fluid to the container through a side-arm (Fig. 13-1 and 13-2). By measuring the amount of liquid required to fill the container and by knowing the volume of the container, the researcher can ascertain the volume of the enclosed part.

Because blood flow rates vary widely with variations in temperature, the fluid within the container must be maintained at a constant temperature. This can be accomplished with servocontrolled heating elements immersed in the fluid or by circulating warm air or water through a jacket surrounding the container. An electric stirrer (not shown in Fig. 13-1 and 13-2) is used to ensure a constant temperature throughout the container.

Potential disadvantages of the water-filled plethysmograph include the hydrostatic pressure of the fluid, which varies with the distance from the air-fluid interface in the chimney to the part immersed below. Ordinarily this pressure is but a few centimeters of water and, consequently, does not seem to affect the recordings appreciably.[2] The necessity for enclosing the part in a rubber sleeve or of immersing the part directly in water alters the ability to sweat and may affect circulatory physiology to some degree. Air bubbles in the system or bulging of the membranes at either end of the container will cushion transient volume changes, thereby lowering the frequency response of the system and decreasing the evident volume change. Moreover, water-filled instruments are somewhat cumber-

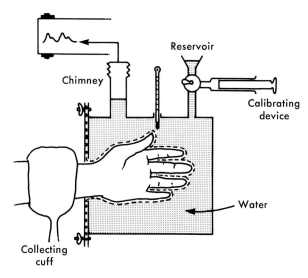

Fig. 13-1. Water-filled plethysmograph. Hand is enclosed in a loose-fitting surgical rubber glove (dashed line).

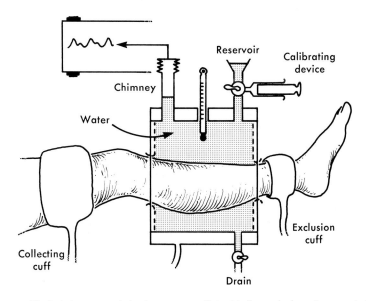

Fig. 13-2. Water-filled plethysmograph for forearm or calf. In this figure, leakage is prevented by sealing rubber diaphragms (dashed lines) to skin at entrance and exit. Rubber sleeve can be used also. Pneumatic exclusion cuff is used around ankle to prevent blood flow to foot from interfering with recordings. During flow measurement this cuff is inflated to supersystolic pressure.

some and cannot be used conveniently to measure flow rates after exercise.

In general, however, this method of plethysmography is quite accurate and has the advantage of being the most direct technique available for evaluating changes in limb volume.

Air-filled plethysmographs

Air-filled plethysmographs measure volume changes indirectly. One class of instruments closely resembles the water-filled devices in that the part being studied is enclosed in a rigid airtight container.[9] An increase or decrease in the volume of the part will produce a similar change in the pressure of the captive air, and this pressure change can be recorded with a suitable transducer. Unlike the water-filled instruments, those filled with air can be constructed of lighter-weight material (such as plastic) and do not require elaborate temperature-regulating features.

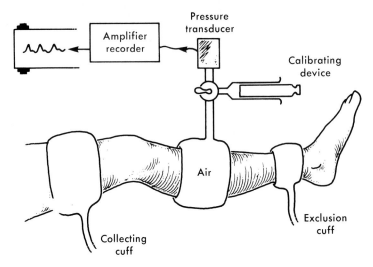

Fig. 13-3. Segmental air plethysmograph. Air-filled cuff is filled to predetermined pressure to maintain good contact with limb. Changes in limb volume produce corresponding changes in air pressure within cuff.

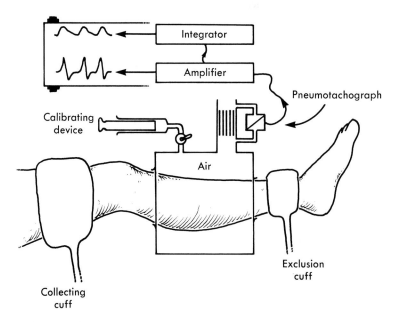

Fig. 13-4. Air-filled plethysmograph that uses pneumotachograph to measure rate of air flow produced by changing volume of enclosed segment. Since flow recording is obtained, it is necessary to integrate resulting curve to obtain volume recording.

An even more convenient adaptation of the air-filled plethysmograph employs a pneumatic cuff that encircles a segment of the part being examined (Fig. 13-3).[14,17,70] The cuff is kept in close approximation to the underlying skin by inflating it with air to some relatively low pressure (for example, 40 to 65 mm Hg). Consequently, volume changes in the enclosed limbs either increase or decrease the pressure of the air entrapped within the cuff. These pressure changes are easily converted to an analog recording by means of an attached pressure transducer. One can calibrate the system by injecting a known quantity of air into the cuff and noting the resulting increase in pressure. Because of the ease with which these devices can be used, they have gained widespread popularity in recent years, particularly for use in diagnostic laboratories. A more detailed description will be given in Chapters 17 and 18.

In general, the frequency response of air-filled plethysmographs is not high, approximately 8 Hz.[18] However, Raines[50] states that his pulse volume recorder functions to 20 Hz without loss of amplitude. Based on harmonic analysis of the frequencies in pulsatile blood flow, a frequency response of 6 to 8 harmonics, or 6 to 8 times the heart rate, should produce an adequate rendition of the pulse contour.[19] Therefore these instruments are capable of providing a satisfactory, if not perfect, tracing of the pulse contour.

When the venous occlusion technique is used with air-filled plethysmographs, errors in blood flow measurement occur because of the high coefficient of expansion of air with temperature changes.[40,65] Because there is little time for the escape of heat from the instrument, expansion of the enclosed part will raise the temperature of the entrapped air as it is compressed. This will produce an inordinately high pressure change for each volume change and yield flow recordings that are too high.

Instruments that allow a free flow of air into or out of the plethysmograph (measuring air flow rather than pressure change) may help to avoid some of these problems.[16] A pneumotachograph attached to the chimney is used to detect air flow. The resulting signal, which resembles an arterial flow pulse, must be integrated to provide a volume pulse recording (Fig. 13-4). According to the inventors, the system has a frequency response of 25 Hz and can record frequencies up to 35 Hz with less than a 20% loss.

Mercury strain gauge

Measurement of limb volume change by means of a mercury-filled rubber tube was first described by Whitney in 1953.[69] More recent models consist of a fine-bore silicone rubber tube completely filled with mercury or an indium-gallium alloy that makes contact with copper electrodes at either end. The tube is wrapped around the part being studied with just enough stretch to ensure good contact. As the part expands or contracts, the length of the gauge is changed by a corresponding amount. Since the resistance of the gauge varies with its length, variations in the voltage drop across the gauge will reflect changes in limb circumference (Fig. 13-5).

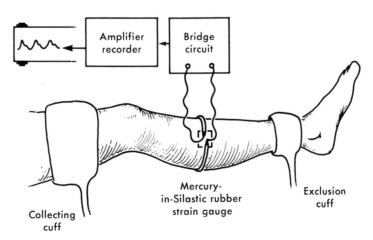

Fig. 13-5. Mercury-in-Silastic rubber strain gauge.

If one assumes that the part is a cylinder with a circular cross section and that the length of the subtended segment remains constant, volume changes bear the following relationship to changes in radius

$$V = \pi r^2 L \tag{1}$$

where V is volume, r is the radius of the segment, and L is its length.

Since L remains constant, equation 1 reduces to

$$V = \pi r^2 \tag{2}$$

With venous occlusion or with each pulse, the radius of the part increases by Δr, so that the new volume becomes

$$V + \Delta V = \pi (r + \Delta r)^2 = \pi (r^2 + 2r\Delta r + \Delta r^2) \tag{3}$$

The increase in volume of the part (ΔV) can be obtained by subtracting its original volume:

$$\Delta V = 2\pi r\Delta r + \pi \Delta r^2 \tag{4}$$

The ratio of the volume change (ΔV) to the original volume (V) is given by dividing equation 4 by equation 2:

$$\Delta V/V = 2\Delta r/r + \Delta r^2/r^2 \tag{5}$$

The circumference (C) of the part is equal to $2\pi r$; hence

$$r = C/2\pi \tag{6}$$

and

$$\Delta r = \Delta C/2\pi \tag{7}$$

If equations 6 and 7 are substituted in equation 5, the following relationship between relative volume change and relative circumference change is obtained:

$$\Delta V/V = 2\Delta C/C + \Delta C^2/C^2 \tag{8}$$

Since all volume changes that occur with pulsatile flow or in response to venous occlusion are minute in comparison with the original volume of the part, $\Delta C^2/C^2$ can usually be neglected. Therefore, for all practical purposes, the relative change in volume of the part is equivalent to twice the relative change in its circumference[69]:

$$\Delta V/V \approx 2\ \Delta C/C \tag{9}$$

Because of these relationships, the volume change of a limb can be calculated easily when the mercury-in-rubber gauge is used. Calibration is accomplished electrically or by stretching the gauge

a known amount. These methods will be discussed in more detail in Chapter 15.

Mercury-in-Silastic rubber gauges are very sensitive and have a high frequency response. The entire system (gauge, amplifier, and recorder) is capable of reproducing the magnitude of periodic stretch without loss up to 100 Hz.[48] The system is free of resonance effects up to 30 Hz, and no significant phase shift between gauge output and stretch is apparent. Thus this instrument is particularly well adapted for accurate rendition of pulsatile phenomena. However, its extreme sensitivity makes it a bit more difficult to use in clinical practice than the air-filled devices.

A potential drawback of the mercury strain gauge is its temperature sensitivity. A change in resistance of about 1% follows a temperature change of 10° C.[32,47] Obviously, this could introduce a measurement error if the gauge is calibrated at a temperature that differs from that existing when the recordings are made. Since correction factors are easily applied, errors related to temperature can be avoided when a high degree of precision is required.

Impedance plethysmographs

Impedance plethysmographs indirectly detect changes in the volume of blood within a limb segment by measuring variations in electric impedance. Impedance (Z) expresses the hindrance to the passage of alternating current (I) through a conductor under the influence of a potential difference (E):

$$Z = E/I \tag{10}$$

Impedance is a vector quantity with resistive, capacitive, and inductive elements. However, in plethysmography the major portion of the impedance is resistive.

In a biologic organism, electricity is transported by the movement of ions in intracellular and extracellular fluids. Since the concentration of ions in these fluids remains relatively constant, the resistive impedance of any segment of the body is inversely proportional to its total fluid content.

In any cylindric conductor, resistance (R) is inversely proportional to its cross-sectional area (πr^2) and directly proportional to its length (L):

$$R = \rho \frac{L}{\pi r^2} \tag{11}$$

In this equation, ρ is the specific resistance of the medium between the electrodes in ohm-cm.

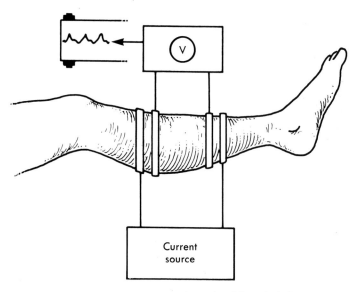

Fig. 13-6. Impedance plethysmograph. Outer two electrodes deliver high-frequency current to limb. Voltage drop across limb is measured between two inner electrodes.

Since volume (V) is the product of the cross-sectional area of the conductor and its length ($\pi r^2 L$), equation 11 becomes

$$V = \rho \frac{L^2}{R} \qquad (12)$$

When the volume changes from V_1 to V_2, equation 12 becomes

$$V_1 - V_2 = \rho L^2 (1/R_1 - 1/R_2) \qquad (13)$$

$$= \rho L^2 \left(\frac{R_2 - R_1}{R_1 R_2} \right)$$

For small changes in volume, the resistances, R_1 and R_2, are almost equal, permitting equation 13 to be simplified:

$$V_1 - V_2 \cong \rho \frac{L^2}{R} \left(\frac{R_2 - R_1}{R} \right) \qquad (14)$$

Equation 12 can be substituted for $\rho L^2/R$ in equation 14 to give

$$V_1 - V_2 \cong V \left(\frac{R_2 - R_1}{R} \right) \qquad (15)$$

$$\frac{\Delta V}{V} \cong -\frac{\Delta R}{R}$$

Thus by measuring changes in resistive impedance, periodic variations in blood volume within a segment can be calculated—at least theoretically.[6,45]

Modern impedance plethysmographs use a high-frequency oscillator (22 to 250 kHz) with low currents. Whereas lower frequencies result in problems of contact resistance and nonuniformity of current distribution, higher frequencies lead to subject-ground artifacts, difficulties in obtaining a high-isolation impedance, and radio-frequency interference.

Basically two forms of instruments have been devised: the two-electrode and the four-electrode types. Because of many problems with the two-electrode system, the four-electrode design is used in most modern instruments (Fig. 13-6).[72] The outer two electrodes send current through the part, and the inner two record the voltage drop.

Although the impedance plethysmograph has proved to be a valuable clinical instrument, there continues to be some controversy concerning what is actually measured. Researchers have gone so far as to suggest that the entire signal is related to electrode artifact rather than volume change.[28] Others discount this theory but acknowledge the complexity of the signal source.[5,39,67] Adding to the complexity is the fact that the electrical resistance of blood is affected by the orientation of red blood cells. Static blood with its random distribution of red cells has a higher resistance in the longitudinal direction than moving blood where the red cells are oriented in the direction of flow.[66] As a result, pulse recordings with the impedance device have a more rapid upslope and a slower downslope than those made with the mercury strain gauge.[5] Similarly the outflow curve in venous occlusion plethysmography tends to be slightly delayed.[4] These distortions are minor and do not adversely affect the clinical use of impedance plethysmography.

Since the specific resistance of blood (ρ_b) is about half that of the surrounding tissues (ρ_t), one might predict that the relative change in resistance as a result of the accumulation of blood during venous occlusion plethysmography would exceed the relative volume change[5,55,73]:

$$\frac{\Delta V}{V} \cong -\frac{\rho_b}{\rho_t}\frac{\Delta R}{R} \qquad (16)$$

$$= -K\frac{\Delta R}{R}$$

While some investigators have confirmed this relationship, reporting values for K ranging from 0.6 to 0.8,[3,73] others, paradoxically, have noted that the impedance method seriously underestimates flow during venous occlusion plethysmography, reporting K values of 1.6 to 3.1.* In most studies, however, simultaneous flows measured with the impedance and mechanical methods (water, air, strain gauge) have been significantly correlated (r = 0.70 to 0.93).[3,43,46,53] This suggests that an experimentally determined conversion factor (K) could be used to provide results that more nearly coincide with volume flow measurements obtained by other means. Although these disparities might prove troublesome to those trying to measure precise volume changes, they are not important when the impedance method is used to diagnose acute venous thrombosis, since this test plots venous outflow versus venous capacitance and cancels any errors resulting from a variable K.[34,68] Indeed, because of its simplicity and reliability, impedance plethysmography has become one of the most popular methods for diagnosing deep vein thrombosis. The theory of impedance plethysmography is more fully developed in Chapter 14.

Photoelectric plethysmographs

Strictly speaking, photoelectric plethysmographs are not true plethysmographs, since they do not measure volume change and are difficult to calibrate.[37] They consist of an infrared light–emitting diode and a photosensor. Blood, which is more opaque to red and near infrared light than the surrounding tissue, attenuates light in proportion to its content in the tissue. In one type of photoplethysmograph, the part being examined is sand-

wiched between the light source and the sensor. Since this variety of plethysmograph depends on transmitted light, its applicability is restricted to thin, relatively transparent organs, such as the earlobe. A more versatile type uses reflected light.[26,62] The light source and photosensor are mounted adjacent to one another on the same face of a small probe, which can be applied quite easily to virtually any area of the body by double-stick transparent tape (Fig. 13-7).

Pulse contours obtained when the output of the photoplethysmograph is amplified through an AC circuit are practically identical to those recorded by other methods. Thus these instruments provide a rapid, simple method for evaluating digital and supraorbital pulses.[8,42,59] DC coupling permits slower changes in the blood content of the skin to be followed. This method of coupling is useful for measuring blood pressure in the limbs, fingers, toes, and penis.[42,52,56] Because the blood content in the skin parallels that in the calf and is correlated with venous pressure, the DC-coupled photoplethysmograph has become a popular instrument for studying limbs with venous valvular incompetence.[1]

VENOUS OCCLUSION PLETHYSMOGRAPHY

Venous occlusion plethysmography can be used to measure the total blood flow to a terminal organ (for example, a hand, foot, finger, or toe) by means of a volume displacement apparatus as in Fig. 13-1. In this illustration the entire hand is enclosed in a watertight container so that any change in its volume can be recorded. A pneumatic cuff is applied to the arm just proximal to the container. When this cuff—often called the collecting cuff—is rapidly inflated well above venous pressure (usually 50 to 60 mm Hg), blood is temporarily trapped in the hand, causing its volume to rise. The initial rate at which the volume of the hand increases is proportional to the blood flow.

The pertinent events in this process are illustrated schematically in Fig. 13-8. In these diagrams the arterial inflow and the venous outflow channels are each represented by a single vessel around which is placed a collecting cuff. Blood pressures within the artery (100 mm Hg) and vein (5 mm Hg) are indicated by attached manometers. (These are added for illustrative purposes and are not necessary for measuring blood flow.) The capacitance vessels within the hand are represented by a bellows.

At rest, with the collecting cuff deflated, the

*References 41, 43, 45, 46, 53, 63.

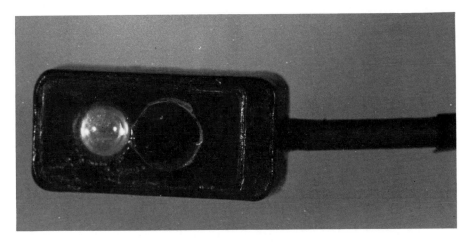

Fig. 13-7. Photoplethysmographic probe showing light-emitting diode and photoelectric sensor. (From Sumner, D.S.: Plethysmography in arterial and venous diagnosis. In Zwiebel, W.J., editor: Introduction to vascular ultrasonography, New York, 1982, Grune & Stratton, Inc.)

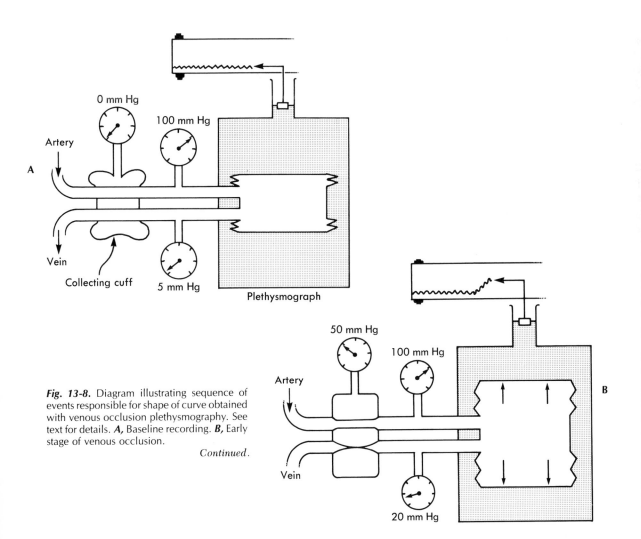

Fig. 13-8. Diagram illustrating sequence of events responsible for shape of curve obtained with venous occlusion plethysmography. See text for details. **A,** Baseline recording. **B,** Early stage of venous occlusion.

Continued.

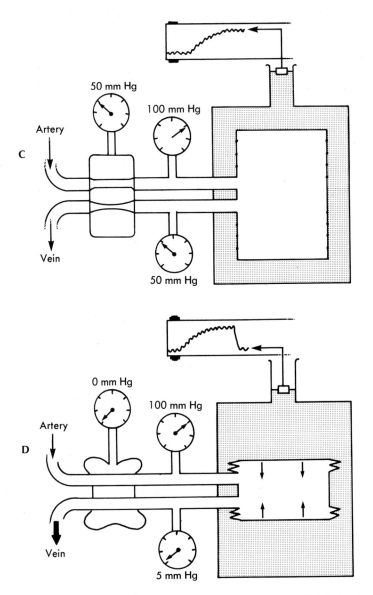

Fig. 13-8 cont'd. C, Late stage of venous occlusion. **D,** Cuff deflation.

baseline of the recording is relatively stable except for the periodic fluctuations caused by the arterial pulse (Fig. 13-8, *A*). When the collecting cuff is suddenly inflated to a level exceeding venous pressure (50 mm Hg), the underlying vein is completely collapsed, thereby preventing the escape of blood from the capacitance vessels (Fig. 13-8, *B*). Because of the shape of the arterial compliance curve, a reduction in transmural pressure (equal to the pressure inside the vessel minus that on the outside) across the artery from 100 to 50 mm Hg will cause relatively little narrowing of the arterial lumen. This small reduction in arterial diameter is far below the critical stenosis limit; consequently, there is little or no initial change in arterial inflow or in arterial pressure. As a result of the unimpeded arterial inflow and a totally blocked venous outflow, the bellows, representing the capacitance vessels, begins to expand. Most of the trapped blood accumulates in the venules and veins. Since the compliance of veins is great at low transmural pressures, a relatively great increase in venous volume is possible without much increase in venous pressure. Thus the initial slope of the line depicting the volume increase of the enclosed part is almost straight, reflecting fairly accurately the arterial inflow before venous occlusion. Later, as venous pressure begins to rise, the arteriovenous pressure gradient across the vascular bed will fall, and the arterial inflow will gradually decrease.

As the veins become more distended, a stiffer portion of the venous compliance curve is reached. Less expansion of the venous wall is possible without a great increase in transmural pressure. Consequently, venous pressure rises to equal (or slightly exceed) the pressures exerted by the collecting cuff. At this point blood again escapes from the veins, and a new equilibrium is attained, with arterial inflow and venous outflow again becoming identical (Fig. 13-8, *C*). Because of the reduction in the pressure gradient across the vascular bed (from 95 mm Hg before occlusion to 50 mm Hg at the new equilibrium point), the total flow rate is reduced. The volume of the part, as depicted by the recording, becomes relatively stable at a new but higher level than that existing before venous occlusion (Fig. 13-8, *C*).

Actually, the volume tracing will continue to rise at a very slow rate as a result of the escape of fluid through the capillary wall into the interstitial space. This is a manifestation of the elevated pressure within the capillaries, which must exceed 50 mm Hg in the present example. The elevated capillary blood pressure upsets the Starling equilibrium; thus fluid will continue to flow into the interstitial space until a new equilibrium is established. Because of the great compliance of the interstitial space, this ordinarily requires a period of many hours.

When the collecting cuff is suddenly deflated, there is a sudden surge of blood out through the veins (Fig. 13-8, *D*). The volume tracing falls rapidly, reaching baseline or near baseline levels.

Fig. 13-9 depicts the events of venous occlusion plethysmography in graphic form.[23] During phase 1 the tracing shows a straight-line rise, indicating a constant inflow of blood into the extremity. As the venous pressure rises in phase 2, the rate of volume increase declines, indicating a decreasing arterial inflow. In phase 3 the curve levels off as the venous pressure rises to exceed the pressure in the collecting cuff. Blood flow through the extremity is reduced as a result of the lowered arteriovenous pressure difference.

Segmental plethysmography

When the entire organ cannot be placed in the plethysmograph or when one wishes to record blood flow to only a segment of a limb, it is necessary to apply a second cuff distal to the plethysmograph (Figs. 13-2 and 13-4). This cuff is inflated to a pressure well in excess of the arterial pressure to exclude flow from those parts of the extremity that are not enclosed in the plethysmograph.

For example, if blood flow to the forearm is being measured and no exclusion cuff has been applied to the wrist, the total arterial inflow destined for both the hand and forearm will be distributed to all the veins distal to the occlusion cuff. Since the rate of blood flow to the hand ordinarily exceeds that to the forearm, failure to apply the distal exclusion cuff will result in a distortedly high recording of forearm blood flow. The same holds true for the lower extremity: an ankle cuff must be applied when calf blood flow is being measured.

When segmental air plethysmographs (Fig. 13-3) or mercury-in-Silastic strain gauges (Fig. 13-5) are used on the forearm or calf, it is also important to apply an exclusion cuff to the wrist or ankle. Although these devices sense flow in only that segment of the limb with which they are in direct contact, it is assumed that flow through the

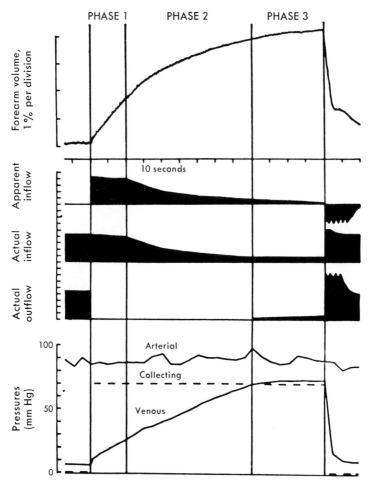

Fig. 13-9. Graph illustrating effect of venous occlusion on forearm volume, arterial inflow, and venous outflow. Simultaneous changes in arterial and venous pressure are also shown. Actual inflow is equivalent to actual outflow plus apparent inflow. Duration of occlusion was 130 seconds. (From Greenfield, A. D. M., and Patterson, G.C.: J. Physiol. [Lond.] 125:525, 1954.)

entire part is fairly uniform. For this reason, it is necessary only to exclude the hand or foot, which have higher flows than the forearm or calf.

Occlusion cuffs, exclusion cuffs, and inflators

The collecting cuff must be inflated rapidly to a preset pressure. This may be accomplished by connecting the cuff to an air reservoir with a wide-bore tube. The capacity of the reservoir must be large in relation to that of the cuff so that sudden inflation of the cuff will not lower the pressure in the system appreciably. Simple inexpensive arrangements that work quite well are easily constructed from odds and ends.

I use a cuff inflator,* which contains a pressure

regulator and two electrically operated solenoid valves. It is connected to an external air pressure source capable of delivering 20 to 100 psi. By means of this instrument, even large cuffs are accurately inflated or deflated to the desired pressure in about a second.

For venous occlusion and arterial flow exclusion, any of a variety of commercially available cuffs are suitable. I prefer to use cuffs with a long bladder (40.5 cm)* so that the entire circumference of the limb will be directly subjected to the air pressure. The width of the cuff can be 10 or 12.7 cm, depending on the diameter of the limb. A large contoured cuff (22 × 71 cm)* shaped to conform to the taper of the thigh is particularly useful for ve-

*Manufactured by Hokanson, Inc., Issaquah. Wash.

*Manufactured by Hokanson, Inc., Issaquah. Wash.

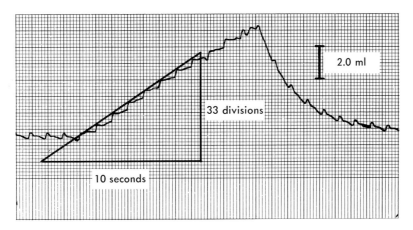

Fig. 13-10. Venous occlusion plethysmographic tracing from human calf at room temperature. Volume for calf enclosed in plethysmograph was 1,200 ml. Calibration signal was 10 divisions for 2.0 ml volume increment. Blood flow is calculated as follows (equations 17 to 19):

$$\frac{33 \text{ div}}{10 \text{ sec}} \times 60 \text{ sec/min} = 198 \text{ div/min}$$

$$\frac{2.0 \text{ ml}}{10 \text{ div}} \times 198 \text{ div/min} = 39.6 \text{ ml/min}$$

$$\frac{39.6 \text{ ml/min}}{1200 \text{ ml}} \times 100 = 3.3 \text{ ml/100 ml/min}$$

nous occlusion during studies of calf blood flow. Digit cuffs of varying lengths constructed of Penrose drains backed with Velcro pile are used for venous occlusion when finger blood flow is being measured.

Venous occlusion pressures should ordinarily be about 50 to 60 mm Hg. The diastolic blood pressure in the arteries underlying the cuff should never be exceeded. When flow studies are conducted on a limb with obstructive arterial disease, it may be necessary to use a lower pressure. Ideally one should experiment with several occlusion pressures to see which gives the steepest slope. In practical terms a wide range of pressures will usually yield identical slopes.

The pressure in the exclusion cuff should always be well above the systolic pressure at the site to which the cuff is applied. Usually a pressure of 200 mm Hg will suffice. The exclusion cuff should be inflated about 30 seconds before any recordings are made.

Calculation of blood flow

Although absolute blood flow in terms of volume of blood per unit time can be measured with water-filled or air-filled plethysmographs, it is the usual practice to express blood flow in terms of volume of flow per unit volume of tissue enclosed in the

plethysmograph per unit time. Depending on the method employed, flow may be expressed as cc/100 cc/min, ml/100 ml/min, or percent volume change per minute. At times one sees flow reported in ml/ml/min, ml/5 ml/min, or ml/L/min. Obviously, if the total volume of the enclosed part is known, any of the latter measurements can be converted into milliliters per minute.

Basically the same methods are used to calculate blood flow whether the entire part or only a portion of it is enclosed in the plethysmograph. To determine the initial rate of filling of the part after the occlusion cuff is inflated, a line is drawn on the recording paper connecting the initial systolic peaks or diastolic valleys (Fig. 13-10). The slope of this line in terms of the arbitrary divisions (div) with which the paper is ruled is determined by measuring the number of divisions the line rises in 1 minute. Usually it is more convenient to measure the rise over a few seconds (t), divide by the number of seconds, and multiply by 60:

$$\text{Div/min} = \frac{\text{Div rise in t sec}}{\text{t sec}} \times 60 \text{ sec/min} \quad \textbf{(17)}$$

Next one uses the calibration signal to convert the arbitrary divisions with which the slope is measured into volume flow per minute. This is done by dividing the calibration volume by the number of corresponding divisions and then multiplying by the division rise per minute from equation 17:

$$\frac{\text{Calibration vol}}{\text{Calibration div}} \times \frac{\text{Div}}{\text{Minutes}} = \text{Vol flow/min} \quad (18)$$

The flow rate per 100 ml of enclosed part can be calculated by dividing the volume flow per minute by the volume of the enclosed part in milliliters and then multiplying by 100:

$$\frac{\text{Vol flow/min}}{\text{Vol of part}} \times 100 = \text{Vol flow/100 ml/min} \quad (19)$$

The volume of the enclosed part can be measured directly by water displacement or it· can be esti-

mated from its dimensions. Calculation of blood flow with the mercury-in-Silastic strain gauge will be discussed in Chapter 15.

Distortion of the tracing

Ideally the initial slope of the plethysmographic tracing following venous occlusion should describe a straight line intersecting the baseline at a definite, sharp angle (Fig. 13-11, *A*). Unfortunately, several artifacts that are commonly seen may prove perplexing.[24] Chief among these is the so-called cuff artifact, which is usually manifested by a sharp upward jump in the tracing preceding the initial slope (Fig. 13-11, *B*). This is usually caused by

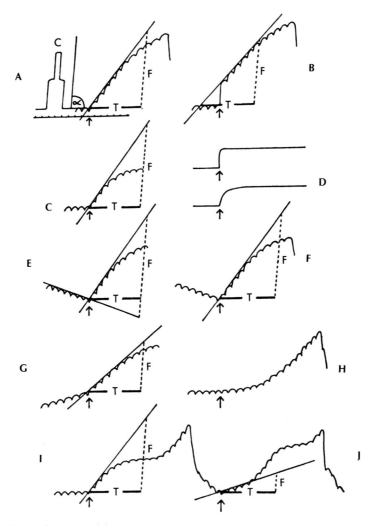

Fig. 13-11. Various distortions of plethysmographic pulse tracing. Arrow indicates point at which occlusion cuff was inflated. *F*, Volume of inflow; *T*, time over which it was measured; baseline, time-trace in seconds; *C*, calibration in two steps of 5 or 10 ml each; α, angle between traverse of recording point and baseline. See text for further explanation. (From Greenfield, A. D. M., Whitney, R.J., and Mowbray, J.F.: Br. Med. Bull. 19:101, 1963.)

the displacement of tissue into the plethysmograph by the inflation of the cuff. If the jump is quite abrupt so that the artifact can be clearly discriminated (Fig. 13-11, *D*, top line), the slope can be constructed in the usual fashion between the initial systolic peaks or diastolic valleys, ignoring the initial jump. If, however, the jump is gradual, it will be difficult to tell artifact from limb swelling (Fig. 13-11, *D*, bottom line). In these cases it is best to discard the tracing and readjust the cuff and strain gauge. To determine the shape of the cuff artifact, a pressure cuff placed proximal to the venous occlusion cuff can be inflated to supersystolic pressure, following which the venous occlusion cuff is inflated. In the absence of arterial inflow, the only change in the level of the tracing will be caused by the cuff artifact (Fig. 13-11, *D*). Sometimes a negative cuff artifact is generated. This may be related to movement of the limb out of the plethysmograph. In these cases there is usually no problem in deciding where to draw the initial slope.

When the rate of arterial inflow is very high or when the venous capacity is limited, there may be no steady upward rise; rather, the pulses describe a curve with a continuously decreasing slope (Fig. 13-11, *C*). Sometimes flow is so great that the part fills within one or two beats. Such curves are rather frequently obtained in digital plethysmography. Since it may not be possible to draw an accurate tangent, flow measurements cannot be made with confidence.

Sometimes the baseline tracing rises or falls between collections. At times this may be caused by a leak in the plethysmograph or movement of the strain gauge (Fig. 13-11, *E*). An alternating baseline may be a result of fluctuation in relative arterial inflow and venous outflow. Such fluctuations can be ignored and the curve constructed as if the baseline were level (Fig. 13-11, *F* and *G*).

When, after venous occlusion, the tracing arises with an ever-increasing slope, the curve is uninterpretable and must be discarded (Fig. 13-11, *H*). Sometimes this artifact can be avoided by decreasing the gap between the plethysmograph and the occlusion cuff.

At times the curve will show differing slopes over the filling period, at first rising rapidly, then more slowly, and finally rapidly again. If this curve is duplicated simultaneously in the opposite limb, it is probably related to periodic fluctuations in blood flow. In such cases the initial slope is still

valid for the flow at the instant of venous occlusion (Fig. 13-11, *I* and *J*).

Accuracy

Venous occlusion plethysmography is perhaps the most accurate noninvasive method for measuring blood flow to the limbs. Several researchers[12,20] have observed little difference between flows measured plethysmographically and those measured directly. In a series of experiments on primate limbs, Raman et al.[51] found plethysmographically measured flow to be about 92% of the undisturbed flow measured electromagnetically.

Applications

Venous occlusion plethysmography finds its major application in physiologic studies of normal and diseased circulation. Although it is used in some clinical laboratories as a diagnostic tool, there are far simpler techniques that will yield equally valuable information. The validity, however, of some of these simpler techniques had to be substantiated by comparison with venous occlusion plethysmography.[60]

Occlusive arterial disease. Resting blood flow measurements are of no value in distinguishing between normal limbs and those with occlusion of major inflow arteries. Because of the capacity of the peripheral vascular bed to dilate as compensation for the increased resistance imposed by the inflow arteries, resting blood flow usually remains within normal limits (Table 13-1).[29,54,57,60] Flow begins to decrease only when there are multiple levels of obstruction and/or involvement of collateral arteries. Thus a decreased flow at normal temperatures would be found in ischemic, pregangrenous extremities. Since blood flow to the tissues (skin in particular) is quite variable, responding to changes in temperature and sympathetic tone, one has to rule out peripheral vasoconstriction in all

Table 13-1. Resting calf blood flow (ml/100 ml/min)*

Normal	3.6 ± 1.3
Iliac occlusion	3.7 ± 2.0
Superficial femoral occlusion	3.9 ± 3.1
Combined iliac and superficial femoral occlusion	4.0 ± 1.9

*Data from Hillestad[29] and Sumner and Stradness.[60]

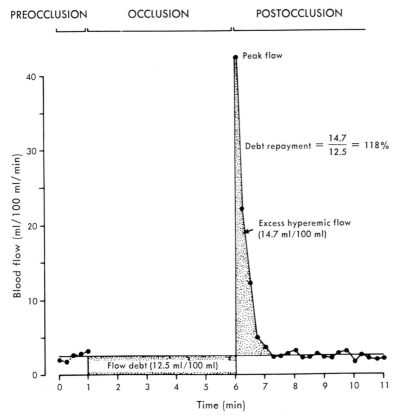

PREOCCLUSION   OCCLUSION   POSTOCCLUSION

Fig. 13-12. Reactive hyperemia response in normal human forearm after 5 minutes of ischemia. (From Strandness, D.E., Jr., and Sumner, D.S.: Hemodynamics for surgeons, New York, 1975, Grune & Stratton, Inc.)

these cases. However, when the circulation is stressed by any mechanism that produces peripheral vasodilatation, the plethysmographic flow pattern in patients with occlusive arterial disease is quite different from that in normal individuals.

Reactive hyperemia and exercise are the two methods most commonly used to achieve maximal or near maximal peripheral vasodilation. Reactive hyperemia is produced by arresting the circulation for 3 to 5 minutes with a pneumatic cuff inflated well above systolic pressure. This cuff is placed on the limb proximal to the venous occlusion cuff and the plethysmograph. Fig. 13-12 shows a typical response in a normal limb. The response in an abnormal limb is obviously quite different in a number of ways (Fig. 13-13). First, the peak hyperemic flow is reduced in the limb with occlusive arterial disease. Also, the time required to reach peak flow is delayed (Table 13-2). Second, the hyperemic response is prolonged. Ordinarily more than three fourths of the excess hyperemia flow is

Table 13-2. Peak reactive hyperemia flow*

	Average flow (ml/100 ml/min)	Time to peak (sec)
Normal	20 to 40	5
Arterial occlusion	3 to 22	10 to 100

*Data from Strandness and Sumner.[58]

confined to the first minute after release of the tourniquet, but in limbs with occlusive disease less than half occurs within the first minute.[29] In spite of the prolonged hyperemic flow, the flow debt is underpaid in abnormal limbs. (Flow debt is the product of the resting blood flow and the period of ischemia.)

The normal flow response to exercise is illustrated in Fig. 13-14. Immediately following exercise, peak flows are attained that are often in excess of 20 to 40 ml/100 ml/min. These flows rapidly decline, usually approaching preexercise values in

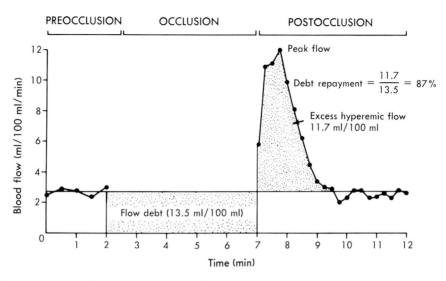

PREOCCLUSION   OCCLUSION   POSTOCCLUSION

Fig. 13-13. Reactive hyperemia response in calf of limb with superficial femoral artery occlusion. Note low peak flow, delay of peak flow, prolonged hyperemic response, and underpayment of flow debt. (From Strandness, D.E., Jr., and Sumner, D.S.: Hemodynamics for surgeons, New York, 1975, Grune & Stratton, Inc.)

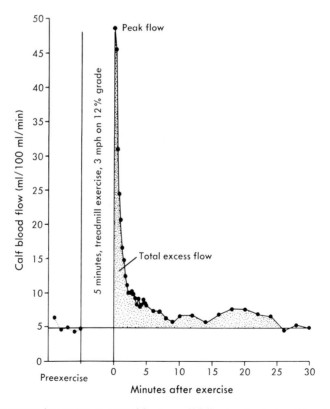

Fig. 13-14. Postexercise hyperemia in normal human calf following 5 minutes of treadmill exercise (3 mph, 12% grade). (From Strandness, D.E., Jr., and Sumner, D.S.: Hemodynamics for surgeons, New York, 1975, Grune & Stratton, Inc.)

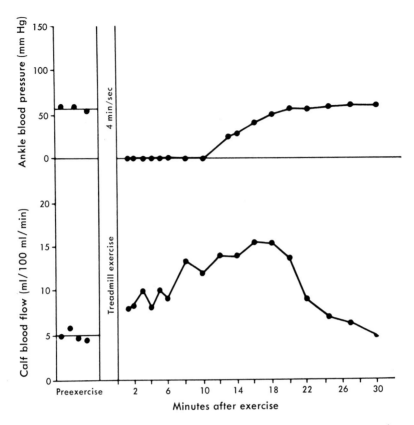

Fig. 13-15. Preexercise and postexercise calf blood flow and ankle pressure in patient with stenosis of iliac artery and occlusion of superficial femoral artery. (From Sumner, D.S., and Strandness, D.E., Jr.: Surgery 65:763, 1969.)

a few minutes. Fig. 13-15 shows the postexercise flow response in a limb with occlusive arterial disease. In these limbs the peak flow is reduced (average: 9 to 20 ml/100 ml/min), the time required to attain peak flow is delayed (average: 3 to 7 minutes), and the hyperemic response may be prolonged well beyond 20 minutes.[30,58,60]

Clearly, these plethysmographic measurements can be used effectively to evaluate the circulation in patients with occlusive arterial disease. However, it is much easier to measure pressures, which vary in much the same way.[60] Accordingly, in my opinion venous occlusion plethysmography has little place in the diagnosis of occlusive arterial disease, although it is of great value to the clinical physiologist.[58] Venous occlusion plethysmography is helpful in evaluating the effects of vasodilators, sympathectomy, or operative procedures on calf, forearm, or finger blood flow.[42]

Vasospastic disease. Hillestad[31] and others[58] have used venous occlusion plethysmography to distinguish between normal, vasospastic, and obliterative arterial disease of the hands and fingers. Whereas at normal local temperatures (32° C) hand blood flow is reduced in patients with peripheral vasospasm, it is normal in patients with other problems that might be confused with this diagnosis. However, when the local temperature is increased to 40° C, there is a great increase in flow in the vasospastic hand, equaling the flow in the normal hand under the same conditions. In obliterative arterial disease flow may remain stable or even drop if there is impending gangrene. A severe drop in flow may occur in the presence of arteritis. Similar studies may also be carried out on the fingers in such patients. Here again, pressure measurements are often easier to perform and may yield equally valuable information.[58]

PLETHYSMOGRAPHY IN VENOUS DISEASE

Plethysmographic techniques have been applied successfully to the diagnosis of acute deep vein

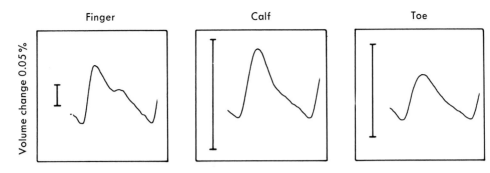

Fig. 13-16. Plethysmographic pulse tracings obtained from normal finger, calf, and toe. Vertical bars indicate 0.05% volume change. (From Strandness, D.E., Jr., and Sumner, D.S.: Hemodynamics for surgeons, New York, 1975, Grune & Stratton, Inc.)

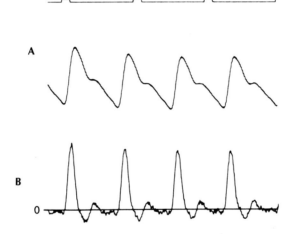

Fig. 13-17. Simultaneous recording of digit volume pulse *(A)* and its electrical differential *(B)*. Note strong resemblance of differentiated pulse to arterial flow pulse. (From Strandness, D.E., Jr., and Sumner, D.S.: Hemodynamics for surgeons, New York, 1975, Grune & Stratton, Inc.)

thrombosis. Systems especially designed for this purpose are commercially available and are in widespread use. Although most employ either impedance measuring devices[34,68] or air-filled cuffs,[11] much of the earlier research was done with water-filled plethysmographs or mercury strain gauges—methods that continue to be used.[7,15,25] The mercury strain gauge and the photoplethysmograph are now frequently used to confirm the presence of chronic venous insufficiency and to evaluate its severity.[1] These methods will be discussed in detail in subsequent chapters.

PULSE PLETHYSMOGRAPHY

Sensitive plethysmographs can be used to record the periodic expansion of an organ, limb, or digit that occurs in response to the arrival of the arterial pulse wave. Because the contour and volume of these pulses have diagnostic significance, particularly in the eye and in limbs with obstructive arterial or vasospastic disease, a number of instruments capable of accurately recording the volume pulse are available commercially. Most popular are the air-cuff and mercury strain-gauge plethysmographs and the photoplethysmograph. Since the application of these instruments to specific disease entities will be dealt with in subsequent chapters, the following discussion of their physiologic implications is brief.

The moment-to-moment magnitude of volume expansion is determined by the rate at which blood flows into the part and the rate at which it simultaneously flows out. During the first part of the cycle, blood enters the part by way of the arteries more rapidly than it leaves by the veins; consequently, there is a rapid swelling of the part pro-

ducing the steep ascending limb of the pulse tracing. After peak volume is reached, blood flows out
of the part more rapidly than it enters, allowing it
to return to its diastolic diameter. Characteristically, the resulting descending limb of the tracing is
much more prolonged than the ascending limb.
Although most of the outflow occurs through venous channels, there is often some retrograde flow
in the arteries early in diastole as a result of the
arrival of a reflected wave from the periphery.

Although it is recognized that these periodic volume fluctuations are largely a result of passive dilation or contraction of the vascular channels, it is
not completely clear which vessels are involved.
Because of the great compliance and large volume
of the veins, much of the volume change may take
place in these vessels.[49] This is especially true in
vasodilated states. When, however, the part is vasoconstricted, most of the volume expansion may
be because of changes in arterial diameter.[33,44]
Also, there is evidence that volume pulsations in
the forearm and calf are largely the result of arterial
expansion.[16,44]

Illustrated in Fig. 13-16 are normal volume
pulses obtained from a finger, calf, and toe. Following a steep systolic upstroke there is a slower
downstroke that is curved toward the baseline. Often there is a prominent dicrotic wave on the downslope. A strong resemblance to the arterial pressure
pulse is evident. In limbs with proximal arterial
obstruction, the volume of the pulse may be reduced, the systolic upslope is less rapid, the peak
may be rounded, and the downslope is bowed away
from the baseline.[58,59]

In any given individual, when measurements are
made serially, the volume of the plethysmographic
pulse correlates well with blood flow.[74] On the
other hand, the relative rate of blood flow from
one individual to the next (or even from the same
individual, when measurements are not continuous), cannot be determined by comparing the volume of the plethysmographic pulse. Too many factors are involved. Disparities in pulse volume are
more likely to be a result of proximal obstruction
changing the shape of the wave rather than major
differences in blood flow. Nevertheless, this does
not obviate the value of measuring the height of
the pulse excursion as a diagnostic tool.[17]

When the volume pulse is electrically or mathematically differentiated, a tracing resembling an
arterial flow pulse is obtained (Fig. 13-17). Theoretically, if venous outflow remained constant and

if a zero flow level could be established, differential
tracings could be used to calculate arterial flow.[64]
Because the shape and magnitude of the differential
tracing may show little change even though the
mean flow varies from almost zero to hyperemic
levels, it is impossible to use the differential tracing
to measure blood flow unless a mean flow level
can be established with venous occlusion plethysmography.[16] Making the assumption—as some
have done—that the flat portion of the diastolic
curve or, alternatively, that the lowest point of the
curve represents zero flow is likely to lead to serious errors.

REFERENCES

1. Abramowitz, H.B., et al.: The use of photoplethysmography in the assessment of venous insufficiency: a comparison to venous pressure measurements, Surgery 86:434,
1979.
2. Abramson, D.I.: Circulation in the extremities, New York,
1967, Academic Press, Inc.
3. Anderson, F.A., Jr., et al.: Evaluation of electrical impedance plethysmography for venous volume measurements,
Proceedings of the twenty-ninth annual conference on engineering in medicine and biology, vol. 18, Chevy Chase,
Md., 1976, The Alliance for Engineering in Medicine and
Biology.
4. Anderson, F.A., Jr., et al.: Comparison of electrical impedance and mechanical plethysmographic techniques in the
human calf, Proceedings of the twelfth annual meeting of
the Association for the Advancement of Medical Instrumentation, Arlington, Va., 1977.
5. Anderson, F.A., Jr., et al.: Impedance plethysmography:
the origin of electrical impedance changes measured in the
human calf, Med. Biol. Eng. Comput. 18:234, 1980.
6. Barendsen, G.J.: Plethysmography. In Verstraete, M., editor: Methods in angiology, The Hague, 1980, Martinus
Nijhoff.
7. Barnes, R.W., et al.: Noninvasive quantitation of maximum venous outflow in acute thrombophlebitis, Surgery
72:971, 1972.
8. Barnes, R.W., et al.: Supraorbital photoplethysmography,
simple accurate screening for carotid occlusive disease, J.
Surg. Res. 22:319, 1977.
9. Black, J.E.: Blood flow requirements of the human calf
after walking and running, Clin. Sci. 18:89, 1959.
10. Brodie, T.G., and Russell, A.E.: On the determination of
the rate of blood flow through an organ, J. Physiol. (Lond.)
32:47P, 1905.
11. Comerota, A.J., et al.: Phleborheography: results of a ten-
year experience, Surgery 91:573, 1982.
12. Conrad, M.C., and Green, H.D.: Evaluation of venous
occlusion plethysmography, J. Appl. Physiol. 16:289,
1961.
13. Cooper, K.E., and Kerslake, D.M.: An electrical recorder
for use with plethysmography, J. Physiol. (Lond.) 114:11,
1951.
14. Dahn, I.: On the calibration and accuracy of segmental calf
plethysmography with a description of a new expansion
chamber and a new sleeve, Scand. J. Clin. Lab. Invest.
16:347, 1964.
15. Dahn, I., and Eiriksson, E.: Plethysmographic diagnosis
of deep venous thrombosis of the leg, Acta Chir. Scand.
(suppl. 398):33, 1968.

16. Dahn, I., Jonson, B., and Nilsén, R.: A plethysmographic method for determination of flow and volume pulsations in a limb, J. Appl. Physiol. 28:333, 1970.

17. Darling, R.C., et al.: Quantitative segmental pulse volume recorder: a clinical tool, Surgery 72:873, 1973.

18. Dohn, K.: Three plethysmographs usable during functional states recording volume changes in ml per 100 ml of extremity, Rep. Steno. Mem. Hosp. 6:147, 1956.

19. Ferguson, D.J., and Wells, H.S.: Harmonic analysis of frequencies in pulsatile blood flow, IRE Trans. Med. Electronics 6:291, 1959.

20. Formel, P.F., and Doyle, J.T.: Rationale of venous occlusion plethysmography, Circ. Res. 5:354, 1957.

21. François-Franck, C.E.: Du volume des organes dans ses rapports avec la circulation du sang, Physiol. Exp. (Paris) 2:1, 1876.

22. Glisson, F.: Tractatus de ventriculo intestinis (1622). In Hyman, C., and Winsor, T.: History of plethysmography, J. Cardiovasc. Surg. 2:506, 1961.

23. Greenfield, A.D.M., and Patterson, G.C.: The effect of small degrees of venous distension on the apparent rate of blood inflow to the forearm, J. Physiol. (Lond.) 125:525, 1954.

24. Greenfield, A.D.M., Whitney, R.J., and Mowbray, J.F.: Methods for the investigation of peripheral blood flow, Br. Med. Bull. 19:101, 1963.

25. Hallböök, T., and Göthlin, J.: Strain-gauge plethysmography and phlebography in diagnosis of deep venous thrombosis, Acta Chir. Scand. 137:37, 1971.

26. Hertzman, A.B.: The blood supply of various skin areas as estimated by photoelectric plethysmography, Am. J. Physiol. 124:328, 1938.

27. Hewlett, A.W., and van Zwaluwenburg, J.G.: The rate of blood flow in the arm, Heart 1:87, 1909.

28. Hill, R.V., Jansen, J.C., and Fling, J.L.: Electrical impedance plethysmography: a critical analysis, J. Appl. Physiol. 22:161, 1967.

29. Hillestad, L.K.: The peripheral blood flow in intermittent claudication. V. Plethysmographic studies. The significance of the calf blood flow at rest and in response to timed arrest on the circulation, Acta Med. Scand. 174:23, 1963.

30. Hillestad, L.K.: The peripheral blood flow in intermittent claudication. VI. Plethysmographic studies. The blood flow response to exercise with arrested and free circulation, Acta Med. Scand. 174:671, 1963.

31. Hillestad, L.K.: Research on peripheral hemodynamics in various disease states, Acta Med. Scand. 188:191, 1970.

32. Honda, N.: Temperature compensation for mercury strain-gauge used in plethysmography, J. Appl. Physiol. 17:572, 1962.

33. Horeman, H.W., and Noordergraaf, A.: Numerical evaluation of volume pulsation in man. III. Application to the finger plethysmogram, Phys. Med. Biol. 3:345, 1959.

34. Hull, R., et al.: Impedance plethysmography: the relationship between venous filling and sensitivity and specificity for proximal vein thrombosis, Circulation 58:898, 1978.

35. Hyman, C., and Winsor, T.: History of plethysmography, J. Cardiovasc. Surg. 2:506, 1961.

36. Hyman, C., and Winsor, T.: An electric volume transducer for plethysmographic recording, J. Appl. Physiol. 21:1403, 1966.

37. Ingle, F.W.: Calibration of the photoplethysmograph (PPG), Proceedings of the thirty-fourth annual conference on engineering in medicine and biology, 1981.

38. Kerslake, D.M.: The effect of the application of an arterial occlusion cuff to the wrist on the blood flow in the human forearm, J. Physiol. (Lond.) 108:451, 1949.

39. Kinnen, E., Hill, R.V., and Jansen, J.C.: A defense of electrical impedance plethysmography, Med. Res. Engl. 8:6, 1969.

40. Landowne, M., and Katz, L.N.: A critique of the plethysmographic method of measuring blood flow in the extremities of man, Am. Heart J. 23:644, 1942.

41. Liebman, F.M.: Electrical impedance pulse tracings from pulsatile blood flow in rigid tubes and volume-restricted vascular beds: theoretical explanations, Ann. N.Y. Acad. Sci. 170:437, 1970.

42. Manke, D.A., et al.: Hemodynamic studies of digital and extremity replants and revascularization, Surgery 88:445, 1980.

43. Mohapatra, S.N., and Arenson, H.M.: The measurement of peripheral blood flow by the electrical impedance technique, J. Med. Eng. Technol. 3:132, 1979.

44. Noordergraaf, A., and Horeman, H.W.: Numerical evaluation of volume pulsations in man. II. Calculated volume pulsations of forearm and calf, Phys. Med. Biol. 3:59, 1958.

45. Nyboer, J.: Electrical impedance plethysmography, ed. 2, Springfield, Ill., 1970, Charles C Thomas, Publisher.

46. O'Donnell, J.A., and Hobson, R.W., II: Comparison of electrical impedance and mechanical plethysmography, J. Surg. Res. 25:459, 1978.

47. Parrish, D.: Appendix to Strandness, D.E., Jr., and Bell, J.W.: Peripheral vascular disease: diagnosis and objective evaluation using a mercury strain-gauge, Ann. Surg. 161(suppl.):3, 1965.

48. Parrish, D., Strandness, D.E., Jr., and Bell, J.W.: Dynamic response characteristics of a mercury-in-Silastic strain-gauge, J. Appl. Physiol. 10:363, 1964.

49. Parrish, D., et al.: Evidence for the venous origin of plethysmographic information, J. Lab. Clin. Med. 62:943, 1963.

50. Raines, J.K.: Diagnosis and analysis of arteriosclerosis in the lower limbs from the arterial pressure pulse, Ph.D. thesis, Massachusetts Institute of Technology, Cambridge, Mass., 1972.

51. Raman, E.R., Vanhuyse, V.J., and Jageneau, A.H.: Comparison of plethysmographic and electromagnetic flow measurements, Phys. Med. Biol. 18:704, 1973.

52. Ramsey, D.E., Manke, D.A., and Sumner, D.S.: Toe blood pressure, a valuable adjunct to ankle pressure measurement for assessing peripheral arterial disease, J. Cardiovasc. Surg. 24:43, 1983.

53. Schraibman, I.G., et al.: Comparison of impedance and strain-gauge plethysmography in the measurement of blood flow in the lower limb, Br. J. Surg. 62:909, 1975.

54. Shepherd, J.T.: Physiology of the circulation in human limbs in health and disease, Philadelphia, 1963, W.B. Saunders Co.

55. Shimazu, H., et al.: Evaluation of the parallel conductor theory for measuring human limb blood flow by electrical plethysmography, IEEE Trans. Biomed. Eng. 29:1, 1982.

56. Støckel, M., et al.: Standardized photoelectric technique as routine method for selection of amputation level, Acta Orthop. Scand. 53:875, 1982.

57. Strandell, T., and Wahren, J.: Circulation in the calf at rest, after arterial occlusion and after exercise in normal subjects and in patients with intermittent claudication, Acta Med. Scand. 173: 99, 1963.

58. Strandness, D.E., Jr., and Sumner, D.S.: Hemodynamics for surgeons, New York, 1975, Grune & Stratton, Inc.

59. Sumner, D.S.: Rational use of noninvasive tests in designing a therapeutic approach to severe arterial disease of the legs. In Puel, P., Boccalon, H., and Enjalbert, A., editors: Hemodynamics of the limbs, ed. 2, Toulouse, France, 1981, G.E.P.E.S.C.

60. Sumner, D.S., and Strandness, D.E., Jr.: The relationship between calf blood flow and ankle blood pressure in patients with intermittent claudication, Surgery 65:763, 1969.

61. Swammerdam, J.: Biblia naturae, vol. 3, edited by Boerhaave (1737). In Woodcock, J.P.: Theory and practice of blood flow measurement, London, 1975, Butterworth & Co. Publishers, Ltd.
62. Uretzky, G., and Palti, Y.: A method for comparing transmitted and reflected light photoelectric plethysmography, J. Appl. Physiol. 31:132, 1971.
63. Van den Berg, J.W., and Alberts, A.J.: Limitations of electric impedance plethysmography, Circ. Res. 11:333, 1954.
64. Van De Water, J.M., and Mount, B.E.: Impedance plethysmography in the lower extremity. In Swan, K.G., editor: Venous surgery in the lower extremities, St. Louis, 1975, Warren H. Green, Inc.
65. Vanhuyse, V.J., and Raman, E.R.: Interpretation of pressure changes in plethysmography, Phys. Med. Biol. 16:111, 1971.
66. Visser, K.R., et al.: Observation on blood flow related electrical impedance changes in rigid tubes, Pflügers Arch. 366:289, 1976.
67. Weltman, G., Freedy, A., and Ukkestad, D.: A field-theory model of blood-pulse measurement by impedance plethysmography, Ann. Biomed. Eng. 1:69, 1972.
68. Wheeler, H.B., et al.: Bedside screening for venous thrombosis using occlusive impedance plethysmography, Angiology 26:199, 1975.
69. Whitney, R.J.: The measurement of volume changes in human limbs, J. Physiol. (Lond.) 121:1, 1953.
70. Winsor, T.: The segmental plethysmograph. A description of the instrument, Angiology 8:87, 1957.
71. Woodcock, J.P.: Theory and practice of blood flow measurement, London, 1975, Butterworth & Co. Publishers, Ltd.
72. Young, D.G., Jr., et al.: Evaluation of quantitative impedance plethysmography for continuous blood flow measurement. I. Electrode systems, Am. J. Phys. Med. 46:1261, 1967.
73. Young, D.G., Jr., et al.: Evaluation of quantitative impedance plethysmography for continuous blood flow measurement. III. Blood flow determination in vivo, Am. J. Phys. Med. 46:1450, 1967.
74. Zweifler, A.J., Cushing, G., and Conway, J.: The relationship between pulse volume and blood flow in the fingers, Angiology 18:591, 1967.

CHAPTER 14

Impedance plethysmography: theoretic, experimental, and clinical considerations

H. BROWNELL WHEELER and BILL C. PENNEY

This chapter describes the theoretic, experimental, and clinical considerations involved in electric impedance plethysmography (IPG), particularly as employed for the extremities. The principles are applicable to use of this technique in other regions of the body as well. Selected clinical applications of IPG are discussed briefly.

BACKGROUND

The first impedance plethysmographic measurements in biologic specimens are generally credited to Cremer in 1907.[19] Noninvasive measurements in humans using skin electrodes were first reported in 1937 by Mann.[62] However, the method received its greatest clinical impetus from several publications by Nyboer, beginning in 1940.[74,76] Nyboer reported several experiments to support his theory that changes in electric impedance were a result of changes in blood volume, electrically in parallel with other tissues in the field. Using this model he converted impedance measurements to blood volume measurements and even to blood flow measurements. Other researchers[63] subsequently employed Nyboer's technique of ''impedance plethysmography,'' as he termed the method.

In IPG, skin electrodes are applied to the body region being studied. A weak, high-frequency AC current is passed through the electrodes. The current strength is so weak that it is imperceptible to the subject, and the frequency is so high that it is incapable of stimulating the heart.

Although other electrode configurations have been employed, the tetrapolar configuration shown in Fig. 14-1 has become more or less standard.[84] Current is passed between two outer electrodes, and voltage changes across the field are measured through two separate inner electrodes. This electrode configuration eliminates the variable of skin resistance.

An accurate and precise theoretic basis for IPG has been described by Geselowitz[31] and others.[56,57,70] Their formulations were derived from basic electromagnetic field theory. These formulations allow prediction of the impedance change caused by a conductivity change in any known location within a four-electrode impedance field, provided the lead vectors from current and voltage electrodes are known.

Sensitivity to conductivity changes is proportional to the scalar product* between two voltage-gradient fields. One voltage-gradient field is produced by the current passing between the current electrodes. The other voltage-gradient field is that which would be created if current were passed between the voltage electrodes (Fig. 14-2). By using this theory the sampling field can be predicted for various electrode configurations in any region of the body. These theoretic predictions can then be subjected to laboratory verifications.

THEORETIC AND EXPERIMENTAL STUDIES

To understand the nature of the impedance signal, two questions must be answered: (1) What

☐ Some of the studies mentioned briefly herein were supported in part by grants from the National Science Foundation (GY 11514 and EPP-75-08986), the National Institutes of Health (HL-19038), the St. Vincent Hospital Research Foundation, and the Max C. Fleischmann Foundation.

*The scalar product between two electric fields is defined as the product of the magnitudes of the two fields multiplied by the cosine of the angle between them.

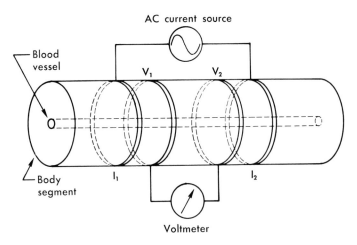

Fig. 14-1. Diagrammatic representation of four-electrode IPG. Weak, high-frequency current passes between I_1 and I_2. Voltage changes are recorded between V_1 and V_2, reflecting blood volume changes in body segment under study.

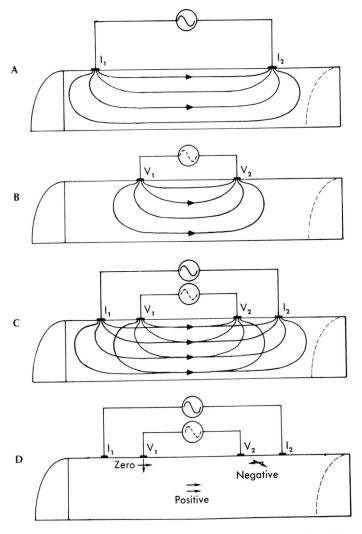

Fig. 14-2. Sampling efficiency of four-electrode IPG can be predicted from knowledge of two electric fields. **A,** Field produced by current passing between current electrodes. **B,** Field that would be produced by current flow between voltage electrodes. Superimposing these fields, **C** shows angles of intersection between them. Depending on these angles, **D** shows that sensitivity will be positive, negative, or null.

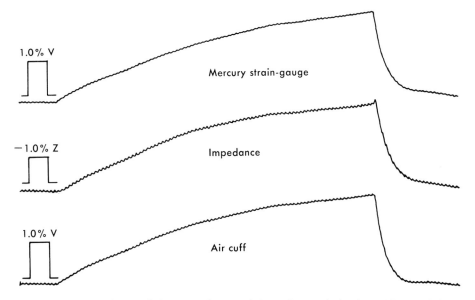

Fig. 14-3. Venous occlusion plethysmography recorded simultaneously by three different plethysmographic techniques.

physiologic changes contribute to segmental conductance changes? (2) What is the sampling field of the instrumentation employed?

At rest, impedance changes are primarily caused by respiratory or cardiac activity. Inspiration and expiration change the volume and flow of air in the chest, producing corresponding changes in the electric impedance. Each heartbeat produces changes in blood pressure, blood volume, and blood flow throughout the body. Synchronous changes can be observed in the conductance of almost any body segment. The question arises as to whether the conductance changes are solely a result of changes in blood volume, as proposed by Nyboer, or may also be influenced by changes in pressure, flow, or some other variable of circulatory physiology. Each of these variables has been evaluated with respect to IPG.

Volume changes

The effect of volume changes on the impedance signal has been studied by making simultaneous IPG and volume plethysmographic measurements. Since blood velocity changes also affect the impedance signal, the relationship between blood volume and impedance changes is best studied during slow changes in venous volume.[4] This relationship has been quantified using air,[3] water,[113] and strain-gauge plethysmography.[1,97]

The responses of impedance, air, and mercury strain-gauge plethysmographs to calf volume changes produced by venous occlusion are compared in Fig. 14-3. During venous filling the curves are essentially identical (mean correlation coefficient of 0.995). The ratio of percent volume change/percent impedance change has been found to equal the ratio of the resistivity of blood/resistivity of tissue.[97] Under most conditions this ratio falls in a narrow range (about 0.75 to 1.0).[1,97] However, a low hematocrit level or excessive tissue fluid will change this ratio.[30,44,103] For example, if the hematocrit level drops to 20% and the tissue resistivity is 165 ohm · cm, this ratio will drop to 0.55 (Fig. 14-4). Conversely, for a hematocrit level of 40% and edematous tissue with a resistivity of 110 ohm · cm, the ratio will be about 1.3. Thus blood volume changes indicated by IPG may be falsely low in markedly edematous limbs and falsely high in severely anemic patients.

Flow changes

The electrical resistance of a tube of blood is known to decrease as the blood starts flowing.[99] This phenomenon is explained by the shape and orientation of the red blood cells.[32,34,47] At the frequencies typically used in IPG (10 to 100 kHz), the red blood cells are essentially nonconducting. Electric current encounters a higher resistance when it "sees" the full front view of a red blood cell than when it "sees" the smaller side view.

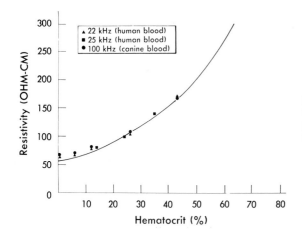

Fig. 14-4. Relationship between hematocrit and resistivity of human blood measured at two different frequencies. Data points for canine blood are similar.[30] Note that resistivity rises with hematocrit.

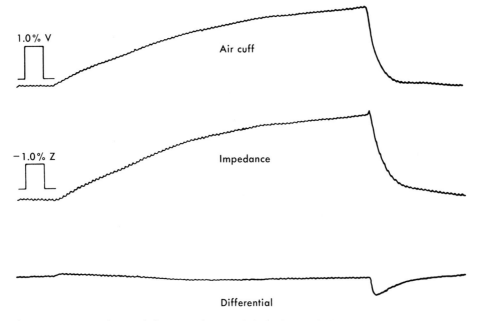

Fig. 14-5. Venous occlusion plethysmography recorded simultaneously by air cuff and impedance techniques. Differential analysis shows slight delay in venous outflow portion of impedance tracing.

Shear forces in flowing blood cause the red blood cells to turn so their long axis is parallel to the flow. An electric current parallel to the flow will then "see" only the side view of the red cells. Thus blood flow reduces the electric resistivity in the direction of the flow. This phenomenon has a noticeable effect on the impedance signal whenever stationary blood begins to flow.

Previously stationary blood begins to flow rapidly when venous occlusion is released. This produces a transient difference between the impedance signal and the volume change signal measured with a mechanical plethysmograph[4] (Fig. 14-5). Similarly, rapid changes in arterial blood velocity occur with each heartbeat. Differences between the pulsatile impedance and mechanical plethysmographic recordings are again noted[4] (Fig. 14-6). These differences appear when rapid changes in blood flow occur.

To quantify the effect of blood flow changes on the arterial impedance signal, an in vitro model was constructed. Blood was pumped in a pulsatile fashion through a bovine carotid artery and a rigid plastic tube assembled in series with a variable

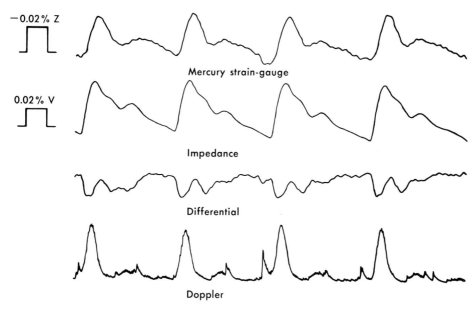

Fig. 14-6. Simultaneous recordings of arterial pulses. The impedance signal is greater in amplitude and breadth than mercury strain-gauge tracing. Signal differences coincide with flow changes shown by Doppler flowmeter (see text).

peripheral resistance.[82] Changes in pressure and flow in the system were measured with a pressure transducer and an electromagnetic flowmeter. Impedance changes were measured both on the artery, which was expansile, and on the rigid plastic tube, which was nonexpansile. Volume changes in the artery were recorded with a mercury-in-Silastic strain-gauge plethysmograph. Volume changes in the rigid tube were assumed to be negligible.

When blood was pumped through the circuit, pulse contours were seen in the impedance and mercury strain-gauge measurements from the artery. A small but definite impedance pulse was also recorded from the rigid plastic tube. This was present despite the fact that a volume change could not occur in the rigid tubing. This signal was only 10% to 15% of the impedance pulse obtained from the artery, but nevertheless, it constituted a discrete signal unrelated to volume change (Fig. 14-7).

When the experiment was repeated with saline solution, pulsations were once again recorded from the artery with both IPG and strain-gauge plethysmography. However, no longer was there a detectable impedance pulse from the rigid tube. The effect previously observed with blood did *not* occur with an electrolyte solution free from red blood cells.

IPG is the only plethysmographic method af-

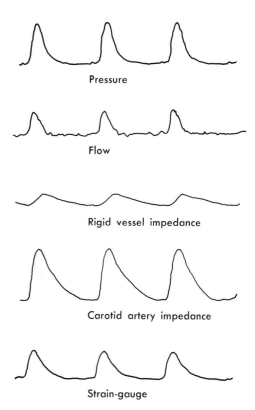

Fig. 14-7. Simultaneous tracings in laboratory model of circulatory system designed to separate effects of volume, pressure, and flow on impedance tracing (see text).

fected by changes in blood velocity. The chief effects encountered in clinical use are (1) a modest augmentation of the arterial pulse waveform and (2) a transient "blip" at the moment venous occlusion is released. This blood velocity effect can be a slight liability when accurate measurement of blood volume is required. It can be an asset in other situations, for example, when measuring volume-restricted vascular beds, such as inside the teeth[63] and skull,[59] or when sampling calcified arteries. This effect also gives a larger arterial pulse signal for analysis.

Pressure changes

The relationship between pressure and impedance changes is an indirect one. Intravascular pressure changes cause volume changes according to each vessel's compliance curve, and these volume changes are sensed by IPG.

Pressure changes between the skin and the electrodes can upset the polarization bilayer and change the electrode contact impedance. While this can affect the impedance measured with the four-electrode technique, the errors produced can be kept small (less than 5% of the signal of interest[79]) through proper instrument and electrode design.[32]

Sampling efficiency

Recognizing that conductance changes measured by IPG are primarily caused by blood volume changes (modified by a variable small component resulting from any rapid change in blood flow within the electric field), the next question that arises in interpreting the results of IPG is the extent of the sampling field. For example, in studying the leg the researcher needs to know if volume changes deep within the leg are measured as efficiently as are those near the surface. The researcher also needs to know if volume changes close to the electrodes are measured more or less efficiently than those in the center of the sampling field. Similar questions are applicable to any indirect form of plethysmography. Since electric IPG has a firm theoretic basis subject to experimental verification, such questions can be answered.

Circumferential electrodes. Quantitative predictions concerning the efficiency of the electric sampling field in the lower leg have been made using theoretic formulations.[80] A uniform cylinder encircled by four narrow electrodes was used as the model for these calculations. An analytic solution for the electric field that would be produced by

current flowing through either pair of electrodes was obtained using conventional mathematical methods. This solution was in a form that allowed numerical evaluation of the two voltage-gradient fields. The sensitivity to a conductivity change at any longitudinal or radial position within the electric field was then predicted by evaluating the scalar product between these two voltage-gradient fields.

The following experiment was conducted to test the predictive ability of this theoretic model for various longitudinal and radial positions within the electric field. Liverwurst and bologna were chosen for laboratory studies because they approximate uniform cylinders and their conductivity is similar to that of the leg. Circumferential electrodes were placed on these sausages, which were then encased in plaster to prevent any volume change. Small holes (0.9 cm in diameter) were drilled at specified radial positions. A conductivity change could be produced in a known location within the electric field by filling these holes with normal saline solution. Filling these holes at a constant rate produced a standard conductivity change at a constantly varying position (Fig. 14-8).

The first derivative of the impedance signal during filling provided the sensitivity as a function of time. This was converted to a function of position using the dimensions of the sausage, the placement of the electrodes, and the filling time. This procedure was followed in nine experiments, with holes in four radial positions. The results were then compared with the theoretic predictions for sampling efficiency as a function of longitudinal position. Typical comparisons are given in Figs. 14-9 and 14-10. Experimental results conformed closely to theoretic predictions (average root-mean-square [RMS] error was 8%).

To determine whether superficial vessels are sampled more efficiently than deep vessels, that is, to determine radial sampling efficiency, an analogous experiment was conducted. Two pairs of electrodes were placed on each of three sausages, with separations proportional to 10 cm (the voltage field) and 18 cm (the current field) on a 37 cm circumference calf—typical electrode placement for impedance phlebography. The sausages were encased in plaster, and holes were bored at four radial positions in each. Filling each of these holes individually with saline solution and measuring the resultant impedance change allowed an experimental definition of the sensitivity-to-conductivity changes in longitudinal vessels as a function of

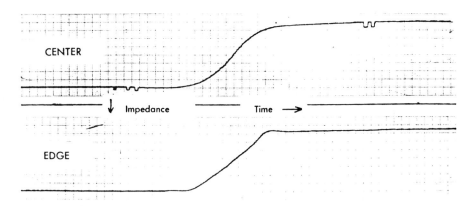

Fig. 14-8. Impedance recordings made while holes in sausages were filled at constant rate (see text). Sampling efficiency at center of field is similar to, but less sharp than, at edge.

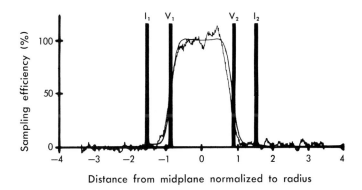

Fig. 14-9. Laboratory studies illustrating longitudinal sampling efficiency for superficial conductivity changes. Solid line represents theoretic prediction.

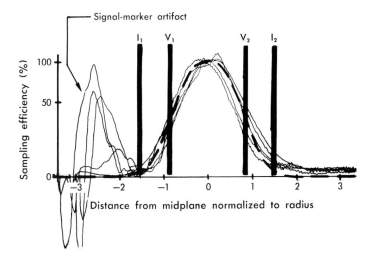

Fig. 14-10. Laboratory studies illustrating longitudinal sampling efficiency for deep conductivity changes. Heavy dashed line represents theoretic prediction.

their radial position. For this particular electrode geometry, the deep vessels are apparently sampled with at least 80% of the efficiency obtained in more superficial vessels. Other experiments showed that if the current electrodes are moved closer to the voltage electrodes, the sampling efficiency for deep vessels is lower. As the current electrodes are moved farther away, the sampling efficiency for deep vessels increases until it approaches 100% (Fig. 14-11).

A researcher might question whether a uniform cylinder model can yield much insight about what

is being measured in the human calf, which is a nonuniform mixture of bone, fat, muscle, and other tissues. To answer this question, normal saline solution has been injected into the calves of cadavers while impedance recordings have been made. Circumferential current and voltage electrodes separated by one-half and one-third the maximum calf circumference, respectively, were used to make these recordings. Saline injections (2 ml) were made at two depths, just below the skin and deep in the muscle mass, and at from seven to nine longitudinal positions. The impedance changes noted in each of the 20 legs were fitted to the theoretic predictions using a least-squares criterion.[5] The theoretic predictions and the experimental results display the same characteristics (Fig. 14-12).

From these and other studies, IPG measurements of the calf have been shown to represent a well-defined region extending only slightly beyond the voltage electrodes. For the electrode configuration typically used in impedance phlebography, this region extends only about 2 cm outside the voltage electrodes (about 0.3 times the radius of the leg) (Fig. 14-13). For this same electrode configuration the sampling efficiency for deep vessels is nearly the same as that for superficial vessels. Thus in its ability to reflect deep volume changes as sensitively as superficial changes and in its ability to sample a distinctly defined region, IPG possesses attributes of an ideal plethysmographic technique. Similar mathematical models and laboratory testing have been applied to IPG in other regions of the body.

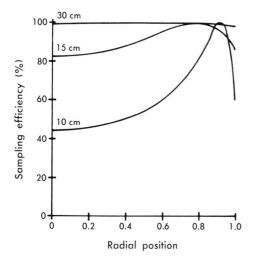

Fig. 14-11. Sampling efficiency as a function of radial position. (0 = center, 1.0 = edge; with V_1 and V_2 separated by 8 cm and I_1 and I_2 separated by 10, 15, and 30 cm.)

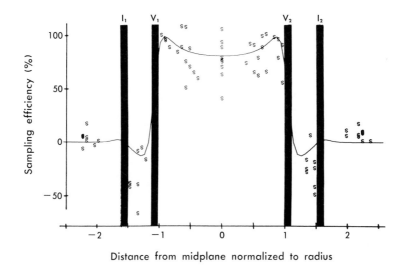

Fig. 14-12. Sampling efficiency for superficial saline injections in lower leg of cadavers. Solid line represents theoretic prediction.

Spot electrodes

For some clinical applications, circumferential electrodes are less suitable than spot electrodes, such as those routinely employed for electrocardiography. The field sampled by any given array of spot electrodes can be predicted from the considerations previously described. Electrode arrays can be designed for specific uses, such as sampling superficial blood vessels.

The sampling fields associated with spot electrodes on the surface of a uniform block[2,79,83,96] or cylinder[111] have been studied. Electrode size and spacing affected how quickly the sampling sensitivity attenuates with depth and position lateral to the electrodes. Two regions of negative sensitivity, each roughly hemispheric and located between a current electrode and the voltage electrode with the same polarity, have a profound influence on the size (and polarity) of the signal from a superficial vessel. By tilting the axis of the electrode array relative to the direction of the vessel, one can avoid having the vessel pass through these regions of negative sensitivity. With such precautions, superficial vessels can be reliably sampled.

Imaging with IPG

Since the electric conductivity of many tissues differs, there is the theoretic possibility of forming tomographic images with IPG. This is appealing, since there would be no hazard from ionizing radiation and the image contrast could be higher than with some other imaging methods. Applications could include detecting pulmonary edema[40] and breast cancer,[46] or planning and monitoring hyperthermia treatment.[69]

Initial studies have had limited success.[9,107] These studies indicate that a method must be developed to confine the electric current to a narrow path.[86] It has also been noted that the calculations involved are more difficult than in computerized tomography (CT), since they require iterative solutions.[85] Despite these problems, interest continues in this area.[72,104,114]

CLINICAL USES

A detailed description of the many proposed clinical applications of IPG is beyond the scope of this publication. The interested reader is referred to more comprehensive publications.[60,63,74] This presentation will be limited to a mention of some areas of recent study.

Cardiac evaluation

Thoracic IPG measurements for cardiac output determination were popularized in 1966 by Kubicek et al.[53] Since then many studies have evaluated its use. Some studies have found good correlations[24,29,87] while others note variability between subjects[7,15,39,93] and dependence on the peripheral resistance and contractile state of the heart.[26,58,90,94,112] Several studies conclude that it is best used for following relative changes in stroke volume in the same individual.[11,25,50,67]

Measurements of the cardiac synchronous

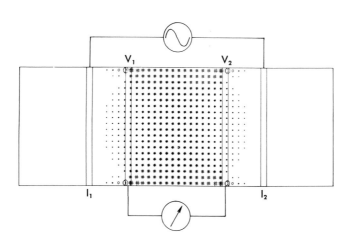

Fig. 14-13. Computer plot of sampling efficiency in four-electrode configuration simulating that used in IPG for diagnosis of deep vein thrombosis.

change in thoracic IPG have been studied for several diagnostic purposes.[41,54,88,101] They have been used to quantify aortic or mitral valve regurgitation.[91,92] A number of researchers have evaluated impedance recordings made during exercise,[21,28,66,68,102] particularly for the determination of systolic time intervals.[33,95]

Changes in the baseline component of the thoracic IPG have been used to detect changes in thoracic fluid volume as a result of changes in pulmonary wedge pressure,[37] fluid overload,[10] and cardiac insufficiency precipitated by exercise.[8] They have also been used to give an early indication of water intoxication during transurethral resection of the prostate.[16]

Pulmonary monitoring

Thoracic IPG measurements have also been used to monitor regional lung perfusion,[17,110] fluid volume,[40,48,49,65,100] and ventilation.[35,38,42,52] However, the rationale used to guide electrode placement has rarely been discussed. Recently, theoretic models that allow calculation of the electric fields produced in the thorax have been developed.[51,114] These models, combined with the theoretic considerations outlined earlier, could aid the design of electrode arrays to sample selected regions of the lungs.

Neonatal monitoring

Thoracic IPG measurements taken on neonates have been used to detect apnea,[73,78,108] to detect and guide treatment of patent ductus arteriosus,[18] and to obtain indices of cardiovascular status.[27] Cephalic IPG measurements have been used to detect hydrocephalus[89] and intraventricular hemorrhage.[98] Again, there is a need for further theoretic study to guide electrode placement and interpretation of results.[61,71]

Cerebrovascular evaluation

In adults, cerebral IPG measurements have been used to detect cerebral atherosclerosis,[36,45] to obtain an index of cerebral blood flow,[43] and to detect certain psychologic disorders that may be associated with altered cerebral circulation.[22] Such measurements have not been used widely, perhaps because there are problems interpreting the signal.[60,64] Individual differences in the high-resistivity skull and low-resistivity scalp cause uncertainty in the proportion of the signal of intracranial origin. While the contribution of the scalp can be made fairly small through proper electrode placement,[109]

the contribution of the skull's circulation remains unknown. At present, these factors make cephalic IPG measurements unsuitable for selectively detecting occlusive disease of the arteries feeding the brain.

Peripheral arterial evaluation

IPG has been used as a convenient method of obtaining waveforms from peripheral arteries.* These waveforms have been used to detect reduced arterial compliance resulting from atherosclerosis[6,44] and to study the effectiveness of drug therapy.[12,13] Combined with venous occlusion during reactive hyperemia, IPG measurements have been used to estimate the severity of proximal arterial obstructions.[77]

Similar measurements can also be made with air, water, or strain-gauge plethysmographs,[23] but these mechanical plethysmographs typically have to encircle the body segment containing the vessels to be sampled. IPG and photoplethysmography can make focal observations without encircling the region. This localized sampling ability may be of particular use in the groin, neck, and trunk.

Detection of venous thrombosis

Perhaps the most widespread use of IPG in recent years has been for the detection of deep vein thrombosis. This technique is described in more detail in Chapter 74.

SUMMARY

Although IPG has been actively studied since the 1930s, a firm theoretic and experimental basis has been developed only recently. It is now possible to predict the sampling efficiency for various electrode arrays in any portion of the body. This has already been accomplished with respect to the lower leg. Methods have been developed to design electrode arrays to sample a specific body region while minimizing the signal from adjacent areas.

In the past, IPG has been employed primarily because of its convenience and sensitivity. The ability to make plethysmographic observations merely by applying electrodes to the skin is appealing to both the patient and the physician. The method is safe and simple. The signal is clean and free of artifacts. It can be calibrated easily, and accurate quantitation of conductance change can be assured.

*References 14, 20, 55, 75, 81, 105.

However, other types of plethysmography have also been simplified and improved. The future of IPG may relate not so much to the desirable characteristics already described, some of which are now shared by other methods of plethysmography, but rather to certain features unique to the impedance technique. These features include the ability to sample a wide variety of anatomic regions, including deep-seated organs and tissues, and to reflect changes in the blood flow as well as blood volume. These features are not shared by conventional volume displacement plethysmographs.

The potential clinical usefulness for a noninvasive technique that can sample visceral hemodynamics has yet to be determined. Enough promising experiments have been reported to generate interest in using IPG to study the brain, heart, lungs, and kidneys, but these applications have not yet been used widely in clinical practice. It seems likely that further research, based on the established theoretic principles outlined herein, will expand the clinical usefulness of IPG considerably in years to come.

ACKNOWLEDGMENT

The authors are particularly indebted to Fredrick Anderson, Jr., and Professor Robert Peura for their contributions to this study. We are also grateful to the biomedical engineering students from Worcester Polytechnic Institute who have participated in studying the experimental and theoretic bases of impedance plethysmography. Their interest and enthusiasm have been constantly stimulating, and their work in the laboratory has been of great technical assistance. We are particularly grateful to Craig Sherman, Steven Pareka, John Mortarelli, and John Arcuri for their participation in some of the laboratory experiments and to Dr. Nilima Patwardhan for her invaluable assistance with the cadaver studies.

REFERENCES

1. Anderson, F.A., Jr.: Impedance plethysmography in the diagnosis of arterial and venous disease, Ann. Biomed. Eng. 12:79, 1984.
2. Anderson, F.A., Jr., Penney, B.C., and Wheeler, H.B.: Regional impedance plethysmography: an experimental method for study of specific blood vessels, Proceedings of the fourteenth annual meeting of the Association for the Advancement of Medical Instrumentation, Arlington, Va., 1979.
3. Anderson, F.A., et al.: Evaluation of electrical impedance plethysmography for venous volume measurements, Proceedings of the twenty-ninth annual conference on engineering in medicine and biology, vol. 18, Chevy Chase, Md., 1976, The Alliance for Engineering in Medicine and Biology.
4. Anderson, F.A., et al.: Comparison of electrical impedance and mechanical plethysmographic techniques in the human calf, Proceedings of the twelfth annual meeting of the Association for the Advancement of Medical Instrumentation, Arlington, Va., 1977.
5. Anderson, F.A., Jr., et al.: Impedance plethysmography: the origin of electrical impedance changes measured in the human calf, Med. Biol. Eng. Comput. 18:234, 1980.
6. Arenson, J.S., Cobbold, R.S.C., and Johnston, K.W.: Dual-channel self-balancing impedance plethysmograph for vascular studies, Med. Biol. Eng. Comput. 19:157, 1981.
7. Bache, R.J., Harley, A., and Greenfield, J.C., Jr.: Evaluation of thoracic impedance plethysmography as an indicator of stroke volume in man, Am. J. Med. Sci. 258:100, 1969.
8. Balasubramanian, V., and Hoon, R.S.: Changes in transthoracic electrical impedance during submaximal treadmill exercise in patients with ischemic heart disease—a preliminary report, Am. Heart J. 91(1):43, 1976.
9. Bates, R.H.T., McKinnon, G.C., and Seagar, A.D.: A limitation on systems for imaging electrical conductivity distributions, IEEE Trans. Biomed. Eng. 27:418, 1980.
10. Berman, I.R., et al.: Transthoracic electrical impedance as a guide to intravascular overload, Arch. Surg. 102:61, Jan. 1971.
11. Boer, P., et al.: Measurement of cardiac output by impedance cardiography under various conditions, Am. J. Physiol. 237:491, 1979.
12. Brevetti, G., et al.: Protective effects of propranolol on the exercise-induced reduction of blood flow in arteriopathic patients, Angiology 30:696, 1979.
13. Brevetti, G., et al.: Propranolol-induced reverse vascular steal in arteriopathic patients, Angiology 33:78, 1982.
14. Brown, B.H., et al.: Impedance plethysmography: can it measure changes in limb blood flow? Med. Biol. Eng. 13:674, 1975.
15. Casthély, P., Ramanathan, S., and Chalon, J.: Considerations on impedance cardiography, Can. Anaesth. Soc. J. 27:481, 1980.
16. Casthély, P., et al.: Decreases in electric thoracic impedance during transurethral resection of the prostate: an index of early water intoxication, J. Urol. 125:347, 1981.
17. Cathignol, D., et al.: Interface for pulmonary exploration by the real-time treatment of curves obtained by transthoracic impedance, Med. Biol. Eng. Comput. 16:459, 1978.
18. Cotton, R.B., et al.: Impedance cardiographic assessment of symptomatic patent ductus arteriosus, J. Pediatr. 96:711, 1980.
19. Cremer, H.: Ueber die Registrierung mechanischer Vorgänge auf electrischem Wege, speziell mit Hilfe des Saitengalvonometers und Saitenelektrometers, Münch. Med. Wochenschr. 54:1629, 1907.
20. Derblom, H., Johnson, L., and Nylander, G.: Electrical impedance plethysmography as a method of evaluating the peripheral circulation. I. Analysis of method. Acta Chir. Scand. 136:579, 1970.
21. Denniston, J.C., et al.: Measurement of cardiac output by electrical impedance at rest and during exercise, J. Appl. Physiol. 40:91, 1976.
22. Dixon, L.M., and Lovett Doust, J.W.: The diagnostic potential of rheoencephalography in psychiatry, Psychiatr. Clin. 11:219, 1978.
23. Doko, S., et al.: Noninvasive evaluation of arterial occlusive disease, Jpn. Circ. J. 47:778, 1983.
24. Edmunds, A.T., Godfrey, S., and Tooley, M.: Cardiac output measured by transthoracic impedance cardiography at rest, during exercise and at various lung volumes, Clin. Sci. 63:107, 1982.

25. Ehlert, R.E., and Schmidt, H.D.: An experimental evaluation of impedance cardiographic and electromagnetic measurements of stroke volumes, J. Med. Eng. Technol. 6:193, 1982.
26. Enghoff, E., and Lövheim, O.: A comparison between the transthoracic electrical impedance method and the direct Fick and the dye dilution methods for cardiac output measurements in man, Scand. J. Clin. Lab. Invest. 39:585, 1979.
27. Freyschuss, U., Noack, G., and Zetterström, R.: Serial measurements of thoracic impedance and cardiac output in healthy neonates after normal delivery and Caesarean section, Acta Paediatr. Scand. 68:357, 1979.
28. Fujinami, T., et al.: Impedance cardiography for the assessment of cardiac function during exercise, Jpn. Circ. J. 43:215, 1979.
29. Gabriel, S., et al.: Measurement of cardiac output by impedance cardiography in patients with myocardial infarction. Comparative evaluation of impedence and dye dilution methods. Scand. J. Clin. Lab. Invest. 36(1):29, 1976.
30. Geddes, L.A., and DaCosta, C.P.: The specific resistance of canine blood at body temperature, IEEE Trans. Biomed. Eng. 20:51, Jan., 1973.
31. Geselowitz, D.B.: An application of electrocardiographic lead theory to impedance plethysmography, IEEE Trans. Biomed. Eng. 18:38, Jan., 1971.
32. Gessert, W.L., et al.: Bioimpedance instrumentation, Ann. N.Y. Acad. Sci. 170:520, 1970.
33. Gollan, F., Kizakevich, P.N., and McDermott, J.: Continuous electrode monitoring of systolic time intervals during exercise, Br. Heart J. 40:1390, 1978.
34. Gollan, F., and Namon, R.: Electrical impedance of pulsatile blood flow in rigid tubes and in isolated organs, Ann. N.Y. Acad. Sci. 170:568, 1970.
35. Grenvik, A., et al.: Impedance pneumography—comparison between chest impedance changes and respiratory volumes in 11 healthy volunteers, Chest 62:439, 1973.
36. Hadjiev, D.: Impedance methods for investigation of cerebral circulation, Prog. Brain Res. 35:25, 1972.
37. Haffty, B.G., Singh, J.B., and Peura, R.A.: A clinical evaluation of thoracic electrical impedance, J. Clin. Eng. 2:107, 1977.
38. Hamilton, L.H., and Rieke, R.J.: Ventilation monitor based on transthoracic impedance changes, Med. Res. Eng. 11:20, 1972.
39. Harley, A., and Greenfield, J.C.: Determination of cardiac output in man by means of impedance plethysmography, Aerospace Med. 39:248, 1968.
40. Henderson, R.P., and Webster, J.G.: An impedance camera for spatially specific measurements of the thorax, IEEE Trans. Biomed. Eng. 25:250, 1978.
41. Hill, D.W., and Lowe, H.J.: The use of the electrical impedance technique for monitoring of cardiac output and limb blood flow during anesthesia, Med. Biol. Eng. 11:534, 1973.
42. Itoh, A., et al.: Non-invasive ventilatory volume monitor, Med. Biol. Eng. Comput. 20:613, 1982.
43. Jacquy, J., et al.: Cerebral blood flow and quantitative rheoencephalography, Electroencephalogr. Clin. Neurophysiol. 37:507, 1974.
44. Jaffrin, M.Y., and Vanhoutte, C.: Quantitative interpretation of arterial impedance plethysmographic signals, Med. Biol. Eng. Comput. 17:2, 1979.
45. Jenkner, F.L.: Rheoencephalographic differentiation of vascular headaches of varying causes, Ann. N.Y. Acad. Sci. 170:661, 1970.
46. Jossinet, J., Fourcade, C., and Schmitt, M.: A study for breast imaging with a circular array of impedance electrodes, Proceedings of the fifth international conference on Electrical Bio-impedance, Tokyo, 1981.
47. Kanai, H., Sakamoto, K., and Miki, M.: Impedance of blood; the effects of red cell orientation, Dig. Int. Conf. Med. Biol. Eng., vol. 11, Ottawa, Ontario, Canada, 1976, National Research Council.
48. Keller, G., and Blumberg, A.: Monitoring of pulmonary fluid volume and stroke volume by impedance cardiography in patients on hemodialysis, Chest 72(1):56, 1977.
49. Khan, M.R., et al.: Quantitative electrical-impedance plethysmography for pulmonary oedema, Med. Biol. Eng. Comput. 15:627, 1977.
50. Khatib, M.T., et al.: The thoracic-impedance and thermal dilution methods of measuring cardiac output—a comparison in the dog, Br. J. Anaesth. 47:1026, 1975.
51. Kim, Y., Tompkins, W.J., and Webster, J.G.: A three-dimensional modifiable body model for biomedical applications. In Cohen, B.A., editor: Frontiers of engineering in health care, New York, 1981, IEEE Publishing Services.
52. Kira, S., et al.: Transthoracic electrical impedance variations associated with respiration, J. Appl. Physiol. 30:820, 1971.
53. Kubicek, W.G., et al.: Development and evaluation of an impedance cardiac output system, Aerospace Med. 37:1208, 1966.
54. Kwoczyński, J., and Palko, T.: A trial of non-invasive diagnosis of muscular subaortic stenosis by the impedance method, Mater. Med. Pol. 11:242, 1979.
55. Lee, B.Y., et al.: Noninvasive hemodynamic evaluation in selection of amputation level, Surg. Gynecol. Obstet. 149:241, 1979.
56. Lehr, J.: A vector derivation useful in impedance plethysmographic field calculations, IEEE Trans. Biomed. Eng. 19:156, Mar., 1972.
57. Lehr, J.L.: Physiological impedance measurements—a theoretical and experimental treatment of guarded electrode and other techniques, doctoral thesis. Pittsburgh, 1972, Carnegie-Mellon University.
58. Lewis, G.K., Peura, R.A., and Singh, J.B.: The quantitative effect of the heart on transthoracic impedance measurement, Proceedings of the 27th conference on engineering in medicine and biology, vol. 16, Chevy Chase, Md., 1974, The Alliance for Engineering in Medicine and Biology.
59. Lifshitz, K.: Rheoencephalography. I. Review of the technique, J. Nerv. Ment. Dis. 136:388, 1963.
60. Lifshitz, K.: Rheoencephalography. II. Survey of clinical applications, J. Nerv. Ment. Dis. 137:285, 1963.
61. Lifshitz, K.: Electrical impedance cephalography, electrode guarding, and analog studies, Ann. N.Y. Acad. Sci. 170:532, 1970.
62. Mann, H.: Study of peripheral circulation by means of an alternating current bridge. Proc. Soc. Exp. Biol. Med. 36:670, 1937.
63. Markovich, S.E., editor: International conference on bioelectrical impedance, New York, 1970. The New York Academy of Sciences.
64. Masucci, E.I., Seipel, J.H., and Kurtzke, J.F.: Clinical evaluation of "quantitative" rheoencephalography, Neurology (Minneap.) 20:642, 1970.
65. Meijer, J.H., et al.: Differential impedance plethysmography for measuring thoracic impedances, Med. Biol. Eng. Comput. 20:187, 1982.
66. Miles, D.S., et al.: Estimation of cardiac output by electrical impedance during arm exercise in women, J. Appl. Physiol. 51:1488, 1981.
67. Miller, J.C., and Horvath, S.M.: Impedance cardiography, Psychophysiology 15(1):80, 1978.

68. Miyamoto, Y., et al.: Continuous determination of cardiac output during exercise by the use of impedance plethysmography, Med. Biol. Eng. Comput. 19:638, 1981.

69. Mochizuki, A., and Takada, H., and Saito, M.: Impedance computed tomography and the design of hyperthermia, Proceedings of the fifth international conference on Electrical Bio-impedance, Tokyo, 1981.

70. Mortarelli, J.R.: A generalization of the Geselowitz relationship useful in impedance plethysmographic field calculations, IEEE Trans. Biomed. Eng. 27:665, 1980.

71. Murray, P.W.: Field calculations in the head of a newborn infant and their application to the interpretation of transcephalic impedance measurements, Med. Biol. Eng. Comput. 19:538, 1981.

72. Nakayama, K., Yagi, W., and Yagi, S.: Fundamental study on electrical impedance CT algorithm utilizing sensitivity theorem on impedance plethysmography, Proceedings of the fifth international conference on Electrical Bio-impedance, Tokyo, 1981.

73. North, J.B., and Jennett, S.: Impedance pneumography for the detection of abnormal breathing patterns associated with brain damage, Lancet 2:213, July, 1972.

74. Nyboer, J.: Electrical impedance plethysmography, ed. 2, Springfield, Ill., 1970. Charles C Thomas, Publisher.

75. Nyboer, J., Kreider, M.M., and Hannapel, L.: Electrical impedance plethysmography, a physical and physiologic approach to the peripheral vascular study. Circulation 2:811, 1950.

76. Nyboer, J., et al.: Radiocardiograms: electrical impedance changes of the heart in relation to electrocardiograms and heart sounds, J. Clin. Invest. 19:963, 1940.

77. O'Donnell, J.A., et al.: Impedance plethysmography—noninvasive diagnosis of deep venous thrombosis and arterial insufficiency, Am. Surg. 49:26, 1983.

78. Pallett, J.E., and Scopes, J.W.: Recording respirations in newborn babies by measuring impedance of the chest, Med. Electron. Biol. Engin. 3:161, 1965.

79. Penney, B.C.: Development of a two channel impedance plethysmograph, signal analysis techniques, and electrode arrays: with application to carotid stenosis detection, doctoral dissertation, Worcester, Mass., 1979, Worcester Polytechnic Institute.

80. Penney, B.C., et al.: The impedance plethysmographic sampling field in the human calf, IEEE Trans. Biomed. Eng. 26(4):193, 1979.

81. Persson, A.V.: Clinical application of electrical impedance for the study of arterial insufficiency, Med. Instrum. 13:95, 1979.

82. Peura, R.A., et al.: Influence of erythrocyte velocity on impedance plethysmographic measurements, Med. Biol. Eng. Comput. 16:147, 1978.

83. Peura, R.A., et al.: Regional impedance plethysmography: experimental and computer model studies for measuring single blood vessels, Proceedings of the fifth international conference on Electrical Bio-impedance, Tokyo, 1981.

84. Plonsey, R., and Collin, R.: Electrode guarding in electrical impedance measurements of physiological systems—a critique, Med. Biol. Eng. Comput. 15:519, 1977.

85. Price, L.R.: Electrical impedance computed tomography (ICT): a new imaging technique, IEEE Trans. Nucl. Sci. 26:2736, 1979.

86. Price, L.R.: Imaging of the electrical conductivity and permittivity inside a patient: a new computed tomography (CT) technique, J. Soc. Photo. 206:115, 1979.

87. Quail, A.W., and Traugott, F.M.: Effects of changing haematocrit, ventricular rate and myocardial inotropy on the accuracy of impedance cardiography, Clin. Exp. Pharmacol. Physiol. 8:335, 1981.

88. Rasmussen, J.P., Sorensen, B., and Kann, T.: Evaluation of impedance cardiography as a noninvasive means of measuring systolic time intervals and cardiac output, Acta Anaesthesiol. Scand. 19:210, 1975.

89. Reigel, D.H., et al.: Transcephalic impedance measurements during infancy, Dev. Med. Child Neurol. 19:295, 1977.

90. Rubal, B.J., Baker, L.E., and Poder, T.C.: Correlation between maximum dZ/dt and parameters of left ventricular performance, Med. Biol. Eng. Comput. 18:541, 1980.

91. Schieken, R.M., et al.: Effect of aortic valvular regurgitation upon the impedance cardiogram, Br. Heart J. 40:958, 1978.

92. Schieken, R.M., et al.: Effect of mitral valvular regurgitation on transthoracic impedance cardiogram, Br. Heart J. 45:166, 1981.

93. Secher, N.J., Thomsen, A., and Arnsbo, P.: Measurement of rapid changes in cardiac stroke volume. An evaluation of the impedance cardiography method. Acta Anaesthesiol. Scand. 21(5):353, 1977.

94. Secher, N.J., et al.: Measurements of cardiac stroke volume in various body positions in pregnancy and during Caesarian section: a comparison between thermodilution and impedance cardiography, Scan. J. Clin. Lab. Invest. 39:569, 1979.

95. Sheps, D.S., et al.: Continuous noninvasive monitoring of left ventricular function during exercise by thoracic impedance cardiography—automated derivation of systolic time intervals, Am. Heart J. 103:519, 1982.

96. Sherman, C.W., et al.: Impedance plethysmography: the measuring field associated with an array of small electrodes. Proceedings of the 13th annual meeting of the Association for the Advancement of Medical Instrumentation, Arlington, Va., 1979.

97. Shimazu, H., et al.: Evaluation of the parallel conductor theory for measuring human limb blood flow by electrical admittance plethysmography, IEEE Trans. Biomed. Eng. 29:1, 1982.

98. Siddiqi, S.F., et al.: Detection of neonatal intraventricular hemorrhage using transcephalic impedance, Dev. Med. Child Neurol. 22:440, 1980.

99. Sigman, E., Kolin, A., and Katz, L.N.: Effects of motion on electrical conductivity of blood, Am. J. Physiol. 118:708, 1937.

100. Smith, R.M., and Gray, B.A.: Canine thoracic electrical impedance with changes in pulmonary gas and blood volumes, J. Appl. Physiol. 53:1608, 1982.

101. Sramek, B.B.: Noninvasive technique for measurement of cardiac output by means of electrical impedance, Proceedings of the fifth international conference on Electrical Bio-impedance, Tokyo, 1981.

102. Takada, K., et al.: Reliability and usefulness of impedance cardiography to measure cardiac response during exercise, Proceedings of the fifth international conference on Electrical Bio-impedance, Tokyo, 1981.

103. Trautman, E.D., and Newbower, R.S.: A practical analysis of the electrical conductivity of blood, IEEE Trans. Biomed. Eng. 30:141, 1983.

104. Uchikawa, Y., Fujimaki, M., and Kotani, M.: Analysis of the distribution of electric potentials on the body surface using electric impedance method, Proceedings of the fifth international conference on Electrical Bio-impedance, Tokyo, 1981.

105. Van de Water, J.M., Laska, E.D., and Ciniero, W.V.: Patient and operation selectivity—the peripheral vascular laboratory, Ann. Surg. 189:143, 1979.

106. Van de Water, J.M., et al.: Monitoring the chest with impedance, Chest 64:597, 1973.
107. Vannier, M.W.: Imaging instruments by CT based on electrical impedance, J. Nucl. Med. 22:95, 1981.
108. Walker, C.H.M.: Impedance respiratory monitoring in the newborn infant, Biomed. Eng. 3:454, 1968.
109. Weindling, A.M., Murdoch, N., and Rolfe, P.: Effect of electrode size on the contributions of intracranial and extracranial blood flow to the cerebral electrical impedance plethysmogram, Med. Biol. Eng. Comput. 20:545, 1982.
110. Weng, T.R., et al.: Measurement of regional lung function by tetrapolar electrical impedance plethysmography, Chest 76:64, 1979.
111. Yamada, N., Sakamoto, K., and Kanai, H.: On the sensitivity of impedance plethysmography, Proceedings of the fifth international conference on Electrical Bio-impedance, Tokyo, 1981.
112. Yamakoshi, K., Togawa, T., and Ito, H.: Evaluation of the theory of cardiac-output computation from transthoracic impedance plethsymogram. Med. Biol. Eng. Comput. 15(5):479, 1977.
113. Yamakoshi, K.I., et al.: Admittance plethysmography for accurate measurement of human limb blood flow, Am. J. Physiol. 235(6):H821, 1978.
114. Yamashita, Y., and Takahashi, T.: Method and feasibility of estimating impedance distribution in the human torso, Proceedings of the fifth international conference on Electrical Bio-impedance, Tokyo, 1981.

CHAPTER 15

Mercury strain-gauge plethysmography

DAVID S. SUMNER

The use of the mercury strain gauge to measure volume changes in human limbs was first reported by Whitney in 1953.[45] Almost 10 years elapsed before the method was applied in the clinical laboratory for the evaluation of peripheral vascular disease. The early reports of Holling et al.[14] and of Strandness et al.[38] established the potential value of the technique. Largely as a result of subsequent work by Strandness and colleagues,[8,31,34,36] the method has become popular in many vascular laboratories throughout the world.

The mercury strain gauge has important advantages not shared by all plethysmographs. First, the apparatus is inexpensive, simple to use, and portable. There is no need to immobilize the patient with his limbs encased in bulky water-filled containers while studies are being carried out. Finally, the technique is quite versatile. Blood flow can be measured by the venous occlusion method, pulse volume and contour can be recorded with accuracy, and segmental blood pressures can be measured even in severely ischemic extremities.

THEORY

The basic theory has been discussed in Chapter 13 and need not be repeated here. It is sufficient to remind the reader that the mercury-in-Silastic strain gauge senses volume changes indirectly by measuring changes in the circumference of the part around which it is placed. Stretching the gauge increases its electric resistance. These variations in resistance can be faithfully recorded with a variety of bridge circuits.

In a cylinder with a circular cross section the ratio of volume change (ΔV) to the original volume (V) has the following relationship with the ratio of change in circumference (ΔC) to the original circumference (C)*:

$$\frac{\Delta V}{V} = \frac{2\Delta C}{C} + \frac{\Delta C^2}{C^2} \qquad (1)$$

or for very small changes:

$$\frac{dV}{V} = \frac{2dC}{C} \qquad (2)$$

Because relative changes in gauge resistance (dR/R) are related to relative changes in gauge length (dL/L) by

$$dR/R = 2dL/L \qquad (3)$$

changes in gauge resistance are related to changes in limb volume by

$$dR/R = dV/V \qquad (4)$$

provided the length of the gauge (L) equals the circumference of the limb (C).[13,20,29,33]

This is a very important relationship, since it allows for direct electric calibration of the system in terms of volume change of the part around which the gauge is stretched.

There are, however, some potential pitfalls that should be considered. The cross section of the limbs may not be truly circular. Whitney[45] dealt with this problem and concluded that the relationship in equation 2 still holds for other geometric configurations provided the shape remains unaltered on expansion or contraction. When the shape is altered with volume change so that the dimensions of only one of the two orthogonal axes changes, errors can be introduced. For example, if

*See Chapter 13 for development of this equation.[45]

the cross section were elliptic with the short axis being 0.8 the length of the long axis and if expansion occurred only in the long axis, formula 2 would become[45]:

$$dV/V = 1.44 \; dC/C$$

On the other hand, if only the short axis changed, the formula would be:

$$dV/V = 3.27 \; dC/C$$

In practice, unidirectional changes seldom, if ever, occur and probably do not contribute significantly to measurement error.

A problem that has not been considered extensively is that of unequal expansion of various parts of the limb. Knox et al.[20] have shown that the skin overlying the muscular compartments of the calf expands more than the skin over the tibia. When the gauge completely encircles the limb without overlap, the unequal expansion does not affect the accuracy of the results. If the gauge were too short and its ends were attached to the skin overlying the muscle, the resistance change (dR/R) would be larger than the actual volume change of the subtended calf segment (dV/V). If the gauge were attached only to the skin over the tibia, the calculated volume change would be too low.

While gauges that are too short are seldom used, gauges that are too long are commonly employed. One commercially available system uses gauges of sufficient length to fit limbs of all sizes. When these gauges are applied to the limb there is invariably some overlap. If the overlap is placed over a muscular portion of the leg, calculated volume changes will be too large; if the overlap is over the pretibial region, calculated volume changes will be too low. According to Knox,[20] results obtained with the overlap in the two positions are appreciably different, usually varying by more than 30%. In tests used to detect deep vein thrombosis, in which the rate of calf volume decrease can be normalized against the increase in calf volume produced by a congesting cuff, the errors tend to cancel each other and absolute accuracy is not required. In most other circumstances, it is desirable to select gauges that completely encircle the limb without overlap (Chapter 73).[5]

INSTRUMENTATION

The strain gauges are constructed of fine-bore silicone rubber tubing (0.020 × 0.037 inch, 0.15 × 0.040 inch, or 0.012 × 0.025 inch) com-

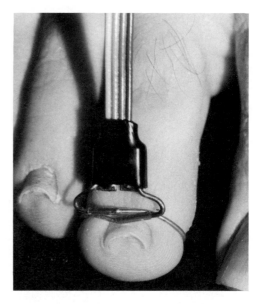

Fig. 15-1. Mercury-in-Silastic strain gauge applied to second toe. (From Sumner, D.S.: Digital plethysmography. In Rutherford, R.B., editor: Vascular surgery, ed. 2, Philadelphia, 1984, W.B. Saunders Co.)

pletely filled with mercury or an indium-gallium alloy. Electric contact is achieved by means of copper electrodes that are inserted a short distance into each end of the tubing. Since calves, forearms, and digits come in all sizes, gauges of differing lengths must be available. Ideally the gauges are applied to the limb or digit with a minimal degree of stretch—about 10 g. Usually this means that limb gauges must be 1 to 3 cm shorter than the circumference of the limb, and digit gauges must be 0.5 cm shorter than the circumference of the finger or toe to which they will be applied.

Digit gauges are usually constructed to form a complete circle to facilitate application to the finger or toe (Fig. 15-1). Limb gauges can be applied as a single strand, in which case the lead wires are not joined (Fig. 13-5), or as a double strand, in which case the lead wires are joined and the mercury-filled silicone rubber tube is looped around the limb and hooked over the terminal (Figs. 15-2 and 15-3). Gauges loosely backed with Velcro are designed to fit multiple limb sizes. Although this arrangement permits easy application, it necessitates a certain amount of overlap, which can be a disadvantage if accurate flow readings are required.

Several matching circuits for plethysmographs

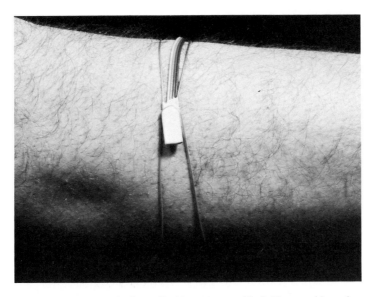

Fig. 15-2. Four-lead limb gauge applied to calf of leg. Mercury-filled silicone rubber tube encircles leg and is held in place by hooking it over "terminal."

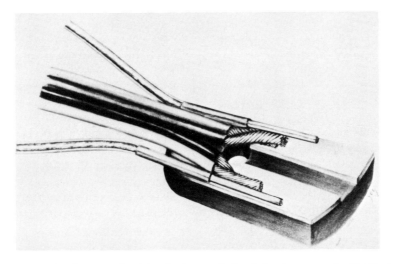

Fig. 15-3. Underside of "terminal" of four-lead gauge before it has been coated with Silastic. (From Hokanson, D.E., Sumner, D.S., and Strandness, E.D., Jr.: IEEE Trans. Biomed. Eng. 22(1):25, 1975.)

are commercially available.* These instruments can be DC-coupled to a recorder to follow both slow and pulsatile volume changes or AC-coupled for pulsatile recordings only. The Hokanson and Medsonics plethysmographs have the advantage of permitting electric calibration. These circuits make use of the relationship of gauge resistance to limb volume given in equation 4.

*Parks Electronics Laboratory, Beaverton, Ore.; D. Eugene Hokanson, Issaquah, Wash.; Medsonics, Mountain View, Calif.

Resistance changes are most accurately measured when the gauge is constructed with four lead wires, as described by Sigdell,[33] Hokanson et al.,[13] and Michaux[25] (Figs. 15-3 and 15-4). Two lead wires are attached to each end of the mercury-filled silicone rubber tube. Current is fed to the gauge through one set of lead wires; the voltage drop is sensed by the other set of wires, which is connected directly to the bridge circuit (Fig. 15-4, *A*). Since there is virtually no current through the wires con-

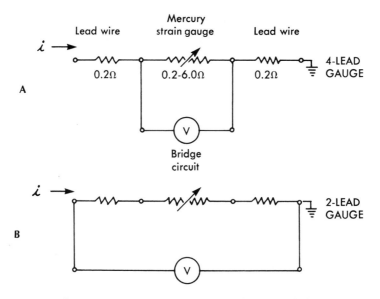

Fig. 15-4. Diagrams illustrating two ways of connecting bridge circuit to mercury strain gauge. **A,** Two lead wires are connected to each end of gauge. One of wires at each end of gauge is connected directly to bridge circuit. This four-lead arrangement effectively places strain gauge at corners of measurement bridge. **B,** When only two leads are employed, lead-wire resistances are incorporated in bridge circuit, making electric calibration impossible.

nected to the bridge circuit, the resistance of the lead wires does not affect electric calibration. If electric calibration were attempted using two-wire gauges with the bridge circuit terminals at the ends of the lead wires (Fig. 15-4, *B*), considerable error would be introduced.

To illustrate this problem, let us assume that the resistance of each lead wire is 0.2 ohm and that of an unstretched digital gauge is 0.2 ohm. With the two-wire arrangement the resistances of the lead wires are in series with that of the gauge, giving a baseline value of 0.6 ohm (0.2 + 0.2 + 0.2). If the volume of the limb increased by 1%, the increase in resistance of the gauge would be (equation 4)

$$dR = 0.2(0.01) = 0.002 \text{ ohm}$$

Consequently, the relative increase in resistance of the entire system of gauge and lead wires (dR/R) would be

$$0.002/0.6 = 0.003$$

or only 0.3%. Therefore electric calibration would imply an increase in volume of only 0.3% rather than the 1% increase that actually occurred–an unacceptable error. However, when the bridge circuit leads are at the end of the mercury-filled tube, the relative increase in resistance would be

$$0.002/0.2 = 0.01$$

or 1%, an accurate value. Obviously, if measurements were made on the calf with a longer gauge having, for example, a resistance of 6 ohms, there would be much less error with the two-wire system. In this case the electric calibration would indicate a 0.9% volume increase.

Electric calibration is performed while the gauge is in situ. This avoids errors resulting from changes in temperature or stretch of the gauge that may accompany mechanical calibration performed after the gauge has been removed from the limb. Regardless of the baseline stretch on the gauge, once the bridge has been balanced, a panel switch can be used to increase the output of the bridge by the same amount as a 1% increase in gauge resistance.[13] This signal is recorded for comparison with the plethysmographic data. Fig. 15-5 illustrates the 1% calibration signals obtained with the two-wire and four-wire systems and a comparison of them with a standard mechanical stretch.

An additional feature of some models of the Hokanson plethysmograph is a follow-and-hold circuit that permits limb volume change to be read directly from a panel meter. In studies of venous outflow, this can eliminate the need for a strip-chart recorder.

Mechanical calibration may be carried out in situ by means of a calibrated screw arrangement to which the gauge is attached.[9,45] With devices of

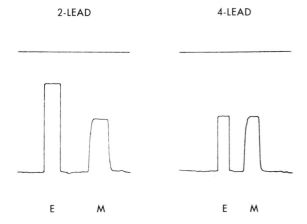

2-LEAD   4-LEAD

E   M   E   M

Fig. 15-5. Comparison of electric calibration with mechanical calibration using two-lead and four-lead (Hokanson) system. *E* designates 1% electric calibration signal, and *M* is signal produced by 0.5% mechanical stretch of gauge (0.5% mechanical stretch is equivalent to 1.0% volume increase; see equation 2). Note that electric calibration signal with two-lead system is far too large. This would lead to significant underestimation of volume change. (From Hokanson, D.E., Sumner, D.S., and Strandness, D.E., Jr.: IEEE Trans. Biomed. Eng. 22(1):25, 1975.)

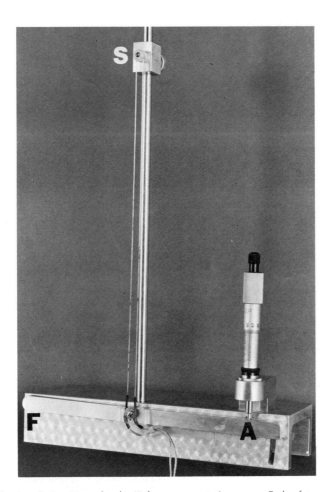

Fig. 15-6. Calibrating device ("stretcher bar") for mercury strain gauges. Ends of gauge are secured at point midway between fulcrum *(F)* and anvil *(A)*. Gauge is looped around spindle *(S)*, which is free to slide up and down on vertical steel shaft. By manually adjusting spindle, one can return gauge to same length that it had on limb. Micrometer is then turned to produce known stretch on gauge. Because of position of gauge halfway between anvil and fulcrum, micrometer reading will be exactly twice stretch on gauge.

this sort the gauge is stretched a known length and the calibration signal recorded. Mechanical calibration in situ has the advantage of avoiding temperature changes (which would affect the resistance of the gauge) and of eliminating errors as a result of the deformability of soft tissues.[9] However, the apparatus is bulky and may not conform precisely to the curvature of the limb to which it is applied.

For most studies it is more convenient to remove the gauge from the limb and attach it to a mechanical stretcher bar (Fig. 15-6). The gauge is stretched manually by means of a slide arrangement on the bar until the pen of the recorder returns to baseline levels, indicating that the length of the gauge is the same as it was when it was in place on the limb. By means of a micrometer, one can then produce an additional known stretch of the gauge. The resulting signal is recorded for calibration purposes.

Because a 10° C change in gauge temperature causes a 1% change in resistance,[6,29] removal of the gauge from a limb where the temperature is 30° C to the surrounding air where the temperature is 20° C will introduce a significant error when absolute limb dimensions are being measured. To avoid these errors, methods for temperature compensation have been devised.[16] However, such devices are not necessary when blood flow or pulse volume are being studied, since the errors introduced by temperature change are negligible under these circumstances.[16]

MEASUREMENT OF BLOOD FLOW

By using the technique of venous occlusion plethysmography, one can measure blood flow in almost any portion of a limb with the mercury strain gauge. The method is particularly applicable to flow studies on cylindric parts such as the calf, forearm, fingers, and toes.

Since the theoretic aspects of venous occlusion plethysmography have been dealt with in Chapter 13, only the practical points specifically related to the use of the mercury strain gauge will be discussed here.

Calf blood flow

All measurements should be conducted in a draft-free room at a comfortable temperature (22° to 25° C). With the patient relaxed in a supine position, the calf is elevated slightly above heart level and maintained in that position with a pillow under the heel. Another pillow must be placed un-

der the thigh to prevent extension of the knee and to ensure that the calf is not resting on the examining table. A large (preferably contoured) venous occlusion cuff (22 × 71 cm)* is wrapped around the thigh just above the knee. Another pneumatic cuff (10 or 12.7 × 40.5 cm)* is wrapped around the ankle (Fig. 15-7). A mercury-in-Silastic strain gauge is positioned so that it encircles the calf at its widest part (Figs. 15-2 and 15-7). To conform precisely to all changes in calf circumference, the gauge should be applied with a slight amount of tension (about 10 g). Excess tension must be avoided, since this will interfere with calf expansion. Ordinarily, the gauge should be 1 to 3 cm shorter than the circumference of the calf.

After the plethysmograph has been balanced so that a relatively stable baseline is evident on the recorder paper, the ankle cuff is inflated well above the systolic blood pressure. At this point it is usually necessary to readjust the baseline. About 30 seconds should elapse before any recordings are made. With the recording paper running, the thigh cuff is rapidly inflated above venous pressure but below arterial diastolic pressure. Immediately, the tracing will rise above the baseline, producing a curve similar to that depicted in Fig. 15-7. When a slope of sufficient length is obtained, the thigh cuff is deflated and the tracing allowed to return to baseline before another flow recording is made. After the series of measurements is completed, the ankle cuff is deflated. A rest period of several minutes may be required before another series of measurements is made to allow the hyperemia of the part to subside.

With the tracing at baseline level, the gauge may be calibrated in situ. As described previously in this chapter, a mechanical stretching device[45] may be used; or if a four-lead (Hokanson) gauge and plethysmograph are being used, electric calibration is employed.[13] Otherwise, the gauge is removed and attached to a ''stretcher bar'' (Fig. 15-6) for calibration.[29]

For most studies a venous occlusion pressure of about 50 to 60 mm Hg will be appropriate. Occasionally it may be necessary to use a lower pressure when the patient has obstructive arterial disease in order not to exceed the arterial diastolic pressure. By trying several different occlusion pressures, the researcher can select that which gives the steepest slope. Usually a wide range of pres-

---

*D. Eugene Hokanson, Issaquah, Wash.

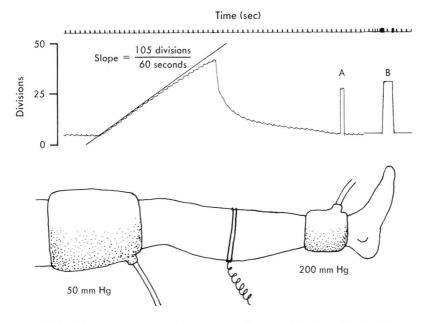

Fig. 15-7. Calf blood flow measurement with mercury strain gauge. Electric calibration *(A)* corresponds to 1% increase in calf volume and equals 22 divisions on recording paper. Mechanical calibration *(B)* with 0.2 cm stretch of gauge produces deflection of 26 divisions on recording paper. Calf circumference was 34.6 cm. (From Strandness, D.E., Jr., and Sumner, D.S.: Hemodynamics for surgeons, New York, 1975, Grune & Stratton, Inc.)

sures will yield similar slopes. The venous occlusion cuff must be filled rapidly within a second or two to the predetermined level. As described in Chapter 13, this can be accomplished with an air reservoir or with an electrically controlled cuff inflator containing a pressure regulator and two solenoid valves.*

Not infrequently, the tracing will rise or fall a short distance almost instantly after the cuff is inflated. This so-called cuff artifact is usually a result of a shift of the calf skin or muscle mass produced by the cuff. If the cuff artifact is sharply defined, it will not interfere with flow measurement. Of course, the slope of the curve must not be drawn to include the artifact. Often the cuff artifact can be eliminated by readjusting the pillows or the occlusion cuff or by elevating the calf slightly.

Reactive hyperemia. To study blood flow under conditions of maximal peripheral vasodilation, hyperemia may be produced by reinstituting blood flow after a period of ischemia. As discussed in Chapter 13, this is an important method for evaluating the functional capacity of the circulation in patients with obstructive arterial disease.[11]

In addition to the apparatus previously discussed,

*D. Eugene Hokanson, Issaquah, Wash.

a second pneumatic cuff (arterial occlusion cuff) must be placed around the thigh proximal to or over the venous occlusion cuff. After control flow measurements have been made, the arterial occlusion cuff is inflated well above arterial systolic pressure and left inflated for 5 minutes. (The proper pressure can be determined with the aid of a Doppler flowmeter.) Thirty seconds before deflating the arterial occlusion cuff, the cuff around the ankle is inflated above systolic pressure. Then 10 seconds before deflating the arterial occlusion cuff, the venous occlusion cuff is inflated to appropriate level (usually 50 to 60 mm Hg). At time "zero" the arterial occlusion cuff is suddenly deflated, whereupon the tracing on the recording paper will rise with a very steep slope. This tracing represents the initial flow recording at time "zero." Usually it is possible to obtain another flow recording at about 5 seconds and every 15 seconds thereafter until resting flow levels are reached (Figs. 13-11 and 13-12).

Exercise hyperemia. Another and perhaps more physiologic way of inducing peripheral vasodilation is through exercise. Calf exercise may be performed with the patient supine by having him flex his ankle against a foot pedal.[12] An even more physiologic way is to have the patient walk on a treadmill for a specified length of time or until forced to stop because of claudication.[42,43]

When studies are performed with the patient supine, all the cuffs and gauges can be left in place so that measurements can be made immediately on cessation of exercise. However, when treadmill studies are performed, the gauge and cuffs will have to be disconnected during the exercise period and then rapidly reconnected after the patient returns to a supine position. Since exercise hyperemia is more prolonged than is reactive hyperemia, the elapsed time is not too critical (Figs. 13-13 and 13-14).

Forearm blood flow

All forearm blood flow measurements are made exactly as described for calf blood flow. The venous occlusion cuff, however, need only be 10 or 12 cm wide. It is placed around the upper arm. The arterial exclusion cuff is placed around the wrist.

Digit blood flow

The procedure for measuring finger or toe blood flow is similar to that employed for calf flow. A pneumatic cuff for venous occlusion is wrapped around the proximal phalanx. Depending on the size of the digit, this cuff may be 1.5 or 2.5 cm wide (Fig. 15-8). Such cuffs are constructed of Penrose drains backed with Velcro. No distal cuff is employed. The strain gauge is placed around the distal phalanx at the base of the nail. Measurements are made with the hand or foot positioned comfortably, with the digits slightly above heart level.

Finger blood flow is often much higher than calf or forearm flow; consequently, the curve may rise from baseline to peak levels in one or two pulse beats, making accurate flow measurements difficult.[22] A cuff artifact is frequently present, and this may be hard to eliminate. If the cuff artifact is "sharp," it is easily recognized and will present no problem. On the other hand, if the artifact is "rounded," it may be difficult to subtract from the actual flow tracing (Fig. 13-10). In these cases the magnitude and slope of the cuff artifact can be determined by first inflating a cuff around the upper arm or leg to above systolic pressure and then inflating the venous occlusion cuff around the base of the digit. With this maneuver the rise in the baseline that occurs with no arterial inflow will become evident, and appropriate corrections can be made.

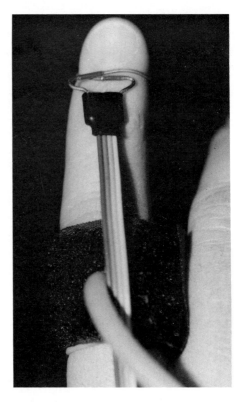

Fig. 15-8. Method for measuring digit blood flow and digit blood pressure with mercury strain gauge and pneumatic cuff applied to proximal phalanx. (From Sumner, D.S.: Noninvasive measurement of segmental arterial pressure. In Rutherford, R.B., editor: Vascular surgery, ed. 2, Philadelphia, 1984, W.B. Saunders Co.)

Calculation of blood flow

Blood flow is calculated from the venous occlusion tracing by connecting the initial systolic peaks or diastolic valleys of the pulsations with a straight line. This represents the slope of the flow curve (Fig. 15-7). The first step is to determine how many arbitrary divisions (div) of the recorder paper the slope rises in 1 minute. In the example shown in Fig. 15-7 the slope is 105 div/min.

When electric calibration is used, the number of divisions corresponding to a 1% resistance change is determined. Because the calibration may have to be performed at a different recorder attenuation than that used for the flow tracing, the appropriate adjustment must be made. Since a 1% resistance change is equivalent to a 1% volume change (equation 4), flow is simply calculated as

$$\text{Flow (ml/100 ml/min)} = \frac{\text{Slope (div/min)}}{\text{Calibration (div/1\% vol change)}} \quad (5)$$

In the example shown in Fig. 15-7 the electric calibration *(A)* is 22 div, and the flow is

$$\frac{105 \text{ div/min}}{22 \text{ div/1\% vol change}} = 4.8 \text{ ml/100 ml/min}$$

The problem is slightly more complicated when mechanical calibration is employed. First, one determines how many divisions on the paper correspond to a given stretch of the gauge. By dividing the stretch by the number of divisions, the stretch per division is obtained. When this is multipled by the slope, the amount of gauge stretch per minute is obtained:

$$\frac{\text{Gauge stretch (cm)}}{\text{Div/gauge stretch}} \times \text{Slope (div/min)} = \qquad (6)$$

$$\text{Gauge stretch (cm)/min}$$

In Fig. 15-7, 26 divisions correspond to a 0.2 cm stretch of the gauge. Accordingly, the gauge stretch per minute is

$$\frac{0.2 \text{ cm}}{26 \text{ div}} \times 105 \text{ div/min} = 0.81 \text{ cm/min}$$

Assuming that the gauge stretch per minute is equal to the circumference increase per minute, the ratio of circumference increase to the original circumference ($\Delta C/C$) can be calculated. Since the ratio of volume change to the original volume ($\Delta V/V$) is equal to twice $\Delta C/C$ (equation 2), blood flow can be calculated as follows:

$$\text{Flow (ml/100 ml/min)} = 2 \times \frac{\Delta C \text{ (cm/min)}}{C \text{ (cm)}} \times 100 \quad (7)$$

It is necessary to multiply by 100 to express the flow in terms of 100 ml of tissue; otherwise flow would be expressed as ml/1.0 ml/min.

In Fig. 15-7 the circumference of the calf is 34.6 cm. Therefore the flow is

$$2 \times \frac{0.81 \text{ cm/min}}{34.6 \text{ cm}} \times 100 = 4.7 \text{ ml/100 ml/min}$$

The small disparity between the flows calculated from the electric and mechanical calibration is a result of the inability to read the calibration signals to a fraction of a division.

Accuracy

Flow measurements made with the mercury strain gauge are subject to the same inaccuracies that occur with other instruments for venous occlusion plethysmography. In addition, the mercury strain gauge does not enclose a large volume of tissues as does the water plethysmograph. Consequently, one has to assume that the events taking place under the strain gauge are duplicated in adjacent portions of the limb.

Despite these objections, flows measured with the mercury strain gauge are remarkably similar to those obtained with the water-filled device.[14,45] However, several studies have indicated that the mercury strain gauge tends to slightly underestimate blood flow. For example, Clarke and Hellon[2] found that the mercury strain gauge tended to underestimate flow by about 9%. Also, Lind and Schmid,[21] who made comparisons during rest and exercise, observed that the mercury strain gauge consistently gave measured flows that were about 1 ml/100 ml/min less than those measured with the water-filled plethysmograph. Eickhoff et al.[7] found that the mercury strain gauge slightly underestimated calf blood flow at rest when compared to the Dohn air-filled plethysmograph; however, during hyperemia the flows measured by the two techniques were virtually identical.

PLETHYSMOGRAPHY IN VENOUS DISEASE

The theory and basic methodology involved in the use of plethysmography to study venous disease will be discussed in Chapter 73.

MEASUREMENT OF SEGMENTAL ARTERIAL BLOOD PRESSURE

Strandness and co-workers[35,39] developed a method for measuring segmental arterial blood pressure that uses the digital mercury strain gauge as a flow sensor. Basically it is a modification of the technique first proposed by Winsor in 1950.[46]

A pneumatic cuff is wrapped around the limb segment being studied, and a mercury strain gauge is placed around the forearm, calf, finger, or toe distal to the cuff. (A digital gauge is sufficient for most purposes; the gauge need only be placed in other locations when digital perfusion is absent.) As mentioned previously, the mercury strain gauge acts merely as a flow sensor.

Measurements are made by inflating the pneumatic cuff above systolic pressure. At this point any pulsations present in the digital plethysmographic record will disappear (Fig. 15-9). As the pressure in the cuff is gradually released, there will be a slow decline in digit volume. When the systolic pressure in the arteries underlying the cuff is reached, the digit volume will begin to increase, often rapidly. At the same time digit pulses, if previously present, will reappear (Fig. 15-9). The

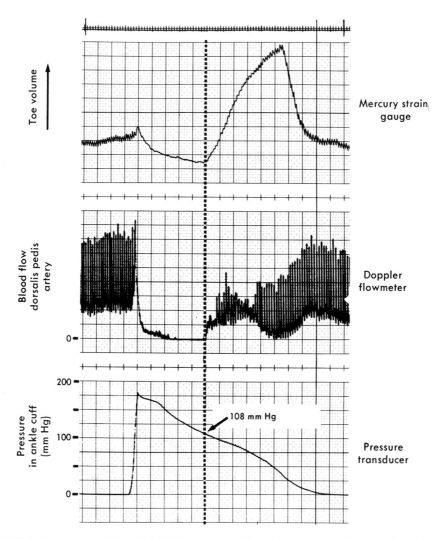

Fig. 15-9. Measurement of systolic blood pressure at ankle with mercury strain gauge placed around second toe. Doppler flow signal is included for comparison. (From Sumner, D.S.: Noninvasive measurement of segmental arterial pressure. In Rutherford, R.B., editor: Vascular surgery, ed. 2, Philadelphia, 1984, W.B. Saunders Co.)

point at which the digit volume increases, or at which digit pulses return, is the systolic pressure.

The mercury strain gauge often is applicable when other methods for sensing flow return cannot be used. For example, the Doppler technique for measuring blood pressure may fail when there are no remaining major arterial channels carrying blood at sufficient velocity to produce a signal. Thus even in highly ischemic extremities a blood pressure can usually be obtained with the mercury strain gauge if the researcher is careful and persistent.

In the usual investigation of arterial disease of the lower extremities the strain gauge is applied to the second toe, and pneumatic cuffs are placed around the ankle, below the knee, just above the knee, and at the upper thigh. Pressures are recorded from all levels, beginning at the ankle. Of these pressures the ankle pressure is the most accurate and the most significant in determining the presence or absence of obstructive arterial disease. In almost all normal limbs the ankle pressure equals or exceeds the arm pressure. On the average, the ankle systolic pressure is about 110% of the arm systolic pressure.[47] Further discussion of the significance of leg pressures will be found in other chapters.

MEASUREMENT OF DIGITAL ARTERIAL BLOOD PRESSURE

Digital blood pressure can be measured by the same technique.[10,26] A pneumatic cuff is placed around the proximal phalanx and a mercury strain gauge around the distal (Fig. 15-8). Although finger pressures are easy to obtain, toe pressure mea-surements are more difficult, since toes are often too short to accommodate both the cuff and the gauge comfortably. The photoplethysmograph is often more useful under these circumstances.[32]

The prognostic significance of toe blood pressures has been investigated by Holstein et al.[15], who reported that only 7 of 24 limbs (29%) with skin lesions healed when the big toe pressure was 20 mm Hg or below; 4 of 8 (50%) healed when the pressure was 30 mm Hg or greater. Similarly, Ramsey et al.[32] found that 95% of distal foot lesions failed to heal when the toe pressure was less than 30 mm Hg, but 86% of such lesions healed when the toe pressure exceeded 30 mm Hg (Fig. 15-10). Thus 30 mm Hg appears to be the pressure above which healing can be anticipated. Since there is no appreciable difference between the results in diabetics and nondiabetics, this test may prove to be more useful than the ankle pressure, which in diabetics is often distortedly high because of the presence of arterial calcification.

In patients with symptoms of cold sensitivity or ischemia of the fingers, it is important to differentiate between fixed arterial obstruction (caused by atherosclerosis, trauma, emboli, Buerger's disease, arteritis, and so on) and that resulting from vasospasm (Raynaud's disease). Digital pressures are often quite helpful in these cases.

Finger pressures in patients with arterial obstruction of the digital, palmar, or forearm arteries are consistently reduced, whereas finger pressures in patients with vasospastic conditions are normal when they are examined in a warm room (25° C). In my experience the finger pressure index (finger pressure divided by the ipsilateral brachial pres-

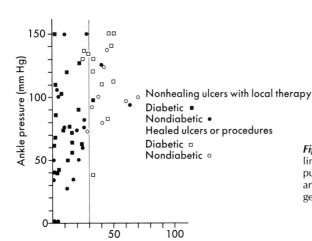

Nonhealing ulcers with local therapy
Diabetic ■
Nondiabetic ●
Healed ulcers or procedures
Diabetic □
Nondiabetic ○

Fig. 15-10. Comparison of ankle and toe pressures in 58 limbs with healed or nonhealing ischemic ulcers or toe amputations. (From Sumner, D.S.: Measurement of segmental arterial pressure. In Rutherford, R.B., editor: Vascular surgery, ed. 2, Philadelphia, 1984, W.B. Saunders Co.)

sure) averaged 0.97 ± 0.09 in normal individuals, 0.96 ± 0.11 in patients with vasospastic conditions, and 0.56 ± 0.27 in patients in whom obstruction was present.[41]

Nielsen and Lassen[27] have introduced an interesting test that uses the mercury strain gauge to measure pressure in fingers that have been locally cooled. As described in Chapter 63, this test appears to discriminate between patients with vasospastic disease, whose finger pressures drop rapidly at temperatures below 20° to 25° C, and normal individuals, whose finger pressures drop only minimally at 10° C. It also provides an objective method for evaluating the severity of the vasospastic process and for measuring the response to therapy.[28]

Digital arterial pressures are also useful in assessing the hemodynamics of arteriovenous fistulas.[39] When a steal is present, the digital arterial pressure is reduced with the fistula open but increases toward normal levels when the fistula is compressed.

DIGITAL PULSE PLETHYSMOGRAPHY

Digital plethysmography is among the more sensitive methods available for studying peripheral vascular disease.[1,35,40] Although almost any form of plethysmograph can be modified to record digit pulses, the mercury-in-Silastic strain gauge and the photoplethysmograph are the most useful. Because of its simplicity and high frequency response, the strain gauge remains a favorite of many clinical researchers and physiologists.

The basic mechanics of the plethysmographic pulse have been reviewed in Chapter 13.

Procedure

Studies should be conducted in a warm room (22° to 25° C) with the patient relaxed, preferably in a supine position. A strain gauge that fits snugly, but not too tightly, around the digit is selected (Fig. 15-1). Because of the extreme sensitivity of the digital blood flow to variations in temperature, it is important that the hands and feet be warm. At times it may be necessary to immerse the hands and feet in warm water for a short period before making the tracings. An electric blanket is also helpful.

The plethysmograph may be AC coupled when the researcher is concerned only with the general morphology of the pulse; however, if total changes in digit volume are being studied, it is necessary to use DC coupling.

Pulse contour

As shown in Fig. 15-11, *C*, the normal digit pulse is characterized by a sharp systolic upstroke that rises rapidly to a peak and then drops off more slowly toward the baseline. The downslope is curved toward the baseline and usually contains a more or less prominent dicrotic wave about midway between the peak and the baseline. This dicrotic wave is caused by the reflection of the arterial pulse from the periphery.

The pulse recorded distal to an arterial obstruction differs in several ways from the normal (Fig. 15-11, *B*). Not only is the general shape more rounded, but the upswing is more gradual and the downslope is bowed away from the baseline. No dicrotic wave is present. In limbs with severe arterial disease (such as ischemic rest pain or multilevel obstruction), the digital pulse may be severely reduced or entirely absent.[34]

A pulse that encompasses some of the features of both the normal and obstructive forms has been identified (Fig. 15-11, *A*).[3,34,44] This so-called peaked pulse is commonly found in patients with cold sensitivity, particularly those with collagen

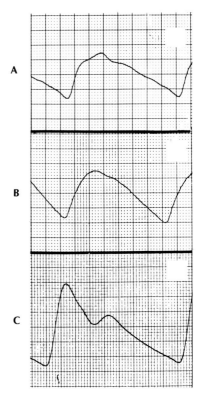

Fig. 15-11. Typical digit pulse contours. *A*, Peaked pulse. *B*, Obstructive pulse. *C*, Normal pulse. (From Sumner, D.S., and Strandness, D.E., Jr.: Ann. Surg. 175:294, 1972.)

vascular problems or some other form of anatomic digital artery disease.[18,44] The peaked pulse has a somewhat slower upswing than does the normal pulse. Near the peak there is an anacrotic notch. On the downslope the dicrotic wave is less prominent than it is in normal pulses and tends to be located closer to the peak.

By using these simple criteria, the clinician can usually diagnose significant arterial obstruction in the vessels located proximal to the site of gauge application. This includes the digital, pedal, and hand arteries as well as those major, more proximally located, arteries that typically are involved with obstructive processes. For example, the finding of an abnormal toe pulse in a patient with a normal ankle systolic pressure would tend to localize the disease to the pedal or digital arteries. Such observations can be of value in assessing the prospects for healing in a patient with ischemic lesions of the toes. If a good pulse is obtained, the prognosis may be favorable; but if pulses are flat or absent, the prospects for healing without reconstructive surgery would be remote.

Also, the finding of a peaked or obstructive pulse in a patient with cold sensitivity is an indication that the patient does not have primary Raynaud's disease but rather some form of obstructive arterial disease producing a secondary Raynaud's phenomenon. Often this will turn out to be one of the collagen diseases. On the other hand, finding a normal pulse in such a patient makes the diagnosis of primary Raynaud's disease more likely.

Analysis of the digit pulse contour

Although a number of complex methods have been devised for describing digit pulse contours, they add little to simple pattern recognition for differentiating between normal and abnormal forms. Various investigators have measured the slope of the ascending and descending limbs of the curve, the pulse width at one half its maximum excursion, the ratio of the amplitude of the dicrotic notch to peak amplitude, and the relative amplitudes at various points along the curve (Fig. 15-12).[19,23,48] Although these parameters may be helpful in comparing pulses statistically, in my opinion they are purely arbitrary measurements with little or no physiologic meaning.

Since the mercury strain gauge has a high-frequency response (flat out to 100 Hz),[30] more rig-

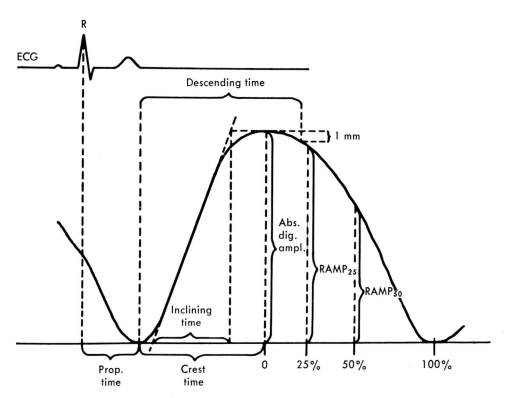

Fig. 15-12. Method for describing morphology of digit volume pulse. (From Zetterquist, S., et al.: Scand. J. Clin. Lab. Invest. 28:409, 1971.)

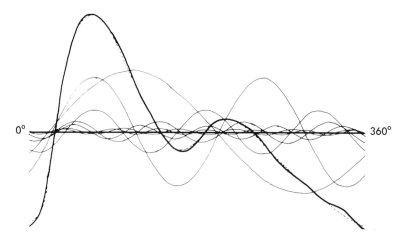

Fig. 15-13. Fourier analysis of normal digit volume pulse. Heavy solid lines indicate plethysmographically obtained pulse-wave; light lines are cosine waves corresponding to first seven harmonics; dotted lines depict pulse contour as reconstructed from first seven harmonics. (From Strandness, D.E., Jr., and Sumner, D.S.: Hemodynamics for surgeons, New York, 1975, Grune & Stratton, Inc.)

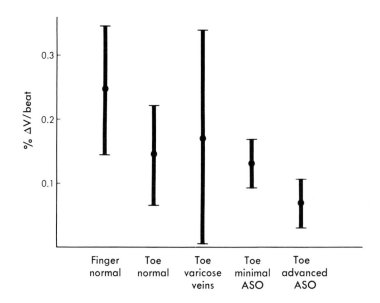

Fig. 15-14. Mean digit pulse volume in normal limbs and in limbs with arterial and venous disease. Vertical bars indicate ±1 standard deviation. (From Strandness, D.E., Jr.: Peripheral arterial disease. A physiologic approach, Boston, 1969, Little, Brown & Co.)

orous analytic techniques are possible. As shown in Fig. 15-13, the pulse wave may be broken down into its harmonic components by Fourier analysis.[3,34,39] Each harmonic can be characterized in terms of its amplitude and phase angle. With progressive proximal obstructive disease the relative amplitudes of all harmonics beyond the first tend to become more attenuated, thereby producing the rounded contour typical of the obstructive pulse. In addition, the first harmonic develops an increased phase lag accounting for the delayed peak. Data such as these can be handled mathematically

and can be compared to similar studies on pressure and flow waves.[24]

Pulse volume

Although the digit pulse may be markedly reduced or even absent in limbs with advanced arterial disease, pulse volume is, at best, only a crude indicator of the extent of arterial obstruction in less severe cases (Fig. 15-14).[4,34,48] Even in normal individuals arterial pulse volume is extremely variable, responding to changes in local temperature and sympathetic nervous activity (Fig. 15-15).

Skin temperature

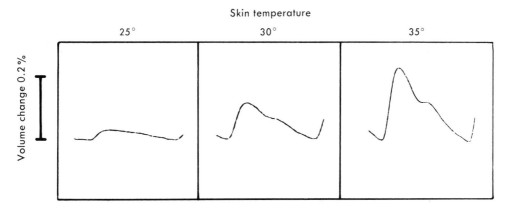

Fig. 15-15. Relationship between digit pulse volume and skin temperature in normal individual. Note that contour of pulse shows little change except during intense vasoconstriction. (From Strandness, D.E., Jr., and Sumner, D.S.: Hemodynamics for surgeons, New York, 1975, Grune & Stratton, Inc.)

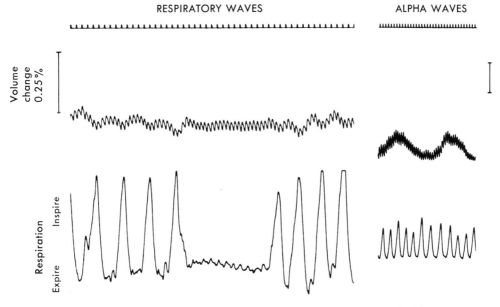

Fig. 15-16. Plethysmographic tracing from normal fingertip. Respiratory waves and alpha waves are present. (From Strandness, D.E., Jr., and Sumner, D.S.: Hemodynamics for surgeons, New York, 1975, Grune & Stratton, Inc.)

In any given digit of the same individual, the volume of the digit pulse varies directly with the blood flow, provided all studies are performed during the same examination period without moving the gauge.[49] Thus the pulse volume provides a convenient method for observing variation in digit blood flow during the reactive hyperemia test or in response to sympathetic nervous activity. However, relative estimates of blood flow from person to person or even from day to day in the same individual cannot be obtained by comparing digit pulse volumes.

Assessing sympathetic activity

Since digit blood flow is quite sensitive to sympathetic nerve impulses, the volume of the pulse may be used to follow changes in sympathetic activity. In addition, vasoconstriction of veins and arteries in response to increased sympathetic outflow will reduce the total volume of the digit.

As shown in Fig. 15-16, fingertip volume varies with respiration in the presence of normal sympathetic tone. Other deflections, known as alpha waves, also occur several times each minute. These waves are considerably larger than the respiratory

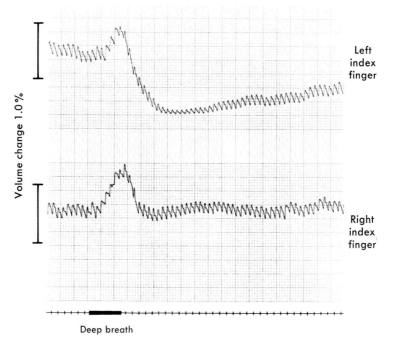

Fig. 15-17. Response of digit volume and digit pulse volume to deep breath. Simultaneous tracings were made from index fingers of both hands in patient who had undergone right cervicothoracic sympathectomy several weeks previously. Brief rise in volume that accompanies deep breath is a result of temporary compression of venous outflow. (From Strandness, D.E., Jr., and Sumner, D.S.: Hemodynamics for surgeons, New York, 1975, Grune & Stratton, Inc.)

waves. Beta and gamma waves have also been described.[1,17] Sympathectomy inhibits these responses.

When a normal individual takes a deep breath, the volume of his digits increases momentarily and then falls precipitously to a much lower level as the total quantity of blood in the finger or toe decreases.[1,35,39] At the same time the pulse volume decreases to a low level, gradually rising to its original amplitude over a period varying from seconds to minutes (Fig. 15-17). In the presence of a surgical sympathectomy or peripheral neuropathy due to diabetes, the inspiratory reflex will be absent.[37,39]

Other ways of testing the integrity of the sympathetic nervous supply to the digits include placing ice cubes on the forehead or chest or creating a painful stimulus such as a needle stick. When sympathetic innervation is intact, these stimuli will cause vasoconstriction. However, in my experience such maneuvers have not proved to be as reliable as the "deep breath" test. Reflex vasodilation may also be used to test for sympathetic activity. Normally when one hand is placed in water at 40° C, the digital volume pulse on the opposite side will increase as a result of reflex inhibition of the sym-

pathetic tone. Thus the absence of dilation indicates absence or reduction of sympathetic innervation.

Reactive hyperemia

Creation of hyperemia following a period of ischemia is an excellent method for assessing the functional severity of peripheral arterial disease. Since acute changes in pulse volume reflect acute changes in digit blood flow with a fair degree of accuracy, digit plethysmography provides a convenient method for qualitatively assessing the reactive hyperemia response.

Reactive hyperemia is produced by inflating a pneumatic cuff placed around the ankle or upper arm to a pressure greater than systolic. After the cuff has been inflated for 3 to 5 minutes, the pressure is suddenly released, and digit volume pulses are followed for the next several minutes. The volume of the largest pulse obtained during the period of reactive hyperemia is compared with the prehyperemic pulse volume.

In normal extremities the volume of the hyperemic pulse will be several times that of the control pulse (Fig. 15-18). This merely reflects the ability of the peripheral arterioles to dilate in response to a period of ischemia. However, in the presence of

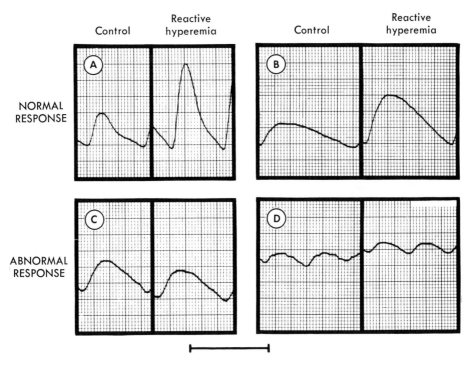

Fig. 15-18. Response of digit volume pulse in second toe to 5-minute period of ischemia (reactive hyperemia test). In normal response, volume of digit pulse more than doubles (upper panels). In abnormal response, there is little change in pulse volume. *A,* Normal circulation (pressure: arm 130, ankle 140). *B,* Superficial femoral occlusion (pressure: arm 100, ankle 80). *C,* Diabetic for 20 years (pressure: arm 135, ankle 135). *D,* Multilevel disease, iliac and superficial femoral (pressure: arm 118, ankle 46). *B* to *D* are recorded at twice sensitivity used in *A.* (From Sumner, D.S.: Digital plethysmography. In Rutherford, R.B., editor: Vascular surgery, ed. 2, Philadelphia, 1984, W.B. Saunders Co.)

significant obstructive arterial disease, there may be little or no increase in pulse volume during the postischemic period (Fig. 15-18). This is explained by the fact that the peripheral arterioles have already dilated to a considerable degree to compensate for the increased resistance imposed by the proximal arterial obstruction. Stated in another way, the magnitude of the pulse volume increase is inversely proportional to the degree of preexisting peripheral vasodilatation. When the peripheral arterioles are already dilated because of a peripheral neuropathy, there will also be little hyperemic response.

Based on previous experience, I believe a surgical sympathectomy is most likely to produce a good result when the pulse at least doubles in volume in response to hyperemia. This merely indicates that the arterioles continue to have the capacity to dilate; it says nothing about the status of the sympathetic innervation. If there is little increase in pulse volume, there is less likelihood that sympathectomy will produce much increase in blood flow.

It must be emphasized that the presence or absence of reactive hyperemia has no direct relation to the integrity of the sympathetic nervous system. Vessels in fully sympathectomized extremities retain the ability to dilate in response to a period of ischemia. Some other methods, such as the "deep breath" test or reflex vasodilatation, must be used when one is concerned about sympathetic activity.

REFERENCES

1. Burch, G.E.: Digital plethysmography, New York, 1954, Grune & Stratton, Inc.
2. Clarke, R.S.J., and Hellon, R.F.: Venous collection in forearm and hand measured by strain gauge and volume plethysmograph, Clin. Sci. 16:103, 1957.
3. Conrad, M.C.: Functional anatomy of the circulation to the lower extremities, Chicago, 1971, Year Book Medical Publishers, Inc.
4. Conrad, M.C., and Green, H.D.: Hemodynamics of large and small vessels in peripheral vascular disease, Circulation 29:847, 1964.
5. Cramer, M., et al.: Standardization of venous flow measurements by strain gauge plethysmography in normal subjects, Bruit 7:33, March 1983.
6. Eagan, C.J.: The physics of the mercury strain gauge and of its use in digital plethysmography, Technical report 60-17, Fairbanks, Alaska, 1961, Arctic Aeromedical Laboratory.

7. Eickhoff, J.H., Kjaer, L., and Siggard-Andersen, J.: A comparison of the strain-gauge and the Dohn air-filled plethysmograph for blood flow measurements in the human calf, Acta Chir. Scand. 502:15, 1980.

8. Gibbons, G.E., Strandness, D.E., Jr., and Bell, J.W.: Improvements in design of the mercury strain gauge plethysmograph, Surg. Gynecol. Obstet. 116:679, 1963.

9. Greenfield, A.D.M., Whitney, R.J., and Mowbray, J.F.: Methods for the investigation of peripheral blood flow, Br. Med. Bull. 19:101, 1963.

10. Gundersen, J.: Segmental measurements of systolic blood pressure in the extremities including the thumb and the great toe, Acta Chir. Scand. (suppl.)426:1, 1972.

11. Hillestad, L.K.: The peripheral blood flow in intermittent claudication. V. Plethysmographic studies. The significance of the calf blood flow at rest and in response to timed arrest of the circulation, Acta Med. Scand. 174:23, 1963.

12. Hillestad, L.K.: The peripheral blood flow in intermittent claudication. VI. Plethysmographic studies. The blood flow response to exercise with arrested and free circulation, Acta Med. Scand. 174:671, 1963.

13. Hokanson, D.E., Sumner, D.S., and Strandness, D.E., Jr.: An electrically calibrated plethysmograph for direct measurement of limb blood flow, IEEE Trans. Biomed. Eng. 22(1):25, 1975.

14. Holling, H.E., Boland, H.C., and Russ, E.: Investigation of arterial obstruction using a mercury-in-rubber strain gauge, Am. Heart J. 62:194, 1961.

15. Holstein, P., et al.: Distal blood pressure in severe arterial insufficiency. Strain-gauge, radioisotopes, and other methods. In Bergan, J.J., and Yao, J.S.T., editors: Gangrene and severe ischemia of the lower extremities, New York, 1978, Grune & Stratton, Inc.

16. Honda, N.: Temperature compensation for the mercury strain-gauge used in digital plethysmography, Technical report 61-28, Fairbanks, Alaska, 1961, Arctic Aeromedical Laboratory.

17. Honda, N.: The periodicity in volume fluctuations and blood flow in the human finger, Angiology 21:442, 1970.

18. Huff, S.E.: Observations on peripheral circulation in various dermatoses, Arch. Dermatol. 71:575, 1955.

19. Koike, S., et al.: The morphology of the digital volume pulse wave in health and hypertension recorded plethysmographically, Jpn. J. Hyg. 23:60, Oct. 1968.

20. Knox, R., et al.: Pitfall of venous occlusion plethysmography, Angiology 33:268, 1982.

21. Lind, A.R., and Schmid, P.G.: Comparison of volume and strain-gauge plethysmography during static effort, J. Appl. Physiol. 32:552, 1972.

22. Manke, D.A., et al.: Hemodynamic studies of digital and extremity replants and revascularizations, Surgery 88:445, 1980.

23. Mathiesen, F.R., et al.: Follow-up study of patients with occlusive arterial disease. Pulse curve morphology and xenon-133 clearance, Acta Chir. Scand. 136:591, 1970.

24. McDonald, D.A.: Blood flow in arteries, ed. 2, Baltimore, 1974, The Williams & Wilkins Co.

25. Michaux, B., et al.: Calibration-free mercury strain-gauge plethysmograph, Med. Biol. Eng. Comput. 17:539, 1979.

26. Nielsen, P.E., Bell, G., and Lassen, N.A.: The measurement of digital systolic blood pressure by strain-gauge technique, Scand. J. Clin. Lab. Invest. 29:343, 1972.

27. Nielsen, S.L., and Lassen, N.A.: Measurement of digital blood pressure after local cooling, J. Appl. Physiol. 43:907, 1977.

28. Nobin, B.A., et al.: Reserpine treatment of Raynaud's disease, Ann. Surg. 187:12, 1978.

29. Parrish, D.: Appendix to Strandness, D.E., Jr., and Bell, J.W.: Peripheral vascular disease: diagnosis and objective evaluation using a mercury strain gauge, Ann. Surg. 161(suppl.):32, 1965.

30. Parrish, D., Strandness, D.E., Jr., and Bell, J.W.: Dynamic response characteristics of a mercury-in-Silastic strain gauge, J. Appl. Physiol. 10:363, 1964.

31. Radke, H.M., et al.: Monitor of digit volume changes in angioplastic surgery: use of strain gauge plethysmography, Ann. Surg. 154:818, 1961.

32. Ramsey, D.E., Manke, D.A., and Sumner, D.S.: Toe blood pressure, a valuable adjunct to ankle pressure measurement for assessing peripheral arterial disease, J. Cardiovasc. Surg. 24:43, 1983.

33. Sigdell, J.E.: A critical review of the theory of the mercury strain-gauge plethysmograph, Med. Biol. Eng. 7:365, 1969.

34. Strandness, D.E., Jr.: Peripheral arterial disease: a physiologic approach, Boston, 1969, Little, Brown and Co.

35. Strandness, D.E., Jr., and Bell, J.W.: Peripheral vascular disease: diagnosis and objective evaluation using a mercury strain gauge, Ann. Surg. 161(suppl.):1, 1965.

36. Strandness, D.E., Jr., Gibbons, G.E., and Bell, J.W.: Mercury strain gauge plethysmography. Evaluation of patients with acquired arteriovenous fistula, Arch. Surg. 85:215, 1962.

37. Strandness, D.E., Jr., Priest, R.E., and Gibbons, G.E.: Combined clinical and pathological study of diabetic and non-diabetic peripheral arterial disease, Diabetes 13:366, 1964.

38. Strandness, D.E., Jr., Radke, H.M., and Bell, J.W.: Use of a new simplified plethysmograph in the clinical evaluation of patients with arteriosclerosis obliterans, Surg. Gynecol. Obstet. 112:751, 1961.

39. Strandness, D.E., Jr., and Sumner, D.S.: Hemodynamics for surgeons, New York, 1975, Grune & Stratton, Inc.

40. Sumner, D.S.: Digital plethysmography. In Rutherford, R.B., editor: Vascular surgery, ed. 2, Philadelphia, 1984, W.B. Saunders Co.

41. Sumner, D.S., Lambeth, A., and Russell, J.B.: Diagnosis of upper extremity obstructive and vasospastic syndromes by Doppler ultrasound, plethysmography, and temperature profiles. In Puel, P., Baccalon, H., and Enjalbert, A., editors: Hemodynamics of the limbs, Toulouse, France, 1979, G.E.P.E.S.C.

42. Sumner, D.S., and Strandness, D.E., Jr.: The relationship between calf blood flow and ankle blood pressure in patients with intermittent claudication, Surgery 65:763, 1969.

43. Sumner, D.S., and Strandness, D.E. Jr.: The effect of exercise on resistance to blood flow in limbs with an occluded superficial femoral artery, Vasc. Surg. 4:229, 1970.

44. Sumner, D.S., and Strandness, D.E. Jr.: An abnormal finger pulse associated with cold sensitivity, Ann. Surg. 175:294, 1972.

45. Whitney, R.J.: The measurement of volume changes in human limbs, J. Physiol. (Lond.) 121:1, July, 1953.

46. Winsor, T.: Influence of arterial disease on the systolic blood pressure gradients of the extremity, Am. J. Med. Sci. 220:117, Aug., 1950.

47. Yao, J.S.T.: Hemodynamic studies in peripheral arterial disease, Br. J. Surg. 57:761, 1970.

48. Zetterquist, S., et al.: The validity of some conventional methods for the diagnosis of obliterative arterial disease in the lower limb as evaluated by arteriography, Scand. J. Clin. Lab. Invest. 28:409, 1971.

49. Zweifler, A.J., Cushing, G., and Conway, J.: The relationship between pulse volume and blood flow in the fingers, Angiology 18:591, 1967.

CHAPTER 16

Air plethysmography in venous disease: the phleborheograph

JOHN J. CRANLEY

The plethysmograph, by definition, is an instrument that measures volume or enlargement. It was originally used to measure swelling of organs. The technique of measuring arterial inflow to an organ by the venous occlusion method was first reported by Brodie and Russell in 1905,[2] and in 1909 Hewlett and van Zwaluwenburg[16] reported the adaptation of this method to study the blood flow in an extremity. After this, many types of plethysmographs using either water or air were devised.* An exhaustive history of plethysmography was published by Hyman and Winsor in 1961.[17]

Although there is a vast volume of literature on the use of the plethysmograph to study the arterial circulation, it is only in recent years that attention has been directed to the study of the venous side by plethysmographic techniques.[20-22,25,28]

Basically four types of plethysmographs have been developed—those using water or air and, more recently instruments using the photoelectric cell[15] or the mercury-in-rubber strain gauge.[26] The advantage of the water plethysmograph is its great accuracy in transmitting both volume and pressure changes. The disadvantages are (1) the cumbersome nature of the devices, making them impractical for routine clinical use; (2) the hydrostatic effect of water, which may inhibit swelling of the part; and (3) the reflected waves that may sometimes be seen. The advantages of air plethysmography are that it is much more convenient to use and is generally simpler in construction. However, the air plethysmograph is subject to Boyle's law, which relates pressure, volume, and temperature of a gas in a closed system, making the system

*References 1, 3, 11-14, 18, 19, 27.

sensitive to changes in temperature. The photoelectric cell cannot be calibrated volumetrically. This is also true of the mercury-in-rubber strain gauge, but this instrument is capable of measuring changes in limb circumference, which can be mathematically related to volume change in the encircled part.

The air plethysmograph is under discussion at present. In the absolute sense, in a closed system there cannot be a volume change without a pressure change and vice versa. Nevertheless, the terms *pressure gauge* and *volume gauge* are useful to describe transducing devices that approach the theoretical ideal for measurement of pressure or volume changes. Thus an ideal pressure transducer would have a rigid diaphragm that is displaced to the smallest possible degree, reflecting pressure changes without corresponding volume changes. On the other hand, the true volume transducer must have a diaphragm that moves with the smallest possible pressure. Fig. 16-1 is a clinical example demonstrating these differences. The tracings are of a normal subject on whose finger an oncometer was placed. The digital pulse was recorded by two different transducers, using air followed by water transmission. In Fig. 16-1, *A*, the digital pulse is shown as recorded by the Statham P 23 AA transducer, an excellent pressure transducer. After the tracing was completed, the gauge was filled with water without moving the cup on the figertip. Note the tremendous increase in amplification at maximum, 15 times that of air transmission (Fig. 16-1, *B*).

In Fig. 16-1, *C*, the water has been drained and the tubing from this cup attached to the Grass PT 5 volume transducer. In Fig. 16-1, *D*, this gauge

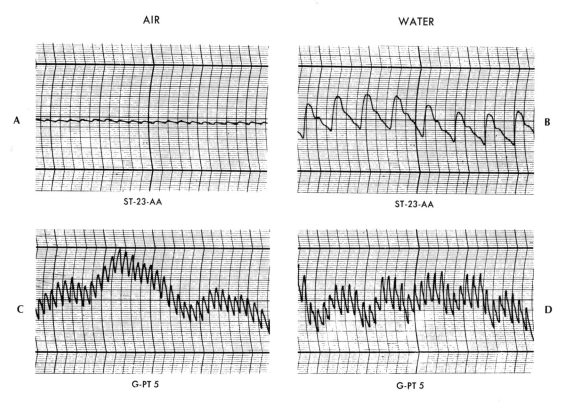

Fig. 16-1. A, Digital pulse of normal subject recorded by Statham P 23 AA transducer using air transmission. **B,** Digital pulse recorded by Statham P 23 transducer using water transmission. Note 15-fold increase in amplification compared with that in **A. C,** Digital pulse recorded by Grass PT 5 transducer using air transmission. **D,** Digital pulse recorded by Grass PT 5 transducer using water transmission. Note minimal increase in amplification compared with that in **C.**

has been filled with water. It is obvious that there is minimal difference between the tracing of the finger in air and in water with the volume transducer. This transducer comes close to the ideal volumetric transducer, which would give the same recording in air or water. Fig. 16-2 indicates the response of this gauge to injection of minute amounts of air and water. It can be seen that for all practical purposes the response to air is similar to the response to water, and thus one has an accurate volumetric transducer. With such a transducer air plethysmography becomes practical, accurate, and convenient to use.

Our study of the use of the air plethysmograph in the noninvasive diagnosis of deep vein thrombosis (DVT) was begun using the research polygraph and the Grass PT 5 volumetric transducer in conjunction with segmental pressure cuffs. This instrumentation was considered to be too sophisticated for widespread clinical use. Consequently, the manufacturer was asked to design an instrument that would be practical, convenient to use, and easy

to master. The instrument progressed through several model changes before the design was considered acceptable for marketing. This final model is called the phleborheograph (Figs. 16-3 to 16-5). The results obtained with the polygraph and the phleborheograph are identical, suggesting that the phleborheograph is qualitatively equal to the research polygraph for these purposes, although it is greatly simplified for use by technicians.

During the developmental period, two, four, and finally six channels were used. When two or four channels were used, the necessity of manually changing the cuffs repeatedly and recalibrating after each change unduly prolonged the duration of the test and made it more complex. The use of six channels makes it possible to apply all the cuffs at once, calibrate into them all simultaneously, and run the test without interruption. It is desirable to have all the changes in the limb recorded simultaneously with respiratory movements measured directly from the thorax. This permits easy detection of breath-holding, exaggerated breathing,

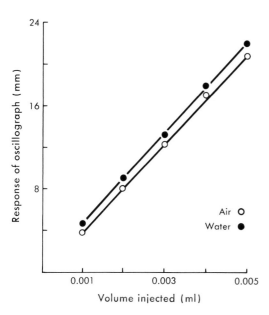

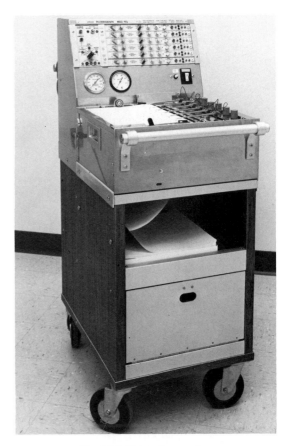

Fig. 16-2. Response of Grass PT 5 volume transducer to injection of minute amounts of air and water. Note minimal variations. This gauge is an accurate volumetric transducer.

Fig. 16-3. Phleborheograph.

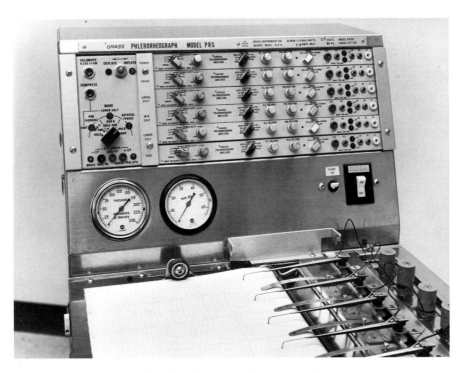

Fig. 16-4. Console of phleborheograph.

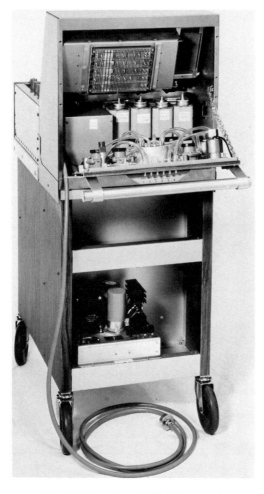

Fig. 16-5. Rear view of phleborheograph.

Cheyne-Stokes respiration, or sudden changes in respiratory movement in the nervous patient. Even though most patients report that the application of pressure is painless, occasionally a patient will take a quick breath each time pressure is applied. If this were not apparent in the respiratory tracing, one might be misled by the significance of the sudden rise in baseline on application of pressure.

Lower extremity technique

The first channel records directly from the thorax. The cuff for the second channel is placed on the thigh just above the knee. Three cuffs are placed in close proximity to each other on the proximal lower leg. The sixth cuff is placed on the foot. The first four channels record only the volume changes. The fifth and sixth channels are alternately used to record volume change or to apply pressure to the limb. Thus when the sixth cuff is being used to apply pressure to the foot, the fifth cuff as well as all those above it are recording volumetric changes. Similarly, when the fifth cuff is being used to apply pressure to the calf, the sixth cuff records volumetric changes in the foot. The cuffs used are all currently available blood pressure cuffs. The strap of the chest cuff has been lengthened to permit its use around the epigastrium. The cuff encircling the upper thigh also has been lengthened. We are currently using a cuff approximately twice as wide as the others for the foot.

After the cuffs have been applied, an automatic inflation sequence is activated that fills the cuffs until 10 mm Hg pressure is obtained, to ensure an adequate coupling between the cuff and the limb. A monitor lamp and a pressure gauge on the instrument panel indicate the inflation process. An additional lamp turns on when proper recording pressure has been reached. A paper speed of 2.5 mm/sec is usually selected for the phleborheogram. For pulse tracings a 25 mm/sec paper speed is used.

Calibration is volumetric. When the calibrating button is depressed, 0.2 cc of air is removed from each recording cuff. Amplification is adjusted so that the 0.2 cc of air results in a 2 cm downward deflection of the recording pen. By calibrating before each recording, one is able to compare the magnitude of the respiratory waves, the emptying of the foot, or the amplitude of the digital pulses accurately when the test is recorded at different periods of time and on different subjects.

Foot compression. There are two recording modes. With the selector switch on *Run A*, the sixth cuff is used for application of pressure to the foot, and all the other cuffs record volume changes. During the first period of the tracing the technician merely observes the respiratory waves then presses the *Compress* button. This delivers three short bursts of air to the sixth cuff. Currently we are using 100 mm Hg applied for approximately 0.5 second at intervals of 0.5 second. This pressure is monitored by a pressure gauge on the instrument panel and is measured at the source in the instrument. Approximately half this pressure is lost in the airway, and only 50 mm Hg pressure is delivered to the foot. This is not uncomfortable for the patient. In the normal subject, the baselines of the tracings of the limb remain level despite the application of pressure to the foot. In the patient with

DVT, compression of the foot cuff will cause congestion of blood in the limb and a rise in the baseline of the tracing.

Recently the baseline elevation has been redefined by Comerota et al. through work done in our laboratory.[4] The *absolute* baseline is defined as a plot of points connecting the minimum volume of each respiratory wave, and the *dynamic* baseline represents the normal volume of the extremity that is expected at any point during the respiratory wave. See Chapter 72 for further discussion on the diagnosis of DVT of the extremities.

Calf compression. At the completion of *Run A,* the cuffs are deflated and the mode switch moved to *Run B.* The cuffs are reinflated and the calibration is repeated. At this time, when the *Compress* button is pressed, pressure is applied to the lower calf. In this case 50 mm Hg is used as the source pressure, and approximately 30 mm Hg is delivered to the calf of the patient. Compression of the calf causes a rise in the baseline of the proximal tracings if there is obstruction of venous outflow. In addition, in the normal subject compression of the calf produces some degree of emptying of the foot, which is lessened or absent in the presence of DVT.

Ankle compression. While still in the *Run B* mode, the midcalf cuff (No. 5) is moved to ankle level and is used to deliver compressions. Cuffs 1 through 4 and 6 are used for recording the same as during calf compression (*Run B₁*). Compressions are identical to those used in *Run B₁* with regard to timing, duration, and pressure.

Once again, emptying of the foot is observed as in *Run B₁.* Unlike *Run B₁,* however, the midcalf recording does not usually fall. The baseline of this recording cuff and the others remains level. If there is obstruction to venous outflow a rise in baseline occurs. In addition, foot emptying may be reduced or absent.

Upper extremity technique

To record volume changes in the upper extremity, certain modifications are necessary. Recording cuffs are placed around the thorax, upper arm, and upper and middle forearm, along with a compression cuff on the wrist. The mode selector is turned to *Run B* and the wrist cuff is rapidly inflated to 50 mm Hg, producing compressions that pump the blood proximally. The proximal arm cuffs record any changes in volume that occur at rest or with these volume challenges. In the upper extremity,

respiratory waves can persist despite complete venous occlusion, probably because of rich venous collaterals around the shoulder. Therefore a diagnosis of upper extremity deep venous occlusion is usually based on the presence or absence of baseline rise alone.[24] Results are reported in Chapter 72.

A six-position *Function* switch on each phleborheograph amplifier adjusts the frequency response of the system to enhance the recording as desired. The *Resp* position enables the technician to effectively filter out the pulse waves and record only the respiratory waves.

The *PRG* position provides frequency response so that pulses and respiratory waves are recorded. In the *Pulse* position the respiratory waves are filtered, and amplification is automatically increased fivefold to detail the pulse contour.

The *ECG* position provides a high-frequency response suitable for reproducing the electrocardiogram, should that be desired. A special ECG amplifier can be obtained to facilitate the ECG recording. Two DC positions are provided to facilitate Doppler studies.

An input receptacle is included that permits the use of special photoelectric transducers for recording pulsations in the fingertip, the ear, or the supraorbital area. This receptacle also accepts a unidirectional or bidirectional Doppler velocity detector.

There has been a recent modification of the phleborheograph to make it more convenient to measure arterial pulsation. Because it measures volume changes accurately, the original phleborheograph was not convenient to measure arterial pulsations. The reason for this is that there are two volumetric changes going on in the normal limb at all times. One is the amplitude of the arterial pulsation, which is what one wishes to measure, and the other is the change in volume of the limb as a result of respiration, which causes the baseline to be unstable. This instability can be controlled by application of sufficient pressure to the proximal thigh to eliminate the respiratory waves.

Recently the phleborheograph was altered to do this. The recording cuff pressure is automatically set to 50 mm Hg and the amplifiers are set to display the arterial pulses. This combination effectively filters out the respiratory waves. The arterial pulse waves recorded are comparable to those obtained by other pulse volume recorders (Fig. 16-6). This

PVR PRG

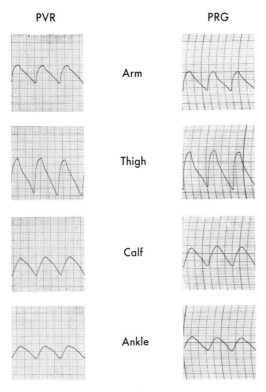

Arm

Thigh

Calf

Ankle

Fig. 16-6. Arterial pulse waves.

change enables the investigator to record from up to six sites simultaneously. The built-in volume calibrator used in the venous mode is also used in the arterial mode.

Other attachments make it possible to record segmental pressures on the phleborheograph by superimposing the arterial pulse, sensed by the Doppler ultrasound flow detector, on the cuff pressure waveform.

Finally, by using a rectal probe it is possible to assess the pulsatility of the arterial waves in the rectum and sigmoid for determination of the patency of the inferior mesenteric and hypogastric arteries (Fig. 16-7, *B*).

Fig. 16-7, *A*, is a tracing of some of the extended uses of the phleborheograph. In the first line it is being used as a digital plethysmograph with a finger oncometer. By this mechanism one can measure the amplitude of the digital pulses and relate them to the size of the enclosed finger by the water displacement method. This also may be used to measure blood flow by the venous occlusion method. The second tracing is that of the phleborheograph

being used in the *Pulse* position. This setting permits one to analyze pulse waves visually and measure the amplitude of the pulse wave volumetrically. The third line is a Doppler tracing with the blood flowing toward the probe in the foot, and the fourth line is a mercury-in-rubber strain-gauge tracing. The fifth line is the tracing of a digital pulse recording using a photoelectric transducer. On the sixth line an ECG module is in use. Fig. 16-7, *B*, shows the rectal probe in use to assess inferior mesenteric and hypogastric arteries.

If desired, the equipment can be used to detect venous occlusion by the maximum venous outflow method (Fig. 16-8). One or more channels may be used for recording the maximum venous outflow.

The maximum calibrated sensitivity of the phleborheograph in the *PRG* mode is 0.25 ml for fullscale pen deflection, or 50 mm. In the *Pulse* mode, sensitivity is increased to 0.05 ml full scale. With the sensitivity controls at maximum the overall system sensitivity can be increased to approximately 0.15 ml full scale in *PRG* mode and 0.03 ml full scale in the *Pulse* mode. Circuitry is also provided to facilitate connection to tape recorders and computers.

During the past 12 years at various stages of development, using first the research polygraph, then the earlier models, and finally the phleborheograph, in excess of 27,000 lower extremities have been studied at Good Samaritan Hospital.[4-10] It has been possible to obtain phlebograms on 748 extremities also studied with the phleborheograph. Our results (reported in Chapter 72) have been closely duplicated by others using the same technique.

The phleborheograph is an instrument specifically designed for the noninvasive diagnosis of DVT of the lower extremity. A modified technique is used for upper extremity diagnosis. It employs state-of-the-art electronics to achieve high sensitivity, is calibrated volumetrically after the cuffs have been applied to the patient, and delivers a uniform stimulus to all extremities simultaneously recording with six channels. It is highly versatile and may be used as an amplifier and direct-writing recorder for digital plethysmography or as a recording oscillometer. It may be used with the Doppler velocity detector, the mercury-in-rubber strain gauge, a photoelectric transducer, an ECG module if desired, or with a rectal probe. It is portable, of rugged construction, can be moved freely about the hospital, and is modular to permit easy servicing.

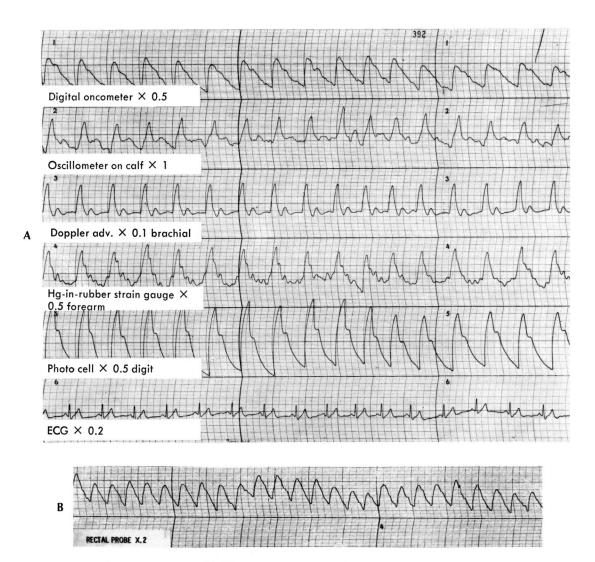

Digital oncometer × 0.5

Oscillometer on calf × 1

Doppler adv. × 0.1 brachial

Hg-in-rubber strain gauge × 0.5 forearm

Photo cell × 0.5 digit

ECG × 0.2

RECTAL PROBE X.2

Fig. 16-7. A, Extended uses of phleborheograph. In line 1 it is being used as digital plethysmograph with finger oncometer. By this mechanism one can measure amplitude of digital pulses and relate them to size of enclosed finger by water displacement method. This may also be used to measure blood flow by venous occlusion method. In line 2 phleborheograph is being used in *Pulse* position to record oscillations of the calf. In line 3 it is connected to bidirectional Doppler velocity detector with blood flowing toward probe. In line 4 phleborheograph is being used with mercury-in-rubber strain gauge recording oscillations of a limb. In line 5 it is being used with photocell placed on fingertip. In line 6 phleborheograph is being used with ECG module. *B,* Rectal probe in use to assess patency of inferior mesenteric and hypogastric arteries.

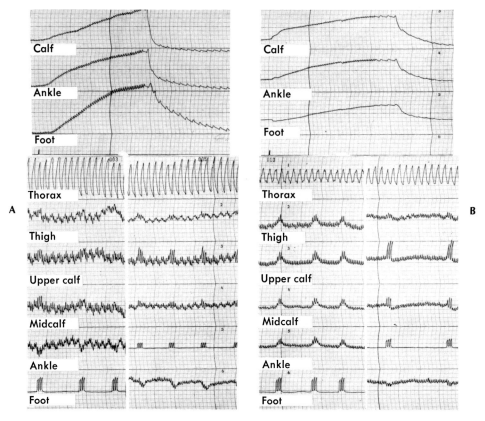

Fig. 16-8. A, Top, maximum venous outflow is shown for asymptomatic limb, with tracings of calf, ankle, and foot. Bottom, phleborheogram of same asymptomatic limb. *B,* Top, maximum venous outflow of patient with DVT involving femoroiliac area. Bottom, phleborheogram of same limb.

ACKNOWLEDGMENT

Throughout the developmental period of phleborheographic technique and instrumentation, consultation has been sought with F.A. Simeone, M.D., and A.M. Grass, Sc.D., on a continuing and active basis.

In addition, the following former and present Kachelmacher Research Fellows in Venous Diseases at Good Samaritan Hospital, Cincinnati, have all actively participated in and made significant contributions to the development of the phleborheograph: A.Y. Gay, Logan, Ohio; W.J. Sull, Sedalia, Missouri; A.J. Canos, Cincinnati; K. Mahalingam, Cincinnati; E.B. Ferris, Honolulu; S.L. House, Quincy, Illinois; A.J. Comerota, Temple University, Philadelphia; S.E. Cook, Bangor, Maine; L.J. Hyland, Dayton, Ohio; P.J. Sippel, Manitowoc, Wisconsin; E.D. Sullivan, New Haven, Connecticut; L.D. Flanagan and W.S. Karkow, Kachelmacher Memorial Laboratory for Venous Diseases, Good Samaritan Hospital, Cincinnati.

REFERENCES

1. Berry, M.R., et al.: A compensating plethysmograph for measuring blood flow in the extremities, J. Lab. Clin. Med. 33:101, 1948.
2. Brodie, T.G., and Russell, A.E.: On the determination of the rate of blood flow through an organ, J. Physiol. (Lond.) 32:47, 1905.
3. Burch, G.E.: A new sensitive portable plethysmograph, Am. Heart J. 33:48, 1947.
4. Comerota, A.J., et al.: Phleborehography—Results of a ten-year experience, Surgery 91:573, 1982.
5. Cranley, J.J.: Phleborheography, R.I. Med. J. 58(3):111, 1975.
6. Cranley, J.J.: Vascular surgery. 2. Peripheral venous diseases, New York, 1975, Harper & Row, Publishers.
7. Cranley, J.J.: Phleborheography. In Kempczinski, R.F., and Yao, J.S.T., editors: Practical noninvasive vascular diagnosis, Chicago, 1982, Year Book Medical Publishers, Inc.
8. Cranley, J.J., Canos, A.J., and Mahalingam, K.: Noninvasive diagnosis and prophylaxis of deep venous thrombosis of the lower extremities. In Madden, J.L., and Hume, M., editors: Venous thrombosis: prevention and treatment, New York, 1976, Appleton-Century-Crofts.
9. Cranley, J.J., et al.: A plethysmographic technique for the diagnosis of deep venous thrombosis of the lower extremities, Surg. Gynecol. Obstet. 136:385, 1973.

10. Cranley, J.J., et al.: Phleborheographic technique for diagnosing deep venous thrombosis of the lower extremities, Surg. Gynecol. Obstet. 141:331, 1975.
11. Ferris, E.B., and Abramson, D.L.: Description of a new plethysmograph, Am. Heart J. 19:233, 1940.
12. Freeman, N.E.: The effect of temperature on the rate of blood flow in the normal and in the sympathectomized hand, Am. J. Physiol. 113:384, 1935.
13. Goetz, R.H.: Plethysmography of the skin in the investigation of peripheral vascular diseases, Br. J. Surg. 27:506, 1940.
14. Grant, R.T., and Pearson, R.S.B.: The blood circulation in the human limb: observations on the differences between the proximal and distal parts and remarks on the regulation of body temperature, Clin. Sci. 3:119, 1938.
15. Herzman, A.B.: Photoelectric plethysmography of fingers and toes in man, Proc. Soc. Exp. Biol. Med. 37:529, 1937.
16. Hewlett, A.W., and van Zwaluwenburg, J.G.: The rate of blood flow in the arm, Heart 1:87-97, 1909.
17. Hyman, C., and Winsor, T.: History of plethysmography, J. Cardiovasc. Surg. 2:506, 1961.
18. Landowne, M., and Katz, L.N.: A critique of the plethysmographic method of measuring blood flow in the extremities of man, Am. Heart J. 23:644, 1942.
19. Lewis, T., and Grant, R.: Observations on reactive hyperemia in man, Heart 12:73, 1925.
20. Mackay, I.F.S., and McCarthy, G.: Measurement of venous valvular competency in the legs, J. Appl. Physiol. 12:329, 1958.
21. Mullick, S.C., Wheeler, H.B., and Songster, G.F.: Diagnosis of deep venous thrombosis by measurement of electrical impedance, Am. J. Surg. 119:417, 1970.
22. Sakaguchi, S., et al.: Functional plethysmography: a new venous function test, J. Cardiovasc. Surg. 9:87, 1968.
23. Simeone, F.A., et al.: An oscillographic plethysmograph using a new type of transducer, Science 116:355, 1952.
24. Sullivan, E.D., Reece, C.I., and Cranley, J.J.: Phleborheography of the upper extremity, Arch. Surg. 118:1134, 1983.
25. Wheeler, H.B., et al.: Diagnosis of occult deep vein thrombosis by a noninvasive bedside technique, Surgery 70:20, 1971.
26. Whitney, R.J.: Measurement of volume changes in human limbs, J. Physiol. (Lond.) 121:1, 1953.
27. Wilkins, R.W., Doupe, J., and Newman, H.W.: The rate of blood flow in normal fingers, Clin. Sci. 3:408, 1938.
28. Winsor, T., and Hyman, C.: Objective venous studies (insufficiency, obstruction and inflammation), J. Cardiovasc. Surg. 2:146, 1961.

CHAPTER 17

Mechanics of air plethysmography in arterial disease: the pulse volume recorder

JEFFREY K. RAINES

Plethysmography may be defined as the measurement of volume change. There are two general classes of plethysmographs: venous occlusion and segmental.

Venous occlusion plethysmography is a more time-consuming procedure that provides an estimate of limb or digit blood flow usually expressed in cubic centimeters per minute per 100 g of tissue.[1,9,10] This procedure is not described further in this chapter.

Segmental (limb and digit) plethysmographic recordings have proved to be important in the clinical evaluation of the peripheral arterial system. The segmental recordings are similar to the arterial pressure-pulse contour and reveal the degree of occlusive disease, an estimate of collateral circulation, anatomic localization of obstructive lesions, and indirectly, the level of perfusion. These measurements should not be confused with absolute blood flow, which segmental plethysmography does not measure. Plethysmographic data combined with clinical findings, segmental limb pressures, and treadmill exercise testing provide useful hemodynamic information necessary for the rational management of patients with peripheral disease.

The pulse volume recorder (PVR)* was developed through the combined efforts of the Massachusetts Institute of Technology and the Massachusetts General Hospital. It is a quantitative segmental plethysmograph designed for high sensitivity and clinical application.[2,6,7] It provides pulse volume recordings and systolic pressure measurements of the extremities, is adaptable to arterial

*Life Sciences, Inc., Greenwich, Conn.

measurements taken before and after exercise, and is capable of producing permanent records for reference. It may also be used to diagnose deep vein thrombosis in major veins of the lower and upper extremities and is now available with an attachment to measure opthalmic systolic artery pressure. Chapter 54 describes the practical clinical use of this instrument and gives examples of PVR recordings; the remainder of this chapter is devoted to describing the mechanics of the PVR.[5]

OPERATING PROCEDURE

To use the PVR, appropriate blood pressure cuffs are placed on the extremity or digit and a measured quantity of air (75 ± 10 cc) is injected until a preset pressure (65 mm Hg) is reached. This procedure ensures that, at a given pressure, the cuff volume surrounding the limb is constant from reading to reading. If this cuff setting (volume and pressure) is not met, the cuff must be reapplied at a slightly different tension. The PVR electronic package measures and records instantaneous pressure changes in the segmental monitoring cuff. Cuff pressure change reflects alteration in cuff volume, which in turn reflects momentary changes in limb volume. Cuffs are available in different sizes for all anatomic locations, including the digital level. They have a neoprene bladder surrounded by a nonelastic nylon Velcro band that allows easy application.

The PVR method is simpler than making volume calibrations with application of the cuff, as has been done with other instruments.[11] Similarly, it obviates mathematical corrections for volume and pressure changes and provides PVR recordings that can be visually compared with those previously obtained. PVR recordings are taken at a chart speed of 25 mm/sec.

The major components of the PVR are illustrated in Fig. 17-1. The electronic circuit includes a pressure-sensitive silicone NPN plantar transistor with its emitter-base junction mechanically coupled to a diaphragm.[4] A differential pressure applied to the diaphragm produces a large reversible change in the gain of the transistor, which has a uniform frequency response up to 150 kHz. Additional electronic components of the PVR include (1) a sample-and-hold circuit that operates in closed-loop fashion to maintain a proper operating point for the pressure sensor, (2) logic circuits that set solenoid valve configuration according to the mode selected by the operator, and (3) a dual-limit comparator that detects and corrects for excessive differential pressures applied to the sensor.

CALIBRATION

The PVR is calibrated so that a 1 mm Hg pressure change in the cuff provides a 20 mm chart deflection. If desired, maximum chart deflection may be translated (by means of cuff dynamics formulas) into volume change per cardiac cycle.

FREQUENCY RESPONSE

The frequency response of the complete device (cuff and electronic package) was tested by strapping a water-filled bladder around a rigid plastic cylinder, which in turn was encircled by an air-filled PVR monitoring cuff. A small piston-in-cylinder pump was then connected to the bladder to produce a sinusoidal pressure change in the monitoring cuff. The amplitude of these oscillations remained constant up to a pump frequency of 20 Hz, which is sufficient to evaluate the higher-frequency components of the human arterial pressure-pulse contour accurately.[3]

LINEARITY

The linearity of the system was tested by measuring cuff pressure changes as a function of cuff volume changes. This was studied over a range of mean cuff pressures varying from 20 to 200 mm Hg and with injected cuff volumes varying from 20 to 125 cc. Within the range studied, cuff pressure change was indeed a linear function of cuff volume change. This study also points out the importance of taking clinical readings at consistent cuff pressures and volumes.

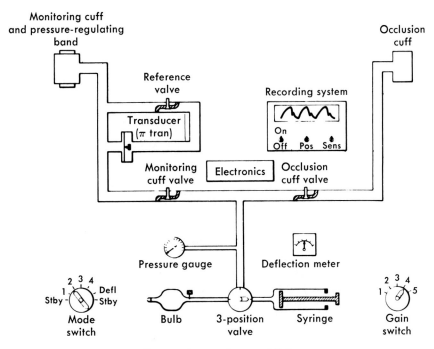

Fig. 17-1. System diagram of PVR.

CUFF DYNAMICS

To aid in the development of the PVR operating procedure and the interpretation of its recordings, it was important to understand how the pressure of the air in the cuff related to the arterial pressure and limb volume changes. To accomplish this a number of experiments and analyses were performed.[5]

First, consider a constant mass of air in the cuff at an absolute pressure p_c in a volume V_c. Furthermore, if it is assumed that the gas undergoes an isentropic process, the following equation may be written

$$p_c V_c^\gamma = \text{Constant} \tag{1}$$

where γ is the ratio of specific heats (for air, $\gamma = 1.4$).

To test the validity of the isentropic assumption, the pressure-measuring components of the PVR were connected to a rigid cylinder (50 cc volume). Also included in the pneumatic circuit was a small piston-in-cylinder pump with a 1 cc stroke volume. The pump was used to oscillate the total volume of the system at various frequencies while measuring the pressure changes. It was found that at frequencies from 0.25 to 20 Hz (highest frequency tested) the pressure amplitude remained constant. The pressure amplitude increased approximately 34% gradually from zero frequency (isothermal) to 0.25 Hz. This experiment suggests that in the range of primary frequencies encountered in clinical use (0.5 to 1.5 Hz) the air in the cuff undergoes an isentropic process, changing from isothermal to isentropic between zero and 0.25 Hz. It can be shown that the identification of the process is not critical to the analysis, since its effect is combined with the elastic expansion of the cuff. Since the volume excursions in the cuff are a small fraction (2% maximum) of its mean volume, equation 1 can be differentiated to give

$$\delta p_c = \frac{-\gamma \bar{p}_c}{\bar{V}_c} \delta V_c \tag{2}$$

where p_c and V_c have been replaced by their time-mean values $\bar{p}_c$ and $\bar{V}_c$, respectively. The time-mean volume $\bar{V}_c$ is also a function of cuff pressure and the injected air mass. If the initial volume of air injected at atmospheric pressure (P_{ATM}) is V_I, the volume of air in the cuff is defined by equation 3:

$$\bar{V}_c = \frac{P_{ATM}}{\bar{p}_c}(V_I + V_1 + V_2) - V_2 \tag{3}$$

Here V_1 is the tube volume from an internal shutoff valve in the PVR to the monitoring cuff; V_2 represents the tube volume from the shutoff valve to the syringe. V_1 and V_2 are 21 and 22 cc, respectively. The compression of the injected air is assumed to be isothermal, since it subsists for a long period of time, much longer than 4 seconds (0.25 Hz). Combining equations 2 and 3 we find

$$\delta p_c = \frac{-\gamma \delta V_c \bar{p}_c}{(P_{ATM}/\bar{p}_c [V_I + V_1 + V_2] - V_2)} \tag{4}$$

To investigate the validity of equation 4 another experiment was performed. The monitoring cuff was connected to the PVR electronics with a 1 cc syringe also in the pneumatic circuit. The syringe was used to change the total air volume in increments of 0.25 cc from 0.25 to 1 cc at different cuff pressures and initial injected volumes. Cuff gauge pressures at 20, 40, 60, 80, and 100 mm Hg were used with injected volumes of 25, 50, 75, and 100 cc. The results of this experiment indicated that the bladder constrained by the nylon Velcro band is not inextensible but instead expands with pressure over the monitoring cycle. The edges and corners of the bladder that are not constrained by the cuff may move and make additional volume available. The actual volume change of the air in the bladder δV_x resulting from the expansion of the cuff is defined by

$$\delta V_x = \delta V - \delta V_c \tag{5}$$

where δV is the volume change applied to the cuff.

The ratio of $\delta V_x/\delta V$ varies with mean cuff pressures and injected volumes.[5] It is interesting to note that the extrapolations of the measurements to $p_c \to 0$ leads to $\delta V_x = \delta V$, and that even at high cuff pressures the expansion is still present but to a lesser degree as the bladder becomes stiffer. The fact that wrapping an inextensible band around the cuff does not change the results suggests that end effects, not the stretching of the bladder, are the dominant factors. This observation suggests that the sensitivity of the PVR may be considerably improved by designing a cuff that absorbs all the limb volume change.

Clinical practice has indicated improved sensitivity is not necessary; slightly modified blood pressure cuffs are adequate. Including the results of the preceding experiment, we rewrite equation 4 as

$$\delta p_c = \frac{-\gamma \delta V \left(1 - \frac{\delta V_x}{\delta V}\right)}{\left[\frac{(P_{ATM}/\bar{p}_c [V_I + V_1 + V_2] - V_2)}{\bar{p}_c}\right]} \tag{6}$$

Equation 6 defines the relationship of limb volume change (δV) and cuff pressure change (δp_c).

It is of interest to continue the analysis and define the relationship of cuff pressure to arterial pressure. Assume that the volume changes of the limb caused by the passage of the pressure pulse are proportional to the changes in the arterial volume δV_a encompassed by the cuff. This has been shown to be true, even in the edematous limb. We write

$$\delta V = \delta V_a = C_a \, \delta p_a \qquad (7)$$

where $C_a = \delta V_a/\delta p_a$ is the compliance of the arterial section surrounded by the cuff and p_a denotes the arterial pressure. Combining equations 6 and 7:

$$\delta p_c = \frac{\gamma C_a \, \delta p_a \left(1 - \frac{\delta V_x}{\delta V}\right)}{\left[\frac{(P_{ATM}/\bar{p}_c \, [V_1 + V_1 + V_2] - V_2)}{\bar{p}_c}\right]} \qquad (8)$$

Since $\delta V_x/\delta V$ is approximately independent of δV, it follows from equation 8 that if C_a remains constant, the variations in the cuff pressure are proportional to the variations in arterial pressure, and the output of the pressure-sensitive transistor will yield a good representation of the arterial pressure-pulse contour. The critical experiment to test the accuracy of this analysis is, of course, the comparison with direct intraarterial measurements. This comparison has been made with excellent correlation and is provided in Chapter 54.

DIAGNOSTIC INDICES

A number of important diagnostic parameters are contained in the pulse volume recordings.

The amplitude of the pulse volume recording with a constant pneumatic and electronic gain is a function of local pulse pressure, segmental arterial compliance, and the number of arterial vessels in the segment under investigation. These are all affected by the development of arteriosclerotic disease. Reduced pulse pressure and obliterated arterial channels are major hemodynamic parameters that affect functional perfusion.

Since the pulse volume contour is linked to the pressure-pulse contour (equation 8), the shape of the pulse volume contour contains useful hemodynamic information. Contour alterations are largely the result of changes in terminal reflection coefficients, which are a function of peripheral resistance. Peripheral resistance changes to compensate for fixed arterial resistance caused by obstructive lesions. This phenomenon has been previously described.[5,7]

SUMMARY

This chapter has described the engineering development and mechanics of the PVR; its clinical application to arterial periperal vascular disease is outlined in Chapter 54.[8]

REFERENCES

1. Clarke, R.S., and Heilon, R.F.: Venous collection in forearm and hand measured by the strain-gauge and volume plethysmograph, Clin. Sci. 16:103, 1957.
2. Darling, R.C., et al.: Quantitative segmental pulse volume recorder: a clinical tool, Surgery 72:873, 1972.
3. Geddes, L.A.: The direct and indirect measurements of blood pressure, Chicago, 1970, Year Book Medical Publishers, Inc.
4. Pitran specifications, Stow Laboratories, 1969, Hudson, Mass.
5. Raines, J.K.: Diagnosis and analysis of arteriosclerosis in the lower limbs from the arterial pressure pulse, doctoral dissertation, Cambridge, Mass., 1972, Massachusetts Institute of Technology.
6. Raines, J.K., Jaffrin, M.Y., and Rao, S.: A noninvasive pressure-pulse recorder: development and rationale, Med. Instrum. 7:245, 1973.
7. Raines, J.K., Jaffrin, M.Y., and Shapiro, A.H.: A computer simulation of arterial dynamics in the human leg, J. Biomech. 7:77, 1974.
8. Raines, J.K., et al.: Vascular laboratory criteria for the management of peripheral vascular disease of the lower extremities, Surgery 79:21, 1976.
9. Strandness, D.E., Jr., and Bell, J.W.: Peripheral vascular disease. Diagnosis and objective evaluation using a mercury strain-gauge, Ann. Surg. 161(suppl.):1, 1965.
10. Whitney, R.J.: The measurement of volume changes in human limbs, J. Physiol. 121:1, 1963.
11. Winsor, T., et al.: Peripheral pulse contours in arterial occlusive disease, Vasc. Dis. 5:61, 1968.

CHAPTER 18

Oculoplethysmography: timed comparison of ocular pulses and carotid phonoangiography

LORIN P. McRAE and MARK M. KARTCHNER

Cerebral ischemia secondary to extracranial carotid occlusive disease is of particular interest among the various causes of stroke because it is often amenable to early detection and surgical correction before the onset of disabling neurologic consequences. Other stroke-causing disease processes such as cerebral embolus, cerebral hemorrhage, and brain tumor are no less significant but may not be as readily detected or managed before the onset of neurologic deficits as is extracranial carotid occlusive disease.

The success of noninvasive tests designed for the early detection and evaluation of extracranial carotid occlusive disease depends on the safety, accuracy, and reproducibility with which they evaluate changes in internal carotid blood flow. Oculoplethysmography has been extensively used in clinical applications, is simple to perform, and is sufficiently accurate to provide considerable assistance in the detection and evaluation of clinically significant carotid occlusive disease. Carotid phonoangiography has been used in conjunction with oculoplethysmography to enhance the overall test accuracy and is particularly helpful in following the progression of carotid lesions.

THEORY

Oculoplethysmography: pulse-wave phase shift

There is a continuous, relatively constant drainage of blood from the eyes through the veins. However, the flow of blood into the globe of the eye is pulsatile, resulting in continuous cyclic variations in the net volume of blood within the globe. These pulsatile variations in volume give rise to oculoplethysmography (OPG), the graphic representation of eye volume changes.

Many medical professionals tend to equate the words *pulse* and *pressure*. It should be emphasized that the pulses recorded by OPG represent volumetric pulsations of the eye that cannot be equated with intraocular, retinal, or ophthalmic artery pressures. Intraocular pressures measured by tonometry[1] and retinal or ophthalmic artery pressures as determined by compression or suction ophthalmodynamometry[10-12] have clinical value but should not be equated with the volumetric pulses obtained by direct OPG.

During diastole the venous outflow from the eye is greater than the arterial inflow, and thus the volume and diameter of the ocular globe decrease. As the heart contracts and the rate of arterial blood flow into the eye increases, the volume of the eye will begin to increase when the rate of inflow exceeds the rate of venous drainage. Furthermore, the rate at which the globe expands or contracts at any instant of time is directly related to the difference in rates of inflow and outflow of blood from the eye. Proximal arterial occlusive disease, which reduces the rate of blood flow into the eye during systole, results in a small delay before inflow exceeds outflow, causing the globe to begin to expand. This also results in prolongation of the total time required for the eye to reach its maximum expansion (Fig. 18-1).

For further clarification it should be noted that the initiation of the movement of blood in both right and left ophthalmic arteries in response to a heart contraction will be virtually instantaneous with no appreciable time difference, regardless of the presence of proximal arterial stenosis. However, the volumetric pulse obtained by OPG is responsive not to this initial movement of blood but only to the expansion of the globe when enough

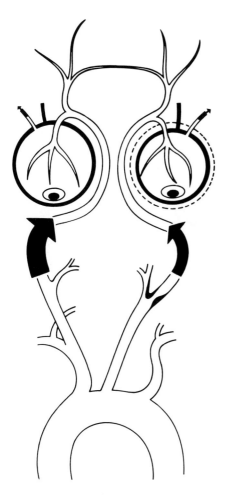

Fig. 18-1. Conceptual representation of slower expansion of left ocular globe during early systole as result of reduced arterial inflow secondary to proximal arterial stenosis.

blood has entered the eye to cause an increase in volume.

Abnormal vascularization within the eye, scar tissue, or other eye pathology that limits the capacity of the eye to expand and contract in response to pulsatile arterial blood flow will limit the size or amplitude of the volumetric variations with each heartbeat. Thus reduction in ocular pulse amplitude is most commonly associated with eye pathology and not with proximal arterial occlusive disease. However, in cases of severe proximal arterial stenosis with poorly developed collateral circulation, insufficient blood may arrive at the eye during the cardiac cycle to cause full expansion; therefore an ocular pulse amplitude reduction will be noted *in association with a marked delay.* In many cases involving the natural evolution of atherosclerotic arterial occlusive disease there is enough collateral

circulation to prevent ocular pulse amplitude reduction, and only delays are noted (Fig. 18-2). Bilateral ocular pulse amplitude reduction most often results from low cardiac output or cerebral edema and cannot be assumed to imply internal carotid stenosis unless noted in conjunction with ocular pulse delay.

Even in the case of total internal carotid or common carotid occlusion, it is not the small additional distance that blood must flow through collateral arteries to reach the eye that causes a delay. The delay in ocular pulses as recorded by OPG is the result of reduced pulsatile flow through the smaller collateral arteries. There are documented cases of congenital absence of a common carotid artery or long-standing total occlusion of an internal carotid artery in which the collateral circulation is adequate to completely eliminate any measurable ocular pulse delay. In a patient with acute occlusion of an internal carotid artery and the capacity to develop collateral circulation, the retinal artery pressures are the first to equalize; next, volumetric pulse amplitudes tend to equalize[18]; and in exceptional cases, enough collateral circulation develops to eliminate ocular pulse delays.

Technical considerations in the measurement and recording of volumetric ocular pulses can and occasionally do cause changes in pulse amplitude and timing. In our experience, changes in volumetric pulse amplitude resulting from technical considerations are much more common than are variations in ocular pulse timing. Since ocular pulse amplitude variations so often result from factors unrelated to carotid stenosis, earlier attempts by others to use pulse amplitude alone as an indication of stenosis have produced inconstant and unreliable results.

Random micro-eye-movement artifact often makes difficult to visually detect and reliably measure ocular pulse delays. With the current method a continuous differential waveform is generated by electronically subtracting the left ocular pulse from the right and amplifying the difference. The pulsatile amplitude and phase shift of this differential tracing is used to identify ocular pulse phase shift or delay that may not be apparent by direct visual examination of the ocular pulses alone. Equally important is the ease with which a *flat* differential trace without cardiac-related pulsation demonstrates the absence of unilateral ocular pulse delay despite apparent time difference resulting from micro-eye-movement artifact (Fig. 18-2).

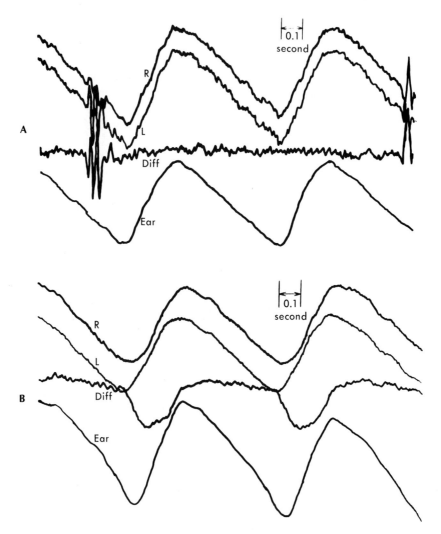

Fig. 18-2. Samples of ocular pulses. *A,* Normal equal amplitudes and timing. *B,* Delay with equal amplitude resulting from severe right arteriosclerotic internal carotid stenosis.

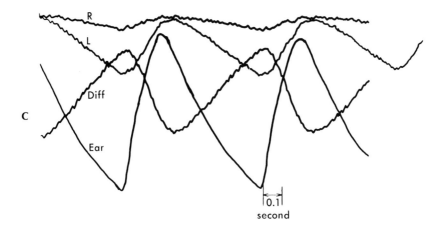

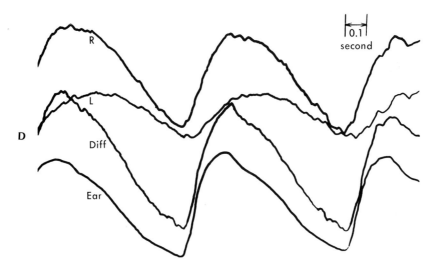

Fig. 18-2, cont'd. C, Amplitude reduction with no delay resulting from old right eye injury. *D,* Delay with amplitude reduction 2 days after total left common carotid occlusion as result of trauma.

The formation of the differential trace is achieved by electronically processing the right and left ocular pulse waveforms in accordance with the equation

$$Diff(t) = 2[R(t) - L(t)] + K$$

where

Diff(t) = Differential as a function of time
R(t) = Right ocular pulse as a function of time
L(t) = Left ocular pulse as a function of time
K = Constant allowing for arbitrary vertical positioning of the differential trace, that is, the reference zero for the differential trace

Thus the differential trace depends on subtraction or the algebraic difference of the amplitude of the simultaneously recorded ocular pulses at every instant of time. The multiplication factor of 2 in the differential equation has been empirically established for emphasis of the commonly encountered variations in ocular pulses. Fig. 18-3 shows the generation of differential traces corresponding to six representative combinations of right and left ocular pulses. The difference, R(t) − L(t), is represented by small arrows, positive values being upward, for specific convenient instances of time. It should be noted that the entire differential pulse can be determined graphically by the use of these arrows at a sufficient number of points along the time axis.

Obviously, there are innumerable differential trace variations corresponding to the different ocular pulse contour, amplitude, and timing combinations. However, as with grossly normal and abnormal ECG traces, the more classic differential traces are readily recognized. The flat differential trace of Fig. 18-3, A, reflects identical ocular pulses without delay or amplitude differences. The markedly skewed differential traces of Fig. 18-3, C and D, occur when pulse amplitudes are equal but one pulse is delayed relative to the other. Greater cau-

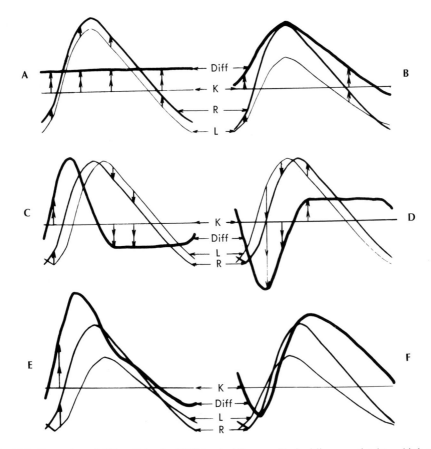

Fig. 18-3. Generation of differential pulse (Diff) by doubling amplitude difference of right and left ocular pulses, 2 × (R − L), about arbitrarily selected baseline (K). **A,** No ocular pulse delay or amplitude difference. **B,** Amplitude reduction of left pulse. **C,** Left pulse delay. **D,** Right pulse delay. **E,** Left pulse delay and left amplitude reduction. **F,** Right pulse delay with left pulse amplitude reduction.

tion is required to distinguish the time-aligned differential pulses of Fig. 18-3, *B,* resulting from ocular pulse amplitude reduction without pulse delay from the differential traces of Fig. 18-3, *E* and *F,* which result when the difference in pulse amplitude and timing are both present. The former are characteristic of ocular pathology or technical error, whereas the latter are indicative of severe internal carotid flow reduction. Similar to ECG analysis, expertise in OPG interpretation can only be achieved by continued use and practice. The continual comparison of ocular pulses represented by the differential trace minimizes the error inherent in a single time measurement.

Carotid phonoangiography: the audiovisual analysis of cervical bruits

Turbulent blood flow occurring at points of narrowing in the arterial system often causes bruits. Generally, for a given rate of blood flow, the greater the degree of localized arterial stenosis, the more intense and high pitched is the resulting bruit. Microphonic auscultation of bruits, oscilloscopic visualization of the audio frequency waveforms of these sounds, and photographic recording of the waveforms over the cervical carotid arteries constitute carotid phonoangiography (CPA).[5,15]

Bruits are primarily noted during systole because of the increased blood flow during cardiac contraction. Since both adequate blood flow and a localized arterial stenosis are required to produce sufficient turbulence to create an audible bruit, bruits often disappear as internal carotid stenosis exceeds 80% to 90%, because of reduced blood flow. Similarly, marked bruits may be noted in arteries with minimal stenosis, because of turbulence caused by increased blood flow secondary to an arteriovenous fistula or contralateral arterial occlusion and greater flow through the patent arteries. Clinically insignificant bruits are often encountered over the arteries of young patients without arterial stenosis and are caused only by the turbulent flow created at arterial bifurcations.

Bruits observed over the carotid bifurcation that extend throughout systole and into diastole represent a marked pressure gradient across an internal carotid stenosis, since external carotid blood flow during diastole is rarely associated with bruits, regardless of the degree of localized stenosis. Carotid bifurcation bruits extending into diastole often reflect more severe contralateral stenosis or total occlusion and greater blood flow on the side of the observed diastolic bruit.

Bruits that are present at all locations along the cervical carotid are often not of carotid origin but rather radiate up from the aortic arch. The relative amplitude or intensity of carotid bruits along the neck is not a good indicator of the source of the bruit. The amplitude of the bruit reflects the placement and proximity of the microphone or stethoscope relative to the underlying artery. An increase in duration or frequency (density) of the bruit as one proceeds up the neck is a good indication that the carotid bifurcation is its primary source (Fig. 18-4).

We have been using *split-trace* CPA recording since 1977, and similar units have been commercially available for several years. With this technique, the upper half of each trace is replaced with a filtered, amplified version of the original trace. This processed signal results in a video trace more representative of what can be heard, a desirable result because the ear is much more sensitive to the higher range of the bruit frequency spectra. Fig. 18-5 shows the same high-pitched bruit recorded with and without the split-trace feature. The split-trace recordings (1) allow clear visualization of some high-pitched bruits that are easily heard but are lost in the baseline artifact of other CPA recordings, (2) clearly demonstrate the extension of some bruits into diastole when the diastolic extension is not obvious by auscultation or standard CPA visual representations, (3) provide definite external carotid identification of some high-pitched, short duration bruits, and (4) help localize the source of bruit in many cases where bruit is found at all positions along the neck.

It will be assumed in subsequent discussions of OPG studies and their interpretation that CPA recordings are available to the physician making the OPG-CPA evaluation.

Light opacity earlobe plethysmography: external carotid volumetric pulses

Since the volume of blood in the earlobe varies cyclically with arterial pulsations, variations in light transmission through the earlobe can be sensed and processed to produce graphic representations of volumetric pulses associated with external carotid flow. In contrast to the eye, in which the vascular bed and initial volume under consideration are well defined, the earlobe produces great variations in light opacity pulses. Variations are observed resulting from earclip placement and varying degrees of vasodilation secondary to temperature, earlobe massage, and even the emotional

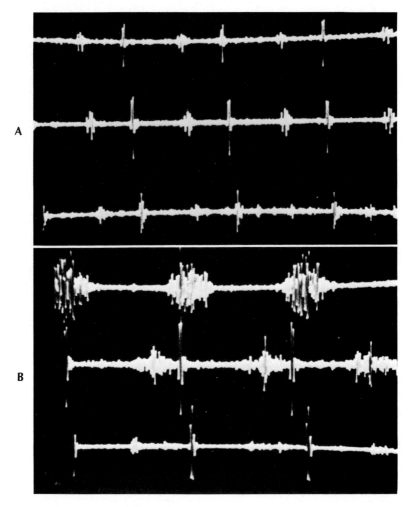

Fig. 18-4. *A,* Samples of normal "lubb-dupp" heart sounds over cervical carotid artery. *B,* Bruit throughout systole indicating significant carotid stenosis.

state of the patient. Because of the wide variations in pulse amplitude, timing of the peaks of the pulses, and the general pulse shape or morphology, these ear pulse features are not generally useful for diagnosing proximal arterial occlusive disease. Therefore only the relative timing of the initial increase in blood volume under the earclip, as indicated by an upswing in the ear pulse, can be used for evaluating external carotid circulation.

Although extensive arteriographic correlation or invasive blood flow measurements have not been performed to determine the correlation of ear pulse timing and proximal arterial occlusive disease, marked ear pulse delays of greater than 40 msec reliably indicate moderate to severe ipsilateral external carotid stenosis. However, stenosis or occlusion of the proximal external carotid artery may not result in a delay of the ipsilateral ear pulse.

This is because of the extremely rich collateral circulation common in the external carotid vascular system.

Ear pulse timing of external carotid circulation was initiated to establish a reference baseline for measuring bilateral ocular pulse delays in patients with severe bilateral carotid flow reduction. Although reasonable success has been achieved in detecting severe bilateral internal carotid flow reduction, an added bonus has been the detection of external carotid stenosis as the source of approximately 5% of asymptomatic carotid bruits.

As with bruits recorded by CPA, it will also be assumed henceforth that bilateral ear pulse recordings are available as an integral part of the study procedure. The complementary values of CPA and ear pulses to OPG are illustrated in the test results shown in Fig. 18-6.

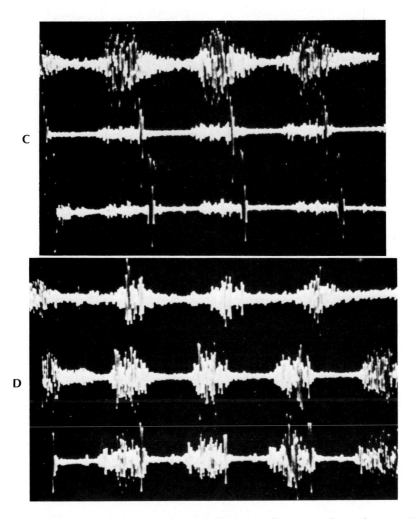

Fig. 18-4—cont'd. C, Bruit extending into diastole indicating significant *internal* carotid stenosis. *D,* Bruit radiating from aortic arch as noted by greatest duration at base of neck (bottom trace).

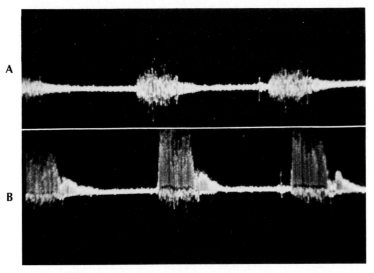

Fig. 18-5. High-pitched bruit extending into diastole recorded *A,* without and *B,* with split-trace high-frequency enhancement.

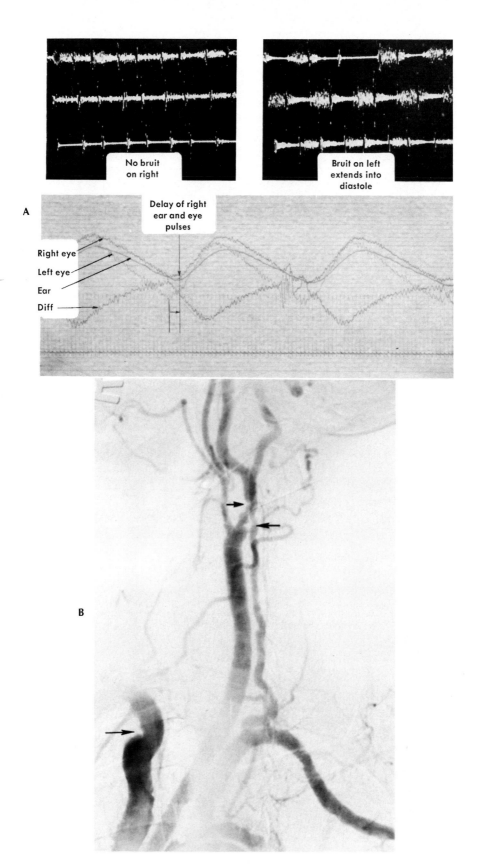

Fig. 18-6, A, Complementary OPG and CPA studies showing right eye and ear pulse delay but diastolic bruit from left carotid. **B,** Confirming arteriograph with arrows identifying severely constricting atherosclerotic lesions.

METHODOLOGY
OPG technique: past and present

The majority of the volumetric ocular pulse waveform recordings used to establish and document the pulse delay concept of OPG have been obtained from fluid-filled corneal suction cups held in place on the cornea by mild suction, varying from 25 to 70 mm Hg.[17] Currently, 40 to 50 mm Hg suction is used. An increase in the volume of the eye causes the cornea to withdraw from the suction cup, producing an increase in negative pressure or suction within the cup. Pressure variations in the suction cups from 1 to 8 mm Hg in response to pulsatile variations of ocular volume are currently recorded at a vertical sensitivity of 0.5 mm Hg/cm (or 1 mm Hg/cm when needed) and at a paper speed of 10 cm/sec. To date, no attempt has been made in our laboratory to establish a correlation coefficient between the incremental pressure changes noted in the suction cup and the corresponding incremental changes in retinal artery pressures or the incremental changes in total eye volume. Although this would be an interesting project with potential rewards, such a correlation is not required when considering the relative timing of the ocular pulses.

Initially using an adaptation of the fluid-filled system in a dry or air-filled mode, several hundred patients were tested using both the fluid-filled and air-filled systems for comparative ocular pulse recordings. The ocular pulses obtained by the two systems were acceptably similar in most patients (Fig. 18-7). Depending on the volume of air space in the closed eyecup system, higher frequency components of the waveforms are filtered and additional electronic amplification is required. Filtering and amplification tend to decrease the micro-eye-movement and increase the artifact from large eye movements in air-system recordings as compared to fluid systems. The high-frequency filtering also diminishes the distinct flattening of the pulse troughs found in cases of severe bilateral carotid stenosis.

The conveniences of an air-filled system (minimal preparation, maximum portability, and supine testing) have led to its common adoption for new installations. An air-filled system with appropriate response and calibration produces ocular pulse and differential waveform recordings sufficiently comparable to a fluid system for diagnostic purposes. Our experience suggests that simplified systems, without recordings, relying on numerical values for pulse delays, are prone to errors that may have significant clinical consequences.

Testing with a fluid-filled OPG system is most

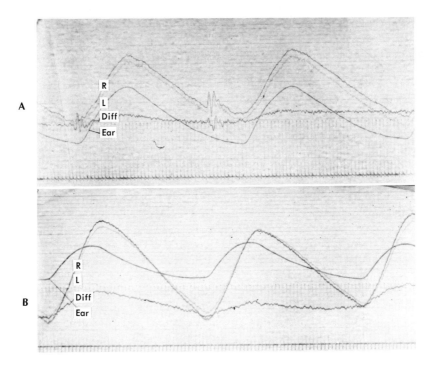

Fig. 18-7. Comparison of ocular pulses recorded from ***A,*** fluid-filled system and ***B,*** air-filled system.

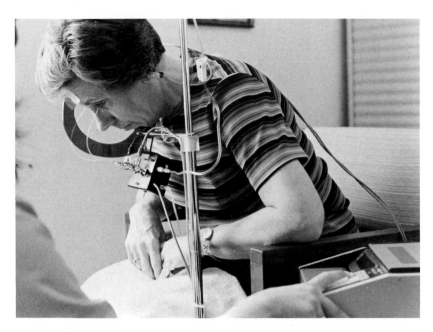

Fig. 18-8. Normal fluid-filled OPG procedure.

easily accomplished when the patient is seated with the head supported in a forward position and the eyes focused downward. This permits the eyecups to be filled with fluid and applied to the corneas with minimum possibility of air bubble entrapment (Fig. 18-8). Testing of supine patients can be performed with only slightly greater inconvenience by flooding the eyewells with fluid as the edge of the cup is placed at the lateral margin of the cornea. The cup is subsequently rotated slowly over the cornea as the fluid forces all air from the inner surface of the cup (Fig. 18-9). By way of contrast, in an air-filled system the cups are most easily applied with the patient in the supine position, since the greatest potential for error is tear or fluid droplets that may be sucked into the tubing and cause amplitude reduction or delay of the corresponding ocular pulses.

Initially, a frequency response of over 200 Hz was used for recording ocular pulses[16] with a subsequent reduction to 30 Hz without noticeable degradation of the diagnostic qualities of the pulses. Also, carbon dioxide was used to preflush the system before filling with fluid to eliminate microbubbles. Subsequently, with the reduction in frequency response, microbubbles were no longer detrimental to test results. Normal saline solution was used as a fluid medium, but subsequent evaluations have revealed no adverse effects when distilled water is employed. The use of distilled water in place of saline solution results in less residual deposit and equipment corrosion. The exact suction level used to hold the corneal cups in place is not critical. It is desirable, however, to use equal suction in both cups on a given patient to minimize differences in the amplitude of the ocular pulses.

Measurements of the absolute time interval from the R wave of the ECG complex to the initiation of the upward deflection of the ocular pulse and to the peak of the ocular pulse have been taken from approximately 2000 patients. The R wave to ocular pulse interval has been so variable and dependent on parameters other than carotid occlusive disease that it is of little value in assessing internal carotid flow reduction.

Temporal artery compression was evaluated and found to be of no particular value in conjunction with the relative timing of the ocular pulses by OPG. Physician-applied carotid compression in conjunction with the OPG phase delay concept has been evaluated for a limited number of patients. In a group of eight patients with unilateral total internal carotid occlusion, OPG with carotid compression revealed the primary source of collateral circulation, that is, ipsilateral external or contralateral internal carotid artery, but the carotid compression also resulted in one case of severe bradycardia. OPG is designed for the detection and evaluation of extracranial carotid occlusive disease in screening patients for carotid arteriography, and

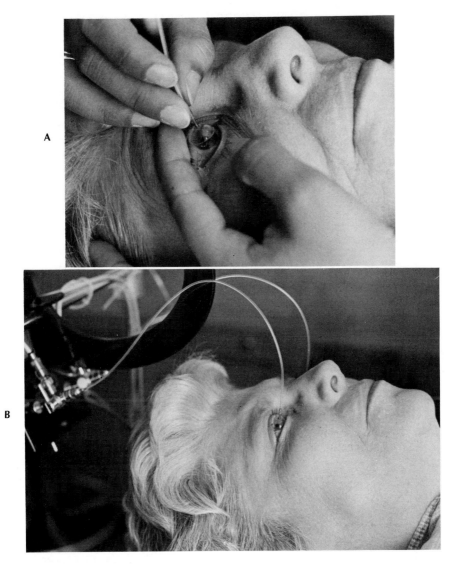

Fig. 18-9. OPG testing of supine patient. ***A,*** Suction cup placement. ***B,*** Both cups applied.

the additional information obtained by arterial compression does not enhance the clinical value of the OPG study. Therefore arterial compression is not recommended in conjunction with this test.

Topical anesthesia is applied to each eye for patient comfort before insertion of the corneal suction cups. Also, in the fluid-filled system, the fluid is warmed to body temperature, since the eyes have a high sensitivity to cool fluid, which produces a tendency to withdraw and blink.

Testing procedure

The normal procedure of OPG testing is to first take bilateral brachial blood pressures to detect those patients in whom a marked reduction of pres-

sure indicates subclavian artery occlusion with a possible subclavian steal. The patient is placed supine without a pillow, with the chin slightly extended and rotated to obtain the best exposure over the cervical carotids for auscultation. With the CPA unit in use, audio and visual scans along the course of the cervical carotid artery reveal the presence and relative degree of bruit. Three traces are photographed from each side of the neck, the first at the highest possible position over the palpable cervical carotid, the second from the estimated site of the carotid bifurcation or maximum bruit, and the third at the base of the neck just above the clavicle. The patient is asked not to breathe during the 5 seconds required for each trace. The three audio

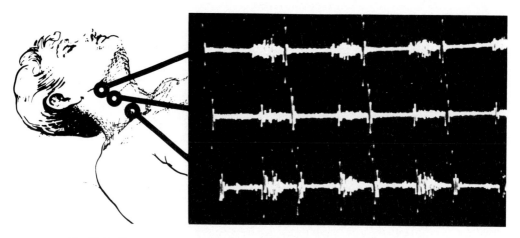

Fig. 18-10. Three traces corresponding to three positions along cervical carotid artery.

frequency waveform traces from one side of the neck are recorded at corresponding positions on a single photograph (Fig. 18-10). The procedure is then repeated on the opposite side of the neck. Since tense neck muscles, breathing, or other patient movement produces noise that degrades the quality of the studies, every effort should be made to provide for patient comfort and to solicit patient cooperation. Hyperventilation assists in helping some patients hold their breath, thereby eliminating breathing artifact during the interval required for photographing the oscilloscopic traces.

On termination of the CPA portion of the test, anesthetic eyedrops are applied and the OPG performed. The patient is generally moved to a chair before fluid OPG, but left in the supine position if air OPG is used. In either case, when the patient sits up on the edge of the bed, support should be provided to avoid patient collapse as a result of momentary cerebral ischemia. This caution is advised because the patients under consideration often experience dizziness on arising from a supine position, especially after having hyperventilated or if experiencing cerebral ischemia as a result of carotid occlusive disease.

A simple ongoing explanation of the procedure is valuable in soliciting patient cooperation throughout the OPG test. The earlobes are briefly massaged to enhance circulation, and the light opacity earclips are applied. After amplitudes of the pulses from the two earlobes are adjusted, a 5-second trace of earlobe pulses is recorded. Variations in ambient light intensity will appear on the ear pulse recording; therefore movement in the vicinity of the patient is to be avoided. Also, there

is a definite strobing effect from most fluorescent light fixtures that may be sensed as artifact by the light opacity detectors.

The patient is then requested to focus on some object to maintain eyeball stability. The eyecups are applied to each anesthetized cornea following the prescribed protocol for the OPG system being used. The two ocular pulses, the right earlobe pulse, and the electronically generated differential trace are simultaneously recorded for approximately 10 seconds. With the patient in the same position the procedure is repeated, but with the eyecups crossed to the opposite eye for confirmation of the technical adequacy of the study. This additional step takes less than a minute for a trained technician and greatly enhances the reliability of the test recordings.

The technical quality of the study is determined by the nurse or technician, and all photographs and recordings are appropriately identified for subsequent physician evaluation. The patient is cautioned to avoid rubbing or abusing the eyes for an hour to allow for complete cessation of the anesthetic effect. The entire testing procedure is generally accomplished in less than 10 minutes.

Patient acceptance of the testing procedure has been excellent with no absolute contraindications. Testing is generally deferred in patients with obvious eye infection, recent eye surgery, or detached retina until cleared by an ophthalmologist.

Interpretation of OPG-CPA studies

To correlate OPG-CPA results with the degree of carotid occlusive disease, it is first necessary to define acceptable criteria for describing the severity

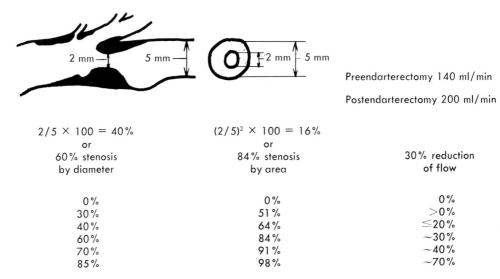

		Preendarterectomy 140 ml/min
		Postendarterectomy 200 ml/min
2/5 × 100 = 40%	(2/5)² × 100 = 16%	
or	or	
60% stenosis	84% stenosis	30% reduction
by diameter	by area	of flow
0%	0%	0%
30%	51%	>0%
40%	64%	≤20%
60%	84%	~30%
70%	91%	~40%
85%	98%	~70%

Fig. 18-11. Correlation between diameter, area, and flow reduction for internal carotid stenosis.

of stenoses. Physicians in clinical practice often relate a stenosis to the degree of diameter reduction of the arterial lumen as viewed arteriographically.[4,8,17,23] In contrast, those involved with animal research and those with direct access to artificially restricted arteries tend to prefer the percentage cross-sectional area reduction of the arterial lumen.[3,6] Fig. 18-11 illustrates the relationship between percentage diameter reduction, percentage area reduction, and approximate *average* reduction of internal carotid flow. This is based on 500 intraoperative electromagnetic blood flow measurements and on the assumption that the arterial lumen remains cylindric. For purposes of this discussion of OPG-CPA interpretations, a percentage stenosis will refer to the reduction in the *diameter* of the arterial lumen.

CPA was initiated by us in late 1966 in an effort to estimate the degree of stenosis to be anticipated if a carotid arteriogram was performed.[15] No precise relationship was found to exist between the bruit waveform and the degree of underlying carotid stenosis. However, a stenosis of 40% to 50% will generally produce a bruit beginning at the first heart sound and tapering off in such a way as to barely extend to the second heart sound. With increasing stenosis the bruit tends to increase and more completely fill the interval between the first and second heart sounds. At approximately 80% stenosis the amplitude of the bruit begins to diminish, and the bruit disappears at less than 90% stenosis (Fig. 18-12).

Fig. 18-12 illustrates the general progression of the bruit with increasing degrees of stenosis. With a split-trace CPA system, only the bottom half of the trace can be compared to the samples of Fig. 18-12, since the upper half (above the baseline) of each trace is distorted by electronic processing. Also the percent of stenosis applies only to carotid bifurcation bruits and should not be used to evaluate bruits transmitted from the base of the neck or heard over other areas of the body. A split-trace bruit at the carotid bifurcation that is larger above the baseline than below and is high pitched, but which terminates abruptly before the end of systole is from tight external carotid stenosis. Extension of the bruit beyond the second heart sound into diastole, either by standard CPA as below the baseline or above the baseline with split-trace CPA, does not always occur with progressive stenosis but is highly significant when observed, as previously discussed.

Successful OPG patient testing was initiated by us in July, 1971.[16] Subsequently, intraoperative electromagnetic blood flow and direct percutaneous arterial pressure measurements were performed before and after endarterectomy on 500 carotid arteries to establish the significance of varying degrees of ocular pulse delay. A consistent lateralized ocular pulse delay, which is visually perceptible in either the peaks or the troughs of the ocular pulses on the OPG recording, generally indicates greater than 40% internal carotid flow reduction corresponding to greater than 70% reduction in the di-

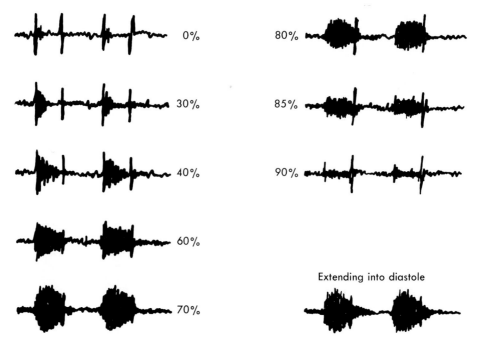

Fig. 18-12. Diagnostic characteristics of carotid bruits.

ameter of the internal carotid artery. The presence of a visually apparent ocular pulse delay without bruit at the middle or high position on the ipsilateral side indicates greater than 85% stenosis, occlusion of the internal carotid, or possibly an obstruction high in the internal carotid or ophthalmic artery. Given greater than 70% stenosis, a tighter stenosis will not necessarily cause a greater delay, since further delay or absence therefore is more a factor of collateral circulation to the eye in question.

A delay demonstrated by the differential waveform but not apparent by visual examination of the ocular pulses generally indicates an internal carotid flow reduction of 20% to 40% corresponding to a reduction of internal carotid artery diameter of 40% to 70%. A relatively flat differential trace, without cardiac-related cyclic pulses, negates the existence of unilateral ocular pulse delay. This is particularly important to remember if an attempt is made to record actual delay measurements, since eye movement artifact may appear as a delay.

The original interpretive criteria just outlined are generally adequate but, because of their subjectivity, may lead to excessive errors. Also, high or low heart rates, large or small pulse amplitudes, and excessive heart arrhythmia make the ocular pulse

delays vary for a given degree of stenosis. These same factors cause errors for those who attempt to use predetermined delays such as 10 or 20 msec to indicate the degree of stenosis without considering heart rate or point of measurement.

Greater objectivity for OPG interpretation is achieved by determining the quotient of the differential deflection resulting from delay divided by the amplitude of the delayed pulse (Diff/Amp ratio). When properly determined the Diff/Amp ratio very simply accounts for heart rate and pulse amplitude variations and can be used even with a cardiac arrhythmia. A Diff/Amp ratio of less than 0.10 implies insignificant unilateral carotid blood flow reduction and a Diff/Amp ratio of greater than 0.20 indicates greater than 40% internal carotid flow reduction from a severe stenosis on the side of the delay.[20]

In brief, the Diff/Amp technique requires determination of the systolic interval as bounded by the first pulse trough and last pulse peak. These two points on the differential trace are joined by a straight line referred to as the *pseudobaseline*. The differential deflection resulting from delay is the vertical displacement of the differential trace from this pseudobaseline at midsystole. The pulse am-

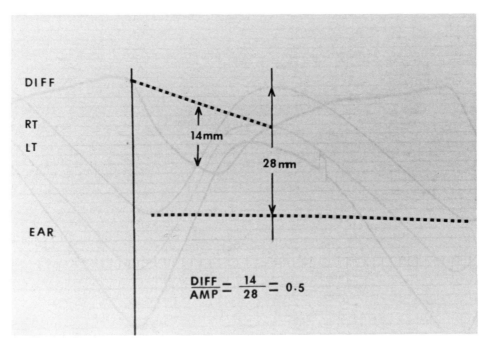

Fig. 18-13. Illustration of Diff/Amp ratio computation on air OPG recording from patient with severe right internal carotid artery stenosis.

plitude used in the ratio is the vertical distance from trough to peak of the delayed pulse (Fig. 18-13). Interpretive expertise requires an awareness of subtle differences in some ocular pulses with dicrotic notching, diastolic delays, flattened troughs, etc.[19] The objectivity achieved using the Diff/Amp ratio has greatly enhanced the interpretation and clinical application of both fluid- and air-filled OPG.

Regardless of the percentage diameter reduction present, it has been determined by us[16] as well as others[2,6] that a stenosis reducing the lumen to less than 2.5 mm diameter is required to cause a reduction in internal carotid flow. In patients with bilateral carotid stenosis, as the arterial lumen is narrowed to less than 1.5 mm, the resulting reduction in internal carotid flow is such that even slight differences in the internal carotid lumen will produce marked delays in the ocular pulse on the side of greater flow reduction. Thus in a patient with bilateral carotid stenoses, a 70% to 80% diameter reduction of one internal carotid artery may be correctly identified on initial OPG evaluation, whereas the only evidence of a 50% to 60% stenosis on the contralateral side may be the presence of a bruit. Bilateral delay of the ocular pulse troughs (or point of rapid ascent) of greater than 40 msec

relative to the earlobe pulse, usually in conjunction with a carotid bruit on at least one side, indicates severe bilateral internal carotid flow reduction. Also, a 40 msec or greater delay of one earlobe pulse relative to the other or of both ear pulses relative to the ocular pulse indicates marked stenosis of the corresponding external carotid artery or arteries. In contrast to ocular pulses, for which both peak and trough timing should be considered, only trough timing of ear pulses is used.

For reporting the results of OPG studies and for convenience in defining the severity of carotid occlusive disease, the scoring chart of Table 18-1 has been developed. Separate categories for those with total occlusion and those with a severe stenosis of 85% to 99% are desirable, but the parameters being evaluated by these tests preclude such a fine distinction. More recently we have used real-time ultrasonic imaging with a pulse-gated Doppler system together with the OPG-CPA tests and have found it very helpful for differentiating a total occlusion from a severe stenosis.

We recommend interpreting all OPG-CPA studies initially without reference to or knowledge of the patient's clinical symptoms. If the interpreting physician then wishes to review the clinical symp-

Table 18-1. Kartchner-McRae scoring chart for internal carotid occlusive disease

Grade	CPA (stenosis)	OPG (flow reduction)	Hemodynamic significance
1	<40%	<20%	Negative
2	40% to 60%	20% to 30%	Mild
3	60% to 70%	30% to 40%	Moderate
4	70% to 85%	>40%	Severe
5	>85%; no bruit	~100%	Very severe or total

toms and render an opinion relating the OPG-CPA test results to these symptoms, this can be accomplished without distorting the OPG-CPA interpretation. However, comparative evaluation of previous studies is valuable in patients with serial OPG-CPA studies.

Test accuracy and limitations

In our experience of over 30,000 studies performed on 20,200 patients, no major complications have been reported nor absolute contraindications encountered. The absence of an eye is a limitation of the test and good judgment may delay test performance because of an eye infection or recent eye surgery. Patient acceptance of the testing procedure has been excellent.

We have reported an overall accuracy of 90% in 936 patients when comparing OPG to carotid arteriography for detecting the presence or absence of significant extracranial carotid occlusive disease,[17] and reports by others using similar criteria generally substantiate this level of accuracy.[7,14,21] Proper use of the Diff/Amp ratio should help dedicated OPG-CPA users achieve similar accuracy, but inherent limitations imposed by using the percent of stenosis measured from arteriograms for the standard of comparison preclude accuracies much closer to 100%.

OPG test results are dependent on actual reduction in internal carotid artery blood flow. This is clearly demonstrated by a patient with a lesion showing a 3 mm lumen in a 7 mm internal carotid artery representing 57% stenosis but with no decrease in internal carotid artery flow. A carotid bruit may be present over such a lesion, indicative of a possible source of emboli, but the OPG study would be negative.

The primary causes of OPG error are marginal ocular pulse delays and mild arteriographic stenoses that do not compromise internal carotid flow. These two sources account for approximately one

half of the 10% incidence of disagreement between arteriography and OPG. Although ear-to-eye pulse comparative timing assists in detecting severe bilateral internal carotid stenoses, the absence of bilateral ocular pulse delay in patients with 40% to 70% bilateral stenosis still accounts for approximately one fourth of the false-negative OPG evaluations. Most patients with greater than 70% stenosis bilaterally will be detected by careful OPG-CPA testing.

Approximately one fourth of false-negative and false-positive OPG studies are unequivocal as to the absence or presence of ocular pulse delay. Even in serial studies or OPG evaluations done after endarterectomy, such results may remain in error. These false studies are assumed to be caused by anomalies of the distal circulation to the eye. One such anomaly is the external carotid origin of the ophthalmic artery in an estimated 3% or 4% of patients.[9,13,22] The unknown parameter or anomaly in these cases could possibly be deciphered using extensive arterial compression maneuvers, other noninvasive diagnostic tests, or high-quality selective cerebral arteriography.

SUMMARY

We now use real-time B-mode ultrasound imaging with range-gated Doppler ultrasound together with OPG-CPA for the noninvasive laboratory evaluation of clinical patients requiring carotid testing. Ultrasound carotid imaging is extremely efficient for detecting small atherosclerotic plaques in the carotid arteries. The great majority of these are clinically insignificant. Some cases of intraplaque hemorrhage and craters can be identified as probable sources of emboli. Using range-gated Doppler ultrasound in association with imaging has also been very helpful for differentiating total occlusion from severe internal carotid stenosis. Ultrasound carotid imaging, however, encounters its greatest weakness in precisely those areas where OPG-CPA is the strongest, that is, with acute progression of occlusive disease and in determining the presence and degree of distal internal carotid blood flow reduction.

CPA is sensitive to changes of the internal configuration of the carotid arteries resulting in noticeable alterations of the bruits even when not detectable by imaging or OPG. The soft plaque or recent thrombus is often transparent to ultrasound imaging and may not cause sufficient change in blood flow to be noted by OPG. The relative efficacy of Doppler spectral analysis for detecting these progressive changes has yet to be demonstrated.

OPG has extensive clinical documentation demonstrating its effectiveness for evaluating the hemodynamic significance of carotid stenosis. Ultrasound imaging is often most limited in determining the hemodynamic significance because of the shadows and tortuous lumen associated with chronic calcific plaque and the nonechogenic nature of fresh atheroma and thrombus. Other noninvasive tests are also reported to have good accuracy compared with arteriography but in contrast with OPG do not have good correlation with positive tests and the incidence of strokes in untreated patients.

In our experience the use of OPG-CPA has doubled the positive yield of carotid arteriography, thus reducing both the risk and cost of unnecessary procedures. Of greatest importance is the potential for reducing strokes with proper patient management facilitated by reliable early detection and dependable evaluation of extracranial carotid occlusive disease.

REFERENCES

1. Barrios, R.R., and Solis, C.: Carotid compression tonographic test: a new method to study the carotid circulation, Acta Neurol. Lat. Am. 9:48, 1963.
2. Berguer, R., and Hwang, N.H.C.: Critical arterial stenosis: a theoretical and experimental solution, Ann. Surg. 180:39, 1974.
3. Best, M., et al.: Ocular pulse studies in carotid stenosis. Relationship to carotid hemodynamics, Arch. Ophthalmol. 85:730, 1971.
4. Blaisdell, W.F., et al.: Joint study of extracranial arterial occlusion. IV. A review of surgical considerations, J.A.M.A. 209:1889, 1969.
5. Braun, H.A., et al.: Auscultation of the neck. Incidence of cervical bruit in 4296 consecutive patients, Rocky Mt. Med. J. 63:51, May, 1966.
6. Brice, J.G., Dowsett, D.J., and Lowe, R.D.: Haemodynamic effects of carotid artery stenosis, Br. Med. J. 2:1363, 1964.
7. Dean, R.H., and Yao, J.S.T.: Hemodynamic measurements in peripheral vascular disease, Curr. Prob. Surg. 12(8):1, 1976.
8. DeWeese, J.A., et al.: Endarterectomy for atherosclerotic lesions of the carotid artery, J. Cardiovasc. Surg. (Torino) 12:299, 1971.
9. Fields, W.S., et al.: Special procedures and equipment in the diagnosis and management of stroke, Stroke 4:113, 1973.
10. Galin, M.A., and Best, M.: Studies in intraocular vascular dynamics, Trans. Ophthalmol. Soc. U.K. 91:279, 1971.
11. Galin, M.A., Baras, I., and Cavero, R.: Ophthalmodynamometry using suction, Arch. Ophthalmol. 81:495, 1969. Cit. no. 4050621.
12. Gee, W., Mehigan, J.T., and Wylie, E.J.: Measurement of collateral cerebral hemispheric blood pressure by ocular pneumoplethysmography, Am. J. Surg. 130:121, 1975.
13. Gillilan, L.A.: The collateral circulation of the human orbit, Arch. Ophthalmol. 65:684, 1961.
14. Gross, W.S., et al.: Comparison of noninvasive diagnostic techniques in carotid artery occlusive disease, Surgery 82:271, 1977.
15. Kartchner, M.M., and McRae, L.P.: Ausculation for carotid bruits in cerebrovascular insufficiency, J.A.M.A. 210:494, 1969.
16. Kartchner, M.M., McRae, L.P., and Morrison, F.D.: Noninvasive detection and evaluation of carotid occlusive disease, Arch. Surg. 106:528, 1973.
17. Kartchner, M.M., et al.: Oculoplethysmography: an adjunct to arteriography in the diagnosis of extracranial carotid occlusive disease, Am. J. Surg. 132:728, 1976.
18. Masland, W.S., Kartchner, M.M., and McRae, L.P.: Evaluation of extracranial occlusive vascular disease by oculoplethysmography and carotid phonoangiography, Contemp. Aspects Cerebrovasc. Dis. 177:185, Dallas, 1976, Professional Information Library.
19. McRae, L.P., Crain, V., and Kartchner, M.M.: OPG/CPA interpretation manual, ed. 2, Tucson, 1978, Tucson Medical Center.
20. McRae, L.P., and Kartchner, M.M.: Oculoplethysmography. In Kempcyinski, R.F., and Yao, J.S.T., editors: Practical noninvasive vascular diagnosis, Chicago, 1982, Year Book Medical Publishers, Inc.
21. Persson, A.V.: New methods for clinical evaluation of carotid artery disease, Lahey Clinic Foundation Bulletin 26:40, Jan.-Mar., 1977.
22. Quisling, R.G., and Seeger, J.F.: Orbital anastomoses of the anterior deep temporal artery, Neuroradiology 8:259, 1975.
23. Thompson, J.E., et al.: Carotid endarterectomy for cerebrovascular insufficiency (stroke): follow-up of 359 cases, Ann. Surg. 163:751, 1966.

CHAPTER 19

Current methods of evaluating vascular disease with radionuclides

KATHRYN F. WITZTUM

FUNDAMENTALS OF RADIOISOTOPE DIAGNOSIS*

To appreciate the applications, limitations, and potential of the various radionuclide imaging and nonimaging techniques in diagnosing vascular diseases it is necessary to understand the essentials of nuclear physics and radioactive decay, radiation detection, and imaging and nonimaging methods of nuclear data acquisition and analysis. Hence, the first portion of this chapter will present a simplified approach to the topics just mentioned, and the final part will contain an overview of current nuclear techniques, with greater emphasis on those tests not covered extensively in other chapters.

Basic nuclear physics

All matter is composed of atoms, and each atom is composed of fundamental subunits, primarily protons, neutrons, and electrons,[21] represented schematically in Fig. 19-1 according to the Bohr atomic model: A central nucleus composed of protons and neutrons is surrounded by electrons moving in fairly discrete orbits of different radii, with each orbit having one or more specific energy shells depending on the orbital distance from the nucleus.

Relation of nucleus and electrons

A nucleus exerts a type of binding energy on its orbiting electrons. The concept is analogous to the differing forces exerted by the sun on each planet

*Modified from Witztum, K.F.: Nuclear cardiology techniques: introductory principles and applications to myocardial imaging in diagnosis of acute myocardial infarction. In Karliner, J.S., and Gregoratos, G., editors: Coronary care, New York, 1981, Churchill Livingstone, Inc.

in our solar system (the farther away from the sun, the less the gravitational pull of the sun on the planet). Similarly, an electron in an inner shell of an atom is attracted or "bound" to the nucleus by a force greater than that which binds an electron in a more distant shell. Conversely, the energy required to *remove* an electron from its shell and completely separate it from the atom may be termed the *binding energy* (E_β) for the electron. The binding force exerted on an electron in a given shell (such as the K shell) is greater from a large nucleus with a large positive charge, than from a small nucleus. Therefore the binding energy for K-shell electrons (or those in any other shell) increases rapidly with increasing atomic (Z) number.

In the stable or *ground* state, electrons occupy the highest binding energy levels (or the lowest possible shells), since nature usually takes the course of least resistance. On the surface it may seem to be a contradictory statement when one juxtaposes the phrases *highest binding energy level*, and *lowest shell* or *least resistance*. However, binding energy must be considered negative energy, in that energy must be "lost" into the system before an electron can be liberated. A K-shell electron requires more input energy (or lost, or greater negative energy) to be freed than does an L-shell or an M-shell electron; whereas from the standpoint of the nucleus, the K-shell electrons are the most easily held because they are closest to the influence of the nuclear positive charge. Consequently, if by some mechanism a "hole" is created in an electron shell of an atom having electrons in more distant shells as well, the vacancy will be promptly filled by an electron "cascade" from energy levels far-

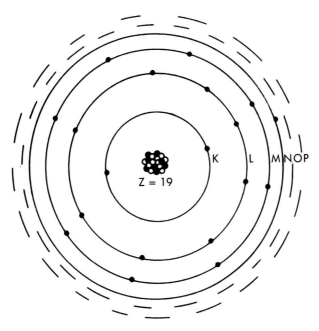

Fig. 19-1. Schematic diagram of Bohr model of atom for potassium (Z = 19). (Reproduced with permission from Hendee, W.R.: MEDICAL RADIATION PHYSICS: Roentgenology, Nuclear Medicine & Ultrasound, 2nd edition. Copyright © 1979 by Year Book Medical Publishers, Inc., Chicago.)

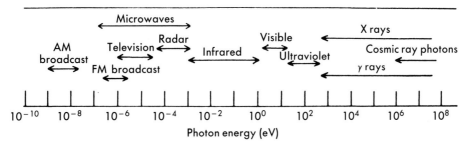

Fig. 19-2. Electromagnetic spectrum. (Ranges are approximate; no exact end points exist.) (Reproduced with permission from Hendee, W.R.: MEDICAL RADIATION PHYSICS: Roentgenology, Nuclear Medicine & Ultrasound, 2nd edition. Copyright © 1979 by Year Book Medical Publishers, Inc., Chicago.)

ther from the nucleus. As a result of this cascade phenomenon, energy is released, usually in the form of *electromagnetic radiation,* and most often as a *photon.* If these photons are not very energetic, they fall on the scale of ultraviolet, visible, infrared, and so on. If they are more energetic (>100 eV*), they are considered x rays. The electromagnetic spectrum is shown in Fig. 19-2. During the transition of a particular electron from one

*The symbol eV means *electron volt,* which is a unit of energy defined as the kinetic energy of an electron accelerated through a potential difference of one volt; 1 eV = 1.6×10^{-19} joule; 1 keV = 10^3 eV; 1 MeV = 10^6 eV.

level to another—for example, from L to K—the energy released equals the difference between the binding energies of the original and final energy levels of that electron. This energy release is termed *characteristic radiation,* because specific photon energies are characteristic of differences in binding energies unique to the electrons of a specific atom. Occasionally the energy emitted when an electron moves to a different level may cause the ejection of another electron from the atom, usually from the same shell as the cascading electron. Such an ejected electron is called an *Auger electron* and occurs more commonly from low Z-number atoms.

Radionuclides: excitation and ionization

To change an atom from ground state to a state in which an electron cascade will occur, energy must first be imparted to an orbital electron so that it will move out of its normal shell. If sufficient energy is supplied only to cause the electron to move from a lower shell to an unoccupied site in a higher shell, the process is called *excitation*. If the absorbed energy equals or exceeds the binding energy for that electron so that it is completely removed from the atom, *ionization* is said to have occurred.

The majority of nuclei with Z numbers above 82 and many with Z numbers less than 82 are unstable either because of the arrangement of protons and neutrons or because of the neutron/proton (n/p) ratio. These unstable nuclides, or *radionuclides,* eventually tend to seek a stable state by undergoing transitions such as *nuclear fission* (separation into two parts) or, more frequently, by *radioactive decay* in which the nucleus emits either electromagnetic radiation, charged particles, or both.

Modes of radioactive decay

The possible modes of radioactive decay include alpha ($_2^4\alpha$); beta (β^- or $_{-1}^0\beta$, also called negatron decay), gamma (γ); positron (β^+ or $_{+1}^0\beta$); electron capture (EC); and internal conversion (IC).

Alpha decay. Alpha (α) decay, or emission of a helium nucleus (two protons and two neutrons in a very stable configuration), was first described by Ernest Rutherford in 1899 and its particulate nature characterized in 1911 by Boltwood and Rutherford. This type of transition occurs in radionuclides with a high Z number, and may be described by the general equation

$$_Z^A X \rightarrow {}_{(Z-2)}^{(A-4)} Y + {}_2^4 He$$

Alpha decay releases nuclear energy as kinetic energy of the α particle, and each α particle from a specific nuclide is ejected with a *discrete energy.*

Negatron decay. Negatron decay (or negative beta, $_{-1}^0\beta$, decay), discovered by Henri Becquerel in 1896, tends to occur in those radionuclides in which the n/p ratio is too high for maximum nuclear stability. Thus during this decay process, the n/p ratio is reduced by transmutation of a neutron to a proton, releasing an electron and energy. This transition may be expressed as

$$_0^1 n \rightarrow {}_{+1}^1 p + {}_{-1}^0\beta + \bar{v}$$

Note that the negatron, $_{-1}^0\beta$, (which is really the same as an ordinary electron, but is denoted by $_{-1}^0\beta$ to indicate its *nuclear origin*) is considered to have essentially *no mass,* compared with the neutron and proton. However, the net mass-energy equivalents must be equal on both sides of the reaction. The fact that during these transitions the *total disintegration energy* almost always exceeds the energy accounted for by the mass-energy equivalent of the negatron, the kinetic energy of the $_{-1}^0\beta$, and any photon energy released simultaneously, gave rise to the postulation that a second ''particle'' must accompany the emission of a negatron. The energy unaccounted for in such transitions is possessed by this particle, called an *antineutrino* (or $\bar{v}$ in the equation just given). This is an uncharged particle with vanishingly small mass, which interacts only rarely with matter. Although negatrons emitted by a particular nuclide have *discrete characteristic maximum energies* ($E_\beta max$), most of the negatrons ejected during a particular transition have energies *less* than $E_\beta max$. As a result, each $_{-1}^0\beta$ decay path has a characteristic $E_\beta max$, a characteristic $_{-1}^0\beta$ *spectrum,* and a characteristic $E_\beta mean$. The $_{-1}^0\beta$ spectrum depicts the relative frequencies of negatrons emitted, with energies ranging from (a theoretic) zero to $E_\beta max$ for that $_{-1}^0\beta$ decay path. The $E_\beta mean$ for that path is usually the most commonly occurring negatron energy and is approximately equal to $E_\beta max/3$.

Positron decay and electron capture. Emission of positively charged electrons, or positrons ($_{+1}^0\beta$), from radionuclides was first discovered by Anderson in 1932 in cosmic rays and was described in conjunction with artificial radioactivity in 1934 by Curie and Joliot. Positron emitters have n/p ratios too low for maximum nuclear stability and, therefore, tend to increase the n/p ratio through the following nuclear change:

$$_{+1}^1 p \rightarrow {}_0^1 n + {}_{+1}^0\beta + v$$

where $_{+1}^0\beta$ indicates the positively charged nature and nuclear origin of the ejected positron, and v represents the accompanying *neutrino.* Also, as with negatron decay, positrons are emitted with *characteristic energy spectra* and $E_\beta max$.

The transition energy of the nucleus must supply at least 1.02 MeV during positron decay. Radionuclides that do not produce this amount of transition energy but still need to increase their n/p ratios for greater stability decay by means of *electron capture* (EC). In this process, an electron is captured from orbit, usually from the K shell, which results in a nuclear transition summarized by:

$$_{+1}^{1}p + _{-1}^{0}e \rightarrow {}_{0}^{1}n + \upsilon$$

Again, a neutrino is released and the K shell vacancy is filled by electron cascade, releasing either x radiation or an Auger electron. If a particular radionuclide decays both by positron emission and by electron capture positron decay generally will occur more often than EC.

Gamma decay. When a loss of energy alone (with no change in n/p ratio) is sufficient to cause a radionuclide to become stable, an *isomeric transition* occurs, with release of *gamma (γ) radiation*. Gamma photons were described first in 1900 by Villard. It may be noted from Fig. 19-2 that x and γ radiation occupy the same general region in the electromagnetic spectrum. Indeed, they may be distinguished in general only by their different origins: γ rays from nuclei; x rays from interactions in or around electron orbits, or from electron-nuclear collisions also resulting in extranuclear photon emissions. Gamma decay may occur in conjunction with any of the described modes of radioactive decay.

Internal conversion

On occasion, instead of releasing γ photons, a nucleus undergoes *internal conversion* (IC), in which the excess nuclear energy interacts with an inner orbital electron, causing it to be ejected as a *conversion electron,* with a kinetic energy equal to the nuclear energy excess minus the binding energy of the electron. No γ radiation is emitted, but subsequent electron cascade produces x rays and/or Auger electrons. The *coefficient of internal conversion* is the ratio of the number of conversion electrons produced by a particular IC pathway to the number of γ rays produced alternatively. IC tends to occur more often with increasing atomic number and with longer-lived excited nuclear states.

MATHEMATICS OF RADIOACTIVE DECAY

The rate of decay of a sample of radioactive material is referred to as the *activity* of the sample and is quantitated in curies, where one curie (Ci) is defined as follows:

1 Ci = 3.7×10^{10} disintegrations per second (dps)
1 millicurie = 1 mCi = 3.7×10^{7} dps = 10^{-3} Ci
1 microcurie = 1 μCi = 10^{-6} Ci

The original definition of the curie was the rate of decay of 1 g of radium, which was initially measured numerically as just shown. More recent determinations of this decay rate have established it as actually 3.61×10^{10} dps; however, the classic numeric equivalent of the curie has been retained.

Every radionuclide has a unique and characteristic fractional rate of decay over time, which has been established and defined as the *decay constant* for that radionuclide. The symbol for a decay constant is lambda (λ), which has units of inverse time (sec^{-1}, min^{-1}, and so on), and may be determined for a given radioactive sample from the following relationship:

$$A = \lambda n$$

where A is the activity (or radioactivity, as discussed previously), which may be measured with various types of counting devices; and n is the number of radioactive atoms in the sample. n may be calculated from the equation

$$n = \frac{(\text{grams in sample}) (\text{atoms/g-atomic mass})}{(\text{grams/g-atomic mass})}$$

$$= \frac{(\text{grams in sample}) (6.02 \times 10^{23})}{(\text{atomic mass number})}$$

where 6.02×10^{23} is Avogadro's number, and by definition one gram-atomic mass of a nuclide is equal to the mass number in grams. The relationship, $A = \lambda n$, indicates that the number of atoms (A) of a particular radionuclide that will disintegrate in a given time interval is dependent on the total number of atoms (n) in the sample and, therefore, λ is a probability factor defining the likelihood that a single radioatom will decay per given unit of time. From this relationship, it may be shown that

$$n_{t1} = n_{t0}\, e^{-\lambda t1}$$

where n_{t0} is the number of atoms originally present in a sample at time zero (t_0), t_1 is a given elapsed time, n_{t1} is the number of atoms left in the sample after time t_1 has elapsed, and e is the exponential quantity 2.7183, which is the base of the natural (or Napierian) logarithm system. It should be carefully noted that t_1 in this equation must be expressed in the same units of time as the inverse time units of λ for the given radionuclide. Therefore if λ is given as hours^{-1}, then t_1 must also be expressed in hours of elapsed time. The equation just given may also be stated as

$$A = A_0 e^{-\lambda t}$$

where A_0 and A are initial and final activity. These relationships are referred to as the *exponential decay equations* and are fundamental to any work requiring the use of radionuclides. A further important term, introduced earlier, is the concept of half-life, or $T_{1/2}$. The *physical half-life* of a particular radionuclide is also unique, like its λ, and is defined simply as the time required for one-half of the atoms of a sample of that nuclide to decay away. The physical $T_{1/2}$ of a nuclide may be determined as follows:

$$n = \tfrac{1}{2}n_0 \text{ when } t = T_{1/2}$$

Therefore, by substitution

$$\tfrac{1}{2}n_0 = n_0 e^{-\lambda T_{1/2}}$$
$$\text{or } (\tfrac{1}{2})\left(\frac{n_0}{n_0}\right) = e^{-\lambda T_{1/2}}$$
$$2 = e^{\lambda T_{1/2}}$$
$$\text{or } \ln 2 = \lambda T_{1/2}$$

Since $\ln 2 = 0.693$, the very important resulting equation may be written:

$$T_{1/2} = \frac{0.693}{\lambda}$$

Both λ and the physical $T_{1/2}$ of this equation are well-established values for all known radioisotopes. The radioisotopes most commonly employed in nuclear vascular studies are shown in Table 19-1 along with their principal modes of decay and their principal useful photons and relative abundances.

The actual $T_{1/2}$ *elimination* of a radioactive substance from the body depends not only on the physical decay of the radionuclide, but also on the biologic elimination of the substance from the body by various potential excretory routes. Therefore, the *effective half-life*, or $T_{1/2 \text{ eff}}$, relates to $T_{1/2 \text{ phys}}$ and $T_{1/2 \text{ biol}}$ as follows:

$$\frac{1}{T_{1/2\text{eff}}} = \frac{1}{T_{1/2 \text{ phys}}} + \frac{1}{T_{1/2 \text{ biol}}}$$

The biologic $T_{1/2}$ is determined by the nature of the particular pharmaceutical to which the radionuclide is attached.

RADIATION INTERACTION WITH MATTER
Particulate radiation interactions

To discuss the basic principles of nuclear medicine instrumentation, radiation safety, and dosimetry, we must introduce the kinds of interactions with matter that are possible for the emitted radiation produced during the decay processes just described. The two major categories of radiation are *particulate* and *nonparticulate (or photon)* radiation. Of the types of radiation discussed earlier, α particles, positrons, and negatrons are all particulate; γ and x radiation are photons, or nonparticulate radiation.

Heavy-charged particles, such as α particles (and also protons, deuterons, and so on), lose kinetic energy rapidly as they penetrate matter. The energy transfer to the absorbing medium is accomplished

Table 19-1. Decay characteristics of some radionuclides used in nuclear vascular studies*

Radionuclide	Physical half-life $(T_{1/2})$	Decay mode†	Principal useful photons (abundance)
^{99m}Tc	6.0 hr	IT	140keV (90%)
^{201}Tl	73.0 hr	EC, (γ)	69-83 keV (93%; ^{200}Hg x rays)
^{133}Xe	5.3 d	β^-, (γ)	81 keV (35%)
^{111}In	2.8 d	EC, (γ)	172 keV (89%) 247 keV (93%)
^{123}I	13 hr	EC, (γ)	159 keV (84%)
^{43}K	22.2 hr	β^-, (γ)	373 keV (85%)
^{81}Rb	4.58 hr	β^+, EC	511 keV‡ (2 photons, 33%) (daughter ^{81m}Kr, 13 sec, 190 keV γ,§ 65%)
^{83}Rb	1.25 min	β^+, EC	511 keV (2 photons, 81%)
^{13}N	10.0 min	β^+	511 keV (2 photons, 100%)
^{11}C	20.5 min	β^+	511 keV (2 photons, 100%)
^{15}O	2.0 min	β^+	511 keV (2 photons, 100%)

*Modified from Budinger, T.F., and Rollo, F.D.: Physics and instrumentation. In Holman, B.L., et al., editors: Principles of cardiovascular nuclear medicine, New York, 1978, Grune & Stratton, Inc.

†EC, Electron capture; IT, isomeric transition; β^+, positron decay; β^-, negatron decay; (γ), secondary γ emission(s)

‡511 keV, 2 photons—emitted as result of β^+ annihilation after β^+ decay (see discussion of annihilation under interactions of radiation with matter).

§γ, Gamma photon emitted during IT of ^{81m}Kr daughter.

primarily by interaction of electric fields, and "physical contact" of particles is not necessary. The energy imparted to the absorber, if sufficient, may produce *excitation* of electrons or ejection of *primary electrons* from orbits, which is *ionization*. The primary electrons may in turn cause the ejection of *secondary electrons*. The excited (non-ejected) electrons will in turn release their energy as *characteristic* or *x radiation*. An ejected electron and its residual positive ion are termed an *ion pair*. The *specific ionization* (SI) is the total number of primary and secondary ion pairs produced per unit length of path of the particle in the absorbing medium. The *linear energy transfer* (LET) of a particle is the average loss of energy per unit path length. The *range* of an ionizing particle in an absorbing medium is the straight line distance it travels before stopping completely, and is defined in terms of initial energy (E) of the particle and its LET. LET is directly related to the density of the absorbing medium (that is, the denser the medium, the more possible interactions can occur per unit path length and, therefore, the higher the SI). However, *range* is *inversely* related to LET. So it follows that the denser the medium, the shorter the range of a particle with a given energy. Thus a high energy particle expending its energy over a short range in a relatively dense material (such as soft tissue) can produce a great deal of ionization and possible damage. The range of α particles of a few MeV or less is only a few microns in soft tissue. Therefore this form of radiation is virtually useless in nuclear imaging but would be of potentially great harm.

Negatrons and positrons impinging on an absorbing medium may interact with either the orbiting electrons or the nuclei of the medium. If the kinetic energy of the incident particle (E_k) is relatively low (approximately 0 to 10 MeV), it is most likely to interact with orbiting electrons of the medium, and the probability of these electron-electron interactions increases proportionally with the Z number of the absorber. Such an interaction may produce one of two effects on the orbiting electron—excitation or ionization. In either case, the impinging electron consequently loses energy and is deflected or *scattered* at some angle with respect to its original path. Excitation is, as usual, followed by characteristic x-ray emission. When ionization occurs the ejected orbital electron has imparted to it a certain total energy, which is divided between the binding energy necessary to cause ejection and

the remaining energy, which becomes the kinetic energy of the ejected electron. Subsequently, secondary electrons may also be ejected, as described under α-particle interactions. The most significant difference between the interactions of these lower energy electrons compared with the lower energy α particles just mentioned is apparent when we consider the relative SI of the two types of particles. For example, for a negatron or positron of energy in the range of 0.1 MeV, the SI in air may be estimated at 150 ion pairs/cm. For α particles, the SI in air averages 30,000 to 70,000 ion pairs/cm. For the electron of about 0.1 MeV

$$LET = 5.06 \text{ keV/cm}$$

For an α particle of about 0.1 MeV (assuming SI = 30,000)

$$LET = 1011 \text{ keV/cm (or about three orders of}$$
$$\text{magnitude greater than for the electron).}$$

When a positron has expended its kinetic energy, it combines with an electron of the absorbing medium, and pair *annihilation* occurs, with their mass-energy equivalents being released as two 511 keV photons emitted in opposite directions. It is this *annihilation radiation* from positron-emitting radionuclides that is used in the positron tomographic imaging devices currently being developed and refined.

When the kinetic energy of an impinging negatron or positron is higher (usually >10 MeV), the particle is more likely to interact with the nuclei of the absorbing medium. The impinging electron may be simply deflected with *reduced energy* away from the nucleus *(elastic scattering);* or the incident particle may interact via *inelastic scattering,* in which case the impinging electron is deflected with *reduced velocity* and the consequent *release of electromagnetic radiation* called *bremsstrahlung* (German for "braking" radiation).

The x rays emitted by an x-ray tube, used for diagnostic radiology, are primarily the result of "boiling" electrons off a tungsten filament by means of an electric current in the filament, accelerating those electrons through a potential difference until they reach an optimum energy, and causing those accelerated electrons to bombard a tungsten target to produce the bremsstrahlung (or x-ray) photons, which are then allowed to exit the shielded tube through a narrow "window." Thus the x-ray beam for production of x-ray images is emitted.

Nonparticulate radiation interactions

There are five major categories of interaction that may occur between a γ-ray or x-ray photon and the medium through which it passes on being emitted from a radionuclide or x-ray source. These are (1) coherent scattering, (2) photoelectric absorption, (3) Compton (incoherent) scattering, (4) pair production, and (5) photodisintegration. Of these potential interactions, photoelectric absorption, Compton scattering, and pair production are of greatest significance in nuclear medicine. Coherent scattering is important only in that it may degrade the resolution of nuclear medicine images obtained from low-energy γ emitters.

During *photoelectric absorption,* the total energy of the incident x photon or γ photon is transferred to an electron of an atom of the absorbing medium, which results in ejection of that electron from the atom with a kinetic energy equal to the original photon energy minus the binding energy of the ejected electron. Most photons interact preferentially with electrons having binding energies nearest to the energy of the incident photon. After such an interaction occurs, the resultant shell vacancy is filled by the usual electron cascade, with emission of characteristic radiation and/or Auger electrons, as previously discussed. Thus if a monoenergetic beam of photons of known energy is aimed at a thin foil of a particular element, and the transmission of that beam of photons is measured while varying the beam energy by known amounts, the transmission of that beam through the foil (or conversely, the photoelectric absorption of the beam) will change dramatically whenever the beam energy closely approximates the binding energy of a particular electron in a particular shell of that element. These dramatic changes are termed *absorption edges* of the K and L electron orbits of a particular element. For example, the K edge of lead is 88 keV. We take advantage of the knowledge of other specific absorption edges routinely in radiology by the use of iodine and barium as contrast media, having K edges of 33 and 37 keV, respectively, which allow a significant number of x-ray photons in the usual diagnostic range of 33 to 88 keV to be absorbed, thus producing opacification on the radiograph of structures filled with such media. Since photoelectric interactions in soft tissue usually occur at photon energies *less* than 0.5 keV, radionuclide emissions ordinarily used in nuclear medicine imaging (with photopeaks of 80 keV or greater) stand a far better chance of having suffi-cient numbers of photons escape the soft tissue barrier to interact with the imaging detector (without being absorbed photoelectrically by the soft tissues). The electron ejected in a photoelectric interaction is called the *photoelectron.* The probability of photoelectric absorption *decreases* as photon energy increases, and *increases* as the Z number of the absorber increases. Therefore:

$$\text{probability of photoelectric event} \propto \frac{Z^3}{(h\upsilon)^3}$$

where *h*υ is the energy of the incident photon, and Z is the atomic number of the absorber. Photoelectrons may undergo secondary interactions of their own with the absorbing medium—the characteristic photons and Auger electrons usually have energies less than 0.5 keV, and are absorbed rapidly by the immediate surrounding medium.

Emitted x photons or γ photons of energy between 30 keV and 30 MeV interact in soft tissue primarily by Compton scattering. Compton interactions are *nearly independent of the Z number* of the absorbing medium, but are more directly related to its *electron density.* Therefore radiographs produced with high-energy photons show very poor contrast because of poor differential absorption in the different body tissues. Compton scatter also contributes very significantly to degradation of nuclear medicine images. The incident photon in a Compton interaction impinges on a loosely bound electron. The electron is ejected as a *Compton electron* with kinetic energy equal to the energy lost by the incident photon. The incident photon is also deflected, with a residual energy equal to the initial energy minus the kinetic energy of the Compton electron. The deflected photon is termed the *Compton photon.* If *h*υ' is the energy of the scattered photon in keV, and *h*υ is the energy of the incident photon, it may be shown that, for a Compton scatter photon scattered at 180 degrees, *h*υ' = 255 keV at maximum, no matter how much we may theoretically increase the energy of the incident photon. Similar calculations may be performed to show that maximum *h*υ' for a photon scattered at 90 degrees is 511 keV. Conversely, for incident photons of relatively low energy, such as the 80 keV photon of ^{133}Xe, if we assume only a 10% energy loss in Compton scatter (or 80 − 8 = 72 keV), it also may be shown that 73 degrees will be the angle of scatter for Compton photon. Whereas, for a slightly more energetic photon such as ^{99m}Tc, assuming a 10% energy loss (140 keV −

14 = 126 keV), 54 degrees will be the Compton photon scatter angle. In a Compton interaction in which the incident photon may lose only 1% of its initial energy, these differences in the scatter angle of the Compton photons become even more significant for the low-energy photon emitters. It is apparent, therefore, that lower-energy photons, which lose relatively little energy in Compton interactions, are scattered at a much larger angle than higher-energy photons, even for the same relative energy loss. This becomes extremely important in the clinical setting, where scattered photons degrade conventional image quality, and the primary process of eliminating scatter is by energy discrimination (as will be discussed further in the section on radiation detection). Therefore energy selection for low-energy photon emitters should be more precise (than for higher-energy radionuclides), to achieve the same conventional image quality relative to scatter radiation.

The third major type of interaction of photons with matter is known as *pair production* and may occur only when the incident photon has at least the mass/energy equivalent of two electrons. As the photon (of at least 1.02 MeV) enters the vicinity of a nucleus of the absorber, the photon is transformed into a negatron and a positron, each having as *kinetic* energy one-half the energy *in excess* of the 1.02 MeV, which was possessed by the incident photon. Both particles then expend their kinetic energy in excitation and/or ionization in the absorber until the negatron comes to rest and the positron annihilates with a "nearby" electron, with the typical release of two 511 keV photons in opposite directions, just as in positron decay.

The final important considerations regarding interactions of nonparticulate radiation in any medium are (1) the mathematics of *attenuation* (defined as the decrement in the amount of radiation emerging from a medium, compared with the incident radiation, which is produced by one or more of the types of absorption or scatter previously described) and (2) the definitions of *attenuation coefficient* (in general), and of *half-value layer*. In a manner similar to radioactive decay, the number of photons passing through the medium may be expressed by the equation

$$A = \mu n$$

where A is the attenuation or rate of removal of photons from an incident beam with n photons initially, while traversing and interacting with an ab-

sorbing medium, and μ is the coefficient of attenuation for the particular medium and photon beam of interest. It should be emphasized that μ is unique and specific to the type of medium *and* to the energy of the photons in the beam (analogous to the uniqueness of λ, the disintegration constant for each radionuclide, as discussed earlier). If the photon beam is essentially monoenergetic (that is, γ or "hardened" x rays), narrow, and contains minimum scatter photons (that is, attenuation occurring under conditions of good geometry), then the following equation pertains:

$$n = n_0 e^{-\mu X}$$

where n is the number of photons *penetrating* (or emerging from) the absorbing medium, n_0 is the original number of photons in the beam as it enters the medium, X is the thickness of the absorbing medium, in units of inches, centimeters, and so on, and μ is the attenuation coefficient for the beam in this medium, which implies that μ has units of in^{-1}, or cm^{-1}, and so on. Therefore μ in this instance is defined as the *linear attenuation coefficient*. In general, μ varies primarily with the energy of the incident x-ray or γ-ray beam, the atomic number of the absorber, and the density of the absorber. The similarity between the *attenuation equation* just given and the previously discussed *decay equation* is obvious. And logically, just as the *half-life* of a radionuclide may be defined in terms of λ, so we may define *half-value layer* in terms of μ as

$$HVL = \frac{\ln 2}{\mu}$$

$$or \quad HVL = \frac{0.693}{\mu}$$

where HVL, or half-value layer, is the thickness of a particular material required to reduce the intensity (or number of photons) of an x-ray or γ-ray beam to one half the initial or incident number of photons. The *HVL of soft tissue* for ^{201}Tl or ^{133}Xe is about 3.8 cm, and for ^{99m}Tc about 4.6 cm. The clinical importance of these values will be evident after we have discussed the constraints of radiation safety and dosimetry, radiation detection, and imaging instrumentation.

RADIATION DETECTION

Inasmuch as the process of nuclear medicine imaging is based on one type of radiation detection, it seems useful to briefly discuss the principles of detecting and counting radioactivity. The most common detection systems are based on the physical interaction of radiation with matter and are classified in one of the three following ways[50]:

1. By the medium in which the interaction occurs, for example, liquid, solid, or gas detectors
2. By the nature of the phenomenon produced, that is, excitation or ionization
3. By the type of electronic pulse generated, that is, amplitude that is constant or proportional to the energy delivered in the interaction

Of the types of detectors just mentioned, gas-filled ionization chambers are common in nuclear medicine and have important uses, such as for personnel dosimetry, dose calibrators, laboratory monitors, proportional counters for measuring charged particles, and Geiger-Müller tubes for measuring ambient radiation. All gas-filled detectors operate on the same principle—the ability of ionized gas within an electrically charged enclosure to alter the voltage potential between two electrodes. Ionizing radiation entering the detector chamber produces negative and positive ion pairs, which are collected by the electrodes of the chamber, based on the direction of the electric field. A capacitor in the circuit between the two electrodes undergoes a change in charge proportional to the number of ions collected. The pulse height thus produced is shown as a function of the voltage applied across the electrodes, for α and β particles, in Fig. 19-3. In the *recombination* region of these curves, the electric field is too weak to attract many ion pairs before they can reform into neutral atoms. As the voltage increases, the fraction of ion pairs collected, and thus charge, increases. With further increases in voltage, all ion pairs produced are collected with no recombination. In this *ionization plateau*, the capacitor charge or pulse height remains relatively constant over a range of applied voltages. The *saturation voltage* is the charge necessary for operation in this region. As voltage is increased beyond saturation, the charge collected is increased by *gas amplification*, resulting from secondary ionization from the primary ions, which may even become an *avalanche* with tertiary ions, and so forth. The pulse height in this range depends on the initial energy of the ionizing radiation and therefore is called the *proportional region*. At the upper end of this region, the two curves come together, such that the pulse height becomes more

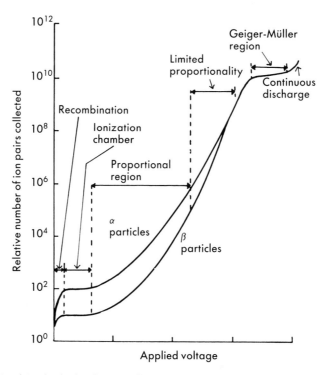

Fig. 19-3. Relationship of pulse height (or total number of ion pairs collected by electrodes) in gas-filled detector, to high voltage between electrodes. (Reproduced with permission from Hendee, W.R.: MEDICAL RADIATION PHYSICS: Roentgenology, Nuclear Medicine & Ultrasound, 2nd edition. Copyright © 1979 by Year Book Medical Publishers, Inc., Chicago.)

dependent on the voltage applied than on the energy of the initial ionizing event. This is the range of *limited proportionality*. In the Geiger-Müller region, the pulse height becomes entirely independent of the energy of the original event, and a plateau is again reached. Above this region, continuous discharge occurs within the chamber.

The most useful of these curve regions are the *ionization, proportional,* and *Geiger-Müller* ranges. Geiger-Müller tubes are highly sensitive for detecting and measuring all types of radiation, including weak x rays (and high energy β particles) and are therefore useful in required low-level radiation surveying such as is encountered in the majority of radiation safety needs and in nuclear medicine usage. However, because of the independence of radiation energy and pulse height in these tubes, discrimination of one type of radiation from another (such as γ vs. β) is not possible.

Solid scintillation detectors: basic prototypes

Compared to gas-filled detectors, solid scintillation detectors have two advantages that make them highly useful in nuclear medicine: (1) they are capable of much higher counting rates and (2)

they are much more efficient for γ-ray detection (while maintaining pulse-height proportionality). The basic components of a solid scintillation detector system, with a thallium-activated NaI(Tl) crystal, are shown in Fig. 19-4. This type of detector is the basis of the design for the Anger-type[2] gamma camera used most commonly for nuclear medicine imaging. As gamma photons enter the crystal they are absorbed by the three processes of photoelectric interaction, Compton interaction, and pair production, in proportion to the energy of the incident photon. Most of the interactions of useful tracer photon energies involve photoelectric or Compton attenuations, because of the 3.67 g/ml density of NaI(Tl) and the Z number of iodide (I), which is 53. As the incident photon strikes the crystal, its energy is imparted to the electrons of the atoms of the crystal lattice. The excited electrons then give off light photons, or *scintillations,* as they return to ground state. The Tl impurities in the crystal greatly speed up this process by acting as electron acceptors. A single gamma photon may produce many ion pairs in the crystal and thus many photons. If the γ-ray energy is completely absorbed within the crystal, the number of light photons

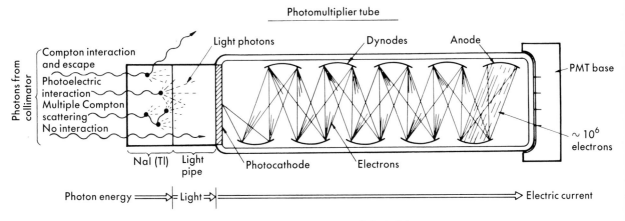

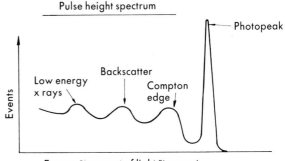

Fig. 19-4. Basic solid scintillation detector consisting of NaI (Tl) crystal optically coupled to photomultiplier tube. Photons absorbed in crystal produce scintillations, light intensity being proportional to amount of energy absorbed. Light photons from crystal striking photocathode of photomultiplier tube liberate photoelectrons, which are multiplied many times by cascading through series of metal grids (dynodes) shown. Pulse height spectrum shows the distribution of photon energies arriving at detector. (From Budinger, T.F., and Rollo, F.D.: Physics and instrumentation, Prog. Cardiovasc. Dis. **20**[1]:19-53, 1977.)

emitted is directly proportional to the energy of the incident photon. This would be true if 100% photoelectric interaction occurred, which is more nearly the case for photons of energy <150 keV. Above this energy, more Compton scatter occurs, and frequently part of the γ energy escapes the crystal, with fewer light photons produced, and the resulting output is less than the input photon energy. This energy loss accounts for the Compton portion of the γ-ray spectrum *(pulse-height spectrum)* shown in Fig. 19-4.

The visible light photons emitted by the scintillation crystal are detected by a photomultiplier (PM) tube, or in the case of a gamma camera, many PM tubes arranged evenly across the crystal surface, as seen in Fig. 19-5.

The pulse-height analyzer is the mechanism that differentiates the primary photoelectric events from scattered or less energetic events, which may also interact with the detector crystal. If less energetic photons were accepted by the system as primary events, significant image degradation would result. Therefore the primary photopeak is specifically selected by means of an *energy window* in the pulse-height analyzer, usually set at 20% *around* the primary photopeak energy.

It is apparent from the pulse-height spectrum in Fig. 19-4 that the most important discrimination function is to eliminate Compton scatter, as was alluded to earlier. The scintigraphic image produced by the accumulation of many such "discriminated" photons from many parts of the camera crystal may be displayed by registering an X and Y pulse for each event (to discern location) and a Z pulse to quantify input energy of the event.

The display device can be a persistence scope or special cathode ray tube (CRT), which may be viewed directly or used to produce images directly on x-ray or Polaroid film, or the signals may be routed to a single or multiple imaging device, such as a Matrix formatter; or the signals may be digitized and stored in computer matrices (or other data format), as described later in this chapter.

In summary, a conventional scintigraphic image is produced when a specific radioactive tracer, localizing in a specific organ in the body, emits γ photons. Of these photons, which may be emitted in any direction from the source organ, only those emitted straight toward the detector will be potentially useful. And while passing through the intervening soft tissue, 50% of these primary photons will be eliminated for each half-value-layer thickness of soft tissue encountered before exiting the body. Of the exiting "good" photons approaching the detector face, some will be eliminated by the camera collimator, a special lead-septated "focusing" device used to improve images by screening out scatter photons from the body (Fig. 19-5).

The total number of good photons (or scatter) reaching the collimator face is also affected in part by the distance that must be traversed through air, from the body surface (and source organ) to the collimator. The further away the collimator is from the body surface, the fewer photons will reach it, according to a modification of the relationship

$$n = n_0/d^2$$

where n_0 is the initial number of photons leaving any point of the source organ or the body surface, n is the number of photons arriving at the detector face, and d is the distance between the point source and the detector (assuming the attenuation of air itself is negligible). This relationship is known as the *inverse square law.*

At relatively close distances to large-diameter detectors, because of geometry, the actual point-source counting efficiency by the $n = n_0/d^2$ relationship must be adjusted according to the following equation:

$$gp = \tfrac{1}{2}(1 - \cos\theta)$$

where gp is geometric efficiency point-source and θ is the angle subtended between the center and the edge of the detector face from the point source.

After photons have passed through the collimator, they may then interact in the crystal partially or totally; or they may not interact at all. Of those interacting photons, ultimately only those passing the "discrimination test" of pulse-height analysis will be used to produce the image. The more photons of ideal energy emitted from the source organ, the better or faster the image will be produced. Therefore, within the dead-time count-rate limitations of the detector, for purposes of creating an image, the higher and more differential the concentration of radioisotope in the organ of interest, the better. However, we must also deal with the realities of radiation dosimetry and safety, both for radiation workers and for patients; therefore, appropriate limits must be set. These considerations spur the constant search for better and more efficient imaging technology, and more ideal radiopharmaceuticals.

There are other types of radiation detection de-

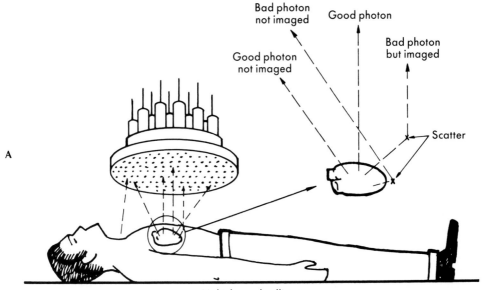

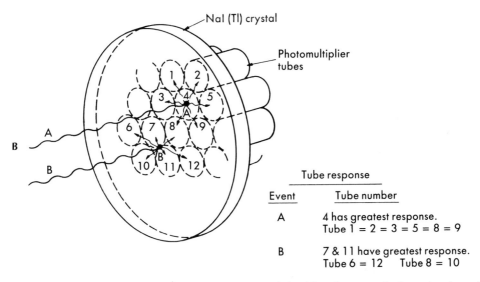

Fig. 19-5. Principle of Anger-type gamma camera. ***A,*** Relationships of organ to be imaged to face of camera collimator, which acts as multihole "lens." Only photons emitted in direction essentially parallel to holes of collimator will be allowed to reach face of camera crystal. Between holes are lead septa that attenuate (or stop) scattered photons entering at unacceptable angles. Some "good" photons will also be attenuated if they strike face of septa; conversely, some lower energy "bad" photons, if they are parallel to holes, will be allowed to enter crystal, but most of these should be screened out via pulse height analysis. ***B,*** Position of good photons (or "good" scintillation events) is deduced by amount of light detected by photomultiplier tubes relative to one another as they are distributed over surface of camera crystal. (From Budinger, T.F., and Rollo, F.D.: Physics and instrumentation, Prog. Cardiovasc. Dis. **20**[1]:19-53, 1977.)

vices, such as liquid scintillation counters and semiconductor or germanium-lithium detectors. Discussion of these, however, is neither within the scope of this chapter, nor currently germane to this topic.

DIGITAL COMPUTER METHODS

The development of current computer technology began in the 1950s after the invention of the vacuum tube.[37] Vacuum tubes permitted much faster operations than mechanical devices but were unreliable and more often down than working. However, transistors, which became available in the early 1960s, proved reliable, conserved power, and were smaller and cheaper. With this innovation, computer capacity increased while costs decreased, and with the advent of integrated circuit technology, dedicated minicomputers became cost-effective and more generally available. Further recent refinements have produced microprocessors, in which the circuitry of a minicomputer has been reduced to the size of a small chip, which may cost as little as a few dollars. Thus computer applications have become extensive in many fields, among them nuclear medicine.

Computer matrices: static and dynamic digital nuclear imaging

Image computer processing methods that have been recently explored range from various background subtraction, contrast enhancement, and cinematic or tomographic methods, to suppression of unwanted anatomical structures, organ-sizing, or absolute count quantification.[9-11] These or other data processing methods for nuclear images appear to have real merit in numerous preliminary clinical trials. These techniques presently are undergoing broader application and validation before definitive statements may be made as to their general utility. Nevertheless, the basic concepts of static digital nuclear imaging bear examining, because they relate to all other methods of computer data acquisition and analysis.

The most common mode of static digital image recording is the *frame* or *histogram* mode, as illustrated in Fig. 19-6. In this method, the digital picture is "built up" in the computer memory as follows: A part of the computer memory is organized as an x, y grid or matrix of digital numbers called *pixels* (contraction of *picture elements*). For illustration purposes, we may imagine that this grid (whatever its x, y dimensions in pixels) is superimposed on the face of the camera crystal, such that x max = y max = the diameter of the crystal face. By way of the camera electronics, a photon interacting with the crystal produces analog signals representing the x and y coordinates of that event on the crystal surface. These analog x, y signals may be converted to digital x, y signals corresponding to the same x, y coordinates (or "address") in the computer matrix by an analog to digital (A/D) converter. Therefore each time the z signal from one of these scintillation events passes the pulse-height analysis test, the appropriate pixel in the computer matrix is incremented by exactly one count. Subsequent events may increment the same address, or any other matrix address, such that by totaling the number of events in each pixel,

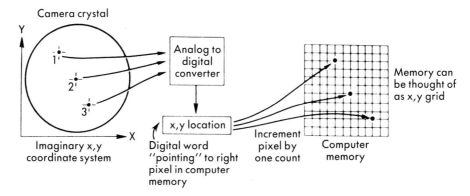

Fig. 19-6. Schematic representation of digital data acquisition in histogram or frame mode. Each acceptable event is routed from camera electronics to computer storage location corresponding to x, y location of that event within camera crystal. Specified area in computer memory is thus created that is a 1 : 1 matrix map of crystal face. (From Lewis, S.E., Stokely, E.M., and Bonte, F.J.: Physics and instrumentation. In Parkey, R.W., et al., editors: Clinical nuclear cardiology, New York, 1979, Appleton-Century-Crofts.)

a digital map of the image is generated. This map may be visually represented in a printout of the *decimal values* of each pixel (even though the actual count information in each pixel is coded in *binary* numbers); or the map may be displayed as a digital image on a video device in which the count information is displayed as shades of a gray or color scale.

In byte mode acquisition, twice as many *images* may be stored for the same number of memory words as compared to word mode, with most nuclear medicine computers. However, in byte mode, since only eight bits per pixel are available for encoding count information, byte mode images may have a maximum count per pixel of 255 counts before pixel overflow would occur (unless automatic rescaling of the entire matrix occurs as directed by the software); in word mode images, with 16 bits per pixel, over 65,000 counts per pixel may be registered before pixel overflow occurs. Thus byte mode acquisition is ideal for dynamic frame mode studies in which rapid sequence images with relatively low count-rate statistics will suffice (such as brain dynamic studies) and, therefore, will require half the space on the bulk storage unit (for example, a disk) as compared to word mode.

The second type of digital data storage is *list* or *serial mode* acquisition. In its simplest form, this method may be thought of as a *direct transfer* of x, y coordinates from the camera crystal face into computer memory (or onto disk or tape) in the *sequential order* in which the events occurred without any effort at constructing image matrices at the time of acquisition. In a somewhat more complex form of list mode data, other types of data may be inserted into the list of x, y addresses, such as clock time markers (or physiologic trigger markers). This method is illustrated in Fig. 19-7. This type of data can be formatted a posteriori into digital image matrices.

Further hardware and software considerations

A few additional points regarding the "mechanics" of the nuclear medicine computer system should be briefly mentioned as desirable features:

Basic software supplied by the manufacturer. With the multiplicity of minicomputer systems currently being marketed, virtually all the necessary programs for acquiring and processing the various dynamic and static studies now commonly employed in nuclear medicine should be available with almost any system. These include smoothing, filtering, contrast enhancement, as well as other image manipulations, profile selection, and dynamic curve generation, display, and manipulation.

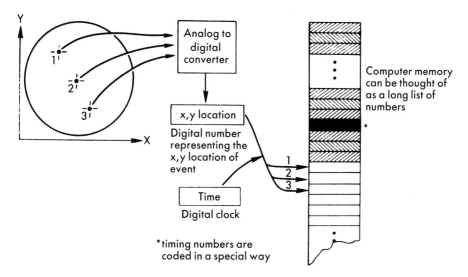

Fig. 19-7. Schematic representation of digital data storage in list or serial mode. Rather than accumulating count data in form of picture in computer memory, x, y location of each acceptable event is stored *as it occurs* in next available spot on either disk or magnetic tape, along with coded timing markers. Images are produced after the fact: Desired time interval is selected, and matrix map for histogram data is created by using list of events from disk or tape as input data (instead of using events directly from camera). (From Lewis, S.E., Stokely, E.M., and Bonte, F.J.: Physics and instrumentation. In Parkey, R.W., et al., editors: Clinical nuclear cardiology, New York, 1979, Appleton-Century-Crofts.)

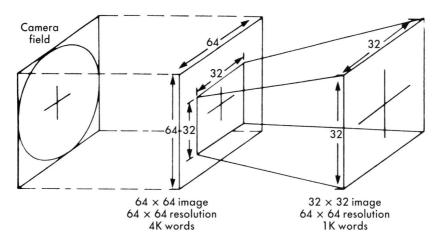

Fig. 19-8. Schematic illustration of principles of hardware "zoom." Field of view of camera shown on left has been digitized in 64 × 64 array of pixels (also called a *4K array,* since 64 × 64 = 4096). Zoom feature allows portion of this array (in this case, 32 × 32 or 1K portion) to be magnified up to same physical size as original 64 × 64 array. Spatial resolution in 32 × 32 array is same as in 64 × 64 array; however, storage of 1K array rather than 4K array takes only 25% as much memory space, with no loss in resolution. (From Bachrach, S.L., Green, M.V., and Borer, J.S.: Semin. Nucl. Med. 9:257, 1979.)

Each system should come with adequate documentation and system-user prompts for ease of use.

Hardware zoom. Hardware zoom is a feature of the A/D converter that allows for higher digital resolution without decreasing the framing rate, by means of amplification of the x, y analog signals.[3] The essence of this feature is in effect to magnify a *portion* of the camera's field of view, so that a smaller matrix array size will have pixel resolution equivalent to that of the original full-field resolution, while at the same time requiring *less memory* for digitization than the full field. This principle is demonstrated in Fig. 19-8. A further useful feature is analog offset controls, which allow the zoomed area to become any portion of the camera's field of view, rather than only a central portion. In many cases this is now both a computer and a camera option.

Display requirements[3,37]

1. Capability of displaying relatively low-resolution images (for example, 32 × 32 or 64 × 64 dynamic acquisition) as visually acceptable images
2. Flicker-free movie format and multiple static image display
3. Between 32 and 256 shades of gray
4. Interpolation, if needed, must be "on-the-fly" hardware interpolation
5. "Gray-scale look-up table," for easy adjustment of gray-scale translation

Region-of-interest (ROI) selection options

1. Lightpen
2. Joystick
3. Automatic

Additional options. Higher level language compilers (such as for Fortran, Assembly, and Basic) are useful when *programming* capability is desired. Hardware multiply and divide and hardware floating point will allow greater speed of repetitive processing. These are also important in expediting filtering or tomographic reconstruction outlines for data processing. Alternatively, array processing and distributive processing may be preferred and are offered by several manufacturers.

NEW DEVELOPMENTS IN NUCLEAR IMAGING TECHNIQUES: SINGLE PHOTON EMISSION COMPUTED TOMOGRAPHY (SPECT)

The primary goal of any tomographic imaging system (whether it uses information obtained via nuclear decay, x-ray transmission, ultrasound reflection, or nuclear magnetic resonance [NMR]) is to produce accurate anatomic (or functional, metabolic, or other parametric data) images of body sections at a selected depth. Thus each of these methods must be able to accurately "dissect out" specific information, from specific tissue types, at specific three-dimensional locations. The classic diagnostic imaging approach to this kind of information was first described by Bocage in 1921, using x-ray transmission and employing the principles of what is now called *focal-plane tomography*. In focal-plane tomography, information from the plane of interest is recorded (in either analog or digital form) in sharp focus, while off-plane information (either above or below) is minimized by blurring. This concept was first applied to nuclear imaging by Anger in 1965. However, another concept of tomography was introduced in 1963 by Kuhl et al. as *image separation radioisotope scanning*[44]; this became the prototype concept that was the basis of x-ray computed tomography (CT), developed by Hounsfield and published in 1973. This concept of *transaxial tomography* depends on computer data analysis for reconstruction of a specific image plane. The impact of x-ray CT systems on the entire practice of medicine has been profound. However, the further development and application of transaxial tomography as SPECT nuclear imaging are only now beginning, and the true impact on medicine, when coupled with new radiopharmaceuticals and improved instrumentation and computer software, remains to be seen.

As noted previously, there are *two fundamental classifications of x-ray or nuclear tomography,*[44] which are based on the general anatomic orientation of the primary body plane being extracted; these are (1) *longitudinal tomography* and (2) *transverse tomography*. Focal-plane tomography is an example of longitudinal tomography (other examples in nuclear tomography include coded aperture imaging and multipinhole, or limited angle, tomographic imaging); transaxial tomography and transverse tomography are equivalent (the major type of SPECT imaging in this class is rotating gamma camera tomography). Another example of nuclear transaxial tomography is positron emission tomography (PET), which is discussed in Chapter 24. In comparing current SPECT systems that employ one of these two types of tomography, the transaxial or rotating camera systems have been found superior because of less interference from planes adjacent to the plane of interest and because thinner planes or sections can be extracted. The *advantages of rotational SPECT* over conventional planar nuclear imaging are as follows:

1. Improved target-to-background contrast
2. Improved delineation of anatomic and pathologic details
3. Accurate measurement of organ or segmental volumes of interest
4. Determination of relative quantity, and po-

tentially of absolute quantity of a specific radioactive tracer in a target volume, and thereby potential measurement of tracer concentration and kinetics (depends on accurate attenuation correction in the reconstruction algorithm)

The *principles of data acquisition for rotating camera SPECT* are based on a gamma camera that rotates in either a 180- or 360-degree arc about an axis parallel and as near as possible to the central long axis of the subject, with the detector face parallel to the axis of rotation.[42,57] The computer controls both data acquisition and camera rotation. Some systems acquire data in relatively short time intervals during slow continuous rotational detector motion (with data stored in discrete computer matrices, each of which is a temporally equal segment of total rotation time); other systems acquire data for both a fixed time interval and at discrete, equally spaced angular increments through the entire arc of detector rotation (with no data collection during the actual rotation from one angular increment to the next). Parallel hole collimation is usually used, so that each detector or image element "sees" only the radioactivity located along a narrow band, or *ray,* which extends from the detector element, through the patient, to the center of rotation. For example, assume a planar source of uniformly distributed radioactivity, located in a three-dimensional volume and oriented perpendicular to the axis of rotation (Fig. 19-9, *A*).[44] If there were *no attenuation* of γ photons originating from any point within this activity plane, then the count rate observed at any detector element would be proportional to the sum of all counts originating along the part of the ray intersected by the activity plane (called the *ray sum*); therefore any such ray sum would also be proportional to the length of ray segment intersected by the activity plane. When a ray is "scanned" across a plane in the subject volume—or conversely, if a linear count profile is obtained by sampling adjacent detector elements along any line on the detector face that corresponds to the plane of interest in the subject volume at a particular angular increment—a *projection* is formed. If there are enough linear data samples taken along all count profiles of all projections and also enough angular samples (or projections) obtained under ideal conditions (that is, no attenuation, and perfect detector response), then it would be possible to reconstruct a perfectly accurate cross-sectional image extracted from any plane lo-

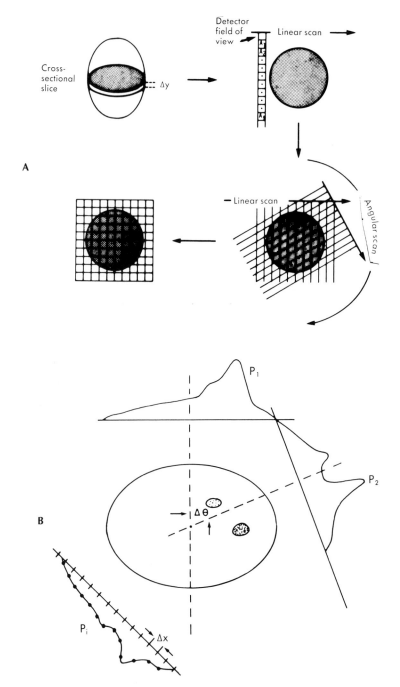

Fig. 19-9. A, Schematic illustration of data collection format for transaxial ECT consisting of linear scans at discrete angles through 180 degrees around object. A_1, A_2, etc. are discrete amounts of activity within detector field of view. **B,** Schematic representation of object cross section containing low background level of radioactivity and two hot lesions (one hotter than the other). Count-rate profiles *(P)* are obtained at multiple angles around object tangent to surface. Angular sampling occurs at increments $\Delta\theta$ that for most ECT systems range between 2 and 10 degrees. Data are digital for collection and manipulation in computer. Linear sampling increment along count profile is ΔX, typically 2 to 10 mm, depending on object size and coarseness of matrix. Peak heights in *P* associated with hot lesions are affected by attenuation between lesion and detector and uniformity of response of detector. Uniformity of response relates to both variations in sensitivity and spatial resolution. The sum of count-rate profiles (P_i) constitutes data set used in reconstruction algorithms for generation of cross-sectional image. (**A** from Murphy, P.H., et al.: Emission computed tomography: a current status report. In Freeman, L.M., and Weissmann, H.S., editors: Nuclear medicine annual 1980, New York, 1980, Raven Press; **B** from single photon emission computed tomography and other selected computer topics, New York, 1980, The Society of Nuclear Medicine.)

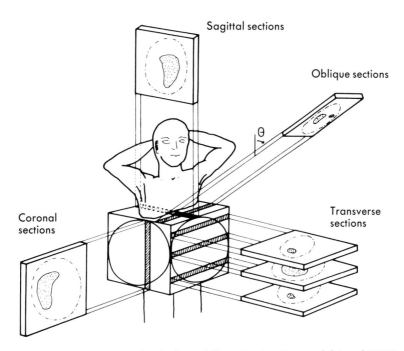

Fig. 19-10. Stack of sections, oriented to body, and illustrating imaging capabilities of SPECT rotating camera system. Because of circular field of view of gamma camera, nonzero values are contained within sphere of cube. Stack is normally oriented to frontal (anteroposterior) view of patient. (From Witztum, K.F.: Nuclear cardiology techniques: introductory principles and applications to myocardial imaging in diagnosis of acute myocardial infarction. In Karliner, J.S., and Gregoratos, G., editors: Coronary care, New York, 1981, Churchill Livingstone, Inc.)

cated within the subject volume subtended by the area (or useful field) of the detector face (Fig. 19-10).[31] If this logic is extended to the situation where (1) activity distribution in the subject volume is *nonuniform,* (2) detector response is not perfect but is corrected as perfectly as possible, (3) attenuation occurs unpredictably throughout the volume of interest but is also compensated as perfectly as possible, and (4) the influence of linear and angular sampling frequencies is limited more by the inherent detector resolution and the subject signal-to-noise ratio (that is, an optimum number of samples is in each case finite and practical), we have an approximation of "reality" (Fig. 19-9, *B*).

The three general types of *mathematical algorithms*[57] that have been of primary *importance in medical tomographic image reconstruction* are (1) simple backprojection, (2) iterative reconstruction, and (3) analytical reconstruction (most commonly used is convolution or filtered backprojection). *Simple backprojection* reconstruction is illustrated in Fig. 19-11.[57] With this method, the observed count-rate or ray-sum activity for any ray is assumed to be in reality distributed evenly over

every image element in that ray; thus the "true composition" of the image at each angular increment is estimated by projecting the ray back across the image matrix at an appropriate uniform intensity, with the rays of each profile then projected through the image matrix from every angular orientation used. This results in a "star" artifact for every point of high activity in the real object from any view, with the number of "star arms" being equal to the number of angular increments used. This method retains most of the qualitative information of the original data, but has a blunting effect on the original relative intensity differences, and so can never yield an accurate reconstruction no matter how many projections are taken.

Iterative reconstruction, which was the fundamental technique used by Hounsfield and by Kuhl, represents systematic successive approximations of the best correction factors to apply to a first guess assumption of the correct image content, which would produce matching profiles compared with the observed profiles. The *analytic reconstruction method* most often used in current x-ray CT and rotating SPECT imaging is *convolution or filtered*

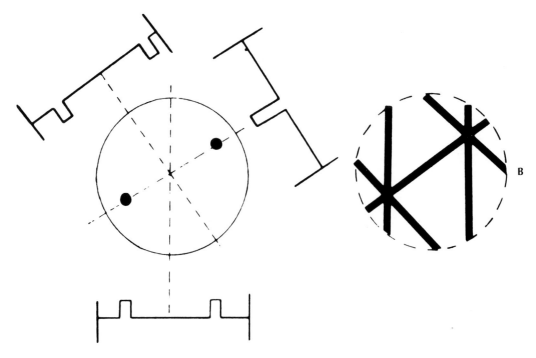

Fig. 19-11. A, Object with two point sources of radioactivity is scanned at three angular orientation, resulting in three projections (profiles) of object. **B,** Three profiles are backprojected across image plane in attempt to reconstruct original distribution. Simple backprojection results in peaks in activity distribution at correct locations. However, severe star artifact is observed. (From single photon emission computed tomography and other selected computer topics, New York, 1980, The Society of Nuclear Medicine.)

backprojection. Basic to this type of reconstruction is the fact that there is a predictable mathematical relationship between the Fourier transform of the *observed projection* from a given angular orientation and the Fourier transform of the *true object activity function* obtained from the same angle. Specifically, the Fourier coefficients of the backprojected image divided by the magnitude of the spatial frequency are equal to the Fourier coefficients of the true image. This implies that accurate reconstruction may be achieved by first applying the proper *filter* to the profiles before backprojecting. The filter in its simplest form is called the *ramp* but is usually modified by a *window function*, which gives a *frequency filter function* characterized by amplitude and *cutoff frequency* values. Typical window functions are the *Shepp-Logan window* and the *Hamming window;* hence the filter nomenclature *Ramp-Hamming filter,* and so on. The inverse Fourier transform of the frequency filter function yields the spatial convolving function, or the *convolution kernel* (Fig. 19-12).[42] In general,

the higher the cutoff frequency, the better the spatial resolution, but also the greater the sensitivity to statistical variation or *noise* (and conversely). Thus the proper filter choice depends on the noise level in the data and the nature of the object being reconstructed (that is, the ramp multiplied by a window function appropriate to the inherent data constraints of noise and required spatial resolution). Most current SPECT software offers several choices of filters and usually an operator-determined cutoff frequency. The final major variables superimposed on this reconstruction technique are the *method* of *attenuation correction,* and the *timing* of its application in the reconstruction algorithm—that is, whether it is done before or after backprojection. (This may vary from one software supplier to another, and the operator usually has no choice in the matter.) The effects of attenuation and of attenuation correction may be appreciated by examining the phantom data for ⁹⁹ᵐTc, shown in Fig. 19-13.[42]

The *important physical factors and assump-*

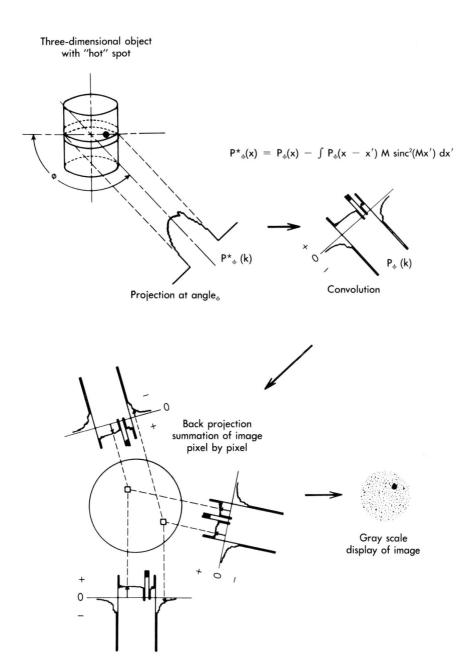

Three-dimensional object
with "hot" spot

$$P^*_\phi(x) = P_\phi(x) - \int P_\phi(x - x') \, M \, sinc^2(Mx') \, dx'$$

$P^*_\phi (k)$

Projection at angle$_\phi$

Convolution

$P_\phi (k)$

Back projection
summation of image
pixel by pixel

Gray scale
display of image

Fig. 19-12. Illustration of filtered backprojection technique for image reconstruction. Original count profile (Pϕ) is convoluted with filter function to yield filtered profile (P*ϕ). Filtered count profiles are backprojected to obtain reconstructed cross-sectional image. (From Murphy, P.H., et al.: Emission computed tomography: a current status report. In Freeman, L.M., and Weissmann, H.S., editors: Nuclear medicine annual 1980, New York, 1980, Raven Press.)

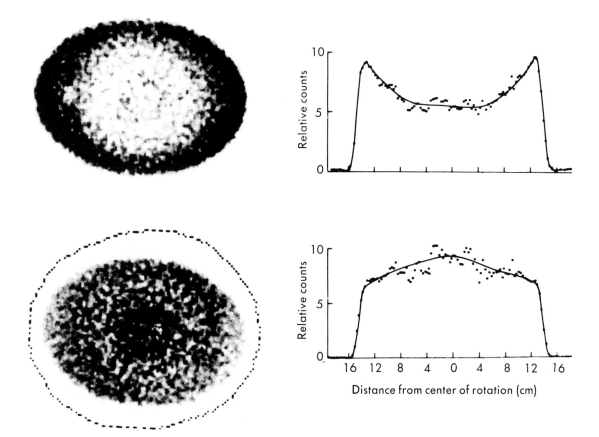

Fig. 19-13. Magnitude of attenuation with ^{99m}Tc can be seen in this transverse tomogram of uniform elliptical phantom, measuring 30 cm × 21 cm. By assuming constant attenuation coefficient throughout object, simple correction factor can be applied, reducing variation in counts along major axis to ±10%. (From Murphy, P.H., et al.: Emission computed tomography: a current status report. In Freeman, L.M., and Weissmann, H.S., editors: Nuclear medicine annual 1980, New York, 1980, Raven Press.)

tions[31,42,44,57] that determine reconstructed image quality in rotational SPECT are as follows:

1. Detector reading proportional to linear sum of activity—dependent on attenuation correction, no scatter radiation detection, and linear response of detector and electronics over the full dynamic range of count rates encountered
2. Uniform detection response with depth
3. High detector efficiency and uniformity to assure acceptable statistical accuracy (require 30 million count floods for uniformity correction even with optimum and continuous self-tuning, stability, PM tube coupling, and magnetic shielding)
4. Linear and angular sampling frequencies consistent with detector resolution, required accuracy in reconstructed image, and desired image resolution
5. Radioactivity, patient, and organ remain in a stationary state during data acquisition time
6. Accurate mechanical positioning in linear and angular directions

A BRIEF OVERVIEW OF RADIOPHARMACEUTICALS, RADIATION DOSIMETRY, AND RADIATION SAFETY

A *radiopharmaceutical,* or *radioactive drug,* is defined as a "radioactive element or labeled compound whose physical, chemical and biological properties render it both safe and useful for administration to humans."[40] The majority of these agents are classified for *diagnostic uses,* which implies that "the amount of drug that must be administered to provide useful information will produce no effects due to chemical toxicity, and that the resultant radiation dose will be much smaller than the levels producing demonstrable somatic radiation damage."[40] Radiopharmaceuticals differ from radiochemicals in that radiopharmaceuticals are considered *drugs,* or *medicinals,* and are therefore by law subject to biologic control testing to avoid any adverse reaction that might result after they are administered (by the appropriate route) to patients.

For the purposes of routine nuclear imaging techniques employing any Anger-type gamma camera, ideally the radioiosotope portion of the radiopharmaceutical should have a primary photon energy between 20 and 600 keV (most ideally about 150 keV) and a physical half-life ($T_{1/2}$) between 1 hour

and 1 year.[40] Nuclides with a physical $T_{1/2}$ longer than 1 year may potentially produce unwarranted radiation to the patient, because even though a short *biologic* $T_{1/2}$ may, in part, compensate, a small fraction of the administered dose is usually retained for a long period. (Exceptions to the rule are the noble gases, such as ^{133}Xe, ^{85}Kr, and ^{81m}Kr, which are readily eliminated via pulmonary excretion into expired air and have a biologic $T_{1/2}$ of 4 to 5 minutes and no excessively long components.) Conversely, an isotope with a physical $T_{1/2}$ shorter than 1 hour is not usually practical for labeling and sterilization of appropriate chemical compounds. The new positron emitters, such as ^{11}C, ^{15}O, and ^{13}N, are currently being explored by centers equipped with cyclotrons (for production of such ultrashort-lived isotopes—$T_{1/2}$ from 2 to 20 minutes) and appropriate imaging devices, such as the positron emission transaxial tomographic camera. These agents appear to offer very exciting new information in the areas of multiorgan metabolism, blood flow, and oxygen consumption. However, general availability of the required production and imaging technology seems unlikely in the near future.

Further ideal characteristics for radioisotope imaging are that the isotope be easily produced, readily available, inexpensive, have a high enough *specific activity* (defined as activity per unit mass of a sample, for example, curies per gram [Ci/g]) so as to produce *no* physiologic or toxic effects (when used in *tracer quantities* for imaging), decay by isomeric transition or electron capture without internal conversion (so that there is *no particulate* radiation produced, thus resulting in lower patient radiation dose), and be easily labeled to a variety of pharmaceuticals, which remain intact after administration to the patient and are readily and specifically localized in particular organ systems.

Technetium-99m (^{99m}Tc) is the radionuclide that most nearly satisfies the list of criteria just given. With the many available "instant" kits for producing a wide variety of ^{99m}Tc-labeled radiopharmaceuticals, it is easy to see why ^{99m}Tc has become the workhorse of nuclear imaging. Technetium is produced either by neutron bombardment of molybdenum-98 (^{98}Mo) or by fission from the neutron bombardment of uranium-235 (^{235}U):

$$^{98}\text{Mo}(n,\gamma) \searrow \\ \xrightarrow{} {}^{99}\text{Mo} \xrightarrow[T_{1/2}\,=\,67\text{ hr}]{\beta^-} {}^{99m}\text{Tc} \xrightarrow[T_{1/2}\,=\,6\text{ hr}]{140\text{ keV}\,\gamma} {}^{99}\text{Tc} \\ ^{235}\text{U }(n,\text{ fission}) \nearrow$$

The most efficient method of maintaining an abundant and readily available supply of ^{99m}Tc is by means of the *generator system,* in which the ^{99}Mo is adsorbed on an alumina column in a lead-shielded container. As ^{99}Mo decays to ^{99m}Tc, a *transient equilibrium* is established in which the activity of ^{99}Mo and the activity of ^{99m}Tc (in an undisturbed system) become equal over time. Once equilibrium is established, the daughter (^{99m}Tc) activity thereafter decreases with an apparent $T_{1/2}$ equal to the physical $T_{1/2}$ of the parent (^{99}Mo). Then, at any point in time, the column may be eluted or "milked" with normal saline, bringing out the available ^{99m}Tc while leaving essentially all ^{99}Mo adsorbed to the column. Thereafter, transient equilibrium may be allowed to become reestablished, the column then "milked" again, and so on. ^{99m}Tc eluted from the generator is in the chemical form of Tc-pertechnetate, ^{99m}TcO$_4^-$, which is Tc VII oxidation state. With few exceptions, this form must be reduced to allow labeling of the various pharmaceuticals with technetium. The reducing agent in most kits is stannous ion, a fact that has been serendipitously advantageous to nuclear imaging using labeled red cells as the intravascular agent.

The theory of calculation of radiation doses to patients resulting from radioisotope imaging procedures is beyond the scope of this chapter; however, it should be noted that the majority of these procedures produce organ and whole-body doses of approximately 0.5 rad or less. (In most cases, the dose is about equivalent to x-ray exposure to the thorax in a standard chest examination.) *Rad* is an acronym for *radiation absorbed dose* and is a measure of the amount of energy absorbed in a medium, such as soft tissue, as the result of exposure to ionizing radiation: 1 rad $= 10^{-2}$ joule/kg. The unit of radiation exposure is the *roentgen* (R), where 1 R $= 2.58 \times 10^{-4}$ coulomb/kg of air. A third commonly encountered term is the *rem,* which is a *dose equivalent* (DE) measurement, based on the fact that the chemical or biologic effect of a particular type of radiation is a function of the *linear energy transfer* (LET) of that radiation. This is reflected in the formula:

$$DE(rem) = D(rad) \times QF$$

where QF is a *quality factor* that varies with the LET of the radiation. The QF for γ-rays is *one.* Therefore for γ radiation, rad = rems. Dose limits for the general public and for occupationally exposed persons have been set at 0.5 rem/yr and 5 rem/yr, respectively, excluding background environmental radiation and medical diagnostic exposure; these are the *maximum permissible doses* (MPD) to the whole body. Such figures are based on concern for the genetic effects of radiation on the population and determination of the dose furnishing a genetic burden that is acceptably low in the population.[21] The radiation dosimetry of nuclear medicine and the radiation wastes resulting from this medical subspecialty are generally considered to be low-level radiation. Although standard procedures in handling any radioactive materials are observed by those who work in the field of nuclear medicine, no special precautions are considered necessary after a patient has undergone a nuclear imaging procedure.

SUMMARY OF NUCLEAR IMAGING VASCULAR EVALUATION PROCEDURES: ASSESSMENT OF REGIONAL CEREBRAL BLOOD FLOW WITH SPECT AND XENON-133 OR IODINE-123 AMPHETAMINES AND USE OF INDIUM-III–LABELED PLATELETS IN DIAGNOSIS OF CEREBROVASCULAR OR OTHER VASCULAR DISEASES

The radiopharmaceuticals and types of nuclear studies (either imaging or nonimaging) that have been applied in the study of central, cerebral, and peripheral vascular diseases are numerous and diverse. The following is a general list of these topics and references:

1. Intraarterial radiolabeled particles for arterial blood flow evaluation
   a. Primarily research use for measurement of tissue arterial supply, in normal or experimental conditions (labeled microspheres, many sizes and labels available)[26]
   b. Infrequent clinical applications include determining patency of *vascular bypass anastomoses,* such as in cerebrovascular disease (^{99m}Tc-labeled microspheres),[15] and assessment of *tumor arterial perfusion* before and after intraarterial chemotherapy (^{99m}Tc macroaggregates)[27,28]
2. Assessment of lower extremity peripheral arterial disease
   a. Rest/stress thallium-201 (^{201}Tl) peripheral perfusion scans for detection and location of significant arterial lesions (intravenous [^{201}Tl]chloride)[8,53,55]

b. Intradermal ^{133}X clearance for preoperative determination of best amputation level[12,41,56]

3. Intravenous evaluation of other vascular diseases with ^{99m}Tc agents
   a. Assessment of presence of peripheral vascular injury in trauma[52]
   b. Diagnosis of iatrogenic arteriovenous malformation (AVM) in the genitourinary system[39]
   c. Demonstration of systemic arterialization in pulmonary AVM[5]
   d. Investigation of vascular tumors of the carotid body and glomus jugulare[30,59]
   e. Evaluation of possible renovascular hypertension with [^{99m}Tc] DTPA or [^{131}I]hippuran renograms; orthostatic induction (supine vs. upright renograms)[10]; stress induction (rest vs. exercise stress renograms)[9,16,54]; quantitative renography (normal vs. abnormal absolute quantitation of renal function)[19]

4. SPECT regional cerebral blood flow analysis:
   a. ^{133}Xe (discussed later in chapter)
   b. ^{123}I-labeled amphetamines (discussed later in chapter)

5. Diagnosis of vascular diseases with ^{111}In-labeled autologous platelets (multiple applications, discussed later in chapter)

Regional cerebral blood flow with SPECT: new pharmaceuticals—^{123}I-labeled amines

The two requirements for imaging brain parenchyma with radiopharmaceuticals are blood-brain–barrier permeability to the tracer under normal conditions (with changes that readily reflect abnormality) and retention of the tracer material in brain parenchyma for sufficient time to obtain the desired images.[22,23,29] Great strides have recently been made with PET imaging in the study of several parameters of regional brain physiology. But these studies are not generally available at this time because of the need for local medical cyclotron support and the expense and complexity of the imaging equipment, and they are unlikely to become generally available in the near future. Hence the recent development of a family of ^{123}I-labeled amines, which satisfy the previously noted requirements for brain imaging, has stimulated considerable interest, especially as they have been shown to be amenable to SPECT multicrystal and rotational transaxial tomographic imaging also. It is the lipophilic

nature of these materials that enables blood-brain–barrier permeability; when given intravenously they are completely cleared during a single brain microcirculatory passage, and therefore the regional distribution of tracer amounts in the brain parenchyma is proportional to regional brain blood flow. (Another radiotracer that has characteristics similar to the ^{123}I-labeled amines for assessing brain blood flow is radioxenon in solution in the blood—usually ^{133}Xe. This will be discussed in the following section.)

Two of these ^{123}I-labeled amines have thus far been evaluated in early-phase human investigations: *N*-isopropyl-*p*-[^{123}I]-iodoamphetamine (*called* [^{123}I]*IMP*) and recently *N,N,N'*-trimethyl-*N'*-[2-hydroxy-3-methyl-5-[^{123}I]iodobenzyl-1,3-propanediamine (called [^{123}I]HIPDM). Whether caused by specific receptor or pH-shift mechanisms of retention, the biodistribution of these compounds 1 hour after an intravenous dose shows the following in monkeys[23,29]:

	Dose in brain (%)	Dose in lungs (%)
[^{123}I]IMP	7	30
[^{123}I]HIPDM	5.2	14

The retention of HIPDM in the brain over time is more stable than of IMP; but the maximum brain uptake is superior with IMP and sufficiently stable from 30 minutes to 1 hour after injection for good SPECT tomographic imaging. To preserve optimum image quality, it is best to use an ^{124}I-free ^{123}I preparation. The clinical applications published thus far with these agents include the following[22]:

1. Cerebrovascular disease
2. Epilepsy focus
3. Primary and metastatic brain tumors
4. Parkinson disease, normal-pressure hydrocephalus, and other neurologic disorders

Figs. 19-14 to 19-16 show [^{123}I]IMP tomographic brain images in normal distributions and in a patient with an acute cerebrovascular accident of less than 12-hours duration (showing earlier acute diagnosis with IMP than with x-ray CT imaging). The clinical potential of these agents is very exciting and certainly warrants broad evaluation, not only for central nervous system disease, but also in relation to pulmonary uptake-metabolism of amines.

Regional cerebral blood flow analysis: ^{133}Xe probe counts or SPECT images

^{133}Xe clearance from the brain monitored with multiple external nonimaging probes has been used

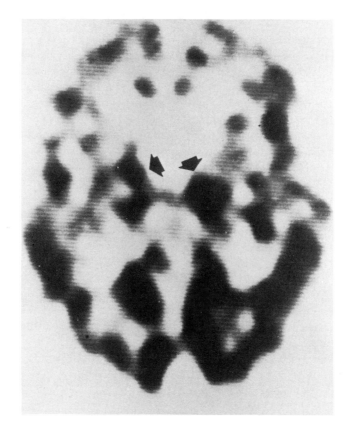

Fig. 19-14. Normal [¹²³I]iodoamphetamine transaxial image. Cortical uptake appears to be related to gray matter blood flow, with good demarcation of interlobar fissure. In this tomographic slice taken 2 cm above orbitomeatal line, basal ganglia and thalamus are clearly defined by arrows. (From Hill, T.C., et al.: Initial experience with SPECT [single-photon computerized tomography] of the brain using N-isopropyl I-123 p-iodoamphetamine: concise communication, J. Nucl. Med. 23:191, 1982.)

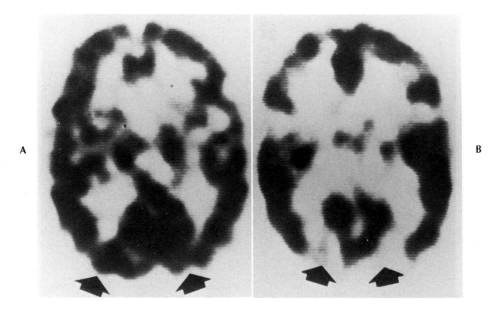

Fig. 19-15. A, Normal [¹²³I]iodoamphetamine scan obtained in patient during visual and auditory stimulation. Note relatively increased blood flow to occipital visual perceptive areas (arrows). **B,** [¹²³I]iodoamphetamine image obtained in patient with eyes closed during and immediately following injection. Note markedly decreased perfusion to occipital visual perceptual areas (arrows). (From Hill, T.C., et al.: Initial experience with SPECT [single-photon computerized tomography] of the brain using N-isopropyl I-123 p-iodoamphetamine: concise communication, J. Nucl. Med. 23:191, 1982.)

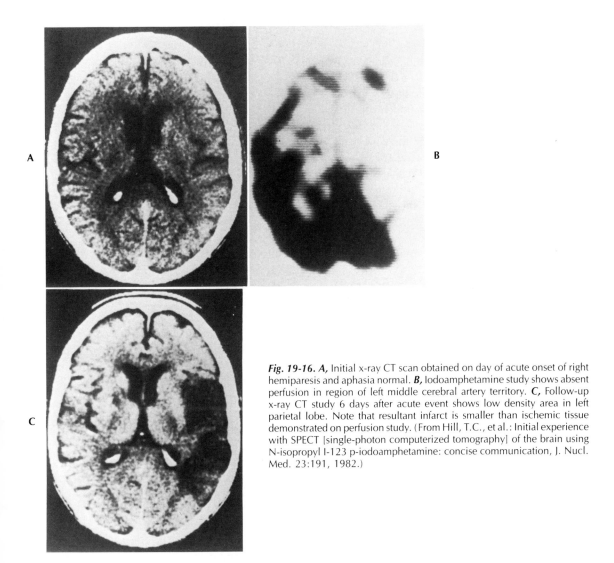

Fig. 19-16. A, Initial x-ray CT scan obtained on day of acute onset of right hemiparesis and aphasia normal. **B,** Iodoamphetamine study shows absent perfusion in region of left middle cerebral artery territory. **C,** Follow-up x-ray CT study 6 days after acute event shows low density area in left parietal lobe. Note that resultant infarct is smaller than ischemic tissue demonstrated on perfusion study. (From Hill, T.C., et al.: Initial experience with SPECT [single-photon computerized tomography] of the brain using N-isopropyl I-123 p-iodoamphetamine: concise communication, J. Nucl. Med. 23:191, 1982.)

to evaluate human regional cerebral blood flow since the mid 1960s.[51] The xenon has been administered either by ventilation or by intracarotid infusion with equal success in diagnostic results. However, this nonimaging approach suffers from inadequate localizing information. Most recently, SPECT imaging of brain ^{133}Xe clearance maps, taken at 1 minute per map slice (three simultaneous slices) during 2 minutes of clearance after a 1-minute rebreathing period with 10 mCi of ^{133}Xe gas per liter of oxygen, has compared quite favorably with the data from the first 10 minutes after an intravenous dose of [^{123}I]IMP in assessing regional brain blood flow.[32] These data were obtained using a highly specialized, rapidly rotating four-faced digital gamma camera SPECT system, which

is not available in the United States market. Further efficacy and cost-effective evaluations seem indicated. These studies obviously could not be attempted with standard single-face rotating camera SPECT systems.

[111]In-labeled autologous platelets in the assessment of cardiovascular and vascular diseases of diverse etiologies

[111]In-labeled platelets (labeled via [^{111}In]oxine) have been studied in connection with a large variety of diseases, beginning with the early oxine-labeling work of Thakur et al. published in 1976.[11] ^{111}In-labeled platelet scintigraphy in humans is now performed in many medical centers for numerous research-related and clinical reasons. The following

is a general survey of the published clinical applications:

1. Platelet survival, aggregation and release studies[11] under various known or suspected conditions, including possible hypersplenism, other causes of thrombocytopenia, diet-induced atherosclerosis in other primates, with aspirin or other drug therapy or during prostacyclin infusion, after acute experimental intimal arterial damage in animals, during active venous thrombosis in both humans and experimental animals (also during animal thromboembolic episodes), or with new pulmonary emboli less than 24 hours old (some of these studies used both blood and imaging tests)

2. Imaging for detection of coronary artery thrombi[4] or platelet deposition in coronary artery bypass grafts[17] (also effect of drug therapy on each of these[11])

3. Imaging to detect platelet accumulation on prosthetic valves or large prosthetic arterial bypass grafts (such as aortofemoral grafts)[11]

4. Imaging abdominal aortic aneurysms[11]

5. Imaging of acute myocardial infarction[13]

6. Imaging subacute, experimental, aortic valvular bacterial endocarditis in animals[48]

7. Imaging human left ventricular mural thrombi (Fig. 19-17)[11,58]

8. Assessment of arterial or venous catheter thrombogenicity[38]

9. Image diagnosis of transplant rejection (primarily renal transplants)[34]

10. Evaluation of cerebrovascular-carotid arterial disease[11,14,25,45,46]

[111]In-labeled platelet imaging evaluation of cerebrovascular-carotid arterial disease: atherosclerosis or thrombosis?

A number of prior radiographic or pathologic studies have demonstrated the strong association between cerebral ischemia or infarction and atherosclerotic disease of the ipsilateral internal carotid artery.[45] Precisely how internal carotid disease relates etiologically to these ischemic cerebrovascular events has not been clearly defined. Two important observations have been made:

1. Fresh intraplaque hemorrhage is the most common finding in atherosclerotic lesions of patients with recent hemispheric ischemia or infarct.

2. Fibrin-platelet thrombi form on arterial plaques in the neck and then embolize distally; such platelet thrombi have been found adherent to resected plaques, and platelet emboli have been observed in retinal vessels during clinical episodes of transient blindness.

Neither of these factors alone appears sufficient to explain all the clinical and pathologic findings in patients with cerebrovascular disease. Noninvasive methods to evaluate the contribution of such individual factors to the pathogenesis of cerebral ischemia would be of obvious value; hence studies of in vivo platelet behavior with ^{111}In-labeled platelets in these patients have generated considerable interest (Figs. 19-18 and 19-19).[11]

Several investigations have shown that ^{111}In-labeled platelets distribute in the circulating platelet pool and maintain essentially normal viability and function without appreciable loss of the radiolabel.

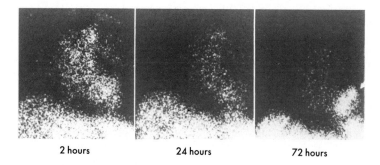

2 hours   24 hours   72 hours

Fig. 19-17. Sequential ^{111}In-labeled platelet scintigrams in patient with left ventricular mural thrombus. Increased activity at cardiac apex is noted at 72 hours. (From Stratton, J.R., et al.: Left ventricular thrombi: in vivo detection by indium-111 platelet imaging and two dimensional echocardiography, Am. J. Cardiol. 47:874, 1981.)

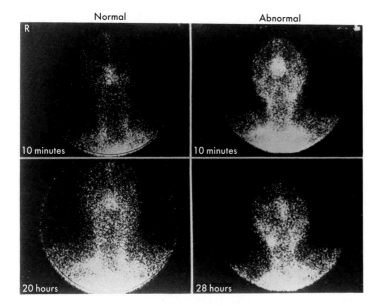

Normal   Abnormal

10 minutes   10 minutes

20 hours   28 hours

Fig. 19-18. Carotid atherosclerotic plaque. Sequential ¹¹¹In-labeled platelet scintigrams show increased activity at 28 hours near bifurcation of right common carotid artery in 42-year-old man (right panel). Angiography demonstrated 80% stenosis at origin of right internal carotid artery and small intraluminal thrombus. Normal sequential images of head and neck are shown on the left for comparison. (From Davis, H.H., II, et al.: Scintigraphic detection of carotid atherosclerosis with indium-111–labeled autologous platelets, Circulation 61:982, 1980.)

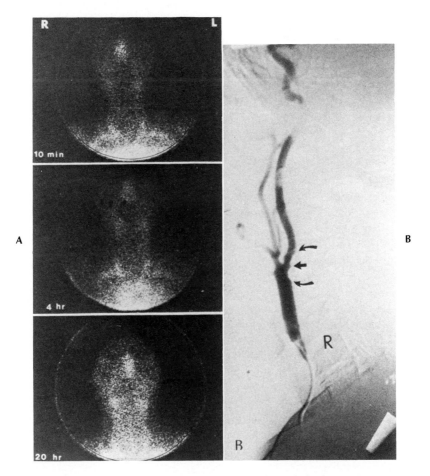

Fig. 19-19. Carotid atherosclerotic plaques. **A,** Sequential ¹¹¹In-labeled platelet scintigrams in a 59-year-old man show progressively increasing activity at the bifurcations of both common carotid arteries. **B,** Right carotid arteriogram shows a small plaque (curved arrows) involving the distal common carotid and proximal internal carotid arteries. There is a small central ulcer (arrow). (From Davis, H.H., II, et al.: Scintigraphic detection of carotid atherosclerosis with indium-111–labeled autologous platelets, Circulation 61:982, 1980.)

Studies of these labeled cells in carotid atherosclerosis (either with or without ^{99m}Tc-labeled red blood cell, blood pool subtraction techniques) have yielded the following general results[11,14,25,45,46]:

1. ^{111}In-labeled platelets accumulate at about 50% of angiographically abnormal sites.
2. They also accumulate at about 25% of angiographically normal sites.
3. In one large series there was no correlation found between the prior or subsequent incidence of transient ischemia or infarction and the findings on ^{111}In-labeled platelet scintigraphy.
4. There was no relation between the scintigraphic result and the degree of angiographic stenosis, the angiographic demonstration of ulceration, or the use of anticoagulant or antiplatelet drugs, either alone or in combination.

The lack of correlation between scintigraphy, angiography, and clinical or pharmacologic factors of apparent pathogenic importance in this study has been given two alternative explanations: (1) Factors other than the formation of platelet thrombi in cervical carotid arteries may be of primary importance in the etiology of cerebral ischemia; (2) Conversely, the ^{111}In-labeled platelet imaging techniques used thus far may not be sufficiently sensitive to detect all clinically significant platelet thrombi. Accordingly, Powers[45] has suggested that other parameters in the ^{111}In-labeled platelet studies may be of greater clinical relevance to stroke than merely the accumulation of obvious platelet thrombi; for example, he has proposed that the *rate of platelet accumulation* in arteries may be calculated using dual-tracer methods. This kind of quantitative index may correlate more closely with clinical events and drug therapy response. On the other hand, it is well known that atherosclerotic pathogenesis probably involves not only platelet–arterial wall interactions, but also platelet–blood cholesterol–arterial wall interactions, the in vivo nature of which has also to be further elucidated. Therefore it is of interest that recent techniques for labeling low-density lipoprotein (LDL) cholesterol (with both iodine and ^{99m}Tc)[24,33] have enabled preliminary positive imaging results in carotid atherosclerosis as well. Thus one might readily speculate that some combination of dynamic parameters involving dual platelet-cholesterol imaging could prove to be the best correlate of clinical disease and therapeutic results in cerebral ischemia. The additional refinement of SPECT imaging and quantitation has also been proposed and will be of great interest in conjunction with the recent development of dual-isotope SPECT imaging software.

REFERENCES

1. Anger, H.O.: Scintillation camera, Rev. Scint. Instruments 29:27, 1958.
2. Anger, H.O.: Gamma ray and positron scintillation camera, Nucleonics 21:56, 1963.
3. Bachrach, S.L., Green, M.V., and Borer, J.S.: Instrumentation and data processing in cardiovascular nuclear medicine: evaluation of ventricular function, Semin. Nucl. Med. 9:257, 1979.
4. Bergmann, S.R., et al.: Noninvasive detection of coronary thrombi with In-111 platelets: concise communication, J. Nucl. Med. 24:130, 1983.
5. Brendel, A.J., et al.: Radionuclide angiographic demonstration of systemic lung arterialization with arteriovenous fistulas, J. Nucl. Med. 24:228, 1983.
6. Budinger, T.F.: Physics and physiology of nuclear cardiology. In Willerson, J.T., editor: Nuclear cardiology, Philadelphia, 1979, F.A. Davis Co.
7. Budinger, T.F., and Rollo, F.D.: Physics and instrumentation. In Holman, B.L., Sonnenblick, E.H., and Lesch, M., editors: Principles of cardiovascular nuclear medicine, New York, 1978, Grune & Stratton, Inc.
8. Burt, R.W., et al.: Leg perfusion evaluated by delayed administration of thallium-201, Radiology 151:219, 1984.
9. Clorius, J.H., and Schmidlin, P.: The exercise renogram: a new approach documents renal involvement in systemic hypertension, J. Nucl. Med. 24:104, 1983.
10. Clorius, J.H., et al.: Hypertension associated with massive, bilateral, posture-dependent renal dysfunction, Radiology 140:231, 1981.
11. Cunningham, D.A., and Siegel, B.A.: Radiolabeled platelets. In Freeman, L.M., and Weissmann, H.S., editors: Nuclear Medicine Annual 1982. New York, 1982, Raven Press.
12. Daly, M.J., and Henry, R.E.: Quantitative measurement of skin perfusion with xenon-133, J. Nucl. Med. 21:156, 1980.
13. Davies, R.A., et al.: Imaging the inflammatory response to acute myocardial infarction in man using indium-111-labeled autologous platelets, Circulation 63(4):826, 1981.
14. Davis, H.H., et al.: Scintigraphic detection of carotid atherosclerosis with Indium-111-labeled autologous platelets, Circulation 61(5):982, 1980.
15. Etani, H., et al.: Demonstrating patency of STA-MCA anastomosis with Tc-99m albumin microspheres, J. Nucl. Med. 24:136, 1983.
16. Fuller, P.J., Kelly, M.J., and Stockigt, J.R.: Unmasking of asymmetrical renal perfusion after exercise in unilateral renovascular hypertension, letter to the editor, J. Nucl. Med. 24(5):488, 1983.
17. Fuster, V., et al.: Noninvasive radioisotopic technique for detection of platelet deposition in coronary artery bypass grafts in dogs and its reduction with platelet inhibitors, Circulation 60(7):1508, 1979.
18. Gottschalk, A.: Radioisotope scintigraphy with technetium-99m and gamma scintillation camera, AJR 97:860, 1966.
19. Gruenewalk, S.M., and Collins, L.T.: Renovascular hypertension: quantitative renography as a screening test, Radiology 149:287, 1983.
20. Harper, P.V., et al.: Technetium-99m as a scanning agent, Radiology 85:101, 1965.

21. Hendee, W.R.: Medical radiation physics: roentgenology, nuclear medicine and ultrasound. ed. 2, Chicago, 1979. Year Book Medical Publishers, Inc.

22. Holman, B.L., et al.: Brain imaging with radiolabeled amines. In Freeman, L.M., and Weissmann, H.S., editors: *Nuclear medicine annual 1983,* New York, 1983, Raven Press.

23. Holman, B.L., et al.: A comparison of two cerebral perfusion tracers, N-isopropyl i-123 p-iodoamphetamine and I-123 HIPDM, in the human, J. Nucl. Med. 25:25, 1984.

24. Isaacsohn, J.L., et al.: Adrenal imaging with Tc-99m-labeled low density lipoproteins (abstract), J. Nucl. Med. 25:72, 1984.

25. Isaka, Y., et al.: Platelet accumulation in carotid atherosclerotic lesions: semiquantitative analysis with Indium-111 platelets and Technetium-99m human serum albumin, J. Nucl. Med. 25:556, 1984.

26. Kairento, A.L., et al.: Regional blood-flow measurement in rabbit soft-tissue tumor with positron imaging using the $C^{15}O_2$ steady-state and labeled microspheres, J. Nucl. Med. 24:1135, 1983.

27. Kantarjian, H.M., Bledin, A.G., and Kim, E.E.: Arterial perfusion with Tc-99m macroaggregated albumin (MAAAP) in monitoring intra-arterial chemotherapy of sarcomas, J. Nucl. Med. 24:297, 1983.

28. Kim, E.E., and Haynie, T.P.: Intraarterial cancer chemotherapy, arterial occlusion, and Tc-99m macroaggregated albumin perfusion scintigraphy, J. Nucl. Med. 24(10):966, 1984.

29. Kung, H.F., Tramposch, K.M., and Blau, M.: A new brain perfusion imaging agent: [I-123]HIPDM:N,N,N′-trimethyl-N′-[2-hydroxy-3-methyl-5-iodobenzyl]-1,3-propanediamine, J. Nucl. Med. 24:66, 1983.

30. Laird, J.D., et al.: Radionuclide angiography as the primary investigation in chemodectoma: concise communication, J. Nucl. Med. 24:475, 1983.

31. Larsson, S.A.: Gamma camera emission tomography. Development and properties of a multi-sectional emission computed tomography system. Acta Radiol. 363:1, 1980.

32. Lassen, N.A., et al.: Cerebral blood-flow tomography: xenon-133 compared with isopropyl amphetamine-iodine-123: concise communication, J. Nucl. Med. 24:17, 1983.

33. Lees, P.S., Lees, A.M., and Strauss, H.W.: External imaging of human atherosclerosis, J. Nucl. Med. 24:154, 1983.

34. Leithner, C.H., et al.: Indium-111 labelled platelets in chronic kidney transplant rejection, Lancet 2:213, 1980.

35. Lewis, S.E., Stokely, E.M., and Bonte, F.J.: Physics and instrumentation. In Parkey, R.W., et al., Clinical nuclear cardiology, New York, 1979, Appleton-Century-Crofts.

36. Lewis, S.E., et al.: Scintigraphic methods for sizing myocardial infarction. In Parkey, R.W., et al., editors: Clinical nuclear cardiology, 1979, Appleton-Century-Crofts.

37. Lieberman, D.E.: The fundamentals of digital nuclear medicine in computer methods, St. Louis, 1977, The C.V. Mosby Co.

38. Lipton, M.J., et al.: Evaluation of catheter thrombogenicity in vivo with Indium-labeled platelets, Radiology 135:191, 1980.

39. Lisbona, R., et al.: Radionuclide detection of iatrogenic arteriovenous fistulas of the genitourinary system, Radiology 134:201, 1980.

40. McAfee, J.G., and Subramanian, G.: Radioactive agents for imaging. In Freeman, L.M., and Johnson, P.M., editors: Clinical Scintillation imaging, ed. 2, New York, 1975, Grune & Stratton, Inc.

41. Moore, W.S.: Determination of amputation level: measurement of skin blood flow with xenon Xe 133, Arch. Surg. 107:798, 1973.

42. Murphy, P.H., et al.: Emission computed tomography: a current status report. In Freeman, L.M., and Weissmann, H.S., editors: Nuclear medicine annual 1980, New York, 1980, Raven Press.

43. Parker, J.A., and Treves, S.: Radionuclide detection, localization and quantitation of intracardiac shunts and shunts between the great arteries. In Holman, B.L., Sonnenblick, E.H., and Lesch, M., editors: Principles of cardiovascular nuclear medicine, New York, 1978, Grune & Stratton, Inc.

44. Phelps, M.E.: Emission computed tomography, Semin. Nucl. Med. 7(4):337, 1977.

45. Powers, W.J.: In-111 platelet scintigraphy: carotid atherosclerosis and stroke, J. Nucl. Med. 25:626, 1984.

46. Powers, W.J., et al.: Indium-111 platelet scintigraphy in cerebrovascular disease, Neurology 32:938, 1982.

47. Radiological health handbook, rev. ed., compiled and edited by the Bureau of Radiological Health and Training Institute, Environmental Control Administration, U.S. Department of Health, Education, and Welfare, Public Health Service, Consumer Protection and Environmental Health Service, Rockville, Md., Jan. 1970.

48. Riba, A.L., et al.: Imaging experimental infective endocarditis with indium-111-labeled blood cellular components, Circulation 59(2):336, 1979.

49. Richards, P.: The technetium-99m generator. In Andrews, G.A., Kinseley, R.M., and Wagner, H.N., Jr., editors: Radioactive pharmaceuticals, Washington, D.C., 1966, U.S. Atomic Energy Commission.

50. Rocha, A.F.B., Harbert, J.C., editors: Textbook of nuclear medicine: basic science. Philadelphia, 1978, Lea and Febiger.

51. Rozenfeld, D., and Wolfson, L.I.: The effects of activation procedures on regional cerebral blood flow in humans, Semin. Nucl. Med. 11(3):172, 1981.

52. Rudavsky, A.Z., and Moss, C.M.: Radionuclide evaluation of peripheral vascular injuries. Semin. Nucl. Med. 13(2):142, 1983.

53. Seder, J.S., et al.: Detecting and localizing peripheral arterial disease: assessment of [201]Ti scintigraphy, AJR 137:373, 1981.

54. Shreiner, D.P.: The exercise renogram: a new approach documents renal involvement in systemic hypertension, letter to the editor, J. Nucl. Med. 24(9):859, 1983.

55. Siegel, M.E., and Stewart, C.A.: Thallium-201 peripheral perfusion scans: feasibility of single-dose, single-day, rest and stress study, AJR 136:1179, 1981.

56. Silberstein, E.B., et al.: Predictive value of intracutaneous xenon clearance for healing of amputation and cutaneous ulcer sites, Radiology 147:227, 1983.

57. Single photon emission computed tomography and other selected computer topics, New York, 1980, The Society of Nuclear Medicine.

58. Stratton, J.P., et al.: Left ventricular thrombi: in vivo detection by Indium-111 platelet imaging and two dimensional echocardiography, Am. J. Cardiol. 47:874, 1981.

59. Zwas, S.T., et al. Diagnosis of jugular paraganglioma by radionuclide angiography: concise communication, J. Nucl. Med. 24:1005, 1983.

CHAPTER 20

Doppler ultrasonic arteriography

ROBERT W. BARNES

The vascular system may be visualized using ultrasound in one of three modes: (1) Doppler ultrasound to image the vascular lumen with a display similar to that of angiography, (2) real-time B-mode ultrasound to visualize the vascular walls, and (3) a hybrid of these two techniques, or so-called duplex (echo-Doppler) scanning. This chapter will review the principles and general applications of Doppler ultrasonic arteriography and duplex scanning.

INSTRUMENTATION

The Doppler ultrasonic arteriographic system consists of three basic components: (1) a Doppler ultrasonic velocity detector, (2) a transducer holder and position-sensing arm (spatial resolver), and (3) a graphic display (Fig. 20-1). The duplex scanner consists of a real-time B-mode ultrasonic imaging system and an integrated pulsed Doppler velocity detector.

Doppler velocity detector

The Doppler component of the imaging system may be either a continuous-wave or pulsed Doppler device. The Doppler unit may or may not have direction-sensing capability.

Continuous-wave Doppler system. A continuous-wave (CW) Doppler ultrasonic imaging system was originally described by Reid and Spencer.[35] The device is currently marketed as *Dopscan*. The instrument has a CW Doppler transducer that permits sampling of blood flow velocity from the common carotid artery and its branches. The transducer is constrained to movement by a position-sensing arm so that the crude image of the carotid bifurcation may be displayed on a storage oscilloscope. The Doppler flow velocity signals may be analyzed by

audible interpretation, analog waveform recordings, or real-time sound spectrum analysis with a color-coded display to represent signal amplitude on a storage oscilloscope.

A CW Doppler ultrasonic arteriograph was developed by Curry and White[12] for two-dimensional display of flowing blood in the carotid bifurcation. The image of the carotid bifurcation is color coded by the peak Doppler frequency shift to reflect three different ranges of carotid flow velocity, which correlate with the severity of carotid stenosis. The instrument is marketed as the *Echoflow* device.

Pulsed Doppler system. The first ultrasonic arteriograph used a pulsed Doppler velocity detector and was developed by Hokanson et al.[19] in 1971. The pulsed Doppler system emits bursts (0.5 to 1.0 μsec) of ultrasound. The receiving crystal is time gated to receive reflected Doppler-shifted ultrasound at variable intervals following the transmitted signal. The range of detected flow from the transducer corresponds to the time interval for the ultrasound to travel to and from the site of detected flow. Use of several gates permits simultaneous detection of flow from multiple points along the path of the sound beam. The resolution of the single sample gate is approximately 1 mm³. The pulsed Doppler arteriograph permits imaging of the vascular lumen to detect sites of atherosclerotic plaque not easily detected with CW Doppler arteriographs. The initial clinical application of pulsed Doppler arteriography was described by Mozersky et al.[29]

Recently the addition of computerized analysis of pulsed Doppler ultrasonic arteriographic information has permitted multiplanar views of imaged vascular segments, as originally described by Miles et al.[26] The instrument produces simultaneous lateral, anteroposterior and transverse views of the

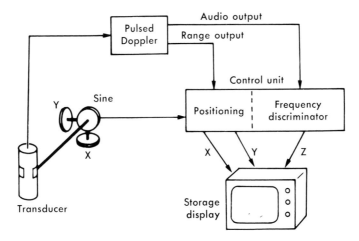

Fig. 20-1. Block diagram of components of pulsed Doppler ultrasonic arteriograph (Hokanson).

carotid bifurcation for the detection of carotid atherosclerosis. The technique is sensitive to vascular diameter reductions of 40% or greater. This technique is particularly important to identify eccentric atherosclerotic plaques that are common at the origin of the internal carotid artery.

A multichannel pulsed Doppler ultrasonic arteriograph, the so-called MAVIS system (Mobile Artery and Vein Imaging System),[13] permits vascular imaging with 30-channel pulsed Doppler signals. Directional flow velocity is color coded.

Initial duplex (echo-Doppler) scanning. The ultrasonic duplex echo-Doppler scanner was originally described by Barber et al.[2] This device provided ultrasonic B-mode displays with a diagnostic scanner that yielded dynamic Doppler information from blood flow in addition to both static and dynamic echo information from stationary and more slowly moving tissues. The effect combined the flow imaging capability of a multigate pulsed Doppler velocity detector with a fast rotational pulsed-echo B-mode scanner. The duplex system was designed for performing ultrasonic echo-Doppler arteriography where the location and geometry of the interface between occlusive atherosclerotic tissue and blood was of prime concern. Although spatial alignment of echo and Doppler images may be obtained using the same transducer and scanning mechanism for both, initial clinical trials suggested that a two-transducer system was more desirable. The ability to superimpose images of both tissue and blood decreases the uncertainties inherent in the display in either image alone. Detailed discus-

sions of B-mode imaging and of the duplex scanner are presented in Chapters 21 and 38.

Position-sensing arm

An integral part of the Doppler ultrasonic imaging system is the mechanical arm that holds the Doppler transducer and translates the position of detected flow information to a storage oscilloscope. The mechanical arm permits the Doppler transducer to move in one or more planes. Angular and rotational movements are detected by means of potentiometers, which in turn provide varying voltage outputs to the display (oscilloscope) output. The mechanical arm of the system incorporates three rotational potentiometers, each one for a different plane of movement. Two of the potentiometers sense movement of the mechanical arm in the x and y directions. The third potentiometer detects rotation of the position-sensing arm. The output of these potentiometers is coupled with the range output of the pulsed Doppler velocity detector to accurately locate detected flow as a spot in an appropriate position on a storage oscilloscope. A linear potentiometer may be used on the position-sensing arm so that three-dimensional information may be obtained. Such information, when coupled to a computerized data processor, permits generation of three-dimensional images in multiple orthographic planes.[26]

The probe-position translator in the CW Doppler imaging system of Reid and Spencer[35] uses a telescoping rho-theta arm mounted on a rotating post and gimbal. The telescoping motion of the arm is linked to the rho potentiometer and the rotating post to the theta potentiometer.

A different method for determining the location and orientation of the ultrasound beam was described by Moritz and Shreve.[28] In this system a microprocessor-based spatial locating system involves measuring the transient times of spark-generated shock waves. A small flexible coaxial cable is used to connect the spark gaps to a spark generator, and the technique imposes minimum constraint on the ultrasound technician in the use of the equipment.

Display system

CW or pulsed Doppler imaging systems provide graphic information about blood vessel morphology, as well as blood flow velocity information from analysis of the Doppler frequency shift signal. Because of inherent problems of imaging blood vessels with arterial wall calcification,[17] velocity analysis has become an important aspect in the detection of vascular disease.

Graphic display. The vascular morphology is displayed on a memory (storage) oscilloscope. The detected loci of blood flow information are appropriately positioned on the storage oscilloscope using the voltage outputs of the potentiometers of the position-sensing mechanical arm. In CW Doppler arteriographs, the resolution of the Doppler probe is insufficient to provide accurate morphology of the vascular lumen. The imaging system is designed to locate sample volumes of Doppler information for subsequent velocity analysis. Thus CW Doppler arteriographs provide vessel images as a map to permit spatial recognition of sites of Doppler sample volumes for inferring vascular disease on a basis of abnormal velocity information.

In contrast, pulsed Doppler arteriographs have sufficient spatial resolution to permit depiction of a morphologic vascular image that may accurately approximate the lumen morphology seen on contrast arteriography (Fig. 20-2). The pulsed Doppler arteriograph also permits voltage output of the range gate of the Doppler probe so that spatial information in three planes may be analyzed.

The memory oscilloscope is unblanked whenever the voltage output of the Doppler frequency detector exceeds a certain threshold (such as above 200 Hz). A low-frequency cutoff is incorporated to minimize artifact from probe movement, vessel motion, and other low-frequency signals that may

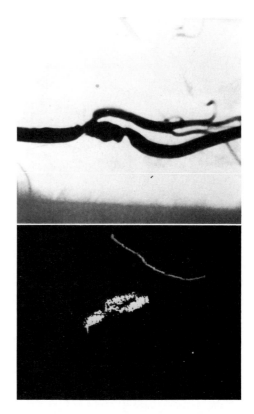

Fig. 20-2. Pulsed Doppler ultrasonic arteriographic image of carotid bifurcation *(bottom)* of patient with stenosis of internal and external carotid arteries documented by conventional contrast arteriography *(top)*.

produce spurious artifact. The Doppler transducer is systematically moved along the course of the underlying vessel with the scanning procedure governed by the audio output of the Doppler instrument, as well as the appearance of stored spots on the oscilloscope, which correspond to loci of detected flow occupying the available area of the vascular lumen. The stored image may then be photographed on Polaroid film or recorded on an automatic printout or videotape for a permanent record.

The ultrasonic image may be displayed in one of three modes: (1) longitudinal cross-section, (2) transverse cross-section, or (3) projectional views. In the longitudinal cross-section, an image is built up in the plane of movement of the Doppler probe as it courses along the length of the underlying blood vessel. Pulsed Doppler arteriographs may permit simultaneous storage of several spots on the oscilloscope equivalent to the number of range gates (up to 30 in the MAVIS scanner). Movement of the transducer longitudinally along the vessel thus permits rapid buildup of the vascular image if the Doppler probe is constrained to move in the plane of the underlying blood vessel. The transverse cross-sectional views provide unique images that cannot be duplicated by conventional contrast arteriography. In the images, the cross-sectional morphology of the blood vessel is displayed in the same plane, as the Doppler transducer is moved at right angles to the longitudinal axis of the vessel. Such views may be particularly important when visualizing eccentric atherosclerotic plaques in vessels such as carotid or femoral artery bifurcations. The projectional view displays an image of the vessel in a plane that is at right angles to the ultrasonic beam. The projectional mode permits views similar to standard contrast arteriograms and is particularly useful when imaging the carotid bifurcation by either the CW or pulsed Doppler technique. A lateral view of the carotid bifurcation is obtained that is similar to images obtained with contrast arteriography. With a computerized interpretation of sampled Doppler velocity information, multiplanar views of the underlying blood vessel may be obtained simultaneously.[26]

Velocity analysis. Both CW and pulsed Doppler imaging systems provide information about blood velocity that cannot be obtained by standard contrast arteriography. The simplest method is to detect blood velocity with the audible interpretation by the observer. The Doppler shift spectrum consists of a wide range of frequencies that form the composite signal that can be heard with a loud speaker or with earphones. With experience, the examiner can readily detect normal and abnormal arterial and venous velocity signals. The observer also may learn to differentiate flow in the internal and external carotid arteries. The audible interpretation permits detection of blood flow disturbances associated with arterial stenosis that reduce the diameter of the lumen by 50% or greater. Lesser degrees of stenosis usually require more sophisticated velocity analysis, such as that provided by real-time sound spectrum analyzers.

The Doppler signal may be processed by a zero-crossing circuit or other technique to produce an analog output on a strip chart recorder. This phasic voltage output usually corresponds to the mean velocity of the blood flow encompassed within the ultrasonic beam. Although the analog output permits recording of normal multiphasic arterial signals, as well as abnormal monophasic signals distal to arterial stenoses or occlusions, the technique does not permit a complete evaluation of all the information in the spectrum of the Doppler frequency shift.

To display different velocities associated with varying degrees of arterial stenoses, Curry and White[12] used a color coding of three different ranges on the image of the CW Doppler ultrasonic arteriograph. Normal velocities are displayed in red, moderately increased velocities in yellow, and the highest peak velocity in blue. The observer can identify areas of increased blood flow velocity associated with localized arterial stenosis from this simple color-coded display of the CW Doppler image of the carotid bifurcation. While this technique permits fairly accurate detection of arterial stenoses of 50% diameter reduction or greater, the technique is insensitive to milder degrees of arterial disease.

To accurately define blood flow velocity aberration associated with minor stenoses, sound spectrum analysis of the Doppler signal has proved to be the most accurate approach.[3] A complete description of sound spectrum analysis techniques is provided in a separate chapter. Spectrum analysis was originally performed with off-line techniques requiring a tape recording of the Doppler signal for subsequent analysis of the component spectra. With the development of real-time sound spectrum analyzers,[37] rapid analysis and display of CW or pulsed Doppler signals may be obtained at the time of Doppler ultrasonic arteriography. The importance of analyzing Doppler velocity information during vascular imaging was emphasized by Hobson et al.,[18] who found that such velocity information was of much greater diagnostic value than morphologic images from real-time echo arteriography, particularly for differentiating moderate or advanced atherosclerotic stenosis from occlusion of the vascular lumen. These workers found that real-time B-mode images alone were accurate only for relatively mild atherosclerotic plaques, but that Doppler velocity information, as obtained from Doppler ultrasonic arteriography or duplex scanning, was necessary for maximal accuracy in the detection of extracranial carotid atherosclerosis. Recent refinements in sound spectrum analysis techniques[21,36,37,43] have enhanced the accuracy of Doppler detection of carotid atherosclerosis, with or without imaging techniques.

APPLICATION

The use of individual Doppler or B-mode imaging techniques will be described in separate chapters of this textbook. The following section will review some of the clinical applications of Doppler ultrasonic arteriographs, so that the reader may understand and appreciate the versatility of this device in the detection of vascular disease.

Arterial disease

Carotid artery disease. The most widespread application of Doppler ultrasonic arteriography has been for the detection of extracranial carotid atherosclerosis. CW Doppler arteriographs are generally sensitive only to more advanced arterial disease that reduces the lumen by 50% diameter reduction or greater. Reported accuracy for the Dopscan CW Doppler arteriograph[7,39,41,44] includes a sensitivity ranging from 63% to 92% and a specificity varying between 53% and 96%. The reported accuracy of detecting or excluding significant (greater than 65%) stenosis or occlusion of the internal carotid artery using the Echoflow CW device[31,32,42] has exceeded 90%. The use of real-time sound spectrum analysis of CW Doppler velocity information permits improved sensitivity of detection of nonobstructing carotid plaques as reported by Rittgers et al.[38]

Pulsed Doppler ultrasonic arteriography provides improved detection of arterial stenoses of less than 50% diameter reduction without sacrificing accuracy in identifying more severe disease. Barnes et al.[3] reported a sensitivity of 96% in detecting carotid stenosis of greater than 25% diameter reduction. However, in the absence of spectrum analysis, the specificity was only 44%, primarily because of abnormal images associated with vascular wall calcification. The addition of sound spectrum analysis to the Hokanson pulsed Doppler ultrasonic arteriograph provided a sensitivity of 90% and a specificity of 92% in detecting or excluding carotid stenosis with greater than 25% diameter reduction. Hobson et al.[18] reported a sensitivity of 78% and a specificity of 73% with the Hokanson pulsed Doppler arteriograph. Using the same instrument, Sumner et al.[40] reported a sensitivity of 89% and a specificity of 86% in detection or exclusion of carotid stenosis of greater than 40% diameter reduction. Using a computerized multiplanar modification of the Hokanson arteriograph, Miles et al.[27] found a sensitivity of 96% and a specificity of 92% in detection of carotid stenosis of 20% diameter

reduction or greater. Lusby et al.[23] employed a MAVIS scanner and documented a sensitivity of 43% and a specificity of 100% in the detection or exclusion of any degree of extracranial carotid occlusive disease.

Recently several investigators* have reported the use of duplex scanning for sensitive detection of extracranial carotid disease. Most of these reports have emphasized the diagnostic value of spectrum analysis of the pulsed Doppler signal, which samples flow from selected areas of the arterial lumen visualized by the B-mode component of the duplex scanner. It should be emphasized that the diagnostic value of duplex scanning primarily relates to the analysis of Doppler flow information and not the imaged lumen. Reported sensitivity to any degree of carotid disease varies between 85% and 99%. The specificity has generally been lower, ranging from 36% to 95%, probably as a result of identifying abnormal flow velocity patterns at the carotid bifurcation in many normal subjects. The addition of computerized pattern recognition of the Doppler velocity information, as reported by Greene et al.,[16] has largely removed the subjective variability of observer interpretation. Using computer-based pattern recognition, they were able to differentiate between normal and diseased vessels with 97.5% accuracy, between greater than and less than 50% stenosis with 98.2% accuracy and between greater than and less than 20% stenosis with 85.9% accuracy. Langlois et al.[22] found that this technique of pulsed Doppler ultrasonic velocity analysis exceeded the accuracy of interpretation of standard contrast arteriograms by two different observers, using the κ statistic.

Vertebral artery disease. Interrogation of vertebral artery blood flow by Doppler ultrasonic arteriography is much more difficult than that of carotid disease detection. However, White et al.[43] found that with the use of either CW Doppler ultrasonic arteriography (Echoflow) or a pulsed Doppler system, the vertebral artery could be visualized in 60% to 75% of patients. Unfortunately, Doppler ultrasonic arteriography fails to provide satisfactory interpretation of vertebral artery disease in a significant number of patients.

Aortofemoral artery disease. Doppler ultrasonic arteriography has recently been applied to the detection of localized arterial stenoses in the peripheral arteries, primarily the iliac and femoral arter-

*References 4, 6, 9, 14, 16, 20, 22, 33.

ies. Baird et al.[1] used the MAVIS scanner to detect stenosis of the profunda femoris artery in 33 limbs of 33 patients. A stenosis of greater than 50% diameter reduction was invariably associated with a damping factor of the maximal Doppler velocity waveform of greater than 1.5. Blackshear et al.[5] have used the duplex scanner to identify normal velocity patterns in the deep femoral artery under conditions of rest and during reactive hyperemia. These studies indicate that transient turbulent flow velocities are induced under conditions of hyperemic blood flow.

Doppler ultrasonic arteriography permits noninvasive assessment of flow velocity disturbances associated with arterial prostheses. Baird et al.[1] used the MAVIS scanner to detect the internal diameter of iliofemoral and iliopopliteal bypass prostheses. They noted a significant reduction in graft diameter just above the popliteal anastomosis when compared with the femoral anastomosis of axillobifemoral bypass grafts. Clifford et al.[11] used both the MAVIS scanner and real-time duplex scanning to evaluate 136 arterial grafts, noting probable neointima formation, graft dilation, graft kinking, and differences in graft compliance using these noninvasive diagnostic techniques.

Visceral arteries. Pulsed Doppler ultrasonic arteriography has recently been extended to more deeply lying visceral arteries. Campbell et al.[10] used a pulse-gated Doppler ultrasonic detector to study blood flow velocity profiles in uterine arcuate arteries during the second and third trimesters of pregnancy. They noted Doppler evidence of increased vascular resistance in 14 of 31 pregnancies associated with complications, with a high frequency of eclampsia, poor fetal growth, and fetal hypoxia. Maulik et al.[25] used a pulsed Doppler velocity detector to evaluate human umbilical hemodynamics in 27 pregnant patients. Using coherent averaging of signals and feature characterization techniques, the authors noted a high pulsatility index in association with three cases of oligohydramnios, indicating the possibility of an elevated placental circulatory impedance. Recently, Norris[30] found that the duplex scanner was useful in detecting significant stenosis of the renal arteries in patients with renovascular hypertension. The pulsed Doppler ultrasonic signal not only correlates well with the presence of significant proximal renal artery stenosis, but also may be an indicator of increased parenchymal renal vascular resistance in patients with secondary nephrosclerosis.

Venous disease

There have been few reports of the use of Doppler ultrasonic arteriography in the detection of venous disease. The use of CW Doppler ultrasound in the absence of imaging capability is a fairly reliable technique to detect acute and chronic venous disease, provided the observer has experience with the technique. However, Doppler ultrasonic arteriography may provide information about patients with acute deep vein thrombosis,[13] and the method may be applicable for deeply lying veins in the abdomen, such as the portal circulation or renal veins.

Arterial physiology and mechanics

Doppler ultrasonic arteriography has been used to noninvasively quantify blood flow[15] and analyze velocity flow patterns in the carotid[5,8,34] and femoral arteries.[5] In addition, these techniques may be used to noninvasively evaluate arterial wall properties and plaque constituents.[24]

REFERENCES

1. Baird, R.N., et al.: Pulsed Doppler angiography in lower limb arterial ischemia, Surgery 86:818, 1979.
2. Barber, F.E., et al.: Ultrasonic duplex echo-Doppler scanner, IEEE Trans. Biomed. Eng. 21:109, 1974.
3. Barnes, R.W., et al.: Noninvasive ultrasonic carotid angiography: prospective validation by contrast angiography, Surgery 80:328, 1976.
4. Bendick, P.J., Jackson, V.P., and Becker, G.J.: Comparison of ultrasound scanning/Doppler with digital subtraction angiography in evaluating carotid arterial disease, Med. Instrum. 17(3):220, 1983.
5. Blackshear, W.M., Jr., Phillips, D.J., and Strandness, D.E., Jr.: Pulsed Doppler assessment of normal human femoral artery velocity patterns, J. Surg. Res. 27:73, 1979.
6. Blackshear, W.M., Jr., et al.: Carotid artery velocity patterns in normal and stenotic vessels, Stroke 11:67, 1980.
7. Bloch, S., Baltaxe, H.A., and Shoumaker, R.D.: Reliability of Doppler scanning of the carotid bifurcation: angiographic correlation, Radiology 132:687, 1979.
8. Breslau, P.J., et al.: Effect of carbon dioxide on flow patterns in normal extracranial arteries, J. Surg. Res. 32:97, 1982.
9. Breslau, P.J., et al.: Ultrasonic duplex scanning with spectral analysis in extracranial carotid artery disease. Comparison with contrast arteriography, Vasc. Diagn. Ther. 3:17, 1982.
10. Campbell, S., et al.: New Doppler technique for assessing uteroplacental blood flow, Lancet 1(8326 Pt.1):675, 1983.
11. Clifford, P.C., et al.: Arterial grafts imaged using Doppler and real-time ultrasound, Vasc. Diagn. Ther. 1:43, 1981.
12. Curry, G.R., and White, D.N.: Color coded ultrasonic differential velocity arterial scanner (Echoflow), Ultrasound Med. Biol. 4:27, 1978.
13. Day, T.K., Fish, P.J., and Kakkar, V.V.: Detection of deep vein thrombosis by Doppler angiography, Br. Med. J. 1:618, 1976.

14. Fell, G., et al.: Ultrasonic duplex scanning for disease of the carotid artery, Circulation 64:1191, 1981.
15. Gill, R.W.: Pulsed Doppler with B-mode imaging for quantitative blood flow measurement, Ultrasound Med. Biol. 5(3):223, 1979.
16. Greene, F.M., Jr., et al.: Computer based pattern recognition of carotid arterial disease using pulsed Doppler ultrasound, Ultrasound Med. Biol. 8:161, 1982.
17. Hartley, C.J., et al.: The effects of atherosclerosis on the transmission of ultrasound, J. Surg. Res. 9:575, 1969.
18. Hobson, R.W., et al.: Comparison of pulsed Doppler and real-time B-mode echo arteriography for noninvasive imaging of the extracranial carotid arteries, Surgery 87:286, 1979.
19. Hokanson, D.E., et al.: Ultrasonic arteriography. A noninvasive method of arterial visualization, Radiology 102:435, 1972.
20. Keagy, B.A., et al.: Comparison of oculoplethysmography/carotid phonoangiography with duplex scan/spectral analysis in the detection of carotid artery stenosis, Stroke 13:43, 1982.
21. Keagy, B.A., et al.: A quantitative method for the evaluation of spectral analysis patterns in carotid artery stenosis, Ultrasound Med. Biol. 8:625, 1982.
22. Langlois, Y., et al.: Evaluating carotid artery disease: the concordance between pulsed Doppler/spectrum analysis and angiography, Ultrasound Med. Biol. 9:51, 1983.
23. Lusby, F.J., et al.: Carotid artery disease: a prospective evaluation of pulsed Doppler imaging, Ultrasound Med. Biol. 7:365, 1981.
24. Lusby, R.J., et al.: Transient ischaemic attacks: the static and dynamic morphology of the carotid artery bifurcation, Br. J. Surg. 69:S41, 1982.
25. Maulik, D., et al.: Doppler evaluation of fetal hemodynamics, Ultrasound Med. Biol. 8:705, 1982.
26. Miles, R.D., Russell, J.B., and Sumner, D.S.: Computerized ultrasonic arteriography: a new technique for imaging the carotid bifurcation, IEEE Trans. Biomed. Eng. 29:378, 1982.
27. Miles, R.D., et al.: Computerized multiplanar imaging and lumen area plotting for noninvasive diagnosis of carotid artery disease, Surgery 93(5):676-682, 1983.
28. Moritz, W.E., and Shreve, P.L.: A microprocessor-based spatial-locating system for use with diagnostic ultrasound, Proc. IEEE 64:966, 1976.
29. Mozersky, D.J., et al.: Ultrasonic arteriography, Arch. Surg. 103:663, 1971.
30. Norris, C.S.: Noninvasive evaluation of renal artery stenosis and renovascular resistance, J. Vasc. Surg. 1:192, 1984.
31. O'Leary, D.H., Persson, A.V., and Clouse, M.E.: Noninvasive testing for carotid artery stenosis: I. Prospective analysis of three methods, AJNR 2:437, 1981.
32. O'Leary, D.H., et al.: Noninvasive testing for carotid artery stenosis. II. Clinical application of accuracy assessments, AJNR 2:565, 1981.
33. Phillips, D.J., et al.: Detection of peripheral vascular disease using the Duplex Scanner III, Ultrasound Med. Biol. 6(3):205, 1980.
34. Phillips, D.J., et al.: Flow velocity patterns in the carotid bifurcations of young, presumed normal subjects, Ultrasound Med. Biol. 9(1):39, 1983.
35. Reid, J.M., and Spencer, M.P.: Ultrasonic Doppler technique for imaging blood vessels, Science 176:1235, 1972.
36. Reneman, R.S., and Spencer, M.P.: Local Doppler audio spectra in normal and stenosed carotid arteries in man, Ultrasound Med. Biol. 5:1, 1979.
37. Rittgers, S.E., Putney, W.W., and Barnes, R.W.: Real-time spectrum analysis and display of directional Doppler ultrasound blood velocity signals, IEEE Trans. Biomed. Eng. 27:723, 1980.
38. Rittgers, S.E., Thornhill, B.M., and Barnes, R.W.: Quantitative analysis of carotid artery Doppler spectral waveforms: diagnostic value of parameters, Ultrasound Med. Biol. 9:255, 1983.
39. Spencer, M.P., and Reid, J.M.: Quantitiation of carotid stenosis with continuous-wave (C-W) Doppler ultrasound, Stroke 10:326, 1979.
40. Sumner, D.S., Russell, J.B., and Miles, R.D.: Are noninvasive tests sufficiently accurate to identify patients in need of carotid arteriography? Surgery 91:700, 1982.
41. Weaver, R.G., Jr., et al.: Comparison of Doppler ultrasonography with arteriography of the carotid artery bifurcation, Stroke 11:402, 1980.
42. White, D.N., and Curry, G.R.: A comparison of 424 carotid bifurcations examined by angiography and the Doppler echoflow, Ultrasound Med. Biol. 4:363, 1978.
43. White, D.N., Curry, G.R., and Stevenson, R.J.: Recording vertebral artery blood flow, Ultrasound Med. Biol. 4:377, 1978.
44. Zweibel, W.J., et al.: Correlation of peak Doppler frequency with lumen narrowing in carotid stenosis, Stroke 13:386, 1982.

CHAPTER 21

Pulse echo ultrasonography for the noninvasive imaging of vascular anatomy

GEORGE R. LEOPOLD

The use of diagnostic ultrasound as an imaging tool has expanded remarkably in the past decade. Since the vascular system consists of fluid-filled tubes rimmed by highly elastic boundaries, it is ideal for study by this method. In general, ultrasonic applications in vascular disorders are divided into two large groups: (1) Doppler ultrasound and (2) pulse echo (reflected) ultrasound. The first of these is designed primarily to provide information about flow within the vessel to be examined, and the second concerns noninvasively producing an actual image of the vessel. This chapter deals only with the latter method.

Recent improvements in the technology of transducers and recording methods have allowed progressively finer detail to be visualized within the neck, abdomen, pelvis, and extremities. These improvements, as well as those anticipated in the next few years, make the future bright for this imaging technique.

FUNDAMENTALS OF ULTRASOUND PRODUCTION AND INSONATION

All currently useful ultrasound techniques are variations of the familiar echo-ranging devices such as sonar (sound navigation and ranging). A pulse is generated and travels through a medium until it strikes a barrier (interface). A portion of the pulse is directed back to the starting point. If the velocity of sound in that medium is known, the elapsed time from emission to reception may be used to calculate the distance of the barrier from the sound source.

In medical diagnostic ultrasound, the frequencies employed are in the range of 1 to 15 million cycles per second (1 to 15 MHz). In general, the lower the frequency, the greater the penetration of the ultrasound beam. As frequency increases, resolution is correspondingly increased. For a particular application, one chooses the highest frequency possible that allows sufficient penetration to the vessel or region to be studied. The carotid artery, for example, since it is relatively superficial, may easily be demonstrated with a 10 MHz transducer, whereas the aorta of a large patient may require a 2 MHz source.

For most applications, the source (usually termed *transducer*) is a lead-zirconate-titanate crystal, a polarized synthetic ceramic material. This material possesses a property known as *piezoelectricity,* which means that external mechanical pressures will cause a slight rearrangement of its crystalline lattice. As a result, small electric voltages are created. Conversely, when an electric current is passed across the crystal, the result is a small mechanical pressure wave, which is called *ultrasound.*

In clinical practice, an alternating current is applied to the transducer from 500 to 1000 times a second. The result is a steady stream of pulses, each of which is approximately a μsec in duration.

Since ultrasound is poorly transmitted through air (in contrast to liquids and solids), the transducer must be coupled with the patient's skin for adequate insonation. This may be done by scanning through an interposed water bath or by applying a substance such as mineral oil to the skin. In the latter case the transducer may be placed directly on the skin. Recently the design of transducers has permitted the inclusion of focusing lenses that help to prevent image-degrading beam divergence. By using a transducer that focuses in the area of interest, the maximum resolution is obtained.

Tissue interaction

Having entered the body, the sound beam travels unimpeded as long as it remains in the initial medium. When the boundary (interface) between two media is reached, a small portion of the initial pulse is reflected back toward the transducer. The greater the change in density and elasticity between the two media, the stronger the resultant echo. If a suitable scale is superimposed on the oscilloscope, the distance of the interface from the transducer may be read directly. In addition to the portion of the initial pulse that is reflected, a tiny amount is absorbed within the interface and produces heat. This phenomenon is the basis for using ultrasound in physical therapy. It should be noted, however, that therapy equipment uses continuous-wave (rather than pulsed) ultrasound and that the energy levels employed are far greater. The portion of the initial ultrasound pulse that is not reflected or lost within the interface passes through to interact with deeper tissues where the same processes are repeated.

At the frequencies mentioned earlier, the ultrasound beam behaves much like a light beam, obeying many of the physical laws that apply to light. As a result, the more perpendicular a beam is to an interface, the stronger the returning echo. If the interface is inclined at more than a few degrees to the beam, it is reflected to some point other than the transducer and is not recorded. This has important implications for the individual performing the examination. As far as can be established by current research, the technique is without hazard for the patient or his offspring. Although it is known that ultrasound of sufficient intensity and duration can produce destructive cavitation in soft tissues, these effects are unknown at the levels employed in diagnostic instruments.

Display format

The returning ultrasound pulse emerges from the body and strikes the transducer during its silent period. As the crystal is compressed by this mechanical energy, each echo is converted to a pulse of electrical energy, the amount of which is proportional to the density difference between the two media involved. These pulses are then transmitted to an oscilloscope, where multiple display formats are possible.

A mode. In the simplest form of display, the echo reflections are shown as vertical deflections along the horizontal time base of the oscilloscope screen.

The echoes thus appear as spikes, the distance of which from the transducer may be accurately determined from the superimposed graticule or grid. Since the strength of the echo on the screen is indicated by its height, this method of display is usually termed *amplitude modulation,* or *A mode.*

A mode is generally useful for making measurements along a single line of sight of the transducer. In vascular ultrasonography, for example, early papers dealing with abdominal aortic aneurysms frequently used A-mode measurements.[10] With this method, the examiner palpated the abdomen to determine the point of maximum pulsation. The transducer was then applied to the abdomen and the angle of inclination was adjusted until the maximal signals of the walls of the aorta were visible. By making many such measurements along the length of the aorta, these investigators reported success in determining its size noninvasively. Apparent limitations, however, are the facts that the maximum diameter may never actually be imaged (incomplete examination) and that it may be in a transverse plane, which is difficult to detect by this method.

A-mode studies are seldom used for this type of application today. For clinical purposes, measurements of sufficient accuracy may be obtained from the B-scan images to be described.

B mode and M mode. The B-mode and M-mode forms of ultrasound recording are designed to record motion characteristics of structures being investigated. To accomplish this, the returning echo pulse is not shown as a spike, but is reduced to a dot on the oscilloscope screen. The strength of the echo is no longer indicated by its amplitude but rather by its brightness. This type of display is usually termed *brightness modulation,* or *B mode.* To incorporate motion into the display, the returning echoes are allowed to drift across the screen at a precisely known rate. Thus structures that are phasically changing their distance from the transducer will appear as undulating lines, whereas those that are not moving will be represented as straight lines. These events may be stored by time-exposure photography, but modern instruments now incorporate a fiberoptic strip chart recorder for this purpose. Such a display is usually termed *motion mode, time-motion mode,* or simply *M mode.*

M-mode display is most commonly used in echocardiography. The motion characteristics of the cardiac valves and myocardium have been extensively studied and have provided enormous insight into a wide variety of cardiac disorders. To a lesser extent, this format has been used in imaging the pulsatile characteristics of the abdominal aorta. This method of imaging suffers from the same limitations as does A mode—chiefly, the disadvantage of a rather limited sampling of the areas of interest. To date, pulsatile characteristics of aortic aneurysms have yielded little information of practical clinical value.

B scan. In the B-scan method of display, the B-mode format of echo presentation is used. In this case, however, the transducer is moved about the surface of the body in a preselected plane, which may have any orientation desired by the examiner. Since many sightings of the transducer are being performed, the information must be accurately coded if an anatomic image is to result. With most articulated arm static scanners employed for creating such images, this is achieved by a series of sine-cosine potentiometers within the scanning arm. This allows the recording device to assign each individual sighting its proper anatomic position. In performing the examination, the transducer is swept across the area of interest but is maintained within a fixed plane by the scanning arm. Some degree of transducer movement is allowed within this plane so that more reflecting interfaces may be struck. As the information from these multiple positions is accumulated, a two-dimensional image is formed. Such displays are termed *B scans,* and a complete examination consists of a variety of scans at closely spaced intervals (typically 1 to 2 cm) in multiple planes through the area of interest.

In the earliest instruments employed, the recording medium was the surface of a phosphor-coated oscilloscope. Individual echoes were converted to small flashes of light that "stuck" to the phosphor. This method soon became unsatisfactory, since the phosphor tended to wear unevenly and rather strong echoes were needed for recording. The resultant images, called *bistable,* were entirely black and white with no opportunity to show gradations of echo strength.[24]

The introduction of gray-scale techniques with expanded dynamic range was pioneered by Kossoff[22] and associates in Australia. Modern gray-scale equipment, which is widely available, uses a television scan converter to produce pictures of remarkable clarity. This device allows the incoming electric pulses from the transducer to be stored on a matrix of silicon dioxide diodes. At the completion of the scan, the stored voltages are read and

transferred to a television monitor. The result of this innovation is a dramatic lowering of the intensity threshold of recording. In addition, it has become possible to recognize multiple shades of gray—a feature that has permitted the assessment of the parenchyma of many organs. Early gray-scale instruments used analog scan converters to form an image. Although quality images were produced, the reliability of such units was seriously in question. More recent units employ digital scan converters with a greatly increased reliability. Additionally, such units allow both preprocessing and postprocessing of the data. This capability can be helpful in bringing out subtle changes that may be difficult to detect with the naked eye.

Storage of the data in digital form is a necessary first step in preparing for the data manipulations that will be present in the ultrasound machines of the future. One of the intended uses of these data is in the important area of tissue characterization. In vascular ultrasound, this capability could mean the ability to recognize fresh thrombus, soft plaques, and ulcerations—all of which are difficult or impossible to demonstrate with the equipment of today.

REAL-TIME ULTRASONOGRAPHY

Since the earlier editions of this book a revolution in ultrasound instrumentation has occurred. As mentioned previously, articulated arm scanners, which produce static scans, have been the standard method of imaging. Another type of scanner, called *real time,* has now begun to assume the preeminent role. Such units derive their name from the fact that the retrieved ultrasound information is updated at a rate that is rapid enough to allow visualization of physiologic motion present within the field of view. Once the frame rate exceeds 15 frames per second, the display is perceived as continuous by the eye. The result is an ultrasound moving picture that is entirely analogous to x-ray fluoroscopy. This type of image may be obtained in a number of ways. Some use an array of transducers that fire sequentially. Others use a few transducers that are moved mechanically to interrogate the desired area. Finally, the most sophisticated units, called *phased arrays,* employ a small transducer composed of many elements (for example, 64 or 128) that remain stationary but move the ultrasound beam around by a process called *electronic beam steering.* While intrinsically more expensive, manufacturers of such equipment point to greater reliability (no moving parts) and better lateral resolution resulting from the ability to eliminate noise-producing side lobe artifact.

Initially the images obtained from real-time instruments were inferior to those produced by static scanners. With the introduction of more sophisticated processing, this objection has been overcome. Most modern ultrasound laboratories use a combination of static and real-time devices. Real-time equipment has become smaller and in many cases can be transported to the bedside of a critically ill patient. This capability is of obvious benefit in locations such as the operating room. A pertinent example of interest to vascular surgeons is the ability to use a high-resolution instrument in evaluating the result of carotid endarterectomy.[33] Since the device can be sterilized, it may be placed directly on the vessel and affords a complete view of the operative site. It is anticipated that this method will soon replace or greatly reduce the need for intraoperative angiography in this situation.

Although most feel that real-time equipment, for the reasons just given, will eventually supplant static equipment, it should be pointed out that some disadvantages do exist. The greatest of these is the fact that the images produced usually display only a small sector of the area of interest. For those not present when the examination was performed, such images may be harder to interpret than the more global images produced by static scanners. A possible solution for this problem is the recording of real-time images on videotape for review by others at a later date. An additional disadvantage is the inability to change transducers with real-time devices. Although most static scanners come with a variety of transducers of differing frequencies and focal depths, most real-time devices are limited to one or two frequencies and often have a fixed focal plane. This objection may soon be overcome by improvements occurring in the design of phased arrays.

Applications

Neck vessels. The vessels of the neck were among the first to be studied by ultrasonic B-scan imaging. Because of their relatively superficial location, they are readily imaged by transducers of 7.5 or 10 MHz. As a result, images of very high resolution may be obtained (Fig. 21-1). To date, most studies have concerned the carotids because of the obvious clinical importance of these vessels.[17,20,41] Refer to Chapter 37 for more infor-

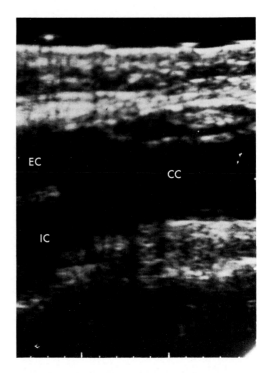

Fig. 21-1. Longitudinal scan of normal patient showing both branches of common carotid artery. (Smallest division is 1 mm.) *CC,* Common carotid; *EC,* external carotid; *IC,* internal carotid.

mation on this subject. Initially it was hoped that these devices might provide a much needed screening test for surgically correctable disease in the region of the bifurcation. Unfortunately, the bulk of clinical evidence now suggests that this is not the case. Although high-resolution imaging alone will detect the great majority of plaques in this area, it is apparent that softer, less echogenic (perhaps newer), lesions may be overlooked. Also disappointing has been the failure to detect all but the grossest of ulcerations. Fresh thrombi are also composed of weakly echogenic material, leading to situations where the vessel looks anatomically normal but is in fact completely occluded. Finally, extensive calcification in the anterior wall of the vessel may render visualization impossible because of total reflection of the ultrasonic beam.

Although these drawbacks seem to speak against the use of this method, this is not the case. By combining the image with the information obtained from range-gated Doppler studies (Duplex scanning), the clinician gains a great deal of information.[6,7] Duplex scanning is of great benefit in detecting fresh occlusions, differentiating between partial and complete obstruction (important in considering surgery), and sorting out the vascular anatomy in complicated situations. Given the variability in orientation of the internal and external carotid arteries to the common carotid, occasions do occur in which it is impossible to correctly identify the branches on the basis of the image alone. Since flow is always forward in the internal carotid artery because of the low resistance of the interval carotid arterial vascular bed, its Doppler signal is quite different from those of the other vessels. Caution is still necessary, however, since in situations where the internal carotid artery is completely occluded, the external carotid artery may assume the flow characteristics normally found in the internal branch.

Duplex scanning is successful in detecting occlusive disease in nearly 95% of cases where lumen diameter is narrowed by greater than 50% (corresponding to an area reduction of 75%). This rate of detection compares favorably with all other methods, including the recently developed intravenous digital angiographic techniques.[40] It should be clear to all who work in this field, however, that only obstructive lesions are being considered. The very important area of detection of small or soft plaques with minimal ulceration, which may be the source of transient ischemic attacks, still eludes modern diagnostic methods (including the standard method, carotid angiography). It is therefore inappropriate to speak of a perfect screening test for atherosclerotic disease of the carotid artery, since none presently exists.

Although little specific attention has been devoted to the jugular veins, there are in fact occasions when valuable clinical information can be gained. Numerous reports exist of detection of complications secondary to insertion of catheters into these vessels. Also, jugular vein thrombosis, which usually occurs as a result of an inflammatory process nearby in the neck, is frequently reported.[38] As with arterial thrombus, these lesions are probably the chronic form of the disorder rather than representing the acute event.

Other peripheral vessels. Studies of other peripheral vessels are possible, and their success is generally related to the size of the patient.[30] With larger patients, study of the femoral arteries may require a much lower transducer frequency, which results in degradation of the image. Such studies are usually requested to evaluate the complications or results of invasive procedures such as surgery

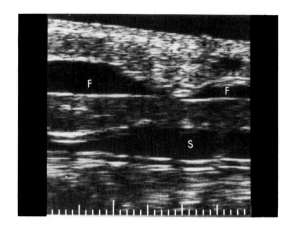

Fig. 21-2. Longitudinal scan of hemodialysis shunt demonstrates complex fluid collection *(F)* external to shunt *(S)* and compressing it.

or percutaneous angiography.[39] Popliteal artery aneurysms are easily diagnosed because of their superficial location.[34] These examinations have been particularly helpful in diagnosing those aneurysms that escape detection on physical examination because of large amounts of thrombus. Similarly, those cases of popliteal cysts masquerading as calf thrombophlebitis are easily diagnosed by this method. This distinction is important, as administration of anticoagulants in the former situation is contraindicated.

One peripheral system that is worthy of special mention is the *hemodialysis access shunt* used in patients with chronic renal disease. Such shunts are subject to frequent mechanical complications that may be life threatening to the patient. Angiography has been the traditional method of evaluating such patients, but it is painful and has inherent risks for damaging the shunt. In many of these situations, ultrasound can adequately identify the problem (Fig. 21-2) and permit definitive therapy.[23,32] It is imperative that those performing such studies have knowledge of the initial surgery performed and any subsequent revisions of it, as well as the type of material used (autologous, synthetic, etc.). Also important is a thorough history indicating whether the problem encountered is one of difficulty in retrieving blood at a rate sufficient to operate the dialysis machine or one of difficulty in reinfusing blood after the dialysis process.

In the situations just mentioned, the clinical problems could be analyzed in large part from the morphologic changes alone. It should be reemphasized, however, that most of these studies would also benefit from the addition of a range-gated Doppler system to simultaneously evaluate flow—just as in the case of carotid artery evaluation.

Vessels of the thorax. Since most of the vessels of the thorax are surrounded by air-filled lung, they are generally not accessible to study by ultrasonography. Although some success in measuring the width of the aortic arch was initially reported with A-mode ultrasound directed caudally in the suprasternal notch,[9] most would concede that study of the thoracic aorta for any reason is better accomplished by radiographic techniques. Computerized tomography (CT) is excellent for this purpose and has the advantage of being able to demonstrate intimal flaps in cases of aortic dissection. On occasion, aneurysms of the descending thoracic aorta are large enough to reach the posterior chest wall. In these rare instances, ultrasonic scanning in a plane along the left paraspinal muscles will succeed in demonstrating the aneurysm.

Vessels of the abdomen and pelvis. Unlike the thorax, the abdominal cavity is well suited to ultrasonic study. Except in those patients with extensive mesenteric fat or bowel gas, most of the major vessels are routinely visualized.[25] Ultrasonic study of these vessels has provided a great deal of useful clinical data. Identification of the vascular structures provides an excellent road map in finding the individual organs. In addition, recognition of characteristic displacement of these vessels often permits a very specific clinical interpretation to be made. Lastly, pathologic conditions involving the vessels themselves may be evident from the scan.

Aorta and branches. Because of its highly elastic walls and proximity to the anterior abdominal wall, the abdominal aorta is easily studied (Fig. 21-3). The major clinical benefit derived from this has been in the detection and serial follow-up of patients with aneurysms.[26] By using both longitudinal and transverse scans, the widest diameter of the aorta is easily located. Measurements made directly from these images have an accuracy of ± 3 mm and are thus sufficient for clinical purposes. Gray-scale imaging has permitted the recognition of thrombi usually present in such lesions (Fig. 21-4).[14] On occasion, real-time ultrasonography has been useful in recognizing the pulsatile intimal flap within a dissecting aneurysm.[3] Although the length of the aneurysmal segment can also be estimated from the sonogram, prediction of involvement of the renal arteries remains problematic. Since ste-

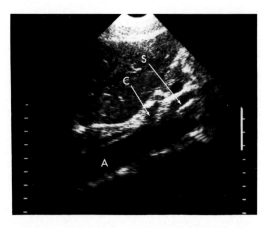

Fig. 21-3. Longitudinal section of abdomen near midline. Abdominal aorta *(A)*, celiac axis *(C)*, and superior mesenteric artery *(S)* are well shown.

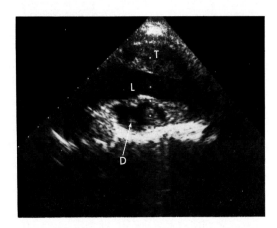

Fig. 21-4. Longitudinal sector scan of abdominal aortic aneurysm. There is considerable thrombus *(T)* both anteriorly and posteriorly. Blood has dissected into posteriorly located component *(D)*, probably at site of ulceration. *L,* Lumen.

nosis of one or more of the major branches of the aorta (in addition to the renal arteries) is common, most surgeons still prefer contrast aortography before surgery. It is conceivable that intravenous digital angiography may soon be capable of fulfilling this need.

In patients with aneurysms not undergoing surgery following initial diagnosis, ultrasound plays a vital role. Serial measurements performed at intervals of 6 months to a year are recommended. Since this technique has now been employed routinely for nearly 10 years, a wealth of data concerning the natural evolution of this disorder is emerging.[1] Preliminary data disclose that an increase in diameter of greater than 4 mm in a single year should be considered presumptive evidence of impending rupture, regardless of the patient's symptoms.

Recently some authors have touted CT as the procedure of choice in evaluating aortic aneurysms.[2] While there is no question that this method can add valuable information, it is unnecessary in the usual case. Since CT scans are ordinarily made perpendicular to the x-ray table without respect to the spine, the anteroposterior measurement is greater than the actual diameter of the vessel. In addition, the inability to easily reformat the image into a longitudinal (sagittal) projection is a major disadvantage. Finally, the cost—particularly if serial studies are to be done—renders this an impractical choice of study.

Increasing use of digital angiography following intravenous injection has also been suggested by some as valuable in this disorder. Unfortunately, just as with direct contrast aortography, those lesions with significant thrombus may appear quite normal or grossly underestimate the size of the aneurysm. Early studies do indicate, however, that such studies are quite accurate in the detection of iliac artery aneurysms, which are often difficult to detect by ultrasonography.[37] It seems quite reasonable to suggest that a combination of these two studies would be an appropriate workup for these patients when surgery is considered imminent.

In the vast majority of patients, the origins of the celiac, superior mesenteric, and renal arteries (Fig. 21-5) may be visualized.[18] Branching of the celiac artery into its hepatic, splenic, and left gastric divisions is also easy to detect. Aneurysms of any of these branches may be identified with this technique.[36] Presently, stenoses of these vessels cannot be detected. Perfection of ultrasound units offering directed Doppler examination at the depths required will add an entirely new dimension to these studies, and noninvasive quantitation of flow within the arteries described is expected to become a reality.

Systemic veins. Like the arteries, most of the major veins within the abdomen are easily visualized. If real-time equipment is employed, the phasic change in the size of these vessels with respiration is quite apparent.[13] Persistent, fixed dilation of them is an indication of elevated systemic venous pressure.[15] For purposes of demonstration, scans are usually conducted in suspended deep inspiration to produce maximum distention.

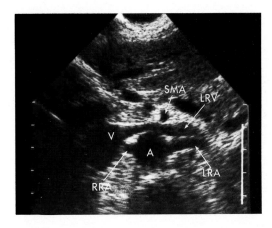

Fig. 21-5. Transverse sector scan, normal patient. In addition to aorta *(A)* and inferior vena cava *(V)*, renal arteries *(RRA, LRA)*, left renal vein *(LRV)*, superior mesenteric artery *(SMA)*, superior mesenteric vein, and portions of splenic vein are also shown.

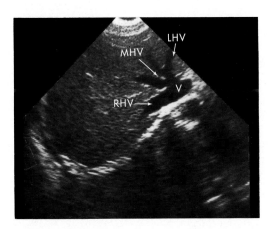

Fig. 21-6. Transverse sector scan of liver, normal patient. Confluence of hepatic veins and inferior vena cava is apparent. *LHV*, left hepatic vein; *MHV*, middle hepatic vein; *RHV*, right hepatic vein.

The inferior vena cava and hepatic and renal veins are easily demonstrated (Fig. 21-6). Study of the hepatic veins is critical in those patients with liver function abnormalities. Dilated intrahepatic veins, without other evidence of abnormality, suggest passive congestion as an explanation (Fig. 21-7). Careful attention is also paid to these veins when segmental resection of the liver is planned for focal lesions. Since the right, middle, and left hepatic veins may be seen at their entrance to the vena cava, the mass may be correctly located on the basis of the ultrasound alone in many cases. Accessory veins draining the right lobe of the liver and entering the vena cava separately may also be

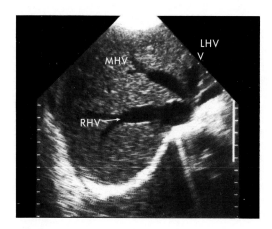

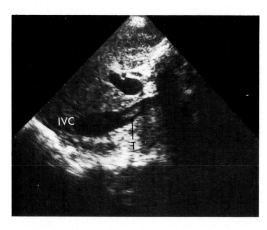

Fig. 21-7. Transverse sector scan of liver in patient with severe right-sided heart failure. Dilation of hepatic veins is obvious. On real-time study, veins failed to show phasic changes with respiration. *LHV,* Left hepatic vein; *MHV,* middle hepatic vein; *RHV,* right hepatic vein.

Fig. 21-8. Longitudinal sector scan of inferior vena cava (IVC) demonstrating intraluminal thrombus *(T)*. In this patient, source is carcinoma of right kidney.

noted, and their recognition assists in planning the operative procedure.[27]

Analysis of the renal veins assumes importance in those cases where tumor is present in the kidneys.[11,35] The method has proven accurate in assessing the extension of tumor into these veins and the inferior vena cava (Fig. 21-8). Although ultrasound is quite successful in detecting tumor thrombus, the bland thrombus responsible for pulmonary emboli usually goes undetected, since it lies distal to the entrance of the renal veins where the vena cava is narrower and often covered by air-filled bowel.

Although thrombus in the inferior vena cava is usually from renal cancer, direct invasion of this vessel is also occasionally seen in primary hepatocellular carcinoma. Assessment of the patency of portacaval shunt is possible in some patients. If the shunt is functional, rather characteristic pseudoaneurysm formation of that portion of the vena cava proximal to the anastomosis is noted. As with most of the vessels discussed in this chapter, the addition of Doppler capability in making this evaluation will be quite welcome. Displacements of the vena cava by extrinsic masses may be quite helpful in narrowing the differential diagnosis. For example, masses in the pancreatic head produce an indentation on the anterior aspect of the vessel. A mass that produces anterior displacement of the vena cava usually arises in the right adrenal gland, which lies directly posterior to it.

The portal venous system. Visualization of this system has obvious clinical significance in the evaluation of a large number of disorders of the liver, spleen, and intestines. The intrahepatic and extrahepatic portal veins, as well as the splenic and superior mesenteric veins, are the branches most consistently seen.

Within the liver the main right and left branches, as well as a number of smaller tributaries, may be seen entering the central portion of their respective lobes. Diminution in the number of these branches is highly suggestive of an infiltrative disorder such as fatty metamorphosis or cirrhosis.[12] When such processes are far advanced, routes of collateral flow such as a recanalized umbilical vein may be seen.[5,8] Tumor invasion of the portal vein by hepatocellular carcinoma is extremely common, and detection of this finding is highly specific for that disorder.[19,31] With regard to the extrahepatic (main) portal vein, failure to visualize it should be regarded as suspicious for portal vein thrombosis.[29] If this lesion is accompanied by abundant periportal collaterals—so-called cavernous transformation of the portal vein—a very characteristic ultrasound appearance is found.[28] Instead of the single, large portal vein seen just anterior to the vena cava, a tangle of tiny vessels resembling a cluster of grapes replaces it (Fig. 21-9). In the normal individual, the main portal vein assists the ultrasonographer in finding the common hepatic duct, since that structure lies adjacent to the anterolateral border of the

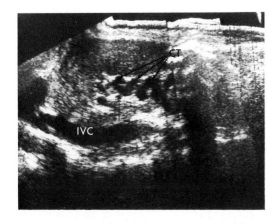

Fig. 21-9. Longitudinal scan of inferior vena cava *(IVC)*. Anterior to the IVC, in expected location of main portal vein, are numerous small fluid-filled structures *(CT)*. This appearance is strongly suggestive of cavernous transformation of portal vein. In this case, etiology is severe pancreatitis.

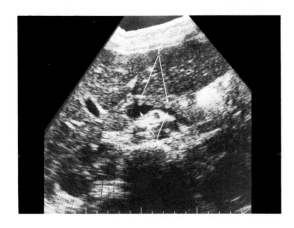

Fig. 21-10. Transverse scan, normal patient. Splenic vein *(SV)* is easily identified and serves as marker for dorsal surface of body and tail of pancreas *(P)*.

vein and parallels it for a considerable distance.[16]

The splenic vein, in addition to being an anatomic marker for the dorsal surface of the pancreas (Fig. 21-10), often provides other useful information. Dilation of the vessel may be an indicator of portal hypertension, but the same finding results from any condition that causes increased blood flow to the spleen. When portal hypertension is present, the collateral routes of flow are often visible on ultrasonic study.[4,21] Varices isolated to the area of the splenic hilus suggest a process causing obstruction of the distal portion of the splenic vein of either inflammatory or neoplastic origin.

The superior mesenteric vein is most easily visualized in longitudinal scans just anterior to the abdominal aorta. In addition to participating in the general dilation of the portal venous system seen in portal hypertension, it may be selectively occluded by neoplasms of the pancreatic head, producing a distinctive appearance on sonograms of this area.

REFERENCES

1. Bernstein, E., et al.: Growth rates of small abdominal aortic aneurysms, Surgery 80:765, 1976.
2. Buscaglia, L.C. Fodor, L.B., and West, W.W.: Use of CT scan in the diagnosis of abdominal aortic aneurysms, CT 4(3):197, 1980.
3. Conrad, M. et al.: Real time ultrasound in the diagnosis of acute dissecting aneurysm of the abdominal aorta, AJR 132:115, 1979.
4. Dach, J., et al.: Sonography of hypertensive portal venous system: correlation with arterial portography, AJR 137:511, 1981.
5. Fakhry, J., Gosink, B., and Leopold, G.: Recanalized umbilical vein due to portal vein occlusion: documentation by sonography, AJR 137:410, 1981.
6. Fell, G., et al.: Ultrasonic duplex scanning for disease of the carotid artery, Circulation 64:1191, 1981.
7. Garth, K., et al.: Duplex ultrasound scanning of the carotid arteries with velocity spectrum analysis, Radiology 147:823, 1983.
8. Glazer, G., et al.: Sonographic demonstration of portal hypertension: the patent umbilical vein, Radiology 136:161, 1980.
9. Goldberg, B.: Suprasternal ultrasonography, JAMA 215:245, 1971.
10. Goldberg, B., Ostrum, B., and Isard, H.: Ultrasonic aortography, JAMA 198:353, 1966.
11. Goldstein, H., Green, B., and Weaver, R.: Ultrasonic de-

tection of renal tumor extension into the inferior vena cava, AJR 130:1083, 1978.

12. Gosink, B., et al.: Accuracy of ultrasonography in diagnosis of hepatocellular disease, AJR 133:19, 1979.

13. Grant, E., et al.: Normal inferior vena cava: caliber changes observed by dynamic ultrasound, AJR 135:335, 1980.

14. Harter, L., et al.: Ultrasonic evaluation of abdominal aortic thrombus, J. Ultrasound Med. 1:315, 1982.

15. Henriksson, L., et al.: Ultrasound assessment of liver veins in congestive heart failure, Acta Radiol. [Diag.] 23:361, 1982.

16. Hoevels, J.: Topographic relation of portal vein to extrahepatic bile ducts. A combined portographic-cholangiographic study in 25 cadavers. ROEFO 129(2):217, 1978.

17. Humber, P., et al.: Ultrasonic imaging of the carotid arterial system, Am. J. Surg. 140:199, 1980.

18. Isikoff, M., and Hill, M.: Sonography of the renal arteries: left lateral decubitus position, AJR 134:1177, 1980.

19. Jackson, V., et al.: Real time ultrasonographic demonstration of vascular invasion by hepatocellular carcinoma, J. Ultrasound Med. 2:227, 1983.

20. James, E., et al.: High resolution dynamic ultrasound imaging of the carotid bifurcation: a prospective evaluation, Radiology 144:853, 1982.

21. Juttner, H., et al.: Ultrasound demonstration of portosystemic collaterals in cirrhosis and portal hypertension, Radiology 142:459, 1982.

22. Kossoff, G.: Gray scale echography in obstetrics and gynecology, Report No. 60, Sydney, Australia, April 1973, Commonwealth Acoustic Laboratories.

23. Kottle, S., et al.: Ultrasonographic evaluation of vascular access complications, Radiology 129:751, 1978.

24. Leopold, G.: Ultrasonic abdominal aortography, Radiology 96:9, 1970.

25. Leopold, G.: Gray scale ultrasonic angiography of the upper abdomen, Radiology 117:665, 1975.

26. Leopold, G., Goldberger, L., and Bernstein, E.: Ultrasonic detection and evaluation of abdominal aortic aneurysms, Surgery 72:939, 1972.

27. Makuuchi, M., et al.: The inferior right hepatic vein: ultrasound demonstration, Radiology 148:213, 1983.

28. Marx, M., and Scheible, W.: Cavernous transformation of the portal vein, J. Ultrasound Med. 1:167, 1982.

29. Merritt, C.: Ultrasonographic demonstration of portal vein thrombosis, Radiology 133:425, 1979.

30. Neiman, H., Yao, J., and Silver, T.: Gray scale ultrasound diagnosis of peripheral arterial aneurysms, Radiology 130:413, 1979.

31. Pauls, C.: Ultrasound and computed tomographic demonstration of portal vein thrombosis in hepatocellular carcinoma, Gastrointest. Radiol. 6:281, 1981.

32. Scheible, W., Skram, C., and Leopold, G.: High resolution real-time sonography of hemodialysis vascular access complications, AJR 134:1173, 1980.

33. Sigel, B., et al.: Comparison of B-mode real-time ultrasound scanning with arteriography in detecting vascular defects during surgery, Radiology 145:777, 1982.

34. Silver, T., et al.: Gray scale ultrasound evaluation of popliteal artery aneurysms, AJR 129:1003, 1977.

35. Slovis, T., et al.: Evaluation of the inferior vena cava by sonography and venography in children with renal and hepatic tumors, Radiology 140:767, 1981.

36. Subramanyam, B., LeFleur, R., and Bosniak, M.: Renal arteriovenous fistulas: sonographic findings, Radiology 149:261, 1983.

37. Turnipseed, W., et al.: Digital subtraction angiography and B-mode ultrasonography for abdominal and peripheral aneurysms, Surgery 92:619, 1982.

38. Wing, V., and Scheible, W.: Sonography of jugular vein thrombosis, AJR 140:333, 1983.

39. Wolson, A., Kaupp, H., and McDonald, K.: Ultrasound of arterial graft surgery complications, AJR 133:869, 1979.

40. Wood, G., et al.: Digital subtraction angiography with intravenous injection: assessment of 1000 carotid bifurcations, AJR 140:855, 1983.

41. Zwiebel, W.: High resolution carotid sonography, Semin. Ultrasound 2(4):316, 1981.

CHAPTER 22

Digital subtraction angiography: methodology

THERON W. OVITT

The history of digital subtraction angiography is relatively short, with the first clinical examinations being performed in early 1979.[2] For the next year examinations were performed at only three centers (University of Arizona, Cleveland Clinic, and University of Wisconsin), and the clinical efficacy of the procedure was established. It is only in the past 2 or 3 years that manufacturers have been able to provide these instruments for general clinical use. Each succeeding commercial instrument introduced into the market is either more sophisticated or cheaper than its predecessor. There continue to be major innovations in the technology, as evidenced by the recent development of the new subtraction techniques of recursive filtering[6] and hybrid subtraction.[4]

The appeal of digital subtraction angiography is that diagnostic studies of large arteries can be obtained with the intravenous injection of contrast medium on an outpatient basis in approximately 90% of cases.[1,3,8,10] At present the clinical indications for intravenous angiography require only slight suspicion of disease, because of low morbidity and cost compared with routine angiography. The only vessels that have been resistant to examination, so far, are small tumor vessels and the coronary arteries.

Digital video subtraction intravenous angiography is an electronic image-enhancement technique designed to amplify low-contrast iodine signals to suitable contrast levels for diagnosis of major vascular abnormalities. The image acquisition system consists of a specially designed x-ray image intensifier–video chain. Images are continuously obtained before and after the intravenous injection of contrast, converted into a digital format by means of an A/D convertor, and stored. Images obtained

before the appearance of contrast are subtracted from those obtained after, so that the resultant image contains contrast only. The image is then electronically contrast enhanced to demonstrate the final image of arterial structures, which is displayed on a video screen (Fig. 22-1, *A* to *D*).

The procedure takes only minutes to perform; however most examinations take about 1 hour to complete because of the time required for setup, venous cannulation, and the multiple projections required for a complete examination.

The study is performed as an outpatient procedure with no premedication. A standard consent form (as for an intravenous pyelogram) is signed. The patient is given breathing instructions (because this is a subtraction technique, no motion is permitted) and then lies on the x-ray table. A catheter is placed in an antecubital vein, contrast is injected, images are obtained over 10 to 20 seconds, final images are immediately displayed, and either the examination is terminated or further runs are made. A small pressure dressing is applied to the puncture site and the patient leaves, free to resume normal activities. The only untoward effects are a "warm flush" after the injection and occasionally nausea and vomiting. Serious reactions to the contrast are rarely seen.

The contrast can be injected peripherally through a short 16-gauge angiocatheter introduced into the antecubital vein or in the superior vena cava after introducing a 5 F pigtail catheter. Contrast is power injected intravenously at the rate of 12 to 25 ml/ sec for a total of 40 to 50 ml. We have had no complications of injection using the catheter technique in more than 1000 patients and only one serious contrast reaction in more than 4000 injections.

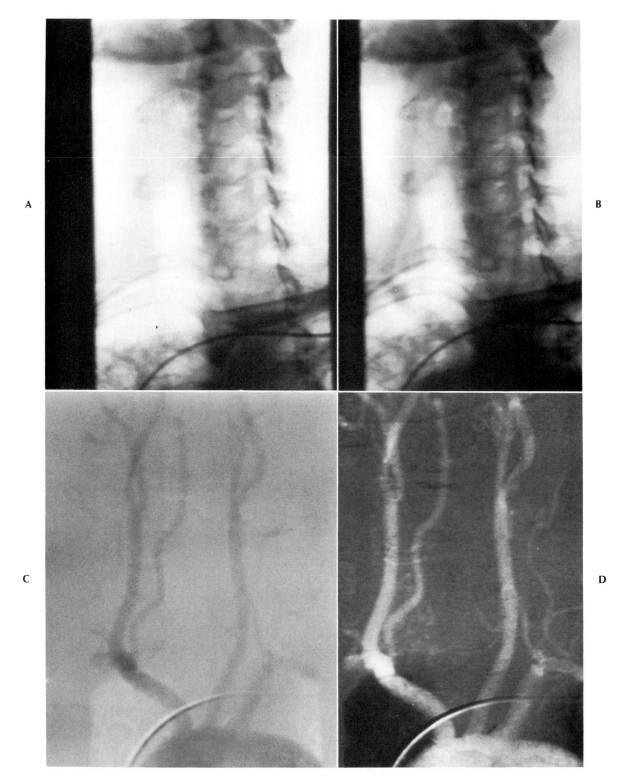

Fig. 22-1. Intravenous angiographic subtraction series. ***A,*** Right posterior oblique view of neck before contrast. ***B,*** Peak arterial concentration. ***C,*** Subtracted, unenhanced image. ***D,*** Subtracted, contrast-enhanced image.

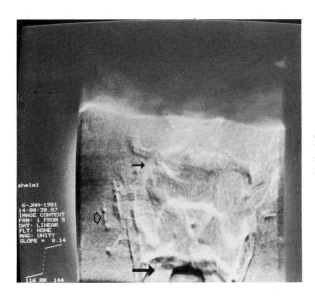

Fig. 22-2. Anteroposterior view of neck. Subtracted image, without contrast, demonstrating motion artifacts caused by swallowing *(large black arrow)*, movement *(small black arrow)*, and vascular pulsations *(open arrow)*.

The major limitations to intravenous angiography are as follows:

1. Susceptibility to motion artifacts. This includes both voluntary and involuntary motion, such as peristalsing bowel gas, involuntary swallowing, and cardiovascular pulsations (Fig. 22-2). It is possible to correct some of these motion artifacts with image manipulation, such as reregistration of the subtraction mask or rubber sheeting the contrast mask to fit the contrast image. Hybrid energy subtraction, a new technique not yet in general clinical practice, addresses this problem by taking two nearly simultaneous exposures, one at low kVp and one at high kVp. By subtracting these two exposures, and with mathematical processing, the iodine-containing structures can be preserved while eliminating soft tissues, even those that have moved. Bone is removed by the conventional subtraction method.

2. Poor arterial opacification. This is usually caused by low cardiac output, but occasionally by poor injection techniques and multiple vessel occlusions (including venous proximal to injection site).

3. Poor spatial resolution compared with direct arteriography. Because of the low concentration of contrast in the arteries, usually 5% to 10%, after a venous injection, considerable noise is present in the final, amplified image.

Another major technical factor limiting the performance of intravenous angiography is the small size and relatively modest resolution of the image intensifier. Most intensifiers used for this procedure have a maximum field size of 9 inches in diameter (compared with 14 × 14 inches for a standard film changer). The intensifier is scanned by a 512 × 512 matrix television system at a 5 MHz band width that limits resolution to approximately 1.8 line pairs at 20% modulation transfer function (compared with 3 to 4 line pairs/mm for screen-film). Because the iodine concentration (signal) is relatively low by the time it reaches the arterial side, considerable amplification of the signal is required to discern the blood vessel. Therefore the remainder of the imaging system is designed to add as little electrical noise to the x-ray image as possible. Most systems incorporate a state of the art television camera with a high signal/noise ratio in order not to further degrade the image from the intensifier.

EQUIPMENT

The equipment for digital intravenous angiography incorporates x-ray and electrical components (Fig. 22-3).

X-ray tube and generator

The x-ray source should be a high-flux, high-heat x-ray tube, so that relatively short exposures can be performed. Calculations indicate that a 1-

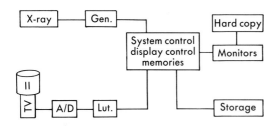

Fig. 22-3. Block diagram of digital subtraction system. *X-ray*, X-ray tube; *Gen.*, x-ray generator; *II*, image intensifier; *TV*, television camera; *A/D*, analog to digital converter; *LUT*, look-up table.

mrad exposure to the intensifier face is needed per exposure to obtain satisfactory images after an intravenous injection. The x-ray generator should be stable and able to produce repeatable exposures so that exact subtractions can be obtained.

Image intensifier

The image intensifier receives the latent x-ray image and converts the invisible x-ray photons to light images, which are then recorded by the television camera. Large-field (12- to 14-inch image intensifiers are preferable to the standard 9- or 6-inch intensifiers for abdominal and peripheral work. The head and neck can be evaluated routinely on the smaller intensifiers.

Television system

A high-quality television system is a must to obtain adequate images for digital subtraction angiography. At present all manufacturers but one use high-quality television cameras with a high signal/noise ratio. Almost no manufacturer of digital equipment recommends, or accepts responsibility for, adapting to existing television systems within present angiography or catheterization laboratories. One important variable among manufacturers is the use of interlaced vs. noninterlaced scanning. Noninterlaced scanning has the ability to produce short pulses with no wasted radiation. Interlaced scanning is advantageous when obtaining images at high temporal rates (such as ventriculography). The television output signal is amplified and then digitized by means of an A/D convertor.

A/D convertor

The A/D convertor is a high-speed instrument, capable of 10 megawords per second at 13-bit accuracy. This allows digitization in real time, at 512 × 512 pixels. The image is digitized and then transferred to a digital image storage unit.

Image processor

The digital image store is a memory device that holds the digitized image before it is transferred to either a digital or analog disk. Memories in sequence can be used for real-time subtraction, and they can also be used to integrate images to decrease noise before transfer.

Image processors range from very simple hard wire configurations, which are cheaper and very reliable and are designed for specific capabilities, to the larger, programmable processors, with the ability to add memory planes, designed for multiple modality use as well as further expansion as new processing techniques develop.

The video image processor accepts the incoming digitized images from the A/D convertor and temporarily stores them in 512 × 512 memories contained within the processor. These memories serve as a temporary holding device, so that incoming images can either be immediately processed or stored on digital disks in raw form. Because digital disks are limited in the rate of information they can receive, an all-digital system at present can accept only approximately seven images per second in the 512 × 512 configuration. If an analog storage system is used, these images can be loaded in real time, 30 images per second, onto the video disk or tape with some degradation of information. Memories can be placed in parallel so that real-time subtraction can be performed, resulting in immediate continuous display and recording of subtracted images. By this method the first image without contrast is stored in a memory and serves as the mask from which all subsequent images are immediately subtracted.

The video image processor is a high-speed digital data acquisition and processing device designed to efficiently handle large volumes of data such as are present in digitized video images. The rapid commercial development of these processors is recent and is in response to the needs of complex image analysis required for space and satellite pictures. This technology is readily applied to digital video x-ray imagery. Memories can also serve to add images together to improve the signal/noise ratio before being unloaded onto a disk or tape. All of these functions are controlled by the acquisition console, which has keyboards, knobs, and joy sticks, similar to computed tomography analysis consoles. Complex image-enhancement techniques, some used in space and satellite image analysis, are being examined and new techniques are constantly being developed, so that a complete, current description of image-enhancement techniques is quickly outdated.

Storage

Images can be stored either in digital form, on digital disks, or in analog form, on analog disks or tape recorders. The advantage of storing images on digital disks (compared with analog storage) is that all information remains digitized and image degradation is eliminated. Images are recalled from storage, sequentially manipulated, and displayed very rapidly until the best subtracted, enhanced image is obtained. The final image is usually recorded on film by a multiformat camera for a permanent record.

There are at least 20 different manufacturers of digital subtraction angiographic modules, no two of which are the same.[11] Some units are designed exclusively for cardiac work, some exclusively for peripheral arterial work, and some units have the capability for both. Therefore, system configurations vary; however, all have the ability to record, subtract, and contrast enhance sequential images.

CLINICAL APPLICATION AND RESULTS
Head and neck

The most common request for intravenous angiography is related to the circulation of the head and neck, particularly for the evaluation of atherosclerotic disease in the cervical carotid arteries.[9] The information obtained is quite comparable to that of conventional aortic arch injection, but with minimal risk, at far lower cost, and as an outpatient procedure. In our experience approximately 90% of examinations are considered diagnostic. Because of the limited spatial resolution, small ulcerating lesions and intracranial vascular stenoses are not expected to be visualized. If the patient has definite symptoms and the intravenous examination yields suboptimal or ''normal'' results, we recommend conventional selective carotid angiography.

Chilcotte, from the Cleveland Clinic, reported 100 consecutive patients who underwent conventional arteriography as well as intravenous angiography.[10] The diagnostic accuracy of the intravenous examination varied from 60% to 95%, depending on the quality of the study (for example, patient

motion, overlapping vessels). This study was performed early in their clinical experience, on equipment that has since been upgraded. If the study were repeated today, better results might be expected.

In our institution the intravenous study has often obviated the need for selective intraarterial examinations by either clearly excluding the suspected disease or accurately delineating the disease process to the satisfaction of both the neuroradiologist and the referring physician. For our standard carotid studies we start with an anteroposterior view using a 14-inch intensifier that demonstrates the carotid arteries from their origins, including the aortic arch, to the bifurcation just below the mandible. We then routinely perform one or two oblique projections in the 10-inch mode to delineate the carotid bifurcations. We then usually perform a fourth projection, an anteroposterior view of the intracranial circulation, to look for major vessel occlusion (Fig. 22-4, *A* to *D*).

The major indications for the carotid intravenous study are asymptomatic bruit, questionable ischemic symptoms, and as preoperative evaluation for patients undergoing coronary bypass surgery or other major vascular surgery where there is a high index of suspicion of significant carotid disease. Other indications for intravenous angiography are the demonstration of aneurysms, glomus jugulare tumors, relationship of carotid arteries to sphenoid sinus and sella before transsphenoidal hypophysectomy, and venous occlusive disease. In addition, we routinely perform postsurgical evaluations with this technique. The major factor leading to suboptimal results is patient motion, including breathing or swallowing. Other poor results arise from venous images superimposed on carotid bifurcation, poor contrast density related to low cardiac output, and positioning errors resulting in overlap of vertebral and carotid arteries.

Renal arteries and abdominal aorta

After initial success with digital intravenous angiography in imaging the carotid arteries we turned our attention to the abdominal circulation. The renal circulation in particular became a central focus of interest, and numerous applications have been found.[5] These include the investigation of renovascular cause of hypertension, characterization of renal masses, evaluation of unexplained hematuria, and evaluation of renal transplant donors and recipients. Our injection and filming technique is

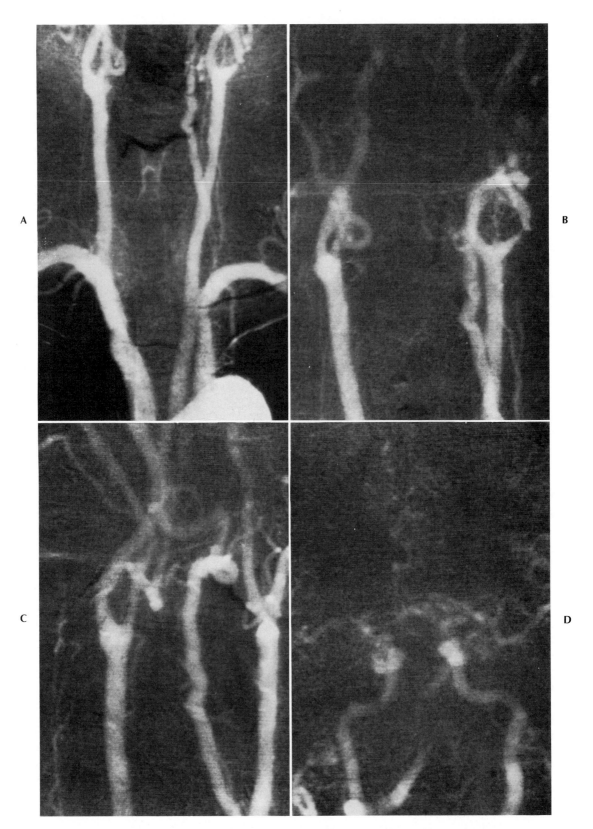

Fig. 22-4. Left carotid bruit. ***A,*** Anteroposterior view with 14-inch field. ***B,*** Right posterior oblique view with 10-inch field. ***C,*** Left posterior oblique view with 10-inch field. ***D,*** Anteroposterior view of head with 10-inch field.

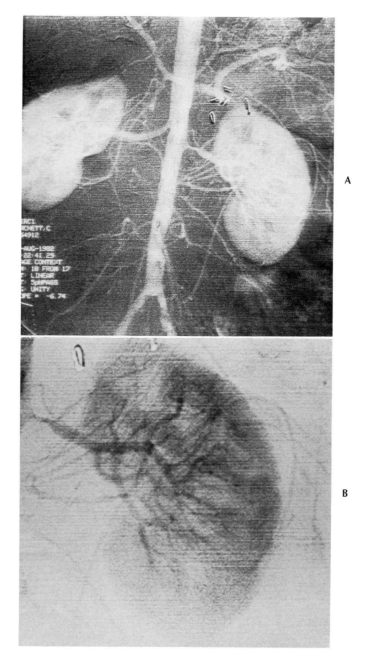

Fig. 22-5. Study in patient with hypertension. Anteroposterior view with 14-inch field *(A)* and 10-inch field *(B).*

similar to that of carotid studies, and again multiple projections are usually required because of overlapping abdominal vessels (Fig. 22-5, *A* and *B*). The technique has accurately detected and quantified renal artery stenoses in hypertensive patients. It has been helpful in characterizing intrarenal lesions and has been especially useful in postoperative studies. All kidney donors are now studied with this technique, because it is an outpatient procedure. We have also examined a large proportion of kidney recipients and have differentiated between renal artery stenosis and renal rejection as a cause of compromised renal function where other studies were inconclusive.

Peripheral vascular disease

The peripheral vascular tree is rather easy to examine by this technique because motion is not a problem. The major limitation is the limited field size, either 9 or 14 inches, which precludes examining an entire leg or arm with one contrast injection. Therefore, our indications have been primarily postoperative or examination of a specific site looking for a specific abnormality.[1] The most common indications are for evaluating localized abdominal or iliac aneurysms, determining sites of arterial occlusion, and evaluating patients after bypass surgery or endarterectomy to determine the cause of diminished pulse (Fig. 22-6). Arterial occlusions and occluded grafts are readily documented. Patent grafts, including small complex graft sites, are well demonstrated by this technique.

Pulmonary disease

Pulmonary intravenous angiography is technically more difficult to perform because of movement created by breathing and by the transmitted cardiac pulsations. As stated above, movement precludes successful subtraction, and inadequate results are obtained. This is more often true in intrathoracic studies than in extrathoracic studies because the transmitted cardiac pulsations preclude exact registration. However, satisfactory pulmonary angiograms demonstrating first-, second-, and in many cases third-order branches are successful in the majority of cases[8] (Fig. 22-7). We have used this technique only to exclude major pulmonary emboli. The technique does not have sufficient discrimination to separate the smaller vessels; therefore, small pulmonary emboli cannot be excluded. Criteria for diagnosis of pulmonary emboli are the same as for conventional arteriography, that is,

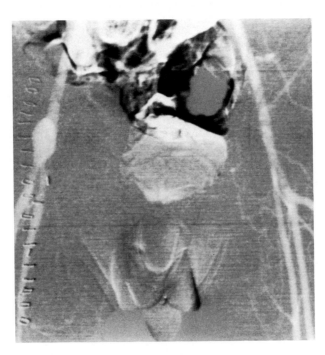

Fig. 22-6. Postoperative vein graft with false aneurysm at proximal anastomosis.

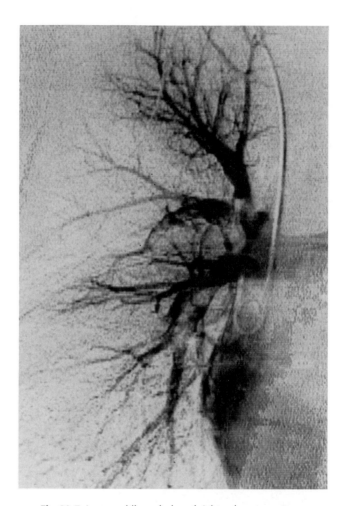

Fig. 22-7. Large saddle embolus of right pulmonary artery.

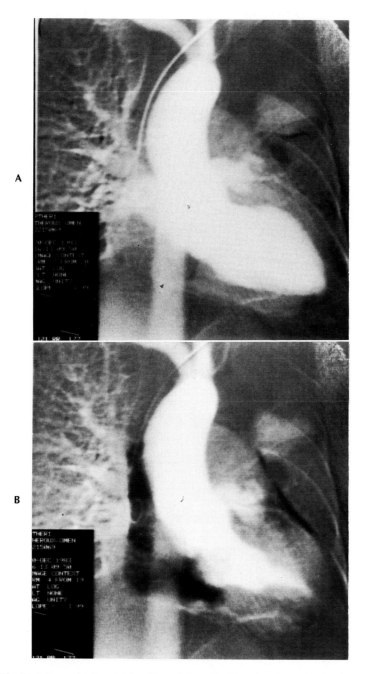

Fig. 22-8. Normal left ventricle with end diastolic *(A)* and end systolic *(B)* phases.

abrupt cutoff of a vessel with a meniscus sign or demonstration of an intraluminal filling defect. The primary usefulness of this procedure is in a patient with an infiltrate and pleuritic pain and few or vague signs of infection. This technique has been valuable in demonstrating normal pulmonary arterial supply to these areas of infiltrate.

Heart disease

Digital intravenous angiography is well suited for the evaluation of left ventricular function and wall motion abnormalities (Fig. 22-8, *A* and *B*). It is more sensitive than nuclear medicine techniques in those centers that perform this study.[7] Heart disease is a relatively new area for digital intravenous angiography, and initial clinical experiences at a limited number of institutions indicate that it will become a major diagnostic tool in evaluation of such disease. A number of centers are focusing on evaluation of postoperative coronary bypass grafts as well as studying the native coronary circulation, and so far the results have been mixed. However, considerable research is under way to improve the technique.

CONCLUSIONS

Digital intravenous angiography has become a major diagnostic tool for the evaluation of major vascular abnormalities. Because it is performed as an outpatient procedure and entails low cost and low morbidity, the indications for angiographic examination have been expanded to include many patients with soft physical findings or symptoms and also for more extensive routine postoperative evaluation. The equipment and software techniques are continually being improved, the technology is still evolving, and more clinical applications can be anticipated in the near future.

REFERENCES

1. Buonocore, E., et al.: Digital subtraction angiography of the abdominal aorta and renal arteries, Radiology 139:281, 1981.
2. Christenson, P.C., et al.: Intravenous angiography using digital video subtraction: intravenous cervicocerebrovascular angiography, A.J.N.R. 1:379, 1980.
3. Clark, R.A., and Alexander, E.S.: Digital subtraction angiography of the renal arteries, Invest. Radiol. 18:6, 1983.
4. Guthaner, D.F., et al.: Clinical application of hybrid subtraction digital angiography: preliminary results, Cardiovasc. Intervent. Radiol. 6:290, 1983.
5. Hillman, B.J., et al.: Renal digital subtraction angiography: 100 cases, Radiology 145:643, 1982.
6. Kruger, R.A., and Liu, P.Y.: Time domain filtering using computerized fluoroscopy: intravenous angiography applications, Proc. SPIE Conf. Dig. Radiog. 314:319, 1981.
7. Mancini, G.B.J., et al.: Cardiac imaging with digital subtraction angiography, Cardiovasc. Intervent. Radiol. 6:252, 1983.
8. Pond, G.D., et al.: Comparison of conventional pulmonary angiography with intravenous digital subtraction angiography for pulmonary embolic disease, Radiology 147:345, 1983.
9. Seeger, J.F., et al.: Digital video subtraction angiography of the cervical and cerebral vasculature, J. Neurosurg. 56:173, 1982.
10. Weinstein, M.A., et al.: Digital subtraction angiography in the evaluation of intracranial and extracranial vascular disease, Cardiovasc. Intervent. Radiol. 6:187, 1983.
11. Zauzmer, D., editor: Applied radiology, 1984 buyer's guide, Los Angeles, 1983, Barrington Publications, Inc.

CHAPTER 23

Quantitative angiography by video dilution technique

BO M. T. LANTZ

In the clinical workup of patients with peripheral arterial disease, angiography is considered mandatory by most vascular surgeons. The exact localization of obstructive lesions, extent of collateral circulation and identification of arteriovenous communications and aneurysms are just a few diagnostic capabilities of angiography that are invaluable for the surgeon in planning appropriate therapy. Unfortunately, pathologic morphology is not always correlated with pathophysiology. A seemingly severe anatomic obstruction of an artery may not cause a significant decrease of blood flow, whereas a smaller lesion may have a severe impact on regional blood flow. Thus, the angiographic appearance of the vascular system does not provide relevant information about hemodynamic parameters such as the blood flow, the most important determinant of arterial adequacy.

The video dilution technique (VDT) is a new radiologic method for the determination of arterial blood flow in conjunction with routine angiography. VDT is a modification of the indicator dilution technique originally described by Stewart[27,28] and by Hamilton et al.[3,4] It uses angiographic contrast medium as the flow indicator. The catheter used for sampling indicator concentration by conventional dilution technique has simply been replaced by an electronic window introduced in the fluoroscopic television image.

The method allows for accurate determination of blood flow in any regional artery where a catheter can be placed. Flow measurements are conveniently performed later, and the procedure takes only a few minutes. It does not significantly add to the patient's cost or risk, and there are no contraindications for VDT other than those for angiography in general. With the use of small catheters (3 to 5 F) and the new nonionic contrast media, angiography is a safe diagnostic method in experienced hands.

Interventional techniques such as embolization and percutaneous transluminal angioplasty (balloon dilation) require arterial catheterization. The immediate effect of such interventions can be determined by VDT immediately. In the event of a successful dilation with an adequate blood flow increase, the patient can be sent home immediately without hospitalization. Inasmuch as angiography is mandatory in the workup of some patients with vascular disease, VDT may be used to acquire valuable physiologic information that cannot be obtained easily by other means. It can be performed in any standard angiographic suite with no additional equipment other than a densitometer. A resumé of the theory, technique, validation, and clinical application of VDT follows.

THEORY

Determination of arterial blood flow at angiography by VDT necessitates the use of a liquid radiopaque indicator with dynamic properties compatible with pulsatile blood flow. It also requires a detector system with high temporal and spatial resolution. Some basic principles of dispersion, dilution, and propagation of liquid indicators in a pulsatile circulatory system are described together with characteristics of the recorded data at the sampling site and the theoretical basis for volume estimates.

Detector system

Two systems with different detector characteristics are available for the study of a liquid flow indicator in vivo: catheter sampling technique and densitometry. The first, the Stewart-Hamilton (S-H) principle, records the concentration of the indicator at the sampling site as a function of time. The second technique, densitometry (VDT), records the mass of the indicator at the sampling site as a function of time (Fig. 23-1).

Concentration of indicator. Determination of blood volumes in the intact circulation was first described by Stewart[27,28] in the 1890s. By recording the dilution of an indicator on the arterial side after a continuous venous injection, Stewart developed the fundamental concepts for the determination of cardiac output. In the 1920s the method was modified by Hamilton et al.[3,4] to a single-bolus technique. Assessment of the cardiac output in the modern cardiovascular laboratory is still based on the classic S-H principle. A bolus of an indicator is injected in a vein and the average dilution of the indicator is determined by sampling on the arterial side. The technique assumes complete mixing of the indicator and the blood and random sampling of the mixture. The integrated concentration-time curves are identical in every artery. They reflect the flow at the injection site and do not give any information about flow at the sampling site (Fig. 23-2). Flow at the injection site can be calculated by determining the mean concentration of multiple samples in a transilluminated cuvette; that is, the technique requires calibration. If the injection is made in an artery such as the thoracic aorta, a sampling from any artery distal to this site will reflect the flow in the thoracic aorta. For accurate calculation of flows after an arterial injection, however, the catheter sampling rate must be high (15 to 20/sec) to record variations of concentration within fragments of the cardiac cycle. Arterial sampling after venous injection does not require a rate of more than one sample per second, because the bolus is spread over 20 to 30 seconds after passage through the pulmonary circulation. Arterial blood flow determination by the S-H principle requires two arterial catheters: an injection catheter and a sampling catheter. In addition, the sampling catheter must have a high-frequency response. Because of these practical inconveniences the S-H principle has not been widely applied for arterial blood flow determination.

Mass of an indicator (VDT). There is one important difference in recording characteristics between the S-H technique and VDT. In addition to indicator concentration c, the densitometer measures the cross-sectional volume v at the sampling site.

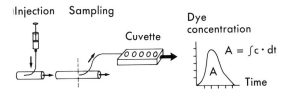

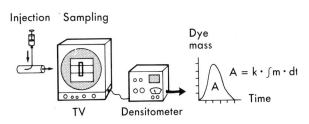

Fig. 23-1. Indicator detector systems with different recording characteristics. With Stewart-Hamilton principle *(top)*, area A represents integral of indicator concentration *(c)* as function of time. With densitometry *(bottom)*, A represents integral of indicator mass *(m)* as function of time. Constant *(k)* accounts for radiographic and electronic conversion factors.

Because concentration times volume represents the mass of contrast,

$$m = c \times v$$

the densitometric recording represents a mass-time curve compared to the concentration-time curve obtained by catheter sampling (Fig. 23-1). Thus the integrated area A under the mass-time curve can be written

$$A = k_1 \int m \cdot dt$$

where the constant k_1 accounts for radiographic and electronic conversion factors. The area reflects the flow at the injection site and the cross-sectional volume at the sampling site (Fig. 23-2).

The integrated area A is the basic parameter for calculating blood flow by VDT. Its dependence on indicator and flow parameters has been extensively studied in a pulsatile hydrodynamic model[8,9] and in an in vivo canine model.[7,10,12,17]

Volume estimates

Densitometry is the detector system used for blood flow determination from angiographic images. It may be the recording of the contrast bolus on films (cine) or in fluoroscopic radiation (video) by analog or digital technique. The densitometric technique is characterized by a frequency response depending on the frame rate of the cine films or

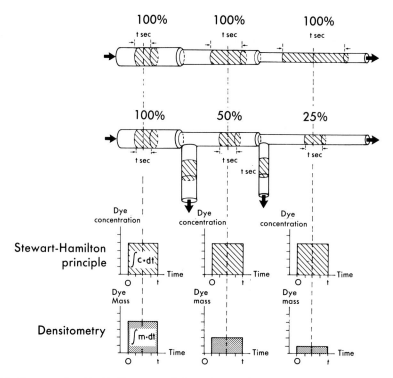

Fig. 23-2. Concentration *(c)* of indicator sample by catheter is the same at any distant site reflecting flow at injection site only. Mass *(m)* of indicator recorded by densitometry. $m = c \times$ volume. The densitometric recording represents a mass-time curve at the recording site analagous to the concentration-time curve.

video images. The densitometric mass-time curves can be used in two ways for blood flow measurements: (1) dimensional techniques (mean transit time technique, MT), and (2) dilution techniques (video dilution technique, VDT).

Dimensional techniques. In the late 1950s and early 1960s attempts were made to estimate blood flow in single arteries by calculating the velocity of an injected contrast bolus on serial films or cine films by densitometric methods.[2,5,24] After the development of the videodensitometer in 1964[29] an accurate determination of x-ray attenuation within an arbitrary area of the fluoroscopic image became possible. The densitometric curve of an iodine contrast medium in the circulatory system was recorded and used for quantitative measurements.[1,20-23,25,26] The technique, known as the mean transit time technique (MT) uses the velocity of contrast volume within the vessel. It is then necessary to know both the volume of the arterial segment and the mean transit time within it. The arterial volume can be estimated from the cine film or the television image, and the transit time can be obtained from two dilution curves upstream and downstream of the arterial segment. MT has two

serious disadvantages. First, it assumes the flow in the artery is constant, which is clearly not true. Measurements obtained vary with the phase of the cardiac cycle. Transit time measured during a complete cardiac cycle would avoid this problem, but only a segment of thoracic aorta is large enough to contain the volume of a complete cardiac cycle. The capacity of all other peripheral arteries restricts the transit time in the segment in the fluoroscopic field to well under one cardiac cycle.

Second, the MT technique requires accurate measurement of the arterial segment volume. Inaccuracies of magnification, vessel diameter, and deviation of the vessel out of the fluoroscopic plane lead to serious errors of calculated flow. Hence, MT has not achieved general clinical acceptance. If applied to intravenous injections for arterial blood flow measurements, this technique would, in addition, suffer from even greater problems in identifying the peak of the indicator bolus, which is spread out over several seconds after passage through the pulmonary circulation.

Video dilution technique. The dependence of the integrated densitometric area A on different hemodynamic parameters can easily be studied in a

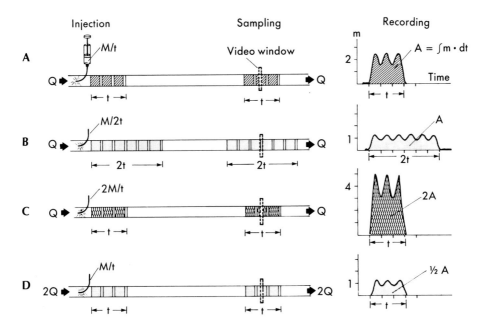

Fig. 23-3. Densitometric recordings of contrast bolus in pulsatile circulatory system with one inlet and one outlet (see text).

pulsatile flow model by changing the parameters independently.

In Fig. 23-3 the mass-time curves were obtained in fluoroscopy by a videodensitometric window covering a cross-section of a single-pipe flow system after contrast injection at a proximal site. At constant rate, M amount of contrast was injected during three cycles in the pulsatile flow Q during the time t (Fig. 23-3, A). All the injected contrast passed the densitometric window during time t, yielding an integrated densitometric area A. If the same amount of contrast was injected into the same flow (Q) at half the rate, the concentration of the indicator at the sampling site would be 50% lower but recorded over a period twice as long (2t). Consequently the integrated area under the curve would be the same (Fig. 23-3, B). If a double amount of contrast (2M) was injected at the same rate in the same flow, the concentration of the indicator at the sampling site and the integrated densitometric area would be two times larger (Fig. 23-3, C). The opposite would occur (Fig. 23-3, D) if M amount of contrast was injected in a flow twice as great (2Q). The indicator would then be diluted to half its concentration, which would be reflected in the size of the integrated area, which would be half of that recorded in Fig. 23-3, A.

If the conditions at the recording site (radiation intensity, videodensitometric window size, posi-

tion of image intensifier and object) are kept constant the integrated densitometric area A is directly proportional to the amount of injected contrast material M and inversely proportional to the flow Q at the site of injection:

$$A = \frac{M}{Q} \cdot k_2$$

Thus,

$$Q = \frac{M}{A} \cdot k_2$$

where k_2 is a calibration constant. The area is independent of the speed of injection, the distance between injection and measuring sites, and the diameter of the pipe at the site of injection. As k_2 cannot be easily determined, the unit for flow Q is expressed in arbitrary units.

Concept of relative flow

Relative flow can be defined as one blood flow measurement expressed as a fraction of another. It might be a comparison of the baseline flow in an artery with the flow in the same artery after dilation or drug therapy. It could also be the blood flow in a regional artery compared with the flow in the aorta. Both options have been extensively studied in the hydrodynamic model comparing VDT with volumetric flow estimates.[8,9] As shown above, the integrated densitometric area A only reflects the

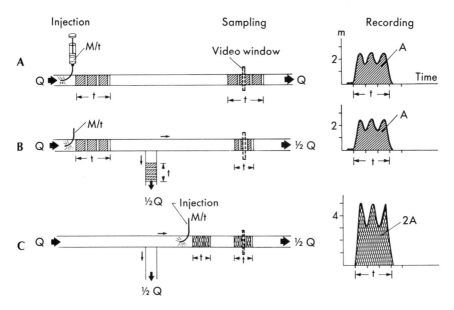

Fig. 23-4. Densitometric recordings of contrast bolus in pulsatile circulatory system with one inlet and two outlets (see text).

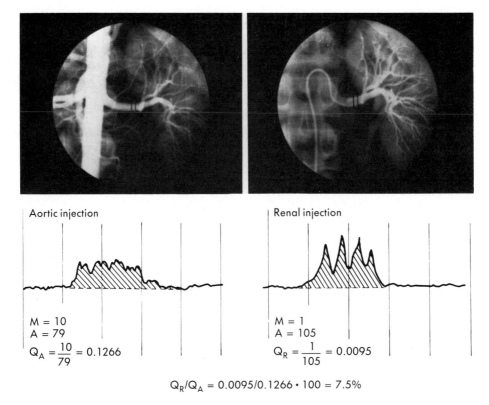

Aortic injection

$M = 10$
$A = 79$
$Q_A = \dfrac{10}{79} = 0.1266$

Renal injection

$M = 1$
$A = 105$
$Q_R = \dfrac{1}{105} = 0.0095$

$$Q_R/Q_A = 0.0095/0.1266 \cdot 100 = 7.5\%$$

Fig. 23-5. Determination of blood flow in left renal artery as fraction of cardiac output. Contrast from aortic 10 ml injection *(left)* and from 1 ml selective injection *(right)*. Videodensitometric window is shown. (From Lantz, B.M.T., et al.: AJR 134:1161, 1980. Copyright 1980, American Roentgen Ray Society. By permission of the Williams & Wilkins Co.)

flow at the *site of injection* and not the flow at the site of recording. Consequently, two recordings obtained at the same site in the circulatory system after contrast injections at two different proximal sites will reflect the flows at these sites. This is illustrated in Fig. 23-4 where a side pipe carries off 50% of the flow in the main pipe. The conditions are otherwise the same as in Fig. 23-3. Observe that the densitometric recording and the integrated area will be identical even when only 50% of the total amount of indicator passes the sampling site (Fig. 23-4, *B*). The concentration of the indicator established at the injection site will be the same throughout the circulatory system. After branching, the length of the contrast column (and the velocity) will be half the original. The time t for the contrast to pass the densitometer window, however, is still the same. If the same contrast amount is injected into the distal portion of the main pipe, which carries half the flow ($Q/2$), the concentration of the indicator will be twice as high (Fig. 23-4, *C*). This is reflected by the mass-time curve where the integrated area will be twice as great ($2A$).

After two contrast injections (M_1, M_2) at two separate sites of a flow system, the integrated areas (A_1, A_2) recorded at the same distal measuring site will reflect the flows (Q_1, Q_2) at the injection sites, respectively:

$$Q_1 = \frac{M_1}{A_1} \cdot k_2$$

and

$$Q_2 = \frac{M_2}{A_2} \cdot k_2$$

where Q_1 and Q_2 are expressed in arbitrary units. The ratio can then be described:

$$\frac{Q_1}{Q_2} = \frac{M_1 \cdot A_2}{M_2 \cdot A_1}$$

This function was studied in the hydrodynamic model and yielded a correlation of $r = 0.9971$, compared with volumetric flows.[8,9]

RECORDING TECHNIQUE

A practical example of relative flow measurements should clarify the details of technique (Fig. 23-5).[10] To determine the blood flow in the left renal artery as a fraction of cardiac output, the catheter tip is placed in the ascending aorta with fluoroscopic guidance. The image intensifier is then centered on the left renal artery, and the kilovoltage and amperage of the radiation are set and locked (automatic brightness control not used). Just before a bolus injection of 10 ml contrast medium, the videotape recorder is started and respirations are suspended. The passage of contrast material is then recorded on videotape (Fig. 23-5, *left*). After an interval of several minutes the catheter is carefully filled with contrast material and the tip selectively positioned in the left renal artery without moving the object or the image intensifier. The videotape recorder is again activated, and 1 ml contrast is injected into the left renal artery (Fig. 23-5, *right*). After the examination the videotape is replayed and the densitometric window is positioned over a cross section of the left renal artery. The dilution curve from the aortic injection of 10 ml is obtained and the integrated area measured as $A = 79$. Hence, $Q = k \cdot M/A$, or $k \cdot 10/79 = k \cdot 0.1266$, in arbitrary units. In a similar manner the area A is obtained from the renal injection of 1 ml contrast. The flow $Q = k \cdot M/A$, or $k \cdot 1/105 = k \cdot 0.009524$, expressed in arbitrary units. Then the left renal flow related to the flow in the ascending aorta (cardiac output) is Q renal/Q aortic $= 0.009524/0.1266 \cdot 100 = 7.5\%$. The constant k cancels out if the sampling site is identical during the two recordings and the size of the densitometric window and the radiation intensity are kept constant. It is equally important that the densitometer output signal be proportional to the logarithm of the incident radiation to maintain linearity of the system (Lambert-Beer law).

VALIDATION IN VIVO

The cerebral, renal, splanchnic, and iliofemoral blood flow was determined by VDT as a fraction of the cardiac output in 389 experiments in 20 dogs (Fig. 23-6).[7] The video dilution values were compared with simultaneous electromagnetic flow measurements of arterial flow expressed as a percentage of cardiac output, which was obtained by a flow meter placed on the regional arteries and around the ascending aorta. A nested random effects analysis yielded a correlation coefficient of 0.99 ($r^2 = 0.98$) for the combined data. The 95% confidence limits for the combined data were -2.8% and $+2.4\%$. This means that if the video dilution technique measured blood flow in an artery as 10% of the cardiac output, there would be a 95% chance that the flow measured by flow meter would be

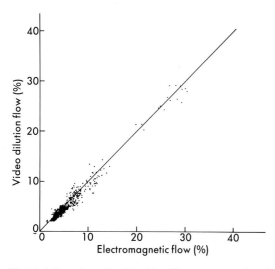

Fig. 23-6. Flow determined by video dilution (Y-axis) plotted against flows determined by electromagnetic flow meter (X-axis) in 20 dogs (n = 389, r = 0.99). Flows expressed as percentage of cardiac output. *Straight line,* Line of identity. (From Holcroft, J.W., et al.: Surg. Forum 31:324, 1980.)

between 7.2% and 12.4%. The 99% confidence limits for the combined data were −3.7% and +3.3%.

CLINICAL APPLICATIONS

Blood flow determination by VDT can easily be applied in the clinical setting in connection with routine arteriography in any area of the circulation where a selective catheter can be placed. It is usually performed while the angiographer is waiting for the serial films to be developed, and the recording procedure is performed within minutes.

Equipment

The examinations are performed on standard angiographic x-ray equipment containing a three-phase generator and a cesium iodide image intensifier connected to a Plumbicon television camera. The contrast injections are recorded on videotape (Sony U-matic ¾ inch) during constant fluoroscopy with locked voltage and amperage. After the angiography is completed, the videotape is replayed and the densitometric window is positioned over a cross section of the artery in the television image. The densitometric curves are frozen on the television monitor, and the flow estimates are automatically calculated by a microprocessor for instant digital readout.*

---

*VDT Mark I, Angiotec Corporation, Berkeley, California.

Clinical considerations

Some steps help avoid unnecessary technical and methodologic errors in clinical applications of VDT. First, it is imperative that the fluoroscopic field is identical when comparing dilution curves from two or more contrast injections. Also, the densitometric window must have the same size and position over the arterial cross section during recordings. Respiration should be suspended during recording (10 to 15 seconds) to avoid baseline fluctuations, and the patient must not move on the table between recordings. It is advisable to lock the voltage and amperage of fluoroscopic radiation to avoid automatic compensation of x-ray intensity when the contrast material passes the radiation field.

Second, it is well known that conventional ionic radiographic contrast material causes vasodilation in peripheral arteries.[6,14-18] Because the increase of local blood flow lasts for about 60 to 90 seconds, waiting at least 2 minutes between injections is recommended to avoid this effect.

Third, incomplete mixing of contrast material with blood, including layering, is a potential source of error. In the aorta good mixing is anticipated because the injection is performed in the direction opposite the flow. In the selective arteries contrast material is injected in the same direction as the flow and perfect mixing cannot be anticipated. This does not seem to be important because the window measures total contrast mass over an arterial cross section rather than the local concentration of contrast within the vessel. To give the contrast an opportunity to mix with the flow, we recommend a distance of at least 2 cm between the tip of the catheter and the recording video window when recording selective injections in regional arteries.

Fourth, it is important to fill the catheter with contrast material before injection to avoid a corresponding volume loss during recording. We use a tuberculin syringe for the manual injection into regional arteries to ensure the delivery of an accurate amount of contrast.

With these precautions, better than 95% of the video dilution measurements are technically satisfactory. The only major disadvantage of the technique is the requirement for patient cooperation.

There are two important modes of application of VDT in the clinical situation: regional blood flow distribution as a fraction of the cardiac output and flow variance in a regional artery as a response to drugs or mechanical interventions.

Regional flow distribution. The distribution of

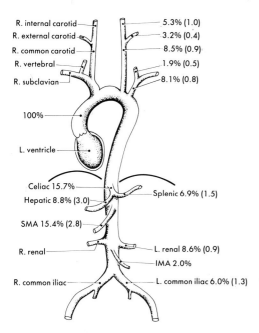

Fig. 23-7. Regional distribution of cardiac output in humans at rest determined by video dilution technique in 70 normal subjects. Standard deviation in parenthesis. *SMA,* Superior mesenteric artery; *IMA,* inferior mesenteric artery. (From Lantz, B.M.T., et al.: AJR 137:903, 1981. Copyright 1981, American Roentgen Ray Society. By permission of the Williams & Wilkins Co.)

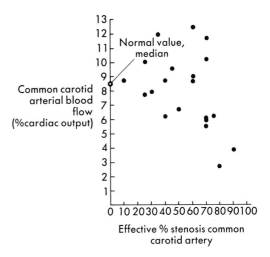

Fig. 23-8. Blood flow in common carotid artery determined by VDT in patients with different stages of stenosis. (From Lantz, B.M.T., et al.: AJNR 3:295, 1982. Copyright 1982, American Roentgen Ray Society. By permission of the Williams & Wilkins Co.)

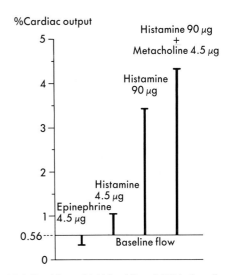

Fig. 23-9. Total bronchial blood flow 0.56% of cardiac output in one sheep weighing 45 kg. Vasoactive effect of some pharmaca shown.

cardiac output to regional arteries in humans at rest has been determined by VDT in 70 normal subjects (Fig. 23-7).[11] We currently use these normal values as standards for the evaluation of patients with a variety of vascular diseases. Regional artery blood flow determination is extremely helpful in determining the significance of questionable lesions in the renal and the carotid circulation. As seen in Fig. 23-8,[13] stenoses of the common carotid artery may have no predictable effect on blood flow until the cross-sectional area has decreased to 70% or more. We have observed several patients with renal artery stenosis undergo apparently successful balloon dilation without flow increase. The technique is also valuable in quantifying the size of shunts and arteriovenous communications expressed as a percentage of cardiac output. Also, in the animal model valuable information about basic physiology can be obtained without explorative surgery. Thus, we have recently assessed the total bronchial blood flow in sheep (less than 1% of cardiac output) and the effect of different drugs on the bronchial circulation (Fig. 23-9). We are currently exploring the hyperemic response in the coronary circulation as a measure of myocardial function.

Flow variance in single arteries. Changes in blood flow in the same artery after mechanical or drug manipulation can easily be determined by VDT. Serial injections are performed in the same vessel, and changes in flow are expressed as a percentage of the initial baseline flow (100%). The vasodilator response to contrast may serve as a simple screening for abnormal peripheral resistance. In patients with peripheral arterial obstructive disease, a reproducable decrease in the peak flow response has

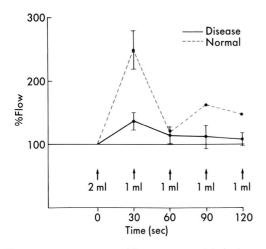

Fig. 23-10. Mean increase of flow (±95% confidence limits) after sequence of contrast injections at 30-second intervals in 23 patients with peripheral arterial obstructive disease compared with normal individuals. Note difference in peak flow at 30 seconds. (From Lantz, B.M.T., et al.: Acta Radiol. [Diagn.] (Stockh.) 23:185, 1982.)

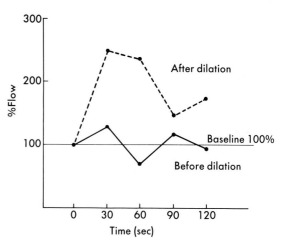

Fig. 23-11. Vasodilator response after a series of test injections in patient before and after successful balloon dilation of superficial femoral artery stenosis. (From Link, D.P., and Lantz, B.M.T.: Acta Radiol. [Diagn.] (Stockh.) 23:81, 1982.)

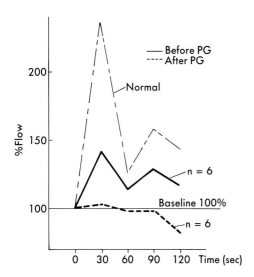

Fig. 23-12. Maximal hyperemia in six patients with severe outflow disease in lower extremities after intraarterial prostaglandin E_1 infusion over 72 hours.

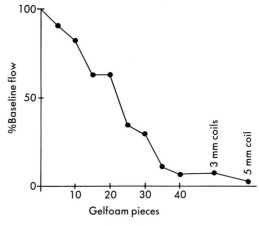

Fig. 23-13. Effect of Gelfoam pieces of emboli during presurgical embolization of spleen as percentage of baseline flow (100%). At end of procedure a 3 mm coil was inserted without effect. A 5 mm coil, however, caused further reduction of flow. (From Porter, B.A., et al.: AJR 141:1063, 1983. Copyright 1983, American Roentgen Ray Society. By permission of the Williams & Wilkins Co.)

been observed (Fig. 23-10).[18] Thus it is possible to instantly record the effect of balloon dilation by a simple test series of contrast injections after angioplasty (Fig. 23-11).[18] Also, the response to vasoactive drugs such as prostaglandin E_1 can be studied (Fig. 23-12). Finally, VDT may also help the angiographer determine the effect of embolic material on blood flow during any phase of a therapeutic embolization procedure (Fig. 23-13).[19]

CONCLUSION

VDT is simple compared with previous densitometric methods because the dimensions of the vessels and the mean transit time of the contrast bolus can be neglected. By using presently available x-ray equipment, VDT has great potential to determine hemodynamic parameters in several areas of the circulation that are not accessible by other techniques. VDT has proved to be important in studying the effect of angiographic intervention techniques, such as embolization and balloon dilation. It can also serve as a valuable functional test in peripheral vascular obstructive disease and can accurately measure the blood flow response to vasoactive drugs. The technique is fast, accurate, and inexpensive. It can be performed in any standard angiographic suite with the addition of a portable densitometer.

REFERENCES

1. Bürsch, J., et al.: Accuracy of videodensitometric flow measurement. *In* Heintzen, P.H., editor: Roentgen-, cine-, and videodensitometry, Stuttgart, 1971, Georg Thieme.
2. Güntert, W., and Zimmer, E.A.: Grundlagen für die Messung der Strömungsgeschwindigkeit des Blutes mittels einer röntgenkymographischen Messmetode, Cardiology Suppl 7:1, 1957.
3. Hamilton, W.F., et al.: Simultaneous determination of pulmonary and systemic circulation times in man and of figure related to cardiac output, Am. J. Physiol. 84:338, 1928.
4. Hamilton, W.F., et al.: Studies on circulation: further analysis of injection method and of changes in hemodynamics under physiological and pathological conditions, Am. J. Physiol. 99:534, 1932.
5. Heuck, F., et al.: Ein röntgenkinematographisches Verfahren zur quantitativen Bestimmung des Blutstromvolumens. R.O.F.O. 98:428, 1963.
6. Hilal, S.K.: Hemodynamic changes associated with the intra-arterial injection of contrast media, Radiology 86:615, 1966.
7. Holcroft, J.W., et al.: Video dilution technique accurately measures blood flow, Surg. Forum 31:324, 1980.
8. Lantz, B.M.T.: A methodologic investigation of roentgen videodensitometric measurements of relative flow, Berkeley, Calif., 1974, University of California Press.
9. Lantz, B.M.T.: Relative flow measured by roentgen videodensitometry in hydrodynamic model, Acta Radiol. [Diagn.] (Stockh.) 16:503, 1975.
10. Lantz, B.M.T., et al.: Determination of relative blood flow in single arteries: new video dilution technique, AJR 134:1161, 1980.
11. Lantz, B.M.T., et al.: Regional distribution of cardiac output: normal values in man determined by video dilution technique, AJR 137:903, 1981.
12. Lantz, B.M.T., et al.: Angiographic determination of splanchnic blood flow, Acta Radiol. [Diagn.] (Stockh.) 21:3, 1980.
13. Lantz, B.M.T., et al.: Carotid blood flow in man determined by video dilution technique. II: Vascular abnormalities, AJNR 3:295, 1982.
14. Lantz, B.M.T., et al.: Vasodilator response in the lower extremity induced by contrast medium. II. Humans, Acta Radiol. [Diagn.] (Stockh.) 23:185, 1982.
15. Lindgren, P., et al.: Vascular effects of metrizoate compounds, Isopaque Na and Isopaque Na-Ca-Mg. Acta Radiol. [Diagn.] (Stockh.) Suppl 270:44, 1967.
16. Lindgren, P., and Törnell, G.: Blood circulation during and after peripheral arteriography: experimental study of the effects of Triurol (sodium acetrizoate) and Hypaque (sodium diatrizoate), Acta Radiol. [Diagn.] (Stockh.) 49:425, 1958.
17. Link, D.P., and Lantz, B.M.T.: Vasodilator response in the lower extremity induced by contrast medium. I. Canine model, Acta Radiol. [Diagn.] (Stockh.) 23:81, 1982.
18. Link, D.P., et al.: Vasodilator response in the lower extremity induced by contrast medium. III. Before and after percutaneous transluminal angioplasty, Acta Radiol. [Diagn.] (Stockh.) 23:381, 1982.
19. Porter, B.A., et al.: Splenic embolization monitored by the video dilution technique, AJR 141:1063, 1983.
20. Rosen, L., and Silverman, N.R.: Videodensitometric measurements of blood flow using cross-correlation techniques, Radiology 109:305, 1973.
21. Rutishauser, W.: Application of roentgen densitometry to blood flow measurement in models, animals, and in intact conscious man. *In* Heintzen P.H., editor: Roentgen-, cine- and videodensitometry, Stuttgart, 1971, Georg Thieme Verlag.
22. Rutishauser, W., et al.: Blood flow measurement through single coronary arteries by roentgen densitometry. I. A comparison of flow measured by a radiologic technique applicable in the intact organism and by electromagnetic flowmeter, AJR 109:12, 1970.
23. Rutishauser, W., et al.: Blood flow measurement through single coronary arteries by roentgen densitometry. II. Right coronary artery flow in conscious man, AJR 109:21, 1970.
24. Scharzkopf, J.H.: Untersuchungen der arteriellen Blutströmungsgeschwindigkeit und des Blutstromvolumens bei Polycythaemia Vera mit der Angiokinematographie, R.O.F.O. 100:479, 1964.
25. Smith, H., et al.: Measurement of flow in saphenous vein–coronary artery grafts by roentgen videodensitometry, Circulation 44(suppl 2):107, 1971.
26. Smith, H., et al.: Roentgen videodensitometric measurement of coronary blood flow: Determination from simultaneous indicator-dilution curves at selected sites in the coronary circulation and in coronary artery–saphenous vein grafts, Proc. Mayo Clin. 46:800, 1971.
27. Stewart, G.N.: Researches on the circulation time in organs and on the influences which affect it, J. Physiol. (Lond.) 15:1, 1894.
28. Stewart, G.N.: Researches on the circulation time and on the influences which affect it. IV. The output of the heart, J. Physiol. (Lond.) 22:150, 1897.
29. Wood, E.H., et al.: Data processing in cardiovascular physiology with particular reference to roentgen videodensitometry, Proc. Mayo Clin. 39:849, 1964.

CHAPTER 24

Positron emission tomography (PET)

JOHN A. CORREIA, NATHANIEL M. ALPERT, and ROBERT H. ACKERMAN

Quantitative physiologic and biochemical information has the potential to provide unambiguous and definitive means of diagnosing and staging disease. Historically, nuclear medicine has, at least in theory, attempted to couple physiologic assessment with imaging to produce "functional" images, or images that show the distribution of a biochemical or physiologic parameter. In practice this has been somewhat limited, both because of the limited number of suitable radiochemicals available and because of limitations associated with physical detection. Other radiologic modalities such as x-ray computed tomography (CT), ultrasound, and digital radiography have shown some potential for physiologic imaging,[18,42,66,76] but for the most part their potential lies in anatomic characterization or in "semiphysiologic" measurements such as the evaluation of vascular dynamics. Nuclear magnetic resonance (NMR) imaging, which has emerged in the last few years, has the potential for physiologic and biochemical imaging, but the NMR signal is related in a very complex and as yet poorly understood way to such information.[72,82] It is therefore unlikely that NMR will provide routine physiologic imaging in the immediate future.

Positron emission tomography (PET) is a nuclear medical imaging technique that takes advantage of a very favorable physical situation. This is the emission of time-correlated pairs of photons, which arise from the decay of certain radioactive nuclei. The net result is that the concentration of radioisotope regionally in an organ can be computed from externally measured signals. Such quantitative activity concentrations, coupled with a physiologic model, in many instances yield quantitative regional physiologic information, which can be presented in image format. Further, a number of light,

biologically active nuclei also happen to be positron emitters, making it possible to chemically synthesize many physiologically active compounds, which can be used in quantitative imaging protocols. In the following sections of this chapter these aspects of positron imaging are reviewed and some applications exemplified. The intent of this review is to give an overall idea of the physical aspects of PET, its current status, and its future potential. The reader is referred to the cited literature for more detailed information on particular aspects of PET.

PHYSICAL ASPECTS OF PET
Detector systems

Certain artificially produced radioactive nuclei that have excess protons decay by the emission of positive electrons called positrons. These positrons are unstable in the sense that, after traveling a small distance (a few microns to several millimeters in tissue, depending on the energy at which they are emitted) they couple with an available electron and undergo an annihilation process. In this process both the positron and the electron disappear and two 0.511 MeV photons, which leave the interaction site in approximately opposite directions, are produced. It is these penetrating photons that are detected in PET.

These time-correlated pairs of photons can be detected in time coincidence as illustrated in Fig. 24-1. Because of limitations in the response times of typical radiation detectors and electronic circuitry, the best that can be done with most PET systems is declare that if two detectors register a signal within a short time, called the coincidence resolving time, they are "simultaneous" and therefore came from the same positron decay. The most commonly used detector material in modern PET devices is bismuth germinate.[20] This material has

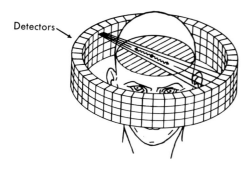

Fig. 24-1. Multiple ring detector geometry for positron emission tomography.

high efficiency for photoelectric interaction of 0.511 MeV photons, acceptable timing properties (typical coincidence resolving time of 20 nsec), and is easy to handle and package. Some very "fast" detector materials such as cesium fluoride (CsF) and barium fluoride (BaF$_2$) allow for more precise determination of the difference in arrival times of two time-correlated photons. Such "time of flight" information can be used to improve the information yield per measured photon in reconstructed PET images.[86,88]

The object to be imaged is surrounded in some fashion by detectors electronically wired in coincidence, as illustrated in Fig. 24-1. The most widely used geometry today is a set of stacked circular rings of detectors with interplane shielding, each ring defining a tomographic plane, and additional tomographic planes being defined by using coincidence pairs from one plane to the adjacent plane. This geometry represents the best compromise between fully surrounding the object with a sphere of detectors and limiting physical factors (for example, scatter), as discussed below. A number of different implementations of this basic geometry have been constructed and are in routine use.*

It should be noted that the overall efficiency of a PET scanner depends upon a number of factors including detector stopping power, detector packing fraction, solid angle subtended by the detector array and electronic considerations such as energy threshold settings. Typical efficiencies for PET scanners are 5-10 times those of the imaging systems used today in nuclear medicine for single photon emission computed tomography.[14]

The resolution of PET reconstructions depends on several factors. The first of these is the size of

*References 10, 12, 16, 17, 46, 59, 68, 78, 85, 86.

the individual detectors. With systems made up of discrete detectors both the in-plane resolution and the plane thickness depend on the detector dimensions. Minimum detector sizes for such systems are defined by the photofraction of the detector and the ability to get out the light produced in scintillation events, both of which decrease with size, and by the necessity to couple photomultiplier tubes of relatively large size to the detectors. Several physical factors, such as the uncertainty in the distance traveled by a positron before annihilation[24] and the fact that the annihilation photons have a small uncertainty in their relative directions because of the atomic motion in the medium in which the decays take place,[23] will probably set the lower limit to practical achievable spatial resolution at 2 to 3 mm. Currently used PET devices have in-plane resolutions of 7.5 to 10 mm and plane thickness of 1 to 2 cm.

The particular physical properties of coincidence detection, as illustrated in Fig. 24-2, give rise to the ability to quantitate regional tissue concentration. The first factor that makes this possible is that the resolution of each detector pair is uniform or depth independent in the volume between the detectors. Second, the individual pairs provide an electronic collimation effect in the sense that pairs of photons produced outside the field of view of the detector cannot both reach the detectors to register. Thus, in principle, no absorbing collimation is necessary to define the volume of origin of a photon pair detected in coincidence. This results in the high detection efficiency cited above. Third, for a pair of annihilation photons traveling along a line in an absorbing medium, the probability of detection of the pair in coincidence depends only on the *total* length of absorber traversed by both photons. Thus a source of positron emitter placed external to the absorber will experience the same absorption effects along a given path as a distributed source within the absorber (Fig. 24-2). We can therefore measure the absorption for each detector pair and for a given absorber with an external source and use this measurement to correct emission data for absorption effects.[8,12,49,51] Obviously the absorption measurement must be made while the object to be imaged contains no radioactivity.

There are also several drawbacks to the coincidence detection of annihilation radiation. The two most important of these involve the detection of coincidence events that carry incorrect information. These events are also illustrated in Fig. 24-2. The first of these is called an "accidental" or "random" coincidence and occurs when two photons from unrelated decays are registered in a pair of detectors within the coincidence resolving time of the system. The count rate from accidental coincidences in a detector pair is given by $\tau N_1 N_2$, where the N_i are the count rates in the individual detectors and τ is the coincidence resolving time of the circuit. The rate of occurrence of these events increases rapidly (approximately as the square of the single detector counting rate) with the amount of radioactivity in the field of view and can reach a significant fraction of the total coincidence events recorded for some imaging situations. These events are not correlated in time; that is, they occur uniformly in time.[44] Because of this they have different properties than the time-correlated "true coincidence" events and can be estimated for each coincidence channel by one of several methods. For example, the single channel rates N_1 and N_2 can be measured electronically and stored along with the coincidence data. Then if the coincidence resolving time for each channel is known, the accidental coincidence rate for that channel can be computed and subtracted from the total measured coincidences for that channel.

A more difficult type of event is called a "prompt scatter" event, and arises when one or both of the pair of annihilation photons emitted in a given decay is Compton scattered in tissue, resulting in the detection of a coincidence event in a detector pair that is different from the pair that would have registered the unscattered photons (Fig. 24-2). Prompt scatter events are not easily distinguished from true coincidences. This is so because scattered events retain their time correlation and often experience an energy loss in scattering that is not large enough to be measured in practical coincidence detectors. The susceptibility of a given system to prompt scatter events can be minimized by proper design of detector shielding. The true coincidence rate is determined by activity in the sensitive volume, whereas activity outside this volume can give rise to prompt scattered coincidences. Thus by restricting the detector acceptance using shielding, the number of scattered events may be minimized. For example, a 50 cm diameter (head sized) detector ring with 1.5 cm plane thickness and unity packing fraction can have a scatter fraction as high as 40% for typical activity distribution. A given PET detector system is usually designed to minimize scatter at some cost in efficiency by reducing accep-

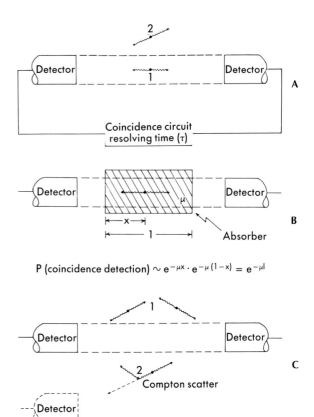

$$P \text{ (coincidence detection)} \sim e^{-\mu x} \cdot e^{-\mu (1-x)} = e^{-\mu l}$$

Fig. 24-2. A, Coincidence detector pair illustrating electronic collimation effect. *Event 1,* within cylinder of sensitivity, will be detected as coincidence, whereas both photons from *event 2* cannot reach detectors. **B,** For source of positron emittor in absorber, probability of detection of coincidence event depends only on total absorber length along line defined by photon path. This is true even if source is outside absorber. Thus a source placed outside absorber can be used to measure total absorption experienced by distributed source within absorber. **C,** Accidental coincidence events *(1)* occur when two photons from different decays arrive at two detectors within coincidence resolving time of detector pair. Such events are not time correlated. Prompt scatter events *(2)* occur when one or both photons emitted in single decay are Compton scattered. Effect of prompt scatter is that coincidence that should have been registered in one detector pair may be "mispositioned" or registered in different detector pair.

tance solid angle. This can be done by increasing the diameter of the detector array, by adding shielding between detectors or between planes, or by a combination of these measures.[45]

To date, only approximate methods for the correction of scattered coincidences have been developed.[7] Usually the scatter response is measured for a standard sized absorber, and the results of this measurement are used to correct the measured coincidence data approximately for the scatter contribution.

Electronic dead time may be a problem in some applications, particularly those with a wide dynamic range of count rates. In most systems dead time can be estimated from measured quantities and accounted for over some range of count rates.[45,59]

Image reconstruction and quantitation

The individual coincidence channel data that cross through a given plane may be sorted into projections or views of either parallel rays or fans. After corrections for detector uniformity variations, accidental coincidences, absorption, prompt scatter, dead time, and radioactive decay (where necessary), these projections may be reconstructed into quantitative transverse section maps of isotope concentration. The reconstruction algorithm usually used is the familiar convolution-backprojection algorithm used in x-ray CT.[9] The resulting reconstructions have been demonstrated to be quantitative to within 5% for a number of different instruments and geometries over a wide range of activity concentrations.* An example of a typical quantitative instrument response is illustrated in Fig. 24-3.

PET, like other nuclear medicine techniques, is photon limited in the sense that the resulting reconstructions have significant statistical imprecision because of the poisson nature of the radioactive decay process. The total number of photons available over reasonable imaging times is limited by subject radiation dose. Also, the reconstruction process amplifies these errors to some degree.[3,39] For example, imaging a uniform brain-sized object at 1 cm resolution requires approximately 2×10^7 photons to achieve 5% statistical precision, whereas imaging the same object at 0.50 cm resolution requires 1.6×10^8 photons for many state of the art instruments. For some newer instrument designs (for example, ECAT III[17]) the use of very small detectors compared with the reconstructed resolution can soften these requirements somewhat (factors of 2 to 4).[70]

Radioisotopes and radiopharmaceuticals

Another set of advantages of PET arise from the fact that several positron emitting isotopes are also light, biologically active atoms. Those of particular interest are ^{11}C (t½ 20.4 minutes), ^{13}N (t½ 10 min-

*References 22, 44, 45, 51, 59, 65, 78.

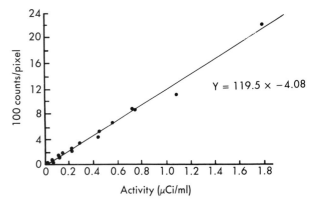

Fig. 24-3. Plot of radioactivity concentration of ^{68}Ga measured by PET versus actual concentration of ^{68}Ga in head-sized phantom containing 3 cm diameter vials, each with different concentration of radioactivity. Projection data were measured with Massachusetts General Hospital positron camera and corrected for random coincidences, absorption effects, prompt scatter, and detector nonuniformities before reconstruction.

utes), ^{15}O (t½ 2 minutes), and ^{18}F (t½ 118 minutes). Because nonradioactive atoms of the same chemical species as these occur in many biologic substances, it is possible to synthesize radiolabeled versions of compounds that directly take part in physiologic processes or analogs of such compounds designed to trace specific parts of a physiologic process. Some examples are ^{15}O-labeled molecular oxygen, which traces the regional rate of oxygen consumption in the brain, or 1-^{11}C-3-methylheptadecanoic acid, which traces the β-oxidation of the myocardium. A more extensive list of compounds that have been synthesized to date and their uses is given in Table 24-1.

Because these isotopes are short-lived, they also have the advantages that compounds labeled with them can be administered to humans with an acceptable radiation dose and that repeat studies or sequential studies with several compounds can be carried out over short periods (minutes to hours). The short half-lives, however, are also the source of a major drawback: isotopes must be produced in close proximity to the imaging site. Thus a cyclotron or other isotope production facility must be located within or near (for practical purposes within 2 km) the hospital complex and appropriate expert staff must be available. Small cyclotrons designed especially for installation in hospitals are commercially available (typically having 50 μA beams of protons at 16 MeV and deuterons at 8 MeV),

Table 24-1. Some radiopharmaceuticals synthesized from positron-emitting isotopes

Compounds	Use
$C^{15}O_2$, $H_2{}^{15}O$, $^{13}NH_3$, ^{18}F-fluoromethane, antipyrine, ^{11}C-alcohols	Cerebral blood flow
$^{15}O_2$	Cerebral O_2 metabolism
^{11}CO, $C^{15}O$	Blood volume
^{68}Ga-ethylenediaminetetraacetic acid	Blood-brain barrier
^{18}F-2-fluoro-2-deoxy-D-glucose, ^{11}C-2-deoxy-D-glucose, ^{11}C-glucose	Brain glucose metabolism, cardiac glucose metabolism
^{82}Rb, ^{11}C-methyl-D-glucose, ^{18}F-3-fluoro-3-deoxy-D-glucose	Heart and brain transport
1-^{11}C-L-lucine, (^{11}C-methyl)-L-methionine	Protein synthesis
^{18}F-spiroperidol, haloperidol, L-dopa; ^{11}C-spiroperidol, pimozide, etorphine	Receptor studies
1-^{11}C-palmitate, 1-^{11}C-3-methylheptadecanoic acid	Cardiac fatty acid metabolism

but they are quite expensive and require a trained operating staff and shielded radioactivity handling areas.[67] Also, provision must be made for safe, automated radiopharmaceutical synthesis.

Several generator-produced short-lived isotopes are also available for PET. The most widely used of these to date are ^{68}Ga from a ^{68}Ge parent[77] and both the parent and the daughter from the ^{82}Rb-^{82}Kr generator.[43]

APPLICATIONS OF PET
Physiologic modeling

The measurement of quantitative regional tissue concentration of radiolabel by PET is the first step in the determination of quantitative regional physiology. To measure a given parameter there must be a physiologic model that relates measurable quantities such as the isotope tissue concentration and concentration of label in various blood fractions to the parameter of interest. This model is often expressed in the form of linear differential equations, derived from a set of compartments, that describe the behavior of the radioactive label in time.[75] The solutions to these equations under a specified set of boundary conditions yields a relationship among measured and physiologic quantities for a given set of experimental conditions.

Such a model also serves as a guide in designing the experimental protocol for a measurement. For example, the choice of the time profile of activity administration, as well as the chemical form of the label, can define the temporal profile of the activity distribution. Under some conditions it is possible to produce a tissue activity distribution that is constant (non–time varying) but still contains physiologic information. In other instances it is necessary to measure a time-varying distribution.

An example of constant distribution is the measurement of regional cerebral blood flow (rCBF) by the continuous inhalation of ^{15}O-labeled CO_2.* The label, ^{15}O, is rapidly transfered to water in the lungs and is circulated throughout the body in arterial blood. After several ^{15}O half-lives (approximately 8 minutes) the distribution of radioactivity in the body becomes constant as a result of an equilibrium established between input to an organ by means of blood flow, output from the organ through blood flow, and radioactive decay. This is illustrated in Fig. 24-4. Because the labeled water is freely diffusible into brain tissue, the flow dependence of the model is on tissue flow. Because the time rate of change of activity in a tissue element is zero when equilibrium is established, neglecting radioactivity in the blood we get the following model operational equation:

$$F/v = \frac{\lambda\, C_T}{C_a - p^{-1}C_T}$$

where

C_T = Radioactivity concentration in tissue element as estimated by PET

C_a = Constant arterial input concentration of radioactivity to be determined by arterial blood sampling

F = Blood flow to tissue element

V = Volume of distribution of water in brain tissue, approximately the tissue volume

= Decay constant of ^{15}O

p = Blood-brain partition coefficient of water.

This expression can be applied on an image element by image element basis to the PET tissue concentration image along with an estimate of the (constant) arterial blood radioactivity to yield an image of rCBF. It should be noted that this requires an independent knowledge of the decay constant of ^{15}O and the blood-brain partition coefficient of water.

If a second continuous inhalation measurement using $^{15}O_2$ is made in the same subject it is possible to combine this measurement with the rCBF mea-

*References 1, 5, 32, 54-56, 83, 92.

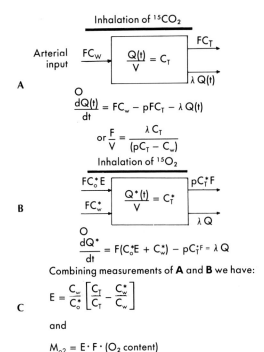

A

$$\frac{O}{dQ(t)}{dt} = FC_w - pFC_T - \lambda Q(t)$$

$$or \quad \frac{F}{V} = \frac{\lambda C_T}{(pC_T - C_w)}$$

Inhalation of $^{15}O_2$

B

$$\frac{O}{dQ^*}{dt} = F(C_o^*E + C_w^*) - pC_T^{*F} = \lambda Q$$

Combining measurements of **A** and **B** we have:

C

$$E = \frac{C_w}{C_o^*}\left[\frac{C_T}{C_T} - \frac{C_w^*}{C_w}\right]$$

and

$$M_{o2} = E \cdot F \cdot (O_2 \text{ content})$$

Fig. 24-4. A, Simple compartmental model for brain tissue element during continuous inhalation of $C^{15}O_2$. After 6 to 8 minutes of inhalation, dynamic equilibrium is established and dQ/dt becomes zero. Relationship among flow, measured tissue concentration, and other quantities is shown. *B,* Simple compartmental model for brain tissue element during continuous inhalation of $^{15}O_2$. Again, dynamic equilibrium is produced, but label is input to tissue from extraction of oxygen (FEC^*_o) and from recirculating labeled water (FC^*_w). *C,* Combining operational equation resulting from this model with that of *A* results in expression shown for extraction fraction of oxygen.

surement to yield images of the regional extraction fraction of oxygen and, if the arterial O_2 content is known, images of the regional rate of cerebral oxygen consumption. The model illustrated in Fig. 24-4, *B,* combined with the rCBF measurement yields the following operational equations for regional oxygen extraction fraction (rOEF) and regional rate of cerebral O_2 consumption (rCMRO$_2$):

$$OEF = \frac{C_w}{C_o^*}\left[\frac{C_T^*}{C_T} - \frac{C_w^*}{C_w}\right]$$

$$rCMRO_2 = F \cdot (OEF) \cdot (O)$$

where

    C_o^* = Concentration of radioactivity in arterial plasma
    C_w^* = Concentration of radioactivity bound to arterial hemoglobin
    C_T^* = Tissue concentration of radioactivity from $^{15}O_2$ measurement
    O = Arterial O_2 content

and the other quantities are as defined above.

There are many other situations in brain and heart where a relationship among PET parameters, arterial blood values as a function of time and physiologic quantities is more complex. Such models often require either the measurement of a dynamic sequence of images or an integrated image of changing activity distribution over some time period and the determination of arterial concentrations of activity as a function of time. Such models

and corresponding radiopharmaceuticals have been developed to measure rCBF and rCMRO$_2$* as well as regional cerebral blood volume (rCBV),[11,38] glucose metabolism,[69,71,74] tissue pH,[19,36,84] protein synthesis,[6,21,71] barrier integrity,[30,94] and receptor density[90] in the brain. In the heart agents and corresponding models to measure blood flow, glucose metabolism, blood volume, and fatty acid metabolism[34,79,80,87] have been developed.

APPLICATIONS IN HUMAN SUBJECTS
Brain studies

An important strength of PET is that it measures physiologic disturbances, which in some disease states, such as epilepsy[27,29,89] and psychiatric disorders,† occur in the absence of anatomic (structural) lesions; in others, such as acute stroke[1,56,92] and Huntington's disease,[53] it anticipates the development of such lesions; and in tumors, where a structural lesion is present, it may serve to metabolically characterize the lesion.[25,54] An additional and very powerful use of PET involves the study of normal physiology, for example the activation of various brain structures in response to sensorimotor or cognitive stimuli such as visual and auditory stimulation.‡

*References 4, 37, 41, 47, 48, 50, 93.
†References 2, 13, 33, 57, 91.
‡References 25, 32, 55, 61-64, 73.

An illustration of the CBF, OEF, and CMRO$_2$ studies discussed above is shown in Fig. 24-5. Fig. 24-5, *A*, shows PET scans at a single level in a subject with a history of left-sided transient ischemic attacks (TIAs) and evincing normal findings on x-ray CT scan. These quantitative images were generated using the Massachusetts General Hospital positron camera, PC-II,[13] and have 1.5 cm inplane spatial resolution and 2.8 cm plane thickness. The quantitative values have a precision in the 5% to 15% range. The measurements were done be-tween attacks. An area of increased OEF is demonstrated on the right middle cerebral artery territory, indicating a mismatch between CBF and CMRO$_2$ in that region. This subject underwent a superficial temporal/middle cerebral artery bypass surgery, and repeat PET studies were carried out after recovery from surgery. The results of the repeat study are shown at the affected level in Fig. 24-5, *B*. After surgery the area of abnormal OEF has resolved, indicating the effect of the bypass surgery and a corresponding cessation of TIAs.

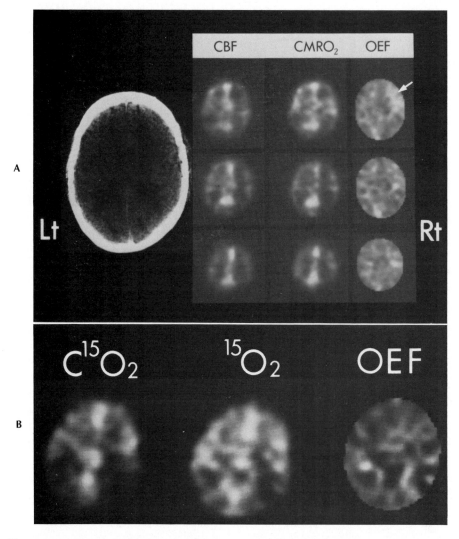

Fig. 24-5. *A*, PET tomographic images of CBF oxygen extraction (OEF) and CMRO$_2$, measured by continuous inhalation of ^{15}O-labeled compounds, in subject with history of transient ischemic attacks (TIA) referent to right middle cerebral artery territory. Images have 1.5 cm resolution. *Arrow*, Region of increased OEF in territory corresponding to TIAs. X-ray CT scan at same level shows normal findings. ***B***, PET images in same subject as in ***A*** after EC/IC bypass surgery. Area of abnormal OEF has resolved, indicating return of normal metabolic function. Subject also evinced cessation of TIAs.

Such studies may in the future be used to select candidates for bypass surgery.

A second example is shown in Fig. 24-6. Shown are CBF studies in a right-handed normal subject. Fig. 24-6, *A,* shows a ''resting study.'' An increased CBF in the left temporal area is observed. This left-right assymmetry is often seen in normal subjects. The subject was then given a fine motor task consisting of sorting two classes of small objects into piles by touch with the left hand. A second CBF study was carried out during the task; the results are illustrated in Fig. 24-6, *B.* We see an increase in CBF (an activation) corresponding to the left-hand activity. Similar types of sensory activation studies have been carried out for motor, visual, and auditory activation by other workers.[25,61-64] This example illustrates the use of PET in normal physiology.

Cardiac studies

A number of research studies of cardiac physiology have also been carried out with PET. These include studies of cardiac blood flow using ^{82}Kr; cardiac metabolism using ^{82}Rb, ^{18}FDG, ^{11}C-labeled fatty acids, and other compounds; and cardiac blood volume using ^{11}CO.*

An example consisting of several cardiac PET studies is shown in Fig. 24-7. This data was obtained at Washington University School of Medicine, St. Louis, using the Super PET I tomograph.[86] Shown are two ECG gated PET studies in the same normal subject at the systolic and diastolic phases of the cardiac cycle. Fig. 24-7, *A,* shows gated images of myocardial fatty acid metabolism measured after the injection of ^{11}C-labeled palmitate.

*References 15, 26, 35, 40, 52, 58, 60, 81.

A   B

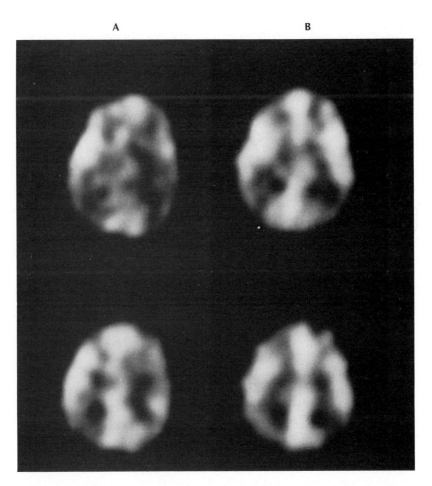

Fig. 24-6. A, PET cerebral blood flow images, measured by continuous inhalation of $C^{15}O_2$, in resting normal right-handed subject. *B,* Cerebral blood flow images in same subject during left-hand fine motor task consisting of separating two classes of small objects by touch. Note increase in cerebral blood flow in left motor area.

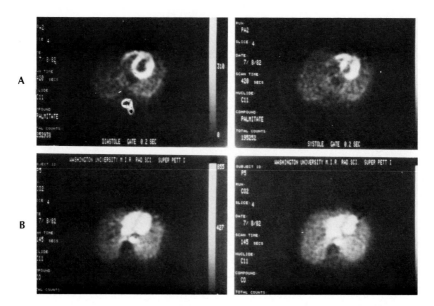

Fig. 24-7. A, Gated PET images of fatty acid metabolism in normal human heart measured with intra-venously injected ¹¹C-palmitate using the Super PET I imaging device. ***B,*** Gated PET blood pool images in the same subject using inhaled ¹¹CO. (Courtesy Dr. M.M. TerPogossian, Washington University, St. Louis.)

Fig. 24-7, *B*, shows blood volume images obtained in the same subject after inhalation of ¹¹C-labeled carbon monoxide.

CONCLUSION

PET presents the capability to measure quantitative regional organ physiology in humans in a relatively noninvasive way. Because of this it has significant potential both as a research tool and a clinical diagnostic modality. Its research use has already been established in heart and brain and is currently being perused in other organ systems. PET may have considerable clinical value in spheres such as: (1) diagnosis and staging of diseases involving physiologic lesions (for example, epilepsy and psychiatric disorders), (2) selection of therapeutic strategies in diseases where a physiologic lesion may later develop into irreversible anatomic damage (TIA, acute stroke, myocardial ischemia), and (3) in monitoring physiologic response to such therapies. Before PET can be used clinically several issues must be resolved: the high cost and limited availability of PET technology,[31] the fact that the complex nature of the technical aspects of PET studies requires a staff of trained experts to carry out studies, and the fact that interpretation of PET studies is subtle and time consuming.

REFERENCES

1. Ackerman, R.H., et al.: PET in ischemic stroke disease using compounds labeled with ¹⁵O: results of clinicophysiological correlations, Arch. Neurol. 38:537, 1981.
2. Alavi, A., et al.: Regional glucose metabolism in aging and senile dementia as determined by ¹⁸F-fluorodeoxyglucose and PET, Brain Res. (Suppl.) 5:187, 1982.
3. Alpert, N.M., et al.: Estimation of the local statistical noise in emission computed tomography, IEEE Trans. Biomed. Imag M1-1:142, 1982.
4. Alpert, N.M., et al.: Strategy for the measurement of rCBF using short-lived tracer and emission CT, J. Cereb. Blood Flow Met. 4:28, 1984.
5. Baron, J.C., et al.: Noninvasive measurement of blood flow, oxygen consumption and glucose utilization in man by PET, J. Nucl. Med. 23:391, 1982.
6. Barrio, J.R., et al.: L(1-¹¹C)-leucine: routine synthesis by enzymatic resolution, J. Nucl. Med. 24:515, 1983.
7. Bergstrom, M., et al.: Correction for scattered radiation in a ring detector positron camera by integral transformation of projections. J. Comput. Assist. Tomogr. 7:42, 1983.
8. Bergstrom, M., et al.: Determination of object contour from projections for attenuation correction in cranial PET, J. Comput. Assist. Tomogr. 6:365, 1982.
9. Brooks, R.A., and DiChiro, G.: Theory of image reconstruction in computed tomography, Radiology 117:561, 1975.
10. Brooks, R.A., et al.: Design considerations for PET, IEEE Trans. Biomed. Eng. 28:158, 1981.
11. Brownell, G.L., and Cochavi, S.: Transverse section imaging with carbon-11 labeled carbon monoxide, J. Comput. Assist. Tomogr. 2:533, 1978.
12. Brownell, G.L., Correia, J.A., and Zamenhof, R.: Positron instrumentation, *In* Lawrence, J.H., and Budinger, T.F., editors: Recent advances in nuclear medicine, New York, 1978, Grune & Stratton, Inc., pp 1-50.

13. Buchsbaum, M.S., et al.: Cerebral glucography with PET: Use in normal subjects and subjects with schizophrenia, Arch. Ger. Psychiatry 39:251, 1982.
14. Budinger, T.F.: Revival of clinical nuclear medicine brain imaging, J. Nucl. Med. 22:1094, 1981.
15. Budinger, T.F., et al.: PET of the heart, Physiolgist 26:31, 1983.
16. Burnham, C.A., et al.: A stationary positron emission ring tomograph using BGO detector and analog readout, IEEE Trans. Nucl. Sci. NS-29:461, 1982.
17. Burnham, C.A., and Brownell, G.L.: A multicrystal positron camera, IEEE Trans. Nucl. Sci. NS-19:193, 1972.
18. Bursch, J.H., et al.: Assessment of arterial blood flow measurements by digital angiography, Radiology 141:39, 1981.
19. Buxton, R.B., et al.: Measurement of brain pH using $^{11}CO_2$ and PET, J. Cereb. Blood Flow Metab. 4:8, 1984.
20. Cho, Z.H., and Farukhi, M.R.: Bismuth germanate as a potential scintillation detector in positron cameras, J. Nucl. Med. 18:840, 1977.
21. Comar, D., et al.: Brain uptake of ^{11}C-methionine in phenylketonuric, Eur. J. Pediatr. 136:13, 1981.
22. Correia, J.A., et al.: Properties of PCII for brain imaging, J. Comput. Assist. Tomogr. 2:652, 1978.
23. DeBeneditti, S.C., et al.: On angular distribution of two photon annihilation radiation, Physiol. Rev. 77:205, 1950.
24. Derenzo, S.E., and Budinger, T.F.: Resolution limit for positron imaging devices, J. Nucl. Med. 18:491, 1977.
25. DiChiro, G., et al.: Glucose utilization of cerebral gliomas measured by ^{18}F-fluorodeoxyglucose and PET, Neurology 32:1323, 1982.
26. Elmaleh, D.R., et al.: Comparison of ^{11}C and ^{14}C labeled fatty acids and their betamethyl analogs, Int. J. Nucl. Med. Biol. 10:181, 1983.
27. Engel, J., Kuhl, D.E., and Phelps, M.E.: Patterns of human local cerebral glucose metabolism during epileptic seizures, Science 218:64, 1982.
28. Engel, J., Kuhl, D.E., and Phelps, M.E.: Regional brain metabolism in humans during seizures. Adv. Neurol. 34:141, 1983.
29. Engel, J., et al.: Local cerebral metabolism during partial seizures, Neurology 33:400, 1982.
30. Eriksson, L., et al.: PET with ^{68}Ga-EDTA and transmission CT in the evaluation of brain infarcts, Acta Radiol. (Diagn.) 22:385, 1981.
31. Evans, R.G., et al.: Cost analysis of PET for clinical use, AJR 14:1073, 1983.
32. Finklestein, S., et al.: PET imaging of normal brain: Regional pattern of cerebral blood flow and metabolism, Trans. Am. Neurol. Assoc. 105:8, 1981.
33. Friedland, R.P., Budinger, T.F., and Ganze.: Regional cerebral metabolism alterations in dementia of the Alzheimer type: PET with ^{18}F-fluorodeoxyglucose, J. Comput. Assist. Tomogr. 7:590, 193.
34. Geltman, E.M., and Sobel, B.E.: Cardiac PET, Chest 83:553, 1983.
35. Giltman, E.M., et al.: Altered regional myocardial metabolism in congestion cardiomyopathy detected by PET, Am. J. Med. 74:773, 1983.
36. Ginos, J.G., et al.: Synthesis of ^{11}C DMO for studies with PET, J. Nucl. Med. 23:255, 1982.
37. Ginsberg, M.D., et al.: A simplified in vivo strategy for the determination of rCBF by PET: Theoretical considerations and validation study, J. Cereb. Blood Flow Metab. 2:89, 1982.
38. Grubb, R.L., et al.: Measurement of regional cerebral blood volume by emission computed tomography, Ann. Neurol. 4:322, 1978.

39. Gullberg, G.T., and Huessman, R.H.: Emission and transmission noise propagation in PET, J. Nucl. Med. 20:609, 1979.
40. Henze, E., et al.: Evaluation of myocardial metabolism with N-13 and C-11 labeled amino acids and PET, J. Nucl. Med. 23:671, 1982.
41. Herscovitz, P., Markham, J., and Raichle, M.E.: Brain blood flow measured with intravenous $H_2^{15}O$.I: Theory and error analysis, J. Nucl. Med. 24:782, 1983.
42. Higgins, C.B., et al.: Quantitation of left ventricular dimensions and function by digital video subtraction angiography, Radiology 144:461, 1982.
43. Hnatowich, D.J.: A method for the preparation and quality control of ^{68}Ga radiopharmaceuticals, J. Nucl. Med. 16:764, 1975.
44. Hoffman, E.J., et al.: Quantitation in PET 4: Effects of accidental coincidences, J. Comput. Assist. Tomogr. 5:391, 1981.
45. Hoffman, E.J., et al.: Performance evaluation of a PET tomograph designed for brain imaging, J. Nucl. Med. 24:249, 1983.
46. Hoffman, E.J., et al.: A new tomograph for quantitative emission tomography of the brain, IEEE Trans. Nucl. Sci. NS-28:99, 1981.
47. Holden, J.F., et al.: CBF using PET measurements of fluoremethane kinetics, J. Nucl. Med. 22:1084, 1981.
48. Huang, S.C., et al.: Quantitative measurement of rCBF in humans by PET and ^{15}O-water, J. Cereb. Blood Flow Metab. 3:141, 1983.
49. Huang, S.C., et al.: A boundary method for attenuation correction in PET, J. Nucl. Med. 22:627, 1981.
50. Huang, S.C., et al.: Measurement of local blood flow and distribution volume with short-lived isotopes: A general input technique, J. Cereb. Blood Flow Metab. 2:99, 1982.
51. Huang, S.C., et al.: Quantitation in PET 2: Effects of inaccurate absorption correction, J. Comput. Assist. Tomogr. 3:804, 1979.
52. Knapp, W.H., et al.: Uptake and turnover of L-(13N)-glutamate in the normal human heart and in patients with coronary artery disease, J. Nucl. Med. 9:211, 1983.
53. Kuhl, D.E., et al.: Cerebral metabolism and atrophy in Huntington's disease determined by ^{18}FDG and PET, Ann. Neurol. 12:425, 1982.
54. Lammertsma, A.A., Wise, R., and Jones, T.: In vivo measurement of rCBF and rCBV in patients with brain tumors using PET, Acta Neurochir. 69:5, 1983.
55. LeBrun-Grande P., et al.: Coupling between rCBF and $rCMRO_2$ in the normal human brain: A study with PET and ^{15}O, Arch. Neurol. 40:230, 1983.
56. Lenzi, G.L., Frackowiak, R.S., and Jones, T.: Cerebral oxygen metabolism and blood flow in human cerebral ischemic information, J. Cereb. Blood Flow Metab. 2:321, 1982.
57. Leon, M.J., et al.: PET studies of aging and Altzheimer's disease, AJNR 4:568, 1983.
58. Lerch, R.A., et al.: Circulation 64:689, 1981.
59. Litton, J., et al.: Performance evaluation of the PC-384 PET camera system for emission tomography of the brain, J. Comput. Assist. Tomogr. 8:74, 1984.
60. Marshall, R.C., et al.: Identification and differentiation of resting myocardial ischemia and infarction in man with PET: ^{18}F-fluorodeoxyglucose and ^{13}N, Circulation 67:766, 1983.
61. Mazziotta, J.C., et al.: Tomographic mapping of human cerebral metabolism: Auditory stimulation, Neurology 32:921, 1982.
62. Mazziotta, J.C., et al.: Tomographic mapping of human cerebral metabolism: Sensory deprivation, Ann. Neurol. 12:435, 1982.

63. Mazziotta, J.C., Phelps, M.E., and Halgran, E.J.: Local cerebral glucose metabolic response to audio-visual stimulation and deprivation: studies in human subjects with PET, Hum. Neurobiol. 2:11, 1983.

64. Mazziotta, J.C., Phelps, M.E., and Kuhl, D.E.: Human cerebral metabolism during limitations in sensory inputs, Trans. Am. Neurol. Assoc. 106:64, 1981.

65. Mazziotta, J., Phelps, M.E., and Plummer, D.: Quantitation in PET 5: Physical anatomic effects, J. Comput. Assist. Tomogr. 5:734, 1981.

66. Meyer, J.S., et al.: Mapping of local blood flow of human brain by CT scanning during stable xenon inhalation, AJNR 1:213, 1980.

67. Nanto, V., and Suolinna, E.M., editors: Medical applications of Cyclotrons II, Medica-Odontologicia 13, 1981.

68. ORTEC, Technical Description, Model 4833 ECAT III, 1983.

69. Phelps, M.E.: PET studies of cerebral glucose metabolism in man: theory and applications in nuclear medicine, Semin. Nucl. Med. 11:32, 1981.

70. Phelps, M.E., et al.: An analysis of signal Amplification using small detectors in PET, J. Comput. Assist. Tomogr. 6:551, 1983.

71. Phelps, M.E., Mazziotta, J.C., and Huang, S.C.: Study of cerebral function with PET. J. Cereb. Blood Flow Metab. 2:113, 1982.

72. Pykett, I.L., and Rosen, B.R.: Nuclear magnetic resonance: In-vivo chemical shift imaging, Radiology 149:197, 1983.

73. Reivich, M., Guv, R., and Alavi, A.: PET studies of sensory stimuli, cognitive processes and anxiety, Hum. Neurobiol. 2:25, 1983.

74. Reivich, M., et al.: The ^{18}F-fluorodeoxyglucose method for the measurement of glucose utilization in man, Circ. Res. 441:127, 1979.

75. Robertson, J.S., editor: Compartmental distribution of radiotracers, Boca Raton, 311., 1983, CRC Press.

76. Rottenberg, D.S., et al.: The measurement of RCBF using stable xenon, J. Cereb. Blood Flow Metab. 1(Suppl. 1):S27, 1981.

77. Ruth, T.J., et al.: Cyclotron isotopes and radiopharmaceuticals. XXX. Aspects of production, elution and automation of ^{81}Rb-^{81}Kr generators, Int. J. Appl. Radiat. Isotope 31:51, 1980.

78. Sank, V.J., Brooks, R.A., and Friauf, W.S.: Performance evaluation of the Neuro PET scanner, IEEE Trans. Nucl. Sci. NS-30:636, 1983.

79. Schelbert, H.R., et al.: Assessment of regional myocardial ischemia by PET, Am. Heart J. 103:588, 1982.

80. Schelbert, H.R., Phelps, M.E., and Shine, K.I.: Imaging metabolism and biochemistry: a new look at the heart, Am. Heart J. 105:492, 1983.

81. Schon, H.R., et al.: ^{11}C labeled palmitic acid for the non-invasive evaluation of regional myocardial fatty acid metabolism with PET myocardium, Am. Heart J. Part 1 103:532, 1983; Part 2 103:548, 1983.

82. Singer, J.R., and Crooks, L.E.: Nuclear magnetic resonance blood flow measurements in human brain, Science 221:654, 1983.

83. Subramanyam, R., et al.: a model for regional cerebral oxygen distribution during continuous inhalation of $^{15}O_2$, $C^{15}O_2$ and $C^{15}O$, J. Nucl. Med. 19:48, 1978.

84. Syrota, A., et al.: Tissue acid base balance and O_2 metabolism in human cerebral information studies with PET, Ann. Neurol 14:419, 1983.

85. Ter-Pogossian, M.M., et al.: PETTVI: a PET tomograph utilizing cesium fluoride scintillation detectors, J. Comput. Assist. Tomogr. 6:125, 1982.

86. Ter-Pogossian, M.M., et al.: Super PET I: a positron emission tomograph utilizing time of flight information, IEEE Trans. Med. Image. MI:179, 1983.

87. Ter-Pogossian, M.M., et al.: Regional asessment of myocardial metabolic integrity in vivo by PET with ^{11}C palmitate, circulation 61:242, 1980.

88. Ter-Pogossian, M.M., et al.: Photon time of flight assisted PET, J. Comput. Assist. Tomogr. 227, 1981.

89. Theodore, W.H., et al.: ^{18}F-fluorodeoxyglucose PET in refractory complex partial seizures, Ann. Neurol. 14:429, 1983.

90. Wagner, H.N., et al.: Imaging dopamine receptors in the human brain by PET, Science 221:1264, 1983.

91. Widen, L., et al.: PET studies of glucose metabolism in patients with schizophrenia, AJNR 4:550, 1983.

92. Wise, R.J., Bernardi, S., and Frackowiak, R.S.: Serial observations of the pathophysiology of acute stroke: the transition from ischemia to infarction as reflected by oxygen extraction, Brain 106:197, 1983.

93. Yamamoto, Y.L., et al.: PET for measurement of rCBF, Adv. Neurol. 30:41, 1981.

94. Yen, C.K., and Budinger, T.F.: Evaluation of blood brain barrier permeability changes in rhesus monkeys and man using ^{82}Rb and PET, J. Comput. Assist. Tomogr. 5:792, 1981.

CHAPTER 25

Nuclear magnetic resonance in vascular imaging

RUSSELL C. REEVES and GERALD M. POHOST

NUCLEAR MAGNETIC RESONANCE

Nuclear magnetic resonance (NMR), a physical phenomenon exhibited by certain atomic nuclei, was independently discovered by Block and by Purcell in 1946.[1,13] NMR has been used as a spectroscopic approach to determine chemical structure. More recently NMR has been applied to medicine, and now permits spectroscopy that can be performed in vivo and high-resolution tomographic and three-dimensional imaging. Because the signal intensity in images produced by NMR depends on the biophysical characteristics and chemical environment of the nuclei in the tissue, there is intrinsic contrast between moving blood and tissue without the need for the administration of foreign substances such as the iodinated contrast agents used in radiologic studies. Accordingly, NMR offers great potential as a noninvasive vascular imaging modality. Additionally, physical characteristics termed relaxation times (T_1 and T_2) can be assessed by NMR imaging and may allow staging of ischemic tissue injury. Phosphorus-31 NMR spectroscopy can be applied in vivo to study high-energy phosphate metabolism (for example, adenosine triphosphate). Such an approach should allow evaluation of the adequacy of blood supply for maintenance of normal skeletal muscle metabolic function and viability. In the future phosphorous 31 imaging may provide a means to study regional high-energy phosphate metabolism. Other NMR-sensitive nuclei in addition to the proton (H-1) and phosphorous (P-31) are listed in Table 25-1.

GENERAL PRINCIPLES

Nuclear magnetic resonance has many facets. As a high-resolution spectroscopic technique, NMR can provide information about the chemical environment of the atomic species (for example, H-1, C-13, Na-23) under investigation. NMR images can be obtained depicting the quantity of nuclei present and their biophysical characteristics (relaxation times). The following simplified description of the principles of NMR is given to provide a basis for understanding the determinants of the spectroscopic signal and of image intensity. Nucleons, the particles that make up atomic nuclei (that is, protons and neutrons) have an intrinsic spin. Certain nuclei, those with an odd number of nucleons, have a net spin. The nucleus is charged, and because moving charges generate magnetic fields, each spinning nucleus generates a magnetic field and behaves like a tiny bar magnet. Normally these nuclear bar magnets are randomly aligned within the weak magnetic field of the earth; however, as the external magnetic field intensity is increased, the "magnetic" nuclei tend to align in the direction of the externally applied field. When tipped out of alignment with an extrinsic field a nucleus will tend to realign by precessing back to the aligned position, as a child's top or a gyroscope precesses back to its position of alignment within

Table 25-1. Medically relevant NMR nuclei

Nucleus	Relative sensitivity constant* (%)	Relative natural abundance (%)
Proton (H-1)	100.0	99.98
Phosphorus 31	6.6	100.0
Sodium 23	9.3	100.0
Carbon 13	1.6	1.1
Flourine 19	83.0	100.0

*Relative sensitivity constant is NMR sensitivity of the nucleus relative to that of an equal number of protons.

261

the earth's gravitational field. Each NMR-sensitive nucleus has a unique (resonant) frequency of precession in a given magnetic field. Radiofrequency (RF) energy at the resonant frequency is used to tilt the nuclei. This resonant frequency is proportional to the strength of the magnetic field and is given by the Larmor equation:

Larmor frequency = Gyromagnetic ratio ×
Magnetic field strength

where the Larmor frequency is the resonant frequency and the gyromagnetic ratio is a constant specific for each sensitive nucleus. When RF energy is applied at the Larmor frequency for protons, the net magnetic vector for the protons is rotated away from its alignment with the externally applied magnetic field. RF irradiation of sufficient strength and duration to rotate the net magnetic vector 90 degrees is referred to as a 90-degree pulse, and irradiation sufficient to rotate the net magnetic vector 180 degrees is referred to as a 180-degree pulse. The signal that occurs after RF irradiation is stopped is called the free induction decay (FID). Mathematical manipulation (that is, Fourier transformation) of the FID generates the spectrum (Fig. 25-1). The net magnetic vector perturbed by the RF pulse will return to its aligned position at a rate described by the relaxation times T_1 and T_2. To better understand T_1 and T_2 consider the coordinate system with the Z-axis parallel to the external magnetic field and the X-Y plane perpendicular to the external magnetic field. The net nuclear magnetic is initially aligned along the Z-axis. The FID is the signal produced in the X-Y plane. If the magnetic vector is rotated by 90 degrees it lies in the X-Y plane and maximum signal intensity will result during relaxation. If it is rotated by 180 degrees there will be no magnetic vector in the X-Y plane and no signal produced.

When the magnetization vector is tilted, for example by 90 degrees, the net magnetization vector will tend to realign in the direction of the Z-axis. The time constant of the rate of growth along the Z-axis is the relaxation parameter T_1. This relaxation process involves transfer of energy from the stimulated nuclei to the surrounding structure or lattice and is referred to as the spin-lattice relaxation time.

After a 90-degree pulse is applied, all of the stimulated nuclei will initially precess in phase and yield a strong signal. However, because the local magnetic field is different for the different nuclei,

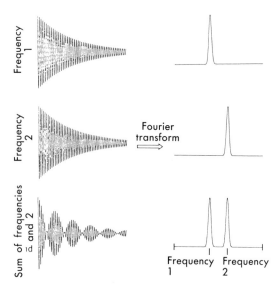

Fig. 25-1. *Left panel,* Two free induction decays (FIDs) resulting after 90-degree radiofrequency stimulating pulse (*freq 1* and *freq 2*), and sum of these two frequencies. Frequencies differ by 10 Hz, so there is "beat" or minimum every 10 cycles. *Right panel,* Result of mathematical operation (Fourier transformation) that converts FID (amplitude vs. time) to spectrum (amplitude or intensity vs. frequency). Location of each peak corresponds to frequency of FID, and area under each peak corresponds to quantity of nuclear species (for example, protons) in sample, giving rise to signal. In imaging system, frequency of peaks corresponds to location of muclei, and area under peaks corresponds to quantity of nuclei at that location.

they will precess at slightly different frequencies and will gradually dephase in the X-Y plane. The time constant that describes the rate of decrease of the magnetization vector in the X-Y plane is T_2. Note that if there was no cancellation of the net magnetization vector in the X-Y plane related to dephasing, T_2 would be equivalent to T_1. Because T_2 is related to interaction between adjacent nuclear spins altering the local magnetic field, it is referred to as spin-spin relaxation. T_2 is generally shorter than T_1, but in certain instances (for example, pure water), T_2 may approach T_1. The following are some of the factors that influence T_1 and T_2 in biologic systems:

1. Compartmental distribution and concentration of water
2. Intercompartmental exchange
3. Distribution and concentration of lipid
4. Presence of metal ions (particularly paramagnetics)
5. Presence and size of macromolecules
6. Temperature.

TISSUE CHARACTERIZATION BY NMR SPECTROSCOPY

Spectroscopy is the term generally applied to the quantitative analysis of a given nuclear species (for example, proton, C-13, P-31). If all nuclei of a given species yielded the same NMR signal, NMR could only be used to measure the overall content of that nuclear species. However, the magnetic field that acts on any nucleus is affected by its surrounding electrons. Thus nuclei in different chemical environments have different resonant frequencies. This shift of frequency is known as chemical shift and is responsible for the capability of NMR to distinguish between different molecular structures. In high-resolution spectroscopy a peak in the spectrum is obtained for each unique chemical environment of the nuclear species being investigated (Fig. 25-2 shows a P-31 spectrum of myocardium). The area under the peak is proportional to the concentration of the species in that chemical environment, and the frequency of the peak, or chemical shift from a known reference point, is determined by the local environment. These characteristics have been used to study intact cellular metabolism, both in vitro and in vivo. In addition the relaxation parameters T_1 and T_2 may be evaluated and used to characterize tissue.

Proton spectroscopy

The proton is an ideal nucleus for NMR studies because it is the most common nucleus in biologic systems and emits relatively intense NMR signals. The relaxation parameters T_1 and T_2 also can be analyzed by both spectroscopy and imaging. Preliminary work on proton relaxation parameters in disease states revealed that T_1 was elevated in malignant tumors,[5] and further studies have demonstrated that this elevation of T_1 is associated with an increase in tissue water content.[17] In studies of the myocardium, significant increases in T_1 have been observed as early as 30 minutes after coronary ligation.[19] Both T_1 and T_2 are elevated after 60 minutes of occlusion. With reflow after 30 or 60 minutes of occlusion both T_1 and T_2 increase significantly. The degree of elevation of T_1 and T_2 is related to the severity of the ischemic insult.[15].

Proton chemical shift spectroscopy

By using proton spectroscopy a number of interesting chemical peaks, especially water and neutral fat, can be demonstrated. In addition, peaks with considerably lower concentration representing

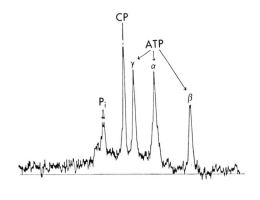

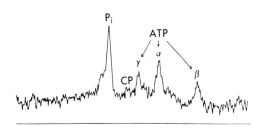

Fig. 25-2. Phosphorus 31 spectra acquired from rat heart under normally perfused *(upper panel)* and ischemic *(lower panel)* conditions. Labeled peaks are Pi, inorganic phosphate *(Pi)*, phosphocreatine *(CP)*, and resonances originating from three chemically distinct phosphorus atoms of adenosine triphosphate *(ATP)*. As anticipated, CP and ATP levels decrease with ischemia.

lactic acid, phosphocreatine, and other relevant metabolites have been observed in vitro. Because these are important tissue metabolites, the ability to monitor them would have obvious importance for determining the presence and severity of tissue ischemia. Because of their low concentration relative to the water and fat present in tissue, substantial progress in NMR techniques will be required before in vivo analysis of these substances with proton NMR will be feasible.

Phosphorus 31 spectroscopy

P-31 spectroscopy is of considerable importance in the assessment of ischemic disease and other disease states of peripheral and cardiac muscle because it can be used to evaluate high-energy phosphate metabolism and intracellular pH. Because of the millimolar cellular concentration, in vivo imaging of the high-energy phosphates has not been done using P-31. P-31 spectroscopy has been applied in the animal laboratory and in humans using topical nuclear magnetic resonance (TMR). TMR has been used by some to refer to the field profiling method of localization of the volume to be studied with or without the additional localization provided by a surface coil. The surface coil is an RF coil placed on the surface of the subject or organ being evaluated. This allows study of tissues to the depth of the radius of the coil. Ross et al.[16] have defined the normal response of human skeletal muscle to anaerobic exercise. They have also used this technique to study patients with McArdle's syndrome, in which lactate is not produced with anaerobic exercise. These techniques may allow the detection and evaluation of tissue ischemia induced by vascular disease. They may be used either at rest or in conjunction with exercise. It should be noted that TMR is not an imaging modality but a technique that generates chemical spectra similar to that produced by an NMR spectrometer.

NMR IMAGING

The principles of NMR imaging were proposed by Lauterbur[11] in 1973. Since then techniques have been developed that allow the acquisition of images with spatial resolution approaching that of x-ray computed tomography, without the need for radiopaque contrast media or ionizing radiation and with a high degree of contrast. Variation of the signal intensity, or contrast, within a proton image is determined by the relaxation properties T_1 and T_2 and the proton density. In addition there is a prominent effect of macroscopic motion such as blood flow, generally to reduce signal. The resonant frequency of a given nucleus is proportional to the local magnetic field that the nucleus experiences. If a magnetic field gradient is imposed on the magnetic field within an NMR spectrometer, nuclei will be sensitive to and emit RF of different frequencies depending on their position; that is, those in the strongest part of the magnetic field will have the highest resonant frequency, whereas those in the weakest part of the field will have the lowest resonant frequency. Because the variation of magnetic field is known to the imaging computer system, the precise position of protons can be derived from the frequency spectrum. NMR imaging systems are capable of acquiring data from one plane, several planes, or in three dimensions. Plane orientation is infinitely flexible. Point-to-point image intensity is determined by the concentration of the proton or other nucleus, its T_1 and T_2, motion, and the imaging pulse sequence (for example, 90-degree pulse followed by a 180-degree pulse, or the con-

verse). The creation of an NMR image requires the repetitive application of a pulse sequence. Time between repeated pulse sequence will influence image appearance because of variations in the completeness of relaxation. The pulse sequence known as *inversion recovery* consists of an initial 180-degree pulse, followed after a variable time τ by a 90-degree pulse. An additional 180-degree pulse is used within 10 to 30 msec to compensate for inhomogeneities in the magnetic field. The inversion recovery pulse sequence produces images related to proton concentration and T_1, and the additional 180-degree pulse adds some T_2 weighting. Another pulse sequence, *saturation recovery,* uses repeat 90-degree pulses separated by an adjustable time. Again a 180-degree pulse shortly after each 90-degree pulse is used to reduce the effects of field nonuniformity. Saturation recovery–generated images also are related to proton concentration and T_1, with less T_1 weighting than inversion recovery. Again these images also have a T_2 component related to the 180-degree, or echo, pulse. A third pulse sequence, *spin-echo,* produces images primarily related to proton concentration and T_2. With spin-echo, T_2 weighting can be varied by changing the time between the 90-and 180-degree pulses.

Aside from morphologic imaging with high resolution, the potential clinical utility of NMR imaging can be considered within four categories largely unique to NMR: noninvasive angiography, tissue perfusion imaging, characterization of tissue using T_1 and T_2, and metabolic studies.

Noninvasive angiography

The decreased signal intensity produced by motion in proton NMR imaging may be used to delineate the internal structure of arterial and venous vasculature where contrast between blood and surrounding tissue is produced by blood motion (Figs. 25-3 to 25-5). The impact of blood motion on image signal intensity is related to blood velocity and the pulse sequence used for imaging. Kaufman et al.[10] have analyzed some of the factors affecting the signal intensity of a moving fluid using a spin-echo pulse sequence.

Tissue perfusion imaging

Preliminary work in myocardium of laboratory animals demonstrates the potential of paramagnetic substances to enhance tissue contrast dependent on the tissue perfusion. Paramagnetic substances have

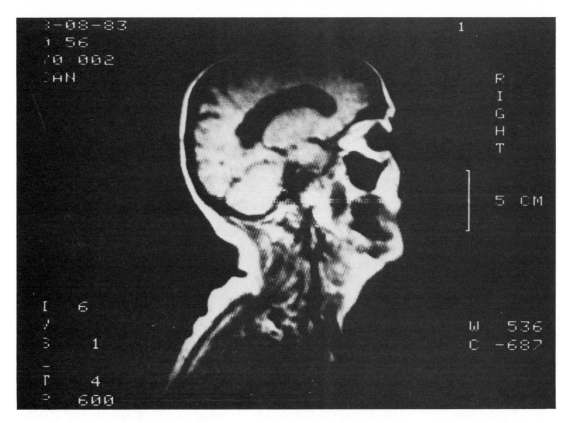

Fig. 25-3. Sagittal plane through common carotid artery and its bifurcation into internal and external carotid arteries is depicted using spin-echo proton NMR imaging method. (Courtesy Siemens Corp.)

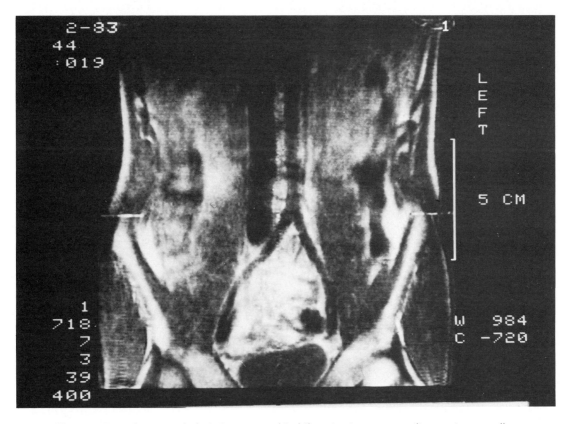

Fig. 25-4. Coronal tomograph depicting aorta and its bifurcation into common iliac arteries, as well as inferior vena cava, using spin-echo proton NMR imaging approach. (Courtesy Siemens Corp.)

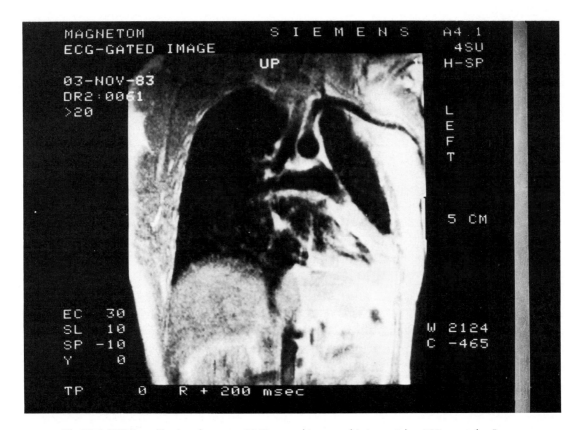

Fig. 25-5. ECG "gated" spin-echo proton NMR coronal tomographic image taken 200 msec after R wave of cardiac QRS complex and approximating mid- or end systole. Cross section of aortic arch and portions of right and left pulmonary arteries are seen. Left ventricular myocardium is well visualized. Lack of signal from blood near mitral valve likely represents residual diastolic flow. Left subclavian artery and portion of left vertebral artery are seen. (Courtesy Siemens Corp.)

unpaired electrons, which when sufficiently close to NMR-sensitive nuclei accelerate relaxation of the NMR-sensitive nuclei, shortening T_1 and T_2. Manganese (Mn + +) is strongly paramagnetic and has been shown in radionuclide studies to distribute in myocardium proportional to blood flow.[4] Lauterbur et al.[12] have demonstrated by spectroscopy that intravenously administered manganous chloride reduced the relaxation times of normal myocardium. Others, using proton NMR imaging in canine studies, have demonstrated that manganous chloride clearly outlined areas of myocardial ischemia or infarction. The area of decreased signal intensity seen in these manganese-enhanced NMR images correlated closely with triphenyl tetrazolium chloride defects as well as thallium defects in both 90-minute and 24-hour coronary ligations.[2,6] Manganous chloride, however, is relatively toxic and will likely not be clinically useful. These paramagnetic metals may be less toxic when administered as chelates, but such chelation may reduce the paramagnetic properties. Gadolinium ethylenediaminetetraacetic acid or gadolinium DTPA is excreted essentially unchanged by the kidney and as such may be useful for providing enhanced images of the kidney.[9] There are stable organic free radicals that are paramagnetic and of low toxicity. Such agents are considerably less paramagnetic than the paramagnetic heavy-metal ions. Nevertheless, such agents may prove clinically useful. Paramagnetic substances extracted by skeletal muscle would be of value in evaluating relative blood flow distribution during exercise in patients being evaluated for significant peripheral vascular disease.[3]

Tissue characterization

Premilinary studies have demonstrated that many disease states cause prolongation of relaxation parameters compared with normal tissue from the same organ. For example, a myocardial ischemic insult produces elevations of both T_1 and T_2 as early as 30 minutes after coronary occlusion.[15,19] Such elevation in T_1 and T_2 may allow differentiation between abnormal and normal tissue by NMR imaging. Wesbey et al.[18] studied dogs 2 to 7 days after coronary artery ligation by in vivo imaging with a gated spin-echo pulse sequence. In six of the seven dogs the signal intensity was increased in the myocardium supplied by the ligated artery as compared with the normally perfused myocardium; the seventh dog was found at postmortem analysis not to have an infarction. The calculated T_2 in the infarcted myocardium was 69% higher

than normal.[18] It is likely that ischemic injury of skeletal muscle can be characterized similarly.

Other NMR approaches may be helpful in characterizing the ischemic insult in skeletal muscle. Altered metabolic function resulting from ischemia may be monitored using in vivo spectroscopy and possibly imaging. For example, in addition to water and fat proton spectroscopy, it can provide a means for assessing lactic acid and phosphocreatine concentration. P-31 NMR studies, especially in conjunction with exercise stress, is another potential avenue for evaluating the metabolic effects of an ischemic insult. The techniques to perform in vivo spectroscopy on localized tissue regions have been reviewed by Radda et al.[14] The impact of ischemia on sodium transport leads to sodium gain in damaged cells and might be quantitated. Recent studies have demonstrated that such sodium accumulation of acute cerebral infarct can be visualized by Na-23 NMR images. A major limitation is the relatively low sensitivity of Na-23. Even though studies were performed at a field strength of 1.5 Tesla, acquisition times were on the order of 1 hour. Further studies will be needed to determine the utility of clinical Na-23 imaging in determining the loss of viability resulting from an ischemic insult.

CONCLUSIONS

NMR has enormous potential for imaging the vasculature and for assessing the effects of ischemic insults or other disease states on skeletal and cardiac muscle. Because of the decreased signal intensity produced by blood motion, angiography without ionizing radiation or contrast materials is possible in three dimensions. In addition, atherosclerotic disease of the arterial wall might be visualized. The effect of ischemia on the tissues might be analyzed in multiple ways including imaging of proton T_1 and T_2 and in vivo spectroscopy and imaging of lactate, pyruvate, or inorganic and high-energy phosphates (ATP or PC).

The ultimate clinical utility of NMR also will be related to its cost, its ability to provide unique information, and its potential hazard. If the promise becomes reality, the ability to quantitate tissue injury produced by vascular disease and to measure the functional significance of vascular lesions by metabolic means will add to the ability to evaluate and treat vascular disease. Because of the expense of NMR imaging, the evaluation of vascular disease alone might not justify its existence but it will add greatly to its usefulness.

REFERENCES

1. Bloch, F., Hanson, W.W., and Packard, M.E.: Nuclear induction, Phys. Rev. 69:127, 1946.
2. Brady, T.I., et al.: Proton nuclear magnetic resonance imaging of regionally ischemic canine hearts: Effect of paramagnetic proton signal enhancement, Radiology 144:343, 1982.
3. Brasch, R.C., et al.: Evaluation of nitroxide stable free radicals for contrast enhancement in NMR imaging, Scientific Program of Society of Magnetic Resonance in Medicine, 1982.
4. Chauncy, D.M., Jr., et al.: Tissue distribution studies with radioactive manganese: a potential agent for myocardial imaging, J. Nucl. Med. 18:933, 1977.
5. Damadian, R.: Tumour detection by nuclear magnetic resonance, Science 171:1151, 1971.
6. Goldman, M.R., et al.: Quantification of experimental myocardial infarction using nuclear magnetic resonance imaging and paramagnetic ion contrast enhancement in excised canine hearts, Circulation 66:1012, 1982.
7. Herfkens, R.J., et al.: Nuclear magnetic resonance imaging of atherosclerotic disease, Radiology 148:161, 1983.
8. Hore, P.J.: A new method for water suppression in the proton NMR spectrum of aqueous solutions, J. Mag Res 54:539, 1983.
9. Huberty, B., et al.: NMR contrast enhancement of the kidneys and liver with paramagnetic metal complexes, Scientific Program, Society of Magnetic Resonance in Medicine, Second Annual Meeting, San Francisco, Aug. 16 to 19, 1983, p. 175.
10. Kaufman, L. et al.: Evaluation of NMR imaging for detection and quantification of obstructions in vessels, Invest. Radiol. 17:554, 1982.
11. Lauterbur, P.C.: Image formation by induced local interactions: examples employing nuclear magnetic resonance, Nature 242:190, 1973.
12. Lauterbur, P.C., Dias, M.H.M., and Rudin, A.M.: Augmentation of tissue water proton spin-lattice relaxation rates by in vivo addition of paramagnetic ions. In Dutton, P.L., Leigh, J.S., and Scarpa, A., editors: Frontiers of biological energies, New York, 1981, Academic Press, Inc., p. 752.
13. Purcell, E.M., Torry, H.C., and Pound, R.V.: Resonance absorption by nuclear magnetic moments in a solid, Phys. Rev. 69:37, 1946.
14. Radda, G.K.: Potential and limitations of nuclear magnetic resonance for the cardiologist, Br. Heart J. 50:197, 1983.
15. Ratner, A.V., et al.: Early detection o myocardial ischemic damage using proton NMR techniques (abst.), Circulation 68, 1983.
16. Ross, B.D., et al.: Examination of a case of suspected McArdle's syndrome by P-31 NMR, N. Engl. J. Med. 304:1338, 1981.
17. Saryan, L.A., et al.: Brief communication: nuclear magnetic resonance studies of cancer. IV: Correlation of water content with tissue relaxation times 1, 2, 3, J. Natl. Cancer Inst. 52:599, 1974.
18. Wesbey, G., et al.: Imaging and characterization of acute myocardial infarction in vivo by gated nuclear magnetic resonance, Circulation 69:125, 1984.
19. Williams, E.S., et al.: Prolongation of proton spin lattice relaxations times in regionally ischemic tissue from dog hearts, J. Nucl. Med. 21:449, 1980.

CHAPTER 26

Local cerebral blood flow imaging with stable xenon

SIDNEY K. WOLFSON, Jr., HOWARD YONAS, and DAVID GUR

Inability to leave the vascular tree renders a radiopaque medium capable of outlining the limits of the vascular space and of estimating transit time of blood across a given vascular bed. The ability to cross the capillary and cell membranes renders a substance useful in estimating the volume flow rate of the blood perfusing and nourishing the tissue itself. Xenon gas, a natural constituent of the atmosphere, is such a substance. Its use in conjunction with computed tomography (CT), xenon may provide highly detailed cerebral blood flow (CBF) measurements. It has been possible to produce anatomic maps in both two and three dimensions with a precision and resolution that may approach that of CT itself. An understanding of the physiologic changes accompanying or preceding morphologic changes is necessary for their correct interpretation, and such knowledge may provide a basis for treatment. As anatomic resolution improves with the advent of devices such as CT and nuclear magnetic resonance (NMR), this is becoming even more significant. We now see elemental functional units and must develop an appreciation of their workings beyond the mere knowledge of their presence and size. The long-existing interest in CBF measurement has been supplemented by efforts to identify metabolic events and relate them to specific anatomic elements. Both blood flow and metabolism have been studied by a variety of newer methods that involve tomographic measurements. Physiologic variations of CBF and its altered patterns in disease remain uncertain at these anatomic levels. This is especially true in relating local CBF (LCBF) to neuroanatomic structures such as gray and white matter, nuclei, ganglia, and specific tracts. Information is needed about flow in specific functional centers in relation to metabolism, nerve transmission, information and motor integration, and projected excitatory and inhibitory influences.

Global and hemispheric measurements[28] and cortical studies[30,34,43] have been performed in humans, but detailed mapping of brain blood flow has been restricted to invasive or acute experiments in animals. These measurements have used radionuclide-labeled microemboli[10,62] or diffusible substances such as iodoantipyrene that equilibrate in tissue.[12,27,47,51] Both require killing the subject after a limited number of measurements. Autoradiography has the advantage of higher resolution but suffers the serious disadvantage of the limited number of measurements (often only one) before the need to kill the subject and perform rapid, crucial manipulation of the brain tissue. Another method used widely in animal research is H_2 clearance.[58,70] This requires the penetration of the region of interest (ROI) by a needle electrode, which, no matter how delicate, of necessity alters local microscopic anatomy and function and also limits the number of simultaneous discrete ROIs in the study.

With these methods valuable information has been obtained about normal CBF, effects of physiologic stimuli on its regulation, and the changes brought about by such conditions as ischemia, edema, altered blood circulation (for example, hemorrhage), tumors, degenerative disease, and specific neurologic insults. Thus we have learned about the autoregulation of CBF and the response to pharmacologic and physiologic stimuli (for example, P_{O_2}, P_{CO_2}) and to neurophysiologic work. We also have been able to appreciate the responses of collateral circulation to ischemia and the pattern of damage or infarction to be expected after a specific vascular accident. LCBF, in fact, is not constant in any region of the brain and varies appropriately as the metabolism and function of a region alter. Motor activation of a hand immediately increases flow within the appropriate region of the motor strip on the opposite side, and visual stimulation activates the occipital region.[24,25] Deprivation of a specific sensory input has also been associated with significant reductions of flow in the appropriate regions. The ability to study normal and diseased brain function by means of a noninvasive and widely available local flow method would appear to have broad application for the study of brain function in both normal and diseased states.

Desirable attributes of a cerebral blood flow method

Both laboratory study and clinical need require repeated precise measurements of blood flow. The method should include measurement of flow in deeply seated structures with equal facility as in superficial structures, have anatomic resolution on a par with the functional elements of interest (for example, tracts and nuclei), and be noninvasive so as not to disturb the organism under study and not impose significant risk or discomfort in the case of human subjects.

The methods discussed thus far do not satisfy these criteria. In this chapter are described several techniques that do meet the criteria, along with brief discussion of the older methods that have contributed so much to present knowledge. The main emphasis is on a technique for measurement of LCBF developed in our laboratories, which we believe fully meets the above criteria and makes use of CT technology, thus imposing minimal increases in cost and technical requirements while significantly improving anatomic resolution and ease of performance. The recent developments include emission tomography of both single-photon[14,31,56] and positron[1,46] varieties and the stable xenon/CT LCBF method as developed in our laboratory and applied by us[9,16-18,64] and by others.[35,44,48,50,53] The older methods are H_2 clearance and [^{14}C]iodoantipyrene autoradiography, which are not clinically applicable, and ^{133}Xe regional cerebral blood flow (rCBF), which has been extensively applied to clinical problems. NMR is not discussed in relation to blood flow because currently its capabilities are very limited at the level of tissue perfusion.[41]

CEREBRAL BLOOD FLOW METHODS
H_2 clearance

H_2 clearance is an invasive laboratory method for monitoring CBF that has had very limited clinical (intraoperative) use. The method is simple and inexpensive, uses easily obtainable equipment, and provides for multiple in vivo determinations of blood flow from any tissue into which small electrodes can be implanted. Much basic physiologic research has been carried out using H_2 clearance. Although Kety,[29] Mishray and Clark,[38] and Hyman[22] contributed the background for this method, Aukland et al.[2,3] described the first use of H_2 polarography in measurement of CBF. The use of the technique rapidly spread.[13,15,40] The H_2 clearance technique has been applied in humans as an adjunct to surgical procedures but has mainly been a laboratory method used for a wide range of blood flow phenomena including middle cerebral artery occlusion,[59] autoregulation, spinal cord trauma,[55] and brain ischemia.[33] Although it was originally believed that the volume of tissue represented by the method was as small as 1 mm^3 (depending on electrode size), evidence exists that H_2 generated as far as 2 to 5 mm from the electrode may contribute to the measured current.[20,57] Disadvantages or restriction of its use include the fact that implantation of electrodes may cause local injury with associated alteration of blood flow[5]; the correct mathematical treatment of the result is not clear because the clearance curves are often polyexponential, raising questions as to whether a single exponential clearance rate is valid[20]; arterial concentration may not fall rapidly to zero as assumed; and platinum electrodes are also sensitive to O_2 concentration, which could cause errors, especially in the case of severely ischemic tissue.[57]

Autoradiography and labeled microspheres

Both of these methods depend on the deposition of a radioactive label in tissue during the early moments after injection into the blood stream. In the case of microspheres, the tracer forms emboli in a small but evenly distributed sample of tissue, which remain in place until the subject is killed.[10,62] The tissue is then cut into volumes of about 1 cm^3 for deep-well counting.

The most widely used autoradiographic method uses [^{14}C]iodoantipyrine, which diffuses into tissue and then remains fixed because blood perfusion is ended by acute decapitation.[47,51] High-resolution autoradiographs are produced by thin sectioning of brain and contact exposure of x-ray film over a period of time. These methods obviously have no clinical or human investigative application, although of importance physiologically.

rCBF with diffusible radioemitters

There is a whole family of methods involving radiolabeled, inert, diffusible gasses.[23,30,34,43,61] These include [85]Kr and ^{133}Xe and depend on the relationship between blood flow and the rate of gas diffusion into or out of tissue. The gas may be administered by intracarotid injection or by inhalation and is monitored by external columnated scintillation counters. These methods usually extract blood flow information from tissue clearance or washout curves after cessation of indicator administration, although they can also use data acquired during absorption or washin. Because of the size of the detectors, such curves from brain contain at least two components having widely different blood flow rates and different indicator solubilities. These components represent gray and white matter. For the method to be noninvasive the indicator must be administered by inhalation and the monitoring must be external to the skin. These methodologic limitations result in restriction on the type of computation and on the precision and resolution of the results. The interaction of the physics of ^{133}Xe photon emission and of the need to detect external to the skin has several undesired effects. Because of self-absorption, the detected signal is limited to relatively superficial levels, and because skin, muscle, and bone are interposed between the detector and tissue of interest, at least one additional flow compartment must be considered when analyzing the measured clearance curves. A serious limitation of this method is the need to define the relative solubility of the indicator (for example, ^{133}Xe) in blood and in tissue. The parameter generally used, λ or blood-brain partition coefficient, must be available from some prior study because it cannot be estimated by the external scintillation counting method. Usually, normative values, either published or determined for gray and white matter in separate cadaver or animal tissue experiments, are applied to the measured tissue and blood clearance data. This is a disadvantage because λ has been found to vary in disease[54] and even may vary among normal individuals. Certainly tumor tissue Xe solubility will not be characteristic of either gray or white matter, so flow estimates for tumor would be subject to serious errors.

A three-compartment model has been proposed,[42] but this requires prolonged periods (40 minutes) of recording clearance of indicators. It has been possible to separate the fast components, or gray matter flow, from the slower components (white matter, bone, muscle, and skin) after only 10 minutes of recording. The fast component then is the only accurate output. Because the tissue of greatest interest with respect to blood flow and metabolism is gray matter, which encompasses nuclei and ganglia as well as cerebral cortex, this approach has considerable merit.

In an effort to obtain more detailed information, as many as 100 or more columnated detectors have been fitted to helmets to record multiple data simultaneously during a single washout curve.[30] These studies have demonstrated correlations in cerebral blood flow with function, such as muscular and mental activity in normal individuals and changes with disease and with aging. There is a general decrease in flow with age, and selected regional reductions are seen with dementias and with localized ischemic disease.

Emission tomography

Single-photon emission computed tomography. The ^{133}Xe tomography technique was described by Lassen et al.[31,56] and by other investigators using the same or other radionuclides such as [81]Kr.[14] This method, generally called single-photon emission computed tomography (SPECT), overcomes two of the major limitations of traditional two-dimensional rCBF methods: restriction to the superficial layer of the tissue under study and occurrence of the error related to counts originating in overlying skin, muscle, and bone. Thus, whereas previous information was available only from cerebral cortex (and only that portion of cortex exposed on the brain convexity to the exclusion of that present in fissures and sulci), it is now possible to apply tomographic techniques and provide information from deeper structures. This is accomplished by choosing appropriate radionuclides and increasing detector sensitivity so as to detect photons reaching the surface from all depths. Inasmuch as the path direction of the photon is known by virtue of the columnated detector and its likelihood of exiting the head depends on its energy and the medium through which it courses, the source of the signal can be established by use of many crossing paths, similar to the approach used in CT. A large number of columnated detectors are placed concentrically about the skull or a smaller array is rotated and computerized methods are used in calculating values at depth. This technique permits use of more traditional radionuclides of longer half-lives without the need to manufacture them on location, as with positron emission tomography (PET). More recently, simplified equipment (rotating gamma camera) has been used that promises to make this method more widely available. It has limitations in resolution but does have the important advantage of use for both blood flow and metabolism. However, positron-emitting radionuclides, also useful for metabolic studies, are more numerous. The SPECT method has been used to study CBF in patients with cerebrovascular disease and tumors.[45] In these and in normal individuals, there has been good agreement with two-dimensional rCBF studies.

Positron emission tomography. PET has received wide interest in recent years because it potentially provides a means of displaying information obtained noninvasively about blood flow and metabolism simultaneously and at varying tissue levels. The method uses as chemical markers certain radionuclides (for example, $^{15}O_2$, $^{13}N_2$, ^{11}C, ^{18}F, ^{77}Kr) that spontaneously disintegrate with the emission of positively charged particles (positron). Positrons travel only very short distances in tissue before losing enough kinetic energy to encounter electrons with which they collide, resulting in the phenomenon of mutual annihilation where the masses of both positron and electron are converted to energy. The result is two photons, each having energy of 0.511×10^6 eV (0.511 meV) and traveling in very nearly opposite directions (180 degrees). A ring of detectors records this event and, because of known path and travel times, can associate the disintegration of the biochemical label with a precise anatomic site within the tomogram, or "slice," under study. The number of such events over time at a given locus reveals the concentration of the specific radionuclide and its chemical substance at that locus. This becomes a very useful tool because it allows the investigator to measure uptake of important metabolites (for example, glucose, O_2) as well as of local blood volume and flow, the information being presented as a functional image of a brain or other tissue slice.

Considerations that limit the usefulness even of this exciting development involve resolution, speed of measurement, availability of evanescent radionuclides, and cost of equipment. In spite of these

limitations, a significant number of units have been installed and an impressive number of very exciting studies are under way. PET does not hold promise, however, for the routine management of clinical problems except at a very limited number of sites. The details of this method are described in Chapter 24.

Stable Xe/CT (local CBF)

The suggestion that Xe gas might be useful as a radio-enhancing agent[63] led to the realization that it could also be used for measurement of CBF if the x-ray device, in this case a CT scanner, was used as a densitometer during a dynamic Xe inhalation sequence. Xe, with an atomic number of 54, has radiodensity characteristics similar to those of iodine (atomic number 53). Unlike I, it is diffusible throughout the body tissues including brain, readily crossing the blood-brain barrier. Kelcz et al.[26] defined the CT enhancement characteristics of stable Xe at approximately the same time that Drayer et al.[9] reported early experiments with blood flow measurements in this laboratory. Subsequently we have continued work to bring this method to an advanced and clinically useful technique for measuring local CBF both in tomographic "slices" and in three-dimensional solid constructions for a series of such slices.[16-18,64] To avoid confusion, we hasten to point out that this solid, or three-dimensional, flow image is not the "three-dimensional" image as referred to in connection with SPECT or PET, where a slice (with thickness) that penetrates completely through the brain is considered three dimensional. We refer to the multilevel "slicing" technique where a solid, of equal (cubic) or near equal (rectangular) dimension, is created from a series of four or more adjacent slices (see below). During the development period a significant number of other investigators have worked in parallel and made substantial contributions to the technique,[35,44,48,50,53] so that we now believe it to be important both for clinical and animal investigation and for the routine management of ischemic or other intracranial disease. A CT manufacturer (General Electric Co., Milwaukee, Wis.) has collaborated with our group to produce a hardware-software package capable of transmitting rapid LCBF measurement with automated flow image generation. This unit, as an option for the Series 9800 scanner, is now undergoing multi-institutional and clinical trial. We briefly describe the method and its principles and provide several illustrations of its use.

Description. In common with other methods, the stable Xe/CT LCBF technique makes use of the Fick principle, which states simply that the quantity of a diffusible indicator present in a tissue at the end of a time period is the difference between the quantity absorbed by the tissue and the quantity removed or washed out of the tissue during that period. From this it follows that the concentration of indicator is a function of its quantity and of the volume of tissue or, at steady state, is the difference between the rate of delivery and the rate of removal. In the case of a highly diffusible indicator (such as Xe gas) transported via the bloodstream, knowledge of the time-dependent changes in blood and tissue concentration and the relative solubility of the indicator in blood and tissue (blood-brain partition coefficient, λ) permits calculation of the blood flow rate to the tissue under scrutiny. This could be a whole brain or hemibrain, or it could be as little as 1 CT unit (voxel). The time-tested equation of Kety and Schmidt[28,43] is used to define the relationship:

$$C(t) = \sum_i w_i \lambda_i k_i \int_0^t C_a(u) e^{-k_i(t-u)} du \qquad (1)$$

$$F = \lambda k \qquad (2)$$

$$F = \lambda_m k \qquad (3)$$

where

$C(t)$ = Indicator concentration in tissue (brain)
w_i = Weight factor
λ_i = Blood-brain partition coefficient
k_i = Flow rate constant
$C_a(u)$ = Indicator concentration in arterial blood
F = Blood flow
m = Equilibration factor (value of 1 implies instantaneous equilibration between blood and tissue).

Because present CT technology permits us to obtain rapid scans of brain (or other tissue) sections 5 mm thick, requires only 4 to 6 seconds per scan, and can be repeated immediately with table incrementation, it is possible to scan three to six levels of brain and repeat at intervals of 1 to 3 minutes. If this is done while the subject breathes a suitable Xe-air or Xe-O_2 gas mixture or after cessation of Xe breathing, the buildup or washout of Xe can be appreciated as a function of the measured enhancement of the CT image. Conveniently, CT now resolves tissue to $0.8 \times 0.8 \times 5$ mm solid elements (voxels), which are presented as an average density on a plane image (pixels), one such image representing each slice taken. Thus interference from overlying skin, muscle, or bone does not disturb

the Xe/CT method, and the anatomic source of each enhancement value is identified by the locus of the voxel.

Fig. 26-1 illustrates the changes in CT enhancement at three locations (ROIs) of a baboon brain while the animal breathes a 61% Xe-O_2 mixture. The cursors were placed so as to sample gray matter (fast-flow region), white matter (slow-flow region), and the center of an experimentally induced cerebral infarction (zero-flow region). The fast-flow ROI equilibrated with blood Xe level within 2 minutes, whereas the slow-flow, or white matter, ROI had not yet equilibrated after 6 minutes. In actuality, complete equilibration of white matter requires about 25 to 30 minutes, as illustrated in Fig. 26-2.

The study is carried out as follows. The awake patient is placed on the CT table with head taped to the plastic headholder. The headholder is lined with a vinyl bag containing polystyrene pellets for immobilization. After the procedure is explained and a comfortable position established, the patient is asked to keep the head perfectly still for about 10 minutes (4 to 6 minutes is essential). One or two baseline sequences of scans are taken in planes parallel to the planum sphenale (similar to the usual CT technique). The patient breathes air or O_2 through a mouthpiece with nose clip or through a mask. The mask or breathing tube is arranged for to-and-fro airway ventilation, as illustrated in Fig. 26-3. If an endotracheal tube is in place, it is simply connected instead of the mouthpiece. A small volume of the last expired air is intermittently aspirated to the thermal conductivity meter calibrated for Xe-O_2 or Xe-air mixtures. When it is established that the baseline scans are good (by radiologic technique, slice orientation), the breathing gas is switched to the predetermined Xe-O_2 or Xe-air mixture (usually 30% to 35% Xe). A preprogrammed scanning sequence is invoked so as to provide scanning series at the desired levels repeated at approximately 1.3, 2, 3, and 5 minutes after the initiation of Xe breathing. At the end of scanning the breathing mixture is switched back to O_2 or air. The entire procedure requires 30 minutes. The actual measurements are made in about 15 minutes, with 5 to 6 minutes of Xe breathing.

At the end of the examination the computer will construct images of the proscribed slices before and four times during Xe inhalation. There are time-dependent Xe enhancement data for each volume unit. Difference between the baseline and Xe-

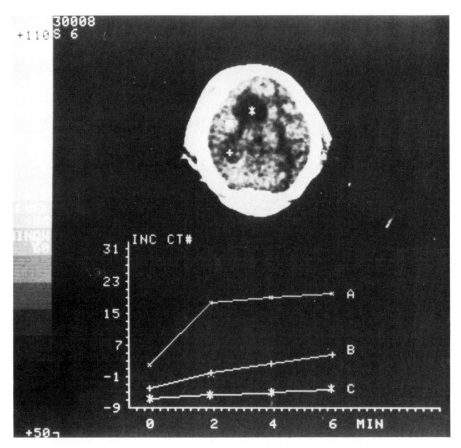

Fig. 26-1. Time-dependent changes in tissue enhancement of baboon brain during 61% Xe inhalation. Curve A plots degree of enhancement (Hounsfield units) from ROI located in fast-flow (gray matter) region. Curve B is ROI selected from slow-flow (white matter) region. Curve C is located within infarct caused by lateral lenticulostriate artery occlusion. Although there is obvious absence of enhancement in infarct, most important point is that equilibration of Xe with tissue is virtually complete in 2 minutes in fast-flow regions but is only partially so after 6 minutes in slow-flow regions.

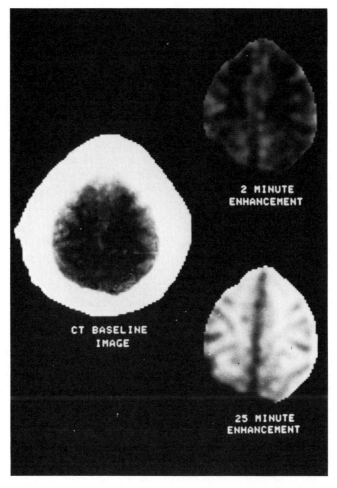

Fig. 26-2. Brain enhancement over time in baboon. Note reversal of more dense regions brought out by 25 minutes equilibration when compared with 5 minutes inhalation of 60% Xe. White matter regions, with greater solubility for Xe but requiring longer to equilibrate, ultimately become more radiodense than more rapidly equilibrating but with lower solubility gray matter regions.

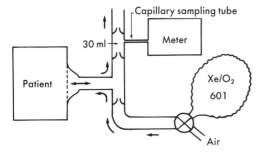

Fig. 26-3. Xe breathing circuit. Sixty-liter bag may contain either Xe-O₂ or Xe-air in concentrations between 30% and 60% Xe. Present clinical protocol calls for 30% to 35% Xe. Expired gas is aspirated at high velocity via capillary and permits thermal conductivity meter to generate expired gas Xe concentration curves. End-tidal Xe levels are easily identified and used for blood flow computations.

enhanced scans is proportional to the tissue Xe concentration. The output of the airway Xe meter is a function of the end-tidal (arterial) Xe concentration. These data may be solved for both λ and for k as defined in equation 1 using multivariable analysis techniques. Blood flow in milliliters per minute per unit volume of tissue is calculated from equation 2. When instantaneous diffusion equilibration cannot be assumed, equation 3 is used. The factor m increases to a maximum value of 1 as the equilibration state is approached. When the method is applied to animal studies, such as a cerebral infarct model in the baboon,[66] the technique is modified because of inability to obtain voluntary cooperation with respect to motion. For example, baboons are anesthetized, an endotracheal tube is inserted, and the animals are paralyzed.

Xe/CT BLOOD FLOW IMAGING
Two-dimensional flow mapping

We have been able to produce blood flow maps with good anatomic correlation between blood flow images and CT anatomy. Goodness of fit studies, comparison of normal with gross anatomic slices, and in the infarct model, the relationship of blood flow values to the pathologically identified infarct boundaries have all contributed to our knowledge of the method's validity. Plate 1 illustrates how flow may be represented on a color scale with values computed for each pixel-sized unit (0.8 × 0.8 mm). When compared with the actual gross pathologic slice the interdigitation of high- and low-flow regions of the map closely follows the distribution of gray and white matter throughout the gyri and central regions of cerebrum and brainstem. Newer image processing methods use smoothing algorithms to further approximate the original anatomy.

Sensitivity to physiologic change. The responsiveness of Xe/CT to physiologic flow variations was assessed in the baboon by increasing the $FiCO_2$ or causing hyperventilation or hypoventilation to alter the $PaCO_2$. The computed blood flow values revealed the wide swings in tissue perfusion expected when going from $PaCO_2$ of 30 torr to 60 torr. A typical response is illustrated in Fig. 26-4, where marked changes are seen in the difference between the upper and lower flow maps corresponding to $PaCO_2$ of 38 and 55. Increases in blood flow with increased $PaCO_2$ are readily appreciated, especially in gray matter regions.

Fig. 26-5 shows flow maps of a normal human subject both at rest and while performing a motor task. Of note in the resting flow map is the even distribution of flow patterns throughout the hemispheres and the fact that the high- and low-flow regions generally follow the gray and white matter distribution of normal anatomy. Zero flow is seen in such structures as ventricles, cysterns, and sulci. Mean flows for an 8.8 × 8.8 × 5 mm region that encompasses the motor cortex dramatically illustrate the sensitivity of the method. At rest, flow was 30.0 ± 8.5 ml/100 g · min (range, 11 to 53 ml/100 gm · min). Rather than implying a lack of

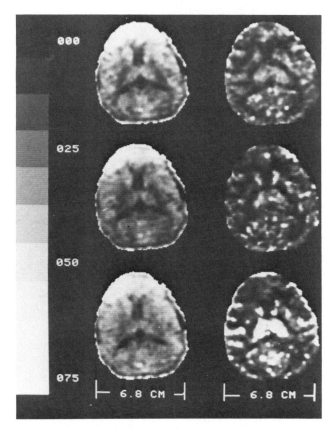

Fig. 26-4. Sensitivity to varying physiologic parameters. Three images to left are Xe-enhanced CT scans of same level of baboon brain. Hyperventilation or hypoventilation was induced to produce $PaCO_2$ of 38, 44, and 55 torr (top to bottom). Corresponding LCBF map is displayed just to right of each CT scan. Readily apparent is change in flow values of various structures, especially in gray matter, caused by varying $PaCO_2$. Gray scale units are milliliters per 100 grams per minute.

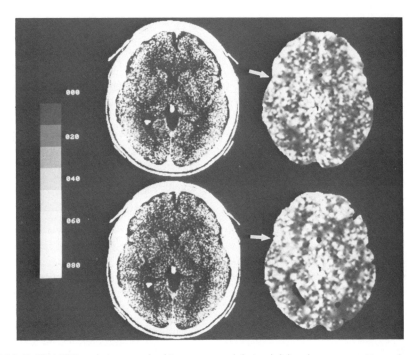

Fig. 26-5. Xe/CT LCBF study in normal subject at rest and during left-hand movement. Upper images of 8a are of CT scan *(left)* and LCBF map *(right)* at rest. In lower images subject is actively opening and clenching left fist. Definite increase in local blood flow is seen in area of motor cortex of lower flow map *(arrows).*

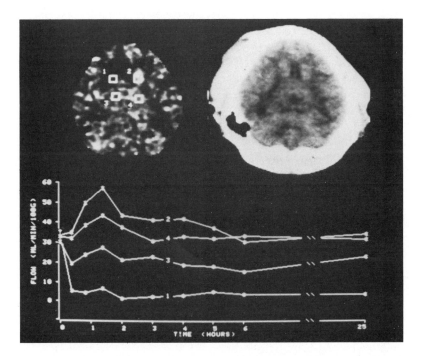

Fig. 26-6. Graphic display of simultaneous blood flow changes. This baboon underwent right lateral lenticulostriate occlusion (method of Yonas[59]) immediately after initial LCBF study. *Upper left* image is flow map from 25-minute postocclusion study, and corresponding baseline CT is shown at right. Four ROIs were chosen so that each pair had approximately same flow before occlusion but represented regions *(1)* within, *(2)* on edge, and *(3, 4)* at varying distances from ischemic zone.

precision, the variations in flow result from high resolution and the fact that the ROI contained both white matter (slow flow) and gray matter (fast flow) components. During hand activity the values increased to 63.4 ± 17.9 ml/100 g · min (range, 24 to 103 ml/100 gm · min). This kind of change has been reported by others[30] using rCBF and PET techniques, but Xe/CT LCBF opens a new dimension in resolution and depth of measurements.

Mapping over time. If good registration (anatomic coincidence of successive studies) is maintained, the computer can seek and plot mean blood flow values for ROIs selected from any flow map data entered. Values are plotted for all ROIs selected and for each study. Thus graphs over time are automatically produced once ROIs are designated[60] (Fig. 26-6). Analysis of this type is helpful in the study of anatomic and temporal blood flow variation associated with an event such as vessel occlusion.

Three-dimensional flow studies

Five or six 5 mm thick slices are taken with a table increment of only 2 or 3 mm providing for considerable overlap. Flow is computed for all slices as usual. The observer may select an ROI on one slice that will be projected through all. Fig. 26-7, *A*, shows how flow values for pixel size units of planes through the Z-axis are calculated using a simple linear interpolation algorithm. Intervening pixels are weighted in favor of the nearest actual slice, and all flow values are stored in a three-dimensional array from which the solid image is constructed. The result is seen in Fig. 26-7, *B*. The computer will cut this solid as desired, to reveal flow maps for interior structures in planes not parallel to the original scans such as coronal or sagittal or at any angle.

LABORATORY APPLICATIONS OF XE/CT

There is a broad application for Xe/CT blood flow studies in the laboratory. Because high Xe concentration and radiation exposure are possible in animals with small heads, such as the baboon, an ideal situation for LCBF determination is presented. Moreover, the subject may be held under rigid immobilization (with muscle relaxants) so that excellent image registration and better resolution are provided. Using 40% to 50% Xe-O_2 mixtures, we have defined exquisite anatomic detail of the normal variation of gray and white matter in nonhuman primates where cortical ribbon normally measures only 2 mm across.[17,19] Disturbances of

flow with experimental stroke caused by embolic or direct vessel occlusive procedures are readily defined, as are variations of flow, as CO_2 is varied.[19] Because of the good control of all experimental parameters, near perfect registration of the successive images may be obtained over a 25-hour period after acute lateral lenticulostriate artery occlusion. The computer can then plot curves of blood flow for multiple ROIs over this period[60] (Fig. 26-6).

CLINICAL APPLICATION OF XE/CT

We have had the opportunity to perform LCBF mapping in more than 350 patients, including multiple studies in many. The method has also been studied at a number of other institutions.* Although the technique has been found useful by virtually all investigators, variations in its application have evolved partly because of individual need and partly because of limitations imposed by the equipment used (for example, resolution and scanning rate). Our efforts over the past 3 years have used GE 8800 or 9800 series equipment. We have been able to scan in 4 to 5 seconds and perform automatic table incrementation under computer control. Thus we can obtain multilevel studies with Xe enhancement data collected for intervals of 30 to 60 seconds. Our most frequent application has been in the area of ischemic cerebrovascular conditions. Other entities studied include brain death, acute and chronic dementia, and multiple sclerosis as well as one arm of a multimodality longitudinal study of Alzheimer's disease.

Xe/CT LCBF is a noninvasive functional or physiologic test and provides information not available from anatomic studies, such as angiography. Factors such as recanalization of previously occluded vessels, microvascular collateralization, and persistence of an ischemic zone late in the course of major vessel occlusion can be assessed by LCBF. The functional aspect of LCBF is helpful in deciding whether blood flow augmentation procedures are indicated. Several illustrative case reports demonstrate the technique and provide examples of its application.

Bilateral carotid disease with internal carotid artery occlusion and inadequate flow reserves

This 62-year-old woman had right internal carotid artery occlusion, with left internal carotid ar-

*References 35, 37, 44, 49, 50, 53, 54, 65, 68.

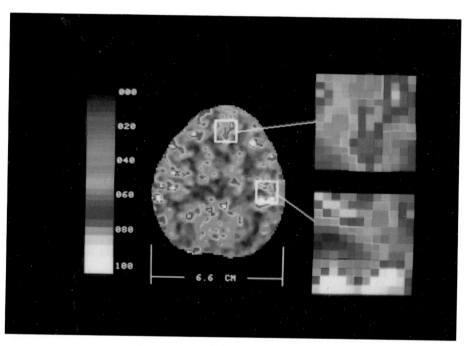

Plate 1. Xe/CT flow map in normal baboon. Flow was calculated for each pixel. Flow scale is given in ml/min/100 gm. Slice is 5 mm thick, and each tissue volume is thus 0.8 × 0.8 × 5 mm. Two selected regions, 9.6 × 9.6 × 5 mm, are displayed magnified six times, clearly illustrating variations between individual volumes measured.

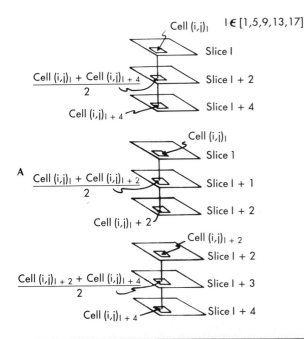

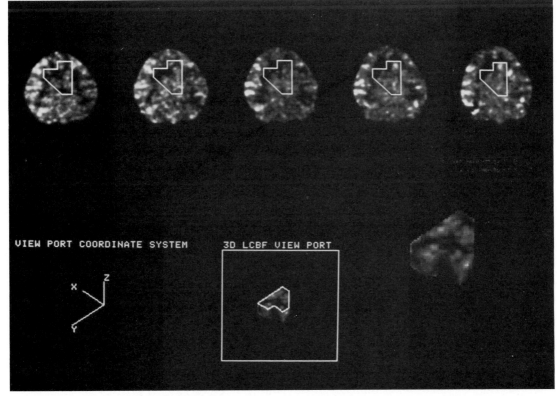

Fig. 26-7. Three-dimensional blood flow images. **A,** Method of weighted linear interpolation used to obtain solid flow image of baboon brain as constructed in **B.** Four to six (five in this case) adjacent and overlapping CT slices are acquired during Xe inhalation using dynamic scanning feature of CT unit. Cerebral infarction caused by lateral lenticulostriate occlusion in this baboon is readily seen as zero to very low-flow region involving basal ganglia and internal capsule.

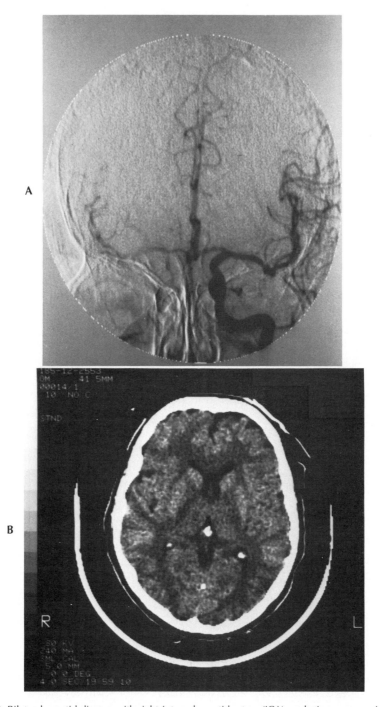

Fig. 26-8. Bilateral carotid disease with right internal carotid artery (ICA) occlusion: poor residual flow. **A,** Left carotid angiogram shows good filling of left middle (MCA) and anterior cerebral arteries in spite of left ICA stenosis below level shown. Right MCA (occluded right ICA) does not receive significant crossover flow from left ICA. **B,** CT scan.

tery stenosis of about 50% at the origin. She had frequent symptoms of right-sided cerebral ischemia, including transient left arm numbness and weakness. Noninvasive tests detected a severe opthalmic artery gradient (31 torr, right lower than left) and clearly demonstrated retrograde ophthalmic artery flow supplied by the right superficial temporal artery. Angiography revealed that the right internal carotid artery was totally occluded and confirmed the retrograde ophthalmic flow. There was no significant crossover circulation via the anterior cerebral complex (Fig. 26-8, *A*). Xe/CT blood flow study showed severe flow reduction in the right middle cerebral artery distribution where the CT anatomy was retained (Fig. 26-8, *B*). There was no infarction. Thus it appeared that this patient would benefit from flow augmentation. A right superficial temporal artery to middle cerebral artery bypass was performed. The frequent symptoms were eliminated, and a postoperative flow study showed a 50% increase in flow in the regions that had been deprived.

Internal carotid occlusion with adequate flow reserves

This 67-year-old man had a left internal carotid artery occlusion two months prior to examination, with improving residual right-sided hemiparesis

and aphasia. The CT scan demonstrated diffuse atrophy of the internal and middle cerebral artery distribution (Fig. 26-9, *A*). A Xe/CT flow study showed adequate gray matter flow levels for all of the areas of retained tissue (Fig. 26-9, *B*). Obviously, in the atrophic areas flow was absent or reduced. Thus there was no apparent compromise of flow reserves to surviving tissue and no benefit to be expected from flow augmentation surgery.

Carotid cavernous fistula

This 25-year-old man had a right carotid cavernous fistula, with severe right-sided proptosis. Although the patient did not have symptoms of cerebral ischemia, angiograms demonstrated the fistula and posed the question of a significant steal from the right cerebral hemisphere. The Xe/CT blood flow study documented high-normal flow in the regions supplied by the right middle cerebral and anterior cerebral arteries (Fig. 26-10). Therefore this arteriovenous fistula was not compromising the cerebral circulation at the time.

Discussion of case reports

Each of these cases illustrates a situation where severe compromise of the internal carotid circulation exists. Inasmuch as the effects of cerebral ischemia are to a great extent dependent on the degree

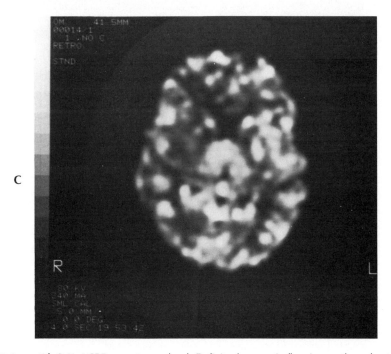

Fig. 26-8, cont'd. C, Xe LCBF map at same level. Definite decrease in flow is seen throughout right MCA distribution.

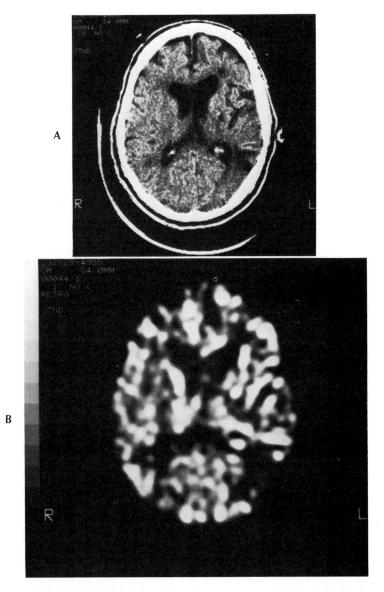

Fig. 26-9. Internal carotid occlusion: good residual flow. *A,* There is obvious cerebral infarct in left ICA distribution, with diffuse atrophy. *B,* Xe LCBF clearly demonstrates adequate flow in these regions with retained tissue per CT. Flow is reduced or absent in obviously atrophic or infarcted regions, as would be expected.

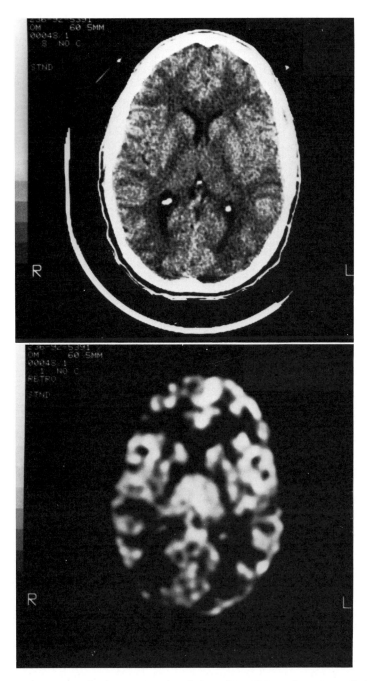

Fig. 26-10. Carotid carvernous fistula: question of steal. CT and Xe LCBF map for patient with right carotid cavernous fistula. Flow map indicates normal or above normal flow in right ICA distribution.

and pattern of blood flow reduction, it is important to understand these variables if efforts are to be made to prevent permanent injury or extension of damage. Vascular occlusive disease may involve the distributing vessels themselves or the extracranial vessels supplying the brain. Collateral channels may or may not be present at the outset or may subsequently develop as disease progresses. This will depend both on anatomic variability and on the pattern and speed with which the flow reduction occurs. Immediately after an occlusive event there may be only a relative reduction of flow because collateral channels exist. Alternatively, there may be virtual absence of flow in a "central" region with a relative decrease in flow in a "border" region. On the other hand, there may actually be increased flow in a region adjacent to severe damage (so called "luxury perfusion"), and metabolism may be "uncoupled" from the flow because of prior neuronal injury.

Where the major disorder is limited to relative blood flow reduction, the patient may be at risk only when there is a temporary further reduction resulting in a so-called transient ischemic attack (TIA). While many TIAs are no doubt the result of small emboli from remote vessel disease, they may also occur as a result of a temporary added reduction in overall flow that brings the affected area into compromise. We have found that LCBF is useful in identifying the latter group where an extracranial to intracranial (EC/IC) bypass procedure will help. Others have used regional blood flow measurements with ^{133}Xe/rCBF[52] and PET.[4] The Xe/LCBF technique is exceptionally appropriate for this task because it can be correlated on a pixel-to-pixel basis with the same anatomic slice of the CT study and enables localization of relative flow reduction in regions of retained anatomic integrity.

When damage is more extensive and profound in a central region, the hyperemic "luxury" area surrounding it may confound rCBF studies, which cannot "see" deeper structures. Xe/LCBF gives a complete section with equal accuracy throughout and permits correct initial analysis as well as accurate tracking of the evolution of the disorder.

Although not illustrated, Xe/CT LCBF has had other clinical utility in our hands and also appears suited for study of a number of pressing problems in clinical research. Patients with closed head injury pose problems when the detected anatomic derangement may be related to the adequacy of tissue perfusion. In children this is especially important, because loss of vasoregulation is more likely to occur with head injury in the very young. The ability to perform multiple-level flow studies with three-dimensional reconstruction through both temporal regions may offer a new approach for the diagnosis and localization of seizure foci, especially when surgical management is required. Many interesting investigative possibilities also exist in this area.

Nervous activity depends on energy-consuming metabolic processes both for impulse transmission and for synthesis of neurotransmitters. Primary failure of blood supply causes secondary failure of these processes. On the other hand, normally the demands of tissue activity regulate the flow of blood, and autoregulatory mechanisms ensure this, (Fig. 26-5). Conditions that are mainly of a functional or even of a degenerative nature might be expected to cause changes in LCBF that precede, coincide, or result from the disease process. Such changes, if present, would aid in diagnosis and in understanding the pathogenesis of such disorders as dementia, depression, and demyelinating disease and metabolically related problems, such as Pick's disease.

PROBLEMS WITH XE/CT
Effects of Xe inhalation

Anesthetic properties. Xe is an inert atmospheric constituent possessing anesthetic properties in concentrations higher than 50% F_1 Xe.[7,32,39] The gas was reasonably well tolerated in a study with healthy volunteers breathing Xe-O_2 mixtures (28% to 47% Xe) for 3 to 6 minutes through a face mask.[67] The most common symptoms were lightheadedness, euphoria, heavy feeling, and tingling of extremities. Other investigators[6,21,36,49] have reported greater tolerance at concentrations up to 70% to 80% in studies in patients as opposed to normal volunteers. In fact, one investigator has reported *no* adverse side effects to 65% Xe breathing in a very carefully monitored study.[8] Our own experience with patients[65,68,69] tends to confirm a very low incidence of significant neurologic side effects.

Effect on blood flow. Prolonged Xe breathing will result in a reducton of blood flow of 10% to 20% from baseline levels.[17] The degree to which this occurs is largely dependent on dose and duration of Xe breathing. We have found that 8 to 10 minutes of 35% Xe may reduce blood flow by 15% to 25%, but no appreciable effect is noticed in the first few minutes. Microsphere studies suggest a small increase (5% to 10%) in the first few minutes.

Motion of subject

The subject's head must remain perfectly still for a minimum of about 10 minutes, because misregistration can occur with an accumulated movement of only 1 to 2 mm. Obtunded and unconscious patients usually present no problem. Similarly, alert and cooperative patients can be easily studied, especially with the aid of evacuable "bean bags" (Vac-Pac; Olympic Medical Supply Co., Seattle). The polystyrene filler material is radiolucent in the scanner. We have also used a thermoplastic material that can be molded to fit the head and fixed to the CT head holder, which has enabled us to obtain good results in some patients who were totally uncooperative and subject to involuntary movement, such as those with advanced Alzheimer's disease. Another approach is the modification of the standard CT head holder to provide noninvasive points of skull fixation, to brace against involuntary movement and to aid the cooperative patient in efforts to remain still. An alternative approach is to increase slice thickness to 1 cm, which would reduce anatomic resolution and decrease the method's applicability to smaller structures. Finally, it is possible to make computational correction for rotational misregistration but not for axial linear motion (craniad or caudad).

Radiation exposure

A trade-off between signal/noise ratio and radiation level certainly exists in work with stable Xe enhancement. Limiting the study to specific slices limits exposure of adjacent structures because the CT beam is well columnated. Repeated scans of the slices under study do result in significant dose to those tissues. Radiation dose is at a minimum with the in vivo autoradiographic technique, but the accuracy of the resulting flow estimate then depends on a single datum for tissue enhancement. As presently done, the usual multilevel study requires a minimum of one baseline and two enhanced scans. We prefer to average two baseline scans and to record at least three or four enhanced scans during Xe inhalation. This results in at least 15 to 20 rad to the slice itself, but much

lower levels are absorbed by organs outside the scan field. The whole-body dose is thus more comparable to that received when a radionuclide study (for example, ^{133}Xe) is carried out.

DISCUSSION

All of the tomographic blood flow methods described have obvious advantages and sometimes more obscure disadvantages. The Xe/CT LCBF method is, in common with the others, completely noninvasive. It cannot be used for rapidly repetitious determinations because it requires a period of gaseous indicator inhalation (washin) and exhalation (washout). Fast phenomena cannot be studied directly. On the other hand, unlike both PET and SPECT, flow changes of small structures can be appreciated (4 mm full width, half maximum, flow values calculated on a pixel-by-pixel basis).

The value of the equilibration factor m for different tissues and techniques, the effect of improving signal/noise ratio, and the interrelationships of the amount of enhancement, Xe concentration, scan sequence, and number of scans, and the merits of single vs. multicompartmental analysis, among other considerations, are of great importance in understanding the significance and anatomic resolving power of the technique. These considerations have been described and analyzed elsewhere by us[18] and by others.[48] The Xe/CT flow method provides the ability to measure and to image blood-brain partition coefficient (λ) as well as blood flow. The λ certainly contains information about the type of tissue, but also may provide clues about the metabolic state and about changes in tissue composition as a result of disease. Although normal metabolism has been inferred from normal CT anatomy, the degree of functional disturbance required to alter radiodensity is unknown, and reduced flow can certainly exist in tissue with a normal CT appearance. These speculations are interesting but remain to be studied. The ability to estimate λ directly from the CBF study also has the advantage of freeing the computation from dependence on "normative" values measured at another time in a different specimen. The use of normative values is an obvious disadvantage when abnormal tissue or foreign tissue such as tumor is involved. The λ for a specific tumor is never available, so tumor blood flow estimated using normal gray, white, or average values is almost always in error.

While the positron-emitting radionuclides of PET can be used as metabolic markers or tracers and can be measured at the same time as blood flow, flow and metabolism are seldom measured simultaneously in practice, apparently because of technical difficulties encountered when this is attempted.

Although free of the need to take precautions with respect to gaseous radionuclides, as with SPECT, the method does expose the patient to ionizing radiation. The dose for thyroid gland, for example, is higher than that absorbed by other blood flow techniques (for example, ^{133}Xe), but the dose to other critical organs (for example, gonads) is comparable or lower. The brain is relatively radioinsensitive, and the more sensitive eyes (cornea and lens) are usually left out of the scan field. Based both on the anesthesia literature of the 1950s and on our experience and that of others, it appears that the concentration of Xe (30% to 35%) required for satisfactory blood flow studies does not cause significant side effects in most subjects.

The cost of sophisticated CT scanners is comparable to costs involved in PET and is greater than those generally encountered with SPECT. Yet only a small portion of these costs is attributable to the LCBF studies because the scanner is already available in most well-equipped medical centers. Equipment that must be dedicated to the CBF application (such as breathing apparatus, recorder, Xe meter) is much less expensive and readily obtained. The development of a commercial package for Xe/CT will make the method available to a very large number of clinical centers at minimal cost.

In theory, the CT slices could be made in any plane. Practical considerations render it difficult to cut scan slices very far from the horizontal, because positioning and holding the patient is difficult. The three-dimensional capability is therefore useful for studying structures whose long axis is in a plane different from the CT slices taken or when blood flow maps are to be compared with pathologic slices made in other planes (for example, coronal or sagittal). Thus, in our blood flow study of senile dementia, we are using data obtained in conventional transaxial planes to construct maps in coronal planes so as to correspond with those to be ultimately studied by the neuropathologist and neurochemist.

In summary, a method of imaging blood flow to the brain, Xe/CT LCBF, is described and discussed in relation to other tomographic blood flow methods. We believe that Xe/CT is an effective blood flow method of high utility and has promise of widespread application because of its relatively high anatomic resolution, low cost, and ease of procedure.

ACKNOWLEDGMENT

The Xe/CT work and methods described have been supported in part by grants from the American Heart Association, Western Pennsylvania Affiliate and Northwestern Pennsylvania Affiliate; USPHS Grant HL 27208 from the National Institutes of Health; by an American Heart Association Established Investigatorship; and by institutional funds of Childrens Hospital of Pittsburgh, Montefiore Hospital Association of Western Pennsylvania, and Presbyterian-University Hospital.

We thank Walter Good, Eugene E. Cook, Richard E. Latchaw, Manfred Boehnke, and Timothy Kerr for help and suggestions, and Janet Fink, Darlene Woomer, and Mary Ann Krupper for manuscript preparation.

REFERENCES

1. Alavi, A., et al.: Mapping of functional activity in the brain with ^{18}F-fluorodeoxyglucose, Semin. Nucl. Med. 11:24, 1981.
2. Aukland, K., Bower, B.F., and Berliner, R.W.: Measurement of local blood flow with hydrogen gas, Circ. Res. 14:164, 1964.
3. Aukland, K.: Hydrogen polarography in measurement of local blood flow: theoretical and empirical basis, Acta Neurol. Scand. 41(suppl 14):42, 1965.
4. Baron, J.C., et al: Reversal of focal "misery perfusion syndrome" by extra-intracranial arterial bypass in hemodynamic cerebral ischemia, Stroke 12:454, 1981.
5. Brock, M., Ingvar, D.H., and Sem Jacobsen, C.W.: Regional blood flow in deep structures of the brain measured in acute cat experiments by means of a new beta-sensitive semiconductor needle detector, Exp. Brain Res. 4:126, 1967.
6. Coin, C.G., and Coin, J.T.: Contrast enhancement by xenon gas in computed tomography of the spinal cord and brain: preliminary observations. J. Comput. Assist. Tomogr. 4:217, 1980.
7. Cullen, S.C., and Gross, E.G.: The anesthetic properties of xenon in animals and human beings with additional observations on krypton, Science 113:580, 1951.
8. Dhawan, V., et al.: Mass spectrometric measurement of end-tidal xenon concentration for clinical stable xenon/computerized tomography cerebral blood flow studies, Biomed. Mass Spectrom. 9:241, 1982.
9. Drayer, B.P., et al.: Xenon enhanced computed tomography for the analysis of cerebral integrity, perfusion, and blood flow. Stroke 9:123, 1978.
10. Dull, W.P., et al.: Relative error and variability in blood flow measurements with radiolabled microspheres, Am. J. Physiol. 243:H371, 1982.
11. Eidelman, B.H., et al.: Cerebral blood flow in multiple sclerosis, Neurology (In press).
12. Eklof, B., Lassen, N.A., and Nilsson, L.: Regional cerebral blood flow in the rat measured by the tissue sampling technique: a critical evaluation using four indicators C[14]-antipyrine, C[14]-ethanol, H[3]-water and xenon[133], Acta Physiol. Scand. 91:1, 1974.

13. Fieschi, C., Boxxao, L., and Agnoli, A.: Regional clearance of hydrogen as a measure of blood flow, Acta Neurol. Scand. 41(suppl 14):46, 1965.

14. Fukuyama, H., et al.: A krypton-81m single photon emission tomography on the collateral circulation in carotid occlusion: the role of the circle of Willis and leptomeningeal anastomoses, J. Cereb. Blood Flow Metab. 3:S143, 1983.

15. Gotoh, F., Meyer, J.S., and Tomita, M.: Hydrogen method for determining cerebral blood flow in man, Arch. Neurol. 15:549, 1966.

16. Gur, D., et al.: Xenon enhanced dynamic computed tomography: multilevel cerebral blood flow studies, J. Comput. Assist. Tomogr. 5:334, 1981.

17. Gur, D., et al.: Progress in cerebrovascular disease: local cerebral blood flow by xenon enhanced CT. Stroke 13:750, 1982.

18. Good, W., et al: Errors associated with single-scan determinations of regional cerebral blood flow by xenon enhanced CT, Phys. Med. Biol. 27:531, 1982.

19. Gur, D., et al.: In vivo mapping of local cerebral blood flow by xenon enhanced CT, Science 215:1267, 1982.

20. Halsey, J.H., Capra, N.F., and McFarland, R.S.: Use of hydrogen for measurement of regional cerebral blood flow: problem of intercompartmental diffusion, Stroke 8:351, 1977.

21. Haughton, V.M., et al.: A clinical evaluation of xenon enhancement for computed tomography, Invest. Radiol. 15:160, 1980.

22. Hyman, E.S.: Linear system for quantitating hydrogen at a platinum electrode, Circ. Res. 9:1093, 1961.

23. Ingvar, D.H., et al.: Normal values of regional cerebral blood flow in man, including flow and weight estimates of gray and white matter, Acta Neurol. Scand. 41(suppl 14):72, 1965.

24. Ingvar, D.H., and Philipson, L.: Distribution of cerebral blood flow in the dominant hemisphere during motor ideation and motor performance, Ann. Neurol. 2:230, 1977.

25. Ingvar, D.H.: Brain activation patterns revealed by measurements of regional cerebral blood flow. In Desmedt, J.E., editor: Cognitive components in cerebral event-related potentials and selective attention progress in clinical neurology, vol 6. Basel; 1979; S. Karger, AG, pp 200-215.

26. Kelcz, F., et al.: Computed tomographic measurement of xenon brain-blood partition coefficient and implication for regional cerebral blood flow: a preliminary report, Radiology 127:385, 1978.

27. Kennedy, C., et al.: Metabolic mapping of the primary visual system of the monkey by means of the autoradiographic [^{14}C] deoxyglucose technique, Proc. Natl. Acad. Sci. USA, 73:4230, 1976.

28. Kety, S.S., and Schmidt, C.F.: The nitrous oxide method for the quantitative determination of cerebral blood flow in man: theory, procedure, and normal values, J. Clin. Invest. 27:476, 1948.

29. Kety, S.S.: The theory and applications of the exchange of inert gas at the lungs and tissues, Pharmacol. Rev. 3:1, 1957.

30. Lassen, N., Ingvar, D.H., and Skinhoj, E.: Brain function and blood flow: changes in the amount of blood flowing in areas of the human cerebral cortex, reflecting changes in the activity of those areas, are graphically revealed with the aid of radioactive isotopes, Sci. Am. 239:62, 1978.

31. Lassen, N.A., Henriksen, L., and Paulson, O.: Regional cerebral blood flow in stroke by ^{133}xenon inhalation and emission tomography, Stroke 12:284, 1981.

32. Lawrence, J.H., et al: Preliminary observations on the narcotic effect of xenon with a review of values for solu-

bilities of gases in water and oils, J. Physiol. 105:197, 1946.

33. Lubbers, D.W., and Leniger-Follert, E.: Capillary flow in the brain cortex during changes in oxygen supply and state of activation. In Cerebral vascular smooth muscle and its control (CIBA Foundation Symposium 56), Amsterdam, 1978, Elsevier-NDU, Excerpta Medica, pp 22-47.

34. Mallet, B.L., and Veall, N.: The measurement of regional cerebral clearance rates in man using xenon-133 inhalation and extracranial recording, Clin. Sci. 29:179, 1965.

35. Meyer, J.S., et al: High resolution three dimensional measurement of localized cerebral blood flow by CT scanning and stable xenon clearance: effect of cerebral infarction and ischemia, Trans. Am. Neurol. Assoc. 104:85, 1979.

36. Meyer, J.S., et al.: Local cerebral blood flow measured by CT after stable xenon inhalation, A.J.R. 135:239, 1980.

37. Meyer, J.S., et al: Multi-infarct and Alzheimer dementias differentiated from normal aging by xenon contrast CT CBF measurements, J. Cereb. Blood Flow Metab. 3:S506, 1983.

38. Misrahy, G.A., and Clark, L.C.: Use of the platinum black cathode for local blood flow measurements in vivo, Proc. Int. Cong. Physiol. (Brussels), 20:650, 1956.

39. Morris, L.E., Knott, J.R., and Pittinger, C.B.: Electroencephalographic and blood gas observations in human surgical patients during xenon anesthesia, Anesthesiology 16:312, 1955.

40. Neely, W.A., et al: Use of the hydrogen electrode to measure tissue blood flow, J. Surg. Res. 5:363, 1965.

41. Nunnally, R.L., Peshock, R.M., and Rehr, R.B.: Fluorine-19 [^{19}F] NMR in vivo: potential for flow and perfusion measurements, Proceedings of the Annual Meeting, Society of Nuclear Magnetic Resonance in Medicine, San Francisco, August 1983; Scientific Program SMRM 266.

42. Orbrist, W.D., et al.: Determination of regional cerebral blood flow by inhalation of 133-xenon, Circ. Res. 20:124, 1967.

43. Obrist, W.D., et al.: Regional cerebral blood flow estimated by ^{133}xenon inhalation, Stroke 6:245, 1975.

44. Ono, H., Ono, K., and Mori, K.: Mapping of CBF distribution by dynamic Xe-enhanced CT scan method, J. Cereb. Blood Flow Metab. 1:50, 1981.

45. Paulson, O.B., et al.: Regional cerebral blood flow distribution evaluated by emission computer tomography with ^{133}xenon and ^{123}I-isopropyl-amphetammine, J. Cereb. Blood Flow Metab. 3:S62, 1983.

46. Phelps, M.E.: Positron computed tomography studies of cerebral glucose metabolism in man: theory and application in nuclear medicine, Semin. Nucl. Med. 11:32, 1981.

47. Reivich, M., et al.: Measurement of regional cerebral blood flow with antipyrine-14C in awake cats, J. Appl. Physiol. 27:296, 1969.

48. Rottenberg, D.A., Lu, H.C., and Kearfott, K.J.: The in vivo autoradiographic measurement of regional cerebral blood flow using stable xenon and computerized tomography: the effect of tissue heterogeneity and computerized tomography noise, J. Cereb. Blood Flow Metab. 2:173, 1982.

49. Rottenberg, D.A., et al: Measurement of regional cerebral blood flow in human subjects using stable Xenon and computerized tomography, Ann. Neurol. 10:102, 1981.

50. Sakai, F., et al.: Xenon enhanced CT method for the measurement of local cerebral blood flow in man, J. Cereb. Blood Flow Metab. 1:29, 1981.

51. Sakurada, O., et al.: Measurement of local cerebral blood flow with iodo[^{14}C]antipyrine, Am. J. Physiol. 234:H59, 1978.

52. Schmiedek, P., et al.: Selection of patients for extra-intracranial arterial bypass surgery based on rCBF measurements, J. Neurosurg. 44:303, 1976.

53. Segawa, H., et al.: CBF study by CT with Xe enhancement: experience in 30 cases, J. Cereb. Blood Flow Metab. 1:52, 1981.
54. Segawa, H., et al.: Computed tomographic measurement of local cerebral blood flow by xenon enhancement, Stroke 14:356, 1983.
55. Senter, H.J., and Venes, J.L.: Altered blood flow and secondary injury in experimental spinal cord trauma, J. Neurosurg. 49:569, 1978.
56. Stokely, E.M., et al.: A single photon dynamic computer assisted tomograph (DCAT) for imaging brain function in multiple cross sections, J. Comput. Assist. Tomogr. 4:230, 1980.
57. Stosseck, K., Lubbers, D.W., and Cottin, N.: Determination of local blood flow (microflow) by electrochemically generated hydrogen: construction and application of the measuring probe, Pflugers Arch. Eur. J. Physiol. 348:225, 1974.
58. Symon, L., Pasztor, E., and Branston, N.M.: The distribution and density of reduced cerebral blood flow following acute middle cerebral artery occlusion: an experimental study by the technique of hydrogen clearance in baboons, Stroke 5:335, 1974.
59. Symon, L.: Regional vascular reactivity in the middle cerebral arterial distribution: an experimental study in baboons, J. Neurosurg. 33:532, 1970.
60. Yonas, H., et al.: Unpublished data.
61. Ueda, H., et al.: External measurement of regional cerebral blood flow in man by common carotid arterial injection of radioactive krypton-85 saline solution, Jpn. Heart J. 9:349, 1968.
62. Wagner, H.N., et al.: Studies of the circulation with radioactive microspheres, Invest. Radiol. 4:374, 1969.
63. Winkler, S.S., et al.: Xenon inhalation as an adjunct to computerized tomography of the brain: preliminary study, Radiology 12:15, 1977.
64. Wolfson, S.K., Jr., et al.: Regional cerebral blood flow by xenon enhanced computed tomography, Proceedings of the Annual Meeting, American Association of Neurosurgeons, New Orleans, 1978, pp 1-3.
65. Wolfson, S.K., Jr., et al.: Two- and three-dimensional imaging of local cerebral blood flow by xenon CT, Ann. Bioeng. (In press.)
66. Yonas, H., et al.: Selective lenticulostriate occlusion in the primate: a highly focal cerebral ischemia model, Stroke 12:567, 1981.
67. Yonas, H., et al.: Side effects of xenon inhalation, J. Comput. Assist. Tomogr. 5:591, 1981.
68. Yonas, H., et al.: Clinical experience with the use of xenon-enhanced CT blood flow mapping in cerebrovascular disease, Stroke 15:443, 1984.
69. Yonas, H., et al.: Clinical applications of xenon/CT blood flow mapping, Proceedings of the International Symposium on Cerebral Blood Flow and Cerebral Metabolism in Man, Heidelberg, Sept. 28 to Oct. 1, 1983. (In press.)
70. Young, W.: H_2 clearance measurement of blood flow: a review of technique and polarographic principles, Stroke 11:552, 1980.

CHAPTER 27

Using the computer in the vascular diagnostic laboratory

DARRELL N. JONES and ROBERT B. RUTHERFORD

Computer use in vascular diagnostic laboratories (VDL) has grown rapidly during the past 5 years. This growth has not primarily been the result of expanding needs or innovative computer applications, but represents applications made practical by advances in computer technology, in particular the development of the microprocessor.

The role of computer applications in any laboratory can be divided heuristically into two broad categories: data management and data analysis. Included in the first category are data acquisition, reduction, organization, storage, and retrieval. The second category includes numeric analysis, automatic interpretations, and statistical inference. These tasks, once identified in general terms, can be appreciated as essential operational components of an efficient VDL. Computer use serves two functions in relation to routine laboratory operation: (1) to increase the efficiency of the work routine and (2) to use information of a scope or complexity that is beyond the reach of manual methods.

This chapter will examine the role of the computer in the VDL with particular emphasis on the microcomputer. Although the majority of applications described are independent of the computer resource employed, microcomputers represent the most practical and likely resource available to the VDL. This discussion will include fundamentals of computer-based data management, a consideration of the limitations of current technology, and speculations on future trends.

MICROCOMPUTERS

The terms *personal computer* and *microcomputer* are often accepted as implying a capability considerably less than a *computer*. The micropro-

cessor employed in these smaller instruments is not conceptually different from the central processing unit (CPU) of full-sized computers used in previous decades. The revolutionary difference is the small size and relatively low cost of the hardware or physical components that comprise a computer. Microcomputers have capabilities of speed, accuracy, and memory that equal the mainframe computers of less than 30 years ago and surpass the laboratory minicomputers of the previous decade.[1,8] High capability at a cost less than the access fees charged for central or mainframe facilities has created a marked increase in computer resources. In addition, these resources are distributed rather than shared. This local user independence presents greater opportunities for instrument applications, that is, smart instrumentation and automated data aquisition, as will be described.

The digital era

Increasingly, digital electronics are being employed in analog instruments. Digital instrumentation means that the continuous voltage produced by a transducer, such as the pressure transducer on a plethysmograph or frequency-voltage converter on a Doppler system, is converted to a series of numeric voltage values at discrete time intervals during the course of the measured event (Fig. 27-1). The accuracy of this analog to digital (A/D) conversion depends on how many discrete intervals are used and the accuracy of each numeric voltage reading. Since any computer has a finite computational speed and finite memory for representing numeric values, there is always an upper boundary on the accuracy of digitizing a continuous event. However, these limitations are usually much

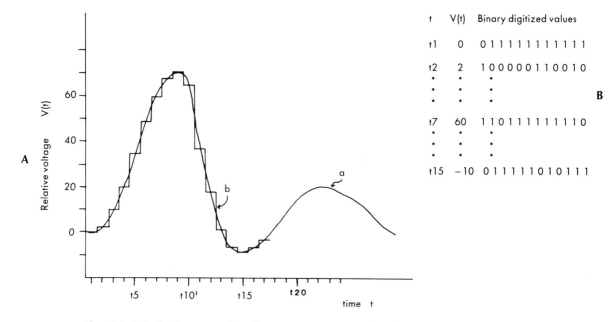

Fig. 27-1. *A,* Stylized representation of A/D conversion. *a,* Analog voltage vs. time plot; *b,* voltage vs. time plot after digitizing. *B,* Partial table of digitized voltage values showing computer representation.

less important than the accuracy of the transducer itself and less limited than human measurement of the same data.

The era of digital electronics implies that all forms of information are being stored, presented, and analyzed in a discrete format. Newer vascular diagnostic instrumentation is likely to be digital and probably microprocessor based.

Smart instrumentation

Once diagnostic data have been reduced to numeric values, microprocessor analysis and feedback are possible. For example, maximum venous outflow (MVO) is being measured under the control of microprocessor-based instruments. A protocol for occlusion cuff inflation and rudimentary analysis of the plethysmographic cuff pressure is specified for microprocessor control. The relatively straightforward calculation of MVO can then be automatically obtained and displayed. Hardware for more complex protocols is not a technically limiting factor. In fact, complex analysis of such directly acquired (digitized) instrument data is possible once software has been written that specifies a particular analysis.

Such instrumentation is both convenient and cost-efficient. The computer control reduces the time involved in laboratory testing, probably in-

creases the accuracy of the test, and, to the extent that the patient has no unusual problems, could reduce the level of necessary competence of the vascular technician. Many manufacturers now market automated laboratories, for example, the Vasculab* system marketed by Medasonics.

The software used in a dedicated, self-contained smart instrument is often called *firmware.* These programs are coded into the hardware in a semipermanent fashion using memory chips. The program is *firm,* since those memory chips must be replaced to change the program. Improvements in analytic processes evolve and protocols change, thereby causing firmware obsolescence. Firmware instruments can create cost-containment problems for the user despite their initially attractive convenience. Additionally, firmware introduces an inflexibility that detracts from the advantages of distributed computer resources, that is, user control. Such instruments can also limit a primary efficiency of microcomputers, that of direct data acquisition into data bases.

Computer-based instrumentation

In contrast, microcomputer-based instruments can be distinguished from microprocessor-based

*Kendall Hospital Company, Mountain View, Calif.

instruments by the flexibility of programming—using software rather than firmware. (*Computer* also implies more flexible peripheral support, such as display screens, printers, and mass storage devices.) Such a distinction may appear trivial, but is important technically and didactically. In the ideal situation, vascular diagnostic instruments would provide digital information to a microcomputer. These data could be analyzed, presented, or stored under evolving formats. Additionally, although the vascular instrument might also be microprocessor based, the measurement and control protocols (such as cuff inflation) would be reprogrammable via the microcomputer host. Vascular diagnostic instruments would be modular adjuncts to the computer-microcomputer system. Truly modular vascular instruments are not currently available. Two potential alternative approaches can be identified as (1) using integrated computer-based systems now available from several manufacturers or (2) modifying existing instruments to interface with a computer. The latter option is not realistic or cost-effective on a clinical basis. The former option avoids interfacing problems and assures compatibility with all instruments supplied by the manufacturer. At least two manufacturers, Life Sciences, Inc.* and Sonicaid, Ltd†, market systems that are in this category. Direct data acquisition is accomplished, but protocol and instrument flexibility is not available with these current systems. However, because marketing control is important to instrument manufacturers, this total-package approach from individual companies may persist for the foreseeable future.

Thus full exploitation of automated data acquisition systems still remains an untapped benefit of microprocessors and microcomputers. Data entry via a keyboard is a major bottleneck for computer applications in the VDL.

SOFTWARE APPLICATIONS

Currently, the potential computer user in a VDL is confronted with more software decisions than hardware considerations. Since most current applications are software based, software compatibility dictates hardware decisions; thus very little vascular-application software is commercially available. This creates a major stimulus for customized in-house software development. The fun-

damental limitation in vascular software development is a lack of sufficient consensus about the needs and protocols of vascular software users. Because of this lack of consensus, commercially defined de facto standards are bound to evolve. Since these standards are not in the best interests of clinical vascular diagnosis, efforts are being made to establish data protocol standards.[4,9]

Data management may be the most prevalent application of computers in medicine. Despite this extensive application, experience suggests that data management is poorly understood by many computer users. Expectations are often unrealistic regarding the computational abilities of applications packages. Undoubtedly, this naïveté is a result of a failure to appreciate the digital or discrete nature of computer-based data.

Computational machines manipulate numbers and indirectly manipulate entities that can be represented by discrete numbers. A direct result of this digital representation is the superficial example that ''Dr. John Jones'' is not equivalent to ''John Jones, M.D.'' In most applications such data are expected to be equivalent, but this expectation can not currently be realized as a function of the computer hardware. The ambiguities of human thought processes require complex analyses written into the applications software. The term *user friendly* can partially measure how well the software program responds to ambiguity; *computer literacy* can mean how well the human can interact with digital machines in an unambiguous fashion.

Software tools for data management

Data management tools are usually incorporated into a single software applications package or Data Base Management Systems (DBMS). These packages are actually an integration of two separate tasks: a data filing system and a data management system. The latter is more user friendly than the former, which is the reason it was created. However, a computer illiterate can specify data files that make management impossible.

Data structures. Primarily there are two types of macrostructures used to store data: hierarchic and relational. Hierarchic is also known as a tree structure. While the hierarchic structure is often praised by system programmers, practicality prefers a relational macrostructure, especially for microprocessor-based systems. Although this view is biased, it is a fact that relational structures are more easily modified and more easily understood. A

*PVR/APL, Life Sciences, Inc., Greenwich, Conn.
†Vasoscan, Sonicaid, Ltd., Fredericksburg, Va.

more detailed discussion of this point can be found in other texts.[6,10]

Relational data bases are often explained by using the analogy of office file cabinets. The data base is a drawer in the cabinet, a file is a folder in the drawer, a record is a page in the folder, a field is a concise item on the page, and a byte is one character of the item. Data relationships are established by this macrostructure and by so-called *keys* or unique data items in each record, as shown below. While this analogy provides a starting point, it does a great disservice to the understanding of the critical aspects of data structure. A data base is never created simply to store numbers and characters. The purpose is to obtain information by retrieval of related data (known as query), so the data base must contain the information expected and the information must be logically unambiguous. This simple observation is usually not fully appreciated.

Data coding. One method for assuring that the data base contains the information to answer any possible query is to store all data available. Although this method is widely attempted, it fails for several reasons. Since any computer is a finite device, there may not be enough storage for all available data. Without planning, all data rarely contain the pertinent information, thus much of the data stored is never accessed and the storage cost is wasted. Also, this method creates data that is difficult to query. The fundamental fallacy is to assume a data base can be created that will provide information to any possible query. Another error is to assume the query process is similar to a human perusing a file folder. Query software often gives the appearance that the process is the same, but when the query results are different than expected the fault is often in the data microstructure and relationship definitions. The human is capable of redefining relationships and extrapolating information content on a continuous ad hoc basis. Digital machines and software are not yet capable of this level of intelligence.

The microstructure of data depends on its discrete nature and the intrinsic properties of numeric systems, primarily that they have intrinsic ordered magnitude. To clarify, the alphabet is stored by numeric representation and thus alphabetic data inherit a microstructure that dictates "B" is numerically larger than "A" (A < B). Fortunately, the humans who specified this convention were not shortsighted, and this structure is appropriate for alphabetic sorting. Similarly since A ≠ B, "iliac stenosis" is not the same as "aortoiliac stenosis"

Fictitious vascular data that demonstrate a relational data base

File A: Laboratory results

Record

Record no.	Field 1 SS no.	Field 2 Name	Field 3 Date	Field 4 (right ankle brachial index)	Field 5 (left ankle brachial index)
1	111-11-1111	Smith, John J.	09/01/83	0.92	1.05
2	222-22-0000	Jones, Darrell N.	10/12/83	0.88	0.95
3	333-33-9999	Rutherford, Robert B.	10/25/83	1.10	0.50
4	111-11-1111	Smith, John J.	10/25/83	0.85	1.00

File B: Therapeutic interventions

Record

Record no.	Field 1 SS no.	Field 2 Name	Field 3 Date	Field 4 Procedure
1	111-11-1111	Smith, John J.	09/02/83	Fem-pop
2	222-22-0000	Jones, Darrell N.	10/28/83	Aortobifem
3	333-33-9999	Rutherford, Robert B.	10/25/83	Fem-tib

In this example, the social security (SS) number (Field 1) serves as the key field, relates records in File A to similar records in File A, and relates records in file B to records in file A. Additionally, Field 1 and Field 3 are used to determine if a record is unique within the file. Two records with the same social security number and the same date would not be allowed in the same file.

even though a logical request may be made for data on stenoses. Without becoming more didactic, storage of descriptive text does not contribute to an informative data base.

Where feasible, data should be broken into discrete units of information and ordering should be logical when query advantage is desired. *Stenosis* can logically be a dichotomous variable, and anatomic location can be ordered by a peripheral segment. Similarly, clinical symptoms can be queried by severity (for example, asymptomatic, nondisabling claudication, or tissue loss). Queries can take advantage of the intrinsic numeric order by requesting all patients with clinical symptoms greater than asymptomatic. This process of controlling the data microstructure is known as data encoding.

Data management summary. When one considers that a data base must be planned and is not simply a direct transfer of existing information routines, the use of computer data bases in vascular diagnosis may be questioned. The answer is an individual decision, but the following criteria remain: (1) increased efficiency of routine and (2) use of more complex or extensive information. Specifically, some uses of data bases include the following:

1. Rapid retrieval or modification of individual patient studies
2. Office automation aid including automated reports, patient scheduling, and billing
3. Rapid retrieval of background information (previous studies and therapeutic interventions) to aid in interpretation of current studies
4. Providing trend analysis of laboratory activity, that is, changing referral sources, changing distribution of study types, and revenue projections
5. Supporting clinical research
6. Monitoring internal laboratory performance standards in comparison with external standards and complementary or competing testing modalities

Initial investments of time will always be relatively large, but the planning necessary to specify a logically coherent data base provides a rarely undertaken analysis of laboratory routine, which has some benefits independent of eventual computer application.

A DBMS should have a relational macrostructure. Other features should include good documentation and screen-mode data entry (Fig. 27-2) and definition. It should also provide for a fairly large number of items per record (greater than 32). These features are noted from experience with two microcomputer DBMS, the DATAEASE* and dBASE II.† DATAEASE is not an optimal software package,

*Software Solutions, Inc., Milford, Conn.
†Ashton-Tate, Culver City, Calif.

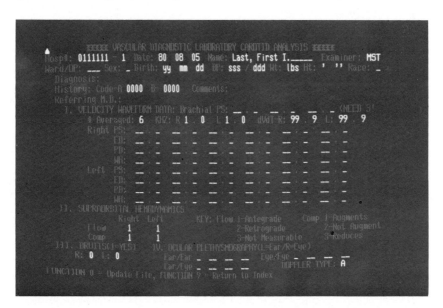

Fig. 27-2. Example of screen-mode data entry. Data are accepted only in highlighted areas. All data on the screen are transmitted to data base with an entry code, that is, function key 0. (From Lowenstein, D.H., et al.: Comput. Biomed. Res. 14:592, 1981.)

but exceeds dBASE II in ease of use and record size restrictions. These observations are not meant to imply that (1) dBASE II will not meet the needs of a particular laboratory or (2) other DBMS are not available and acceptable. (DATAEASE has some significant shortcomings, primarily its inability to incorporate or be incorporated in a sequence of non-DBMS programs, such as A/D conversion or complex data reduction and its lack of conditional program flow.) The number of office automation and business application software packages commercially available is very large. This fact does not make software decisions easy or enjoyable. Potential users should be aware that the computer software industry is constantly evolving toward more user friendly applications packages. By the time this is published, many of the comments on specific products may no longer be appropriate.[2] The goal (and problem) is the selection of a system that will not only meet current needs, but will also have the flexibility to be changed in several years without loss of data and personal investment.

Data analysis software

Data analysis is the historic foundation of computer applications, and the majority of existing software is directed to some analytic process. However, the specific nature of data analysis has fostered specific applications software. These can be arbitrarily classified as (1) firmware for smart instruments, (2) special purpose programs, and (3) analytic tools like a DBMS.

Although the end user can usually specify very little independently from instrument selection, firmware analysis is becoming the rule rather than the exception in vascular laboratory instruments. Special purpose programs are the most abundant class of software and the least likely to be available or usable by the general vascular laboratory. This class includes the large number of programs created by individual researchers or laboratories. It is important to put these programs in the perspective of the computerization of the VDL. Rapid growth of individual computer resources is very recent. Clinical research will respond to this shift in audience within the next few years, and the vascular-specific software will become available for widespread use and validation. Until this occurs, in-house development and adaptation will depend on user expertise and the commercially available analytic software tools.

General purpose analytic software includes the spread-sheet and graphics programs. The Lotus 1-2-3* and VisiCalc† are among the better known. Most good DBMS are also capable of significant numeric analysis. Since numeric analysis is a logical adjunct of data management, the distinction between DBMS and spread-sheet software is becoming rather indistinct. The combination of these tasks was once prohibited by relatively small machine memories, but advances in technology are reducing the cost of microcomputer memory capacity.

Automatic interpretation. To achieve a major saving of clerical and technical paperwork, there is a need for automated output from VDL examinations. This output should identify not only the abnormality, but the degree of abnormality and combine the results of several tests aimed at the same underlying process. The report should also note significant changes between the previous and current studies and include therapeutic interventions and angiographic findings. Comprehensive reports such as this cannot be achieved with standard DBMS software or data analysis packages; such a project is clearly a complex union of a DBMS, analytic programs, and word processing.

In the late 1970s we were involved in the development of a program for automated VDL data analysis and interpretive test generation.[5] The program employed an alogorithmic approach based on both statistical analysis and the thought process of an experienced physician. The program strategy coupled a lexicon of phrases with the diagnostic algorithm to structure a natural language report that imitated the physician's usual diagnostic summary (Fig. 27-3). Although this program met many of the goals previously stated, it is instructive to examine its shortcomings with the perspective of current computer resources.

First, this program certainly falls into the category of special purpose software relying extensively on both the hardware and system-specific software that was available in the institution. This constraint alone predetermined that the program was unlikely to find application outside our laboratory and suggests that the project was a feasibility exercise or just intended for in-house use. Before the microcomputer revolution, most special appli-

---

*Lotus Development Corp., Cambridge, Mass.
†Visicorp, San Jose, Calif.

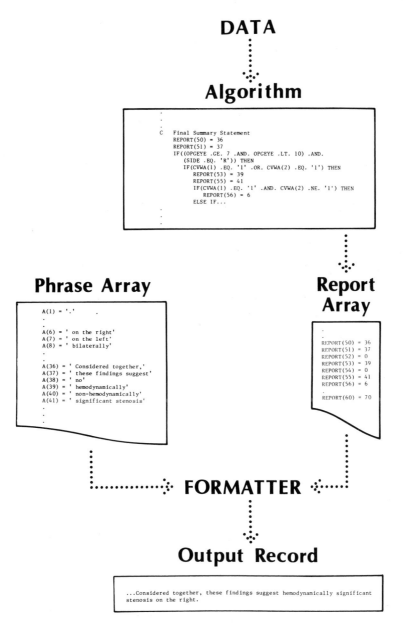

Fig. 27-3. Graphic depiction of methodology for summary report generation. Data are interpreted algorithmically into coded report array that formats standard phrase array into diagnostic summary. (From Lowenstein, D.H., et al.: Comput. Biomed. Res. 14:592, 1981.)

cation programs were developed primarily for in-house use; hardware and software compatibility considerations presented unreasonable constraints.

The program produces a paragraph summary of the observed test results but does not correlate these findings with previous tests or adjunctive information. The phrase array strategy (Fig. 27-3) was typical of very early attempts to program artificial

intelligence.[3] However, the summaries and statements are completely deterministic. Researchers in the field of artificial intelligence would not consider this application in the same class as the rather primitive *Eliza* program that imitated conversation.[3] Thus the second shortcoming is one of inflexibility to changing protocols and diagnostic standards.

Finally the program produces a statement regarding the categoric classification of disease found to be consistent with the test results. This tactic would have been unwise if the program were developed commercially, because it gives the appearance of considerably more capabilities than are actually encoded in the algorithms and could tend to remove the clinician from the decision-making process. It should be clear that computer use has been considered as strictly an aid to vascular diagnosis. The automated interpretive program cannot currently exceed this capability.

An attempt is in progress to widen the scope of the automated interpretive program in our laboratory. The DBMS will be a commercially available product (DATAEASE). Analytic software will be written in BASIC, and reports will be structured for printing and modification by a word processing program (WORDSTAR*). In addition to data summaries, categoric disease classifications will be printed, but with estimates of probability of accuracy. Finally, previous related tests, therapeutic interventions, and angiographic findings will be incorporated. This latter function will be realized by incorporating a file in the data base that contains one record for each patient and is a record of all encounters for that patient including VDL, angiography, and therapeutic interventions. From the viewpoint of data base methodology, this record is a key record pointing to all other related records. Data entry and interpretation will be controlled exclusively by the analytic program language (BASIC). Other query functions will be done using the DBMS query structure. Such a separation of tasks recognizes that DBMS software is currently task specific and cannot support the complexity of analysis inherent in automated interpretation.

Artificial intelligence and diagnostic software. Current medical research depends on a belief in statistical inference. This outlook is mirrored in the common belief that diagnosis is an exercise in probabilities. This view asserts that decisions in the face of uncertainty, that is, insufficient information, require inferences or assumptions to be drawn using prior probabilities or experience. It should not be surprising that current trends are to use the computer to draw prior probabilities from data bases and extrapolate posterior probabilities and diagnostic inferences. When one adds the ability to update the data base based on current outcomes, the process takes on the attributes of artificial in-

telligence. The additional requirements for artificial intelligence are a subject of wide dispute,[7,12] but the potential impact of such software remains the same. The fundamental danger is no different from any computer application, but is perhaps more recognizable. The inferences are only as good as the data base and algorithm used to extrapolate from that data. If the basis and reasoning path employed in the software are not understood by the user, no credence should be given to the result.[11] As the data base becomes larger and the statistical techniques become more complex, this caveat will become more difficult to heed.

SUMMARY

It is clear that microcomputers have opened the door to extensive computer use in VDL. The major impact of the microcomputers to date has been in vascular instrumentation, but the firmware used limits flexibility and the ability to integrate various components into an automated vascular laboratory. Some automated vascular laboratories are commercially available, but the user is forced to use a system that may not fit his needs. Commercial pressures will likely perpetuate these limitations. Specialized software for VDL use beyond smart instrumentation and general purpose DBMS has not yet been developed; the major holdback is a lack of agreement among users on specific needs and standardized protocols. Customizing is possible using current computer resources, but it requires considerable time and expertise and is not likely to be transferable. Standardized reporting practices, defined analytic protocols, and hardware communication compatibility are all needed before we can take full advantage of current computer capabilities, reduce the time and cost of vascular laboratory operations, and increase the speed and sophistication of data analysis.

*Micropro, San Rafael, Calif.

REFERENCES

1. Bell, C.G., Mudge, J.C., and McNamara, J.E.: Computer engineering: a DEC view of hardware systems design, Bedford, Mass., 1978, Digital Equipment Corp.
2. Edwards, S.: Why is software so hard to use? Byte 8(12):127, 1983.
3. Feigenbaum, E.A.: Artificial intelligence, IEEE Spectrum 20(11):77, 1983.
4. Gordon, R.D., Rutherford, R.B., and Jones, D.N.: Workshop sessions of the Vascular Computer Symposium, Aspen, Colo., May 18, 1982.
5. Lowenstein, D.H., et al.: Computer diagnosis in a vascular diagnostic laboratory, Comput. Biomed. Res. 14:592, 1981.

6. Martin, J.: Principles of data-base management, Prentice-Hall, Englewood Cliffs, N.J., 1976.
7. Miller, M.C., Westphal, M.C., and Routt, J.R.: Mathematical models in medical diagnosis, New York, 1981, Praeger Publishers.
8. Pournelle, J.: The next five years in microcomputers, Byte 8(9):233, 1983.
9. Rutherford, R.B., Baker, J.D., and Ernst, C.B.: Preliminary report of committee on standardized reporting in vascular surgery, Presented to the Society for Vascular Surgery/International Society for Cardiovascular Surgery Joint Council, Atlanta, Oct. 17, 1983.
10. Snyders, J.: New trends in DBMS, Computer Decisions, p. 100, Feb. 1982.
11. Szolovits, P.: Providing intelligent medical advice by computer. In Eden, H.S., and Eden, M., editors: Microcomputers in patient care, Parkridge, N.J., 1981, Noyes Publications.
12. Waltz, D.A.: Helping computers understand natural languages, IEEE Spectrum 20(11):81, 1983.

PART TWO

AREAS OF APPLICATION: DETECTION, QUANTITATION, AND PREDICTION

CHAPTER 28

The clinical spectrum of ischemic cerebrovascular disease

EUGENE F. BERNSTEIN

Stroke is the third leading cause of death in the United States, just after heart disease and cancer. It is the second leading cause of death in patients over the age of 70. However, stroke is more greatly feared than most other serious diseases, because only about 25% of patients who have a stroke die and three times as many patients survive with varying and often greatly disabling degrees of neurologic deficit. Both physically and emotionally, a major stroke that results in permanent hemiplegia and aphasia drains the most important qualities of life. Frequently the patient is committed to a nursing home or has a bedridden existence with little hope of significant improvement or recovery. In the last 3 decades a great deal of new information has been obtained concerning the pathogenesis of this disease. Emphasis has shifted from the recognition and treatment of the advanced state of major neurologic involvement to those conditions which precede a major stroke episode and to those diagnostic and management tools that may be used to significantly reduce the likelihood of a major stroke.

Pathogenesis

Ischemic cerebrovascular disease is usually the end result of progressive atherosclerosis in the arterial system leading to the brain. Thus all of the factors known to be significant in the pathogenesis of atherosclerosis are pertinent to this problem, including heredity, high cholesterol and triglyceride levels, obesity, diabetes, smoking, and high anxiety and stress states. The development of an intimal plaque containing atheromatous material is usually the first recognizable pathologic evidence of this disease and is now a frequent finding in

young adults in Western society. Progression of the intimal atheromatous lesion then occurs, followed by necrosis of some central contents of the atheroma. This is presumably because inadequate nutrition results in an increasing diffusion barrier that prevents oxygen and glucose from reaching the depths of the lesion. In addition, subintimal hemorrhage contributes to the development of thicker lesions in the necrotic interior of the atheroma. Such necrotic deeper portions of the plaque may then break through the intimal lining, which results in the release of plaque contents to the arterial bloodstream. This atheroembolic material is then deposited at a distant site that, if in the central nervous system, may provoke neurologic signs or result in physical findings that are indicators or warnings of the future potential of a major stroke. The resulting cavitary lesion in the plaque, which results from the release of atheroembolic plaque material, is referred to as an ulcer and may then be the site of swirling blood, leading to the deposition of platelet fragments and thrombi. Subsequent embolic episodes may therefore contain not only atheromatous material but also varying amounts of platelet clumps and fibrin clots. It is this triad of embolic contents—atheroma, platelets, and fibrin—that justifies the current medical approach to the treatment of this condition.

In addition to the embolic mechanism that is felt to be the most common cause of a stroke and the warning episodes of a future stroke, the atheromatous lesion may progress to obstruct most or all of the lumen of the artery. Larger plaques are more likely to become ulcerated, cavernomatous, and associated with subintimal hemorrhage and eventually lead to thrombosis. Thus an ischemic stroke may result either from inadequate blood flow to the brain or from a large embolus. Early detection of stroke potential has centered around the identification of evolving atherosclerotic lesions in vessels that feed the brain and the detection of symptoms caused by such lesions, although they may appear insignificant or may be entirely transient.

Although atherosclerosis is generally considered to be a diffuse systemic arterial disease, there is a clear predisposition to more severe localized disease at certain selected sites, including the coronary arteries, the branches of the aortic arch, the bifurcations of the carotid arteries, the infrarenal abdominal aorta, and the superficial femoral arteries. Of these the bifurcation of the carotid arteries is an area in which atherosclerotic disease tends to be particularly severe and segmentally localized. Recent research has confirmed the concept that ischemic cerebrovascular stroke is most frequently a result of atherosclerosis in the neck or the arch of the aorta. The precise location and segmental nature of this process is the basis for the surgical approach to the treatment of these conditions, since effective surgical procedures can be performed on well-localized, discreet lesions.

Temporal classification

The clinical stages of ischemic cerebrovascular disease are summarized in the top box on p. 303, ranging from the asymptomatic patient with only a minimally detectable shallow plaque or shallow ulceration in an artery leading to the brain, to the patient with a full, complete, and permanent stroke. Asymptomatic disease may be defined as an identifiable pathologic state associated with the increased likelihood of a future stroke. Such patients are identified by the presence of a cervical bruit or by noninvasive vascular or angiographic procedures that document the existence of carotid bifurcation stenosis or ulceration.

A transient ischemic attack (TIA) is an episode of focal, visual, motor, or sensory loss that persists for less than 24 hours. Most of these episodes are much shorter, usually lasting for 5 to 30 minutes. They are painless, involve no loss of consciousness, are generally associated with a rapid onset and resolution, and may be a result of one of a variety of factors (see middle box on p. 303). If the neurologic symptoms persist more than 24 hours, but eventually resolve completely, the event is referred to as a reversible ischemic neurologic deficit (RIND). If the deficit persists permanently,

the patient has had a stroke. During the time interval that neurologic symptoms are changing, the condition is described as a progressing stroke or stroke in evolution. Once the patient's neurologic condition has become stable with a persisting neurologic deficit the condition is referred to as a completed stroke.

Differential diagnosis of acute cerebral deficit

Although the vast majority of acute cerebrovascular problems are of vascular etiology, a number of systemic, neurologic, and cardiogenic diseases may also produce such symptoms (see bottom box on p. 303). Since the specific identification of a large number of these entities can lead to a satisfactory management and therapy plan, the physician should undertake a methodical and complete workup of any patient with an abrupt cerebral deficit.

THE TIA

Symptoms associated with transient ischemic episodes may generally be classified by the arterial circulation involved. In the anterior circulation from the carotid system, the most frequently observed symptoms include amaurosis fugax (transient monocular blindness) and numbness, weakness, or paralysis of an arm or leg or both (Table 28-1). In addition, lesions in this portion of the brain may be accompanied by dysphasia or aphasia, headache, dizziness, blackouts, buzzing noises, mental deterioration, memory loss, coma, and convulsions. In contrast, patients whose pathologic condition resides in the vertebrobasilar or posterior portion of the brain frequently complain of bilateral visual disturbances, dysarthria, dysphasia, drop attacks, and bilateral sensory deficits. In addition, they may experience vertigo, headaches, bilateral visual disturbances, loss of consciousness, monoparesis, shifting paralysis, or cerebellar ataxia. The relative frequency of these complaints, as assessed in the Canadian Cooperative Study Group,[18] is in Table 28-1. A further localization of the symptom complexes associated with carotid artery distribution and the middle cerebral artery is summarized in Table 28-2, although occlusions of other vessels with variable collateral circulatory compensation may yield similar symptom complexes. The symptom complex associated with the lenticulostriate branches of the internal capsule is important. This complex results in lacunar infarction, which is generally manifested by unilateral motor and sensory findings in the face, arm, and

---

CEREBROVASCULAR DISEASE—TEMPORAL CLASSIFICATION

Asymptomatic—bruit, stenosis, ulceration
Transient ischemic attack (TIA)
Reversible ischemic neurologic deficit (RIND)
Progressing stroke
Completed stroke

---

leg and explains the absence of large-vessel atherosclerotic disease on an angiogram.

Natural history of a TIA. The natural history of patients who have experienced a TIA has been intensively studied in the last 2 decades. Outcome for such patients is based primarily on the symptom complex and on the full spectrum of causes in the box at the bottom of this page that lists the differ-

Table 28-1. Frequency of symptoms in TIA

CAROTID ARTERY DISTRIBUTION	
Symptoms	**Patients (%)**
Paresis (monoparesis, hemiparesis	61
Paresthesia (monoparesis, hemiparesis)	57
Monocular visual	32
Paresthesia (facial)	30
Paresis (facial)	22

VERTEBROBASILAR DISTRIBUTION	
Symptoms	**Patients (%)**
Binocular visual	57
Vertigo	50
Paresthesia	40
Diplopia	38
Ataxia	33
Paresis	33

ETIOLOGY OF ACUTE CEREBRAL DEFICIT

All patients
   → Nonvascular (tumor, etc.)—5%
Vascular etiology—95%
   → Hemorrhagic—14%
Ischemic—81%
   → Cardiogenic—12%
     Other—4%
Cerebrovascular
disease—65%

After Easton, J.D., et al.: Curr. Probl. Cardiol. 8:1, 1983.

Table 28-2. Arterial classification of symptomatic cerebrovascular disease

Artery	Symptoms
Ophthalmic	Amaurosis fugax
Middle cerebral	
Anterior cortical branch	Contralateral sensory and motor loss of face, arm and hand
	Nonfluent aphasia (dominant hemisphere)
Posterior cortical branch	Contralateral sensory loss
	Homonymous hemianopsia
	Fluent aphasia (dominant hemisphere)
Proximal middle cerebral or lenticulostriate branch	Internal capsule
	Unilaterial motor and sensory findings of face, arm, and leg
Vertebrobasilar	Diplopia
	Bilateral facial sensory loss
	Bilateral extremity weakness
	Vertigo
	Ataxia

DIFFERENTIAL DIAGNOSIS OF ACUTE CEREBRAL DEFICIT

Cerebrovascular atherosclerosis
Cardiogenic embolism—valvular, ventricular cavity, tumor, and paradoxic
Arteriopathy—inflammatory (systemic collagen diseases, Takayasu's disease, or infections)
   —noninflammatory (fibromuscular hyperplasia, spontaneous and traumatic dissection, cerebral angiopathies, or neoplasm)
Vasospasm—migraine or hypertensive encephalopathy
Subarachnoid hemorrhage
Coagulopathies and hyperviscosity syndromes
Trauma
Systemic hypotension
Metabolic disturbances
Drug reactions

PROGNOSIS FOLLOWING DETECTION OF RETINAL CHOLESTEROL EMBOLI

208 patients, mean age 64 years of age, 86% males
97% followed for 6 + 2 years, 70 followed for 10 + years
75% (157) had TIA or stroke
45% (94) had stroke
28% (58) had stroke ipsilateral to the retinal embolus

From Pfaffenbach, D.D., and Hollenhorst, R.W.: Am. J. Ophthamol. 75:66, 1973.

Table 28-3. Prognosis following TIA without treatment

Author and year	Patients (No.)	Average follow-up (months)	Stroke (%)
Fisher,[42] 1958	23	?	34
Baker,[7] 1962	20	20	25
Siekert,[102] 1963	160	60	32
Acheson,[1] 1964	151	48	62
Marshall,[73] 1965	158	60	43
Pierce,[81] 1965	20	11	10
Baker,[7] 1966	30	41	23
Baker,[5] 1968	79	41	22
Friedman,[44] 1969	23	27	35
Goldner,[47] 1971	111	?	38
Ziegler,[126] 1973	135	36	16
Whisnant,[120] 1973	198	60	32
Toole,[115] 1975	56	66	19
Olsson,[85] 1976	124	21	15
Canadian Cooperative,[18] 1978	139	26	14
Loeb,[70] 1978	94	78	12
Sorenson,[103] 1983	102	25	11
Bousser,[13] 1983	204	36	18

ential diagnoses of acute cerebral deficits. Approximately one third of the patients with a TIA will have sustained a complete stroke episode within 5 years (Table 28-3). The likelihood of stroke is greatest within the first month after a TIA, during which approximately 5% of the patients will sustain a stroke. The incidence of stroke then decreases gradually with an overall likelihood of 12% within 1 year and 20% within 2 years. The ominous nature of these data dictates the need for an urgent and complete workup of the patient who has experienced a TIA.

The box on the left identifies the even more severe implications of finding retinal cholesterol crystals (Hollenhorst's plaques).[90] Although these patients are technically asymptomatic and since many have not experienced transient monocular blindness, they are clearly at high risk for stroke and should undergo a similar workup.

Twenty-five percent of patients who sustain a permanent stroke and do not die are then faced with the likelihood of further stroke episodes, resulting in the progressive loss and deterioration of their residual neurologic function. Table 28-4 summarizes the available data regarding the incidence of ischemic strokes following a single stroke episode, from which it appears that the likelihood of recurrent stroke varies from 6% to 11% per year. Thus the continuing risk for further neurologic erosion argues for identifying a course of management that will minimize future strokes. The practical problem, however, is that many of these patients have already lost so much neurologic function that they are no longer independently capable of managing their lives. Under these circumstances the additional risks required to attempt to preclude further strokes often do not appear justifiable. Nevertheless, those patients who have recovered from

Table 28-4. Likelihood of recurrent stroke

Author	Patients (No.)	Mean follow-up (months)	Ischemic strokes (%/year)	Lethal strokes (%/year)
Baker[4]	62	13	6%	3%
Baker[5]	60	11	11%	9%
Hill (phase I)[57]	71	10	7%	0%
Hill (phase II)[57]	65	31	11%	1%
McDowell[76]	99	34	8%	2%
Enger[34]	49	23	11%	3%

a stroke with a small permanent deficit that has left them relatively capable of functioning independently are at as great a risk of further stroke as after a TIA and should be considered in the same workup category as patients who have sustained a TIA or RIND.

Workup of the symptomatic patient

The evaluation of patients with a single TIA, RIND, or small stroke should include a complete history, physical examination, and basic workup for systemic, cardiac, and neurologic disease. This workup should include a complete blood count, urinalysis, prothrombin time, partial thromboplastin time, chest x-ray examination, cerebrospinal fluid examination, antinuclear antibody (ANA) level, erythrocyte sedimentation rate, and computerized tomographic (CT) scan (Fig. 28-1). All patients with evidence of cardiac disease that may be a potential embolic source should also have cardiac consultation and appropriate cardiac evaluation. Patients with evidence of systemic disease, including an increased erythrocyte sedimentation rate,

anemia, or thrombocytosis, should be subjected to further studies including ANA, cerebrospinal fluid examinations, and protein electrophoresis levels. A CT scan should be performed in all patients with symptomatic cerebrovascular disease, because it may provide information regarding the presence of a mass lesion, such as a tumor. The CT scan may also permit identifying an ischemic infarction (as a hypodense area) or a hemorrhagic lesion (a hyperdense area). It may also demonstrate a mass effect secondary to edema surrounding an embolic lesion and may permit the diagnosis of a lacunar stroke.

In the absence of evidence of cardiogenic emboli or systemic disease, a presumptive diagnosis of cerebrovascular disease should be made.[31] Cerebrovascular disease is responsible for the transient episode in approximately 65% of patients with such symptoms. A decision must then be made regarding the suitability of the patient as a candidate for carotid surgery with the further workup directed toward that goal. Patients considered at inordinately high risk for cerebrovascular surgery should

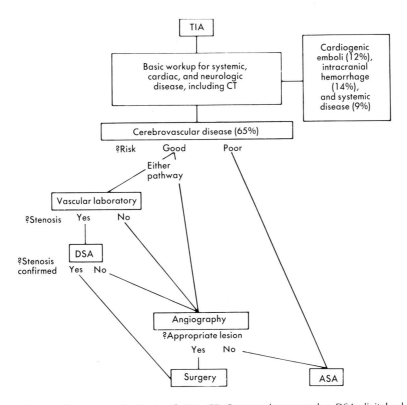

Fig. 28-1. Scheme for workup of patient with TIA. *CT,* Computed tomography; *DSA,* digital subtraction angiography (intravenous); *ASA,* acetyl salicylic acid.

be treated with antiplatelet or anticoagulant therapy, as will be described. Good-risk patients should continue on the management algorithm path in Fig. 28-1. Two equally satisfactory options exist for their further workup. In the first, the patient is sent to the vascular laboratory to obtain evidence of a carotid artery lesion producing significant hemodynamic stenosis. In the presence of such data, intravenous digital subtraction angiography (DSA) will confirm the presence of carotid stenosis in approximately 85% of the patients. This sequence of vascular laboratory data confirmed by DSA has been accepted by many surgeons as an adequate basis for surgery on an anatomically appropriate lesion. If the DSA fails to confirm a vascular laboratory diagnosis of significant carotid disease, the patient should undergo formal contrast angiography.

A second approach for the good-risk patient is to bypass the vascular laboratory and proceed directly with formal contrast angiography. Under these circumstances DSA would be inadequate, since small shallow ulcers or minimal plaquelike lesions would not be diagnosed. Thus formal contrast studies, including the arch of the aorta, great vessels, selective biplane studies of the carotid arteries, and intracerebral angiograms are considered necessary. Patients with anatomically appropriate lesions found under either of these pathways are candidates for surgical therapy.

Role of angiography. Carotid angiography is the appropriate, definitive diagnostic procedure for all patients with a symptomatic acute cerebrovascular event with complete or nearly complete recovery. In addition, selected patients with chronic cerebral ischemia (based on multivessel occlusive disease) or with asymptomatic carotid stenosis (defined by a vascular laboratory study) are also candidates for angiography.

Formal cerebrovascular angiography is generally performed through a femoral puncture with a catheter placed in the arch of the aorta, after which injections are performed and x-ray films are obtained in two planes. Selective injections into both carotid arteries are also routine. In addition, the subclavian arteries are selectively injected for vertebral artery symptoms. All studies should also include intracranial views to identify the possibility of tandem lesions in the upper portion of the internal carotid artery and other intracranial lesions that may be the cause of the patient's symptoms. With modern techniques the risks of cerebral an-

Table 28-5. Complications of cerebral angiography

Author	Year	Patients (no.)	Stroke (%)	Mortality (%)
Swanson[106]	1977	464	1.1	?
Mani[72]	1978	1702	0.1	0
Faught[37]	1979	147	5.4	0
Link[69]	1979	162	0	0
Allen[2]	1981	154	2.0	0
Harrison[51]	1982	188	1.1	?

giography for the evaluation of cerebrovascular symptoms are quite low and carry an expected stroke rate of approximately 1% and an anticipated mortality of a small fraction of 1% (Table 28-5).

The clinical correlation of significant symptoms with the angiographic demonstration of appropriate carotid bifurcation stenosis or occlusion is very high.[10,32,38,48,52] Symptoms such as amaurosis fugax or the presence of retinal emboli have a likelihood of a significant carotid artery lesion in over 90% of the patients. On the other hand, when all patients with carotid system TIAs are subjected to angiography, fully 25% of the angiograms appear normal (Table 28-6). In these patients the workup for other causes, including systemic collagen disease, neurologic conditions, and cardiogenic emboli, should be intensified. Twenty percent of these patients have a minimal irregularity on angiography, and these lesions are consistent with an embologenic pathogenesis. Such patients should be candidates for carotid endarterectomy. Approximately 10% of patients with TIA will have occlusion of the appropriate internal carotid system on angiography. Under these circumstances a careful search must be made for the possibility of embologenic lesions from the contralateral carotid bifurcation or symptoms associated with chronic cerebral ischemia that might benefit by an extracranial-to-intracranial bypass. Although such patients do constitute a higher risk group for surgery, in good hands the surgical approach still offers the best outlook in the prevention of recurrent stroke.

The most important and largest source of data concerning the diagnostic rewards of complete cerebrovascular angiography in patients with stroke symptoms was presented by the Joint Study,[39] which included four-vessel angiography in 4748 patients with stroke symptoms. In 19.4% of the patients no lesions were identified. However, in 74.5% significant and appropriate lesions in a sur-

Table 28-6. Angiographic correlations in carotid TIA

	Angiographic classification			
Author and year	Normal (%)	Minimal disease (%)	Stenosis ≥ 25% (%)	Occlusion (%)
Ramirex-Lassepas, 1973[95]	17	←————69————→		14
Lemak, 1976[67]	43	←————49————→		8
Harrison, 1976[51]	45	10	40	5
Pessin, 1977[89]	←————42————→		46	12
Eisenberg, 1977[33]	9	0	73	15
Marti-Vilalta, 1979[74]	27			
Link, 1979[69]	8	←————89————→		3
Ueda, 1979[117]	11	14	59	16
Van Oudenarrden, 1980[118]	24	32	←————44————→	
Thiele, 1980[110]	13	40	←————47————→	
Barnett, 1980[10]	22	27	35	13
Russo, 1981[99]	55	19	15	11
Muuronen, 1981[83]	49	10	37	4
ESTIMATED MEAN	27%	19%	44%	10%

Adapted from Easton, J.D., et al.: Curr. Probl. Cardiol. 8:1, 1983.

Table 28-7. Distribution of extracranial arterial occlusive diseases in 4748 patients with stroke symptoms

	Stenosis (%)	Occlusion (%)
Innominate	4.2	0.6
Common carotid (Left)	4.8	4.4
Subclavian (Left)	12.4	2.5
Carotid bifurcation (Right)	33.8	8.5
Carotid bifurcation (Left)	34.1	8.5
Vertebral (Right)	18.4	4.0
Vertebral (Left)	22.3	5.7

gically accessible area were identified, although multiple lesions were present in two thirds of the patients (Table 28-7).[39] Carotid bifurcation stenosis was the most common localized lesion associated with stroke symptoms, followed by vertebral origin stenosis and left subclavian stenosis. On the other hand, occlusion of any of these vessels was relatively uncommon.

Therapeutic alternatives. The major alternatives available to patients who have had a transient ischemic episode or a mild episode with good recovery include anticoagulation therapy, antiplatelet aggregation therapy, and surgery. Anticoagulation therapy is suggested as appropriate for patients with a TIA, because it would inhibit the development and propagation of thrombi in association with plaques and ulcers.[32,75,78,108] A summary of the major trials of anticoagulation therapy in the treatment of TIA is presented in Table 28-8. The data indicate that anticoagulation therapy was beneficial in most, but not all, of the studies. However, the incidence of cerebral hemorrhage associated with anticoagulation therapy increases with time and is estimated to be at least 2% per year. Therefore the general consensus has been that anticoagulation is appropriate only in patients requiring a short period of therapy, perhaps up to 6 months, during which the likelihood of stroke is greatest following a TIA episode.[32,46] In general, anticoagulation therapy is limited to those patients who are not surgical candidates or those who refuse surgery. Data regarding use of anticoagulation therapy in patients with progressing stroke also suggest benefits (Table 28-9) and justify advocating the use of these drugs during the immediate period of stroke in evolution.[19] On the other hand, anticoagulation therapy for completed stroke clearly has an adverse effect on outcome, since the risks of serious hemorrhage exceed the benefits of minimizing recurrent stroke (Table 28-10).

Platelet antiaggregation agents have also been used in the treatment of patients with TIA and have been evaluated in a number of prospective randomized trials. The United States and Canadian multicentered studies, which are summarized in Table 28-11, are considered the most valid. In the U.S.

study, when the incidence of TIA, stroke, or death was used as an end point, there was a significant benefit for the patient group treated with aspirin.[39] However, when stroke alone was evaluated, the benefits were not significant. In the Canadian study the results were similar.[18] When TIA, stroke, and death were evaluated, the results indicated some benefit for the aspirin treatment group, at a borderline significance. However, when stroke alone was evaluated, there was no difference between the control group and the treated group. This was also true when stroke alone was evaluated for males. The major benefits of aspirin therefore appear to be in inhibiting the likelihood of further TIA and in decreasing the incidence of death from cardiac disease. Additional studies involving the use of sulfinpyrazone or dipyridamole alone or together with aspirin did not appear to significantly improve the end results for TIA, stroke, or death.

Surgery is the third alternative for the treatment of cerebrovascular occlusive disease. The goals of carotid surgery are to prevent future strokes and prolong life. It also may relieve symptoms, particularly in those patients who are subject to continuing TIAs. Currently accepted indications for surgery include TIAs (plus reversible ischemic neurologic deficits) and prior stroke with significant recovery and a current minimal neurologic deficit.[104,105,112,119] Other indications include symptomatic subclavian steal, chronic cerebral ischemia from multivessel occlusive disease, and select asymptomatic carotid stenosis.[52,88,94] Recent data concerning the risk of carotid endarterectomy for patients with TIAs indicate that the procedure

Table 28-8. Anticoagulation for TIA

Source (author and year)	Ischemic stroke (%)	
	Treatment	Control
Randomized studies		
Baker, 1961[4]	5	0
Baker, 1962[7]	6	25
Pierce, 1965[81]	6	10
Baker, 1966[6]	7	23
MEAN	5	17
Nonrandomized studies		
Fisher, 1958[43]	3	35
Siekert, 1963[102]	7	32
Friedman, 1969[44]	0	35
Toole, 1975[115]	29	13
Olsson, 1965[86]	0	6
Gallhofer, 1979[45]	8	21
Link, 1979[69]	0	—
Terent, 1980[108]	8	31
Olsson, 1980[85]	2	—
Buren, 1981[15]	3	—
MEAN	6	28

Table 28-9. Anticoagulation for progressing stroke

Type of study	Ischemic stroke (%)		
	Patients (No.)	Treatment	Control
Randomized	304	23	46
Nonrandomized	269	21	57

From Easton, J.D., et al.: Curr Probl Cardiol 8:1, 1983.

Table 28-10. Anticoagulation for completed stroke

Author and year	Ischemic stroke (%)		Serious hemorrhage (%)	
	Treatment	Control	Treatment	Control
Baker, 1961[4]	5	6	13	4
Baker, 1962[7]	17	25	24	0
Hill, Phase I, 1962[57]	13	6	1	0
Phase II, 1962	33	29	18	0
McDowell, 1965[76]	21	21	12	2
Enger, 1965[34]	10	20	6	0

should be performed when the mortality is approximately 1% and stroke risk is 5% or less (Table 28-12). In addition, data regarding the late results of carotid endarterectomy for patients with TIAs indicate a reduction of the expected natural history stroke rate of 5% to 7% per year to less than 2% per year (Table 28-13).[8] Such results assume morbidity and mortality data in the currently reported ranges.

Whether carotid endarterectomy is appropriate in asymptomatic patients is clearly more controversial.* Since such patients are at less risk than patients who have sustained a TIA (Table 28-14), the tolerance for perioperative morbidity and mortality must be less, and the responsibility of the

*References 14, 16, 21, 23, 49, 53, 82, 98, 107.

surgical team therefore greater. Data addressing the risk of carotid endarterectomy in asymptomatic patients are presented in Table 28-15 and indicate that the acceptable mortality range should be 1% or less and the acceptable operative stroke range 2% or less. Long-term results of such procedures in asymptomatic patients appear to justify their continued use by selected teams. The available data (Table 28-16) suggest the stroke rate after prophylactic carotid surgery is approximately 1% per year, significantly less than would be expected using other forms of treatment. However, it seems clear that survival following carotid endarterectomy for any of these indiciations is significantly less than that for the general population (Fig. 28-2), primarily as a result of myocardial disease.[55,96,116]

In summary, the three alternative therapeutic

Table 28-11. Aspirin for TIA

Source	Patients (No.)	End point events	Events (%)		
			Treatment	Control	p
U.S. Multicenter Study, 1977[39]	178	TIA, stroke, death	17	38	.01
		Stroke, death	7	16	NS*
		Stroke	5	11	NS
Canadian Cooperative Study 1978[18]	585	TIA, stroke, death	57	66	.05
		Stroke, death	18	22	.05
		Stroke	15	14	NS
		Stroke, death (males)	17	24	.01
		Stroke (males)	14	16	NS

*NS, Not significant.

Table 28-12. Risk of carotid endarterectomy for TIA

Author and year	Operations (No.)	Mortality (%)	Stroke (%)
Schechter and Acinapura,* 1979[101]	200	1.0	1.0
Duke, 1979[28]	70	1.4	5.7
Bouchier-Hayes, 1979[12]	34	—	5.9
Haynes and Dempsey,* 1979[54]	276	1.1	4.0
Pinkerton and Gholkar,* 1979[92]	100	0	4.0
White, 1981[122]	104	1.0	1.9
Whisnant, 1982[121]	151	1.0	3.0
Asiddao, 1982[3]	94	0	4.3
Modi, 1983[79]	249	0.4	1.6
Bernstein, 1983[11]	152	0	2.6
AVERAGE		1.2	4.8

*Minority of patients had small strokes, most had TIAs.

Table 28-13. Late results of carotid endarterectomy for TIA

Author and year	Patients (No.)	Average follow-up (months)	Late stroke* (%)	Late death* (%)
Young, 1969[125]	95	12 to 60	3.2	10.5
Fields, 1970[39]	150	42	4.0	15.3
Thompson, 1970[111]	289	6 to 156	5.4	27.3
Wylie, 1970[124]	129	48	5.7	14.6
DeWeese, 1973[25]	102	60	10.6	34.3
Chung, 1974[20]	58	48	—	20.1
Nunn, 1975[84]	168	39	7.7	31.0
Toole, 1975[114]	77	46	6.9	18.2
McNamara, 1977[77]	52	10	0.0	7.7
Fields, 1977[41]	60	24	13.3	—
Cornell, 1978[22]	65	32	3.1	—
Pinkerton, 1979[92]	85	25	0.0	?
Bouchier-Hayes, 1979[12]	57	12 to 72	3.5	7.0
Ericsson, 1980[36]	143	22	7.0	?
Whisnant, 1982[121]	150	72	—	—
Harrison, 1982[50]	58	50	17.2	?
Bernstein, 1983[11]	152	45	6.0	19.0

*The aggregate estimates were as follows: stroke, 1.8% per year; death, 5% per year.

Table 28-14. Prognosis of asymptomatic carotid artery disease

Author and year	Patients (No.)	Mean follow-up (years)	TIA (%)	Stroke (%/yr)
BRUIT				
Kagan, 1976[62]	124	4	?	1
Kartchner, 1977[64]	1130	2	1.5	1.5
Thompson, 1978[114]	138	4	6.5	4.5
Heyman, 1980[56]	72	6	?	2.3
Dorazio, 1980[27]	97	7	1.6	2.7
Wolf, 1981[123]	171	4	1	3
Busuttil, 1981[17]	58	2.5	8.2	2.1
STENOSIS				
Kartchner, 1977[64]	143	2	2.5	6.0
Moll, 1979[80]	29	2	0	0
Barnes, 1981[9]	19	1	8	2.5 (1.9%)
Busuttil, 1981[17]	45	2.5	11.6	3.0
Humphries, 1976[58]	168	2.6	15	2
Johnson, 1978[61]	22	2	9	0
Levin, 1980[68]	147	0 to 20	12	1 (0%)
Podore, 1980[93]	28	5	14	7
Durwood, 1982[29]	67	4	13	3
ULCERATION				
Type A (small single ulceration)				
Kroener, 1980[65]	63	3		1
Dixon, 1982[26]	72	4		0.9
Type B (larger ulcers)				
Kroener, 1980[65]	24	3		0
Dixon, 1982,[26]	54	4		4.5
Type C (compound ulcers)				
Dixon, 1982[26]	27	4		7.5

Table 28-15. Risk of carotid endarterectomy in asymptomatic patients

Author and year	Operations (No.)	Operative mortality (%)	Perioperative stroke (%)
Young, 1969[125]	33	3	0
Javid, 1971[60]	56	4	2
DeWeese, 1973[25]	50	0	4
Kanaly, 1977[63]	21	0	0
Easton, 1977[30]	11	0	18
Thompson, 1978[112]	167	0	1
Moore, 1979[81]	78	0	3
Crowell, 1981[23]	30	0	0
White, 1981[122]	44	0	0
Assidao, 1982[3]	13	0	15
Burke, 1982[16]	70	3	1
Modi, 1983[79]	74	3	3
Bernstein, 1983[11]	87	0	3

Table 28-16. Late results of carotid endarterectomy for asymptomatic disease

Author and year	Operations (No.)	Mean follow-up (years)	Stroke (%)	Death (%)
Javid, 1971[60]	49	3	4	31
Lefrak, 1974[66]	34	5	3	44
Kanaly, 1977[63]	9	2	0	36
Thompson, 1978[112]	132	4.5	5	33
Moore, 1979[81]	72	6	1	42
Jausseran, 1979[59]	47	2.5	4	4
Thevenet, 1979[109]	92	4.5	4	18
Burke, 1982[16]	57	3.5	2	26
Bernstein, 1983[11]	87	3.8	3	25

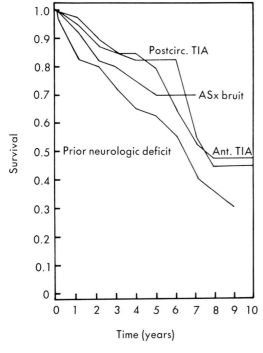

Fig. 28-2. Life table analysis of survival following carotid endarterectomy for variety of indications, showing lower survival rate in patients with prior neurologic deficit. *ASx,* Asymptomatic.

modalities for threatened stroke include anticoagulation therapy, aspirin, and carotid artery surgery.[32,97] Each appears to have its own specific role and indication. Good-risk patients suffering a TIA with appropriate carotid artery lesions should undergo angiography and surgery. Poor-risk patients or those who refuse surgery should be considered candidates for anticoagulation therapy, particularly in the period of time during an acute progressing stroke or in the first few months following a TIA. Antiplatelet aggregation therapy remains the mainstay for other nonoperative patients, although the data justifying its widespread use for the suppression of strokes are not statistically significant or convincing.

CONCLUSION

Ischemic stroke is a major life-threatening and disabling event. Recent information implicates atherosclerotic disease of the aortic arch and carotid arteries as a major source of atheroembolic and flow-inhibiting factors that are the most important pathogenic mechanisms for stroke. An appropriate workup must include efforts to detect systemic, hematologic, neurologic, and cardiogenic causes of such episodes, particularly when the patient has significant residual independent neurologic capability. Identification of a specific clinical entity should permit a treatment plan designed to minimize future neurologic destructive episodes. For the patient with atherosclerotic carotid bifurcation disease a management plan that includes complete cerebrovascular angiography and selects appropriate patients for surgery seems to provide the greatest potential for minimizing future risk from stroke.

REFERENCES

1. Acheson, J., and Hutchinson, E.C.: Observations of the natural history of transient cerebral ischemia, Lancet 2:871, 1964.
2. Allen, G.S., and Preziosi, T.J.: Carotid endarterectomy: a prospective study of its efficacy and safety, Medicine 60:298, 1981.
3. Asiddao, C.B., et al.: Factors associated with perioperative complications during carotid endarterectomy, Anesth. Analg. 61:631, 1982.
4. Baker, R.N.: An evaluation of anticoagulant therapy in the treatment of cerebrovascular disease: report of the Veterans Administration cooperative study of atherosclerosis, Neurology 11:132, 1961.
5. Baker, R.N., Ramseyer, J.C., and Schwartz, W.: Prognosis in patients with transient cerebral attacks, Neurology 18:1157, 1968.
6. Baker, R.N., Schwartz, W., and Rose, A.S.: Transient ischemic attacks—a report of a study of anticoagulant treatment, Neurology 16:841, 1966.
7. Baker, R.N., et al.: Anticoagulant therapy in cerebral infarction, Neurology 12:823, 1962.
8. Bardin, J.A., et al.: Is carotid endarterectomy beneficial in prevention of recurrent stroke? Arch. Surg. 117:1401, 1982.
9. Barnes, R.W., et al.: Natural history of symptomatic carotid disease in patients undergoing cardiovascular surgery, Surgery 90:1075, 1981.
10. Barnett, H.J.M.: The pathophysiology of transient cerebral ischemic attacks, Med. Clin. North Am. 63:649, 1979.
11. Bernstein, E.F., et al.: Life expectancy and late stroke following carotid endarterectomy, Ann. Surg. 198:80, 1983.
12. Bouchier-Hayes, D., DeCosta A., and MacGowan, W.A.L.: The morbidity of carotid endarterectomy, Br. J. Surg. 66:433, 1979.
13. Bousser, M.G., et al.: "AICLA" controlled trial of aspirin and dipyridamole in the secondary prevention of athero-thrombotic cerebral ischemia, Stroke 14:5, 1983.
14. Brewster, D.C., et al.: Rational management of the asymptomatic carotid bruit, Arch. Surg. 113:927, 1978.
15. Buren, A., and Ygge, J.: Treatment program and comparison between anticoagulants and platelet aggregation inhibitors after transient ischemic attack, Stroke 12:578, 1981.
16. Burke, P.A., et al.: Prophylactic carotid endarterectomy for asymptomatic bruit: a look at cardiac risk, Arch. Surg. 117:1222, 1982.
17. Busuttil, R.W. et al.: Carotid artery stenosis—hemodynamic significance and clinical course, JAMA 245:1438, 1981.
18. Canadian Cooperative Study Group: A randomized trial of aspirin and sulfinpyrazone in threatened stroke, N. Engl. J. Med. 299:53, 1978.
19. Carter, A.B.: Anticoagulant treatment in progressing stroke, Br. Med. J. 2:70, 1961.
20. Chung, W.B.: Long-term results of carotid artery surgery for cerebrovascular insufficiency, Am. J. Surg. 128:262, 1974.
21. Cooperman, M., Martin, E.W., and Evans, W.E.: Significance of asymptomatic carotid bruits, Arch. Surg. 113:1339, 1978.
22. Cornell, W.P.: Carotid endarterectomy: results in 100 patients, Ann. Thorac. Surg. 25:121, 1978.
23. Crowell, R.M., and Ojemann, R.G.: Carotid endarterectomy. In Hoff, J.T., editor: Practice of Surgery, Hagerstown, Md., 1981, Harper & Row Publishers, Inc.
24. Crowell, R.M., et al.: Carotid endarterectomy in high risk patients with cardiopulmonary disease (abstract), Stroke 12:123, 1981.
25. DeWeese, J.A., et al.: Results of carotid endarterectomy for transient ischemic attacks five years later, Ann. Surg. 178:258, 1973.
26. Dixon, S., et al.: Natural history of nonstenotic asymptomatic ulcerative lesions of the carotid artery, Arch. Surg. 117:1493, 1982.
27. Dorazio, R.A., Ezzet, F., and Nesbit, N.J.: Long-term follow-up of asymptomatic carotid bruits. Am. J. Surg. 140:212, 1980.
28. Duke, L.J., et al.: Carotid arterial reconstruction: ten-year experience, Am. Surg. 45:281, 1979.
29. Durwood, Q.J., Ferguson, G.G., and Barr, H.W.K.: The natural history of asymptomatic carotid bifurcation plaques, Stroke 13:459, 1982.
30. Easton, J.D., and Sherman, D.G.: Stroke and mortality rate in carotid endarterectomy: 228 consecutive operations, Stroke 8:565, 1977.

31. Easton, J.D., and Sherman, D.G.: Management of cerebral embolism of cardiac origin, Stroke 11:433, 1980.
32. Easton, J.D., et al.: Diagnosis and management of ischemic stroke. I. Threatened stroke and its management, Curr. Probl. Cardiol. 8:1, 1983.
33. Eisenberg, R.L., et al.: Relationship of transient ischemic attacks and angiographically demonstrable lesions of carotid artery, Stroke 8:483, 1977.
34. Enger, E., and Boyesen, S.: Long-term anticoagulant therapy in patients with cerebral infarction: a controlled clinical study, Acta Scand. 178(suppl. 438):1, 1965.
35. Ennix, C.L., et al.: Improved results of carotid endarterectomy in patients with symptomatic coronary disease: an analysis of 1,546 consecutive carotid operations, Stroke 10:122, 1979.
36. Ericsson, B.F., and Takolander, R.J.: Operative treatment of carotid artery stenosis, Lakartidningen 77:893, 1980.
37. Faught, E., Trader, S.D., and Hanna, G.R.: Cerebral complications of angiography for transient ischemia and stroke: prediction of risk, Neurology 29:4, 1979.
38. Fazekas, J.F., Alman, R.W., and Sullivan, J.F.: Management of patients with vertebral-basilar insufficiency, Arch. Neurol. 8:215, 1963.
39. Fields, W.S., et al.: Joint study of extracranial artery occlusion. V. Progress report of prognosis following surgery or non-surgical treatment for transient ischemic attacks and cervical carotid artery lesions, JAMA 211:1993, 1970.
40. Fields, W.S. et al.: Controlled trial of aspirin in cerebral ischemia. II. Surgical results, Stroke 9:308, 1978.
41. Fields, W.S., et al.: Controlled trial of aspirin in cerebral ischemia, Stroke 8:301, 1977.
42. Fisher, C.M.: Use of anticoagulants in cerebral thrombosis, Neurology 8:311, 1958.
43. Fisher, C.M.: Anticoagulant therapy in cerebral thrombosis and cerebral embolism: a national cooperative study, interim report, Neurology 11:119, 1961.
44. Friedman, G.D., et al.: Transient ischemic attacks in a community, JAMA 210:1428, 1969.
45. Gallhofer, B., Ladurner, G., and Lechner, H.: Prognosis of prophylactic anticoagulant treatment in ischemic stroke, Eur. Neurol. 18:145, 1979.
46. Genton, E., et al.: Report of the Joint Committee for Stroke Facilities. XIV. Cerebral ischemia: the role of thrombosis and antithrombotic therapy, Stroke 8:150, 1977.
47. Goldner, J.C., Whisnant, J.P., and Taylor, W.F.: Long-term prognosis of transient cerebral ischemic attacks, Stroke 2:160, 1971.
48. Goldstone, J., and Moore, W.S.: A new look at emergency carotid artery operations for the treatment of cerebrovascular insufficiency, Stroke 9:599, 1978.
49. Grotta, J., Fields, W.S., and Kwee, K.: Prognosis in patients with asymptomatic carotid bruits due to nonstenotic lesions (abstract), Ann. Neurol. 12:85, 1982.
50. Harrison, M.J.G., and Marshall, J.: Angiographic appearance of carotid bifurcation in patients with completed stroke, transient ischemic attacks, and cerebral tumor, Br. Med. J. 1:205, 1976.
51. Harrison, M.J.G., and Marshall, J.: Prognostic significance of severity of carotid atheroma in early manifestations of cerebrovascular disease, Stroke 13:567, 1982.
52. Hart, R.G., et al.: Diagnosis and management of ischemic stroke. II. Selected controversies, Curr. Probl. Cardiol. 8:1, 1983.
53. Harward, T.R.S., et al.: Natural history of asymptomatic ulcerative placques of the carotid bifurcation, Am. J. Surg. 146:209, 1983.
54. Haynes, C.D., and Dempsey, R.L.: Carotid endarterectomy: review of 276 cases in a community hospital, Ann. Surg. 189:758, 1979.
55. Hertzer, N.R., and Lees, C.D.: Fatal myocardial infarction following carotid endarterectomy, Ann. Surg. 194:212, 1981.
56. Heyman, A., et al.: Risk of stroke in asymptomatic persons with cervical arterial bruits: a population study in Evans County, Georgia, N. Engl. J. Med. 302:838, 1980.
57. Hill, A.B., Marshall, J., and Shaw, D.A.: Cerebrovascular disease: trial of long-term anticoagulant therapy, Br. Med. J. 2:1003, 1962.
58. Humphries, A.W., et al.: Unoperated asymptomatic significant carotid artery stenosis: a review of 182 instances, Surgery 80:695, 1976.
59. Jausseran, J.M., et al.: Justification des indications chirurgicales dans les arteriopathies cerebrales extracraniennes asymptomatiques. In Courbier, R., editor: Arteriopathies cerebrales extracraniennes asymptomatiques, Lyons, France, 1979, Documentation Medicale Oberval.
60. Javid, H., et al.: Carotid endarterectomy for asymptomatic patients, Arch. Surg. 102:389, 1971.
61. Johnson, N., et al.: Carotid endarterectomy: a follow-up study of the contralateral nonoperated carotid artery, Ann. Surg. 188:748, 1978.
62. Kagan, A., et al.: Epidemiologic studies on coronary artery disease and stroke in Japanese men living in Japan, Hawaii, and California. In Scheinberg, P., editor: Cerebrovascular disease, New York, 1976, Raven Press.
63. Kanaly, P.J., et al.: The asymptomatic bruit, Am. J. Surg. 134:821, 1977.
64. Kartchner, M., and McRae, L.P.: Non-invasive evaluation and management of the ''asymptomatic carotid bruit,'' Surgery 82:840, 1977.
65. Kroener, J.M., et al.: Prognosis of asymptomatic ulcerating carotid lesions, Arch. Surg. 115:1387, 1980.
66. Lefrak, E.A., and Guinn, G.A.: Prophylactic carotid artery surgery in patients requiring a second operation, South. Med. J. 67:185, 1974.
67. Lemak, N.A., and Field, W.S.: The reliability of clinical predictors of extracranial artery disease, Stroke 4:377, 1976.
68. Levin, S.M., Sondheimer, F.K., and Levin, J.M.: The contralateral diseased but asymptomatic carotid artery: to operate or not? Am. J. Surg. 140:203, 1980.
69. Link, H., et al.: Prognosis in patients with infarction and TIA in carotid territory during and after anticoagulant therapy, Stroke 10:529, 1979.
70. Loeb, C., Priano, A., and Albano, C.: Clinical features and long-term follow-up of patients with reversible ischemic attacks (RIA), Acta Neurol. Scand. 57:471, 1978.
71. Manelfe, C., et al.: Investigation of extracranial cerebral arteries by intravenous angiography: report of 1,000 cases, Am. J. Neuroradiol. 3:287, 1982.
72. Mani, R.L., and Eisenberg, R.L.: Complications of catheter cerebral arteriography: analysis of 5,000 procedures. II. Relation of complication rates to clinical and arteriographic diagnoses, AJR 131:867, 1978.
73. Marshall, J.: Treatment of completed stroke. In Millikan, C.H., Siekert, R.G., and Whisnant, J.P., editors: Cerebral vascular diseases: Fourth Princeton Conference, New York, 1965, Grune & Stratton, Inc.
74. Marti-Vilalta, J.L., et al.: Transient ischemic attacks: retrospective study of 150 cases of ischemic infarct in the territory of the middle cerebral artery, Stroke 10:259, 1979.
75. McDevitt, E., et al.: Use of anticoagulants in treatment of cerebral vascular disease, JAMA 166:592, 1958.

76. McDowell, F., and McDevitt, E.: Treatment of the completed stroke with long-term cerebral vascular diseases. In Millikan, C.H., Siekert, R.G., and Whisnant, J.P., editors: Cerebral Vascular Diseases: Fourth Princeton Conference, New York, 1964, Grune & Stratton, Inc.

77. McNamara, J.O., et al.: The value of carotid endarterectomy in treating transient cerebral ischemia of the posterior circulation, Neurology 27:682, 1977.

78. Millikan, C.H.: Anticoagulant therapy in cerebrovascular disease. In Millikan, C.H., Siekert, R.H., Whisnant, J.P., editors: Cerebral vascular diseases, New York, 1961, Grune & Stratton, Inc.

79. Modi, J.R., Finch, W.T., and Sumner, D.S.: Update of carotid endarterectomy in two community hospitals: Springfield revisited (abstract), Stroke 14:128, 1983.

80. Moll, F.L., Eikelboom, B.C., and Vermeulen, F.E.E.: The value of OPG-Gee in a prospective follow-up study of patients with asymptomatic carotid bruits. In Courbier, R., editor: Arteriopathies cerebrales extracraniennes asymptomatiques, Lyons, France, 1979, Documentation Medicale Oberval.

81. Moore, W.S., et al.: Asymptomatic carotid stenosis: immediate and long-term results after prophylactic endarterectomy, Am. J. Surg. 138:228, 1979.

82. Moore, W.S., et al.: Natural history of non-stenotic, asymptomatic ulcerative lesions of the carotid artery, Arch. Surg. 113:1352, 1978.

83. Muuronen, A., and Kaste, M.: Outcome of 314 patients with transient ischemic attacks, Stroke 13:24, 1982.

84. Nunn, D.B.: Carotid endarterectomy: analysis of 234 operative cases, Ann. Surg. 182:733, 1975.

85. Olsson, J.E., Muller, R., and Berneli, S.: Long-term anticoagulant therapy for TIAs and minor stroke with minimum residuum, Stroke 7:444, 1976.

86. Olsson, J.E., et al.: Anticoagulant vs. antiplatelet therapy as prophylactic against cerebral infarction in transient ischemic attacks, Stroke 11:4, 1980.

87. Ortega, G., et al.: Postendarterectomy carotid occlusion, Surgery 90:1093, 1981.

88. Patterson, R.H.: Risk of carotid surgery with occlusion of the contralateral carotid artery, Arch. Neurol. 30:188, 1974.

89. Pessin, M.S., et al.: Clinical and angiographic features of carotid transient ischemic attacks, N. Engl. J. Med. 296:358, 1977.

90. Pfaffenbach, D.D., and Hollenhorst, R.W.: Morbidity and survivorship of patients with embolic cholesterol crystals in the ocular fundus, Am. J. Opthamol. 75:66, 1973.

91. Pierce, J.M.S., Gubbay, S.S., and Walton, J.M.: Long-term anticoagulant therapy in transient cerebral attacks, Lancet 1:6, 1965.

92. Pinkerton, J.A., and Gholkar, V.: Carotid endarterectomy: 100 consecutive operations, Mo. Med. 76:585, 1979.

93. Podore, P.C., et al.: Asymptomatic contralateral carotid artery stenosis: a five-year follow-up study following carotid endarterectomy, Surgery 88:748, 1980.

94. Prioleau, W.H., Aiken, A.F., and Hairston, P.: Carotid endarterectomy: neurologic complications as related to surgical techniques, Ann. Surg. 185:678, 1977.

95. Ramirez-Lassepas, M., Sandok, B.A., and Burton, R.C.: Clinical indicators of extracranial carotid artery disease in patients with transient symptoms, Stroke 4:537, 1973.

96. Riles, T.S., Kopelman, I., and Imparato, A.M.: Myocardial infarction following carotid endarterectomy: a review of 683 operations, Surgery 85:249, 1979.

97. Roden, S., et al.: Transient cerebral ischemic attacks—management and prognosis, Postgrad. Med. J. 57:275, 1981.

98. Ropper, A.H., Wechsler, R., and Wilson, L.S.: Carotid bruit and the risk of stroke in elective surgery, N. Engl. J. Med. 307:1388, 1982.

99. Russo, L.S.: Carotid system transient ischemic attacks: clinical, racial and angiographic correlations, Stroke 12:470, 1981.

100. Sandok, B.A., et al.: Guidelines for the management of transient ischemic attacks, Mayo Clin. Proc. 53:665, 1978.

101. Schechter, D.C., and Acinapura, A.J.: Panoperative safeguards for carotid endarterectomy, N.Y. State J. Med. 79:54, 1979.

102. Siekert, R.G., Whisnant, J.P., and Millikan, C.H.: Surgical and anticoagulant therapy of occlusive cerebral vascular disease, Ann. Intern. Med. 48:637, 1963.

103. Sorenson, P.S., et al.: Acetylsalicylic acid in the prevention of stroke in patients with reversible cerebral ischemic attacks: a Danish cooperative study, Stroke 14:15, 1983.

104. Stanford, J.R., Lubow, M., and Vasko, J.S.: Prevention of stroke by carotid endarterectomy, Surgery 83:259, 1978.

105. Sundt, T.M., Sandok, B.A., and Whisnant, J.P.: Carotid endarterectomy: complications and preoperative assessment of risk, Mayo Clin. Proc. 50:301, 1975.

106. Swanson, P.D., et al.: A cooperative study of hospital frequency and character of transient ischemic attacks. II. Performance of angiography among six centers, JAMA 237:2002, 1977.

107. Taylor, G.W., et al.: Doppler detection of carotid disease in patients with peripheral vascular disease. In Courbier, R., editor: Arteriopathies cerebrales extracraniennes asymptomatiques, Lyons, France, 1979, Documentation Medicale Oberval.

108. Terent, A., and Andersson, B.: The outcome of patients with transient ischemic attacks and stroke treated with anticoagulants, Acta Med. Scand. 208:359, 1980.

109. Thevenet, A.: Resultats a longue terme de l'endarterectomie carotidienne pour stenose asymptomatique. In Courbier, R., editor: Arteriopathies cerebrales extracraniennes asymptomatiques, Lyons, France, 1979, Documentation Medicale Oberval.

110. Thiele, B.L., et al.: Correlation of arteriographic findings and symptoms in cerebrovascular disease, Neurology 30:1041, 1980.

111. Thompson, J.E., Austin, D.J., and Patman, R.D.: Carotid endarterectomy for cerebrovascular insufficiency: long-term results in 592 patients followed up to 13 years, Ann. Surg. 172:663, 1970.

112. Thompson, J.E., Patman, R.D., and Talkington, C.M.: Asymptomatic carotid bruit: long-term outcome of patients having endarterectomy compared with unoperated controls, Ann. Surg. 188:308, 1978.

113. Thompson, J.E., and Talkington, C.M.: Carotid endarterectomy, Ann. Surg. 184:1, 1976.

114. Toole, J.F., et al.: Transient ischemic attacks due to atherosclerosis: a prospective study of 160 patients, Arch. Neurol. 32:5, 1975.

115. Toole, J.F., et al.: Transient ischemic attacks: a prospective study of 225 patients, Neurology 28:746, 1978.

116. Turnipseed, W.D., Berkoff, H.A., and Belzer, F.O.: Postoperative stroke in cardiac and peripheral vascular disease, Ann. Surg. 192:365, 1980.

117. Ueda, K., Toole, J.F., and McHenry, L.C.: Carotid and vertebrobasilar transient ischemic attacks: clinical and angiographic correlation, Neurology 29:1094, 1979.

118. van Oudenaarden, W.F., Tans, J.T.J., and Hoogland, P.H.: Angiographical findings and risk factors in cerebral ischemia, Eur. Neurol. 19:376, 1980.

119. Whisnant, J.P., Matsumoto, N., and Elveback, L.R.: Transient cerebral ischemic attacks in a community, Mayo Clin. Proc. 48:194, 1973.
120. Whisnant, J.P., Matsumoto, N., and Elveback, L.R.: The effect of anticoagulant therapy on the prognosis of patients with transient cerebral ischemic attacks in a community, Mayo Clin. Proc. 48:844, 1973.
121. Whisnant, J.P., Sandok, B.A., and Sundt, T.M.: Endarterectomy for transient cerebral ischemia: long-term survival and stroke probability (abstract), Stroke 13:113, 1982.
122. White, J.S., et al.: Morbidity and mortality of carotid endarterectomy: rates of occurrence in asymptomatic and symptomatic patients, Arch. Surg. 116:409, 1981.
123. Wolf, P.A., et al.: Asymptomatic carotid bruit and risk of stroke: The Framingham Study, JAMA 245:1441, 1981.
124. Wylie, E.J., and Ehrenfeld, W.K.: Extracranial occlusive cerebrovascular disease: diagnosis and treatment, Philadelphia, 1970, W.B. Saunders Co.
125. Young, J.R., et al.: Carotid endarterectomy without a shunt, Arch. Surg. 99:293, 1969.
126. Ziegler, D.K., and Hassanein, R.: Prognosis in patients with transient ischemic attacks, Stroke 4:666, 1973.

CHAPTER 29

Distribution of intracranial and extracranial arterial lesions in patients with symptomatic cerebrovascular disease

BRIAN L. THIELE and D. EUGENE STRANDNESS, Jr.

In any evaluation of the accuracy of noninvasive methods used to identify extracranial vascular disease, arteriography remains the standard against which these techniques are compared. The current study was conducted to determine the frequency, distribution, and types of lesions in a group of patients with symptomatic cerebral ischemia. These arteriograms were reviewed not only to determine the frequency of hemodynamically significant lesions at the carotid bifurcation, but also to perform a more detailed examination of the location of identifiable atherosclerotic disease in the intracranial and extracranial vessels, with particular reference to the presence or absence of potential embolic sources. While the distribution of atherosclerotic disease in patients with cerebral ischemia was addressed by a national cooperative study,[3] a correlation between arteriographic findings and symptoms was not possible, and no data were presented regarding the morphology of the arteriographic lesions.

Lesion morphology has become increasingly important with the recognition that embolization from the carotid bifurcation may be responsible for symptoms of cerebral and retinal ischemia in a higher proportion of patients than was previously envisaged.[6] Not only have potentially embolic lesions assumed greater attention in symptomatic patients, but Moore et al.[8] have presented evidence to suggest that the presence of ulcerated lesions is a significant factor in predicting which asymptomatic lesions will subsequently become symptomatic.

The widespread use of the indirect, noninvasive methods designed to detect hemodynamically significant lesions has focused attention on the role of such lesions in producing transient or permanent neurologic deficits. Since the relative roles of potentially embolic and hemodynamically significant lesions in the pathogenesis of cerebral ischemia can only be determined by prospective studies, this evaluation represents an attempt to assess the relative importance of these two processes in producing symptoms.

We also examined the frequency of tandem lesions or abnormalities of the intracerebral collateral circulation in the various patient groups. Although the role of the collateral circulation and tandem disease is well recognized in limb ischemia, the importance of these abnormalities in the pathogenesis of cerebral ischemia remains to be documented. Evidence for the importance of isolated siphon lesions in producing symptoms of transient cerebral ischemia is accumulating from the published reports of the relief of such symptoms in patients who have undergone extracranial-intracranial bypass. In addition, observations of the frequency of deficiencies of the circle of Willis made from autopsy dissections have also served as a basis for speculating on the importance of this anomaly in contributing to cerebral ischemia.

METHODS OF STUDY

All patients with symptoms suggesting cerebral ischemia underwent arteriographic study of the extracranial and intracranial vasculature via the percutaneous Seldinger technique. Initially, views were obtained of the arch and origins of the extracranial arteries; then selective catheterization of the carotid arteries was performed, and biplane views of the cervical carotid and intracranial vessels were obtained. Injection was also performed at the arch level with lateral head films to visualize the anterior and posterior intracranial circulation. The radiographs were independently examined by two radiologists who reported stenoses in one of five grades. Grade I represented a normal carotid bifurcation, grade II represented stenoses with less than 10% diameter reduction, grade III represented stenoses of 10% to 49% diameter reduction, grade IV represented stenoses of 50% to 99% reduction, and grade V represented complete occlusion. The radiologists were also asked to comment on the presence or absence of irregularity, ulceration, and specifically whether plaques were smooth. This evaluation was performed for all areas of both the extracranial and intracranial vessels. The presence or absence of the anterior and posterior communicating arteries was also determined from the anteroposterior and lateral head studies. On the basis of these reports, lesions were classified as occlusions, hemodynamically significant lesions (greater than 50% diameter reduction), or potentially embolic lesions (irregular or ulcerated).

Only patients who had well-documented classic symptoms of transient or permanent cerebral ischemia were included in the study. Using this classification, four groups of patients were available for study: the first group had amaurosis fugax alone; the second group had hemispheric symptoms, with or without amaurosis fugax; the third group had vertebrobasilar symptoms; and the final group had fixed neurologic deficits. This latter group consisted of patients whose neurologic deficits had initially exceeded 24 hours but subsequently resolved partially or completely before their studies. The time span between onset of symptoms and arteriography varied from 4 weeks to 1 year.

DISTRIBUTION OF SYMPTOMS

Included in the study were 109 patients with well-documented symptoms who underwent arteriography. The distribution of symptoms is shown in Table 29-1. Nine patients initially had amaurosis fugax alone, and 19 patients had a combination of amaurosis fugax and hemispheric symptoms. By combining these two groups, 28 arteriograms of patients with amaurosis fugax were available for study. Forty-seven patients had symptoms of tran-

sient hemispheric ischemia alone, and with the 19 patients in the preceding group, provided a total of 66 arteriograms for evaluation of the transient hemispheric symptoms. Also studied were 29 patients who had experienced fixed neurologic deficits and 5 patients with vertebrobasilar symptoms.

RESULTS
Amaurosis fugax

The arteriographic findings in the group of patients with amaurosis fugax are summarized in Table 29-2. In all cases the findings were those in the carotid bifurcation appropriate to the patient's symptoms. Of the 28 patients studied, only two (7% of the group) had no lesion demonstrated at the bifurcation. Ten patients (36% of the group) had lesions that were considered potentially embolic but not associated with flow-reducing stenoses. Of the remaining 16 patients, 5 (18%) had smooth, hemodynamically significant lesions and 11 (39%) had a combination of hemodynamically significant and potentially embolic lesions. By combining the second and fourth groups, the num-

Table 29-1. Distribution of symptoms in 109 patients with symptomatic cerebrovascular disease

Symptoms	No. of patients
Amaurosis fugax only	9
Amaurosis fugax plus hemispheric symptoms	19
Hemispheric symptoms only	47
Fixed neurologic deficits	29
Vertebrobasilar symptoms	5

Table 29-2. Distribution of angiographic lesions in 28 patients with amaurosis fugax

Type of lesion	Patients (No.)	Percentage
No lesion	2	7
Potentially embolic only	10	36
Hemodynamically significant*	16	57
Potentially embolic†	21	75

*Includes 5 smooth (18%) and 11 ulcerated or irregular (39%) hemodynamically significant lesions (50% or greater diameter reduction).
†Includes all ulcerated or irregular lesions regardless of degree of stenosis.

ber of potentially embolic lesions in this group of patients totaled 21 (75%), and by combining the third and fourth groups, 16 patients (57%) had hemodynamically significant stenoses. In view of the small number of negative arteriograms, it could be concluded that amaurosis fugax is a highly specific symptom for carotid bifurcation disease and also that potentially embolic lesions are more common than hemodynamically significant lesions.

Hemispheric symptoms

The results obtained from the group of patients with hemispheric symptoms are listed in Table 29-3. There were 47 patients in the group, and in 6 (13%) no lesion was demonstrated at the bifurcation. Nineteen patients (40%) had potentially embolic lesions not associated with flow-reducing lesions. Four patients (9%) had smooth stenoses that were considered hemodynamically significant, whereas the remaining 18 patients (38%) had sten-

Table 29-3. Distribution of angiographic lesions in 47 patients with hemispheric symptoms

Type of lesion	Patients (No.)	Percentage
No lesion	6	13
Potentially embolic only	19	40
Hemodynamically significant*	22	47
Potentially embolic†	37	79

*Includes 4 smooth (9%) and 18 ulcerated or irregular (38%) hemodynamically significant lesions.
†Includes all ulcerated or irregular lesions regardless of degree of stenosis.

oses of greater than 50% diameter reduction associated with irregularity or ulceration. In a form of analysis similar to that of the preceding group, by combining the second and fourth groups, the number of patients with potentially embolic lesions totaled 37 (79% of the group), and by combining the third and fourth groups, the number of patients with hemodynamically significant lesions was 22 (47%). Thus hemispheric symptoms were not as specific for carotid bifurcation disease as amaurosis fugax was, but potentially embolic lesions occurred more frequently than hemodynamically significant ones.

Hemispheric symptoms and amaurosis fugax

The types and distribution of lesions in the group with hemispheric symptoms and amaurosis fugax are summarized in Table 29-4. Of the 66 patients with this symptom complex, 6 (9%) had no lesion visualized at the bifurcation, 27 (41%) had potentially embolic lesions only, 5 (8%) had smooth, hemodynamically significant lesions only, and 28 (42%) had a combination of hemodynamically significant and potentially embolic lesions. Further breakdown of this group revealed that 56 (85%) had potentially embolic lesions, and 33 (50%) had hemodynamically significant lesions of the appropriate carotid bifurcation.

Fixed neurologic deficits

Patients with fixed neurologic defects were characterized by diffuse atherosclerotic changes in both the intracranial and extracranial vessels (Table 29-5). Eight patients (28%) had hemodynamically significant lesions only, and in 7 of these patients complete occlusion of the appropriate internal ca-

Table 29-4. Distribution of angiographic lesions in 66 patients with both hemispheric symptoms and amaurosis fugax

Type of lesion	Patients (No.)	Percentage
No lesion	6	9
Potentially embolic only	27	41
Hemodynamically significant*	33	50
Potentially embolic†	55	84

*Includes 5 smooth (8%) and 28 ulcerated or irregular (42%) hemodynamically significant lesions.
†Includes all ulcerated or irregular lesions regardless of degree of stenosis.

Table 29-5. Distribution of angiographic lesions in 29 patients with fixed neurologic deficits

Type of lesion	Patients (No.)	Percentage
No lesion	0	
Potentially embolic only	5	17
Hemodynamically significant*	21	72
Potentially embolic†	18	62

*Includes 7 occlusions and 1 smooth and 13 ulcerated (45%) hemodynamically significant lesions.
†Includes all ulcerated or irregular lesions regardless of degree of stenosis.

rotid artery was present. Thirteen patients (45%) had ulcerated lesions associated with a stenosis of greater than 50% diameter reduction, and 5 patients (17%) had ulcerated or irregular lesions associated with minimal degrees of stenosis. The incidence of hemodynamically significant lesions was 72%, whereas that of potentially embolic lesions was 62%. A surprising finding was the relative infrequency of complete occlusions of the internal carotid artery (7 of 29 patients or 24%). Compared with those patients who experienced transient ischemic symptoms, the fixed neurologic deficit group had a higher proportion of hemodynamically significant lesions.

Vertebrobasilar symptoms

There were only five patients with vertebrobasilar symptoms, so no significant conclusions could be drawn from an analysis of the location and distribution of lesions. In addition, because of the nonlocalizing nature of their symptoms, it would be impossible to attach significance to a lesion in either carotid artery. Therefore they have been excluded from this analysis.

RELATIONSHIP BETWEEN ULCERATION AND STENOSIS

The results from the preceding study were then evaluated to determine whether ulcerated lesions were more commonly associated with hemodynamically significant lesions. Tables 29-6 and 29-7 detail the relative frequency of ulceration and its relationship to hemodynamically significant lesions. Of the 104 arteriograms examined, 56 patients (54%) were considered to have hemodynamically significant lesions on the appropriate side. Ulcerated lesions predominated in this group and were three times as common as smooth lesions (41% versus 13%). Table 29-7 details the frequency of ulcerated lesions in all the arteriograms with the degrees of stenosis divided into two groups, hemodynamically significant or insignificant. Potentially embolic lesions occurred in 74% of the patient population, but surprisingly, irregularity or ulceration occurred with almost equal frequency whether the degree of stenosis was considered hemodynamically significant or not (41% versus 33%). Thus although ulceration was a frequent accompaniment of hemodynamically significant lesions, it occurred with almost equal frequency regardless of the degree of stenosis.

Finally, the frequency of smooth lesions as identified arteriographically was determined in the total patient population; these results are depicted in Table 29-8. Only 18% of the patients had smooth lesions, and in this group hemodynamically significant lesions were twice as common as nonhemodynamically significant lesions were (13% versus 5%). The remaining 8% of the total patient sample had no lesions identified by arteriography.

INTRACEREBRAL VASCULAR ANOMALY OR DISEASE

In addition to the type and location of lesions in the extracranial vessels, the frequency of intracerebral atherosclerotic lesions and anomalies of the collateral circulation was also assessed. The prevalence of intracerebral disease or anomaly was determined in each of the patient groups, namely, patients with transient ischemia, patients with fixed neurologic deficits, and patients with vertebroba-

Table 29-6. Relationship between ulceration and hemodynamically significant lesions

Type of lesion	Degree of stenosis	Percentage
Smooth lesions	>50% diameter reduction	13
Irregular lesions	>50% diameter reduction	41
ALL LESIONS	>50% diameter reduction	54

Table 29-7. Relationship between ulceration and degree of stenosis

Type of lesion	Degree of stenosis	Percentage
Irregular lesions	>50% stenosis	41
Irregular lesions	<50% stenosis	33
TOTAL POTENTIALLY EMBOLIC LESIONS		74

Table 29-8. Distribution of smooth lesions in patients with symptomatic cerebrovascular disease

Type of lesion	Degree of stenosis	Percentage
Smooth lesions	>50% diameter reduction	13
Smooth lesions	<50% diameter reduction	5
TOTAL SMOOTH LESIONS		18

Table 29-9. Incidence of intracerebral disease or anomaly in patients with symptomatic cerebrovascular disease

Type of symptom	Percentage
Transient ischemia	29
Fixed neurologic deficits	90
Vertebrobasilar symptoms	100

Table 29-10. Incidence of contralateral disease of the carotid bifurcation in 104 patients with symptomatic cerebrovascular disease

Type of lesion	Percentage
Potentially embolic	30
Hemodynamically significant (internal carotid disease)*	29
Hemodynamically significant (external carotid disease)	17

*Occlusions of 12 patients were complete.

silar symptoms (Table 29-9). In the 66 patients with hemispheric and/or ocular transient ischemia, 29% had intracerebral abnormalities, as evidenced by siphon disease or the absence of one or more communicating arteries. In contrast, in the 29 patients with fixed neurologic deficits, the same abnormality was found in 90% of the patient group. All 5 patients with vertebrobasilar symptoms either had anomalies of the intracerebral collateral circulation or evidence of siphon disease.

CONTRALATERAL DISEASE

A similar analysis of the location and type of lesions in the contralateral carotid bifurcation was performed to determine the frequency of hemodynamically significant lesions that could adversely affect the results of the indirect, noninvasive tests. The frequency of hemodynamically significant lesions in the ipsilateral external carotid artery was also determined because of the potential of these lesions to interfere with the testing. Hemodynamically significant lesions were present in the contralateral internal carotid artery in 29% of the 104 patients studied (Table 29-10). Of these hemodynamically significant lesions in the internal carotid artery, 41% (12 patients) were complete internal carotid occlusions. A further 17% had hemodynamically significant lesions of the contralateral

external carotid artery. Potentially embolic lesions occurred in 30% (31 patients). Fifteen percent (15) of the patients also had hemodynamically significant lesions of the ipsilateral external carotid artery. In 40 patients (39%) a hemodynamically significant lesion existed in one or more of the extracranial vessels that would function as collaterals for a lesion in the internal carotid artery.

DISCUSSION

Although the foregoing study was initiated as part of the assessment of the accuracy of noninvasive methods of detecting extracranial vascular disease, it also serves as a means of studying the detailed distribution and morphology of atherosclerosis in these vessels. Not only can these data be used for this purpose, but they may also be used to examine some additional questions. The first area addressed by these studies is the appropriateness and potential accuracy of the indirect, noninvasive tests currently used in evaluating extracranial vascular disease. In the well-documented symptomatic patients studied, we were interested in the frequency of hemodynamically significant lesions, since many indirect methods are designed to detect only such stenoses. In half of the patients with transient hemispheric symptoms with or without ocular ischemia, hemodynamically significant lesions were found on the side appropriate for the symptoms. Thus if one disregarded all the factors that may influence the pressure and flow direction in the retina and periorbital vessels and also assumed that the noninvasive methods used were 100% accurate, only half of the patients with symptom-producing lesions could be identified. The hemodynamics of the ocular and periorbital vascular system are also influenced by flow-reducing lesions in the contralateral carotid system and the ipsilateral external carotid artery. In our patient population with localizing cerebral ischemia, one third (39%) had potential flow-reducing lesions in these sites. Since it is not possible to accurately predict the hemodynamic disturbances that occur as the result of lesions visualized arteriographically, these findings remind us of the diffuse distribution of atherosclerosis in patients with cerebral ischemia and also question the validity of those tests in which distant changes are used to identify the location of proximal lesions. Thus although the indirect tests may tell us that there is an abnormality in the orbital circulation, the inference that it is a result of ipsilateral carotid disease will be valid if this is the only pathologic condition involved. An analogy to this situation can readily be drawn from the non-invasive assessment of lower limb ischemia where reductions in ankle pressure are an extremely reliable guide to the presence of hemodynamic disturbance[2] but are inaccurate in predicting the location of the responsible lesion. On the basis of these findings, we were not surprised at the lack of sensitivity and specificity of these indirect methods.

The next question raised by these studies relates to the pathogenesis of cerebral ischemia and its relation to abnormalities in the intracranial circulation. The demonstration by Moore et al.[8] of the importance of the overtly ulcerated lesion as a major factor predisposing the development of cerebral ischemia is confirmed by these studies. Meaningful statistical analysis cannot be applied to these figures because of the number of variables involved, although some of the results do warrant an attempt at interpretation. If one compares the frequency of potentially embolic lesions between the asymptomatic and symptomatic sides (30% versus 75%), the difference strongly suggests that ulceration or irregularity is associated with the presence of symptoms. When a comparison of the frequency of smooth lesions and potentially embolic lesions on the symptomatic side is made, embolic lesions were four times as common as smooth lesions (74% versus 18%); this further reinforces the view that the pathogenesis of cerebral ischemia is strongly related to the presence of potentially embolic lesions of the carotid bifurcation. Attempts at statistical analysis of these results are hampered by the frequency of overlap of hemodynamically significant and ulcerated lesions and the influence that unknown variables may have. Nevertheless, this study suggests it is the ulcerated lesion that is of major significance in symptomatic cerebral ischemia.

The current treatment of asymptomatic carotid lesions may also be influenced by these arteriographic findings, since high-grade stenoses generally are thought to predispose to occlusion of the internal carotid artery and the production of fixed neurologic deficits. Of the 29 patients with fixed neurologic deficits in this study, only 7 had internal carotid occlusions. While these patients did have a higher frequency of hemodynamically significant lesions than the group with transient ischemic symptoms, the major difference in the two groups was the presence of siphon disease or an abnor-

mality of the collateral vessels in the circle of Willis. It is recognized that traumatic internal carotid occlusion can occur without the production of neurologic deficits, particularly in patients with adequate collateral circulation. Conversely, the development of neurologic deficits in such patients is thought to be related to a congenital absence of communicating vessels in the circle of Willis. It therefore seems reasonable to suggest that disease or abnormality of the intracerebral circulation plays a major role in determining which patients will develop transient ischemic attacks and which patients will develop fixed neurologic deficits with atherosclerosis. We would therefore suggest that a factor needing evaluation in future studies of the natural history of cerebrovascular disease is the role of disease or anomalies of the intracerebral vessels. This is particularly important in view of one current approach to patients with asymptomatic lesions, where the decision for surgical treatment is influenced almost solely by the angiographic demonstration of a high-grade stenosis.

Finally, the demonstration that only 24% of those patients with fixed neurologic deficits had complete occlusions of the appropriate internal carotid artery highlights the need for identification of the patients who still have patent internal carotid arteries that may subsequently be responsible for the development of recurrent symptoms. The observation that 76% of the patients with fixed neurologic deficits still have patent internal carotid arteries on the appropriate side may in part explain the mechanism of recurrent strokes.

SUMMARY

This detailed arteriographic study suggests that in patients with symptoms of cerebral ischemia, isolated disease of a single cervical carotid artery is unusual, and as in other areas of the body, the atherosclerotic process is usually diffuse by the time symptoms occur. It is this diffuse location of lesions that limits the use of indirect test methods as a means of accurately identifying bifurcation disease. This study also provides presumptive evidence to support the view that the majority of symptoms of transient cerebral ischemia occur as a result of embolization from the carotid bifurcation.

In patients with fixed neurologic deficits, the demonstration of a high frequency of siphon lesions or abnormalities of the vessels in the circle of Willis suggests that the status of the intracranial collateral circulation may be a significant factor in the pathogenesis of fixed neurologic deficits associated with carotid bifurcation atherosclerosis.

ACKNOWLEDGMENTS

We acknowledge the assistance of the following: Dr. P.M. Chikos, Assistant Professor, Dr. J.D. Harley, Associate Professor, and Dr. J.H. Hirsch, Assistant Professor, of the Department of Radiology, University of Washington School of Medicine; and Dr. J.V. Young, Research Fellow, Department of Surgery, University of Washington School of Medicine. We also acknowledge the help of the Departments of Surgery and Radiology, Veterans Administration Medical Center and University Hospital, Seattle, Washington.

REFERENCES

1. Blackshear, W.M., et al.: A prospective evaluation of oculoplethysmography and carotid phonoangiography, Surg. Gynecol. Obstet. 48:201, 1979.
2. Carter, S.A.: Response of ankle systolic pressure to leg exercise in mild or questionable arterial disease, N. Engl. J. Med. 287:578, 1972.
3. Hass, W.K., et al.: A joint study of extracranial arterial occlusion. II. Arteriography, techniques, sites, and complications, JAMA 203:961, 1968.
4. Horenstein, S., et al.: Arteriographic correlates of transient ischemic attacks, Trans. Am. Neurol. Assoc. 97:132, 1972.
5. Janeway, R., and Toole, J.F.: Vascular anatomic status of patients with transient ischemic attacks, Trans. Am. Neurol. Assoc. 97:137, 1972.
6. Kollarits, C.R., Lobow, M., and Hissong, S.L.: Retinal strokes. I. Incidence of carotid atheroma, JAMA 222:1273, 1972.
7. Millikan, C.H.: The pathogenesis of transient cerebral ischemia, Circulation 32:438, 1965.
8. Moore, W.S., et al.: Natural history of nonstenotic asymptomatic ulcerative lesions of the carotid artery, Arch. Surg. 113:1357, 1978.
9. Pessin, M.S., et al.: Clinical and angiographic features of carotid transient ischemic attacks, N. Engl. J. Med. 296(7):358, 1977.

CHAPTER 30

Oculoplethysmography and carotid phonoangiography

ARNOST FRONEK

Carotid artery phonoangiography (CPA) and oculoplethysmography as introduced by Kartchner and McRae, represented one of the first methods to evaluate objectively the status of the extracranial carotid artery system.[11,14,15] Although newer techniques have been described, the combination of two methods based on two different principles represented a significant improvement in the detection of carotid artery disease. Since the publication of the first papers by the Tucson group,[11,14,15] laboratories have used this technique, and reports reflecting the growing experience with this approach have appeared in print. As expected, the results are not equivocal, and an attempt will be made to describe them using the advantage of retro-analysis—that is, from a historic viewpoint.

QUALITATIVE CAROTID ARTERY PHONOANGIOGRAPHY
Principle

Bruits (acoustical phenomena caused by flow disturbances) are picked up by a suitable microphone and after appropriate filtering and amplification are displayed on a cathode ray tube (CRT). A Polaroid camera attached to a second CRT in parallel to the monitoring screen provides a hard copy phonoangiogram. A more detailed description is provided in Chapter 18.

Interpretation

Carotid phonoangiograms are evaluated on the basis of the location of maximum bruit amplitude (to identify the approximate site of bruit generation), but more important criteria are the duration and envelope curve of the recorded signals.[11,14] The diagnostic value of these criteria are based not only on systematic comparison studies with angiography[12,13,15] but also on a simple hemodynamic consideration of circumstances influencing the timing and relative changes of bruit amplitude throughout the cardiac cycle. If the signs of flow disturbance extend into diastole or if the amplitude does not diminish significantly at the end of systole, the best explanation is that the stenosis is so severe that even the reduced flow velocity at the end of systole or during diastole generates a high enough Reynolds number[29] to cause a significant flow disturbance. Well-defined systolic and diastolic heart sounds without intervening acoustic phenomena reflect the absence of flow disturbance, whereas a short systolic bruit ending in midsystole is compatible with a flow disturbance originating in a hemodynamically insignificant stenosis (<40% diameter reduction) or may be induced by the presence of a rough surface plaque. A pansystolic bruit that lasts until the end of systole indicates a 40% to 60% diameter obstruction. With increasing stenosis the duration of the bruit plateau is prolonged and starts to spill over into diastole. Although exact correlation studies between bruit duration and degree of stenosis are not available, bruits extending throughout systole or even into diastole reflect hemodynamically significant stenoses.[27,28] McRae et al.[23] recommend using a scoring chart (Table 30-1) to grade the CPA tracings and relate them to the degree of stenosis.

Difficulties arise mainly in the very severe category where, because of extreme loss of energy (produced by a very tight stenosis), false-negative results may distort the phonoangiogram (that is, short and low energy bruits in the presence of very tight stenosis). This is one reason

Table 30-1. Scoring chart for relating CPA tracings to degree of stenosis

Grade	CPA stenosis (% diameter reduction)	Hemodynamic significance
1	<40	Negative
2	40-60	Mild
3	61-70	Moderate
4	71-85	Severe
5	>85 No bruit	Very severe or occlusion

CPA is recommended in conjunction with OPG.[12]

In a separate evaluation of CPA and OPG, Satiani et al.[31] divided the examined arteries into those with hemodynamically significant (>40% stenosis) and with insignificant (<40%) or no stenosis. CPA-detected bruits were found in 79.6% of arteries with >40% stenosis and in 43.4% of cases with insignificant stenoses or normal arteries. Unfortunately, no information is given regarding whether an attempt was made to differentiate the severity of stenosis on the basis of the diagnostic criteria described by Kartchner and McRae. In a similar study, a high rate of false negative results (40%) was reported by Keagy et al.,[16] but only the combined OPG-CPA results are described. Blackshear et al.[3] reported the CPA results separately and found a high false negative rate (66%) for the flow-limiting stenosis group (50% to 99% diameter reduction). However, a surprising 60% false positive rate was found in occluded arteries, that is, a bruit was detected even though the internal carotid artery was occluded, presumably because of flow into the external carotid artery.

A special difficulty may arise in postendarterectomy follow-up. The presence of a bruit after carotid endarterectomy may be related to the newly established mechanical properties of the endarterectomized arterial wall. However, a pansystolic bruit extending into diastole may reflect important hemodynamic disturbances signifying residual or recurrent disease, especially if progression of this finding is observed (Chapter 46).

Another source of false positive results is seen in cases of bilateral carotid disease. Contralateral severe obstruction leads to increased flow rates on the opposite side, resulting in a higher Reynolds number and more severe bruit than warranted by the actual degree of stenosis. However, this condition does not apply only to phonoangiography but also pertains to other diagnostic techniques

based either on changes of flow velocity or the development of a pressure drop.

Differential evaluation of qualitative and quantitative phonoangiography

Both the qualitative and quantitative techniques have the advantage of being relatively simple to learn. Quantitative phonoangiography (QPA)[19] provides a more objective evaluation (determination of break frequency, f_o), whereas carotid phonoangiography (CPA)* permits only a rough estimate of the severity of the stenosis by evaluating the duration of the bruit and configuration of the bruit envelope curve.[11,14] However, it can be argued that this advantage is questionable, because the correlation between the percent of stenosis and vessel diameter is not very close ($r = 0.76$).[17] In addition, the cost-effectiveness factor is also important, since CPA requires less expensive instrumentation. On the other hand, there are two additional factors in favor of QPA. First, significant differences in f_o help identify multiple sources of flow disturbance in the common, internal, and external carotid vessels. Second, a new commercially available spectral analysis device (Spectraview 500) also permits performing power frequency spectrum analysis of the Doppler velocity signals, thus increasing the usefulness of the instrument. A more detailed discussion of QPA can be found in Chapter 33.

The limited accuracy of diagnosing extracranial carotid artery stenosis only on the basis of bruit analysis is underlined by the results of Riles et al.,[30] who reported an increasing incidence of bruit with increasing stenosis, ranging from 25% to 70% of arteries corresponding to a degree of stenosis from 40% to 80%, but with few bruits associated with very tight stenoses. In addition, in 33% of cases with occluded internal carotid arteries there were bruits present, probably related to flow disturbances in the external carotid artery or caused by an oscillating volume of blood hitting the internal carotid arterial cul-de-sac.

In view of the many factors contributing to the genesis of bruits (with regard to their amplitude and frequency components as described previously), phonoangiography should be used in conjunc-

*Although "qualitative phonoangiography" would be a more consistent description, carotid phonoangiography (CPA) is used here to prevent confusion in accordance with the author's original terminology.

tion with another noninvasive technique, for example, OPG[13,14] or duplex Doppler scanning.[20]

OCULOPLETHYSMOGRAPHY
(OPG-KARTCHNER-McRAE)
Principle

Phase shift differences between ocular volume pulses (right and left) are enhanced by amplifying the electronically derived difference between both pulses. As described in Chapter 18, there is evidence that hemodynamically significant obstructions result in a deflection of the differential tracing, whereas a flat tracing is produced if there is no obstruction or if the stenosis is not hemodynamically significant.[12-15,23,24] An additional ear pulse recording helps to identify stenoses in the external carotid artery as well as some cases of bilateral internal carotid artery stenosis. A detailed description of the principle and methodology is given in Chapter 18.

Interpretation

First, the right and left ear lobe tracings are examined for any sign of time delay between these two pulses. A significant delay (>40 msec) indicates the presence of an external or common carotid artery stenosis. The next step is an analysis of the differential tracing (DT). If DT is flat, there is no stenosis, or at least no flow-limiting stenosis, in the right or left internal (ICA) or common (CCA) carotid artery. Quite often, however, there is a heartbeat-synchronous DT deflection that still indicates a normal lumen or insignificant stenosis in the ICA or CCA system, provided there is no deflection from a reference pseudobaseline connecting the trough and peak of one of the ocular pulses (Fig. 30-1). To facilitate reading and interpreting the tracings, McRae et al.[23] recommend using the ratio of the maximum differential deflection (Diff$_{max}$) to pulse amplitude (A):

$$\frac{\text{Diff}_{max}}{A}$$

The following relationship is given between this ratio and the percentage diameter reduction of the internal carotid artery[23]:

$\dfrac{\text{Diff}_{max}}{A}$	ICA diameter reduction (%)
<0.1	<40
0.1-0.2	40-60
>0.2	>61

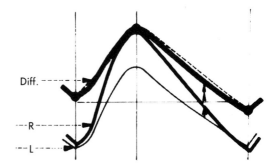

Fig. 30-1. Generation of reference pseudobaseline (interrupted line). *R*, Right ocular pulse; *L*, left ocular pulse; diff., differential tracing.

As can be expected, bilateral ICA obstruction may pose a serious diagnostic problem, because the amplitude of the differential tracing is based on the difference between the right and left ocular volume pulses. Often there is a significant differential deflection in the presence of bilateral lesions. This indicates a hemodynamic predominance of one stenosis. A suspicion of a bilateral lesion is raised if a double-sloped ocular pulse is observed. In the absence of a double slope, a significant bilateral bruit or a contralateral bruit (for example, differential deflection indicates a right ICA obstruction and a bruit is recorded from the left side of the neck) also should suggest the diagnosis of a bilateral obstruction.

The OPG-Kartchner-McRae method is quite sensitive to stenoses greater than 50% diameter reduction, but the severity of the obstruction is sometimes underestimated because ocular pulse delay does not increase beyond 70% diameter reduction. On the other hand, a localized stenosis of the opthalmic artery may represent a source of false positive findings, but this is rare. The same argument is, however, applicable to ocular pneumoplethysmography (OPG-Gee) (Chapter 31). The combined application of OPG and CPA (as we recommended) therefore improves the accuracy of the method.

Contraindications and complications

Direct application of the eyecups to the cornea and the mild negative pressure that keeps the cups in place raises the possibility of complications. The test should not be performed in the presence of a local infection (even if limited to the conjunctiva). Although corneal abrasions are very rare and, even if produced, they heal uneventfully, an infection may lead to undesirable complications. Corneal abrasion is usually caused by poor technique. There are practically no absolute contraindications to the use of this technique; however, a number of situations do suggest a delay in the examination.

1. Recent eye surgery or injury—at least 6 weeks' deferral; preferably consult with an ophthalmologist.
2. Eye infection—wait until infection has cleared. Conjunctivitis should be considered as a relative contraindication because it is sometimes difficult to rule out an infectious cause.
3. Detached retina—wait at least 6 months and preferably consult with an ophthalmologist.
4. Uncooperative patients—if the patient is either under the influence of some toxic substance or affected by an impairment of the central nervous system, light sedation may be needed.
5. Intraocular lens implantation—delay 6 weeks.

Patients with glaucoma can be examined with OPG-Kartchner-McRae without any adverse effects.

A negligible percentage of patients may be sensitive to a safe local anesthetic (0.5% proparacaine HCl used presently). If the patient confirms an allergic reaction to local anesthetics, consultation with the patient's ophthalmologist may help, or, in an exceptional case, an experienced technologist may perform the test without local anesthesia if the test is urgent. Otherwise, antiallergic premedication is suggested.

Combined OPG-CPA evaluation

For reasons described earlier, the accuracy of the examination is significantly improved if both techniques are used, mainly because they use different principles. Kartchner and McRae suggested a scoring chart[23] that can be modified as in Table 30-2.

Comparative accuracy of OPG-CPA

The application of a combination of tests is particularly justified when the methods are based on different principles. A decision must be made, however, as to the criterion for positivity or negativity. If both tests have to be positive to label the result a positive one, specificity is enhanced while sensitivity is reduced. On the other hand, if only one of the tests used is sufficient to label the overall test as positive, then sensitivity is increased at the expense of specificity. In most OPG-CPA publications the latter approach was used, and it is therefore of interest to analyze first the sensitivity and specificity of OPG and CPA separately. This helps in evaluating the contribution of each test to the overall accuracy. It can be seen from Table 30-3

Table 30-2. OPG-CPA scoring chart

Grade	CPA	OPG	Summarized conclusion	Descriptor
1	No bruits or short bruits	Differential tracing flat, or flat pseudobaseline	Normal or less than 40% diameter reduction; not hemodynamically significant	Normal if no bruit; not significant if short bruit
2	Bruit extending throughout systole with decreascendo envelope	Differential deflection about 20% of ocular pulse amplitude	Stenosis of hemodynamic significance (about 55% diameter reduction)	Mild stenosis
3	Bruit extending throughout systole with flat envelope (no decrescendo)	Differential deflection more than 20% of ocular pulse amplitude but no visible ocular pulse delay	Stenosis of moderate hemodynamic significance (about 65% diameter reduction)	Moderate stenosis
4	Bruit extending into diastole	Significant differential deflection more than 30% of ocular pulse amplitude with visible ocular pulse delay	Stenosis of severe hemodynamic significance (about 80% diameter reduction)	Severe stenosis
5	No bruit	Same as above	Occlusion or preocclusion stenosis (about 95%)	Occlusion or extremely severe stenosis

that the overall sensitivity of OPG is higher than that of CPA, while CPA offers a better specificity.

Overall accuracy

As to overall accuracy (Table 30-4) Kartchner et al.[15] originally described the accuracy for OPG with only 8% false positive and 12% false negative results and an overall accuracy of 90% when comparing OPG-CPA to carotid arteriography. Similar results were reported by Dean and Yao,[7] Gross et al.,[9] Persson,[27] and Ginsberg et al.[8] An overall accuracy of about 85% was reported by McDonald et al.[22] and O'Leary et al.[26]

However, some investigators observed less encouraging results. Blackshear et al.[3] found a sensitivity of only 52% in patients with stenoses >50% diameter reduction. Satiani et al.[31] found an overall accuracy of 86% in differentiating significant from insignificant carotid artery stenosis, but in the clinically important group (patients with a 40% to 70% diameter reduction) the accuracy was not reassuring (48.8%). The relatively high rate of false negative findings in this category (40% to 70% diameter reduction) was also emphasized by Keagy et al.[16] and Meade.[25] Kapsch et al.[10] reported an overall accuracy of 63% with a low false negative rate (9.6%) but a high false positive rate (50%), reflecting a high sensitivity but poor specificity. In a very careful analysis, Sumner et al.[34] identified only 64% lesions exceeding 40% diameter reduc-

Table 30-3. OPG-CPA: comparison of overall accuracy

Reference	Criterion % diameter reduction	OPG		CPA	
		Sensitivity (%)	Specificity (%)	Sensitivity (%)	Specificity (%)
Kartchner et al., 1973[12]	>40	90	97	81	91
Satiani et al., 1979[31]	>40			80	96
Blackshear et al., 1979[3]	>50	43	81	34	93
Sumner et al., 1979[34]	>40	64	85	52	82
Kapsch et al., 1981[10]	>50	63		74	
Cebril and Ginsberg, 1982[6]	>40	80	91	67	79
Sumner et al., 1982[34]	>40	46	90	50	81
	>60	61	89	54	77

Table 30-4. Combined evaluation

Reference	Criterion % diameter reduction	Sensitivity (%)	Specificity (%)	Accuracy (%)
Kartchner et al., 1976[15]	>40			90
Kartchner et al., 1977[12]	>40			89
Persson, 1977[27]	>40			90
Gross et al., 1977[9]	>76			90
Satiani et al., 1978[31]	40-75			49
	>75			86
McDonald et al., 1978[22]	>60	87	94	86
Ginsberg et al., 1979[8]	>60			90
Meade, 1979[25]	>40			96
Keagy et al., 1980[16]	40-70	60		
	>70	73		
O'Leary et al., 1981[26]	>65	84	85	84
Kapsch et al., 1981[10]	50-75	74		
	75-95	83		
	>95	91	50	63
Bone et al., 1981[4]	50-74	48		
	>75	94	91	
Cantelmo et al., 1981[5]	>50	66	87	

tion. The results were far better in the 80% to 100% diameter reduction category, with a 94% sensitivity.

The reported results with these tests vary widely, with several factors to explain the discrepancies. The diameter reduction considered as a positive or negative result is one of the most important factors and varies from 40% to 60%. The patient pool is also important. If many normal subjects are examined the results appear to improve. The expertise and technical background of the technician are also critical. Another aspect is whether results are reported ''per artery'' or ''per patient.'' It is true that the ultimate result refers to the patient (for example, to recommend angiography), but the method in question should be considered on its own merit, that is, the capability to identify an arterial lesion.

PULSE WAVE DELAY TIMING (CHRONOPULSE AND ZIRA)
Principle

Pulse wave delay timing modifies the previously described OPG-Kartchner-McRae technique by timing the difference between the pulse arrival time—eye to eye or eye to ear.

Description

The detecting systems are essentially the same as in the OPG-Kartchner-McRae method. Air transmission is used instead of a liquid-filled system, making it possible to perform the study while the patient is in the horizontal position and eliminating the meticulous avoidance of air bubbles that was required in the original OPG-Kartchner-McRae. (An air-transmission OPG-Kartchner-McRae system is now also commercially available, although the potential adverse effect of increased damping has not been reliably analyzed.)

Two commercially available systems (Chronopulse and ZIRA) use a readout of the difference in arrival times (either peak or foot of the curve) between the right and left eye and eye to ear. Archie et al.[1] have identified a delay of 8 msec as optimal to separate negative from positive results (>50% diameter reduction). An eye-to-ear delay of 30 msec or more was considered pathologic. Under these conditions, an overall accuracy of 88% was reported. The results were worse for bilateral lesions. Similar results were reported by Malone,[21] Baker,[2] and String.[32] However these investigators could not confirm Archie's good correlation between the delay time and severity of the lesions.

Baker emphasizes that this method can be used only to identify a unilateral lesion with >60% diameter reduction, although there is no correlation between the delay time and severity of the stenosis.[2]

Evaluation

Although this technique was originally designed to increase the efficiency of the OPG examination, the low reported accuracy does not compensate for this advantage. In addition, there are theoretic reasons that may explain the reported results. The differential tracing in OPG-Kartchner-McRae represents a continuously recorded difference between the recorded pulses, whereas in the pulse wave delay timing technique the time difference is only between two preselected points. The difficulty of diagnosing bilateral disease is compounded because no ''double slope'' criterion exists as in the OPG-Kartchner-McRae method, although a significant eye-to-ear delay may raise one's suspicion. This criterion, however, is not very reliable.[2,32]

Differential evaluation. Pulse delay OPG-Kartchner-McRae vs. OPG-Gee. Both pulse delay OPG-Kartchner-McRae and OPG-Gee fulfilled historically important roles at the birth of noninvasive diagnostic procedures in the area of extracranial carotid artery disease. Currently, however, a more critical approach is needed because several other direct diagnostic alternatives have been developed, such as ultrasonic imaging, direct carotid artery Doppler velocity, and spectral analysis.

The OPG-Gee has an advantage because it offers a more reliable identification of bilateral disease, and the drop in ophthalmic pressure is a very useful hemodynamic index readily transferable to circulatory considerations of the extracranial carotid artery system. The double slope observed in the eye pulse tracings of the OPG-Kartchner-McRae system is not very reliable and is easily identifiable only in very advanced degrees of disease. The adjunct CPA that is often used in conjunction with the plethysmographic technique is indeed helpful and improves the accuracy of the OPG-CPA technique. It should be pointed out, however, that CPA can be used separately with any method, and therefore it is only fair to compare OPG-Kartchner-McRae with OPG-Gee. There are two minor advantages of the OPG-Kartchner-McRae method: its slightly higher sensitivity and the lower negative pressure used throughout the examination. These should tilt the balance of safety slightly, but in view of the absence of significant complications related to either procedure, the weight of this argument is reduced. One common negative aspect of both methods is the fact that they only identify obstructions starting with a diameter reduction of 50% or more. This limits the application of both methods in studies of the natural history of the disease or the effects of nonsurgical therapeutic intervention. Both methods, however, do offer a noninvasive answer to an often-asked question regarding the hemodynamic significance of a suspected stenosis. Finally, the question of cost-effectiveness is favorable for both cases when compared with many other currently available imaging systems.

REFERENCES

1. Archie, J.P., Poser, P.H., and Goodson, D.S.: Accuracy of digitalized differential pulse timing oculoplethysmography, Surg. Gynecol. Obstet. 152:259, 1981.
2. Baker, J.D., Kaufman, M., and Machleder, H.I.: Evaluation of internal carotid stenosis with the Chronopulse, an automated ocular pulse arrival time recorder, Am. J. Surg. 142:212, 1981.
3. Blackshear, W.M., et al.: A prospective evaluation of oculoplethysmography and carotid phonoangiography, Surg. Gynecol. Obstet. 148:201, 1979.
4. Bone, G.E., Dickinson, D., and Pomajzl, M.J.: A prospective evaluation of indirect methods for detecting carotid atherosclerosis, Surg. Gynecol. Obstet. 152:587, 1981.
5. Cantelmo, N.L., et al.: Noninvasive detection of carotid stenosis following endarterectomy, Arch. Surg. 116:1005, 1981.
6. Cebul, R.D., and Ginsburg, M.D.: Noninvasive neurovascular tests for carotid artery disease, Ann. Intern. Med. 97:867, 1982.
7. Dean, R.H., and Yao, J.S.T.: Hemodynamic measurements in peripheral vascular disease, Surgery 12:1, 1976.
8. Ginsberg, M.D., Greenwood, S.A., and Goldberg, H.I.: Noninvasive diagnosis of extracranial cerebrovascular disease: oculoplethysmography-phonoangiography and directional Doppler ultrasonography, Neurology 29:623, 1979.
9. Gross, W.S., et al.: Comparison of noninvasive diagnostic techniques in carotid artery occlusive disease, Surgery 82:271, 1977.
10. Kapsch, D., et al.: Use of combined oculoplethysmography, carotid phonoangiography and Doppler in the noninvasive diagnosis of extracranial carotid occlusive disease, Stroke 12:317, 1981.
11. Kartchner, M.M., and McRae, L.P.: Auscultation for carotid bruits in cerebrovascular insufficiency. Further advances, JAMA 210:494, 1969.
12. Kartchner, M.M., and McRae, L.P.: Noninvasive evaluation and management of the "asymptomatic" carotid bruit, Surgery 82:840, 1977.
13. Kartchner, M.M., and McRae, L.P.: Carotid phonoangiography and oculoplethysmography. In Nicolaides, A.N., and Yao, J.S.T., editors: Investigation of vascular disorders, London, 1981, Churchill Livingstone.
14. Kartchner, M.M., McRae, L.P., and Morrison, F.D.: Noninvasive detection and evaluation of carotid occlusive disease, Arch. Surg. 106:528, 1973.
15. Kartchner, M.M., et al.: Oculoplethysmography: an adjunct to arteriography in the diagnosis of extracranial carotid occlusive disease, Am. J. Surg. 132:728, 1976.
16. Keagy, B.A., et al.: Oculoplethysmography/carotid phonoangiography: its value as a screening test in patients with suspected carotid artery stenosis, Arch. Surg. 115:1199, 1980.
17. Knox, R., Breslau, P., and Strandness, D.E., Jr.: Quantitative carotid phonoangiography, Stroke 12:798, 1981.
18. Krause, H., et al.: Power frequency spectrum analysis in the diagnosis of carotid artery disease, Stroke 15:351, 1984.
19. Lees, R.S., and Dewey, C.F., Jr.: Phonoangiography: a new noninvasive diagnostic method for studying arterial disease, Proc. Natl. Acad. Sci. USA 67:935, 1970.
20. Lees, R.S., Kistler, J.P., and Sanders, D.: Duplex Doppler scanning and spectral bruit analysis for diagnosing carotid stenosis, Circulation 66(suppl. I):102, 1982.
21. Malone, J.M., et al.: Diagnosis of carotid artery stenosis. Comparison of oculoplethysmography and Doppler supraorbital examination, Ann. Surg. 191:347, 1980.
22. McDonald, P.T., et al.: Doppler cerebrovascular examination, oculoplethysmography and ocular pneumoplethysmography, Arch. Surg. 113:1341, 1978.
23. McRae, L.P., Crain, V., and Kartchner, M.M.: Oculoplethysmography and carotid flow angiography, OPG/CPA Interpretation manual, ed. 2, Tucson, Ariz. 1978, Tucson Medical Center.
24. McRae, L.P., and Kartchner, M.M.: Carotid phonoangiography. In Kempezinski, R.F., and Yao, J.S.T., editors: Practical noninvasive vascular diagnosis, Chicago, 1982, Year Book Medical Publishers, Inc.
25. Meade, J.W.: OPG/CPA noninvasive tests for extracranial vascular disease, Contemp. Surg. 15:57, 1979.
26. O'Leary, D.H., et al.: Noninvasive testing for carotid artery stenosis. II. Clinical application of accuracy assessments, A.J.R. 138:109, 1981.
27. Persson, A.V.: New methods for clinical evaluation of carotid artery disease, Lahey Clin. Foundation Bull. 26:40, 1977.
28. Persson, A.V., et al.: Clinical use of noninvasive evaluation of the carotid artery, Surg. Clin. North Am. 60:513, 1980.
29. Reynolds, O.: An experimental investigation of the circumstances which determine whether the motion of water shall be direct or sinuous, and of the law of resistance in parallel channels, Philos. Trans. R. Soc. Lond. 174(III):935, 1883.
30. Riles, T.S., et al.: Symptoms, stenosis and bruit, Arch. Surg. 116:218, 1981.
31. Satiani, B., et al.: Assessment of carotid phonoangiography and oculoplethysmography in the detection of carotid artery stenosis, Am. J. Surg. 136:618, 1978.
32. String, S.T.: Zira oculoplethysmography. In Kempczinski, R.F., and Yao, J.S.T., editors: Practical noninvasive vascular diagnosis, Chicago, 1982, Year Book Medical Publishers, Inc.
33. Sumner, D.S., Russell, J.B., and Miles, R.D.: Are noninvasive tests sufficiently accurate to identify patients in need of carotid arteriography? Surgery 91:700, 1982.
34. Sumner, D.S., et al.: Noninvasive diagnosis of extracranial carotid arterial disease: a prospective evaluation of pulsed-Doppler imaging and oculoplethysmography, Arch. Surg. 114:1222, 1979.

CHAPTER 31

Ocular pneumoplethysmography

BERT C. EIKELBOOM

Ocular pneumoplethysmography (OPG-Gee) is one of the most widely used tests in noninvasive cerebrovascular evaluation because of its valuable principle of pressure measurement for evaluating the hemodynamic significance of a carotid artery lesion. Its background is described in Chapter 12; the following will give practical details on technique, interpretation, and applications.

TECHNIQUE

Before OPG is performed, the patient's medical history is taken with particular regard to the reason for referral, the presence of hypertension, allergies, and ophthalmologic contraindications to the test. These contraindications include a history of retinal detachment, unstable glaucoma, recent eye surgery, lens implants, and conjunctivitis. If there is any doubt, the patient's ophthalmologist should be contacted. The patient is informed that the procedure causes little discomfort although a dimming or loss of vision for several seconds may be experienced. While the test is performed the patient should be instructed to focus on a fixed point and to avoid blinking. The patient is placed in a supine position, and 2 drops of a topical anesthetic agent are applied to each eye. Excess fluid is wiped off with a tissue to avoid aspiration of fluid into the tubing of the eyecups. The blood pressure is measured in each arm by an ordinary sphygmomanometer, and the side with the highest pressure is taken as reference. An automatic blood pressure monitor may be used for measuring the systemic blood pressure and ophthalmic artery pressure simultaneously. The OPG instrument offers the possibility of simultaneous electrocardiogram (ECG) recording, but this is only rarely helpful in routine OPG testing. The eyecups are placed on the sclera, lateral to the cornea. Slight pressure is maintained man-

ually to keep the eyecups in proper position until the vacuum is applied by activating the foot switch. A choice must be made between 300 and 500 mm Hg vacuums. The former is used in normotensive patients and the latter in hypertensive patients. After reaching the chosen vacuum, the record switch is pushed and the vacuum is automatically released in about 30 seconds. Then the technician or physician must evaluate whether the tracings for both the left and right eyes show an appropriate onset of pulsations. The first ocular pulsations are taken for measurement of the ophthalmic artery pressure from the calibrated ruler overlay. In extremely hypertensive patients even a 500 mm Hg vacuum may not obliterate the ocular pulsations, and no real ophthalmic artery pressures can be determined. Blinking artifacts can make it difficult to determine the first two arterial pulsations. The test should then be repeated with the eyes closed, which will solve this problem in most patients. Occasionally, several small pulsations may be present before progression in amplitude of pulsations occurs. In that case, the first pulse that is followed by a pulse of greater amplitude should be taken for ophthalmic artery pressure calculation. One should also be aware of another artifact caused by incorrect placement of the eyecup. This may result in an initial pulse with a large amplitude, not preceded by the usual gradual progression in amplitude (Fig. 31-1). The test should be repeated while care is given to proper eyecup placement.

OPG may be performed with carotid compression to obtain information about the collateral circulation. We have experience in more than 8000 tests that carotid compression is a safe maneuver if it is performed low in the neck to avoid dislodging of atheromatous debris from the carotid bifurcation and stimulation of the baroreceptors.

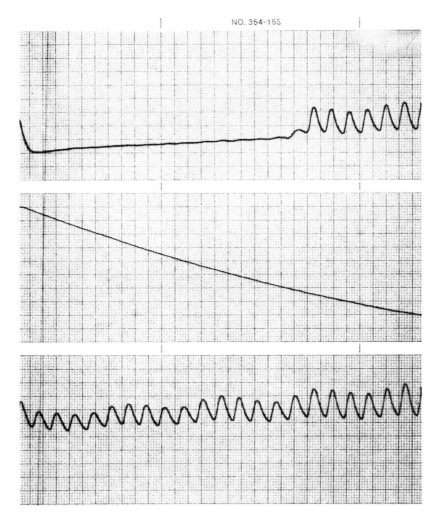

Fig. 31-1. Artifact resulting from incorrect eyecup placement. Initial pulse on right side (top) is not preceded by usual gradual progression in amplitude. (Reproduced with permission from Gee, W.: Ocular pneumoplethysmography [OPG-Gee]. In Kempczinski, R.F., and Yao, J.S.T., et al.: PRACTICAL NON-INVASIVE VASCULAR DIAGNOSIS. Copyright © 1982 by Year Book Medical Publishers, Inc., Chicago.)

Ophthalmic artery pressures are measured in the same way as previously described; the pressure on the side of compression is called the collateral ophthalmic artery pressure (COAP). Some experience is needed to perform carotid compression reliably. A photoplethysmograph on the earlobe on the side of compression is helpful in checking whether complete occlusion is achieved and maintained. Compression should be released gradually to avoid a sudden return of blood flow. The OPG instrument offers the possibility of recording ocular pulsations at high paper speed, which makes the determination of pulse arrival times possible, as with the OPG-Kartchner technique. The value of this procedure is limited. After finishing the test, some scleral erythema may be encountered in the area that has been under the eyecup. We explain to the patient that this does not require treatment and that it will disappear spontaneously. The patient is also told that his eyes may remain anesthetic up to 2 hours after the test and that he should therefore not rub his eyes.

CRITERIA FOR INTERPRETATION

Criteria for the interpretation of the OPG include differences in ophthalmic artery pressure (OAP) between the two sides, the ophthalmic/systemic pressure (OP/SP) ratio, and the pulse amplitude. There has been a lack of unanimity in the literature concerning the criteria that should be used to classify the test as normal or abnormal. Different criteria have been published by several laboratories, creating confusion among the users of the instrument. The choice of criteria is important as it greatly influences the accuracy of the test. We therefore applied these different criteria to the OPG results of 200 patients with angiographically evaluated carotid arteries and found McDonald's criteria to be the most suitable for clinical use.[5] The OPG result is considered abnormal if there is a left to right OAP difference of 5 mm Hg or more, or if the OP/SP ratio is less than 0.66. These criteria result in the best balance between sensitivity and specificity, as can be seen in the receiver operating characteristic (ROC) curve for the different criteria (Fig. 31-2). Better sensitivities can only be reached at the cost of lower specificities, which is not acceptable, since the test has its greatest value in patients with asymptomatic bruits and vague or nonhemispheric symptoms. The application of Gee's criteria will also give good results but is more cumbersome. He considers a left to right difference of 5 mm Hg or more or an OAP $< 39 + 0.43$ SP as abnormal. Quick interpretation is accomplished more easily by using the 0.66 ratio than by Gee's formula.

The pulse amplitude should only be used as a criterion in those hypertensive patients in whom even a vacuum of 500 mm Hg does not obliterate the ocular pulsations. In these cases no OAP can be measured. If a difference in amplitude of 2 mm or more is noted between the first pulsation of the left and that of the right eye, a hemodynamically significant carotid lesion can be expected on the side of the lower amplitude. The pulse amplitude should not be used as a diagnostic criterion if the actual OAPs can be determined. Although the amplitude is lower for carotid arteries with hemodynamically significant lesions than for those without such lesions, application of this criterion will result in a decrease of the test's specificity.[6]

RESULTS

Results obtained with OPG in detecting hemodynamically significant carotid lesions are not only dependent on the criteria used for interpretation of the test, but also on the criteria used for classification of the angiogram as either normal or abnormal. Reading angiograms is more subjective than reading OPG curves, as confirmed by the high intraobserver and interobserver variability of angiography. Accurate measurement of the degree of stenosis is difficult to accomplish. Moreover, many authors do not state whether the vessel diameter within the stenosis is compared to the estimated diameter of the bulbus or to the distal internal carotid artery. Confusion exists about transverse diameter stenosis as compared to cross-sectional area stenosis. How should a stenosis of 60% in the lateral projection with no stenosis present in the anterior-posterior (AP) projection be classified? Also, how should weblike stenoses be classified? Are the hemodynamic consequences of a 60% lesion in the common carotid artery the same as those of a 60% lesion in the siphon, which is a much smaller vessel? Did the angiogram always visualize the whole pathway from aortic arch to ophthalmic artery? Obviously, innominate artery lesions, as well as siphon lesions, may cause a reduction in OAP. Nevertheless, this is only rarely taken into consideration in the literature on OPG results. Degrees of stenosis varying from 50% to 75% have been used as the threshold between normal and abnormal. The results of OPG are influenced by the stenosis threshold that is chosen. The sensitivity will be higher when the threshold is high, but specificity will be low. This relationship is shown graphically in the ROC curve in Fig. 31-2. A comparison of results obtained by different researchers is also hampered by the fact that some researchers present data in terms of patients and others in terms of arteries. Nevertheless, a survey of the existing literature on OPG has been performed, and indicates that sensitivities range from 70% to 92% and specificities from 80% to 100%.[4] The mean sensitivity is 68%, and the mean specificity is 92%. An overall accuracy of approximately 90% is what may be expected of OPG if a fixed angiographic threshold is used as the standard. In our opinion this fixed threshold does not exist, and OPG may sometimes reflect the significance of a lesion more clearly than angiography.

Unfortunately, in the case of an abnormal OPG result no distinction can be made between hemodynamically significant stenosis and occlusion. An interesting observation was made in patients with carotid occlusion on one side and significant stenosis on the other side. As expected, the OAP was mostly lower on the side of the occlusion, but this was not always the case. We documented several cases of lower OAP on the side of the stenosis. This is also an indication that OPG reflects the functional significance of a lesion better than angiography.

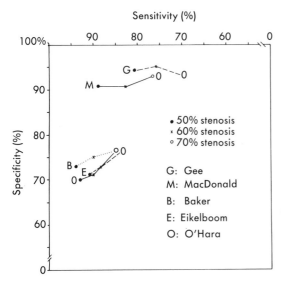

Fig. 31-2. Sensitivity and specificity using different criteria for interpretation of OPG and different angiographic thresholds for hemodynamically significant stenosis. (From Eikelboom, B.C., et al.: Arch. Surg. 118:1169, Copyright 1983, American Medical Association.)

AREAS OF APPLICATION

The primary application of OPG is the assessment of the presence or absence of hemodynamically significant carotid lesions. Symptoms of cerebrovascular insufficiency or asymptomatic bruits can be indications for testing. It is well known, however, that carotid stenosis may be present in the absence of bruits. We have used OPG as a screening device for hemodynamically significant carotid disease regardless of the presence or absence of bruits in 500 consecutive patients with symptoms or peripheral obstructive arterial disease. Carotid bruits were found in 130 patients (26%). The OPG was abnormal in 86 patients (14%) and half of them had no bruit, so abnormal OPG results were present in 43 of 370, or 12% of the patients with peripheral arterial disease who had no bruits. A similar screening study has been published for 500 patients scheduled for cardiac operations.[1] Bruits were present in 32 patients (6%), while 18 patients (3%) had abnormal OPG measurements. It is interesting that, similar to our peripheral arterial disease group, 50% of these patients had a bruit and 50% did not. Therefore 9 out of 468 cardiac patients (2%) without bruits had abnormal OPG findings. Thus normal OPG findings occur much more often in patients with peripheral arterial disease than in patients with cardiac disease. When hemodynamically significant carotid disease is confirmed by angiography, it is our policy to perform carotid and cardiac surgery simultaneously.

OPG is an excellent tool for documentation of the natural history of carotid disease. We are performing a prospective follow-up study on 400 patients with asymptomatic carotid bruits. At the first examination a pressure-reducing lesion was identified by OPG in 47 patients (11.8%); nine of these patients proved to have carotid occlusion. During a mean follow-up period of 3 years, 44 patients (11%) changed from normal to abnormal.

Several researchers have shown that patients with an abnormal OPG are at a much higher risk of stroke compared to those with a normal OPG. Busuttil[2] followed 215 patients with a history of stroke, TIA, or asymptomatic bruits. In patients with hemodynamically significant stenosis, the incidence of stroke and death was 16.2%, but it was only 2.2% in patients with nonhemodynamically significant OPG-negative lesions. A further step in recognizing stroke-prone patients can be made by performing OPG with carotid compression. Those patients who show clinical signs of cerebral ischemia during compression and those who have COAPs less than 60 mm Hg are at high risk when stenosis progresses to occlusion. Aggressive surgical therapy is indicated in these patients.

OPG and electroencephalogram (EEG) with carotid compression make it possible to predict preoperatively which patients will need a shunt during carotid endarterectomy.[9] We performed these tests in 126 patients. Insertion of a shunt was based on intraoperative test clamping with EEG control and was necessary in 11 patients (8.7%). The sensitivity of preoperative OPG and EEG was 100% and the specificity 76%. Preoperative prediction of the stump pressure is also of great value when carotid ligation or resection is planned to identify those patients who are vulnerable to cerebral ischemia.[3]

After carotid endarterectomy has been performed, OPG is used to document early patency. A recovery room OPG is indicated in case of an immediate postoperative neurologic deficit. It allows differentiation between early thrombosis and intracranial hemorrhage. If the OPG is abnormal on the operated side, thrombosis has probably occurred and the patient is immediately taken back to the operating room without losing time with angiography. However, special criteria for interpretation of OPG in this period may have to be applied.[10] The reasons for this phenomenon have not yet been established. After carotid endarterectomy, OPG is performed once a year to detect restenosis. We found 5% restenoses and occlusions after a mean follow-up of 2.5 years.

The effect of a extraintracranial bypass operation for carotid occlusion can also be evaluated by OPG. OAPs are determined without and with compression of the bypass. The difference between these pressures represents the contribution of the bypass to the intracranial perfusion pressure. It averaged 12.8 mm Hg in 13 patients who underwent this operation for unilateral internal carotid occlusion.

OPG can be used to determine the ocular blood flow. Its calculation is the product of pulse rate, calibrated ocular pulse amplitude, and a constant of 0.0016.[8] The ocular blood flow is a reflection of the stroke volume of the heart, and its measurement by OPG can be used for hemodynamic assessment of cardiac pacing.[7] It offers a simple method for documentation of the effect of ventricular versus atrioventricular sequential pacing. A final application of OPG is that used in comatose patients with head injuries. Ocular blood flow reflects cerebral blood flow and alterations in brain compliance as a result of cerebral edema. A bilateral reduction of ocular blood flow below 0.53 mm/min may be incompatible with cerebral survival.[8] Serial OPG studies may be useful for simple documentation of changes in brain compliance and may influence therapeutic decisions.

REFERENCES

 1. Balderman, S.C., et al.: Noninvasive screening for asymptomatic carotid artery disease prior to cardiac operation, J. Thorac. Cardiovasc. Surg. 85:427, 1983.
 2. Busuttil, R.W., et al.: Carotid artery stenosis hemodynamic significance and clinical course, JAMA 245:1438, 1981.
 3. Ehrenfeld, W.K., Stoney, R.J., and Wylie, E.J.: Relation of carotid stump pressure to safety of carotid artery ligation, Surgery 93:299, 1983.
 4. Eikelboom, B.C.: Ocular pneumoplethysmography (OPG-Gee) and oculoplethysmography (OPG-Kartchner): review and perspectives, Int. Angiol. (In press.)
 5. Eikelboom, B.C., et al.: Criteria for interpretation of ocular pneumoplethysmography (Gee), Arch. Surg. 118:1169, 1983.
 6. Eikelboom, B.C., et al.: Pulse amplitude as a diagnostic criterion in OPG-Gee, Bruit 7:50, 1983.
 7. Gee, W.: Ocular pneumoplethysmography in cardiac pacing, PACE 6:1268, 1983.
 8. Gee, W., et al.: Ocular pneumoplethysmography in head-injured patients, J. Neurosurg. 59:46, 1983.
 9. Moll, F.L., Eikelboom, B.C., and Ackerstaff, R.G.A.: The value of electroencephalography and ocular pneumoplethysmography in carotid shunting, Neth. J. Surg. 34:53, 1982.
10. Ortega, G., et al.: Postendarterectomy carotid occlusion, Surgery 90:1093, 1981.

CHAPTER 32

Periorbital Doppler velocity evaluation of carotid obstruction

EDWIN C. BROCKENBROUGH

Obstruction to blood flow through the internal carotid artery invokes collateral blood supply from the circle of Willis and from reversal of flow in the ophthalmic artery. These collateral pathways serve to ameliorate the effects of the restricted carotid blood flow. In addition, they provide a simple means by which the diagnosis of carotid obstruction may be suspected. Using a Doppler ultrasonic velocity detector, flow in these vessels may be examined and the presence or absence of functioning collateral pathways determined. The technique for this examination has been developed over a period of years and has proved to be a reliable method of screening for significant carotid obstruction.

My first experience in this area began in 1967 with the advent of the early commercial models of the Doppler velocity detectors.[2] The concept of the supraorbital Doppler test for carotid obstruction was developed in conjunction with another diagnostic technique for carotid disease, which we called ocular plethysmography.[3] Both these tests were based on the principle of compressing collateral vessels feeding the ophthalmic artery as a means of recognizing the abnormal flow patterns associated with internal carotid obstruction. The Doppler test became more refined when direction capability was added to the instrument in 1968. As our experience grew, it became apparent that the frontal, supraorbital, and angular arteries were each important to an understanding of the vagaries of collateral circulation, hence the more descriptive term *periorbital Doppler examination.*

A number of other investigators have made observations similar to ours and produced their own contributions in this area. Maroon et al.[5] independently described "ophthalmosonometry" in 1969, Müller[6] expanded on this concept in 1972 and stressed the importance of retrograde flow in the frontal artery as a diagnostic sign for internal carotid occlusion. Machleder and Barker[4] used the periorbital test in 1972 and emphasized its usefulness in recognizing unsuspected carotid obstruction. In 1975 Barnes and Wilson[1] contributed a very comprehensive treatment of this subject, adding many of their own observations as well as reviewing in detail the principles involved. Following is a status report on the periorbital test—the anatomy and principles on which the test is based, the technique of the examination, what information can be derived, and the role of the test in the spectrum of noninvasive diagnostic tests of the cerebrovascular system.

ANATOMIC BASIS OF THE PERIORBITAL EXAMINATION

Blood flow through the internal carotid artery is distributed almost entirely to intracranial vessels. The one exception to this is the ophthalmic artery. This artery passes into the orbit, gives rise to a number of intraorbital branches, and then terminates in three branches that surface on the face. These are the nasal, frontal, and supraorbital branches (Fig. 32-1). The nasal artery becomes the angular artery, which descends along the lateral border of the nose and communicates with the facial branch of the external carotid artery. The frontal and supraorbital arteries turn upward and pass into the subcutaneous tissue of the forehead where they communicate with branches of the superficial temporal artery. These communications serve as collateral pathways in the event of internal carotid obstruction. Other communications between the

□ Supported in part by NIH grant no. HL19341.

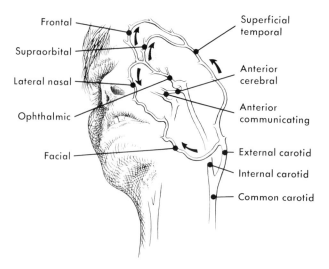

Fig. 32-1. Arteries of significance to periorbital Doppler test. Normal flow pattern is shown by arrows.

ophthalmic artery and branches of the external carotid artery occur through the ethmoid and lacrimal branches. Although these are not accessible for Doppler examination, they should be considered because of their contribution to the collateral blood supply. In addition to the periorbital anastomoses, the other major collateral pathway is the anterior communicating artery of the circle of Willis. It is through this pathway that crossover circulation occurs from the opposite internal carotid artery.

TECHNIQUE OF EXAMINATION

The examination consists of detecting flow in the periorbital vessels, noting the quality and direction of the velocity signals, and determining the response of these signals to compressions about the face and neck.

The Doppler equipment for the examination should have directional capability, and the probe should be small enough to permit separate examination of each of these vessels.* The examination is begun with the patient in the supine position and the eyes gently closed. The probe is then placed at the inner canthus of the eye and the maximum flow signal identified. It is then moved along this signal toward the rim of the orbit. This is the point of examination of the frontal artery. The probe is then moved laterally to the supraorbital notch, where the supraorbital signal is identified. The angular artery may be located over the lateral aspect

of the nose. It is the smallest of the three vessels and is usually accompanied by a large vein, making examination more difficult than in the preceding vessels. Furthermore, this vessel is often absent in patients whose eyeglasses rest on this portion of the nose. For these reasons examination of the angular artery is reserved for the patient in whom the frontal and supraorbital flow signals are abnormal.

If the Doppler probe is held in the proper angle, the direction of flow can usually be determined reliably. In some instances, however, a tortuous artery may alter the geometry of the probe angle in relation to the vessel, and the observed direction of flow may be reversed. Compression techniques help to minimize errors of this sort.

After the examiner has located the frontal and supraorbital arteries and noted the direction and quality of the flow signals, he compresses the superficial temporal artery in front of the ear, just above the zygoma. In most patients there will be slight augmentation of the frontal and supraorbital signals, but in some normal individuals there will be no change. If the signals are diminished or obliterated by temporal artery compression, the flow may be assumed to be retrograde. The facial artery is then compressed along the lower border of the mandible and the effect of this compression on the frontal artery is noted. These maneuvers are then repeated on the opposite side. Finally, common carotid compression is performed to identify crossover circulation. This compression is accomplished low in the neck, well away from the carotid bifurcation, and is maintained for only one or two

*Directional Doppler 806, Parks Electronics Laboratory, Beaverton, Ore.

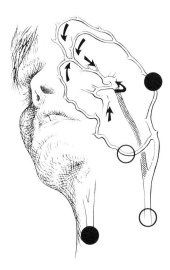 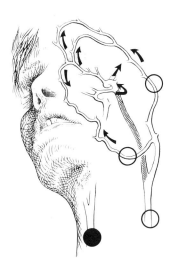

Fig. 32-2. Carotid occlusion, or high-grade stenosis—dominant periorbital collaterals. This is flow pattern seen in over 90% of patients with this condition.

Fig. 32-3. Carotid occlusion, or high-grade stenosis—dominant crossover collaterals. This pattern is sometimes seen in long-standing carotid obstruction. Key diagnostic maneuver is contralateral carotid compression.

heartbeats. During this compression the probe is usually held at the inner canthus of the eye where the maximum flow signal is located. Normally, the signal at this point is obliterated or greatly diminished by ipsilateral carotid compression and is not affected by contralateral carotid compression. With the ipsilateral carotid compressed, the residual flow signals on both sides should be about the same. Although there is undoubtedly some inherent risk of dislodging an embolus during carotid compression, the risk is low if the compression is deft and brief. We have not recognized any complications in over 4000 patients in whom the compressions have been carried out.

During the examination it is important that the examiner hold the probe in a steady position, facilitated by resting the hand holding the probe on the patient's forehead and bridge of the nose. It is also important that the probe be held lightly, since even a modest pressure from the tip of the probe can obliterate flow in these small vessels. In this regard the examiner must resist the tendency to press with the probe at the same time he is compressing the temporal or facial vessels with the opposite hand.

PATTERNS OF COLLATERAL BLOOD FLOW

A variety of patterns of collateralization are seen around the orbit in the presence of internal carotid obstruction. Following are representative examples.

Dominant periorbital collaterals (Fig. 32-2). The most common pattern of collateralization, constituting over 90% of all abnormal examinations, the pattern of dominant periorbital collaterals is usually associated with high-grade stenosis or total occlusion of the internal carotid artery. The examiner first notices that there is asymmetry between the two sides. The signal on the obstructed side is dampened and has only a single component, or it may be loud and continuous. The direction indicator on the Doppler instrument shows that the direction of flow in the periorbital vessels is reversed. Furthermore, the periorbital signals are obliterated or diminished with temporal and facial artery compressions. In some instances a reversed signal may be converted to a normal directional signal by these compressions. Finally, there is usually evidence of some crossover flow with common carotid compression. Ipsilateral common carotid compression results in a prominent residual signal that may be either antegrade or retrograde, depending on whether the dominant collateral supply travels through the opposite internal carotid or the opposite external carotid artery. Compression of the contralateral carotid artery will usually increase the retrograde flow in the periorbital vessels.

Dominant crossover collaterals (Fig. 32-3). The pattern of dominant crossover collaterals is the next most common condition and is usually seen in patients with long-standing occlusion of the internal carotid artery or in patients with a common carotid

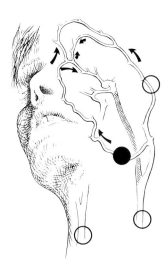

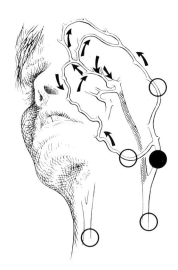

Fig. 32-4. Carotid occlusion, or high-grade stenosis—dominant facial artery collateral. This is variant of pattern in Fig. 23-2. Key diagnostic maneuver is facial artery compression.

Fig. 32-5. Carotid occlusion, or high-grade stenosis—dominant intraorbital collaterals. This is rare cause for diagnostic error. Key diagnostic maneuver is selective compression of external carotid artery.

artery occlusion. The examiner first notices asymmetry between the two sides and usually detects an abnormal signal on the affected side. The flow is noted to be coming from within the orbit, but with compression of the common carotid artery on the affected side, there is augmentation of the periorbital flow signals in a normal direction. The diagnosis is confirmed with contralateral common carotid compression, which eliminates the crossover supply and usually produces a reversal of flow in the periorbital vessels.

Dominant facial artery collateral (Fig. 32-4). Dominant facial artery collateral is a variant of the pattern seen in Fig. 32-2, in which the facial artery not only supplies retrograde flow to the angular artery but also supplies flow to the frontal, and sometimes the supraorbital, vessel. This results in normal directional flow in the latter vessels so that the response to temporal artery compression may be normal. The diagnosis is made by compressing the facial artery and noting that it diminishes or obliterates the frontal and supraorbital signals as well as the angular signal.

Dominant intraorbital collaterals (Fig. 32-5). Occasionally communications within the orbit may provide sufficient flow to produce normal directional signals in the periorbital vessels. These anastomoses probably occur between the orbital branches of the ophthalmic (anterior and posterior ethmoid, lacrimal) and branches of the internal maxillary (sphenopalatine, middle meningeal) arteries. This variant has been observed on several occasions in patients with long-standing internal carotid artery occlusion. It is fortunate that this is a rare condition, since the standard compression techniques may suggest normal blood supply. If suspected, the diagnosis can be made by selective compression of the external carotid artery, which will obliterate or diminish the periorbital signals. With a little practice this compression can be accomplished satisfactorily while the temporal artery is monitored with the Doppler probe for completeness.

Balanced internal carotid/external carotid artery supply (Fig. 32-6). Usually a sign of early hemodynamic obstruction of the internal carotid artery, the balanced internal carotid/external carotid artery supply occurs in patients in whom the stenosis has not progressed to the point of producing complete periorbital reversal. The examiner first notices asymmetry between the two sides. The signal on the affected side will be in a normal direction during the systole and reversed in late diastole. In this balanced state small changes in collateral flow or in peripheral resistance may shift the periorbital flow from one direction to the other. Compression of the contralateral common carotid artery, for example, may result in periorbital flow reversal. Nitroglycerin, if administered sublingually, will produce a progressive reduction in the normal directional component and progressive increase in the reversed component. Occasionally this balanced

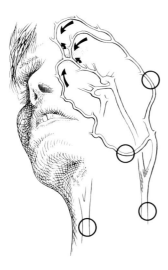

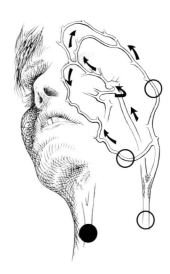

Fig. 32-6. Carotid stenosis—critically balanced flow in periorbital vessels. Bidirectional flow may be identified.

Fig. 32-7. Combined internal and external carotid stenosis—normal directional periorbital flow may be present. Key diagnostic maneuver is contralateral carotid compression.

state is produced by stenosis of the external carotid artery as well as of the internal carotid artery or by a stenosis in the common carotid artery at the bifurcation (Fig. 32-7). In either of these situations, however, there is usually evidence of collateralization from the opposite side that may be demonstrated with contralateral carotid compression.

DIAGNOSTIC CRITERIA

From the observations made during the periorbital Doppler examination one can be reasonably confident about the presence or absence of collateral blood flow. If collateral circulation is present, the diagnosis of carotid obstruction may be inferred. However, no distinction can be made between total occlusion of the carotid artery and high-grade stenosis; it must be emphasized that clinically significant, but nonobstructing, lesions cannot be detected by this method. Collateralization around the orbit can usually be recognized when the diameter of the internal carotid is reduced by 65% to 70%. This corresponds to a 2 mm or smaller channel as seen on the angiogram. We prefer to quantitate the obstruction in terms of the diameter at the narrowest point, since this is the measurement obtained most easily and agreed on most readily.

The most reliable signs of collateralization are *retrograde flow* from the temporal and facial arteries and evidence of *crossover flow* from the op-

posite carotid artery. Doppler changes that are not diagnostic but strongly suggestive include *asymmetry* between the two sides, *dampened* velocity signals, and change from a normal two-component signal to either a *systolic* signal or a *continuous* signal.

Retrograde flow. Retrograde flow is recognized from the direction indicated on the Doppler instrument as well as from compressing the facial and temporal arteries. Occasionally the periorbital vessels will be supplied from the contralateral temporal and facial arteries, which must be compressed to confirm the source.

Crossover flow. Abnormal supply via the anterior communicating artery is diagnosed by compressing the contralateral common carotid artery. If there is *normal directional* periorbital flow, the Doppler signals will be diminished or will become reversed by this maneuver. Likewise, compression of the ipsilateral common carotid artery will not obliterate the periorbital signals and may augment them.

If there is reversed periorbital flow, opposite carotid compression will augment the reversed flow. Compression of the ipsilateral carotid artery results in normal directional periorbital flow.

Asymmetric signals. Although asymmetry between the two sides is not diagnostic, it is suggestive of abnormal flow and warns the examiner to look carefully for other signs of collateralization. The asymmetry is caused by one of the following signal abnormalities.

Dampened flow signal. Whether normal directional or reversed, the periorbital signals on the side of an obstructed carotid will be less brisk than on the opposite normal side.

Single-component flow signal. As an obstructing lesion begins to reduce flow in the internal carotid artery, one of the first Doppler changes observed is elimination of the diastolic component of the periorbital signal.

Bidirectional flow signal. With further progression of the stenosis the flow signal becomes bidirectional, with reversed flow detectable at the end of diastole. In this balanced state changes in peripheral resistance may shift the flow in either direction. This can be demonstrated by administering sublingual nitroglycerin to the patient. Over a period of 1 or 2 minutes the antegrade component will diminish and the retrograde component will increase. Flow can be completely reversed by this technique, which may be useful as a provocative test for lesions of borderline significance. This response is considered to be a result of lowering the peripheral resistance in the intracranial distribution more than the resistance in the external carotid distribution.

Continuous flow signal. Occasionally a nearly continuous signal will be heard in the periorbital vessels, resembling the sound of an arteriovenous fistula. This is often observed in the presence of an acute internal carotid occlusion and suggests that a high-pressure gradient exists between the external and internal carotid arteries.

DIAGNOSTIC ACCURACY

The purpose of the periorbital Doppler examination is to recognize functioning collateral pathways around the orbit and, by inference, hemodynamically significant carotid obstruction. We believe that an accuracy of 95% or better is realistic and readily achieved by a careful, reasonably astute examiner. Using essentially the same method of approach, Barnes and Wilson[1] recently reported a 98.7% overall accuracy of diagnosis in a series of 76 patients undergoing angiography. These investigators had two false negative diagnoses (5%) in a group of 38 carotid arteries, with occlusion or stenosis of 75% or greater.

There are a number of possible sources of error in the examination, and the examiner should be aware of these to obtain the highest degree of accuracy. It is important that the anatomy of the periorbital vessels be well understood and that at least the frontal and supraorbital vessels be identified in each examination. The flow signals should be located just beneath the rim of the orbit and the probe angled toward the direction of flow so that a correct direction assessment can be made. The probe must be held steadily, particularly when the compressions are performed. It is essential that the examiner avoid pressing too firmly with the probe and obliterating the flow signal.

Anatomic variants that might lead to diagnostic errors have been illustrated. Occasionally normal individuals will exhibit a reversed flow in the supraorbital artery, even when care is taken to identify the vessel in this supraorbital notch. The reason for this is not certain, but this single abnormality should not lead to an error of interpretation if the remainder of the examination is normal. The lateral palpebral artery may sometimes be misidentified as the supraorbital artery, and since the palpebral artery arises from a branch of the temporal artery, a false-positive compression response may result.

In interpreting the results of the examination it is important for the examiner to resist the temptation to give a precise anatomic diagnosis. The observed data are concerned with collateralization about the orbit, and the basis for this collateralization can only be inferred. Whereas most patients with periobital collateralization will have carotid obstruction in the neck, obstruction at the level of the carotid siphon or of the ophthalmic artery will also produce positive findings. In fact, as it has already been pointed out, the distinction between total occlusion of the internal carotid and high-grade stenosis cannot be made from these observations alone. It must also be emphasized that the diagnosis is almost never based on a single abnormal finding. There are usually two or more abnormalities, and these abnormalities must be consistent with one another. If there is an unexplained finding, or if the findings are inconsistent, the examiner should persist with compressions, that is, contralateral, facial, or temporal compressions, until the collateral pathways are delineated.

ROLE OF THE PERIORBITAL DOPPLER EXAMINATION

The primary advantages of the periorbital Doppler examination are that it is a relatively simple examination and it can be performed with portable equipment at the bedside or in the office. It is inexpensive and involves minimal risk. We have found it to be a valuable adjunct to carotid surgery.

It is particularly reassuring in the recovery room to find that the previously abnormal signals have reverted to normal in a postoperative patient. The patient may later be followed on an outpatient basis and the continued patency of the vessel confirmed on subsequent visits.

It must be reemphasized that fewer than one half of the patients with *clinically significant* atherosclerotic disease at the carotid bifurcation will have Doppler signs of collateralization about the orbit. For this reason a normal periorbital examination, by itself, should not be relied on to rule out disease in a symptomatic individual who might be a candidate for carotid surgery. Our primary use of the periorbital examination, therefore, is as a component of a comprehensive noninvasive cerebrovascular evaluation. We have designed a technician-administered study that begins with a pertinent history and physical examination and includes audio and analog recordings of the vertebral signals, the ophthalmic artery signals in the posterior orbits, and Doppler imaging of the carotid bifurcation.[7] As a part of this study the periorbital examination helps to distinguish obstructing from nonobstructing lesions and to estimate the size of the lumen at the stenosis site. The periorbital Doppler findings should be consistent with the other findings and serve to increase the confidence by which the diagnostic interpretation is made. During the past 3 years approximately 2800 patients have been examined in this manner. This combined approach provided an overall diagnostic accuracy of 98%, when compared with angiographic stenoses of 50% or greater.[7] As a result of the experiences gained from Doppler imaging of the carotid bifurcation and analysis of the Doppler signal characteristics along these vessels, we have found it possible to derive considerable information from a direct examination of the bifurcation area with a simple handheld Doppler probe. The internal and external carotid artery signals can usually be recognized with confidence, and signal abnormalities, such as the increased frequency seen with stenosis, can be readily identified. The significance of this is that using the same relatively simple directional Doppler equipment with which the periorbital examination is performed, the examiner may carry out a reliable screening examination of the carotid bifurcation.

SUMMARY

The periorbital Doppler test is a relatively simple method by which functioning collateral pathways around the orbit may be identified. The presence of carotid obstruction may be inferred from these findings. Using the techniques described, the correlation between the Doppler evidence for collateralization and the angiographic evidence for significant obstruction should be 95% or better. The periorbital Doppler test does not detect nonobstructing lesions that may be of clinical significance, and, for this reason, is used to best advantage as a component of a more comprehensive noninvasive cerebrovascular evaluation. In this setting the periorbital Doppler information distinguishes between obstructing and nonobstructing lesions and adds to the confidence of the overall diagnostic interpretation. The periorbital Doppler test by itself is useful as an office or bedside screening test for carotid obstruction and is valuable for serial follow-up on patients after carotid surgery.

REFERENCES

1. Barnes, R.W., and Wilson, M.R.: Doppler ultrasonic evaluation of cerebrovascular disease, Iowa City, 1975, University of Iowa Press.
2. Brockenbrough, E.C.: Screening for the prevention of stroke: use of a Doppler flowmeter, 1969, Information and Education Resource Support Unit, Washington/Alaska Regional Medical Program.
3. Brockenbrough, E.C., Lawrence, C., and Schwenk, W.G.: Ocular phlethysmography: a new technic for the evaluation of carotid obstructive disease, Rev. Surg. 24:299, 1967.
4. Machleder, H.I., and Barker, W.F.: Stroke on the wrong side: use of the Doppler ophthalmic test in cerebral vascular screening, Arch. Surg. 105:943, 1972.
5. Maroon, J.C., Pieroni, D.W., and Campbell, R.L.: Ophthalmosonometry, an ultrasonic method for assessing carotid blood flow, J. Neurosurg. 30:238, 1969.
6. Müller, H.R.: The diagnosis of internal carotid artery occlusion by directional Doppler sonography of the ophthalmic artery, Neurology 22:816, 1972.
7. Spencer, M.P., et al.: Cerebrovascular evaluation using Doppler C-W ultrasound. Proceedings of the World Federation of Ultrasound in Medicine and Biology, San Francisco, August, 1976.

CHAPTER 33

Quantitative carotid phonoangiography

ROBERT S. LEES, J. PHILIP KISTLER, ARNOLD MILLER, and GARY R. JOHNSON

Atherosclerosis is a progressive disease that is usually clinically silent until late in its course. Noninvasive methods for its detection, localization, and quantitation are therefore particularly important; the lack of adequate methods has hampered not only the care of afflicted patients but also knowledge of the natural history of the disease. In carotid artery disease a rich collateral blood flow makes it possible for high-grade obstructive disease of one or both internal carotid arteries to develop before symptoms appear. When the symptoms occur, transient cerebral ischemia may precede stroke, but catastrophic cerebral infarction, embolic or thrombotic, may occur with little or no warning to the patient. Fortunately, the physician detects the presence of carotid atherosclerosis in many of these patients through the presence of cervical bruits. Bruits occurring over the carotid artery have long been recognized as an indication of disease,[18] although until recently, further diagnosis of carotid disease required invasive x-ray contrast angiography. Recently a number of methods have been proposed for noninvasive diagnosis of carotid stenosis (Chapter 3).[1,2] Most of these are indirect and give only a qualitative assessment of the extent of disease. Ultrasound methodology is still evolving rapidly but has so far been unable to provide accurate quantitative diagnosis of carotid stenosis.[1] Quantitative carotid phonoangiography, in contrast, is a method for direct estimation of the location and extent of carotid stenosis. It is based on quantitative spectral analysis of carotid bruits, which allows accurate numerical estimation of the residual lumen diameter at the stenosis.[5,7,8,11-15]

In this report, the principles and methodology of quantitative carotid phonoangiography will be described in detail, and our ongoing experience in its use will be summarized. The results of over 1100 studies in 1000 patients will be reviewed. Of these patients, 271 had x-ray angiography, giving us the opportunity to compare phonoangiograms with x-ray angiograms of 268 carotid bifurcations, in addition to those reported in our initial clinical trial.[5] Finally, the results of quantitative phonoangiography used in combination with other techniques will be evaluated.[14-16]

METHODS
Theory

Quantitative phonoangiography involves the qualitative spectral analysis of arterial bruits.[13] The theoretic basis for this analysis has been worked out over the past 10 years in our laboratories at the Massachusetts Institute of Technology, the Massachusetts General Hospital, and the New England Deaconess Hospital.[4-8,12-17] We have demonstrated that normal laminar "streamline" blood flow breaks down as blood flows through a significant stenosis, and an unstable turbulent jet is produced.[13] The unstable flow sets the vessel wall in motion; transmission of this motion to the skin surface produces the sound that we recognize as a bruit. The frequency spectrum of the sound produced depends on the effective diameter of the turbulent jet of blood flowing through the stenosis (Fig. 33-1), that is, the bruit itself contains information as to the severity of the stenosis that produced it. Although our early theoretic analysis suggested that the relationship between bruit frequency and amplitude and stenosis geometry was complex,[6-8,13] it proved possible to define a simple algorithm[5] that was clinically applicable. The basis of this algorithm is the Strouhal number (S), an empirical constant that obeys the relationship $S = f_0 d/U$, where f_0 is the *break frequency* characteristic of the sound produced by turbulent flow,

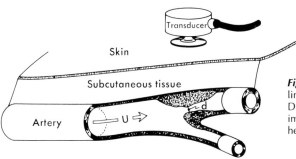

Fig. 33-1. Sketch of stenotic arterial bifurcation. Shown are linear flow velocity, U, and residual lumen diameter, d. Displacement transducer is shown placed over area of maximal stenosis, where sounds transmitted to skin surface are heard with maximal amplitude.

d is the residual lumen diameter at the stenosis, and U is the linear flow velocity through the vessel in the area beyond the stenosis (Fig. 33-1). We have shown in studies with induced stenosis of the dog aorta, where both blood flow and residual lumen diameter could be varied at will, that this relationship holds true for the arterial tree in vivo.[16] The form in which the equation is used to solve for residual lumen diameter is $d = SU/f_0$, and we found empirically that correct results were obtained for the human carotid bifurcation when $SU = 500$, that is, that 500 divided by the break frequency in hertz gave an accurate estimate of the residual lumen diameter in millimeters.[5,11,12,14] The bruits are recorded as described later and analyzed so as to display a frequency-intensity spectrum of that bruit (Fig. 33-2). When a bruit is caused by turbulent flow through a stenosis, we have almost uniformly found spectra that fulfill certain criteria:

1. The intensity of sound increases with frequency, in what may be a regular or irregular fashion, to a single discrete maximum, beyond which it falls off as frequency increases further.[5,13-16] The fall referred to is smooth or nearly so and has a characteristic slope.
2. The frequency at which peak bruit amplitude occurs is the break frequency, f_0 (Fig. 33-2).

Equipment

Bruits are recorded at the skin surface with a standard piezoelectric displacement transducer.* The transducer signal is fed into a commercially produced electrocardiographically gated spectral analyzer that contains an analog to digital (A/D) converter and several powerful microprocessors, which perform a fast Fourier transform (FFT) within a few seconds (Fig. 33-3) (Spectraview, American Edwards Laboratories). The results from six

*Hewlett-Packard 21050A.

cardiac cycles are measured and displayed on the instrument's cathode ray oscilloscope. The Spectraview also generates a permanent copy on paper of the spectrum of the bruit and the estimated residual lumen diameter of the stenosis.

Procedure

The study is usually carried out in a special laboratory with sound-absorbent tile on the walls and ceiling but can be performed in an ordinary hospital room or even an emergency ward if the ambient noise level is not too high. For portable studies, the Spectraview can be mounted on a small trolley cart and easily wheeled around.

The patient is studied while lying comfortably supine on a stretcher or bed. It is often advisable to have the patient lie flat without a pillow so that the neck is not flexed. After we listen carefully over the heart, upper chest, and neck with the stethoscope, the examination is repeated using the Spectraview and its headphones. Then the bruit or bruits are recorded in held expiration so that respiratory noise does not obscure vascular sounds. Ordinarily, multiple recordings are made over the base of the heart (if there is a basal heart murmur), the suprasternal notch, the subclavicular and supraclavicular areas, the sternal insertion of the sternomastoid muscle, and the inferior and superior borders of the thyroid cartilage; halfway between the thyroid cartilage and the angle of the mandible; at the angle of the mandible; over the preauricular artery (if the bruit is audible there); and over any other location at which the bruit can be heard.

For each recording location of interest, recordings are made until the same frequency spectrum is obtained on three separate analyses. This usually takes only 2 to 3 minutes to perform.

Analysis

As might be expected, our interpretive procedure has changed as we gain greater experience in ana-

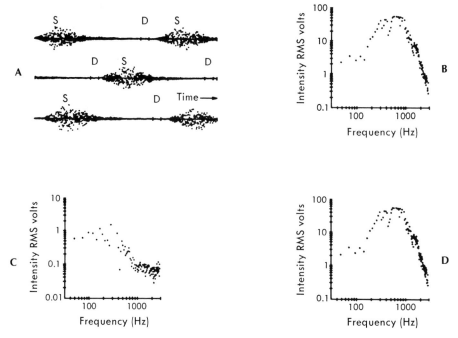

Fig. 33-2. Time display and spectral analysis of typical carotid bruit. **A,** Time display of bruit. Letter *S* between two vertical marks indicates portions of systole selected for analysis. Portions marked *D* indicate sections of diastole to be analyzed. **B,** Frequency-intensity spectrum of peak systolic bruit; analysis of areas marked in Fig. 33-1. **C,** Frequency-intensity spectrum of diastole. Note that intensity is almost two orders of magnitude lower than that of systole. **D,** Difference spectrum, which is very similar to uncorrected systolic spectrum because background noise is of low amplitude. We have found it unnecessary in clinical practice to obtain difference spectrum.

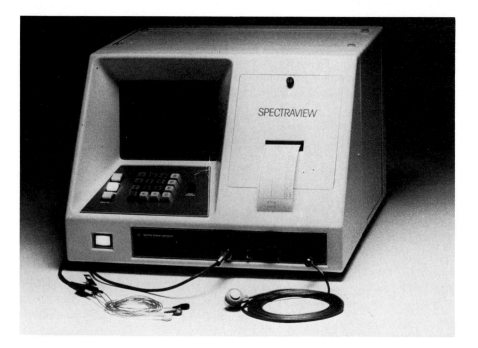

Fig. 33-3. Electrocardiographically gated sound spectral analyzer, designed for use for carotid bruit analysis (Spectraview). Instrument contains high-gain low-noise audioamplifier, high-speed A/D converter, and powerful microcomputer programmed to perform spectral analysis. Incoming signal and spectral analysis may be displayed on instrument's CRT screen and hard copy produced on its dot matrix printer. Heart sounds and Doppler ultrasound returns can also be analyzed by Spectraview.

lyzing bruits that arise between the aortic outflow tract and the base of the skull. Although we concentrated at first on the spectra of bruits recorded over the carotid bifurcation itself,[5] it has become clear with experience that greater accuracy can be achieved even in the analysis of bruits arising from the carotid bifurcation if we explore the entire upper chest and neck.[11] We now recommend comparing the intensity and spectral shape of the basal heart murmur, if present, and its radiation up the great vessels, with bruits arising from the innominate and subclavian arteries, the common carotid artery, and the carotid bifurcation.

DISCUSSION

Quantitative spectral phonoangiography remains an accurate noninvasive method for assessment of carotid stenosis. The results of 98 consecutive studies performed between 1975 and 1977 are shown in Fig. 33-4. The correlation between independent phonoangiographic and radiographic estimates of residual lumen diameter is shown in the figure. In only 7 instances of 98 correlations performed during that period did the phonoangiogram suggest significantly greater stenosis than was present radiographically, and in only 3 cases of the 98 did the test suggest that a lesion of 2 mm or less was not present when such a lesion was later surgically or radiographically demonstrated. The figure includes the results reported at the time the study was performed and therefore underestimates our present ability to make accurate phonoangiographic diagnosis, since our learning curve has been steep. For instance, of the 7 false positive results shown in Fig. 33-4, we would now recognize 5 as the results of bruit radiation, which is discussed later in this chapter. Following is a summary of our most recent results, a comparison of phonoangiographic and radiographic residual lumen diameters in 170 carotid stenoses. Bilateral carotid stenosis had occurred in 47 patients. Six (3.5%) of the bruits studied represented external carotid stenosis only. The residual lumen diameter was estimated by spectral phonoangiography and by x-ray angiography by independent observers who had no knowledge of the results of the other test. These data represent all comparison studies performed in our laboratory subsequent to the data graphed in Fig. 33-4.

Number of patients	123
Number of carotid bruits	170
Number (%) of studies agreeing to within 0.5 mm by the two methods	140 (83%)
Number (%) of studies agreeing to within 1 mm by the two methods	157 (93%)

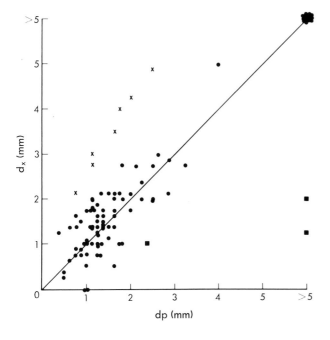

Fig. 33-4. Relationship between residual lumen diameter determined by phonoangiography (d_p) and that determined by x-ray angiography (d_x). In one instance where surgical specimen was obtained that differed markedly in residual lumen diameter from the patient's angiogram, former was used (see text). Instances in which phonoangiographic value was significantly less than radiographic value are represented by X, whereas those in which the converse was true are marked with solid squares.

Reproducibility, like accuracy, is an essential parameter of a useful diagnostic test. In carotid stenosis, good reproducibility enables a noninvasive test to be used to follow the natural history of the disease and to reserve surgical intervention for patients with hemodynamically significant lesions. In our experience over periods ranging from 6 months to 2 years, 86% to 88% of the carotid bruits subjected to multiple phonoangiographic analyses had break frequencies that varied less than 100 Hz, an amount that represented for most patients a change of less than 1 mm in residual lumen diameter. The patients whose bruit had a change of greater than 100 Hz within 13 to 24 months after the initial study had clinical evidence of progression of their disease. These data suggest that quantitative spectral phonoangiography is a highly reproducible test.

It is worthwhile to consider some of the possible sources of difference in the comparison of phonoangiography with standard radiographic carotid angiography. Where a long and complex lesion is present, the phonoangiogram gives an effective residual lumen diameter, whereas the radiographer generally reports the narrowest residual lumen. Similarly, when the lesion is oval or crescentic in cross section, as is often the case, the phonoangiogram gives the diameter of an equivalent round cross section, whereas the diameter may be overestimated or underestimated by x-ray examination, depending on the angle at which the vessel lies with respect to the film. Even when x-ray films are taken in two planes, as is usually the case, it is difficult to reconstruct the true cross section of the stenosis. The radiographic diameter may be considerably in error on occasion for reasons still unclear. For instance, in one of our patients the internal carotid origin had a radiographic diameter of 3.5 mm and a phonoangiographic diameter of 1 mm. At surgery the latter was found to be correct. When we compared the accuracy and applicability of spectral phonoangiography and contrast angiography in a blind series of 36 consecutive patients, comparing both tests with direct measurement of the pathologic specimens,[12] both methods gave comparable results.

Three specific situations in which confusion may arise in interpretation of the phonoangiogram are (1) when complete occlusion of the internal carotid artery is present, (2) when bruits from below (for example, from the common carotid origin, the innominate artery, or the aortic valve) are radiated up the carotid artery, and (3) when the external carotid artery is stenotic and produces a bruit.

The bruit arising from the carotid bifurcation when the internal carotid artery is occluded, as occurred in two of our studies of individual vessels (Fig. 33-4), is usually faint, with a break frequency inconsistent with its amplitude, for example, a low-amplitude bruit with a break frequency of 300 Hz. We know from experience that a 1.7 mm lesion, for instance, generally produces a loud bruit over the carotid bifurcation with a break frequency of about 300 Hz. When a low-amplitude, barely recordable bruit with break frequency of 300 Hz or greater is present, it often represents complete carotid occlusion, although it may also occur in critical carotid stenosis with a pinpoint residual lumen. In the case of complete carotid occlusion, the sound spectrum sometimes does not disclose a discrete peak characteristic of turbulent flow. Not infrequently a bruit, perhaps arising from collateral flow, is equally loud over a wide area and does not have maximum intensity over the carotid bifurcation—a requirement for the diagnosis of carotid stenosis.[5,6] Bruits on the side of a virtual or complete carotid occlusion are also often inconstant, heard one day but not the next. They are not changed by motion of the head or by the Valsalva maneuver, and this helps to differentiate them from cervical venous hums, which are often quite loud and sensitive to postural change, head rotation, and the phase of the respiratory cycle.

Phonoangiography is useful in the analysis of bruits arising from below the carotid bifurcation. In our early clinical experience,[5] when we did not record over the base of the heart and the neck, radiated murmurs and bruits were responsible for most of the bruits that we considered uninterpretable at that time. Some bruits, which we now recognize as radiated from below, were read as suggesting a moderately severe stenosis, that is, they were false positives. We have recently studied both the radiation of bruits arising from the heart and great vessels[11] and the sound spectrum of aortic stenosis.[10] The diagnosis of carotid stenosis can now be made with relative ease, even in the presence of bruits arising from lower in the arterial tree. These generally decrease in intensity as one ascends toward the skull, while carotid bruits are loudest over and above the carotid bifurcation. Occasionally basal heart murmurs are louder near the superior border of the thyroid cartilage than lower in the neck, probably because the carotid artery is

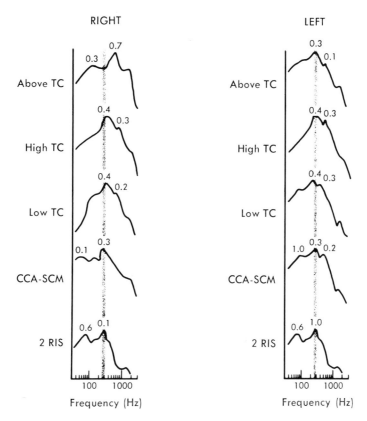

RIGHT

Above TC

High TC

Low TC

CCA-SCM

2 RIS

LEFT

Above TC

High TC

Low TC

CCA-SCM

2 RIS

Frequency (Hz)

Frequency (Hz)

Fig. 33-5. Montage of frequency-intensity spectra at multiple locations in patient with aortic valve stenosis and internal carotid stenosis. Intensity of major systolic frequency peak in aortic area *(2 RIS)* is represented as *1,* with intensity of the other major peaks shown in proportion to it. Shaded area represents approximate frequency of major peak seen in aortic area. At right, aortic murmur decreases in intensity as one ascends to common carotid artery at base of sternocleidomastoid muscle *(CCA-SCM)* and along thyroid cartilage *(Low TC and High TC)* to area over carotid bifurcation *(Above TC),* while higher frequency peak, arising from internal carotid lesion with residual lumen diameter of ≤1 mm, becomes louder as one approaches bifurcation. At left, by contrast, only radiated sound from aortic valve murmur can be seen at all levels.

closer to the skin surface there. This does not usually cause confusion, however, as the bruit is still louder where it originates—over the base of the heart—and the break frequency and shape of the sound spectrum of the heart murmur and the bruit are recognizably similar. A typical instance of the diagnosis of carotid stenosis in the presence of a loud aortic murmur is shown in Fig. 33-5.

When the external carotid artery is stenotic at its origin and the internal carotid is occluded (or widely patent), a bruit over the carotid bifurcation may not signify internal carotid stenosis. Fortunately, as mentioned earlier in this section, this is a relatively rare occurrence, making up less than 4% of all carotid bruits in our recent experience. The radiation of the bruit may be an index of its source.[11] Bruits arising from the external carotid artery tend

to be conducted up its branches and can be heard over the preauricular artery, whereas internal carotid bruits are not usually audible there.

Exact diagnosis of all locations and combinations of lesions around the carotid bifurcation has been greatly facilitated by the development of a commercial instrument for duplex B scan and Doppler assessment of the carotid bifurcation (Chapter 38). When the Spectraview was used in combination with duplex ultrasound scanning in patients with *and* without carotid bruits, accurate diagnosis of carotid stenosis or occlusion was made in 95% of the vessels studied.[14]

Phonoangiography is theoretically applicable wherever a stenotic artery creates a bruit.[17] It has been applied, with apparent success, to other branches of the aortic arch besides the carotid arteries[19] and the aortic valve.[9] An important requirement is that arterial flow velocity either be relatively constant, as is the case with the carotid artery,[3,16] so that an estimated value can be used, or that it be measured by independent means, for example, range-gated pulsed Doppler ultrasound.[10] With the aid of the latter, which is also a noninvasive method, we believe that bruits arising from most of the heart valves and major blood vessels can be analyzed.

Rosen et al.[19] have suggested that the percentage of patients with carotid disease and noticeable bruits is relatively small. Our experience has been quite the opposite; perhaps because our institutions are regional referral centers for cerebrovascular surgery, the majority of our patients with carotid disease have audible and recordable bruits.

Besides being noninvasive, relatively rapid, and painless for the patient, phonoangiography is simple in terms of analysis. Our present commercially available analytical equipment uses a microprocessor and costs relatively little both in time and in money. We think that it should be used in noninvasive evaluation of every patient with cervical bruits.

ACKNOWLEDGMENTS

We are grateful to the neurologic staffs of the Massachusetts General and New England Deaconess Hospitals for referring patients for study, and to Dr. Jay P. Mohr, Dr. Robert G. Ojemann, and Dr. C. Miller Fisher for helpful discussions.

REFERENCES

1. Ackerman, R.H.: A perspective on noninvasive diagnosis of carotid disease, Neurology 29:615, 1979.
2. Barnes, R.W.: Noninvasive diagnostic techniques in peripheral vascular disease, Am. Heart J. 97:241, 1979.
3. Desser, K.B., Harris, C.L., and Benchimol, A.: Carotid blood velocity during cough studies in man, Stroke 7:416, 1976.
4. Dewey, C.F., Jr., Metzinger, R.W., and Lees, R.S.: A small replicable computer system for clinical analysis, Proc. San Diego Biomed. Symp. 15:41, 1976.
5. Duncan, G.W., et al.: Evaluation of carotid stenosis by phonoangiography, N. Engl. J. Med. 293:1124, 1975.
6. Fredberg, J.J.: Pseudo-sound generation at atherosclerotic constrictions in arteries, Bull. Math. Biol. 36:143, 1974.
7. Fredberg, J.J., Lees, R.S., and Dewey, C.F., Jr.: How to listen to your arteries (or what your doctor would hear if he were a fluid dynamicist), Paper no. 70-144, Proceedings of the American Institute of Aeronautics and Astronautics Aerospace Sciences Meeting, New York, 1970.
8. Gurll, N., Dewey, C.F., Jr., and Lees, R.S.: Phonoangiography: a noninvasive technique for diagnosis of arterial disease, Circulation 43(2):173, 1971.
9. Johnson, G., Adolph, R.J., and Campbell, D.J.: Estimation of the severity of aortic valve stenosis by frequency analysis of the murmur, J. Am. Coll. Cardiol. 1:1315, 1983.
10. Keller, H.M., et al.: Noninvasive measurement of velocity profiles and blood flow in the common carotid artery by pulsed Doppler ultrasound, Stroke 7:370, 1976.
11. Kistler, J.P., et al.: The bruit of carotid stenosis versus radiated basal heart murmurs. Differentiation by phonoangiography, Circulation 57:975, 1978.
12. Kistler, J.P., et al.: Correlation of spectral phonoangiography and carotid angiography with gross pathology in carotid stenosis, N. Engl. J. Med. 305:417-419, 1981.
13. Lees, R.S., and Dewey, C.F., Jr.: Phonoangiography: a new noninvasive diagnostic method for studying arterial disease, Proc. Natl. Acad. Sci. USA 67:935, 1970.
14. Lees, R.S., Kistler, J.P., and Sanders, D.: Duplex Doppler scanning and spectral bruit analysis for diagnosing carotid stenosis, Circulation 66(1):102, 1982.
15. Lees, R.S., Miller, A., and Kistler, J.P.: Quantitative carotid phonoangiography. In Nicolaides, A., and Yao, J., editors: The investigation of vascular disorders, Edinburgh, 1981, Churchill Livingstone.
16. Lees, R.S., and Myers, G.S.: Noninvasive diagnosis of arterial disease, Adv. Intern. Med. 27:475, 1982.
17. Miller, A., et al.: Spectral analysis of arterial bruits (phonoangiography):experimental validation, Circulation 61:515, 1980.
18. Mohr, J.P., Fisher, C.M., and Adams, R.D.: Cerebrovascular diseases. In Isselbacher, K.J., et al., editors: Harrison's principles of internal medicine, ed. 9, New York, 1980, McGraw-Hill, Inc.
19. Rosen, R.M., et al.: Phonoangiography by autocorrelation, Circulation 55:626, 1977.

CHAPTER 34

Doppler ultrasonic arteriography and flow velocity analysis in carotid artery disease

DAVID S. SUMNER, DERMOT J. MOORE, and RICHARD D. MILES

Early in the past decade, it became evident that indirect physiologic tests had a limited role in the evaluation of symptomatic cerebrovascular disease. These tests were never expected to identify low-grade lesions, such as ulcerated plaques or stenoses that narrowed the carotid lumen by less than 50%, but it was disconcerting to find that they were highly sensitive only to high-grade lesions and that many moderate stenoses in the 50% to 75% range were being missed.[23] Moreover, the indirect tests were incapable of distinguishing high-grade stenoses from total occlusions. Prompted by a growing dissatisfaction with the indirect tests, several groups who were searching for a practical noninvasive method for imaging the carotid bifurcation independently and almost simultaneously came up with the idea of using the Doppler-shifted signal to map the flow stream.[11,14,18,19] These methods relied on the motion of blood to serve as a contrast medium, somewhat analogous to the use of iodinated compounds in conventional arteriography. The resulting images resembled those obtained with conventional arteriography; hence the name *ultrasonic arteriography* (Fig. 34-1).

The method introduced by Hokanson et al.[14] in 1971 employed pulsed Doppler ultrasound.[18] Although other investigators favored continuous-wave (CW) devices, it was felt that the pulsed technique—though more complicated and perhaps somewhat more difficult to use—had certain advantages. Because of the ability to select the depth of flow recording, the pulsed Doppler arteriograph was more discriminating than the CW devices and was capable of providing both longitudinal and horizontal, cross-sectional views.

From the outset, the diagnostic superiority of the ultrasonic arteriograph, compared with indirect testing, was apparent.[2,25] Not only was the device capable of accurately identifying hemodynamically significant lesions, it also frequently detected low-grade lesions, distinguished between total occlusion and severe stenosis with moderate accuracy, and permitted some estimate of the degree of stenosis. There were, however, some deficits that proved troublesome. Calcification, which severely attenuates ultrasound, led to confusing blank areas in the image—precluding the accurate estimation of stenosis. Areas in which flow was severely reduced, reversed, or stagnant could not be imaged. Even in normal individuals, the outer aspects of the carotid bulb, where flow is sluggish or reversed, were not well outlined. For the same reason, roughened or ulcerated plaques along the arterial wall were seldom visualized. Patent arteries with very tight stenoses at their origins were not imaged, leading to the erroneous assumption that the arteries were occluded. Finally, unless scanning was done in multiple planes, asymmetric stenoses were missed. Thus the flow-map image was at times misleading.

Because astute technicians quickly learn to distinguish normal and abnormal Doppler flow signals, some of these problems were avoided by the simple expedient of listening to the audible output. To make the interpretations of flow signals more objective, however, it became our practice—and that of others—to incorporate real-time spectral analysis into the routine scanning procedure.[3,5,22] In addition, by interfacing a microcomputer with the basic ultrasonic arteriographic instrument, we were able to obtain simultaneous images in multiple planes—an approach that decreased the likelihood of missing asymmetric lesions.[16,17,21]

349

Presently, the only viable noninvasive alternative to the flow-mapping method is the real-time ultrasonic echo technique. Part of the appeal of echo imaging is the real-time aspect itself, which (rightly or wrongly) is perceived by many as a definite advantage. Under ideal circumstances and at the proper focal length, the resolution of the echo image is potentially much greater than that of the Doppler flow map, permitting identification of small plaques and ulcers. Characterization of plaque morphology may also be possible. Nevertheless, superior accuracy is attained only when the echo image is combined with spectral analysis of the Doppler flow signal.[20] Studies are time-consuming, highly dependent on the technician, and often difficult to interpret, and they must be visualized in real time to obtain the maximum information. Moreover, the instruments are quite expensive. Pulsed Doppler arteriographs, on the other hand, are relatively inexpensive; studies can be performed rapidly; the images are easily recorded and can be interpreted after the study has been completed; and the overall accuracy is reasonably good. For these reasons, ultrasonic arteriography remains popular and, in our laboratory, continues to be the mainstay of our diagnostic approach to extracranial carotid arterial disease.

METHODOLOGY

The design of the pulsed Doppler ultrasonic arteriograph and the theoretic rationale governing its application are described in Chapter 20.

Studies are accomplished with the patient lying supine, with the head turned slightly away from the side of the examination. Guided by the audible output, the technician begins the scan in the common carotid artery. The six gates of the Hokanson pulsed Doppler arteriograph are adjusted to the proper depth and are separated sufficiently to provide optimum insonation of the lumen of the underlying artery. The technician then gradually moves the probe up the neck, sweeping it slightly from side to side to ensure complete interrogation of the interface between the flow stream and the vascular wall. Whenever flow in the proper direction is encountered, a dot appears on the oscilloscope screen—its position being determined by the spatial location of the position-sensing arm. After reaching the bifurcation, the technician continues the scanning process up the internal carotid artery, adjusting the depth of the gates to optimize the signal, until further progress is precluded by the mandible. At that point, the probe is shifted anteriorly and medially to identify the more pulsatile signal arising from the external carotid artery. The

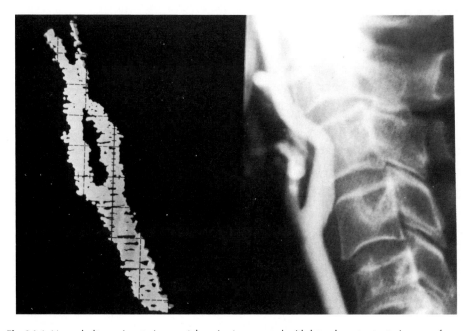

Fig. 34-1. Normal ultrasonic arteriogram (plan view) compared with lateral contrast arteriogram of same bifurcation.

external carotid is then traced back to its origin from the carotid bifurcation, thus completing the scan. In a normal individual, the entire image can be produced in 3 to 5 minutes. When disease is present, the process is more time-consuming but seldom requires more than 10 minutes.

Every effort is made to avoid the temptation to retrace the image to fill in blank areas or smooth out rough edges. Since the patient may have moved slightly, such attempts to clean up the image may obscure small plaques and result in false negative studies. If the image is of poor or questionable quality or if there is any doubt about the presence of a lesion, it is far better to repeat the entire procedure.

During the scanning process, the Doppler signal is continuously fed through a real-time spectral analyzer. This enables the technician to identify those areas in which the spectrum is distorted so that appropriate hard-copy recordings can be made. It also sharpens the technician's ability to interpret the audible Doppler signal. When recordings are made, as mentioned earlier, the depth of the recording gate is carefully adjusted to optimize the signal. In all cases, Doppler spectra are obtained from the common carotid artery just proximal to the bifurcation, from the internal carotid just distal to the bulb, and from any area in which stenosis is suspected. At the end of each scan, the technician records the extent and location of the disease, based on both the audible signal and the appearance of the image.

INTERPRETATION OF THE IMAGE

The images obtained by the procedure just described are called *plan views*. They correspond roughly to a lateral projection of the carotid bifurcation. Because the posterior wall of the carotid artery is the most common site of disease, the plan view is the single best projection. In our experience, the image itself has proved to be of considerable diagnostic value, often correlating very well with conventional angiograms (Figs. 34-1 to 34-3). In practice, however, the technician's assessment of the audible Doppler flow signal is taken into account when the final interpretation is made. For example, finding a high-pitched, harsh signal just distal to the point where the lumen appears narrowed tends to support the diagnosis of severe stenosis. On the other hand, finding a normal signal just distal to a blank area suggests that the blank area represents sonic opacity caused by calcification rather than an occlusion or severe stenosis. An abrupt cutoff of the image with an equally abrupt

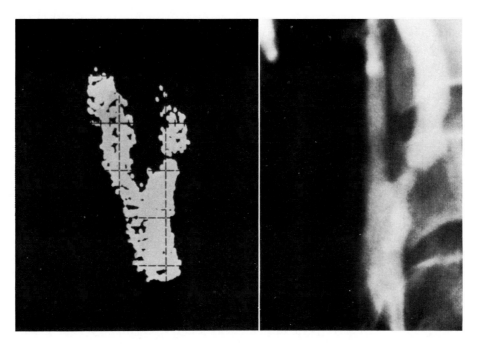

Fig. 34-2. Ultrasonic arteriogram and lateral contrast arteriogram showing 90% stenosis of internal carotid artery.

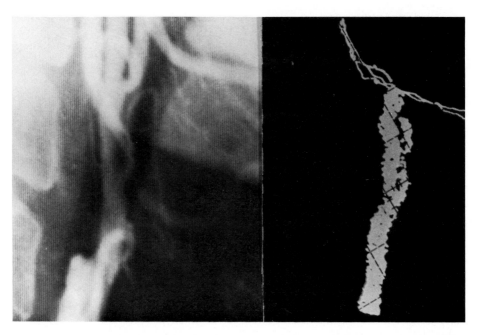

Fig. 34-3. Ultrasonic arteriogram and lateral contrast arteriogram showing occluded internal carotid artery. External carotid artery and two of its branches are visualized. This particular study was misinterpreted by initial reader as showing patent internal and external carotid arteries. Reference to angle of mandible (which had been "drawn" on screen) would have clarified situation. (From Sumner, D.S., et al.: Noninvasive diagnosis of extracranial carotid artery disease: a prospective evaluation of pulsed-Doppler imaging and oculoplethysmography, Arch. Surg. 114:1222, 1979. Copyright 1979, American Medical Association.)

reconstitution distal to a blank area also suggests calcification. Real stenoses, in contrast, usually show a tapering of the image both proximal and distal to the site of the greatest narrowing of the arterial lumen.

The audible signal also helps distinguish the internal, external, and common carotid arteries. Thus the audible signal is particularly important when only one vessel can be outlined distal to the bifurcation. In fact, it may provide the only way of identifying which of the two branches is occluded and which is patent—or which is stenotic and which is normal. Although the internal carotid artery usually lies posterior to the external carotid artery and its image is usually directed posterior to the angle of the mandible, in some patients the arrangement is reversed.

An experienced technician seldom has difficulty deciding on the origin of the signals. Since the internal carotid artery feeds the low-resistance cerebrovascular bed, flow rates are high even during diastole; consequently, signals from this artery normally have a higher frequency than those from the common or external carotid arteries and are con-

tinuous throughout the cardiac cycle. The signal from the external carotid artery, which supplies the face, neck, and other vascular beds that have a relatively high resistance, is typically quite pulsatile, with the biphasic or triphasic signal resembling that obtained from the radial or other peripheral arteries. Reversed flow is not uncommon in the external carotid artery during diastole. Some confusion may arise, however, when the internal carotid artery is occluded and the external carotid artery is called on to function as a major collateral channel, supplying blood to the intracranial tissues. In this event the external carotid signal may assume some of the characteristics of the internal carotid signal. Although signals from the common carotid share the attributes of signals from both of the other arteries, they more commonly resemble those of the internal carotid; when the internal carotid artery is occluded, the common carotid signal approaches that of the external. Because flow disturbances are normally present at the carotid bifurcation, signals from this area commonly have a rough or harsh quality. A cautious technician will, therefore, avoid overinterpretation of signals derived from the vi-

Table 34-1. Accuracy of pulsed Doppler ultrasonic arteriography for detecting any disease in the internal carotid artery that is visible on conventional arteriography

Authors	Sensitivity (%)	Specificity (%)	PPV (%)	NPV (%)	Accuracy (%)
Blackshear et al., 1979[5]	39/56 (70)	7/8 (88)	39/40 (98)	7/24 (29)	46/64 (72)
Sumner et al., 1979[25]*	95/123 (77)	70/86 (81)	95/111 (86)	70/98 (71)	165/209 (79)
Hobson et al., 1980[12]	37/45 (82)	30/34 (88)	37/41 (90)	30/38 (79)	67/79 (85)
Warlow and Fish, 1980[26]	25/33 (76)	16/17 (94)	25/26 (96)	16/24 (67)	41/50 (82)
Cardullo et al., 1982[7]	180/247 (73)	67/77 (87)	180/190 (95)	67/134 (50)	247/324 (76)
Sumner et al., 1982[24]	246/345 (71)	167/226 (74)	246/305 (81)	167/266 (63)	413/571 (72)
Doorly et al., 1982[9]	109/114 (96)	60/76 (79)	109/125 (87)	60/65 (92)	169/190 (89)
Wasserman et al., 1983[27]	56/71 (79)	41/44 (93)	56/59 (95)	41/56 (73)	97/115 (84)
Cumulative	692/911 (76)	388/482 (80)	692/786 (88)	388/607 (64)	1080/1393 (78)

*Not included in cumulative values, since same studies are duplicated in Sumner et al. (1982).

Table 34-2. Accuracy of pulsed Doppler ultrasonic arteriography for distinguishing hemodynamically and nonhemodynamically significant disease of the internal carotid artery

Authors	Sensitivity (%)	Specificity (%)	PPV (%)	NPV (%)	Accuracy (%)
Barnes et al., 1976[2]	23/25 (92)	37/57 (65)	23/43 (53)	37/39 (95)	60/82 (73)
Blackshear et al., 1979[5]	23/26 (88)	32/38 (84)	23/29 (79)	32/35 (91)	55/64 (86)
Sumner et al., 1979[25]*†	60/69 (87)	127/140 (91)	60/73 (82)	127/136 (93)	187/209 (89)
Wolf, 1979[28]†	87/94 (93)	100/109 (92)	87/96 (91)	100/107 (93)	187/203 (92)
Hobson et al., 1980[12]*	25/27 (93)	49/52 (94)	25/28 (89)	49/51 (96)	74/79 (94)
Cardullo et al., 1981[7]	129/141 (91)	153/183 (84)	129/159 (81)	153/165 (93)	282/324 (87)
Hobson et al., 1981[13]	47/54 (87)	127/156 (81)	47/76 (62)	127/134 (95)	174/210 (83)
Bodily et al., 1981[6]	22/23 (96)	22/23 (96)	22/23 (96)	22/23 (96)	44/46 (96)
Sumner et al., 1982[24]†	185/209 (89)	313/362 (86)	185/234 (79)	313/337 (93)	498/571 (87)
Doorly et al., 1982[9]	50/53 (94)	130/137 (95)	50/57 (88)	130/133 (98)	180/190 (95)
Wasserman et al., 1983[27]	39/45 (87)	69/70 (99)	39/40 (98)	69/75 (92)	108/115 (94)
Cumulative	605/670 (90)	983/1135 (87)	605/757 (80)	983/1048 (94)	1588/1805 (88)

*Not included in cumulative values, since same studies are duplicated in Sumner et al. (1982) and Hobson et al. (1981).
†Dividing line between positive and negative studies set at 40% stenosis, others set at 50% stenosis.

Table 34-3. Accuracy of pulsed Doppler ultrasonic arteriography for distinguishing occluded and nonoccluded internal carotid arteries

Authors	Sensitivity (%)	Specificity (%)	PPV (%)	NPV (%)	Accuracy (%)
Barnes et al., 1976[2]	14/14 (100)	65/68 (96)	14/17 (82)	65/65 (100)	79/82 (96)
Hobson et al., 1980[12]	17/17 (100)	59/62 (95)	17/20 (85)	59/59 (100)	76/79 (96)
Warlow and Fish, 1980[26]	6/6 (100)	43/44 (98)	6/7 (86)	43/43 (100)	49/50 (98)
Cardullo et al., 1981[7]	31/37 (84)	280/287 (98)	31/38 (82)	280/286 (98)	311/324 (96)
Sumner et al., 1982[24]	30/49 (61)	505/522 (97)	30/47 (64)	505/524 (96)	535/571 (94)
Doorly et al., 1982[9]	18/20 (90)	170/170 (100)	18/18 (100)	170/172 (99)	188/190 (99)
Wasserman et al., 1983[27]	22/25 (88)	86/90 (96)	22/26 (85)	86/89 (97)	108/115 (94)
Cumulative	138/168 (82)	1208/1243 (97)	138/173 (80)	1208/1238 (98)	1346/1411 (95)

cinity of the carotid bifurcation or the carotid bulb.

In this chapter, unless otherwise indicated, when we speak of the interpretation of the pulsed Doppler image, it is assumed that the interpretation is based on both the image and the audible Doppler signal.

Accuracy

Several independent groups have assessed the accuracy of pulsed Doppler ultrasonic arteriography, using conventional arteriography as the standard. As shown in Tables 34-1 to 34-3, the results have been fairly consistent from one institution to another and have not changed appreciably with time.

It appears that a negative ultrasonic arteriogram cannot be depended on to rule out the presence of all angiographically detectable disease of the internal carotid artery, since the cumulative data show a negative predictive value (NPV) of only 64% (Table 34-1). In other words, 36% of the internal carotid arteries reported to be free of disease on ultrasonic arteriography actually are not. On the other hand, a positive study has a reasonably good chance of being correct; the combined data in Table 34-1 show a positive predictive value (PPV) of 88%. The test reliably rules out hemodynamically significant disease (94% NPV) but less accurately identifies those arteries with disease of this magnitude (Table 34-2). In reality, 20% of the internal carotid arteries reported to have diameter reductions exceeding 50% have less severe disease (80% PPV). If the ultrasonic arteriogram reveals an artery thought to be the internal carotid, there is an excellent chance that the internal carotid is patent (98% NPV); but 20% of the internal carotid arteries that are thought to be occluded actually turn out to be patent (80% PPV) (Table 34-3).

In five reports the data were sufficiently complete to permit categorization of the ultrasonic and x-ray results into four disease categories: normal, <50% stenosis, ≥50% stenosis, and total occlusion.[7,9,12,24,27] Sixty-nine percent of the 1279 studies agreed. The κ value, a measure of the degree of correlation[8], was 0.569 ± 0.018, which is somewhat inferior to the κ values of both digital subtraction angiography (Chapter 40) and duplex scanning.[10,20]

Table 34-4 shows the predictive value of the ultrasonic arteriographic scans divided into the four categories just mentioned. Of 559 internal carotid arteries whose scans were interpreted as being normal, 65% had entirely normal x-ray results; 30% had nonhemodynamically significant disease; and only 5% had diameter stenosis exceeding 50%. Although one fourth of the arteries whose scans indicated <50% stenosis were normal, few had hemodynamically significant lesions. When the ultrasonic arteriogram indicated severe stenosis or total occlusion, only 7% to 8% of the arteries were normal; in other words, 92% to 93% had at least some disease.

To see whether accuracy could be improved by a stricter or more lenient reading of the ultrasonic image, we used the receiver operating characteristic (ROC) curve format to plot our results.[15,24] The three curves in Fig. 34-4 represent data developed when *any* stenosis visible on the arteriogram was called positive (>0%), when any stenosis greater than 20% was called positive, and when only those lesions with stenoses greater than 40% were called positive. As expected, accuracy was greatest for the 40% curve and least for the >0% curve. Although reading the tests leniently (calling the image positive if any degree of stenosis was visible on the ultrasonic scan) improved sensitivity somewhat, specificity suffered. Reading the tests strictly (calling only those images positive that appear to have a 60% stenosis or greater) improved specificity but had a detrimental effect on sensitivity. It appeared that the optimum balance between

Table 34-4. Predictive value of ultrasonic arteriography for disease of the internal carotid artery[7,9,12,24,27]

Ultrasonic arteriographic reading	Number of arteries	Distribution according to conventional arteriographic reading			
		Normal	1%-49% Stenosis	50%-99% Stenosis	Occluded
Normal	559	65.3%	29.7%	3.6%	1.4%
1%-49% Stenosis	202	25.2%	65.3%	8.9%	0.5%
50%-99% Stenosis	369	8.4%	12.5%	73.4%	5.7%
Occluded	149	6.7%	2.0%	12.1%	79.2%

sensitivity and specificity was achieved when the same criteria were used for both the ultrasonic and the conventional arteriographic image. In other words, overreading or underreading the image will not increase accuracy.

Uninterpretable studies

In six reports the incidence of uninterpretable studies varied from 3% to 7%, the cumulative value being 6% (85 cases out of 1406 studies).* Some of the uninterpretable studies were ascribed to technical factors, usually related to a short thick neck, scar tissue, a high bifurcation, or patient motion; but the majority were caused by calcification. Wasserman et al.[27] observed that echo-free areas were significantly more likely to be found in arteries with hemodynamically significant stenoses than in arteries with less severe disease.

SOURCES OF ERROR

The accuracy of ultrasonic arteriography ultimately depends on the skill, concentration, and experience of the technician. Probably the single most important cause of poor results is lack of expertise on the part of the examiner. Results rap-

*References 5, 7, 12, 24, 25, 26.

idly improve as the technician becomes more familiar with the procedure, learns to recognize and cope with anatomic variations, and develops an ear for the Doppler signal.

Errors in technique include retracing the image to smooth out rough edges. This procedure tends to obscure small lesions and to lessen the apparent severity of larger ones. Moving the probe too rapidly along the course of the artery can leave ragged edges that simulate lesions. Failure to explore the neck adequately or to adjust the depth of the flow gates may lead to serious false positive errors.

Tortuosity of the internal carotid artery, low or high bifurcations, and reversal of the positions of the internal and external carotid arteries are among the anatomic variations that might confuse an examiner. False negative studies occur when the disease lies either proximal or distal to the area scanned. While such errors may be unavoidable, they are more frequent when the scan is hastily performed and when only those areas in the immediate vicinity of the carotid bifurcation are interrogated. Misinterpreting a patent external carotid for the internal carotid artery, which may be occluded or severely stenotic, is a particularly treacherous cause of false negative errors (Fig. 34-3). As mentioned previously, the external carotid ar-

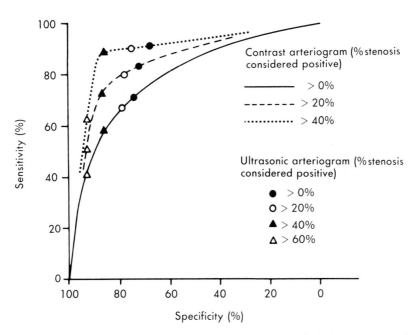

Fig. 34-4. Receiver-operating characteristic curves comparing accuracy of ultrasonic arteriography with conventional arteriography. (From Sumner, D.S., Russell, J.B., and Miles, R.D.: Surgery 91:700, 1982.)

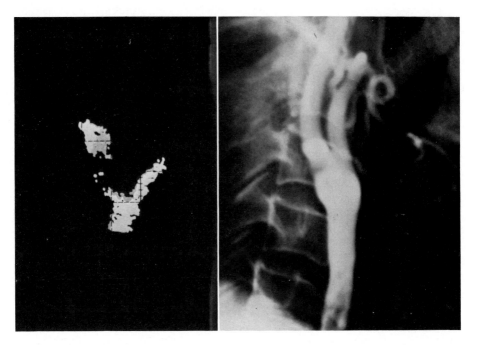

Fig. 34-5. Sonic opacification resulting in blank area on ultrasound scan. Bifurcation appeared normal on x-ray film.

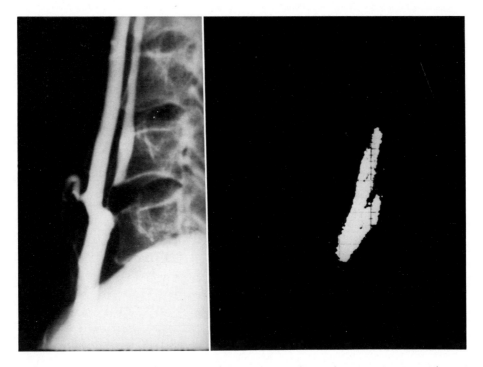

Fig. 34-6. Contrast arteriogram showing severely stenotic internal carotid artery (string sign). Ultrasonic arteriogram implied total occlusion.

tery under these circumstances may enlarge and its signal may come to resemble that of the internal vessel.

Other causes of error are less technician dependent. Sonic opacity resulting from calcification is not only a frequent cause of uninterpretable studies but also may mask a stenosis, mimic an occlusion, or exaggerate the extent of the disease—even in scans of acceptable overall quality (Fig. 34-5). Small lesions, nonstenotic plaques, and wall irregularities are more difficult to recognize than the more stenotic lesions because the resolving power of the instrument is limited by the dimensions of the pulsed Doppler sample volume (about 1 to 2 mm). The area sampled by the Doppler gates almost invariably overlaps the edges of the lumen. Whether a Doppler signal powerful enough to unblank the oscilloscope screen is received depends on the extent of the overlap and the velocity and direction of flow. It is easy to see, therefore, how the flow map may either overestimate or underestimate the degree of stenosis.

Ulcers are incapable of being delineated, since blood at the base of the ulcer cavity moves too slowly to activate the Doppler velocity detector. Reduced, absent, reversed, or disturbed flow—as mentioned earlier in the chapter—cannot be im-

aged and may be responsible for both false positive and false negative errors. For example, beyond a very severe stenosis the velocity and quantity of flow may be too low to be detected, leading to the mistaken impression that the artery is occluded (Fig. 34-6). Because flow separation (an area of stagnant or reversed flow) occurs in the proximal internal carotid artery near the wall opposite the flow divider, the image seldom outlines the entire lumen of the carotid bulb; consequently, plaques in this area may escape detection. On the other hand, distorted audible signals caused by the flow disturbances common in this area may suggest the presence of a lesion when none is present. Low cardiac output, stenoses at the origin of the carotid arteries, or severe intracranial stenoses occasionally compromise the ability to obtain a good image.

Projection errors

Arteriosclerotic plaques are usually assymmetric. Surgeons and radiologists have long emphasized the need to obtain views in more than one plane to avoid missing, overestimating, or underestimating lesions (Fig. 34-7). Because the *plan view* produced by the ultrasonic arteriograph roughly corresponds to a lateral x-ray projection and since most plaques involve the posterior wall of

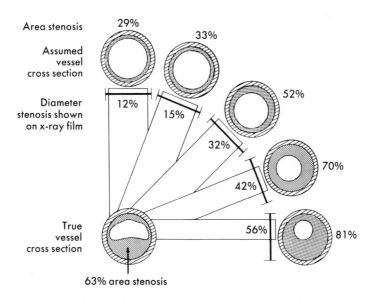

Fig. 34-7. Apparent degrees of area and diameter stenosis when asymmetric lesion is visualized in different projections. (From Sumner, D.S., Russell, J.B., and Miles, R.D.: Pulsed-Doppler arteriography and computer assisted imaging of the carotid bifurcation. In Bergan, J.J., and Yao, J.S.T., editors: Cerebrovascular insufficiency, New York, 1983, Grune & Stratton, Inc.)

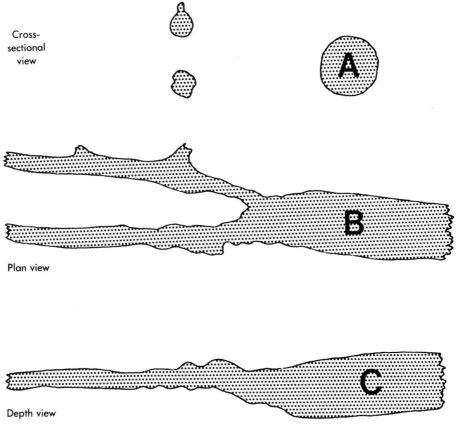

Cross-
sectional
view

Plan view

Depth view

Fig. 34-8. Projection planes that can be obtained with pulsed Doppler ultrasonic arteriograph. *A,* transverse cross section; *B,* plan (lateral) view; *C,* longitudinal (depth) view (roughly corresponds to anteroposterior projection). (From Sumner, D.S., Russell, J.B., and Miles, R.D.: Pulsed-Doppler arteriography and computer assisted imaging of the carotid bifurcation. In Bergan, J.J., and Yao, J.S.T., editors: Cerebrovascular insufficiency, New York, 1983, Grune & Stratton, Inc.)

the carotid arteries, the majority of lesions at the carotid bifurcation should be detected. A few, however, will be missed.

As described in Chapter 20, the pulsed Doppler ultrasonic arteriograph is capable of providing longitudinal (depth) and transverse cross-sectional views (Fig. 34-8). In the plan view, the long axis of the probe is aligned with the position-sensing arm. To obtain longitudinal and transverse cross-sectional views, the probe must be reoriented so that its long axis is perpendicular to the position-sensing arm. Scanning with the probe in this position is more difficult. Moreover, to obtain both plan (lateral) and longitudinal, cross-sectional (depth) views, it is necessary to perform two separate studies, thereby increasing the time required for each examination. For these reasons, longitudinal and cross-sectional views are rarely obtained in most laboratories. Thus the full potential of the pulsed Doppler arteriograph is seldom realized.

COMPUTER INTERFACE

To obtain simultaneous plan and longitudinal views of the carotid bifurcation, we interfaced the pulsed Doppler ultrasonic arteriograph to a microcomputer.[16,17,21] The computer is programmed to digitize the x-y position of the transducer, input binary flow signals from the six range gates, and output a signal that controls the depth of the gates (Fig. 34-9).

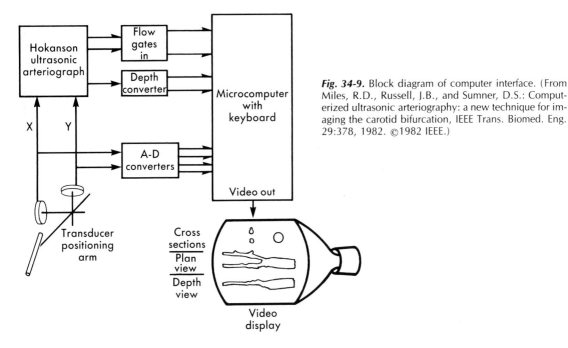

Fig. 34-9. Block diagram of computer interface. (From Miles, R.D., Russell, J.B., and Sumner, D.S.: Computerized ultrasonic arteriography: a new technique for imaging the carotid bifurcation, IEEE Trans. Biomed. Eng. 29:378, 1982. ©1982 IEEE.)

The procedure requires no shift of the position of the probe and no more time and little more expertise than required for conventional plan-view scanning. Both the lateral and depth images appear simultaneously on the video display. In most scans the depth image corresponds roughly to an anteroposterior view. After the common and internal carotid arteries have been examined, the video display is turned off before examining the external carotid artery. This avoids confusing superimposition of the images of the external and internal carotid arteries. At any point during the scanning routine, a transverse cross section can be obtained by activating the proper control button on the keyboard of the computer.

But even simultaneous orthogonal views can overestimate or underestimate the reduction in cross-sectional area (Fig. 34-10).[17] To provide a histogram depicting the cross-sectional areas of the common and internal carotid arteries, the x, y, and z coordinates of the insonated tissue are used to develop a three-dimensional matrix in the computer memory. When flow is detected by a sample gate, a bit in the memory matrix is changed from 0 to 1. As the probe is swept across the long axis of the vessel, the contents of the matrix are summed at 1.0 mm intervals. The resulting area histogram appears on the video monitor simultaneously with the lateral and anteroposterior views (Fig. 34-11).

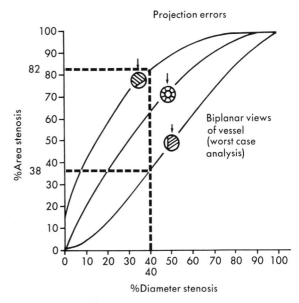

Fig. 34-10. Relationship between area stenosis and diameter stenosis when artery is asymmetrically narrowed *(upper and lower lines)* and when it is symmetrically narrowed *(middle line)*. Two orthogonal projections are assumed. Arrows indicate direction of x-ray beam in projection showing greater degree of narrowing. An apparent 40% diameter stenosis could correspond to 38% to 82% area reduction. (From Sumner, D.S., Russell, J.B., and Miles, R.D.: Pulsed-Doppler arteriography and computer assisted imaging of the carotid bifurcation. In Bergan, J.J., and Yao, J.S.T., editors: Cerebrovascular insufficiency, New York, 1983, Grune & Stratton, Inc.)

After the examination is completed, the data table is used to generate a diameter histogram by taking the square root of the area plot. This histogram depicts the diameter of the vessel as if it were symmetrically narrowed.

The images can be photographed directly from the video screen, stored on diskettes, or reproduced rapidly and inexpensively with a thermal printer.

SPECTRUM ANALYSIS

Valuable additional information can be obtained by analyzing the audio output of the pulsed Doppler system with a real-time fast Fourier transform (FFT) spectral analyzer.[1,3,5,22] The sites at which the spectra are recorded are indicated on the plan view by a vertical bar. The same computer used to generate the histograms and the orthogonal images can also be employed to store frequency data and to calculate peak and mode frequencies, band widths, and other parameters. The spectra and the calculated parameters are displayed simultaneously on the video screen with the images (Figs. 34-12 to 34-14).

Unlike the duplex scanner, the ultrasonic arteriograph does not depict the position of the sample volume within the vessel lumen. It is necessary, therefore for the technician to adjust the depth of the recording gate until the best signal is obtained. This should approximate the center of the flow stream. Also, the angle at which the sound beam intersects the flow stream cannot be determined from the pulsed Doppler image. This results in some lack of standardization of the recorded frequencies. However, by adjusting the probe to optimize the signal, the technician can minimize this variability.

Results

Spectra have been classified into four categories based on the presence or absence of a systolic window and the peak systolic frequency[1,5,20]:

Category I—spectra with windows and peak frequencies of less than 4 kHz

Category II—spectra with reduced or absent windows but peak frequencies of less than 4 kHz

Category III—spectra with or without windows but with frequencies exceeding 4 kHz

Category IV—pulsatile spectra typical of an external carotid signal

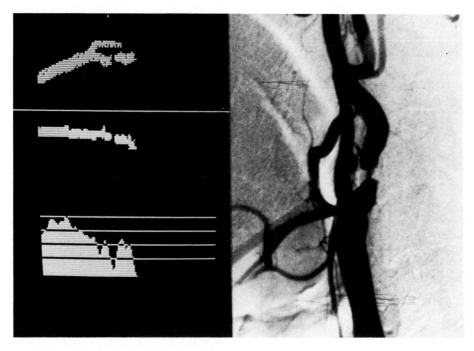

Fig. 34-11. Computerized ultrasonic arteriogram and lateral contrast arteriogram of same bifurcation. Upper panel shows lateral, or plan view; middle panel shows anteroposterior or depth view; lower panel shows area histogram. Histogram indicates 90% area reduction. (From Miles, R.D., et al.: Surgery 93:676, 1983.)

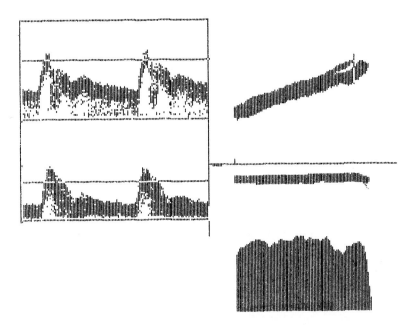

Fig. 34-12. Thermal printout of normal computerized ultrasonic arteriogram and spectral analysis. In lateral view, internal and external carotid arteries are superimposed near bifurcation. Spectra from bifurcation (dark line, lower panel) and from proximal internal carotid artery (light line, upper panel) show good systolic windows.

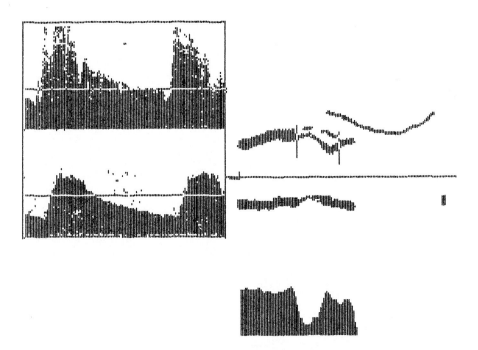

Fig. 34-13. Thermal printout of computerized ultrasonic arteriogram showing severely stenotic internal carotid artery. X-ray examination indicated 60% diameter reduction. Spectra show increased frequencies, disturbance of frequency envelope, and absence of systolic window.

Table 34-5. Internal carotid disease: accuracy of spectrum analysis

Signal characteristics			Number of arteries	Distribution according to conventional arteriographic reading			
Category	kHz	Window		Normal	1%-49% Stenosis	50%-99% Stenosis	Occluded
I	<4	Yes	123	94	28	0	1
II	<4	No	50	23	23	4	0
III	>4	Yes or No	52	6	5	40	1
IV	External signal		16	3	0	1	12
Uninterpretable			5	0	2	1	2

κ = 0.534 ± 0.046.

Table 34-6. Internal carotid disease: accuracy of computerized ultrasonic arteriography (CUA)

CUA reading	Number of arteries	Distribution according to conventional arteriographic reading			
		0	1%-49% Stenosis	50%-99% Stenosis	Occluded
Normal	111	92	18	1	0
1%-49% stenosis	56	22	30	3	1
50%-99% stenosis	43	2	5	35	1
Occluded	22	3	2	4	13
Uninterpretable	14	7	3	3	1

κ = 0.593 ± 0.044.

Results obtained with these criteria are shown in Table 34-5. Of the 246 internal carotid arteries studied, 5 (2%) of the spectra were felt to be uninterpretable.

Table 34-6 shows the results obtained with the computerized scan (results that reflect the technicians' comments regarding the scan) in the same group of patients who were studied by spectrum analysis. Fourteen of the 246 scans (6%) were uninterpretable. In this particular group of patients, the PPV for total occlusion was 59%, that is, out of 22 arteries that were shown to be totally occluded by computerized ultrasonic arteriography (CUA), only 13 were found to be occluded by conventional arteriography. This very low PPV was primarily the result of difficulties encountered with imaging large necks and failure to detect flow beyond severe stenoses.

Accuracy parameters from these studies are summarized in Tables 34-7 and 34-8. When the readers were blinded to the technicians' comments (image only), the results with the CUA were inferior to those reported when the technician's comments were also considered. In other words, the image alone had diagnostic value, but the input of the technician added considerably to its accuracy.

For distinguishing between hemodynamically significant and nonhemodynamically significant disease, the spectrum appeared to be equally as good as the image plus comments and was better than the image alone (Table 34-7). For detecting any disease, the spectrum was a little less sensitive than the image plus comments but was equally as good as the image alone (Table 34-8). The two modalities are complementary, however, and the results of both were considered in arriving at a final diagnosis. When the image and the spectrum agreed, as they did in 89% of the studies for hemodynamically significant disease and in 80% of those for any disease, all of the accuracy parameters were improved. If the overall result was called positive when either of the two tests were positive and negative when both were negative, sensitivity was improved; but specificity suffered—especially for identifying the absence of hemodynamically significant disease.

Table 34-7. Accuracy of CUA and Doppler spectrum analysis for distinguishing hemodynamically significant and nonhemodynamically significant disease of the internal carotid artery

Modality	Sensitivity (%)	Specificity (%)	PPV (%)	NPV (%)	Accuracy (%)
Image only	83	86	63	95	85
Image + comments*	91	93	82	97	93
Spectrum†	92	92	79	97	92
Image + spectrum					
Agree (89%)	98	94	84	99	95
Either positive	96	83	63	99	86

*Derived from data in Table 34-6.
†Derived from data in Table 34-5.

Table 34-8. Accuracy of CUA and Doppler spectrum analysis for identifying any (≥1% stenosis) disease of the internal carotid artery

Modality	Sensitivity (%)	Specificity (%)	PPV (%)	NPV (%)	Accuracy (%)
Image only	74	73	70	77	73
Image + comments*	83	77	78	83	80
Spectrum†	75	75	73	76	75
Image + spectrum					
Agree (80%)	88	93	91	90	91
Either positive	91	74	79	90	82

*Derived from data in Table 34-6.
†Derived from data in Table 34-5.

Both of the tests, separately and combined, had a high NPV for hemodynamically significant disease (Table 34-7). Therefore a negative result effectively ruled out lesions of this magnitude. The NPV for any disease was also acceptable when both tests were considered together (Table 34-8). PPVs, on the other hand, were insufficiently accurate to comfortably identify the presence of hemodynamically significant lesions (Table 34-7). Only when both tests agreed and both were positive could one be reasonably confident that some angiographically detectable lesion was present (Table 34-8). Nonetheless, if the scan suggested the presence of a hemodynamically significant lesion, only 8% (5 out of 65) of the arteries were entirely normal (Table 34-6).

These same data were used to determine to what extent different readers vary in their interpretation of test results. Correlations between three readers ranged from 93% to 95% for the spectrum, from 88% to 92% for the image alone, and 93% to 97% for the image plus technicians' comments. Two of the three readers were significantly more accurate in their interpretations of the spectrum than they were in their interpretation of the image alone. Accuracies were virtually the same when the readings of the spectrum were compared with those based on the image plus technicians' comment. Thus the raw images appear to be more difficult to interpret than the spectra; but this difference disappears when the technicians' comments are considered.

Application

In patients with lateralizing symptoms such as a transient ischemic attack (TIA), stroke, or amaurosis fugax, any lesion that could serve as an embolic focus should be identified. This includes not only severely stenotic plaques but also low-grade stenoses and ulcers. On the other hand, patients with ill-defined nonhemispheric symptoms or asymptomatic carotid bruits are considered to have an appreciably increased risk of stroke only when the internal carotid artery is narrowed by more than 50%. Therefore to provide effective noninvasive screening a test should be capable of identifying

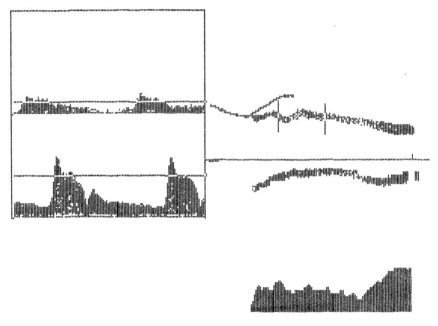

Fig. 34-14. Thermal printout of computerized ultrasonic arteriogram showing occluded internal carotid artery. In this example, external carotid image was recorded in depth view, and its area is depicted in histogram. Bottom spectrum, which was obtained near origin of external carotid, shows configuration typical of this vessel. Upper spectrum, which was obtained more distally, indicates decreased flow velocity.

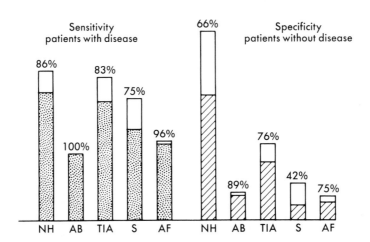

Fig. 34-15. Accuracy of ultrasonic arteriography for identifying patients with surgically correctable lesions of internal carotid arteries. Stippled areas indicate number of patients with positive studies in group with disease; cross-hatched areas indicate number of patients with negative studies in group without disease. *NH,* nonhemispheric; *AB,* asymptomatic bruit; *TIA,* transient ischemic attack; *S,* stroke; *AF,* amaurosis fugax. (From Sumner, D.S., Russell, J.B., and Miles, R.D.: Surgery 91:700, 1982.)

any and all lesions of the internal carotid artery in patients with lateralizing symptoms and be capable of distinguishing between hemodynamically significant and nonhemodynamically significant lesions in asymptomatic patients or patients with nonhemispheric symptoms.

In a previous study we found that the ultrasonic arteriograph correctly identified the presence of hemodynamically significant disease in all patients with asymptomatic bruits and in 86% of those with nonhemispheric symptoms (Fig. 34-15).[24] Any lesion that could have caused a TIA was identified in 83% of the patients with this symptom. In patients with amaurosis fugax, 96% of the potentially operable lesions were detected; only 75% of those that could have caused stroke were found. The specificity in all the diagnostic groups was less satisfactory, averaging 68% and ranging from 42% to 89% (Fig. 34-15). This, of course, is reflected by the rather low PPV of the test. Of those patients who actually underwent carotid endarterectomy, the ultrasonic arteriogram correctly identified the presence of an operable lesion in all patients with amaurosis fugax, 95% with TIA, 84% with stroke, 83% with nonhemispheric lesions, and in all with asymptomatic bruits.[24]

If arteriography were performed on only those patients with positive noninvasive tests, the data in Fig. 34-14 imply that 17% of the patients with TIAs and potentially operable lesions would have been inadequately studied. On the other hand, 76% of those without operable lesions would have been spared unnecessary arteriography. Estimates based on these and similar data suggest that the use of ultrasonic arteriography to select patients for conventional arteriography (rather than performing arteriography on all patients with TIAs) would not adversely affect 3- to 5-year mortality but would increase the long-term stroke rate from 5% to 9%.[23,24] Although the stroke rate is almost doubled, in terms of absolute numbers the increased risk is not large (only 4 of 100 patients). While one cannot justify the routine use of ultrasonic arteriography to determine which patients with lateralizing symptoms should undergo conventional arteriography, the risk of missing an operable lesion is low enough to be acceptable under adverse circumstances. In view of its high NPV for hemodynamically significant disease, preliminary ultrasonic screening does seem to be justified in patients with asymptomatic bruits or nonhemispheric symptoms. Moreover, in the rare patient with well-defined hemispheric symptoms who is also allergic to contrast material, a clearly positive scan and spectrum can be used as the definitive diagnostic study before endarterectomy.[4]

SUMMARY

Pulsed Doppler arteriography has proved to be a reliable method for noninvasive screening of extracranial carotid arterial disease. Instrumentation is relatively inexpensive, and studies can be performed rapidly by experienced personnel. The image itself has considerable diagnostic value, but accuracy is enhanced by the technician's interpretation of the audible Doppler signal and by the incorporation of real-time spectrum analysis into the examination routine. Computerization of the scan to provide simultaneous lateral and anteroposterior images, together with an assessment of the cross-sectional area, has proved to be technically feasible. Whether the additional information will contribute significantly to the overall diagnostic accuracy remains to be seen.

Ultrasonic arteriography, especially when performed in conjunction with spectral analysis, accurately rules out the presence of hemodynamically significant disease and, therefore, is valuable for screening patients with nonhemispheric symptoms or asymptomatic bruits. The combination is also fairly effective for identifying or ruling out any disease perceptible on conventional arteriography. Its accuracy is sufficiently high to justify its use in certain elderly, poor-risk patients, especially when the symptoms are ill-defined or when there is a history of allergy to contrast material. Unfortunately, in our experience, neither ultrasonic arteriography or spectral analysis has been reliable in the assessment of the totally occluded internal carotid artery. Therefore confirmatory arteriography is recommended in all cases of suspected occlusion.

REFERENCES

1. Barnes, R.W., Rittgers, S.E., and Putney, W.W.: Real-time Doppler spectrum analysis. Predictive value in defining operable carotid artery disease, Arch. Surg. 117:52, 1982.
2. Barnes, R.W., et al.: Noninvasive ultrasonic angiography: prospective validation by contrast arteriography, Surgery 80:328, 1976.
3. Blackshear, W.M., Jr.: Pulsed Doppler ultrasonic arteriography and spectrum analysis for quantitating carotid occlusive disease, Paper presented at the Vascular Research Forum, Boston, June 1982.
4. Blackshear, W.M., Jr., and Connor, R.G.: Carotid endarterectomy without angiography, J. Cardiovasc. Surg. 23:477, 1982.

5. Blackshear, W.M., Jr., et al.: Detection of carotid occlusive disease by ultrasonic imaging and pulsed Doppler spectrum analysis, Surgery 86:698, 1979.

6. Bodily, K.C., et al.: Ultrasonic arteriography: implications in patient management, West. J. Med. 135:183, 1981.

7. Cardullo, P.A., et al.: Noninvasive detection of carotid disease: an evaluation of oculoplethysmography, carotid phonoangiography and pulsed Doppler ultrasonic arteriography, Bruit 5:26, December 1982.

8. Cohen, J.: Weighted kappa: nominal scale agreement with provision for scaled disagreement or partial credit, Psychol. Bull. 70:213, 1968.

9. Doorly, T.P.G., et al.: Carotid ultrasonic arteriography combined with real-time spectral analysis: a comparison with angiography, J. Cardiovasc. Surg. 23:243, 1982.

10. Eikelboom, B.C., et al.: Digital video subtraction angiography and duplex scanning in assessment of carotid artery disease: comparison with conventional angiography, Surgery 94:821, 1983.

11. Fish, P.J.: Visualizing blood vessels by ultrasound. In Roberts, C., editor: Blood flow measurement, London, 1972, Sector Publishing, Ltd.

12. Hobson, R.W., II, et al.: Comparison of pulsed Doppler and real-time B-mode echo arteriography for noninvasive imaging of the extracranial carotid arteries, Surgery 87:286, 1980.

13. Hobson, R.W. II, et al.: Oculoplethysmography and pulsed Doppler ultrasonic imaging in diagnosis of carotid occlusive disease, Surg. Gynecol. Obstet. 152:433, 1981.

14. Hokanson, D.E., et al.: Ultrasonic arteriography: a new approach to arterial visualisation, Biomed. Eng. 6:420, 1971.

15. Metz, C.E.: Basic principles of ROC analysis, Semin. Nucl. Med. 8:283, 1978.

16. Miles, R.D., Russell, J.B., and Sumner, D.S.: Computerized ultrasonic arteriography: a new technique for imaging the carotid bifurcation, IEEE Trans. Biomed. Eng. 29:378, 1982.

17. Miles, R.D., et al.: Computerized multiplanar imaging and lumen area plotting for noninvasive diagnosis of carotid artery disease, Surgery 93:676, 1983.

18. Mozerksy, D.J., et al.: Ultrasonic arteriography, Arch. Surg. 103:663, 1971.

19. Reid, J.M., and Spencer, M.P.: Ultrasonic Doppler technique for imaging blood vessels, Science 176:1235, 1972.

20. Roederer, G.O., et al.: Ultrasonic Duplex scanning of extracranial carotid arteries: improved accuracy using new features from the common carotid artery, J. Cardiovasc. Ultrasonography 1:373, 1982.

21. Russell, J.B., Miles, R.D., and Sumner, D.S.: Computerized ultrasonic arteriography: a noninvasive technique for producing multiplanar images of the carotid bifurcation, Bruit 4:27, September 1980.

22. Russell, J.B., Miles, R.D., and Sumner, D.S.: Pulsed-Doppler ultrasonic arteriography with sound spectral analysis for evaluation of the carotid bifurcation, Bruit 6:23, March 1982.

23. Sumner, D.S.: Noninvasive methods for preoperative assessment of carotid occlusive disease. I. Statistical interpretation of test results, Vasc. Diagn. Ther. 2:41, June/July 1981.

24. Sumner, D.S., Russell, J.B., and Miles, R.D.: Are noninvasive tests sufficiently accurate to identify patients in need of carotid arteriography? Surgery 91:700, 1982.

25. Sumner, D.S., et al.: Noninvasive diagnosis of extracranial carotid arterial disease: a prospective evaluation of pulsed-Doppler imaging and oculoplethysmography, Arch. Surg. 114:1222, 1979.

26. Warlow, C.P., and Fish, P.J.: Pulsed Doppler imaging of the carotid artery, J. Neurol. Sci. 45:135, 1980.

27. Wasserman, D.H., et al.: Ultrasonic imaging and oculoplethysmography in diagnosis of carotid occlusive disease, Arch. Surg. 118:1161, 1983.

28. Wolf, E.A., Jr.: Discussion of Sumner, et al.: Noninvasive diagnosis of extracranial carotid arterial disease, Arch. Surg. 114:1229, 1979.

CHAPTER 35

Continuous-wave Doppler imaging of the carotid bifurcation

MERRILL P. SPENCER

Atherosclerosis of the carotid artery bifurcation represents the source of many problems of cerebral circulation, producing local brain ischemia, stroke by embolism from ulcerated plaques, and global hypoperfusion from flow-reducing obstructions. Continuous-wave (CW) Doppler ultrasound excels in detecting hemodynamically significant lesions that are associated with transient ischemic attack (TIA) and stroke. Because TIAs are considered harbingers of stroke and are associated with stenotic lesions on the origin of the carotid bifurcation, it is generally agreed that stenotic plaques should be surgically removed by endarterectomy. If a nonstenotic plaque is found, antiplatelet medication offers an alternative to surgery. CW ultrasound offers a noninvasive method of detecting the surgically amenable stroke-producing lesion.

CW imaging of the carotid bifurcation[8-11,17,20] represents a technique for thorough investigation of the critical region of the origin of the internal carotid artery. Diagnostic signals of interest found there include those of arterial stenosis, turbulence, and calcium deposits. The image represents a rough map of hemodynamic arterial flow channels and is not a direct morphologic representation. Information concerning luminal morphology is deduced from local hemodynamics represented in the spectrum of Doppler-shifted frequencies.

The imaging system is illustrated in Fig. 35-1. The transducer is held in a scanning arm directing the ultrasound beam at a fixed angle (usually about 60 degrees) with respect to the long axis of the body, while the patient is lying down. A supportive pad is placed behind the neck, causing the chin to be slightly elevated. The scanning arm allows the probe to move in three dimensions while tracking only two dimensions in a plane parallel to the body axis and translating the probe position, in this plane, to the x-y coordinates of a television screen.

With acoustic jelly sealing the contact between probe and skin surface, scanning is performed by passing the sound beam back and forth across the arteries in the anteroposterior direction. The blood velocity–shifted CW signal activates the z axis of the television tube, which stores an image of the location of arterial blood velocity signals. By repeated passes across the common carotid artery while gradually following it superiorly to its bifurcation, a *flow map* is developed. Reverse flow signals from the veins are rejected from the image. Simultaneously, the frequency spectrum of the Doppler[16,18] signals is continuously represented. The source of the spectrum is keyed to a cursor showing the position of the probe and spectrum on the arterial image.

The spectrum is developed from a fast Fourier transform (FFT) of both flow direction signals (A and B quadrature signals of the Doppler circuits). Appropriate circuits allow color coding of the flow map for selected spectral features such as maximum frequency (f_{max}) or direction of the Doppler signal. The complete display of Doppler information frequency spectrum and its source in a video-reproducible format provides an objective and quantitative record of all hemodynamic features for diagnostic and teaching purposes (Fig. 35-2).

The probe for CW carotid imaging operates optimally with 5 MHz ultrasound focused with a plastic lens to a depth of 2.5 cm. The piezoelectric crystal, 10 mm in diameter, is split into D-shaped halves, one for transmitting and the other for receiving. If the 5 MHz probe angle is held in the

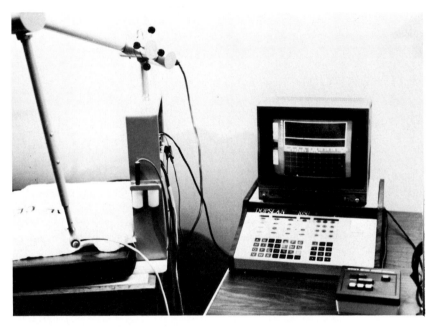

Fig. 35-1. Apparatus for CW Doppler imaging of carotid bifurcation. Left, Mechanical arm holding 5 MHz probe. Right, Control console and fast Fourier transform spectral analyzer.

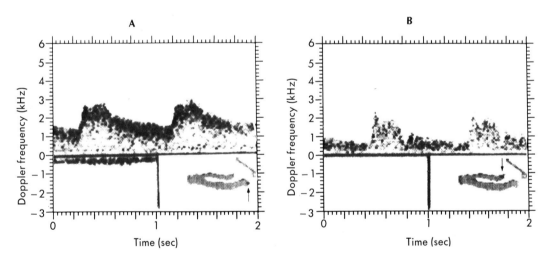

Fig. 35-2. A, Normal CW spectrum from internal carotid artery at distance of 6 cm from carotid bifurcation. Note concentration of energies near upper edge, indicating laminar blood flow. Below zero line, reverse flow frequency signals are seen from underlying jugular vein. **B,** Normal CW spectrum of Doppler frequencies in external carotid artery of same patient. Pulsatility is greater and effects of compliance, caused by early systolic acceleration and early diastolic deceleration of velocities, are seen.

scanning arm at a 60-degree angle with the vessel axis, a Doppler frequency of 1 kHz represents a blood velocity of 30 cm/sec.

CW, rather than pulsed, Doppler ultrasound was chosen for carotid interrogation because with CW it is easier to locate the carotid arteries, and one can follow the highest velocities found within segmental stenoses.[15] With pulsed Doppler ultrasound it is more difficult to find the artery because the limited sample volume and pulse repetition rate produces aliasing, making it impossible to resolve the highest velocities of arterial stenosis.[13] The depth focusing capability of pulsed Doppler ultrasound is not necessary for finding the clinically significant information so well represented by a CW system.

FINDINGS WITH CW DOPPLER IMAGING

Fig. 35-2 illustrates the CW spectrum found at different points around the normal carotid bifurcation. Normal systolic f_{max} ranges from 0.5 to 2.5 kHz at the origin of the internal carotid and 2 to 3 kHz distally. The internal carotid distal frequencies are higher than those at the origin because the normal "bulb" found at the origin has a larger diameter and cross-sectional area. The presence of higher diastolic frequencies arising from the internal carotid artery, as compared with the external carotid, is normal and characterizes the difference in the vascular beds supplied by these two arteries. Higher diastolic velocity and flow are produced by the lower vascular resistance in the brain, compared with other cephalic tissues. This difference assists in identifying the two branches if they are close together or if they overlay each other. The differences in waveform have been formalized by calculation of a pulsatility index.[2,5,8] When the CW images of the two branches are superimposed, the two spectra are also superimposed and readily identified as representing separate arteries (Fig. 35-3).

A useful additional technique for positively identifying the external and internal carotid arteries consists of applying finger oscillation where the superficial temporal artery crosses the supraorbital artery while observing the spectrum at a given image position. A retrograde flow modulation, in response to varying finger pressure, passes down the superficial temporal artery to the external carotid artery, producing undulations on the spectrum recorded there.[17] These undulations are not passed around the bifurcation into the internal carotid artery except when the response in the external carotid artery is very strong. Likewise, the response

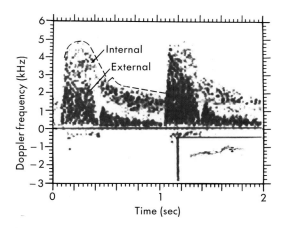

Fig. 35-3. Superimposed spectra of internal and external carotid arteries when CW imaging does not separate these two branches at carotid bifurcation. Elevated frequencies indicate compensatory blood flow from obstruction on opposite side.

is not seen in the common carotid artery unless the internal carotid is occluded. This temporal artery modulation technique is also useful to confirm stenosis of the external carotid artery when high diastolic components produced by stenosis simulate an internal carotid waveform.

The CW diagnosis of occlusion of the internal carotid artery is made not by the absence of that branch in the image, but by the character of the common carotid signal (Fig. 35-4) and by evidence of functioning collaterals around the homolateral eyes,[1,6] as well as increased velocities along the opposite internal carotid and the vertebral arteries. When the internal carotid artery is occluded, the f_{max} waveform of the common carotid, normally a summation of both branches, loses its diastolic component and is asymmetric compared with the opposite common carotid signal (Fig. 35-4).

Fig. 35-5 represents typical CW signals indicating stenosis at the origin of the internal carotid artery. In Fig. 35-5A, f_{max} within the stenotic segment (f_1) is increased above the normal range, whereas in the more distal segment (Fig. 35-5, B), $(f_{max} (f_2)$ decreases and evidences turbulence. If the interpreter relies only on elevated f_1 frequencies, this frequency must exceed 5 kHz to assure an accurate diagnosis of stenosis greater than 50%.[15] The alternative use of the ratio of frequencies f_1/f_2 allows one to diagnose stenosis of less than 50%.[19] The formula to be used in this ratio method is as follows:

$$\% \text{Stenosis} = 100 \ (1 - f_2/f_1)$$

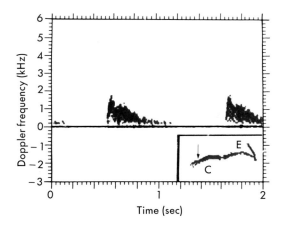

Fig. 35-4. Common carotid CW spectrum in patient with occlusion of internal carotid artery. Pulsatility is increased because diastolic components are considerably reduced.

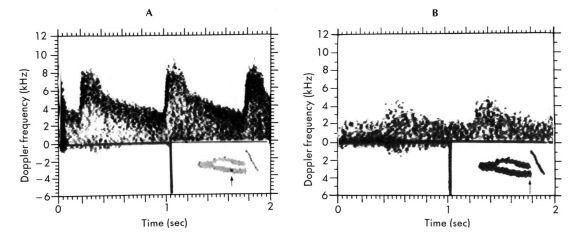

Fig. 35-5. A, CW spectrum diagnostic of stenosis 3 cm above origin of internal carotid artery from carotid bifurcation. **B,** CW spectrum indicating turbulence 2 cm downstream from stenotic signals illustrated in **A.** Spectral broadening is present, as well as some reversal of frequencies and "feathering" of upper edge of spectrum.

Morphologic quantitation of carotid artery stenosis

Since blood flowing into a segmental stenosis must accelerate, there is a necessary relationship between the severity of the stenosis and the increase in the blood velocity. Fig. 35-6 illustrates the theoretic relationships found between velocity and diameter at the origin of the internal carotid artery. Fig. 35-7 shows the relationship found between the smallest diameter measurable on x-ray films of carotid arteries selectively injected through the aortic arch and the CW signal at that site. Artery diameters were measured from arterial injection arteriograms using a micrometer. To obviate film magnification errors, the diameters are expressed as ratios of proximal (stenosis) diameter (d_1) to distal

diameter (d_2) at the level of the mandible. The percent of stenosis can be calculated as follows:

$$\%\text{Stenosis} = 100\,(1 - d_1/d_2)$$

The variations from the theoretic curve are produced by variations in collateral channels from patient to patient, as well as the limitations of arteriography in accurately defining the luminal diameters within the stenotic segment. Despite variations in f_{max} as it relates to angiographically measured diameters, the accuracy of CW Doppler ultrasound is high for several ranges of stenosis when analyzed by decision matrix analysis (Fig. 35-7).

Fig. 35-8 illustrates a variation between microm-

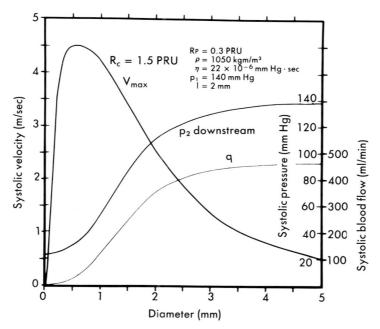

Fig. 35-6. Computer simulation of various degrees of stenosis of internal carotid artery beginning from normal 5 mm diameter to total occlusion. Velocities reach maximum of 4.5 m/sec at diameter of 0.5 mm when collateral resistance Rc is five times that of brain vascular resistance. R_p, Peripheral resistance units; ρ, density of blood; η, viscosity of blood; p_1, central arterial systolic pressure; q, systolic blood flow; l, stenosis length. Velocities, pressures, and flow calibrations are in terms of peak midsystolic maxima.

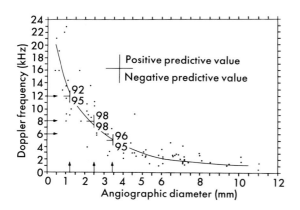

Fig. 35-7. Relation of minimal angiographically measured carotid stenosis diameter to corresponding Doppler frequency using 5 MHz at 60-degree angle. Positive and negative predictive values are shown for three degrees of stenosis.

eter measurements and radiologists' interpretations of stenosis. This comparison demonstrates the casualness with which many radiologists interpret their films. Judging by the general acceptance of the radiologist's interpretations, which are not based on objective measurements, the exact degree of stenosis is not as clinically important to the managing physician as the justifiable recognition that embolization can occur from plaques with any degree of stenosis. It is important, however, to identify those lesions that are hemodynamically significant and particularly to differentiate trickle flow

in preocclusive stenosis (that is, stenosis with 90% diameter reduction) from total occlusion (Fig. 35-9).

The accuracy figures given in this chapter use all patient data regardless of the confidence of the Doppler interpreter in the data presented. A 100% positive predictive value can be achieved if rigid requirements for diagnosis are applied at the time of data interpretation. For example, if f_{max} frequencies greater than 5 kHz on the internal carotid are coupled with collateralization signs around the homolateral eye, this is 100% predictive of a ste-

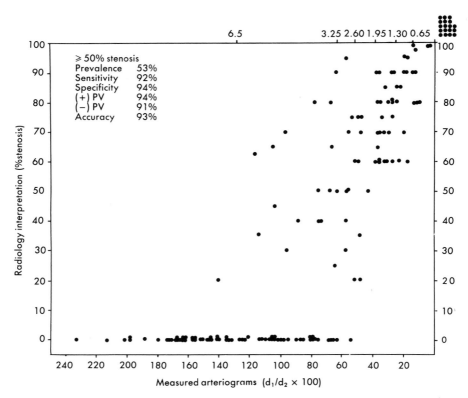

Fig. 35-8. Comparison of radiologist's interpretation with micrometer-measured arteriograms. Abscissa represents percent diameter of proximal internal carotid artery compared with distal internal carotid artery. Insert represents decision matrix analysis of radiologist's interpretations for stenoses ≥50%. *PV,* Predictive value.

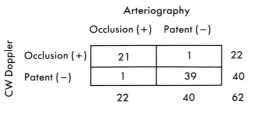

Arteriography

	Occlusion (+)	Patent (−)	
Occlusion (+)	21	1	22
Patent (−)	1	39	40
	22	40	62

CW Doppler

Prevalence 35%   (+)PV 95%
Sensitivity 95%   (−)PV 98%
Specificity 98%   Accuracy 97%

Fig. 35-9. Decision matrix analysis of CW Doppler diagnosis of occlusion vs tight stenosis of internal carotid arteries.

nosis greater than 50% present on the internal carotid. Also, all patients with clear-cut TIA who display f_{max} greater than 5 kHz on the appropriate internal carotid have a stenotic lesion at the origin of that artery. Even though such high levels of confidence in noninvasive diagnosis of carotid stenosis may be achieved, carotid endarterectomy in patients with TIAs is rarely justified without prior arteriography.[7,10] However, computed x-ray tomography is advisable before the decision for surgery, to rule out major intracranial lesions.

Physiologic quantitation of carotid artery stenosis

Holen[4] has demonstrated the pressure drop (Δp) across a stenotic mitral valve can be calculated from the blood velocity (v) determined from the maximum Doppler frequency detected within the stenosis. This idea has been confirmed by Hatle and Angelsen[3] in stenosis of the mitral, aortic, and tricuspid valves.[10] Conditions exist in carotid artery stenosis to apply the same principle and calculate the pressure drop from CW imaging with spectral analysis.[12] The circle of Willis pressure can then be estimated noninvasively by subtracting Δp from the brachial artery pressure measured by sphygmomanometry. Two conditions must be met to assure accuracy of the calculation; (1) the angle between the ultrasonic beam and the direction of the stenotic jet must be known and (2) turbulence downstream from the stenosis must be present. Fig.

35-10 illustrates the relationship between Δp and v. The simplified relationship is as follows:

$$\Delta p = kv^2max$$

where Δp is expressed in millimeters of mercury and v_{max} in meters per second. For the cardiac valves, Holen recommends a k value of 4. For carotid stenosis, a k value of 4 appears to be appropriate, but further validation is necessary.

In terms of hemodynamic significance, the pressure drop and therefore the CW frequency is a far better indication of the effect of stenosis on brain circulation than is detection of collateralization. This is because increased velocity is produced by both increasing stenosis and the limitations of collaterals. Both factors reduce the residual intracranial arterial pressure beyong the obstruction. With trickle flow conditions and total occlusion, however, one must rely on collateralization effects. It must also be said that the patient's symptoms of cerebrovascular insufficiency represent the final indicator of hemodynamic significance.

CW imaging is of assistance in determining the angle of the ultrasound beam and the stenotic jet. By first producing two images at two different angles with the body axis, the two actual angles to the jet can be determined from the cosine relationship. From the known angles between the jet and the ultrasound beams, the true velocity and pressure can be calculated.

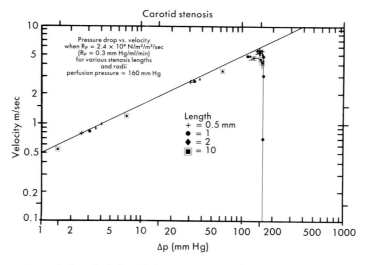

Fig. 35-10. Computer prediction of relationship between pressure drop across stenosis and velocity within stenosis. R_p, Peripheral vascular resistance expressed in both European and American units. Relationship is not greatly influenced by length of stenotic channel.

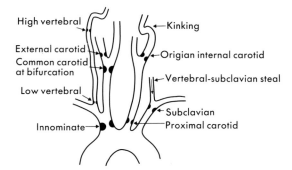

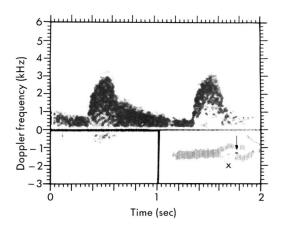

Fig. 35-11. Range of diagnoses of extracranial arterial obstructions using CW Doppler ultrasound.

Fig. 35-12. Nonimaging segment at origin of internal carotid artery produced by calcified plaque. Spectrum represents laminar flow signals detected just downstream from plaque. This effect is used to diagnose nonstenotic plaques and causes no problem in detecting underlying stenosis because modification of probe beam angle, finds way through to signals beneath plaque. Turbulence and collateral effects are also helpful.

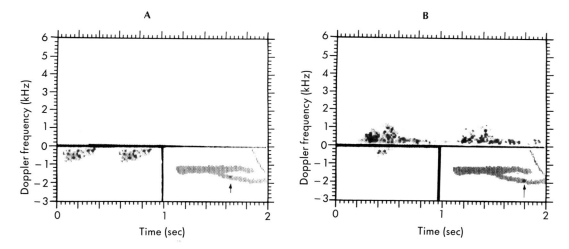

Fig. 35-13. A, Inverted CW spectrum on origin of internal carotid artery representing dispersed deposits in nonstenotic plaque. **B,** Normally directed signals downstream from calcium deposit in same carotid artery.

Auxiliary information from CW

In addition to direct interrogation of the carotid bifurcation, CW allows evaluation of the vertebral artery circulation from its origin at the subclavian artery to the atlas loop at the base of the skull. Since symptoms of vertebrobasilar insufficiency are sometimes dissipated by endarterectomy of a carotid stenosis, it is important to diagnose obstructions to blood flow in both the anterior and the posterior cerebral circulations. Fig. 35-11 diagrams the range of obstructions of the extracranial arteries that can be diagnosed with CW Doppler ultrasound.

Since stroke can be produced by embolism from the left side of the heart, the capability of CW ultrasound with frequency spectral analysis[14] to diagnose stenosis and regurgitation of the aortic and mitral valves provides valuable information in searching for an explanation of brain perfusion symptoms.

Nonstenotic plaques, ulceration, and thrombosis

Since the early use of CW imaging of the carotid bifurcation, regions of abruptly disappearing or inverted signals were found (Figs. 35-12 and 35-13) where the normal polarity of signals indicating expected headward flow was paradoxically reversed. These inversions are most frequently found on the origin of the internal carotid artery but are also seen on the common and external carotid arteries near the bifurcation. They are found both with and without high-frequency signals of stenosis. Evidence[16] suggests that these signals, as well as segmented CW silent zones along the carotid arteries, represent calcium deposits. When found, the presence of inverted and nonsounding segments represent a mature plaque with a necrotic and calcified core.

The presence of ulceration (denuded intima), cratering, or ruptured plaque cannot be directly diagnosed with CW ultrasound, though some hope is held out that multigate pulsed Doppler ultrasound can detect vortices within wall craters. Two-dimensional imaging occasionally demonstrates cratering or thrombosis and is sensitive to calcium deposits. Deep craters seen on arteriography may be covered with a complete intima and are often seen on the carotid artery opposite the side of brain damage. Unfortunately, no accurate method exists today for detecting ulceration. The detection of ulceration and thrombus remains an urgently needed noninvasive technology.

SUMMARY

CW imaging of the carotid bifurcation, when combined with frequency spectral analysis, provides physiologic information to diagnose the severity of morphologic stenosis and its hemodynamic significance. The use of various degrees of plaque and stenosis detection in the clinical management of patients is illustrated in Fig. 35-14.

Carotid Doppler / Symptoms	Asymptomatic	Dizziness	Vertebral-basilar	Focal	Transient ischemic attack	Stroke
Normal	0	0	0	APM	APM	0
Nonstenotic plaquing	0	0	APM	APM	APM	0
Stenosis — Mild	F	F	F	A&E	A&E	A&E
Stenosis — Moderate	F	F	F	A&E	A&E	A&E
Stenosis — Severe	A&E	A&E	A&E	A&E	A&E	A&E
Occlusion	0	F	F	F	A&E	0

Fig. 35-14. Patient management decisions available from carotid Doppler imaging diagnoses. *O,* No special action; *F,* follow with repeat Doppler; *A & E,* arteriogram and endarterectomy; *APM,* antiplatelet medication.

REFERENCES

1. Brockenbrough, E.C.: Screening for the prevention of stroke: use of a Doppler flowmeter, Information and Education Resource Support Unit, Washington/Alaska Regional Medical Program, 1969.
2. Gosling, R.G., Beasley, M.G., and Lewis, R.R.: Noninvasive demonstration of disease at the carotid bifurcation by ultrasound. In Reneman, R., and Hoeks, A.P.G., editors: Doppler ultrasound in the diagnosis of cerebrovascular disease, New York, 1981, Research Studies Press.
3. Hatle, L., and Angelsen, B.: Doppler ultrasound in cardiology. Physical principles and clinical applications, Philadelphia, 1982, Lea & Febiger.
4. Holen, J., et al.: Determination of pressure gradient in mitral stenosis with a noninvasive ultrasound Doppler technique, Acta Med. Scand. 99:455, 1976.
5. Mol, J.M.F.: The clinical use of Doppler hematographic investigation in cerebral circulation disturbances. In Reneman, R., and Hoeks, A.P.G., editors: Doppler ultrasound in the diagnosis of cerebrovascular disease, New York, 1981, Research Studies Press.
6. Muller, H.R.: The diagnosis by directional Doppler sonography of the ophthalmic artery, Neurology 22:816, 1972.
7. Pollak, E.W.: Noninvasive cerebrovascular evaluation: a prerequisite for angiography? Am. J. Surg. 144:203, 1982.
8. Pourcelot, L.: Continuous wave Doppler techniques in cardiovascular disturbances. In Reneman, R., and Hoeks, A.P.G., editors: Doppler ultrasound in the diagnosis of cerebrovascular disease, New York, 1981, Research Studies Press.
9. Reneman, R.S., and Spencer, M.P.: Local Doppler audio spectra in normal and stenosed carotid arteries in man, Ultrasound Med. Biol. 5:1, 1979.
10. Sandman, W., et al.: Carotid artery surgery without angiography: risk or progress? In Greenhalgh, R.M., and Rose, F.C., editors: ed. 2, Progress in stroke research, London, 1983, Pitman Publishing, Ltd.
11. Spencer, M.P.: Using carotid imaging and hand-held probing Doppler evaluation of the aortocranial circulation. In Reneman, R., and Hoeks, A.P.G., editors: Doppler ultrasound in the diagnosis of cerebrovascular disease, New York, 1982, Research Studies Press.
12. Spencer, M.P., and Arts, T.: Carotid stenosis and the Bernoulli principle, Fed. Proc. 40(3):444, 1981.
13. Spencer, M.P., and Fujioka, K.: C.W. Doppler with spectrum analysis in acquired valve disease. In Spencer, M., editor: Cardiac Doppler diagnosis, The Hague, 1983, Martinus Nijhoff.
14. Spencer, M.P., and Hileman, R.E.: Le Doppler à l'emission continué avec analyse spectrale de frequence pour le diagnostic cardiologique en pathologie valvulaire acquisé, Journal D' Imagerie Medicale 1:17, 1983.
15. Spencer, M.P., and Reid, J.M.: Quantitation of carotid stenosis with continuous-wave (CW) Doppler ultrasound, Stroke 10(3):326, 1979.
16. Spencer, M.P., and Reid, J.M.: Cerebrovascular evaluation with Doppler ultrasound, The Hague, 1981, Martinus Nijhoff.
17. Spencer, M.P., and Zwiebel, W.J.: Frequency spectrum analysis Doppler diagnosis. In Zwiebel, W.J., editor: Introduction to vascular ultrasonography, New York, 1982, Grune & Stratton, Inc.
18. Spencer, M.P., et al.: Cervical carotid imaging with a continuous wave Doppler flowmeter, Stroke 5:145, 1983.
19. Spencer, M.P., et al.: On line dual-directional spectral display in Doppler diagnosis of stenotic and non-stenotic plaques. Proceedings of the 25th Annual Meeting of the American Institute of Ultrasound in Medicine, New Orleans, 1980.
20. Thomas, G.I., et al.: Noninvasive carotid bifurcation mapping, Am. J. Surg. 128:168, 1974.
21. West, F.W., Clark, S.J., and Spencer, M.P.: Continuous wave Doppler evaluation of severe carotid occlusive disease, J. Ultrasound Med. 1(7):50, 1982.
22. West, F.W., Clark, S.J., and Spencer, M.P.: Differentiation of tight stenosis from occlusion of the common-internal carotid artery with Doppler ultrasound, Bruit 6:46, 1982.

CHAPTER 36

Color-coded Doppler carotid imaging

DENIS N. WHITE

Techniques developed for the investigation of carotid vascular disease, especially those noninvasive techniques aimed at the carotid bifurcation, always have been restricted by the difficulty of distinguishing the external carotid artery, which supplies the tissues of the face, from the more vital internal carotid artery, which supplies the brain. Auscultation and bruit analysis are of limited value for this reason.

The two-dimensional spatial displays made with contrast angiography had never suffered from such difficulties, and the certainty with which they distinguished between the internal and external carotid systems was one of the reasons that this technique became so successful and definitive. It was therefore only natural that two-dimensional spatial displays should be developed with the ultrasonic nonintrusive techniques.

Direct ultrasonic spatial displays of the carotid system have developed along two lines. The conventional pulse-echo scanning techniques can image the carotid arteries directly. With the development of real-time systems with high-resolution gray-scale displays, it is now possible to explore systematically the carotid arteries and search the images for evidence of occlusive disease. The second approach displays, congruously in two spatial dimensions, not the reflections from the arterial walls and atheromatous plaques, but the back-scattered ultrasonic energy from the moving red cells in the arteries, which is distinguished from other reflected signals by the fact that it is Doppler shifted in frequency by an amount proportional to its velocity relative to the generator-receiver.

The first two-dimensional ultrasonic Doppler displays were made by Hokanson et al. in 1971[3] with pulsed energy and thus were capable of producing two-dimensional tomograms across the long

or short axes of the arteries imaged. The following year Reid and Spencer[11] described a simpler system using continuously generated energy, which made images of the arteries in profiles parallel to the surface-scanning plane. Since the course of most arteries lies parallel to the skin, this system was capable of displaying the vessels over a considerable length, down to depths limited by the attenuation of the generated and reflected energy. With this system, occlusions are made manifest by their failure to appear on the display. Initially it was hoped that it would also be possible to display regions of arterial stenosis by appropriate narrowing of the vessel image. However, the beam width of the generated and received energy was approximately the same size as the arterial lumen. This fact, combined with a 5 mm degree of uncertainty in the spatial sensing mechanisms of the scanning arm,[2] made it difficult to achieve the necessary spatial resolution. It became apparent that the operator was relying more on the accompanying audio signal than on the video display in diagnosing such stenoses. As a region of stenosis was scanned, the audio signal clearly showed that blood was flowing through the stenotic region in a turbulent fashion at increased velocities by an increase in the pitch of the Doppler shift. For this reason it seemed worthwhile to develop a system that could image such regions of increased velocity directly on the video display. This purpose was most easily accomplished by the use of color. Originally we envisaged the use of a large number of different colors, each corresponding to a different Doppler-shift frequency. However, after developing our original system using only three separate frequency filters with corresponding colors, it appeared that such a further development would be confusing and unnecessary.

INSTRUMENTATION

The original system we described[2] has been further developed both by ourselves and by the manufacturer.* The description given here is confined to those developments made since our original publication.

The device generates ultrasonic energy continuously at 4.0 MHz. The generating and receiving crystals are combined in a single probe with the axis of their faces intersecting at a depth of approximately 4 cm to enable recordings to be made from the deeper arteries, such as the vertebral arteries, which usually lie 3 cm beneath the skin. The consequent loss in resolution of the more superficial arteries does not appear to be deleterious.

A special scanning system has been devised with freedom of movement in two dimensions. The plane of scan can be adjusted so that it lies parallel to the skin surface overlying the artery to be imaged. The arm holding the transducer can be rotated in the plane perpendicular to the scanning plane to enable the operator to scan the artery on the other side of the body without adjusting the scanning plane. The transducer is fixed in this arm so that its long axis is at a 45-degree angle to the surface of the skin and the scanning plane.

*Diagnostic Electronics Corp., Lexington, Mass.

The receiving system is no longer a commercial flowmeter, since these did not prove reliable. It has been designed by the manufacturer but still uses the zero-crossing technique and is direction resolving and direction indicating. While both directions of flow can be indicated simultaneously on the time-velocity strip chart recorder incorporated in the machine, the video display only shows flow in one predetermined direction. The audio display, which is also incorporated in the system, is bidirectional. The generating and receiving systems are designed to incorporate an additional pulse-mode facility if desired.

A microcomputer with an associated analog-to-digital converter has now been incorporated into the system and controls both the original DC-to-raster scan converter, which sensed the position of the probe during the scan-by-DC sampling, and also the autoscanner-to-display circuit, which now uses digital memory techniques to center the video display on that smaller region of the scanning plane that was the area of interest. The microcomputer also provides for a much more interactive system than originally described.

The ultrasonic Doppler velocity color-coding circuit (Fig. 36-1) comprises the necessary circuitry for sampling the ultrasonic Doppler-shifted signals and recording this information spatially on a

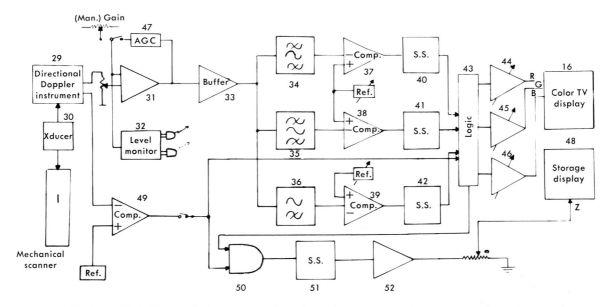

Fig. 36-1. Block diagram of ultrasonic Doppler color-coding circuit. For description see text. *Ref.,* Reference signal; *Man.,* manual; *AGC.,* automatic gain control; *Comp.,* comparator; *S.S.,* single shot multivibrator; *R,* red; *G,* green; *B,* blue. (From Curry, G.R., and White, D.N.: Ultrasound Med. Biol. 4:27-35, 1978.)

colored storage video display from which hard-copy color Polaroid prints can be made.

The directional Doppler instrument is interfaced by blocks 29 through 31 and provides the filter banks (34 through 36) with a spectrum of audio signals, which represent the complex back-scattering velocity components from the moving blood.

If any or all filters are detected, that is, if they have sufficient signal strength present, this information is input to the logic unit on a beat-to-beat basis and is further stored in memory.

It is the logic unit (43) that performs the necessary processing of the filtered information and drives the appropriate weighted output amplifiers to a color matrix and finally to a color monitor.

The Echoflow displays blood flowing at normal peak velocities by the color red (Plate 2, *A,* and Fig. 36-2). Blood flowing at increased velocity, as it will through the narrowed segments of a stenosis, is displayed in yellow (Plate 2, *B,* 1 and 2, and *C,* 1 and 2, and Fig. 36-2); blood at markedly increased velocity through an even tighter stenosis is shown in blue (Plate 2, *B,* 2, and Fig. 36-2). The Echoflow does not attempt to display stenoses as appropriately narrowed segments of the arteries, since the width of the beam prevents this being apparent in many cases. This system also makes occluded vessels manifest, since they do not appear on the display (Plate 2, *B,* 1 and 2, and *C,* 1 and 2, and Fig. 36-2). Plate 2, *D,* 2 and Fig. 36-2 show a high-grade stenosis of the left internal carotid artery before endarterectomy and Plate 1, *E* shows the same pair of bifurcations after endarterectomy.

RESULTS

This technique has been in clinical use at our noninvasive vascular unit for the last 9 years, during which time we have performed about 17,500 carotid scans on approximately 8750 patients. During this time it has been operated by three different persons. The first designed and built the system, the second was a technician with training and experience in ultrasonic techniques, and the present operator has had no previous medical or technical training. Despite these variations in background, the three different operators obtained approximately the same accuracy in normal, stenosed, and occluded arteries. This fact can be verified by comparing our previous results[14-17] with those presented here.

Not every patient scanned had an angiogram, but we reported our results in comparison with the angiographic findings in increasing numbers of consecutive cases[14-17] until the first 1001 consecutive carotid scans with angiographic validation were completed 4 years ago.[13] These results are summarized in this chapter.

Since the accuracy of our technique did not change appreciably as we reported an increasing number of angiographically validated scans up to the 1001 described in this chapter, we have not extended this series further. In the last 4 years the results we have obtained conform to those in our various earlier validated series and we have seen no need to alter our conclusions. More importantly, before 1980 we were the only group who had used the Echoflow over a sufficient period of time to report on its accuracy and inaccuracy. Since that time other workers have used the system, and it seemed more valuable to compare their results with our own rather than to extend our own series indefinitely.

It should be clearly understood that the results reported here and in earlier series *refer to the Echoflow Doppler scan alone.* A greater degree of accuracy can be achieved in examining the carotid bifurcation if the continuous-wave (CW) Doppler scan is combined with other noninvasive procedures. In particular, the periorbital Doppler examination combined with simple CW frequency-time Doppler investigation of the brachial, carotid, and vertebral arteries increases the accuracy of the interpretation of the color-coded spatial scans, as does the use of on-line spectral analysis during the performance of the spatial scan. Our results, however, were based solely on the interpretation of the color-coded spatial scan by means of its video display and the hard copy of the video display. This restriction on the accuracy of the results obtained by the Echoflow system was made deliberately, since it was the performance of this system that we were anxious to investigate and not its accuracy when combined with other techniques.

Table 36-1 compares the results of the Doppler examination with the angiogram in 1001 carotid bifurcations. The areas outlined in the boxes indicate *good* correlation, and those areas with bold-face type indicate acceptable correlation. The degree of angiographic stenosis is estimated as a percentage of the *diameter* (not area) of the internal lumen of the artery compared with a neighboring unoccluded diameter of the same vessel. From Ta-

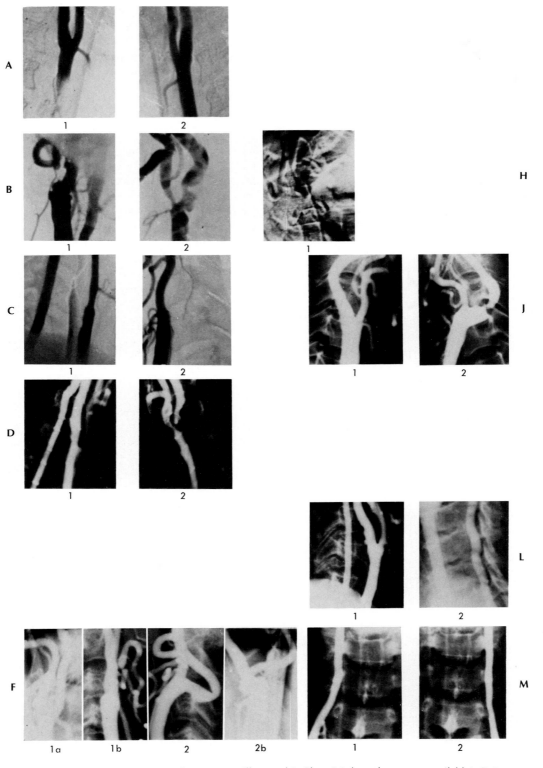

Fig. 36-2. Angiograms corresponding to scans illustrated in Plate 2 (where these were available). *F, 1a* and *1b* and *2a* and *2b*, show anteroposterior and lateral projections, respectively, of right (1) and left (2) carotid bifurcations.

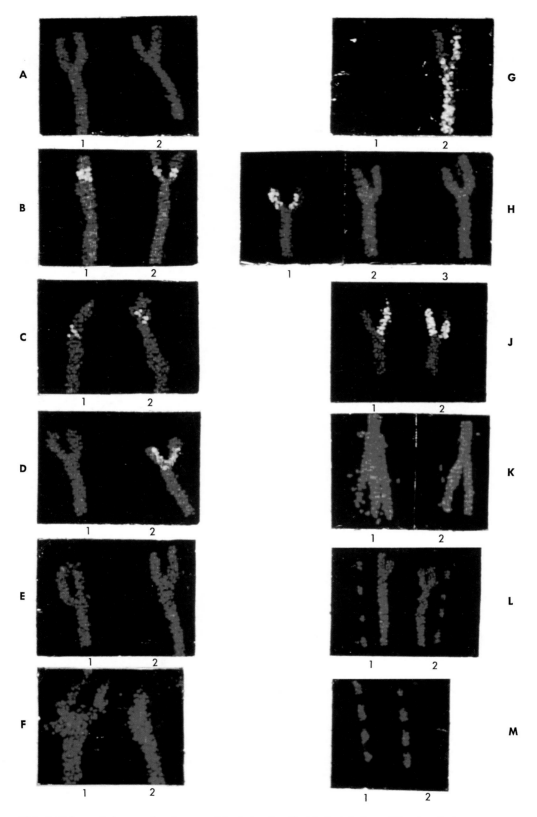

Plate 2. Color-coded scans of various carotid arteries described in text. Left carotid system is shown on right of pairs displayed, and right system is shown on left. **G,** 2, shows left carotid bifurcation; right carotid system was not displayed because of common carotid artery occlusion, **H,** 1, shows left carotid bifurcation; right was not displayed (see text). **H,** 2, and 3, show right and left carotid bifurcations in this patient following repair of innominate occlusion. **K,** 1, shows right femoral trifurcation and **K,** 2, brachial artery bifurcation. **L** is display of right and left carotid and vertebral arteries made with continuous-wave system and **M** shows two vertebral arteries only, made with pulsed and time-gated system.

Table 36-1. Comparison of the Doppler scans and angiograms in 1001 consecutive carotid bifurcations examined by both techniques

Carotid scans*	Angiogram					
	No stenosis	Mild stenosis <24%	Moderate stenosis		Marked stenosis >74%	Occlusion
			25-49%	50-74%		
Normal (red)						
CC	845	**21**	3	0	0	0
IC	486	**123**	11	3	0	2
EC	719	**12**	3	0	1	1
Moderate stenosis (yellow)						
CC	**25**	**11**	20	4	**2**	0
IC	**29**	**55**	41	8	**3**	0
EC	**63**	**34**	29	11	**2**	0
Severe stenosis (blue)						
CC	2	1	**2**	**5**	39	0
IC	0	2	**6**	**21**	88	4
EC	4	1	**4**	**12**	59	0
Occlusion						
CC	1	0	0	0	0	13
IC	9	2	1	1	25	75
EC	1	0	0	0	0	15
High velocity throughout vessel						
CC	7					
IC	6					
EC	30					

*The bifurcations are divided into their three components—common (CC), external (EC), and internal (IC) carotid arteries. The degree of angiographic stenosis is given as a percentage of the diameter of the vessel occluded. The areas outlined by a box represent good agreement between the two techniques; the areas with numbers set in boldface type represent acceptable agreement.

ble 36-1 it will be seen that there was good agreement in 82% of the three segments of the 1001 carotid bifurcations and acceptable agreement in 96%.

Normal carotid bifurcations. There was good agreement between the two techniques when the carotid bifurcations were normal. When the angiogram was normal, the Doppler scan had a specificity of 94% and a negative predictive accuracy of 92%. If scans containing regions of yellow are considered to be within normal limits, then both the specificity and the negative predictive accuracy rise to 99%.

As a result of the confidence our fellow clinicians have developed in the reliability of a normal ultrasonic Doppler scan, there has been a marked decline in the number of normal angiograms performed in Kingston, Ontario, during the last several years. We feel that even if this technique had no other advantages, development of a noninvasive technique that reduces the numbers of patients submitted to the hazards of angiography is an important contribution to patient care.

Occlusions. Of 110 radiologically demonstrated occlusions, the Doppler scan correctly identified 103. In 3 of the cases not diagnosed by the Doppler scan there is fairly good evidence that the occlusion developed in the internal carotid artery after the Doppler scan and before angiography was performed. Thus the true incidence of false negative Doppler scans in cases of carotid occlusion would appear to be 4 out of 110, yielding a sensitivity of 97%. In 3 of these cases we mistook a large collateral branch developed by the external carotid artery shortly after its origin for the common carotid bifurcation. In the fourth case the angiogram was in error. The injection had been made into the internal carotid artery, and the external carotid artery, which did not fill, was falsely diagnosed as being occluded. This error of the angiogram would not have been identified without the preceding Doppler scan.

There were 40 arteries in which the Doppler scan was thought to demonstrate an occlusion not shown to be present radiologically. In 25 of these 40 arteries a very high grade stenosis (98% or more) of the internal carotid artery was present. Presumably the amplitude of the signals from the blood flowing through the hair-thin stenosis and the velocity of the blood in the patent vessel proximal and distal to the stenosis were below the respective thresholds for display by our system.

In 11 of the remaining 15 arteries, stenotic or occlusive lesions were present outside the region scanned, such as the carotid siphon. These lesions slowed flow through the artery being scanned so that it could not activate the display. One of these cases is illustrated in Plate 2, *H,* and corresponding Fig. 36-2. In this case an occlusion of the innominate artery resulted in the right carotid system being filled by retrograde flow from the right vertebral artery. Flow in the right common, internal, and external carotid arteries was of insufficient velocity to activate the Doppler display. Following the excision of the innominate occlusion, the Doppler scan was repeated (Plate 2, *H,* 2 and 3), and both bifurcations were seen to be normal, which had not been apparent from the angiogram (Fig. 36-2, *H,* 1). The normality of the bifurcation was subsequently verified at operation. In the 4 remaining cases arteriosclerotic disease had so deformed the course of the origin of the internal carotid artery that it lay at a 90-degree angle to the beam (Plate 2, *F,* 2, and Fig. 36-2) and hence could return no Doppler-shifted signals. Plate 2, *F,* 1, and Fig. 36-2 also show that arteriosclerosis may sometimes reverse the normal position of the internal and external carotid arteries displayed on the scans. Such deformities can be identified by the different characteristics of flow in the two arteries heard on the audio display and seen on the time-velocity strip chart recording, flow in the internal carotid artery being less pulsatile than that in the external carotid artery.

Stenoses. The Doppler scans were also accurate in displaying severe arterial stenoses. In 219 cases where the angiogram showed a stenosis occluding more than 74% of the arterial diameter, the Doppler scan showed a similar severe stenosis—color coded blue—in 85% of the arterial segments, or 88% if the segments displayed as yellow are also included. There were 25 cases with a very high grade stenosis and hair-thin lumen of the artery, in which the artery was not displayed and an occlusion falsely diagnosed, as previously mentioned. The positive predictive accuracy of the scans for severe stenoses is therefore 74%; however, if the cases with high-grade stenoses that were diagnosed as occlusions

are excluded, the positive predictive accuracy rises to 96%.

Of 65 arterial segments where the angiogram showed a stenosis occluding between 50% and 74% of the arterial diameter, the Doppler scan showed a region color-coded either blue or yellow in 94%. Of 120 arterial segments where the angiogram showed a moderate stenosis (occluding between 25% and 49% of the arterial diameter), the Doppler scan showed a region appropriately color-coded yellow in 75%. Of 262 segments in which the angiogram showed stenosis of less than 24% of the arterial diameter, the Doppler scan showed an appropriate yellow region in only 38%; the majority (60%) had normal Doppler scans.

Collateral flow. There were 42 arterial segments that differed in their Doppler scans from those previously described insofar as the whole arterial segment was color-coded yellow or blue. These were cases in which occlusive disease had resulted in development of a collateral circulation with increased velocities of flow through the arterial segments concerned. Since the external carotid circulation is usually involved in such collateral compensation, 30 of these 43 segments were in the displayed portion of the external carotid artery. In Plate 2, *J,* and Fig. 36-2, a stenosis of the left internal carotid artery is displayed, but another stenosis of the right internal carotid artery at the level of the siphon is outside the range of our scan and is not seen. As a result of these two marked stenoses of both internal carotid arteries, collateral circulation has developed via both external carotid arteries, both of which show increased peak velocities of flow as denoted by the yellow coloration throughout their displayed courses. In Plate 2, *G,* and Fig. 36-2, increased velocities of flow are shown throughout the entire course of the left common and internal carotid arteries as a result of complete occlusion of the right common carotid artery, which does not appear on the display.

RESULTS OF OTHER WORKERS

The first results reported by other workers originated from O'Leary et al.[4] and Persson et al.[10]; these authors also went on to publish further reports.[5,6,8,9] It should be noted that they considered all stenoses of less than 65% as normal. Initial results on 81 patients[4] showed an overall accuracy, sensitivity, and specificity of 96%, and the researchers concluded that the technique was more sensitive and accurate than the periorbital directional Doppler examination and oculopneumo-plethysmography. The two false positive results were caused by a 45% stenosis and kinking of the artery while the one false negative result was caused by imaging branches of the external carotid artery when the internal carotid was occluded. In a later series of 216 patients,[6] O'Leary et al. found that the accuracy of the color-coded Doppler system was 94% in comparison with 84% for oculo-plethysmography combined with carotid phonoangiography and 80% for periorbital directional Doppler sonography. They also found that when the Doppler scans agreed with the periorbital directional Doppler examination an accuracy of 99% was achieved, and when it agreed with oculoplethysmography and phonoangiography the accuracy was 98%. These findings reinforce the statement made earlier in the chapter, that greater degrees of accuracy can be obtained if the Echoflow examination is combined with other noninvasive tests. In more recent results,[9] Persson et al. stated that "the status of the carotid bifurcation in over 97% of the patients" could be predicted using a combination of the Echoflow, auditory spectrum analysis, and common carotid waveforms "to determine the status of the carotid bifurcation," and oculoplethysmography and carotid phonoangiography to assess the hemodynamic implications of the lesions demonstrated by the three other techniques.

Italian workers[7] have also reported good results with the technique and have pointed out that they used it with equal success on 23 supraaortic arch vessels, 21 arteries to the leg, and five to the arm. In Germany[1] there was good correlation between the angiograms and carotid scans in 200 patients. These workers reported that the system provided "reasonable" information for stenoses of between 50% and 75% of the arterial diameter and became "quite accurate" for stenoses of 85% to 90%.

REFERENCES

1. Aichner, F., and Gerstenbrand, F.: Der Dopplerechoflow als neue screeningmethode der extrakraniellen karotiserkrankung, Akt. Neurol. 8:62, 1981.
2. Curry, G.R., and White, D.N.: Color-coded ultrasonic differential velocity arterial scanner (Echoflow*), Ultrasound Med. Biol. 4:27, 1978.
3. Hokanson, D.E., et al.: Ultrasonic arteriography: a new approach to arterial visualization, Biomed. Eng. 6:420, 1971.
4. O'Leary, D.H., Persson, A.V., and Clouse, M.E.: Prospective analysis of the comparative accuracy of various non-invasive modalities in the detection of extracranial carotid vascular disease (abstract), Proceedings of the eighteenth meeting of the American Society of Neuroradiologists, 1980.
5. O'Leary, D.H., Persson, A.V., and Clouse, M.E.: Noninvasive testing for carotid stenosis. Prospective analysis of three methods, AJNR 2:437, 1981.
6. O'Leary, D.H., et al.: Noninvasive testing for carotid artery stenosis. II. Clinical application of accuracy assessments, AJR 138:109, 1982.
7. Oliva, L., et al.: L'arteriografia ultrasonica ad effeto Doppler con analisi colorimetrica morfo-funzionale delle frequenze (Echoflow), Minerva Med. 72:2465, 1981.
8. Persson, A.V., and Dyer, V.A.: Explorations noninvasives des arteres carotides, J. Mal. Vasc. 6:263, 1981.
9. Persson, A.V., Robichaux, W.T., and Griffey, S.P.: Use of Doppler ultrasound in clinical interrogation of carotid bifurcation, J. Cardiovasc. Ultrason. 1:87, 1982.
10. Persson, A.V., et al.: Clinical use of noninvasive evaluation of the carotid artery, Surg. Clin. North Am. 60:513, 1980.
11. Reid, J.M., and Spencer, M.P.: Ultrasonic Doppler technique for imaging blood vessels, Science 176:1235, 1972.
12. Spencer, M.P., et al.: Cerebrovascular evaluation using Doppler CW ultrasound. In White, D.N., and Brown, R., editors: Ultrasound in medicine, vol. 3B, New York, 1977, Plenum Publishing Corp.
13. White, D.N.: The angiographic correlations of 1001 carotid bifurcations examined with a color-coded Doppler scanner (Echoflow). In Diethrich, E.B., editor: Non-invasive cardiovascular diagnosis III, Bristol, England, 1982, John Wright & Sons, Ltd.
14. White, D.N., and Curry, G.R.: Clinical results with a color-coded differential velocity carotid bifurcation tomographic scanner. In White, D.N., and Brown, R., editors: Ultrasound in medicine, vol. 3B, New York, 1977, Plenum Press.
15. White, D.N., and Curry, G.R.: Color-coded differential Doppler ultrasonic scanning system for the carotid bifurcation: results on 486 bifurcations angiographically confirmed. In Kurjak, A., editor: Recent advances in ultrasound diagnosis, Excerpta Medica International Congress Series No. 436, Amsterdam, 1978, Excerpta Medica.
16. White, D.N., and Curry, G.R.: A comparison of 424 carotid bifurcations examined by angiography and the Doppler Echoflow.* In White, D.N., and Lyons, E.A., editors: Ultrasound in medicine, vol. 4, New York, 1978, Plenum Press.
17. White, D.N., and Curry, G.R.: Noninvasive ultrasonic Doppler techniques for the diagnosis of occlusive carotid artery disease and results of the spatial displays of the Echoflow* on 667 carotid bifurcations angiographically confirmed. In Diethrich, E.B., editor: Noninvasive cardiovascular diagnosis, vol. 2, Littleton, Mass., 1981, PSG Publishing Co., Inc.

CHAPTER 37

Ultrasonic imaging for carotid occlusive disease

ANTHONY J. COMEROTA, JOHN J. CRANLEY, and WILLIAM G. HAYDEN

During the past 10 years many noninvasive screening techniques have been developed for the detection of carotid occlusive disease. Since 40% to 50% of all strokes are secondary to atherosclerotic disease of the cervical carotid arteries,[10] it is appropriate that noninvasive vascular laboratory testing be directed toward the detection of the responsible lesion.

Many previously developed noninvasive tests attempt to detect abnormalities of vascular physiology (pulse arrival time, ophthalmic pressure, or collateral flow patterns) that occur only after a 40% to 50% diameter reduction stenosis (70% to 80% area reduction) of the involved carotid artery. Although these physiologic methods imply carotid artery stenosis, they are indirect and in truth detect only that an abnormality exists somewhere between the aortic arch and the orbit of the eye. Techniques that image the carotid bifurcation have grown in popularity and are becoming an established part of the noninvasive cerebrovascular evaluation.

The Doppler imaging devices diagrammatically recreate the vessel lumen on a storage oscilloscope when the flow velocity exceeds a threshold value. An audible analysis of the flow signal, analog waveform analysis, or sound spectral analysis can be included to supplement the visual display. These techniques evaluate the carotid artery directly; however, they are physiologic studies and the image obtained is based on flow.[1,13,14,23] Real-time B-mode ultrasonic imaging provides structural detail of the vessel wall and atherosclerotic plaque. Structures are visualized by sound-wave reflection from the interfaces of tissues with different acoustic impedances, hence providing true anatomic detail. There are many studies that report preliminary results of this technique. Findings range from qualitative statements of excellent correlation, to data

that reflect varying results depending on the grade of disease.* Opinions differ as to how the technical quality of the scan affects accuracy and whether the totally occluded carotid artery can be reliably diagnosed.[5,13] It is difficult to draw conclusions from previously published reports because the transducers used were of varying frequency, there was no standard for performing the technique or interpreting the results, and the numbers of vessels studied were small. It cannot be determined whether these reports represent preliminary data or lasting results that can be achieved with experience. Therefore the definitive role of real-time B-mode carotid imaging was not established, and its true place in the diagnosis of cerebrovascular disease was not yet found.

Potentially this diagnostic technique may have direct influence on patient management; however, it cannot be intelligently used nor can its impact on patient care be assessed until its reliability is clearly defined. This report is an attempt to establish the place of real-time B-mode carotid imaging in the diagnosis of carotid artery disease through analysis of the results of 3 years of experience in three major noninvasive vascular laboratories. During that time, 7031 patients were studied in these laboratories. Bilateral carotid arteriography was performed on 869 patients, and 8 patients received unilateral carotid arteriograms. Inadequate arteriographic visualization resulted in the elimination of 23 vessels. A total of 1723 vessels were studied both noninvasively and arteriographically and form the basis of this report. The noninvasive studies were performed by 11 technicians and interpreted by three physicians. Each laboratory used similar equipment, studied patients according to an estab-

*References 2, 5, 6, 9, 13, 15, 16, 20, 25

lished technique, and interpreted the results using standardized criteria. During the analysis, the influence of scan quality, technical experience, intercenter variability, and addition of indirect physiologic studies was specifically addressed.

Materials

The imager used in the studies just mentioned was the Biosound real-time ultrasonic imager with the 4 cm, 8 MHz transducer. The scan field is 4 cm deep by 3.5 cm wide with an axial resolution of 0.3 mm at 2 cm focal length (Fig. 37-1). The focal zone of the transducer can be modified by a depth control switch. The gray-scale image is viewed on a video monitor at 60 frames/sec. The transducer, which has a small self-contained water bath, consists of a transmitting and receiving piezoelectric crystal with a high-speed shutter and mirror mechanism that directs the beam. The images on the video monitor incorporate 256 shades of gray and represent 6-power magnification of actual vessel size. Videotapes were made for physician interpretation and kept for at least 6 months for further study and analysis. Hard copy reproductions were obtained with the Dunn camera unit or via Polaroid photographs. The reproduction process, however, results in loss of image quality compared to the video image.

Methods

All patients were scanned in the supine position with a pillow beneath their shoulders and with their head rotated away from the side being studied. The transducer was placed immediately superior to the clavicle in a longitudinal plane at the medial border of the sternocleidomastoid muscle. The carotid arteries were visualized in a cephalad direction until the probe was limited by the mandible. The patients were similarly scanned from the lateral, posterolateral, and transverse projections. Between each position, the probe was "rocked" by the technician to more clearly delineate plaques and the intervening portion of the vessel wall. Considering the various angles of evaluation, only a fraction of the vessel wall circumference is "blind" to the ultrasonic beam (Fig. 37-2). Simultaneous identification of the internal and external carotid arteries in longitudinal profile (Fig. 37-3, A) was the exception rather than the rule, since these vessels frequently lie in different planes.

The transverse view is routinely obtained (Fig. 37-3, B). This view was frequently unsatisfactory because of technical artifacts and distortion of sound-wave reflection resulting in poor visualization of part of the vessel wall. When good visualization was obtained on the transverse view, it was invaluable in assessing the amount of disease and degree of stenosis.

The *time-gain control* (TGC) setting was varied and generally adjusted to higher levels to increase visibility of soft plaque and thrombus. Although the high TGC setting increases sensitivity, it likewise tends to promote artifacts observed during scanning and will increase false positive readings.

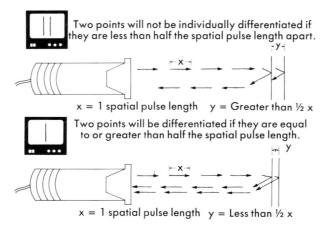

Fig. 37-1. Schematic drawing of ultrasound waves reflecting from tissue interfaces with resultant image produced. Schematic drawing also represents principle of axial resolution. (From Comerota, A.J., Cranley, J.J., and Cook, S.E.: Surgery 89:718, 1981.)

Schematic of right carotid examination

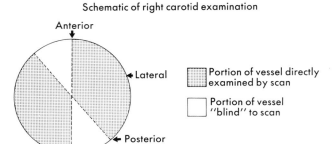

Fig. 37-2. Shaded area represents circumference of vessel wall examined by real-time ultrasound technique. White area represents portion of vessel wall that was "blind" to examination. (From Comerota, A.J., Cranley, J.J., and Cook, S.E.: Surgery 89:718, 1981.)

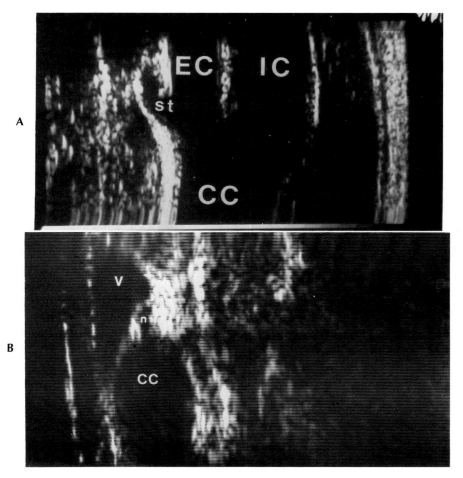

Fig. 37-3. A, Normal longitudinal scan. *CC,* common carotid artery; *IC,* internal carotid artery; *EC,* external carotid artery; *st,* superior thyroid artery. **B,** Normal transverse scan of carotid sheath. Note flattening of jugular vein *(V)* resulting from probe pressure. Also visualized are common carotid artery *(CC)* and vagus nerve *(n).* (From Comerota, A.J., Cranley, J.J., and Cook, S.E.: Surgery 89:718, 1981.)

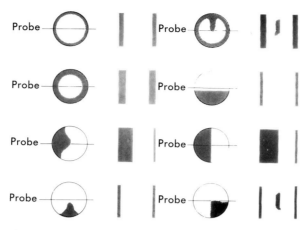

Fig. 37-4. Concepts of interpretation. Representations of plaque configurations as they would appear in longitudinal scan. (From Comerota, A.J., Cranley, J.J., and Cook, S.E.: Surgery 89:718, 1981.)

The low TGC settings maximize contrast between tissue interfaces and minimize or eliminate contrast differences between thrombus and soft plaque with flowing blood.

Interpretation

Ultrasonography and arteriography measure separate but related disease characteristics. The arteriogram reveals a shadow encroaching on the lumen, whereas ultrasound directly visualizes the vessel wall and its abnormality. When correlating the two studies, one must consider the dynamic multiplanar information available with real-time ultrasound vs. the uniplanar or biplanar static views of arteriography. The best ultrasonic image may be at right angles to the best x-ray view that is used for comparison. The varying planes of *sonic section* may reveal different degrees of diameter stenosis (Fig. 37-4), depending on the plane of interrogation and the degree of plaque asymmetry.

All noninvasive studies were interpreted without knowledge of the contrast arteriogram. The carotid branches can be reliably identified, since the external carotid artery is more anterior and medial, is usually smaller, contains the superior thyroid branch, and has minimal diastolic flow. The internal carotid artery is generally more posterior and lateral, has no branches, is frequently bulbous and of larger size than the external, is in apposition to the jugular vein, and normally has significant diastolic flow.

Table 37-1. Scan quality criteria

Quality	Criteria
Excellent	Sharp tissue interfaces, all walls visualized on all views, longitudinal and transverse
Good	Lumen and walls well visualized, intraluminal contents generally distinguishable from wall or surrounding tissue in same projection
Fair	Lumen and walls visualized, but not always in same projection, and some inference required to maintain vessel continuity
Poor	Vessel located and lumen identified, but boundary between wall and lumen is unclear
Nonvisualized	Vessel not visualized

The scan of each internal carotid artery was assigned a quality according to that described in Table 37-1. To assess whether experience affected reliability, the study was divided into two time periods. The first 12 months represent the learning period during which technical familiarity was gained and interpretation criteria established. During the next 24 months, the technique was standardized and should represent the current status of this diagnostic technique.

Each ultrasonic scan and each arteriogram was divided into one of four grades of disease based on the diameter reduction stenosis. The percentage of stenosis indicated by the scan and x-ray films was determined by caliper measurement of the narrowest portion of the lumen within the area of the greatest disease, compared with the most normal portion of the internal carotid artery distal to the stenosis. The four categories were grade I (0% to 39% stenosis), grade II (40% to 69% stenosis), grade III (70% to 99% stenosis), and grade IV (total occlusion).

Specificity refers to the correct identification of normal vessels and those with less than 40% stenosis. It was initially hoped that the normal vessel could be identified separately from the vessel with minimal disease. Because the resolution of the arteriogram would not permit consistent identification of minor vessel wall abnormalities, the 0% to 39% range was accepted as a singular grade. The sensitivity for each of the grades II through IV is defined as the percentage of scans in which the grade of disease identified corresponded with the arteriographic findings. The negative predictive value (NPV) is the percentage of scans indicating normal arteries or disease in the grade I range that were verified by arteriography, and the positive predictive value (PPV) is defined as the percentage of scans correctly identifying disease in the range of grades II through IV. All scans that did not agree with the arteriogram and those that did not visualize the internal carotid artery were considered errors.

Results

The global distribution of scans compared with arteriograms is presented in Table 37-2. The four groups of numbers accompanied by footnote citations represent exact correlation of the scan with the arteriogram.

The specificity of the scan for detecting arteries with little or no stenosis was 86.5% (985/1139). The sensitivity for detecting grade II disease was 72.3% (193/267); for grade III disease, 66.2% (133/201); and for grade IV disease, 63.8% (74/116). The NPV of grade I scans was 93.4% (985/1055). The PPV of grade II scans was 54.2% (193/359); grade III scans, 70.7% (133/188); and grade IV scans, 85.1% (74/87).

There were 168 false positive scans, 136 false negative scans, and 34 internal carotid arteries were not visualized.

In this report, the term *accuracy* has been avoided, since it can often be misleading, depending on the sample population studied and disease distribution within that sample.

Quality. The relationship of the quality and the predictive value of the scans is presented in Table 37-3. A consistent relationship is observed; the

Table 37-2. Results of real-time B-mode carotid imaging compared with those of conventional arteriogram

Ultrasonic scan results	No. of arteries	Distribution according to arteriogram			
		Grade I	Grade II	Grade III	Grade IV
Grade I	1055	985 (86.5)* (93.4)†	42	18	10
Grade II	359	113	193 (72.3)‡ (54.2)§	39	14
Grade III	188	18	24	133 (66.2)‡ (70.7)§	13
Grade IV	87	3	2	8	74 (63.8)‡ (85.1)§
Not visualized	34	20	6	3	5
TOTAL		1139	267	201	116

*Specificity (%).
†NPV (%).
‡Sensitivity (%).
§PPV(%).

better the quality of the scan, the higher its predictive value. When relating quality and predictive value for each scan grade (Table 37-4), it is uniformly observed that the better the quality of the scan, the more reliable the result. The predictive values and the accompanying 95% confidence intervals for excellent or good quality scans for each grade are listed in Table 37-5. Larger 95% confidence intervals are noted with smaller patient groups.

Experience. The specificity and sensitivity per disease grade for each vascular laboratory are represented by the graphs in Fig. 37-5, *A* (first period) and *B* (second period). In each period there are extremely consistent data shared by each vascular laboratory. There are no significant differences between laboratories for any disease grade or between either time period. Analyzing Fig. 37-5, *A* and *B*,

it is apparent that there is improvement in the diagnostic sensitivity for grade III and grade IV disease.

Fig. 37-5, *C*, represents the cumulative data obtained from the three vascular laboratories comparing results of the first time period with the second time period. The improvement in the sensitivity for detecting grade III disease is not statistically significant (p = .12).* However, there is a significant improvement in the ability to diagnose grade IV disease (total occlusion) (p < .002).* It is evident that experience did not improve the ability to detect a normal, mild, or moderately diseased vessel.

Total occlusion. The criteria for diagnosis of the totally occluded vessel (Fig. 37-6) are as follows:
1. A technically good quality scan
2. Visualization of significant disease
3. The absence of radial wall pulsation distal to the area of disease
4. The absence of Doppler flow signals in the diseased segment and distally
5. Abnormal common carotid Doppler signals with loss of the normal diastolic flow pattern[4]

The sensitivity of diagnosing the occluded carotid was low during the first period; however, it was significantly improved during the second period. Additionally, 47% (54/115) of patients with total occlusion were found to have greater than 50% stenosis of the contralateral carotid artery; 78% (42/

Table 37-3. Relationship of quality and predictive value of ultrasonic scans*

Quality of scan	Correct†	Incorrect	Total
Excellent	27 (100)	0	27
Good	747 (87.4)	107	854
Fair	556 (79.1)	147	703
Poor	55 (52.4)	50	105
Not visualized	0	34	34
TOTAL	1385 (80.4)	338	1723

*Figures include all grades of disease detected.
†Numbers in parentheses denote predictive value (%).

*Corrected χ^2 analysis.

Table 37-4. Relationship of quality and predictive value for each scan grade

Quality of scan	Grade I*			Grade II†			Grade III†			Grade IV†		
	Correct	Incorrect	Total	Correct	Incorrect	Total	Correct	Incorrect	Total	Correct	Incorrect	Total
Excellent	24 (100)	0	24	1 (100)	0	1	1	0	1	1 (100)	0	1
Good	545 (97.1)	16	561	94 (61.0)	60	154	77 (75.5)	25	102	31 (83.8)	6	37
Fair	375 (91.5)	35	410	90 (52.0)	83	173	52 (69.3)	23	75	39 (86.7)	6	45
Poor	41 (68.3)	19	60	8 (25.8)	23	31	3 (30.0)	7	10	3 (75.0)	1	4
TOTAL	985 (93.4)	70	1055	193 (53.8)	166	359	133 (70.7)	55	188	74 (85.1)	13	87

*Numbers in parentheses denote NPV.
†Numbers in parentheses denote PPV.

Table 37-5. Real-time B-mode carotid imaging: predictive value and 95% confidence interval for each scan grade (good quality scans)

Scan grade	No. of scans	Predictive value (%)	Confidence interval (%)
I	585	97.3	96/99
II	155	61.3	53/69
III	103	75.7	65/83
IV	38	84.2	68/95

Table 37-6. Real-time B-mode carotid imaging: cumulative frequency of errors

Type of error	No. of errors*
1. Interpretation error	90 (26.6)
2. Scan-arteriogram mismatch	79 (23.4)
3. Technically poor or inaccurate scan	75 (22.2)
4. ICA† not visualized high enough to see stenosis	25 (7.4)
5. ICA-ECA misidentification	21 (6.2)
6. Poor scan—cause uncertain	19 (5.6)
7. Red thrombus or soft plaque not detected	11 (3.3)
8. Poor technique	8 (2.3)
9. Artifact	4 (1.2)
10. Anatomic variation	4 (1.2)
11. Plaque orientation	2 (0.6)
TOTAL ERRORS	338 (19.6)
NO ERRORS	1385 (80.4)
TOTAL VESSELS	1723

*Expressed as a percentage of the total errors.
†ICA, Internal carotid artery; ECA, external carotid artery.

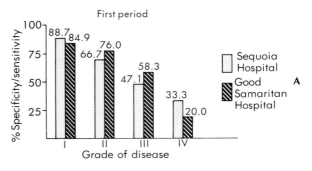

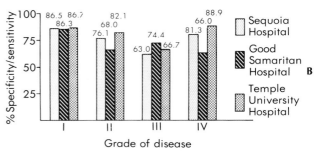

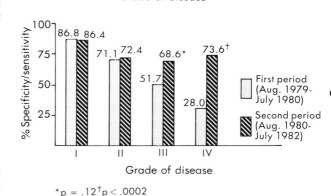

$^*p = .12$ $^†p < .0002$

Fig. 37-5. A, Bar graph representing first period data for each scan grade in each laboratory. **B,** Bar graph representing second period data for each scan grade from each laboratory. **C,** Bar graph representing combined data comparing first and second periods from three vascular laboratories. (From Comerota, A.J., et al.: J. Vasc. Surg. 111:84, 1984.)

54) of the contralateral carotid arteries were accurately identified noninvasively.

Errors. Each false positive and false negative scan was reviewed and the error placed into one of 11 categories (Table 37-6). In some scans there were obviously several contributing factors leading to the error; however, the dominant factor was identified and listed. Interpretation errors, scan-arteriogram mismatch, and technically poor scans secondary to disease were responsible for the overwhelming majority of the errors. In 7.4%, the internal carotid was not visualized high enough to see the stenosis. This was suspected in several in-

stances when the direct carotid Doppler examination was abnormal and an OPG was positive. In such situations, however, it was difficult to determine if the lesion was located in the high cervical or intracranial internal carotid artery. Improvement of the direct carotid Doppler examination should minimize this problem. Misidentification of the external carotid artery for the internal carotid artery was responsible for 6.2% of the errors, and it appeared to be a larger problem in the early part of this study. The inability of the B-mode carotid imager to detect red thrombus or soft plaque has been recognized as a major weakness of the technique and has contributed to diagnostic errors in over one third of the patients in a previous report.[20] These problems were responsible for only 3.3% of the errors in this series. Artifact, anatomic variation, and plaque orientation were infrequent causes of error.

Mismatch. A good quality scan that identified more disease than the arteriogram is called a *mismatch* (Fig. 37-7). When these false positive results were reviewed, no technical, anatomic, or interpretive error could be found. Although it was our impression that these scans were representative of the existing disease and that the arteriogram underestimated the disease present, the mismatch scans are reported as false positive errors. Of the 79 mismatched vessels, 16 underwent carotid endarterectomy. In 14 the operative findings could be compared to the preoperative studies. In 12 out of 14 (86%) the scan was judged correct, and in 2 out of 14 (14%) the arteriogram more accurately represented the disease present. An additional interesting observation was that 70% of the OPGs in the mismatch group were positive, indicating a stenosis of greater than 40% diameter reduction.

Discussion

The disease classification was chosen because it appeared that this imaging technique could provide information that would further refine our ability to identify and quantify atherosclerotic disease of the carotid bifurcation. At the beginning of this study it was anticipated that the completely normal vessel could be differentiated from the vessel with minimal disease. Quickly it became evident that a large number of vessels that were shown to be normal by arteriography showed at least minimal disease on the scan. Using arteriography as the standard to judge noninvasive studies is mandatory. However, it would be unjust to call good quality scans that showed wall plaque erroneous if the same lesion was not indicated on the arteriogram. Many biplane carotid arteriograms result in a single good planar view of the carotid bifurcation because of vessel or bone overlap. The variability and inconsistency of carotid arteriographic interpretations have been documented.[7,24] Although the relationship of accuracy and quality of arteriographic studies has not been documented, data support the fact that contrast arteriography does not reliably identify moderate disease.[8] It was not the intent of this report to evaluate arteriography; however, in the evaluation of any noninvasive technique that uses arteriography as the standard, one must appreciate the shortcomings of the contrast arteriogram.

When identifying the role of any noninvasive test, we must attempt to extract as much information as is available from that test. An objective analysis of the information should reveal areas of strength and weakness of the test, thus allowing its most appropriate clinical use. Since the technology in noninvasive vascular diagnosis is rapidly advancing and becoming more refined and since the therapy for cerebrovascular atherosclerotic disease is in evolution, it follows that noninvasive cerebrovascular diagnosis should become more detailed. It is clear that the implications of asymptomatic disease in a patient with a 50% stenosis of the internal carotid artery are different than those in a patient with a 95% stenosis, yet many reports continue to classify disease as greater than or less than 50%. Data suggest that symptomatic patients with hemodynamic lesions are at greater risk for stroke than symptomatic patients without hemodynamic stenoses.[3,19] Compiling data from several centers, it can be argued that selected asymptomatic patients with hemodynamically significant lesions have a higher risk of developing conditions leading to stroke than symptomatic patients without hemodynamically significant stenoses.[3,18,19] Although we routinely obtain carotid arteriograms on all patients with symptoms of cerebrovascular disease, it is well established that not all patients remain symptomatic and not all patients have a stroke.[21] The question remains as to which of these patients are at high risk, and which, if any, are at low risk and can be treated with platelet inhibitors. Although definitive data are not available, it seems reasonable to suggest that symptomatic patients with minimal cervical carotid disease would be appropriately treated with platelet inhibitors, whereas patients with carotid atherosclerosis associated with a significant stenosis should undergo carotid endarterectomy. If this therapeutic approach is correct, then a noninvasive technique that reliably identifies the normal and minimally diseased vessel will be of particular value, since many patients could be spared carotid arteriography.

An unexpected finding from this study was the high NPV of the good quality grade I scans (97.3%), with the 95% confidence interval being 96% to 99%. The emphasis previously placed on cerebrovascular testing was the detection of the hemodynamically significant lesion. Yet when one evaluates the arteriographic distribution of disease in the patients of this study as well as others, one finds that most vessels are normal or contain min-

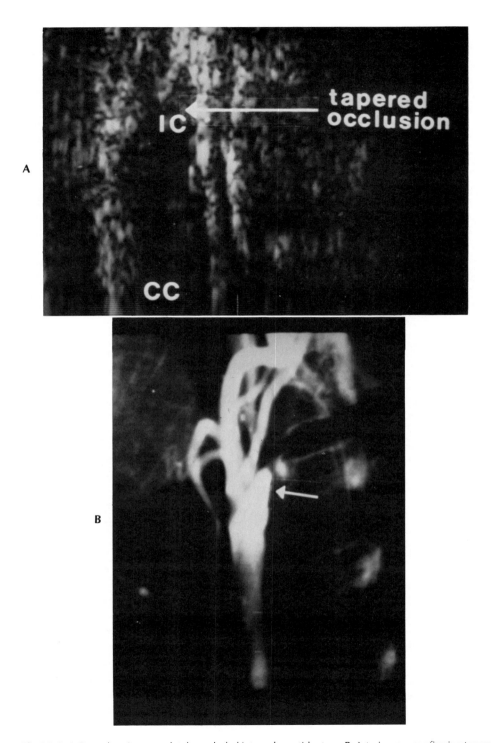

Fig. 37-6. A, Scan showing completely occluded internal carotid artery. **B,** Arteriogram confirming tapered occlusion of internal carotid artery.

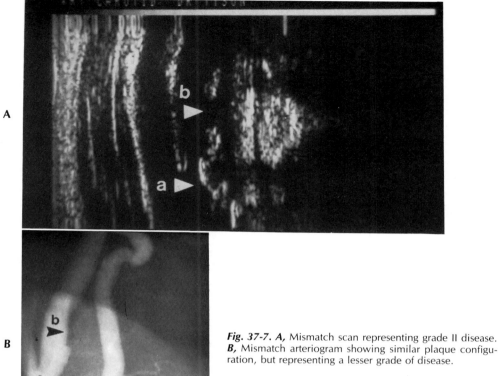

Fig. 37-7. A, Mismatch scan representing grade II disease. **B,** Mismatch arteriogram showing similar plaque configuration, but representing a lesser grade of disease.

imal disease. An additional finding of interest is that of the 869 patients who underwent bilateral carotid arteriography, 438 had arteriograms classified as grade I bilaterally. The good quality B-mode carotid image can be of particular value in identifying these patients, thereby diminishing or eliminating the need for arteriography. The narrow 95% confidence interval indicates that the (97.3%) accurately represents the true value for scans in this category.

The consensus among vascular surgeons is that if a noninvasive technique could reliably identify an occluded internal carotid artery, it would obviate the need for arteriography. It was evident that during the first period of this study the sensitivity for diagnosing total occlusion was extremely low (28%). However, with the integration and improvement of a pulsed Doppler system and the estab-

lishment of defined criteria for the ultrasonic diagnosis of total occlusion, the sensitivity improved significantly during the second period to 74% (p < .0002). The PPV of the good quality scan that diagnoses total occlusion was 82%. Since the number of occlusions was relatively small, the 95% confidence interval was relatively large (68% to 95%).

Patients with totally occluded carotid arteries may be at higher risk of stroke, particularly if there is a contralateral stenosis.[12,22] Therefore the disease status of the contralateral internal carotid artery must be accurately assessed if these patients are to be appropriately treated. An anatomic technique has the greatest potential for reliable assessment, since hemodynamic parameters will be variably affected depending on the collateral flow patterns. In this study, 78% of the contralateral carotid arteries were correctly graded. There is obvious need for improvement; however, with the increasing sensitivity for diagnosing total occlusion, heightened awareness of the need for accurate assessment of the contralateral carotid artery, and technical refinements, reliable noninvasive assessment of this important subset of patients should become the rule.

Previous investigators have considered the mismatching of scans with arteriograms and have accepted the ultrasonic image as a superior study.[9] If we accept that 86% of scans in the mismatch category were truly correct (based on operative data), then in fact there would be 68 fewer errors, resulting in an improved overall specificity to 91% (985/1079) and an improved sensitivity for grade II disease to 77%.

Difficulty in defining degrees of stenosis often arises when evaluating scans and arteriograms showing disease in the carotid bifurcation. Since this is a bulbous area anatomically, a greater volume of atheroma will be required to produce a stenosis as previously defined. In selected instances, 50% of the bulb may be narrowed; however, relative to the distal internal carotid artery there may actually be minimal or no luminal narrowing. In such cases, does a stenosis truly exist? This was a major interpretive stumbling block in this study and remains a constant problem in all correlative studies of cerebrovascular diagnosis.

Understanding the pathophysiology of atherosclerosis and the changes in vessel wall morphology as atheroma develop will also shed some light on the reason for the large mismatch category and the low predictive value of the grade II scans. In the formative stages of atheroma deposition there are degenerative changes occurring in the elastic lamina with resultant dilation of the vessel. Although the atheroma progress, the lumen area is preserved, at least for a time. Since the B-mode ultrasound technique is directed toward evaluation of the vessel wall, it will tend to draw attention to the disease contained within the wall. On the other hand, arteriography shows the residual lumen and does not address actual quantity of atherosclerosis present. When comparing these two techniques it becomes evident that the inherent nature of what is visualized by each image will prevent exact correlation.

The data presented in this report represent as objective an analysis as possible of this diagnostic technique. The results obtained indicate several weaknesses of this technique, as well as the difficulties involved in evaluating the technique. For any diagnostic study it is important to know the reliability of that particular test in an individual patient. A major benefit of this direct anatomic evaluation is that if the study is technically poor, the physician knows that additional investigation will be required.

It was our observation that the three types of atherosclerotic plaque could be characterized by real-time B-mode carotid imaging.[17] The fatty streak, fibrous plaque, and complicated lesions have been identified and assigned ultrasonic characteristics. Direct evaluation of endarterectomy specimens and the corresponding real-time B-mode carotid scan was possible for fibrous lesions and complicated lesions retrospectively. Craters and plaques, calcification, tail-like projections, small ulcerations, and areas of subintimal hemorrhage have been identified. It was only after reviewing the operative specimens and the scans that these direct correlations were made. Although these observations seem to be correct, they are retrospective, and it remains to be seen if this technique can accurately and consistently characterize the various types of atherosclerotic lesions. If it is possible to characterize the type of lesion in addition to quantifying it, then a definite advance will have been made.

SUMMARY

This chapter attempts to evaluate the place of real-time B-mode carotid imaging in the diagnosis of carotid artery disease. It is an analysis of the results of 3 years of experience in three major noninvasive vascular laboratories. During this period over 7000 patients were studied noninvasively with real-time B-mode carotid imaging. Arteriographic comparison of 1723 vessels formed the basis of this study. Angiographic interpretation and interpretation of the noninvasive studies were performed separately and without knowledge of the other. The arteriograms and ultrasonic scans were classified by diameter reduction stenosis—grade I (0 to 39%), grade II (40% to 69%), grade III (70% to 99%), and grade IV (total occlusion). The effect of the experience and technical familiarity that was gained as the imaging studies progressed was determined by segmenting the study into two time periods. The relationship of image quality and predictive value was also evaluated.

The overall data show a specificity of 86.5%

(985/1139) for detecting arteries with little or no stenosis; sensitivity for grade II disease was 72.3% (193/267); sensitivity for grade III was 66.2% (133/201); and sensitivity for grade IV was 63.8% (74/116).

As experience was gained, each center showed improvement of the imaging technique in the diagnosis of grade III disease (p > .1) and grade IV disease (p < .0002). There was no improvement in specificity and sensitivity for detecting grade II disease. All scan errors were categorized and listed. The majority of errors were interpretation errors 26.6% (90/338), scan-arteriogram mismatch 23.4% (79/338), or poor quality scans secondary to significant disease 22.2% (75/338). It was evident that a direct correlation existed between scan quality and predictive value. There was a 97.3% NPV for grade I scans of good to excellent quality. Out of 79 scan-arteriogram mismatch vessels, 16 were operated on, and from the 14 vessels in which the operative findings could be compared to the preoperative studies, the scan proved more reliable in 86%.

Real-time B-mode carotid imaging is a reliable technique for defining the normal carotid artery and is becoming increasingly sensitive in identifying existing disease. There are retrospective data to support its use in the characterization of atherosclerotic lesions; however, prospective studies are pending. Realizing the limitations of this technique, as well as its strong points, will make it more valuable as a clinical tool.

Several important conclusions can be drawn from this study:

1. The accuracy of real-time B-mode carotid imaging is directly related to the quality of the image and the severity of the disease, that is, the grade of stenosis. It was found that as the disease increases, the quality of the scan decreases. However, it was also demonstrated that a scan of good quality has a high predictive value no matter what the grade of disease.

2. The normal vessel can be reliably identified within narrow confidence limits when a good quality scan is obtained.

3. Significant improvement has been made in the diagnosis of the totally occluded carotid artery. Factors leading to the improved sensitivity include experience with the technique, defined diagnostic criteria, and an improved integrated pulsed Doppler system.

4. High carotid bifurcations and red thrombus within the vessel lumen may not be visualized; however, these represent a relatively small percentage of the false negative studies.

5. The resolution of the scan was better than that of the arteriogram in several cases with operative documentation. Therefore when a good quality scan shows disease not apparent on the arteriogram, the arteriogram is probably falsely negative.

6. The indirect physiologic cerebrovascular studies are complimentary to the direct anatomic study of real-time carotid imaging. Doppler spectrum analysis of flow through the carotid bifurcation will add detailed direct physiologic information, and the investigator interested in and experienced with the combined techniques should be able to significantly improve and refine these data.

7. Comparable results can be obtained by other centers when similar techniques and interpretation criteria are used.

8. The qualitative evaluation of atherosclerotic lesions may be possible with this technique, which will open new avenues of research for the natural history of atherosclerotic lesions and their response to therapy.

ACKNOWLEDGMENT

The author expresses his appreciation to Mira L. Katz and Francene Meinhold for their assistance in the preparation of this manuscript.

REFERENCES

1. Blackshear, W.M., et al.: Detection of carotid occlusive disease by ultrasonic imaging and pulsed Doppler spectrum analysis, Surgery 86:698, 1979.
2. Blue, S.K., et al.: Ultrasonic B-mode scanning for study of extracranial vascular disease, Neurology 22:1079, 1972.
3. Busuttil, R.W., et al.: Carotid artery stenosis—hemodynamic significance and clinical course, JAMA (14)245:1438, 1981.
4. Breslau, P.J., et al.: The role of common carotid artery velocity patterns in the evaluation of carotid bifurcation disease, Arch. Surg. 117:58, 1982.
4a. Chikos, P.M., et al.: Observer variability in evaluating extracranial carotid artery stenosis, Stroke 14:885, 1983.
5. Comerota, A.J., Cranley, J.J., and Cook, S.E.: Real-time B-mode carotid imaging in diagnosis of cerebrovascular disease, Surgery 89:718, 1981.
6. Cooperberg, P.L., et al: High resolution real-time ultrasound of the carotid bifurcation, J. Cardiovasc. Ultrasound 7:13, 1979.
7. Cranley, J.J., Presidential address: Stroke—a perspective, Surgery (5)91:537, 1982.
8. Croft, R.J., Ellam, L.D., and Harrison, M.G.: Accuracy of carotid angiography in the assessment of atheroma of the internal carotid artery, Lancet 1:997, 1980.

9. Evans, T.C.: Ultrasound B-scan imaging of atherosclerosis in carotid arteries. In Budinger, T.F., et al.: Noninvasive techniques for assessment of atherosclerosis in peripheral, carotid and coronary arteries, New York, 1982, Raven Press.

10. Fields, W.S., et al.: Joint study of extracranial arterial occlusion as a cause of stroke. I. Organization of study and survey of patient population, JAMA 203:153, 1968.

11. Gee, W.: Ocular pneumoplethysmography. In Bernstein, E.F., editor: Noninvasive diagnostic techniques in vascular disease, ed. 2, St. Louis, 1982, The C.V. Mosby Co.

12. Grillo, P., and Patterson, R.H.: Occlusion of the carotid artery: prognosis (natural history) and the possibilities of surgical revascularization, Stroke 6:17, 1975.

13. Hobson, R.W., et al.: Comparison of pulsed Doppler and real-time B-mode echo arteriography for noninvasive imaging of the extracranial arteries, Surgery (3)87:286-93, 1980.

14. Hobson, R.W., et al: Oculoplethysmography and pulsed Doppler ultrasonic imaging in diagnosis of carotid arterial disease. Surg. Gynecol. Obstet. 152:433, 1981.

15. Humber, P.R., et al.: Ultrasonic imaging of the carotid arterial system, Am. J. Surg. 140:199, 1980.

16. Johnson, J.M.: Angiography and ultrasound in diagnosis of carotid artery disease: a comparison, Contemp. Surg. 20:79, 1982.

17. Katz, M.L., Comerota, A.J., and Cranley, J.J.: Characterization of atherosclerotic plaque by real-time B-mode carotid imaging, Bruit 4:17, 1982.

18. McRae, L.P., Crain, V., and Kartchner, M.M.: In oculoplethysmography and carotid phonoangiography, Tucson, 1978, Tucson Medical Center.

19. Mendelowitz, D.S., Limmins, S., and Evans, W.E.: Prognosis of patients with transient ischemic attacks and normal angiograms, Arch. Surg. 116:1587, 1981.

20. Mercier, L.A., et al.: High-resolution ultrasound arteriography: a comparison with carotid angiography. In Bernstein, E.F., editor: Noninvasive Diagnostic Techniques In Vascular Disease, ed. 1, St. Louis, 1978, The C.V. Mosby Co.

21. Muuronen, A., and Kaste, M.: Outcome of 314 patients with transient ischemic attacks, Stroke 13:24, 1982.

22. Riles, T.S., Imparato, A.M., and Kopelman, I.: Carotid artery stenosis with contralateral internal carotid occlusion: long-term results in fifty-four patients, Surgery 87:363, 1980.

23. Sumner, D.S., et al.: Noninvasive diagnosis of extracranial carotid arterial disease, a prospective evaluation of pulsed-Doppler imaging and oculoplethysmography, Arch. Surg. 114:1222, 1979.

24. Reference deleted in proofs.

25. Vagnini, F.J., et al.: Real-time carotid ultrasonography. In Diethrich, E.B., editor: Noninvasive assessment of the cardiovascular system, Littleton, Mass., 1982, John Wright•PSG, Inc.

CHAPTER 38

Duplex scanning: practical aspects of instrument performance

DAVID J. PHILLIPS and D. EUGENE STRANDNESS, Jr.

The purpose of this chapter is to present a review of ultrasound Duplex scanner concepts along with discussions of practical considerations of instrument use. Discussion will be limited to the use of Duplex scanning in detection of extracranial peripheral vascular disease; however, the concepts and techniques employed apply equally to Duplex studies performed in other areas of the cardiovascular system.

The Duplex concept was first described by Barber.[2] The development of this concept is a direct result of the need to detect intraluminal disease that might not be visualized by imaging techniques. Some plaques exhibit acoustic properties similar to blood and therefore would not produce a detectable reflection when such an interface was encountered. The Duplex concept is the combination of pulse-echo imaging and pulsed Doppler ultrasound. The sample volume or region over which blood flow can be detected is moved about by the operator to detect blood flow while using the ultrasound cross-sectional image as an anatomic "road map." Thus although an intraluminal plaque might not be seen, its presence is recognized when the sample volume is clearly placed within the lumen and no blood flow is detected.

The original research prototype Duplex scanner alternated pulse repetition frequency (PRF) lines between the echo and pulsed Doppler modes and provided simultaneous imaging and Doppler capability.[2,9] Since the highest Doppler frequency in a pulsed system can be no greater than the PRF divided by two, it was recognized that the PRF for the pulsed Doppler system must be increased to faithfully detect the higher velocities in stenoses.

□ This work is supported by NIH grant no. HL-20898.

This trade-off was realized and accounted for in the first commercially available scanner. Fig. 38-1 shows the Duplex scanner and a typical image of the common carotid artery (CCA). Three 5 MHz transducers are sequentially activated as they pass by the skin surface, generating real-time images at 30 frames per second. When the operator reaches an anatomic area of interest, the scan head is held still, a foot switch is pressed, and one of the transducers is employed in the pulsed Doppler mode. The selected transducer can be positioned in range and angle by the operator to place the white dot (sample volume) at desired intraluminal sites. In Fig. 38-1 the operator controls the sample volume placement by the articulated arm. Fig. 38-2 shows that the scanner operates in either the pulse-echo mode or the pulsed Doppler mode. The image is electronically stored and displayed when the foot switch is activated. This display provides a spatial map for sample volume placement. If the scan head moves, it is easy to switch back and forth between the two operating modes to ensure desired sample volume placement. For the carotid artery application, the maximum depth of interest is 4 cm, which means that the maximum PRF can be 19 kHz. For a 5 MHz system and a standard Doppler angle of 60 degrees the maximum Doppler frequency is 9.5 kHz, which translates from the Doppler equation into a blood cell speed of 293 cm/sec before aliasing occurs. This value is high enough to recognize severe disease states in the human carotid bifurcation.

Fig. 38-3 shows a simplified block diagram of the pulse-echo system. Fig. 38-4 shows a block diagram for the pulsed Doppler system. Additional details of Doppler electronics can be found in Atkinson and Woodcock.[1] The synthesized Doppler

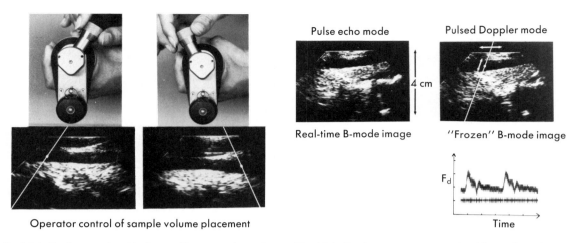

Operator control of sample volume placement

Fig. 38-1. Duplex scan head is shown. Three transducers in rotating wheel generate 90 degree circular sector images at 30 frames/sec. Articulated arm permits operator to position pulsed Doppler sample volume (white dot) anywhere within region defined by image.

Fig. 38-2. Duplex system operates in either pulse-echo or pulsed Doppler mode. Imaging mode permits soft tissue interfaces to be visualized within 4 cm of skin surface. In Doppler mode, sample volume may be positioned as desired. Doppler signal is then subjected to frequency analysis with output displayed on gray-scale paper.

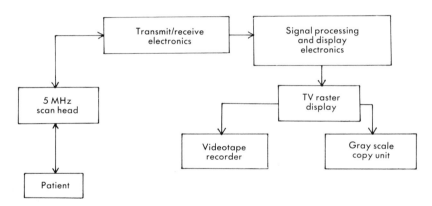

Fig. 38-3. Simplified pulse-echo block diagram of electromechanical instrumentation required to generate an ultrasound image.

signal is sent to a speaker for audio interpretation and to a frequency analyzer to appreciate the subtle features of the Doppler signal. The audio speaker permits an appreciation of increased Doppler frequencies present in high-grade stenoses, but does not permit the ear to perceive the increased distribution of lower frequencies associated with minimal and moderate states of disease. Although there are many types of frequency analyzers, the one used in our laboratory employs a fast Fourier transform algorithm. A spectral line consisting of amplitude versus frequency is generated every 2.5 msec, providing 400 spectral lines per second. To

meaningfully display the three parameters of Doppler frequency, time, and amplitude, the amplitude is encoded as a gray-scale intensity in a chart recorder gray-scale output (Fig. 38-4). An amplitude range of 18 dB is displayed in a normalized format, which means that the maximum amplitude for each spectral line is set to the black level with a linear scaling of all other amplitudes. This gray-scale output permits the distribution of Doppler frequencies to be appreciated as a function of time and forms the basis for diagnostic assessment.

With the sample volume placed at specific sites along the carotid pathway, the pulsed Doppler sig-

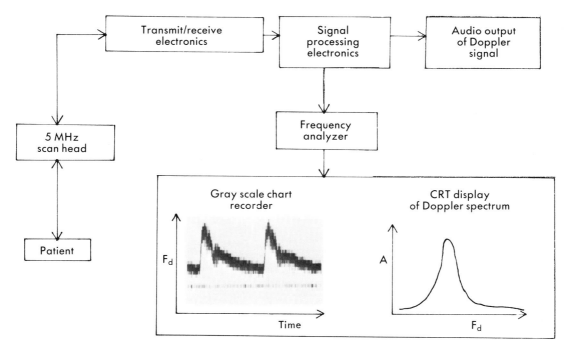

Fig. 38-4. Essential blocks comprising pulsed Doppler system.

nal is subjected to a frequency analysis whose waveform features are compared with contrast arteriography. Good correlation between the flow velocity waveforms and arteriographic assessment has been established over the past 3 years.[3-5,8] Visual assessment of a gray-scale spectra has been used to qualitatively place the artery into one of five categories: A, normal; B, 1% to 15% diameter reduction; C, 16% to 49% diameter reduction; D, 50% to 99% diameter reduction; and E, occlusion. The waveform features used for discrimination are mainly related to peak frequency and spectral broadening parameters. It is important to remember that the Doppler waveform provides functional information about the ability of a vascular segment to conduct blood. The imaging capability provides complementary information about anatomy. Since the clinical validation trials are fully described in the references cited, the present discussion is focused on acquisition and interpretation of flow velocity signals.

The center stream flow velocity patterns that are observed for various states of disease are illustrated by diagram in Fig. 38-5. In large peripheral vessels such as the CCA, as a result of the pulsatile nature of flow and the relatively short entrance lengths, the flow velocity profile is nearly blunt with ve-

locity gradients occurring near the vessel walls. For the sample volume placed at a center stream site, the corresponding flow velocity waveform exhibits a relatively narrow spectrum through the cardiac cycle. The diastolic frequency is well above the zero baseline, since the carotid artery supplies the low-impedance vascular bed of the brain. For early stages of disease, plaque formation at the vessel walls produces velocity gradients well into the vessel lumen that can be detected as an increase in spectral width during the deceleration phase of systole. In the proximal internal carotid artery (ICA), such increases in spectral broadening are seen without an increase in peak Doppler frequency. For disease states greater than 50% diameter reduction in the proximal ICA, there is an increase in peak Doppler frequency at the stenosis, with a dramatic increase in spectral broadening distal to the stenosis with or without elevated frequencies. An empirically derived dividing point indicating disease greater than 50% diameter reduction is a blood cell speed greater than 120 cm/sec in the ICA. The increase in spectral content distal to a stenosis is a result of poststenotic eddies and flow disturbances that often exhibit both forward and reverse flow components.

Fig. 38-6 shows two examples of images where

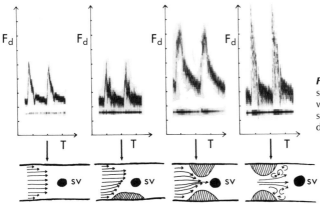

Fig. 38-5. Several Doppler spectral waveforms with corresponding flow velocity profiles thought to produce flow waveforms. Waveform parameters of peak velocity and spectral width are main features extracted from gray-scale display for disease classification. *SV,* Sample volume.

total occlusions have occurred. From the B-mode image a complicated plaque is generally seen at the origin of the ICA with diffuse intraluminal echoes at distal sites. From the real-time image there is usually a loss of radial pulsatility replaced sometimes by a longitudinal pulsatility. From a clinical standpoint, however, it is important to distinguish 100% stenosis or occlusion from a very small residual flow channel. A patient with a residual flow channel is still a surgical candidate, since the disease will remain within the first few centimeters of the ICA, but a total occlusion is inoperable because of an occluded vessel to at least the level of the ophthalmic artery. The Duplex concept is necessary to make this distinction. Using the image as a reference the sample volume is carefully probed throughout the region of suspected occlusion. If a residual flow channel exists, the pulsed Doppler system will detect it as long as the blood flow is greater than 3 cm/sec.

Fig. 38-7 illustrates how the CCA would typically appear in a subject with an occluded ICA on one side and a patent ICA on the other. On the occluded side, the diastolic flow usually goes to zero, since this reflects the relatively high-impedance vascular bed perfused by the external carotid artery (ECA). The contralateral CCA with a patent ICA exhibits diastolic flow well above the zero baseline, which can appear elevated because that artery provides collateral flow to the brain. It is important to compare the two carotid arteries in such cases. A diastolic flow of zero by itself does not positively indicate an internal carotid occlusion, since a cardiac defect, such as aortic insuf-

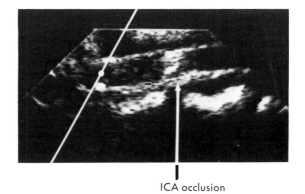

ICA occlusion

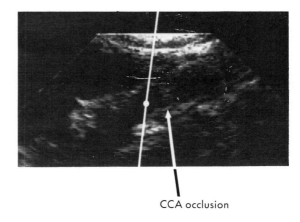

CCA occlusion

Fig. 38-6. Images of ICA and CCA occlusion. Point of occlusion is often characterized by bright intraluminal echoes indicating highly reflective complicated plaque. Diffuse intraluminal echoes distal to this point are also noted, but it is important to probe pulsed Doppler sample volume throughout suspected region to confirm that no flow is present. Threadlike flow channel, if present, is highly significant from patient management standpoint.

A   B

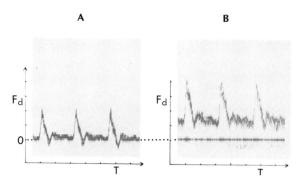

Fig. 38-7. Difference in flow waveforms between CCAs in an individual with, **A,** occluded ICA on one side and **B,** patent ICA on the other. Occluded side exhibits CCA diastolic waveform returning to zero baseline resulting from primary influence of ECA. Contralateral side shows CCA diastolic flow well above zero baseline. Caution should be used, however, since bilateral diastolic flow to zero can also indicate aortic insufficiency.

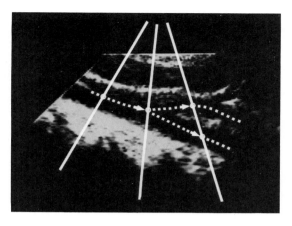

Fig. 38-8. Carotid bifurcation region shows how the sample volume is swept along flow channels to establish patency and detect high-grade stenoses. Procedure is followed in initial survey of carotid system in patient studies.

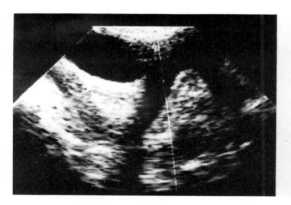
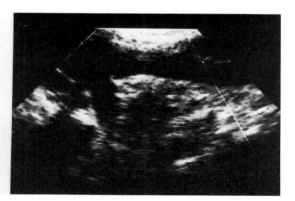

Fig. 38-9. B-mode imaging capability is used to identify kinked and tortuous arteries. This aspect must be appreciated to distinguish high-frequency Doppler signal as result of favorable Doppler angle from high-grade stenosis.

ficiency, can produce a carotid diastolic zero flow bilaterally.

Other uses of the B-mode image in clinical studies are also important. When scanning a patient, the technician first surveys the carotid pathway and local anatomy to establish bifurcation location and to identify tortuosity or any other anatomic variant that would influence the study. In Fig. 38-8 the image is used as a road map while the sample volume is swept along the carotid pathway to establish patency and to identify significant stenoses.

Image identification of tortuous vessels is shown in Fig. 38-9, and atherosclerotic plaques containing calcium are detected in Fig. 38-10 by the bright

intraluminal echoes with posterior shadowing. Following the initial survey, the image is used to locate specific anatomic stations of the carotid pathway where data are recorded. For the left and right sides, the sample volume is placed at center stream sites: the high CCA, the proximal ICA or bulb, the distal ICA (distal to the bulb), and the ECA. These anatomic sites are illustrated in Fig. 38-11 for a young, presumed normal subject.

When recording blood flow velocity signals, the Doppler angle (the angle formed by the transducer and blood vessel axes, Θ) is kept near 60 degrees. The image is used to establish this relationship as illustrated in Fig. 38-12. It should be recalled that

Anterior wall

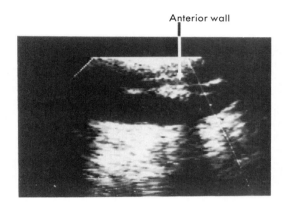

Posterior wall

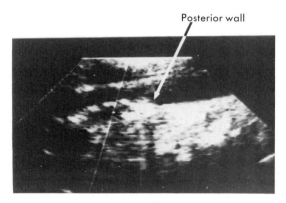

Fig. 38-10. Calcium deposits in atherosclerotic plaque are recognized by bright targets indicating nearly complete reflection and posterior shadow in image.

the Doppler frequency (f_d) is defined by the Doppler equation as follows:

$$f_d = \frac{2f_0}{C} |\bar{v}| \cos\Theta$$

where f_0 is the ultrasound center frequency, c is the speed of sound in soft tissue, and $|\bar{v}|$ is the magnitude of the blood velocity. The 60-degree Doppler angle has been found empirically to provide a favorable Doppler return from human carotid arteries. It is also of tremendous practical convenience to collect data at a standard angle, since when this is done, f_d is directly proportional to the blood cell speed times the constant ($2f_0$/c)cosΘ. This makes it possible to employ diagnostic criteria for flow waveform features directly without having to go through normalizing factors to account for the Doppler angle. For example, Fig. 38-13 shows blood flow velocity recordings from CCA using

different Doppler angles. The amplitudes of the Doppler frequencies are scaled by cosΘ, as predicted by the Doppler equation. Acquiring the flow data at a 60-degree angle at all sites along the carotid pathway is usually easy and of practical convenience in the visual assessment from gray-scale waveforms.

Several practical aspects related to the acquisition and analysis of the pulsed Doppler signal are also important. The main advantage of the "pulsed" approach to Doppler is that discrimination is provided in range or depth. In the continuous-wave (CW) Doppler system, if flow is detected, it is present somewhere along the transducer axis, but its origin is unknown. However, it is more important that the signal from a CW Doppler system represents a composite of all the velocity signals along the line of site. For example, Fig. 38-14 shows a CCA flow velocity waveform from a young, normal individual obtained with a CW Doppler system. Fig. 38-15 shows velocity waveforms obtained with the pulsed Doppler at the same CCA site. The differences are marked and are important if the flow velocity field is to be appreciated. With the sample volume placed near the walls in Fig. 38-15, the Doppler waveforms obtained from sites 1 and 4 exhibit a broad spectrum of frequencies and fill in the entire velocity waveform. At the centerstream sites of 2 and 3, there is a relatively narrow band of Doppler frequencies indicating laminar uniform flow within the sample volume at these sites. Thus a flow velocity field exhibiting a blunt flow velocity profile with gradients near the walls is appreciated with the pulsed Doppler. The CW output of Fig. 38-14 shows a "composite" of these waveform features, but they cannot be appreciated from a spatial standpoint. Since our laboratory has found that early and moderate states of disease may be recognized by increases in spectral broadening without concurrent increases in peak velocity, it is imperative to use a pulsed Doppler system to ensure that normally existing wall gradients are not confused with intraluminal disease.

Such subtle increases in spectral broadening are important in detecting carotid bifurcation disease, and a pulsed Doppler system should be used if minimal and moderate disease states are to be detected. If only the peak Doppler frequency is of interest, a CW Doppler system can be used. A CW Doppler device is easier to use than a pulsed Doppler device for peak frequency detection, since an

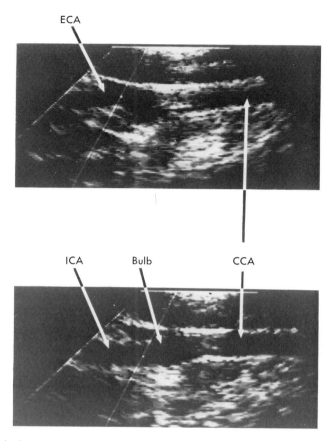

Fig. 38-11. Standard anatomic sites where pulsed Doppler data are acquired in carotid system. Sample volume is placed at center stream sites to eliminate wall gradients. Stenosis detected at nonstandard site is also recorded.

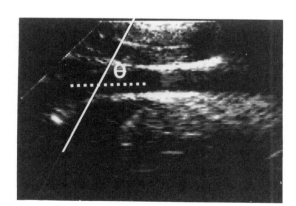

Fig. 38-12. Doppler angle, Θ, is defined by angle formed by transducer and blood vessel central axes. It is assumed that blood flow velocity vector is parallel with vessel axis. If this is not a good assumption, then Θ must be defined by another method. Note that Θ is kept near 60 degrees in studies of carotid arteries.

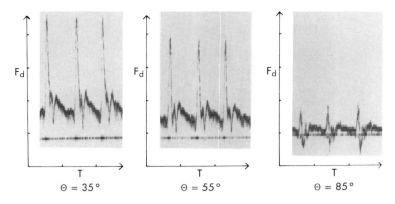

Fig. 38-13. Several blood flow velocity waveforms obtained from same vessel but at different Doppler angles. Note that Doppler peak frequency is directly proportional to $\cos\Theta$ as predicted by Doppler equation ($F_d = k \times \cos\Theta$). If Doppler signal is always acquired at 60 degrees, then Θ becomes a proportionality constant.

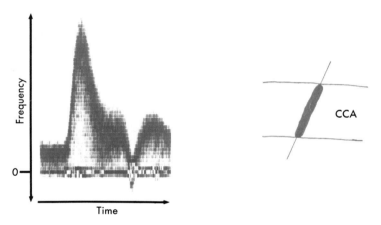

Fig. 38-14. Doppler waveform from CCA using CW Doppler system. Flow waveform is composite or superposition of all flow velocities detected along axis of transducer.

entire "line" is interrogated at once. A good application of the CW technique is in assessing aortic stenosis, where the peak velocity squared correlates well with the pressure gradient across the value.[7]

The importance of sample volume placement is further emphasized in Fig. 38-16. A sample volume placed at three different locations in a carotid artery is shown. With the sample volume at a center stream site, the velocity spectrum is a relatively narrow band. A broad spectrum is seen throughout the cardiac cycle with the sample volume placed near the wall, thus detecting the steep velocity gradient as flow goes to zero at the wall. The last sequence shows both the arterial velocity gradients near the wall in the CCA, and the reverse flow components in the jugular vein in close proximity.

The ability to discriminate velocities in range is a great advantage of the pulsed Doppler system.

An interesting waveform is shown in Fig. 38-17, *B*. During the systolic portion of the waveform, there is a high-amplitude Doppler return that is so strong that "clipping" of the signal occurs and "mirror" imaging results in the spectral output. However, the fundamental frequency is 1 kHz with all other harmonics being multiples of this fundamental. The origin of this interesting signal is especially interesting. The sample volume was found to detect the waveform shown in Fig. 38-17, *B*, only in a very localized region of the proximal ECA shown in Fig. 38-17, *A*. This patient had an endarterectomy with the subsequent thromboendarterectomy arteriogram (TEA) showing a distinct

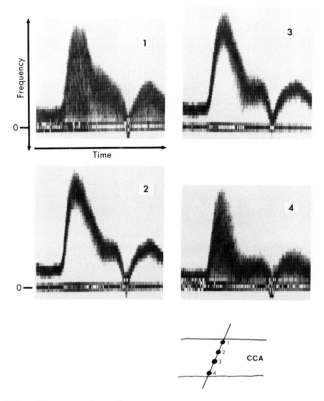

Fig. 38-15. Pulsed Doppler system is used to acquire flow velocity signals in CCA as in Fig. 38-14. Waveforms 1 and 4 exhibit spectral broadening as a result of velocity gradients that exist near vessel walls. More centerline sites of 2 and 3 exhibit relatively narrow-band spectra, reflecting blunt flow velocity profiles known to exist in peripheral vessels of this size. Pulsed Doppler approach is essential if spatial aspects of flow velocity field are to be appreciated.

shelflike structure in the proximal ECA where the plaque was removed. The phonoangiogram shown in Fig. 38-17, *C*, shows a peak at 200 Hz and another one at 1 kHz. The peak at 1 kHz is thought to represent a vibration of the shelflike structure resulting in a bruit in this patient. The 1 kHz vibration appears to occur only in systole and is localized to a small region in the proximal ECA. Thus in some cases the pulsed Doppler system can be used effectively not only to detect but also to localize bruits. This hypothesis is strengthened by our ability to detect and pinpoint several other vibrations in patients with bruits. The region over which the strong Doppler signals could be detected were localized, although the frequencies in the Doppler waveforms were always lower, such as 200 to 400 Hz. Thus the pulsed Doppler system might provide an excellent means to detect and pinpoint the spatial origin of bruits.

Since important diagnostic criteria exist in an increase in the spectral width of the velocity waveform, an effort was undertaken to perform ensemble averaging of the Doppler waveform to see if the process of averaging made these features more apparent. A computer program and hardware interface were constructed[6] that permitted an arbitrary number of waveforms to be ensemble-averaged while using the electrocardiogram (ECG) as a timing reference. In Fig. 38-18 gray-scale spectra are shown for 1 heart cycle and ensemble averages of 4 and 16 heart cycles. The Doppler signal was acquired from the CCA of a patient with a 20% diameter reduction by arteriography. During the systolic phase of the waveform, there is a marked increase in spectral width. The onset of the flow disturbance appears to be better defined when more heart cycles are used in the average.

Another example is illustrated in Figs. 38-19 and

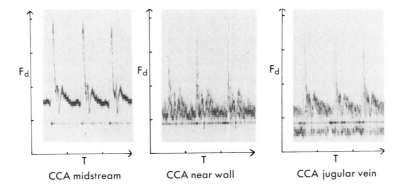

| CCA midstream | CCA near wall | CCA jugular vein |

Fig. 38-16. Importance of sample volume placement. At CCA midstream, spectrum is relatively narrow band. Near wall, velocity gradients exist as noted by broad spectra during both systole and diastole. With sample volume placed at vessel wall, both arterial and venous flow are detected as noted by positive and negative flows.

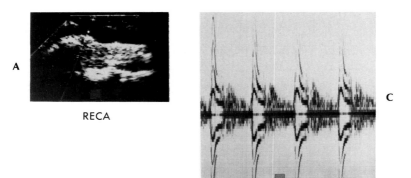

RECA

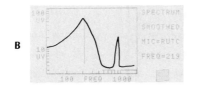

Fig. 38-17. Flow velocity waveform in **B** was obtained from localized region at origin of right external carotid artery (RECA) **A.** Mirrored waveform occurring during systole has fundamental peak frequency of 1kHz. It is thought that high-amplitude vibration during systole is caused by shelflike structure (detected by angiography). Phonoangiogram detects 2 peaks in audible range: one at 200 Hz and one at 1 kHz in **C.** Pulsed Doppler may be useful in detection and localization of bruits in cardiovascular system.

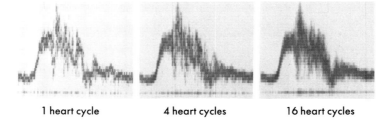

| 1 heart cycle | 4 heart cycles | 16 heart cycles |

Fig. 38-18. Gray-scale output for flow velocity of 1 heart cycle and ensemble averages of 4 and 16 heart cycles. Onset of flow disturbance and central tendency of waveform appear more evident as number of heart cycles used in average increases. Flow waveforms were collected from CCA of patient with 20% diameter reduction as determined by arteriography.

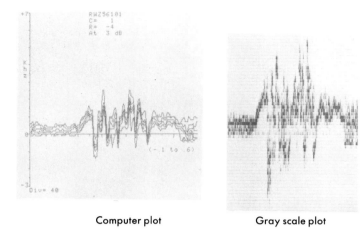

Computer plot   Gray scale plot

Fig. 38-19. Comparison between computer-generated contour plot and the gray-scale plot from frequency analyzer for one heart cycle. Forward and reverse oscillations seen on computer plot are also seen in gray-scale output when viewed edgewise. It is thought that forward and reverse flow components represent vortexes or eddies passing through sample volume during systole.

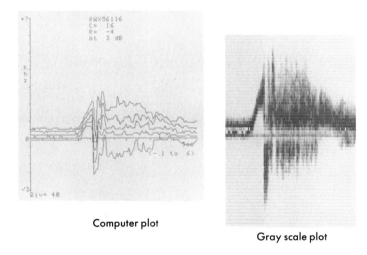

Computer plot

Gray scale plot

Fig. 38-20. Ensemble average of 16 heart cycles obtained from same site as in Fig. 38-19. Prominent reverse flow component is seen at onset of flow disturbance, but at other times during systole broad spectrum is observed. Eddylike structures seen in single heart cycles are not coherent from beat to beat with respect to ECG and will tend to average out over many heart cycles. Thus ensemble averaging enhances waveform features indicating central tendency, although averaging process may also mask important higher frequency structures that are incoherent from cycle to cycle but may provide important information about nature of local hemodynamics and plaque structure. Both instantaneous and ensemble average waveforms appear to provide important information.

38-20. Fig. 38-19 shows a computer contour plot and corresponding gray scale plot of a single heart cycle obtained in the ICA distal to disease. The computer plot shows marked forward and reverse oscillations that can also be seen from the gray scale plot when viewed "edge on." Fig. 38-20 shows the ensemble average of 16 heart cycles and does not exhibit the forward and reverse oscillations except at the onset of the flow disturbance. It is thought that the forward and reverse oscillations shown in Fig. 38-19 represent eddy or vortex structures passing through the sample volume. Since the sample site is distal to the stenosis, the temporal and spatial character of these structures would not be expected to be coherent from heart cycle to heart cycle except for the onset of the disturbance. This is why the ensemble average of 16 heart cycles shows only the first vortex generated, while the others are averaged out over time and are thus seen as a marked increase in spectral width. These examples point out the important observation that ensemble averaging, although bringing out the central tendency of the waveform, may tend to mask or obscure some of the higher frequency flow velocity events that are incoherent from cycle to cycle. It is probable that these hemodynamic aspects are significant in characterizing atherosclerotic lesions. Only by careful documentation of flow velocity waveforms and correlation with a standard will the significance of observed flow velocity waveform features be appreciated.

In summary, this chapter has reviewed ultrasound Duplex concepts to provide insight into the application and interpretation of both imaging and pulsed Doppler modalities. Clinical validation is well documented in other studies. A Duplex scanner is able to provide hemodynamic information from humans. Application of a Duplex scanner is most beneficial to the user who has the time to get to know the instrument's capabilities and limitations.

ACKNOWLEDGMENTS

We wish to acknowledge the efforts of our experienced technologists Jean Primozich and Ramona Lawrence. It has been through their daily efforts that meaningful clinical data have been acquired and used to direct patient management.

REFERENCES

1. Atkinson, P., and Woodcock, J.P.: Doppler ultrasound and its use in clinical measurement, New York, 1982, Academic Press, Inc.
2. Barber, F.E., et al.: Duplex Scanner II: for simultaneous imaging of artery tissues and flow, Proceedings of the Ultrasonic Symposium, IEEE 74CH0896-ISU, New York, 1974, Institute of Electrical and Electronic Engineers, Inc.
3. Blackshear, W.M., Jr., et al.: Detection of carotid occlusive disease by ultrasonic imaging and pulsed Doppler spectrum analysis, Surgery 86:698, 1979.
4. Breslau, P.J., et al.: Ultrasonic Duplex scanning with spectral analysis in extracranial carotid artery disease—comparison with contrast arteriography, Vasc. Diagn. Ther. p. 17, Oct./Nov. 1982.
5. Fell, G., et al.: Ultrasonic Duplex scanning for disease of the carotid artery, Circulation 64:1191, 1981.
6. Greene, F.M., Jr., et al.: Computer-based pattern recognition of carotid arterial disease using pulsed Doppler ultrasound, Ultrasound Med. Biol. 8:161, 1982.
7. Hatle, L., Angelsen, B.A., and Tromsdal, A.: Noninvasive assessment of aortic stenosis by Doppler ultrasound, Br. Heart J. 43:284, 1980.
8. Langlois, Y., et al: Evaluating carotid artery disease: the concordance between pulsed Doppler/spectrum analysis and arteriography, Ultrasound Med. Biol. 9:51, 1983.
9. Phillips, D.J., et al.: Detection of peripheral vascular disease using the Duplex Scanner III, Ultrasound Med. Biol. 6:205, 1980.

CHAPTER 39

Carotid artery velocity waveform analysis

KIRK W. BEACH and D. EUGENE STRANDNESS, Jr.

Because it is now believed that lesions at the carotid bifurcation are responsible for the majority of preventable strokes, a great deal of attention has been focused on efforts to detect those lesions. Although invasive methods for carotid artery evaluation have been developing for more than three decades and noninvasive methods have been evolving for nearly two, a single set of goals for carotid artery evaluation has never been uniformly established. Some practitioners want to identify vessels that exhibit reduced flow rates or introduce a pressure drop. Other practitioners wish to identify small disruptions in the intimal lining of the vessel. Still others hope to detect atherosclerotic plaques that obstruct some specific percentage of the diameter or cross-sectional area of the lumen and identify occluded vessels. The former goals are physiologic, the latter are anatomic. To add to the confusion, arteriography, the standard for evaluating new methods of carotid artery disease diagnosis, although graphic, is a gross anatomic method with limited spatial resolution.

Although the development and evaluation of all diagnostic methods for carotid artery diagnosis have been slowed by this confusion, the impact has been greater on carotid artery Doppler waveform analysis than on other methods. The source of the problem lies in the wide variety of velocity waveforms that may appear in the carotid bifurcation associated with anatomic and physiologic variation. Some of the factors that affect Doppler velocity waveform shape are of local carotid origin and others are of remote intracranial and cardiac origin.

Before commenting on the published methods of carotid Doppler waveform analysis, we will comment on instrumentation and the anatomic and hemodynamic factors that play a role in shaping the waveform. Many of these topics will be covered in more detail in other sections of this book.

DOPPLER SYSTEMS

Although other methods could be used to monitor the arterial velocity waveforms, such as magnetic (magneto-hydrodynamic) flow meters and tracer contrast systems, the most common methods of monitoring the flow in the carotid arteries involve the use of ultrasonic Doppler devices. The devices are popular because of their low cost, ease of use, and apparent safety as well as the large quantity of information available through their use.

Pulsed vs continuous-wave Doppler systems

Ultrasonic Doppler systems are discussed elsewhere, but it is important to emphasize a few features of the systems here. Doppler systems are frequently divided into two classifications, pulsed systems and continuous-wave (CW) systems. The two systems are similar: both operate according to the Doppler equation, both operate at similar ultrasonic frequencies, and both produce similar audio signals. However, the pulsed systems are able to obtain velocity information from a small volume in space, whereas CW systems cannot differentiate between motion signals arising from different distances from the Doppler probe along its axis.

Thus with a pulsed Doppler system the blood velocity can be sampled in midstream or near the artery wall. A CW Doppler system, in contrast, will observe all of the velocities across the vessel width. Of course, the focusing of the ultrasonic beam also has a great effect on the region of flow that is sampled. With a tight focus, a CW system can sample a thin line (the vessel diameter) across the vessel to give a quasi-midstream sample of the blood velocities.

A depth ambiguity is intrinsic to the CW Doppler system, whereas a frequency ambiguity is intrinsic to the pulsed Doppler system. If the expected Doppler frequency shift exceeds half of the pulsed Doppler system pulse repetition frequency (PRF), the Doppler frequencies displayed by the pulsed Doppler system appear to demonstrate lower velocity flow in the direction opposite to the flow under investigation (Chapter 5).

Doppler systems are only capable of monitoring the blood velocity component directly approaching or receding from the Doppler transducer. It is common to use the Doppler equation to correct for angle, assuming that the flow velocity vector is actually parallel to the axis of the artery. In axial laminar flow, this practice works well; however, in the complex helical, disturbed, and turbulent flows that occur in the carotid bifurcation, such a correction has limited value.

Frequency analysis

A variety of frequency analysis methods has been made available for Doppler signal processing. These methods range from analysis by ear through zero-crossing frequency estimators and bandwidth followers to real-time spectral waveform analyzers. The choice of display format on these devices and display range is arbitrary, but the choice greatly affects the appearance of the display.

Although these devices are discussed in detail elsewhere in this book, a few comments about them may be helpful. All are frequency analysis methods and provide records with similarities, yet the time resolution, frequency resolution, sensitivity to noise, and display formats are quite different. It is essential, when reading the literature, to know which type of frequency analyzer was used if quantitative analysis is to be applied.

CW zero-crossing waveforms

Because CW ultrasonic Doppler instruments with zero-crossing frequency analyzers were the first instruments available for vascular diagnosis, until recently the majority of carotid artery waveform research has been done with these systems. Published reports of CW Doppler studies have several features in common. The studies were all performed without ultrasonic imaging, thus the angle between the Doppler probe and the vessel could not be determined. In addition, the exact location from which the waveform was taken, with respect to the carotid bifurcation could not be determined.

Thus the analysis methods have usually been based on waveforms from the common carotid artery (CCA) and the features used are often selected so that they are independent of the Doppler angle.

ANATOMY AND PHYSIOLOGY OF THE CAROTID BIFURCATION

Doppler examination of the velocity waveform in the carotid bifurcation is a physiologic examination. The results of the examination are determined by the resistance to flow of the distal arterial beds, by the shape of the pressure pulses supplied by the heart, and by the effects of the local anatomy as it interacts with the inertial and viscous forces of flow. The fundamental basis of waveform analysis is widely known. The external carotid artery (ECA) feeds high-resistance capillary beds in skin and muscle in the normal person, which results in an arterial waveform characteristic of peripheral arteries, that is, a forward systolic component sometimes followed by an early diastolic flow reversal, which is possibly followed by another forward component and no flow in late diastole. The normal internal carotid artery (ICA) supplies a low-resistance bed in the brain and thus has a velocity waveform like arteries supplying other low resistance beds, that is, a high-velocity forward systolic component followed by sustained forward flow in diastole. This type of waveform is also found in arteries supplying the kidneys, muscles after exercise, vascular tumors, intestines during digestion and the pregnant uterus. Thus to verify that the CCA supplies the brain, it is sufficient to identify (and possibly quantify) forward flow in late diastole. This concept forms the basis of many carotid waveform analysis schemes.

Examination of a local stenosis by obtaining velocity waveforms at the stenosis, as well as proximal and distal to the stenosis, will produce a characteristic set of tracings that reveal high velocities over the narrow portion of the stenosis because of conservation of matter. If the same quantity of blood must flow through an arterial segment of normal diameter and of narrowed diameter, the ratio of the velocities in the segments will be inversely proportional to the cross-sectional areas of the segments (which is approximately equal to the square of the ratio of the residual lumen diameters).

Recent detailed examinations of the flow patterns in the normal carotid bifurcation have revealed that the flow, when examined in detail, is quite complex. The complexities of the flow can manifest in the Doppler waveforms. Some insight into the flow can be obtained from model studies by Ku and Giddens[19] Pulsatile flow was observed in an anatomically accurate glass model of the carotid bifurcation. Within the normal carotid bulb, inertial effects created helices and stagnant vortices that resulted in high resident times for the blood, true reverse flow in part of the ICA cross-section, and associated physiologic stenoses. The stagnant vortices are so severe that some blood is trapped in the bulb for three or more cardiac cycles. The physiologic stenosis occurs when the inertial forces of blood flow divert the main-flow stream from midvessel to a path along the vessel margin. In the case of the carotid bifurcation, this effect causes blood to flow from the middle of the CCA to a path along the ICA wall adjacent to the flow divider between the ICA and ECA. The resultant narrow path of blood flow is a physiologic stenosis that leaves the rest of the carotid bulb, the dilation in the proximal ICA, with a stagnant eddy that rotates and produces simultaneous forward and backward flow in the bulb. Although the Ku and Giddens glass model system[19] was illustrative, it does not have the compliant characteristics of the arteries. Fortunately, Phillips et al.[25] have found Doppler velocity waveforms in the human carotid bifurcation that are consistent with the findings of Ku and Giddens.

Examination of the bifurcation is complicated by the variations in carotid anatomy coupled with variations in physiology. The relative positions of the ICA and ECA are frequently switched in the neck.[24] Identification is aided by the audible character of the signals from the vessels above the bifurcation, the ICA having a monophasic signal and the ECA a signal that is essentially zero in diastole.[4] Since the branches of the ECA are frequently not identified during the carotid Doppler examination and great variations may occur in the velocity waveforms, especially in patients with disease, a great potential exists for error. Errors in vessel identification can be reduced with careful use of compression maneuvers and by combining the direct Doppler examination of the carotid bifurcation with other noninvasive examinations, such as periorbital examinations.

MEASUREMENT OF VOLUMETRIC FLOW RATES

Many investigators have expressed an interest in diagnosing extracranial and intracranial arterial disease by the use of volume flow measurement in the carotid arteries. The quantitative effect of a carotid artery lesion on carotid artery blood flow rate is not immediately obvious. For instance, in the legs, a pressure-reducing arterial stenosis may have no effect on the resting blood flow rate because arteriolar dilation will compensate for the arterial stenosis to maintain blood flow. In the case of the carotid circulation, four parallel arteries, the two ICAs and the two vertebral arteries, join in a collateralizing loop, the circle of Willis. In this case it may be possible to introduce a small resistance to flow in one of the vessels supplying the circle of Willis, which would greatly reduce the flow in that vessel, because the collateral connections make rerouting the blood flow to the other vessels easy.

Attempts to measure the volumetric flow rate in the carotid arteries have not worked well. A Doppler flow-measuring system has been developed by Uematsu[31] that has been shown to compute flow from real-time vessel diameter measurements and fixed-angle CW Doppler velocimetry. The velocity measurement was shown to be independent of the Doppler angle on theoretic grounds; however, the validity of the proof is not obvious. Some features of the instrument have been verified in the laboratory, but the clinical usefulness of the method has not been shown.

CW Doppler systems with zero-crossing waveform analysis

Velocity waveforms have been obtained from both the CCA and the ICA for correlation with severity of disease. Numerous qualitative and quantitative waveform analysis methods have been derived to identify disease. In general, the qualitative methods are similar to the quantitative methods but include the additional factor of experience. Only the quantitative methods will be discussed here.

Two ratios include the brachial diastolic blood pressure as a parameter: the pressure perfusion index and the carotid distensibility index.[10] The pressure perfusion index (PrPI) is defined as follows:

$$PrPI = \frac{\text{Brachial diastolic pressure}}{\text{Carotid diastolic velocity} + 1}$$

where the velocity is from the CCA. Based on the physiology, as ICA stenosis increases, diastolic velocity decreases and thus PrPI increases. The carotid distensibility index (CDI) is defined as:

$$CDI = \frac{\text{Systolic velocity} - \text{Diastolic velocity}}{\text{Systolic pressure} - \text{Diastolic pressure}}$$

where the pressures are obtained from the brachial artery and the velocities from the CCA. As the ICA stenosis increases, both the numerator and the index increase. In both cases, of course, the angle between the Doppler velocitymeter probe and the vessel must be known to find the velocities. Although described as a distensibility index, the ratio does not express distensibility from a physical point of view.

The PrPI has units of pressure divided by velocity, whereas the CDI has units of velocity divided by pressure. The number "1" in the PrPI must also have units of velocity and may take on different values depending on the velocity units used. The "1" is present, of course, because the CCA diastolic velocity may be zero; in the absence of the "1" the PrPI would become infinite.

Three other indices are based on the velocity waveforms alone, the carotid ratio,[10] the Pourcelot pulsatility index,[22,23] and the Archie carotid index.[1] The carotid ratio uses single velocities from the CCA and ICA and thus requires a knowledge of the angle of the Doppler probe with the vessel axis. The other two use ratios from a single waveform and are Doppler-angle independent. The carotid ratio (CR) is defined as follows:

$$CR = \frac{\text{Diastolic velocity (ICA)}}{\text{Diastolic velocity (CCA)}}$$

As ICA stenosis increases, the CCA diastolic velocity decreases and the ICA diastolic velocity increases, causing the CR to increase. The Pourcelot pulsatility index is the earliest angle-independent ratio. It can be defined in two ways (Fig. 39-1); the earliest definition was the ratio of the areas under the velocity waveform using the lowest diastolic flow as a base divided by the area using zero velocity as a base. This relationship is monotonically related to the peak-to-peak difference divided by the systolic peak-to-zero distance. As

both numbers are obtained from the same vessel during the same examination period, the same Doppler angle is used and the ratio should be angle independent. As ICA stenosis increases, CCA diastolic velocity decreases and the ratio increases toward a value of 1.0. The more recent and more useful Pourcelot index is the radio S = D/S. The Archie index (AI) extends the Pourcelot method to compare right and left sides.

$$AI = \frac{\dfrac{\text{Right CCA systolic velocity}}{\text{Right CCA diastolic velocity}}}{\dfrac{\text{Left CCA systolic velocity}}{\text{Left CCA diastolic velocity}}}$$

If the right ICA has a stenosis, the right CCA diastolic velocity will be low, the numerator will be high, and the ratio will be much greater than 1.0. If the left ICA has a stenosis, the left CCA diastolic velocity will be low and the ratio will be much less than 1.0. This method is not only angle independent but it accounts for differences in cardiac function between patients. It does have the disadvantage of being confounded by symmetric bilateral stenoses.

The Pourcelot index, the CR, and the AI are all dimensionless numbers; they are formed by dividing one velocity by another. Therefore the measurements could be made in centimeters per second, in kilohertz, or in any other convenient units. The results are independent of units, unlike the previous ratios that were dependent on the units of measure. The use of dimensionless ratios that are angle independent allows direct comparisons of numeric results by laboratories with different versions of the same basic equipment.

CW Doppler systems with zero-crossing and computerized waveform analysis

In addition to the measurement of the maximum and minimum velocities or frequency shifts, a large

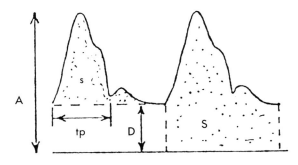

Fig. 39-1. Pourcelot pulsatility index for CCA. Ratio predicts ICA occlusion from CCA waveform. Patent ICA will have forward flow in diastole, reflected in CCA diastole. Since Doppler angle is not known, ratio D/A tells fraction of forward velocity that persists during diastole. Ratio is dimensionless and angle independent, thus is not dependent on Doppler angle or ultrasonic Doppler frequency. Pourcelot ratio is equal to $1 - D/A$. *A,* Zero to peak systolic frequency; *D,* zero to minimum diastolic frequency; *S,* area under Doppler frequency waveform bounded by zero line; *s,* area under Doppler frequency bounded by minimum velocity line; *tp,* systolic period.

number of other measurements can be made on waveforms, including slopes, peak widths, number of up-down cycles per cardiac cycle, and heights of the points of zero slope. Rutherford[29] has subjected parameters derived from velocity waveforms from the common carotid artery to a computerized discriminant analysis. The waveforms were gathered with a CW Doppler system with a zero-crossing waveform display from the CCA. Five parameters were identified that contributed significant discriminating power to an expression for severity of disease (Fig. 39-2). The parameters are as follows:

$$pSV = \text{Peak systolic velocity}$$
$$eDv = \text{End diastolic velocity}$$
$$pDv = \text{Peak diastolic velocity}$$
$$w/h = \frac{\text{Half peak velocity systolic peak width}}{\text{Peak velocity}}$$
$$\frac{dVs}{dT} = \text{Systolic upslope rate}$$

The classification score is derived from the following expression:

$$0.07\,(PSV) + 0.5\,(EDV) - 0.1\,(PDV) - 7.1\,(w/h) + 0.1\,(dVs/dT) - 6.8$$

A score of zero is most common in patients with carotid artery disease but less than 50% diameter reduction stenosis. Young people who are normal have scores around +6, whereas patients with occlusions have scores around −8. Using this method, ICA disease can be separated into four groups using data from the CCA waveform: normal, less than 50% diameter reduction, greater than 50% diameter reduction, and occlusion.

Whereas the first three terms of the waveform expression are in units of velocity (or frequency), the fourth term is in units of distance divided by velocity and the fifth is velocity divided by time. The value of the expression is therefore dependent on the units of measurement.

Examining the expression can give some insight into qualitative analysis of Doppler waveforms, even if the quantitative method is not used. Increased EDV suggests a normal waveform, as does a low peak diastolic velocity (PDV has a negative coefficient). A normal waveform also would have a narrow systolic peak (w/h has a negative coefficient) and a steep systolic upstroke (dVs/dT). These features are all accepted as characteristic of normal waveforms.

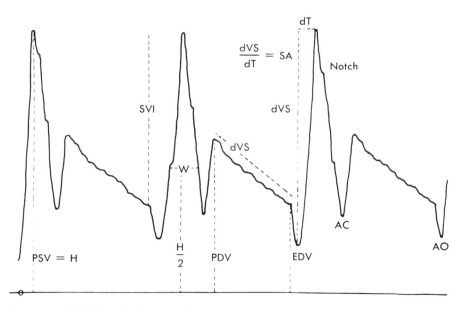

Fig. 39-2. Rutherford pulsatility score for CCA. Velocity waveforms obtained from CCA at estimated Doppler angle of 45 degrees with 10 MHz CW ultrasonic Doppler probe. Score is dependent on both Doppler frequency and Doppler angle. Parameters used to compute score are peak systolic velocity *(PSV)*, systolic velocity increase *(SVI)*, end diastolic velocity *(EDV)*, peak diastolic velocity *(PDV)*, systolic width index *(W/H)*, systolic acceleration *(SA)*, diastolic velocity slope *(DVS)*, and aortic valve opening and closing artifacts *(AO* and *AC)*. (From Rutherford, R.B., Hiatt, W.R., and Kreutzer, E.W.: Surgery 82:695, 1977.)

CW Doppler systems with real-time spectral analysis

The zero-crossing frequency analyzer has several characteristics that limit its applicability to complicated Doppler signals. The zero-crossing analyzer and all other frequency estimators provide a tracing of a single characteristic frequency for each point in time. Often, however, multiple frequencies are present simultaneously in a Doppler signal. It is possible for a CW Doppler probe to be oriented so that it obtains signals from both an artery and a vein at the same time. The result is two simultaneous frequencies, in which case a single characteristic frequency does not fairly represent either the arterial or the venous signal. However, such confusion is rare with direction-sensitive devices in the carotid arteries where arterial unidirectional cephalad and jugular flow is unidirectional caudad. Less obvious is the case of turbulent flow in an artery in which each fluid element is traveling at a different velocity (strictly, velocity includes the speed and the direction). In this case the mean frequency is a logical choice to characterize the Doppler signal. Unfortunately, the statistical variability is so great in such signals and the mean (average) is so sensitive to noise that the mean does not produce a satisfactory result. At this point there is no accepted method to characterize the frequency. A display of the details of the frequency spectrum in time in the form of a spectral waveform has become quite popular and useful (Fig. 39-3). The frequencies displayed on a zero-crossing waveform tracing of the arterial Doppler signal (Fig. 39-3, *A*) cannot be extracted in an obvious way from the real-time spectral waveform of the same arterial signal.

Spectral waveforms resemble zero-crossing waveforms in the general trends displayed. The major

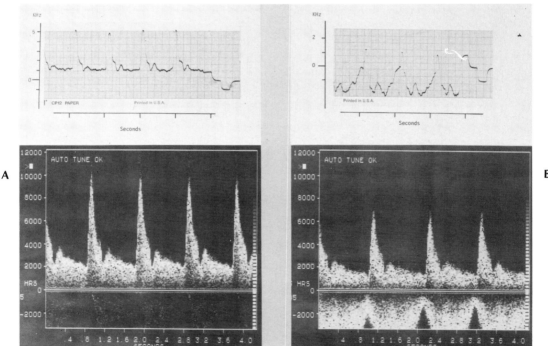

Fig. 39-3. Comparison of real-time spectral waveform and zero-crossing waveform tracing. On left, upper envelope of real-time spectral waveform and zero-crossing tracing display similar wave shapes, but magnitudes are different. Zero-crossing tracing appears to have same magnitude as lower edge of spectral waveform, while it follows contours similar to upper boundary. On right, pulsatile venous flow causes distortion and downshifting of velocity trace. Maximum velocity shift displayed by zero-crossing is tracing 1 kHz, near bottom of arterial spectral waveform. *A,* Arterial signal; *B,* mixed arterial and venous signal.

difference, on first observation, is that the spectral waveform shows the distribution of frequencies present at each time, whereas the zero-crossing waveform does not. Thus waveform features that indicate stenoses, such as increased peak velocity[2,12] are apparent on both types of frequency analysis. The spectral waveform is capable of providing additional information about the distribution of velocities at each point in time. In systole, when inertial forces dominate the flow profile, plug flow is present in the carotid arteries; all of the erythrocytes are moving at the same velocity rather than forming a parabolic velocity profile across the vessel. At that point the spectral waveform is very narrow, leaving a "window" below the waveform. If the flow were parabolic, all velocities between zero and a maximum would be present in the velocity profile and the spectral waveform would consist of an "envelope" that indicates the maximum frequency from midvessel and equal intensities at all frequencies between the envelope and zero frequency. Thus a lower peak velocity with a systolic "window" is characteristic of a normal carotid spectral waveform. As with the zero-crosser tracings, diastolic flow should be greater than zero.

CW Doppler systems with computerized spectral waveform analysis

It is difficult to perform quantitative measurements on spectral waveforms by hand. Since the images consist of a full gray-scale display and there is considerable statistical variability in the individual spectra, it is not possible to measure to a well-defined point. Computer analysis of the spectral waveform is therefore convenient. Although the statistical variability of the spectra will also cause some uncertainty in the parameters measured, several averaging techniques have been able to deal successfully with the problem. Rittgers et al.[26] have extracted five parameters from averaged, computer-extracted, mode, and peak frequency waveforms. The parameters tested were as follows;
1. Systolic mode frequency (Fm)
2. Systolic upper 12 dB band (Fubw)
3. Systolic lower 12 dB band (Flbw)
4. Systolic upper 18 dB frequency (F)
5. Systolic window (SW)

Each of these parameters requires some special comment. The mode frequency is used as the typical or representative frequency from the spectrum. The mode is the frequency of greatest intensity at the time under consideration. Alternate choices for

this frequency are mean, midpoint, and median. If the distribution of frequencies in an individual spectrum was "normal" (Gaussian), or at least symmetric around mode, then the mean, median, midpoint, and mode would all be identical. It would not matter which value was chosen. The spectra, by their statistical nature, are derived from such small data samples by necessity that a robust characteristic frequency must be chosen. The only two that have been tested as yet are the mean and the mode. The mean or average frequency, as stated earlier, is sensitive to noise (Fig. 39-4). The mode is also noise sensitive, but not sensitive to low-level outlying frequencies, as the mean is. Thus the mode is more robust than the mean. The 12 and 18 dB down contour lines provide an estimate of spectral width. The window calculation (SW) is the ratio Fubw/Flbw over a specified region. This is an indication of spectral width.

The parameters just discussed were obtained from locations in the CCA and the ICA. A test of various combinations of parameters revealed three ratios as being most useful:

$$\frac{\text{Peak (18 dB) proximal ICA frequency}}{\text{Peak (18 dB) distal ICA frequency}} > 1.1$$

$$\frac{\text{Mode proximal ICA frequency}}{\text{Mode distal ICA frequency}} > 0.38$$

$$SW = \frac{\text{Upper (12 dB) distal ICA frequency}}{\text{Lower (12 dB) distal ICA frequency}} < 0.38$$

While all three ratios are dimensionless, the first two involve values taken from different sites and therefore require correction for the different Doppler angles at the two sites. The SW takes both values from the same waveform and therefore does not require an angle adjustment. It is also notable that Rittgers[26] uses only ICA systolic data; Rutherford[29] used CCA data from both systole and diastole. Again, these parameters can be used as reported or as a guideline to improve visual interpretation of waveforms.

CW Doppler systems with real-time spectral analysis in models of the carotid bifurcation

In the hope of increasing understanding of carotid waveforms, several researchers have created models of carotid stenoses.[3,8,9] These systems have included both symmetric (coaxial) and nonsymmetric stenoses. Doppler investigations of these

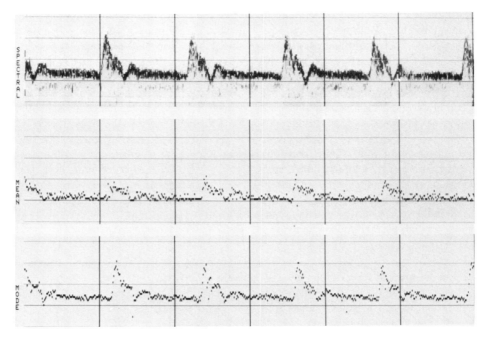

Fig. 39-4. Spectral, mean, and mode waveforms of normal carotid artery. Upper tracing is real-time spectral waveform. Middle tracing is point-by-point plot of mean frequency from each spectrum in spectral waveform. Lower tracing is point-by-point mode plot from each spectrum in spectral waveform. Although mean tracing indicates same heart rate in spectral waveform, few other similarities are shown. Mode gives more plausible waveform. Both characteristics are subject to variation in presence of noise.

models have focused on stenoses with 10% to 50% diameter reduction (expressed in area reduction).

Brown[8] and Douville[9] used pulsatile pumps to force pulsatile flow through a stenosed tube with varying hydraulic resistances at the termination. CW Doppler signals obtained proximal to, at, and distal to stenoses of various grades resembled those seen in the carotid system. The ratio between peak systolic frequency at the stenosis and that proximal to the stenosis (at fixed angles of 60 degrees) correlated with the inverse of the cross-sectional area ratio. Spectral broadening was quantified as follows:

$$SB = \frac{\text{Peak frequency} - \text{Mean frequency}}{\text{Peak frequency}}$$

Spectral broadening was linearly correlated with percent of stenosis in the model system. Flow disturbance associated with the stenosis did not extend more than 3 cm beyond the stenosis in any case. Asymmetric stenoses were associated with the appearance of flow disturbances, including simultaneous reverse flow in the poststenotic region.

Douville[9] implies that quantitative flow rate be-

gins to decrease as a carotid stenosis exceeds 50% diameter reduction, which is a higher grade stenosis than required to cause velocity increases. The result comes from the model that does not include parallel, low-resistance fluid conduits to model the contralateral CCA and vertebral arteries.

A stenotic model in the dog carotid bifurcation was investigated by Bendick.[3] Collars were placed around canine CCAs to create a series of stenoses with 10% to 50% diameter reduction. The stenoses resulted in changes in carotid pressure drop from 0 to 4 mm Hg and flow reductions of from 0% to 5%. Peak Doppler frequency measurements were obtained proximal to and over the stenosis. The ratio of the frequencies was linearly correlated with the percent of stenosis. A stenosis of 20% diameter reduction could be reliably detected by the method.

Pulsed Doppler systems with real-time spectral analysis

As technology progressed, three advances in ultrasonic interrogation of carotid artery velocities occurred concurrently and thus were often used together: carotid B-mode imaging, pulsed Doppler ultrasound and real-time spectrum analysis. Occasionally, pulsed Doppler flow map imaging and real-time spectrum analysis were used, and sometimes pulsed Doppler ultrasound and B-mode imaging were used with zero-crossing waveform analysis. Other alternatives such as B-mode imaging with CW Doppler ultrasound are virtually absent in the literature. Common features of the B-mode imaging, pulsed Doppler ultrasound, and real-time spectrum analysis methodology included setting the Doppler angle at 60 degrees with the vessel axis and performing the real-time spectrum analysis using the fast Fourier transform (FFT) method.

As with some CW algorithms, the velocity ratio between the ICA and the CCA (at fixed angle established with B-mode imaging) was used[5,11,13-15,30] and found to be more accurate at predicting high-grade stenoses (greater than 50% diameter reduction) than a similar ratio from a CW Doppler system (without imaging). An index of spectral broadening[5,30] as follows added little to the accuracy of predicting percent stenosis:

$$SB = 0.47 \times$$

$$\frac{\text{Maximum frequency} - \text{Minimum frequency}}{\text{Maximum frequency} + \text{Minimum frequency}} = \frac{\text{Standard deviation}}{\text{Mean}}$$

Spectral broadening can be quantitated by other methods. Keagy[14,15] examined the diastolic spectral broadening by summing the spectral width at several points in time over the cardiac cycle and by measuring the area of the spectral tracing. The spectral area measurement and the sum of widths are both effective methods of solving the problem of statistical variability in the individual spectra that comprise the spectral waveforms. Keagy's method can discriminate patients with high grades of stenosis from those with lower grades of disease.

A method based on qualitative evaluation of spectral broadening and quantitative measurements of peak systolic frequency in the ICA was reported by Langlois[20] and Breslau.[6] The method separates carotid disease into five categories: (1) normal, (2) 1% to 10% diameter reduction, (3) 11% to 49% diameter reduction, (4) 50% to 99% diameter reduction, and (5) occluded (Fig. 39-5). If ICA peak frequency with a 5 MHz pulsed Doppler signal at 60 degrees to the vessel exceeds 4 kHz (120 cm/sec), the vessel is classified as 50% to 99% di-

ameter reduction. If the ICA peak frequency is lower, qualitative evaluation of the spectral broadening is used to classify the vessel as normal, 1% to 10% diameter reduction, or 11% to 49% diameter reduction. Occlusion is identified by the inability to locate an ICA velocity signal and a finding of zero diastolic flow in the ipsilateral CCA.

Although the ratio of the systolic velocities in the ICA divided by the systolic velocity in the CCA had been used before, another possibility was tested by Knox.[15] With an ICA stenosis, the ICA systolic velocity should increase and the CCA diastolic velocity should decrease. Thus a ratio of ICA systolic velocity (taken with a pulsed Doppler device at 60 degrees) to CCA diastolic velocity should be more sensitive to stenoses than the ratio of the systolic velocities. The parameter showed a good monotonic relationship with ICA percent diameter reduction on angiography, but the slope of the relationship in the zero to 50% diameter reduction stenosis region is too low to allow differentiation of disease. The slope in the 50% to 100% stenosis range allows estimation of the angiographic result from the Doppler system with a resolution of about 10% diameter reduction.

Since the majority of carotid lesions are located in the ICA, it seems unlikely at first that velocity data from the CCA proximal to the ICA could be used to identify and characterize minor lesions in the ICA. The attempts to use CCA waveforms to diagnose carotid disease with a CW Doppler system without imaging were directed at high-grade ICA stenoses and occlusions. They were popular because it is difficult to reliably gather consistent data from the ICA with a CW Doppler probe, but easy to gather data from the CCA. CCA waveform analysis was able to identify those patients with higher grades of ICA disease because of the difference in diastolic flows in the internal and external carotid arteries.

On careful examination of the problem, however, even minor lesions (10% to 49% diameter reduction) in the ICA may affect the CCA waveform because of upstream reflections of wave pulses. Such reflections are seen in other wave transmission systems. The changes in waveform used by Rutherford[29] support this idea, since he was able to see differences in his index between the normal results and the 1% to 49% diameter reduction case. Roederer[27] and Langlois[21] have reported a finding consistent with this idea that does

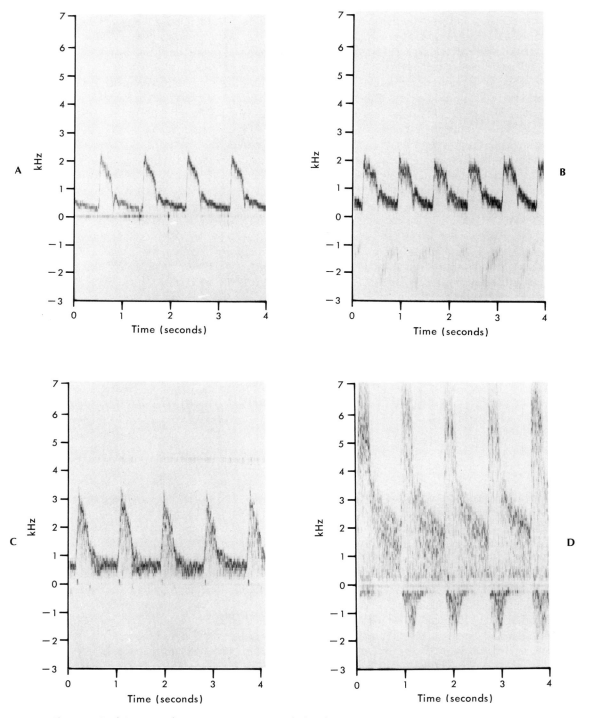

Fig. 39-5. Real-time waveforms representing spectral classification method. **A,** Normal has neither high frequencies nor spectral broadening. **B,** 1% to 10% has minimal spectral broadening. **C,** 11% to 49% has gross spectral broadening. **D,** 50% to 99% has velocities greater than 120 cm/sec.

not require the complicated detail of the Rutherford method. The method depends on the identification of the first zero slope encountered after peak systole. This is a plateau or relative minimum on the descending phase of the systolic peak. It is, however, consistent with Rutherford's method, since an increase in the width of the systolic peak indicates increased severity of disease.

Estimating from the figure provided in Langlois' study,[21] this first zero slope occurs about 80 msec after peak systole in normal vessels and about 50 msec after systole in diseased vessels. If the ICA contained a hydraulic reflector (a lesion) at its proximal end, such a reflection would occur early and manifest as a dicrotic wave. In a normal vessel the reflection from the terminal end of the ICA would appear later. These studies do not cast the issue in the form of a timing parameter, but in the form of a frequency ratio. The suggestion that the true parameter might be the time between the systolic peak and the first zero slope is pure speculation.

Pulsed Doppler systems with real-time spectral waveform and computer analysis

Even though qualitative evaluation of the carotid artery Doppler velocity waveforms has resulted in tremendous success in the ability to predict the results of carotid angiography, the training required to read the waveform tracings is extensive. In addition, there is a certain variability from time to time and from observer to observer in reading the waveforms. To allow a more uniform reading of the waveforms and to detect new velocity waveform characteristics that might help differentiate the grades of disease, several attempts have been made to develop a viable computerized method of reading the waveforms. Keagy[16] has used a commercially supplied microcomputer to perform such analysis, and Greene[18] has developed an in-house hardware and software system to analyze waveforms.

Automatic analysis of raw real-time spectral waveforms as they are generated by the analyzer is difficult, if not impossible. The problem rests in the great statistical variability within these signals. Doppler signals contain sufficient variability that an individual spectrum taken from a spectral waveform is never representative of the spectra in the surrounding time period. This can be appreciated by closely examining a Doppler spectral waveform. Overall, from a distance the trends of frequency

changes and spectral width can be easily recognized; however, up close the individual pixels of the spectra vary tremendously in density. Although the eye and mind can see the trends within the spectral tracing, a computer program would have to be very sophisticated to sort out the statistical variability from the true trends in the data.

The source of the problem is that a single spectrum contains data on the magnitude of perhaps 128 frequency components. These conclusions were generated from Doppler data gathered at a rate of 25.6 kHz over a time of 10 msec, or 256 data points. If there is some statistical variability in the input data (256 values), that variability will appear as a variability in the output values. The propagation of variability is linear from the 256 input values to the 128 pairs of output values. Each pair of output values, representing the real and imaginary components of a single frequency vector, is combined and displayed as a single frequency bin of the output spectrum. As the input variability cannot be reduced, variability of the output can only be reduced by increasing the ratio of input data to output data. The output frequency bins will then contain an average magnitude for each frequency, which will have its variability reduced by approximately the square root of the ratio of input data numbers to output data numbers.

A microcomputer capable of obtaining 2.5 seconds of data was used to obtain and analyze data spectral waveforms from the ICA.[16] To accomplish the required averaging, the area of the spectral waveform record during the first half of the cardiac cycle and the area taken over the entire cardiac cycle were evaluated in addition to the mean of the highest frequencies seen in the diastolic time period. Assuming a heart rate of 60 beats per minute and a spectral transform rate of 100 spectra per second, the computation of the spectral area over the first half of the cardiac cycle (0.5 seconds) averaged the results of 50 spectra. Whereas time resolution within the cardiac cycle is not preserved by this method, the statistical variability (standard deviation) of the results is reduced by a factor of seven (the square root of 50). All three parameters derived by Keagy correlated with percent diameter reduction stenosis. The feature that best correlated with carotid artery stenosis was the peak diastolic frequency.

To solve the problem of statistical variability while preserving the time resolution in the cardiac cycle, Knox et al.[18] have used a method of generating an average spectral waveform of a single cardiac cycle by ensemble averaging the spectral waveforms from 20 cardiac cycles. This increases the number of data points used to generate each spectra from about 250 to about 5000. With ensemble averaging, the standard deviation of the magnitude of a single frequency bin in a spectrum should be reduced by more than a factor of 4.

Using this ensemble waveform, Knox et al.[18] (29) divided signals from nonoccluded carotid arteries into four groups ranging from normal to greater than 50% diameter reduction stenosis. The normal vessels were identified using characteristics of the CCA. The characteristics were a steep downslope after peak systole, the presence of high-frequency components in the velocity waveform (sharp upslopes and downslopes in the range 4 to 10 per second), and a uniform spectral width from peak systole to early diastole. The vessels with greater than 50% diameter reduction stenoses were identified using characteristics of the ICA waveform. They had gross spectral broadening in both systole and diastole. The remaining vessels were divided into those with greater than 20% diameter reduction and those with less than 20% diameter reduction. Spectral widths from both the CCA and the ICA were used for this separation.

EFFECTS OF ALTERED ANATOMY AND PHYSIOLOGY

The methods of carotid artery Doppler waveform analysis previously discussed have been attempting to classify untreated carotid artery disease. The methods may not apply to vessels that have been altered by endarterectomy. Rutherford[29] tested his CCA algorithm on CCA waveforms obtained before and after endarterectomy and found, as expected, that the score increased markedly after surgery as hoped.

Intraoperative monitoring before and after endarterectomy has been used by Zierler[32] to detect technical errors in the surgical procedure. Using a 20 MHz Doppler system, the ICA waveform was examined for increased systolic frequencies and for spectral broadening to classify the lesions as mild, moderate, or severe. Of course, normal and occluded vessels were not subjected to surgery. In all cases with a technically satisfactory result, peak frequencies and spectral broadening were decreased after surgery.

Waveforms obtained with a pulsed Doppler system and spectrum analyzer in the 12-month post-endarterectomy period have the same characteristics related to disease categories as those obtained from untreated vessels.[28] This suggests that Doppler waveform analysis is a convenient method for follow-up of endarterectomy in the early and late postoperative periods.

In addition to the possible effect of anatomic changes resulting from surgery on the velocity waveforms, physiologic changes may also affect Doppler waveforms. Breslau[32] examined the effect of intracerebral vasodilation introduced by breathing a 6.8% mixture of carbon dioxide in air on the carotid waveforms of five young, healthy volunteers. The amount of carbon dioxide used was sufficient to cause a doubling of the ICA flow rate. Diastolic velocities and spectral broadening increased in both the CCA and the ICA with carbon dioxide. Such changes are similar to those indicating a 1% to 10% or a 10% to 49% diameter reduction stenosis.

CONCLUSION

The history of carotid artery velocity waveform analysis has been consistent over the last decade; there have been a series of reports of successively more sophisticated methods of waveform analysis attempting to divide the disease classification into a larger number of categories compared to angiography, with each category reflecting the current clinical practice of the research group. In the beginning, carotid disease was divided into two categories: less than 50% diameter reduction and greater than 50% diameter reduction. Now six classifications may be reported as follows:

1. Normal
2. 1% to 10% (or 15% or 19%) diameter reduction
3. 11% (or 16% or 20%) to 49% diameter reduction
4. 50% to 79% diameter reduction
5. 80% to 99% diameter reduction
6. Occluded

The ultrasonic Doppler equipment used to obtain carotid velocity waveforms has also evolved. Doppler equipment has progressed from nondirectional CW Doppler systems through directional CW Doppler systems to directional pulsed Doppler systems. Since the carotid arteries exhibit little reverse flow, directionality may not appear as an essential feature; however, in a few cases detection of direction was the key to correct evaluation of the arterial status. In an early case in our laboratory, the examining technician detected forward flow in the ECA, reverse flow in the ICA, and no CCA signal. The correct evaluation of CCA occlusion was easy, but without the directional information the diagnosis may have been missed.

Frequency analysis has also evolved from analysis by ear to zero-crossing waveform tracing and finally to real-time spectrum analysis. The additional information about velocity distribution that comes from the spectral waveforms is essential to reliable carotid evaluation. The method of obtaining the real-time spectral waveform, whether it be fast Fourier transform (FFT), time compression, chirp Z, or lambda processor, has little relevance to the user. The time and frequency resolution of the spectrum analyzers probably exceed the requirements of present applications. Thus in the future there will probably be a trend to averaging that reduces the frequency resolution and the time resolution in favor of reducing the statistical variability of the data. In parallel, there will probably be more effort placed on ensemble averaging, but not over the 30-second data acquisition times used by the most aggressive group in this area. Attempts to derive a characteristic frequency will probably continue with the most noise-sensitive statistic, the mean or average frequency, being completely replaced by more robust statistics like the mode. The mode will be replaced by the midpoint. The midpoint will be replaced by the even more robust characteristic frequency, the median.

The number of waveform features has grown (the 80% division is soon to be published), but the same features continue to appear as indicators of lower grades of disease:

CCA:
1. High diastolic velocity
2. Flat diastolic velocity segment
3. Narrow systolic peak:
   a. Sharp upslope
   b. Sharp downslope
   c. Low first zero slope in downslope
ICA:
1. Systolic velocity in the proximal ICA less than:
   a. 1.1 × CCA systolic velocity
   b. 1.1 × distal ICA systolic velocity
   c. 120 cm/sec
   d. 3 × CCA diastolic velocity
2. Systolic spectral width in the distal ICA within the period just after peak systole less than:
   a. 1.1 × spectral width in the CCA
   b. Spectral width in the presystolic ICA waveform
   c. 0.2 × systolic velocity

Although the exact parameters and the way they are expressed vary, the meaning of the features are constant and consistent with the hydrodynamic concepts on which they have been based.

With the apparent complexity of velocity waveforms, some investigators are inclined to suggest that Doppler waveform analysis is too complicated to be practical. Especially since direct visualization of anatomic lesions seems to be easy with angiographic and ultrasonic imaging methods. Unfortunately, a review of the literature does not support this view. Imaging techniques have not been subjected to the critical scrutiny that Doppler methods have. The scrutiny that has occurred has been less than reassuring. First, to diagnose a lesion with imaging, the examiner must be able to see the lesion and thus must choose a view in which the lesion is visible. To be assured of seeing an ulceration of the intima in an artery, high-resolution quadraplanar techniques are required. Second, to discuss the results of such studies, a reproducible interpretation protocol must be established. Third, an evaluation of the results of the studies must be compared to an independent diagnostic standard.

Against such methodologic requirements, Doppler waveform analysis is quite successful. It has never been suggested that Doppler diagnosis requires the lesion to be visualized or that data be gathered from the immediate vicinity of the lesion. In contrast, considerable effort has been directed toward gathering the data from several centimeters proximal and distal to the lesions, and the effort has been successful. Also, the interpretation protocols have been quantitative or semiquantitative for all classifications of disease, to which the waveforms easily lend themselves. In addition, the methods have been consistently compared to an independent standard that was regarded as more respectable. Those comparisons, at the present stage of development, have shown that the ability of an examiner using pulsed Doppler systems with real-time spectral analysis to predict angiography is as accurate as the ability of angiographers to read angiograms after they are taken[28] and thus *Doppler waveform analysis as applied to carotid arteries has equaled or outrun the imaging standard of selective biplanar conventional contrast angiography for identifying and grading carotid artery disease.*

REFERENCES

1. Archie, J.P., Jr.: A simple, non-dimensional, normalized common carotid Doppler velocity wave-form index that identifies patients with carotid stenosis, Stroke 12:322, 1981.
2. Barnes, R.W., Rittgers, S.E., and Putney, W.W.: Real-time Doppler spectrum analysis: predictive value in defining operable carotid artery disease, Arch. Surg. 117:52, 1982.
3. Bendick, P.J., Glover, J.L., and Dilley, R.S.: Transcutaneous detection of subcritical arterial stenoses by Doppler signal spectrum analysis, J. Ultrasound Med. 2:445, 1983.
4. Berry, S.M., O'Donnell, J.A., and Hobson, R.W.: Capabilities and limitations of pulsed Doppler sonography in carotid imaging, J. Clin. Ultrasound 8:405, 1980.
5. Bodily, K.C., et al.: Spectral analysis of Doppler velocity patterns in normals and patients with carotid artery stenosis, Clin. Physiol. 1:365, 1981.
6. Breslau, P.J.: Ultrasonic duplex scanning in the evaluation of carotid artery disease, medical thesis, Maastricht, Holland, 1981, Rijksuniversiteit Limburg te and Seattle, Wash., 1981, University of Washington.
7. Breslau, P.J., et al.: Effect of carbon dioxide on flow patterns in normal extracranial arteries, J. Surg. Res. 32:97, 1982.
8. Brown, P.M., et al.: A critical study of ultrasound Doppler spectral analysis for detecting carotid disease, Ultrasound Med. Biol. 8(5):515, 1982.
9. Douville, Y., et al.: An in vitro model and its application for the study of carotid Doppler spectral broadening, Ultrasound Med. Biol. 9(4):347, 1983.
10. Franceschi, C.: L'investigation vascular par ultrasonographie Doppler, Paris, 1977, Masson.
11. Garth, K.E., et al.: Duplex ultrasound scanning of the carotid arteries with velocity spectrum analysis, Radiology 147:823, 1983.
12. Johnston, K.W., et al.: Cerebrovascular assessement using a Doppler carotid scanner and real-time frequency analysis, J. Clin. Ultrasound 9:443, 1981.
13. Keagy, B.A., et al.: Evaluation of the peak frequency ratio (PFR) measurement in the detection of internal carotid artery stenosis, J. Clin. Ultrasound 10:109, 1982.
14. Keagy, B.A., et al.: Objective criteria for the interpretation of carotid artery spectral analysis patterns, Angiology 33(4):213, 1982.
15. Keagy, B.A., et al.: A quantitative method for the evaluation of spectral analysis patterns in carotid artery stenosis, Ultrasound Med. Biol. 8(6):625, 1982.
16. Keagy, B., et al.: Direct evaluation of internal carotid artery spectral analysis data using a microcomputer, Bruit 7:4, 1983.
17. Knox, R.A., Breslau, P.J., and Strandness, D.E., Jr.: A simple parameter for accurate detection of severe carotid disease, Br. J. Surg. 69:230, 1982.
18. Knox, R.A., et al.: Computer based classification of carotid arterial disease: a prospective assessment, Stroke 13:589, 1982.
19. Ku, D.N., and Giddens, D.P.: Pulsatile flow in a model carotid bifurcation, Atherosclerosis 3(1):31, 1983.
20. Langlois, Y., et al.: Evaluating carotid artery disease—the concordance between pulsed Doppler/spectrum analysis and angiography, Ultrasound Med. Biol. 9(1):51, 1983.
21. Langlois, Y.: The use of common carotid waveform analysis in the diagnosis of carotid occlusive disease, Angiology 34(10):679, 1983.
22. Planiol, T., and Pourcelot, L.: Doppler effect study of the carotid circulation. In de Vlieger, M., White, D.N., and McCreedy, V.W., editors: Proceeding of the second world congress on Ultrasonics in Medicine, New York, 1975, American Elsevier Publishing Co., Inc.
23. Planiol, T., and Pourcelot, L.: Etude de la circulation carotindienne au moyen de l'effet Doppler, Tours, Universite D'Orleans.
24. Prendes, J.L., et al.: Anatomic variations of the carotid bifurcation affecting Doppler scan interpretation, J. Clin. Ultrasound 8:147, 1980.
25. Phillips, D.J., et al.: Flow velocity patterns in the carotid bifurcations of young, presumed normal subjects, Ultrasound Med. Biol. 9(1):39, 1983.
26. Rittgers, S.E., Thornhill, B.M., and Barnes, R.W.: Quantitative analysis of carotid artery Doppler spectral waveforms: diagnostic value of parameters, Ultrasound Med. Biol. 9(3):255, 1983.
27. Roederer, G.O., et al.: Ultrasonic duplex scanning of extracranial carotid arteries: improved accuracy using new features from the common carotid artery, J. Cardiovasc. Ultrasonography 1(4):373, 1982.
28. Roederer, G.O., et al.: Post-endarterectomy carotid ultrasonic duplex scanning concordance with contrast angiography, Ultrasound Med. Biol. 9(1):73, 1983.
29. Rutherford, R.B., Hiatt, W.R., and Kreutzer, E.W.: The use of velocity wave form analysis in the diagnosis of carotid artery occlusive disease, Surgery 82(5):695, 1977.
30. Thiele, B.K., et al.: Current status of ultrasonic imaging and spectral analysis in the detection of arterial stenosis, In Smoking and arterial disease, Marshfield, Mass., 1981, Pitman Medical.
31. Uematsu, S.: Determination of volume of arterial blood flow by an ultrasonic device, J. Clin. Ultrasound 9:209, 1981.
32. Zierler, R.E., et al.: Intraoperative pulsed Doppler assessment of carotid endarterectomy, Ultrasound Med. Biol. 9(1):65, 1983.

CHAPTER 40

Digital subtraction angiography

DAVID S. SUMNER and JAMES B. RUSSELL

Intravenous digital subtraction angiography (DSA), which was introduced only a few years ago, has already had a great impact on the diagnostic approach to cerebrovascular disease. Although it was developed at a time when conventional arteriography had become reasonably safe and noninvasive tests were coming into their own as effective diagnostic tools, it appealed to the medical community and was rapidly and enthusiastically accepted. To those seeking a screening device, the familiar angiographic image provided a welcome alternative to the arcane scans, waveforms, and graphs furnished by noninvasive tests. The ability to visualize not only the carotid bifurcation but also the aortic arch, the vertebral arteries, and the intracranial vasculature was perceived as a definite advantage. To those seeking a definitive diagnostic study, DSA promised a less invasive, less dangerous, and less expensive method for obtaining x-ray–quality images. But DSA has its inherent limitations. Compared with conventional arteriography, its resolution is poor, its format is small, and its images are frequently degraded by motion artifact. Like conventional arch studies, intravenous DSA images are plagued by overlapping vessels and the inability to obtain selective views of the extracranial arteries. Moreover, DSA requires as much or more contrast medium than conventional arteriography.

As DSA sweeps out of the larger medical centers into the community hospitals and as it encroaches on the domain of other diagnostic tests, it is important to examine critically its advantages and disadvantages. Issues such as accuracy and cost-effectiveness must be addressed before this powerful new tool can be assigned its proper place in the diagnostic armamentarium.

IMAGE QUALITY

Chilcote et al.[10] at the Cleveland Clinic reported that the quality of DSA examinations of the carotid bifurcation was good or excellent bilaterally in 60% of patients, good or excellent on one side in 23%, and poor in the remaining 17%. Quality was considered good or excellent when the vessels were well opacified and when the separate origins of the internal and external carotid arteries were well visualized without being superimposed and without overlap by the vertebral arteries. At the Mayo Clinic, Earnest et al.[14] found that 33% of the studies were excellent, 42% were good, and 25% were deficient in one view. The results from UCLA were less encouraging. Both carotid bifurcations were adequately visualized in more than one projection in only 26% of the patients, and only 58% of the studies from individual carotid arteries were felt to be diagnostic.[26] The incidence of totally uninterpretable studies ranges from about 6% to 16%.[10,17,28,44]

A major cause of poor or unsatisfactory images is motion artifact.[10,26,51] Any movement occurring between the time that the initial contrast-free image is stored for the mask and the time that the contrast-containing images are obtained causes misregistration of the bony and soft-tissue shadows (Figs. 40-1 and 40-2). Therefore agitated or uncooperative patients cannot be studied. In otherwise cooperative patients, swallowing is the primary cause of motion artifact. In the oblique views, movement of the larynx and the hyoid bone tends to obscure the carotid bifurcation. Various measures designed to inhibit swallowing, such as having the patient hold his breath, bite on a block, or exhale through a straw, have generally been unrewarding.[10,26] Pulsatile motion of a calcified atheroma at the carotid

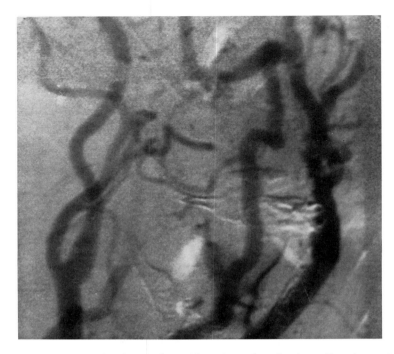

Fig. 40-1. Overlapping external and internal carotid arteries and swallowing artifact obscure left carotid bifurcation.

bifurcation is a less frequent cause of motion artifact.[51] Although selecting another image for the mask (remasking) may decrease misregistration and permit some otherwise unsatisfactory studies to be salvaged, motion artifact continues to be one of the principal unsolved problems of intravenous DSA.

Almost equally disturbing is the problem of vessel overlap.[10,26,51] Because the intravenously administered contrast medium fills all the cervical arteries almost simultaneously, it is impossible to obtain selected views of individual arteries. Superimposition of carotid images precludes lateral views of the bifurcation. The challenges faced by the angiographer are therefore similar to those presented by conventional arch studies. It is the practice of most radiologists to secure an anteroposterior view and both a right and left posterior oblique view. While these angles tend to separate the origins of the external and internal carotid arteries, not uncommonly they are overlapped on one or more views (Figs. 40-1 and 40-3). In some cases the vertebral arteries also overlap the bifurcation (Fig. 40-3). Consequently, in a disturbing number of studies only one good view of the bifurcation is obtained. Except for making more pictures at different angles (which, of course, increases the contrast load), there is little that can be done to circumvent this problem.

In the series reported by Hoffman et al.[26], contrast density was good in 42%, fair in 44%, and poor in 14% of the patients studied. Inadequate opacification is usually associated with a low cardiac output and a prolonged circulation time.[26,53] Although it is a relatively infrequent cause of poor visualization, it can be a problem in some of the elderly patients who comprise a large portion of the referrals for DSA.[26] By positioning the catheter tip in the superior vena cava, the radiologist can deliver a bolus of contrast medium more rapidly than when the tip of the catheter is in an arm vein. In most cases, the resulting increase in opacification is adequate to provide good images. Indeed, many institutions routinely use the central approach and no longer perform peripheral injections.[8,43]

To digitize the projected image, the fluoroscopic screen is divided into a 256 × 256 or 512 × 512 matrix. The latter, by providing more pixels, improves the definition of the image. Nevertheless, the resolution of current DSA instrumentation is limited to only 1 to 2 line pairs/mm, which is much less than the 5 to 10 line pairs/mm capability of conventional arteriography.[13,29,35] In other words, DSA images appear fuzzy in comparison to con-

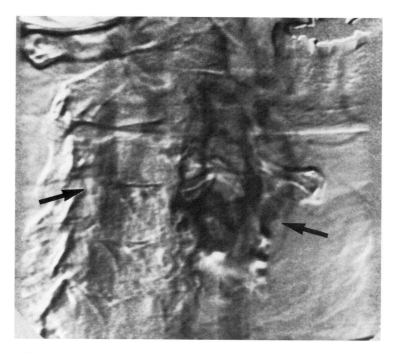

Fig. 40-2. Totally uninterpretable study resulting from severe bony and soft tissue misregistration artifacts. Arrows indicate location of carotid bifurcation.

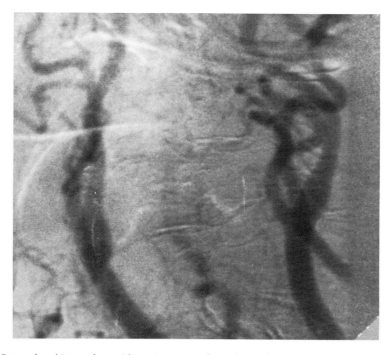

Fig. 40-3. External and internal carotid arteries are overlapped on right side and vertebral artery partially obscures left carotid bifurcation.

Table 40-1. Comparison of DSA and conventional arteriography: radiologists' interpretation of 142 internal carotid arteries*

DSA results (%stenosis)	No. of arteries	Distribution according to conventional arteriography					
		0%	<25%	25%-49%	50%-74%	75%-99%	100%
0	50	38	5	2	4	1	—
<25	8	1	3	3	1	—	—
25-49	18	2	2	8	3	3	—
50-74	19	2	—	2	10	5	—
75-99	24	—	—	—	2	19	3
100	9	—	—	—	—	—	9
Uninterpretable	14	6	—	3	2	3	—

From Russell, J.B., et al.: Surgery 94:604, 1983.
*κ = 0.588 ± 0.053.

ventional x-ray images when similar magnification is employed.[6,29] If the level of contrast is adequate, the clinically important extracranial arteries are satisfactorily depicted, but fine detail is lost.[8] Wall irregularities, small ulcers, and thrombi may escape detection.[51] Only the larger intracranial arteries can be studied.

When the injection is made into a peripheral arm vein, the contrast medium may reflux up into the jugular vein and obscure the picture.[10] Reflux is more likely to happen when the patient performs a Valsalva maneuver. Introducing the contrast medium directly into the superior vena cava via a long catheter obviates the problem.

CAROTID BIFURCATION STUDIES
Accuracy

Despite the widespread use of DSA to diagnose extracranial carotid disease, relatively few studies comparing the accuracy of DSA to conventional arteriography have been published. The early literature and the majority of recent reports are largely anecdotal. In contrast, the accuracies of most noninvasive tests have been exhaustively investigated. This disparity results, perhaps, from the perception that DSA is a radiographic technique and, as such, constitutes its own standard.

During a recent 12-month period, DSA of the extracranial carotid arteries was performed on 688 patients at one of the two major hospitals in our community, and 78 of these patients subsequently underwent conventional arteriography, providing 142 carotid bifurcations for comparison (14 of the studies were unilateral). All DSA images and conventional arteriograms were evaluated by staff radiologists, and their interpretations, as documented

in written reports, were compared. Although not all conventional arteriograms were performed by the same individual or even in the same hospital, the radiologists had access to the interpretation of the DSA. Nonetheless, we felt that this comparison was of interest, since the radiologist's interpretation often influences the decisions of physicians responsible for patient care.

The data from this portion of the study are shown in Table 40-1. The extent of the disease in the internal carotid arteries was classified into one of six categories (normal; minimal, <25% diameter stenosis; mild, 25% to 49%; moderate, 50% to 74%; severe, 75% to 99%; and total occlusion, 100%). Fourteen (10%) of the DSA images were considered uninterpretable. Of the 128 interpretable studies, 87 (68%) agreed exactly with conventional arteriography and 113 (88%) agreed within ± one category. If the uninterpretable studies were included, 61% agreed exactly and 80% agreed within ± one category. The κ statistic for the six categories of interpretable vessels was 0.588 ± 0.053.[11]

Sensitivity, specificity, positive predictive value (PPV), negative predictive value (NPV), and overall accuracy figures for the interpretable data are given in Table 40-2. When any disease was noted on the conventional arteriogram (>0% stenosis), the NPV was only 76%, implying that 24% of all internal carotid arteries with DSA findings reported as being negative were actually stenotic. Moreover, 16% of the arteries reported as having diameter reductions less than 50% actually had hemodynamically significant lesions (84% NPV). On the other hand, a positive DSA was highly reliable (91% to 94% PPV).

Table 40-2. Accuracy of DSA: radiologists' interpretation of 128 internal carotid arteries

Positive criterion* (%stenosis)	Prevalence (%)	Sensitivity (%)	Specificity (%)	PPV (%)	NPV (%)	Accuracy (%)
>0	85/128 (66)	73/85 (86)	38/43 (88)	73/78 (94)	38/50 (76)	111/128 (87)
≥25	75/128 (56)	64/75 (85)	47/53 (89)	64/70 (91)	47/58 (81)	111/128 (87)
≥50	60/128 (47)	48/60 (80)	64/68 (94)	48/52 (92)	64/76 (84)	112/128 (88)

From Russell, J.B., et al: Surgery 94:604, 1983.
*Degree of stenosis considered positive for both DSA and conventional arteriography.

Table 40-3. Comparison of DSA and conventional arteriography: retrospective review of 139 internal carotid arteries*

DSA results (%stenosis)	No. of arteries	Distribution according to conventional arteriography					
		0%	<25%	25%-49%	50%-74%	75%-99%	100%
0	43	31	8	3	1	—	—
<25	14	3	7	4	—	—	—
25-49	16	—	2	11	3	—	—
50-74	16	2	—	3	9	2	—
74-99	20	—	—	1	4	13	2
100	8	—	—	—	—	1	7
Uninterpretable	22	5	2	3	5	5	2

From Russell, J.B., et al.: Surgery 94:604, 1983.
*κ = 0.581 ± 0.055.

Table 40-4. Accuracy of DSA: retrospective review of 117 internal carotid arteries

Positive criterion (%stenosis)*	Prevalence (%)	Sensitivity (%)	Specificity (%)	PPV (%)	NPV (%)	Accuracy (%)
≥0	81/117 (69)	69/81 (85)	31/36 (86)	69/74 (93)	31/43 (72)	100/117 (85)
≥25	64/117 (55)	56/64 (88)	49/53 (92)	56/60 (93)	49/57 (86)	105/117 (90)
≥50	42/117 (36)	38/42 (90)	69/75 (92)	38/44 (86)	69/73 (95)	107/117 (91)

From Russell, J.B., et al.: Surgery 94:604, 1983.
*Degree of stenosis considered positive for both DSA and conventional arteriography.

If uninterpretable findings were included in the analysis, 20 (31%) of the 64 internal carotid arteries with negative or uninterpretable DSA results actually had some degree of stenosis; 17 (19%) of the 90 studies in which the DSA was uninterpretable or showed less than 50% disease actually had hemodynamically significant stenoses (Table 40-1).

A blind retrospective review of the same set of studies produced similar data (Tables 40-3 and 40-4.[44] We felt that three of the internal carotid arteries were inadequately visualized on conventional arteriography and that 22 (16%) of the DSA images were uninterpretable; therefore comparisons were limited to 117 sides. Conventional arteriography revealed disease in 29 (45%) of the 65 internal carotid arteries with negative or uninter-

pretable DSA images and hemodynamically significant disease in 16 (77%) of the 95 internal carotid arteries with DSA images that were uninterpretable or that showed less than 50% stenosis (Table 40-3). Receiver operating characteristic (ROC) curves for the retrospective data confirm the increasing accuracy of DSA for the more severe stenoses and demonstrate that the optimum balance between sensitivity and specificity for identifying any specific degree of stenosis was obtained when the positive criteria for DSA and conventional arteriography were the same (Fig. 40-4).[33]

Listed in Tables 40-5 and 40-6 are accuracy figures from other reports in which the data were complete enough to calculate statistical parameters.[10,17,28,50,53] The cumulative figures did not differ

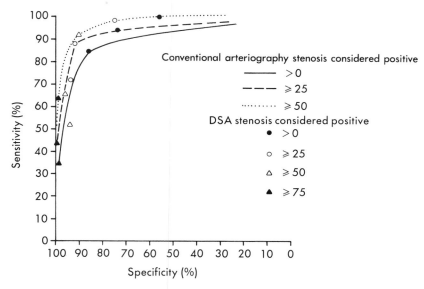

Fig. 40-4. ROC curves for retrospective DSA data. Uninterpretable studies are excluded. (From Russell, J.B., et al.: Surgery 94:604, 1983.)

Table 40-5. Accuracy of diagnostic-quality DSA for detecting any stenosis of the internal carotid artery: correlation with 454 conventional arteriograms

Reference	Prevalence (%)	Sensitivity (%)	Specificity (%)	PPV (%)	NPV (%)	Accuracy (%)
Chilcote et al., 1981[10]	122/179 (68)	106/122 (87)	49/57 (86)	106/114 (93)	49/65 (75)	155/179 (87)
Turnipseed et al., 1982[50]	59/72 (82)	56/59 (95)	13/13 (100)	56/56 (100)	13/16 (81)	69/72 (96)
Eikelboom et al., 1983[17]	94/108 (87)	84/94 (89)	12/14 (86)	84/86 (98)	12/22 (55)	96/108 (89)
Wood et al., 1983[53]	80/95 (84)	70/80 (88)	11/15 (73)	70/74 (95)	11/21 (52)	81/95 (85)
Cumulative	355/454 (78)	316/355 (89)	85/99 (86)	316/330 (96)	85/124 (69)	401/454 (88)

Table 40-6. Accuracy of diagnostic-quality DSA for detecting hemodynamically significant lesions of the internal carotid artery: correlation with 515 conventional arteriograms

Reference	Positive criterion (%stenosis)	Prevalence (%)	Sensitivity (%)	Specificity (%)	PPV (%)	NPV (%)	Accuracy (%)
Chilcote et al., 1981[10]	≥40	70/179 (39)	61/70 (87)	96/109 (88)	61/74 (82)	96/105 (91)	157/179 (88)
	≥60	43/179 (24)	41/43 (95)	125/136 (92)	41/52 (79)	125/127 (98)	166/179 (93)
Turnipseed et al., 1982[50]	≥50	43/72 (63)	44/45 (98)	27/27 (100)	44/44 (100)	27/28 (96)	71/72 (99)
Eikelboom et al., 1983[17]	≥50	60/108 (56)	57/60 (95)	44/48 (92)	57/61 (93)	44/47 (94)	101/108 (94)
Wood et al., 1983[53]	≥40	38/95 (40)	36/38 (95)	55/57 (96)	36/38 (95)	55/57 (96)	91/95 (96)
	≥60	30/95 (32)	28/30 (93)	61/65 (94)	28/32 (88)	61/63 (97)	89/95 (94)
Kempczinski et al., 1983[28]	≥50	25/61 (41)	21/25 (84)	33/36 (92)	21/24 (88)	33/37 (89)	54/61 (89)
Cumulative*	≥50	221/515 (43)	205/221 (93)	272/294 (93)	205/227 (90)	272/288 (94)	477/515 (93)

*Chilcote and Wood: values for ≥50% criterion estimated by averaging ≥40% and ≥60% data.

significantly from our data. Basically they show that sensitivities and specificities of diagnostic quality DSA are in the 85% to 90% range for detecting or ruling out any degree of stenosis and that they are in the 90% to 95% range for differentiating hemodynamically significant from nonhemodynamically significant disease. A positive test result is likely to be valid (high PPV), but a negative test result has about a 30% chance of missing low-grade stenoses (low NPV for any disease). On the other hand, DSA images interpreted as showing less than 50% stenosis are likely to be valid (high NPV for hemodynamically significant disease).

As one would expect, the better the DSA image, the more accurate the results become. For example, when the DSA quality was good or excellent, Chilcote et al.[10] noted sensitivities and specificities of 91% and 94%, respectively, for detecting any disease and 97% and 93% for differentiating between stenoses greater or less than 60%. Poor images, however, yielded sensitivities and specificities of 73% and 50% (any disease) and 80% and 87% (≥60% disease).

Perfect agreement between the DSA image and conventional arteriography occurred in 58% to 96% of the studies (Table 40-7). Much of this disparity can be attributed to the way in which the individual investigators categorized the degree of stenosis, those using small categories (for example, 1% to 19%, 20% to 39%, etc.)[10,14,44,53] reporting lower values than those using large categories (such as 1% to 49%, 50% to 99%.[8,17,50] The κ statistic, which should provide a better way of measuring agreement between DSA and conventional arteriography, also suffers from the lack of consistency

between the number and size of the stenosis categories (Table 40-7)[11] If the data are grouped into four standard categories (no disease, hemodynamically insignificant, hemodynamically significant, and total occlusion), κ values range from 0.68 to 0.94, with the cumulative value for the 517 studies being 0.755 ± 0.022. Like the Pearson correlation coefficient, perfect correlation gives a κ value of 1.00, and no correlation gives a κ value of 0. Therefore a κ of 0.755 suggests that DSA is substantially useful for group-type predictions and some individual predictions.

Investigators who have directly compared DSA results with operative findings report accuracy data that differ little from those summarized in Table 40-6.[30]

Total occlusion. Total occlusions of the internal carotid artery are quite accurately identified by DSA. A review of six reports reveals that 85 of 89 total occlusions were identified (96% sensitivity).* All 85 internal carotid arteries that appeared to be occluded on DSA were confirmed by conventional arteriography (100% PPV). Our retrospective results were not as good (Table 40-3). We found that 2 (9%) of 22 uninterpretable studies were occluded and that 2 (18%) of 11 occluded arteries had uninterpretable studies.[44] Only 7 of 9 occlusions were correctly interpreted (78% sensitivity), and 1 of 8 thought to be occluded was actually patent (88% PPV).

Ulcers, web stenoses, and thrombosis. In our study, DSA identified 11 of 32 irregularities of the internal carotid arteries that were interpreted as ul-

*References 10, 17, 28, 44, 50, 53.

Table 40-7. Agreement of diagnostic-quality DSA and conventional arteriography (internal carotid arteries)

Reference	Uninterpretable studies excluded (%)	Perfect agreement (%)	Agreement ± one category (%)*	κ ± σ	Normalized‖ κ ± σ
Chilcote et al., 1981[10]	11	65	91	0.572 ± 0.044†	0.718 ± 0.43
Turnipseed et al., 1982[50]	?	96	99	0.942 ± 0.30‡	0.943 ± s 0.032
Eikelboom et al., 1983[17]	12	81	94	0.739 ± 0.051‡	0.778 ± 0.049
Wood et al., 1983[53]	8	58	99	0.497 ± 0.061†	0.690 ± 0.062
Russell et al., 1983[44]	16	67	94	0.581 ± 0.055§	0.675 ± 0.055
Earnest et al., 1983[14]	6	73	95	—	—
Celesia et al., 1983[8]	9	84	?	—	—

*Authors' stenosis categories vary from ±20 to ±49.
†Seven stenosis categories.
‡Five stenosis categories.
§Six stenosis categories.
‖Four stenosis categories (0%, 1%-49% or 1%-59%, 50%-99% or 60%-99%, 100%).

cerated plaques on conventional arteriography (34% sensitivity).[44] Out of 16 ulcers that were identified by DSA, 5 were false positives (69% PPV). Turnipseed et al.[50] report a sensitivity of 67%, with 5 of the 6 false negative studies being in internal carotid arteries with a stenosis less than 50%. Of the ulcers observed on conventional arteriography in Chilcote's series[10] all were detected by good to excellent quality DSA examinations, but none were detected by poor DSAs. The overall sensitivity was 50%. In a report from the Mayo Clinic, 6 out of 11 ulcers of the internal carotid artery visualized by DSA were confirmed at surgery (55% PPV).[14] One fourth of the diagnostic errors studied by Turski et al. resulted from overlooking ulcerations.[51]

Weblike stenoses and thrombi are also frequently overlooked.[2,14,51]

Causes of diagnostic error

The major cause of diagnostic error is poor image quality resulting from any of the problems mentioned earlier in this chapter. In a series of 18 diagnostic errors reported by Turski et al.,[51] 8 (44%) were caused by misregistration artifacts, 5 (28%) by vessel overlap, 4 (22%) by failure to profile the lesion, and 1 (6%) by poor contrast. Vessels seen in only one projection cannot be assumed to be normal; indeed, Hoffman et al.[26] have chosen to label such studies nondiagnostic. Of 126 carotid arteries visualized in more than one projection, 19 (15%) appeared normal in at least one projection, but abnormal in another. Had the views been restricted to the normal projection, these lesions would have been missed.

A particularly unfortunate drawback of DSA examinations is the inability to obtain a true lateral view of the carotid bifurcation.[51] Lesions on the posterior wall of the internal carotid artery—the most common site of atheroma and ulceration— are apt to be obscured in oblique views by an overlapping external carotid artery.[48] According to Kaseff,[27] a lateral view is necessary in 37% of carotid bifurcations to adequately display the anatomy.

Even when contrast is adequate and there is no motion artifact, the fine detail necessary to visualize ulcerations, weblike stenoses, and thrombi is difficult to attain, not only because of limited resolving power but also because of restricted viewing angles. The detections of ulcers, however, is difficult by any angiographic technique and therefore is not a problem unique with DSA.[16] Using the operative specimen as the standard for the pres-

ence or absence of ulceration, Eikelboom et al.[18] found conventional arteriography to have a sensitivity of 73% and a specificity of 62%. The PPV was 63%, and the NPV was 72%. In other words, ulceration was absent in 37% of those arteries thought to be positive by arteriography and was present in 28% of those arteries that showed no ulcer on the arteriogram, figures that differ little from those reported by Earnest et al.[14] with DSA.

Finally, DSA has usually been compared with conventional arteriography, which itself is not a completely reliable standard.[7] In a well-designed postmortem study, Croft et al.[12] found that conventional arteriography was only about 67% to 70% sensitive and 87% to 97% specific for detecting any atherosclerotic lesion at the carotid bifurcation. The sensitivity and specificity were better (100% and 96%, respectively) when the observers were requested to differentiate between diameter stenoses greater or less than 20%. Moreover, different observers reviewing the same series of arteriograms may arrive at somewhat different estimations of the degree of carotid stenosis. Even the same observer viewing the same films at a later date may arrive at different conclusions. Chikos et al.[9] found that different observers' estimations of the degree of internal carotid stenosis varied by 8.6% $\pm$ 9.5% and that percent agreement for stenoses of 50% or greater was only 85%. Perfect agreement occurred in 75% of their studies when the percent stenoses were categorized into five groups—a figure similar to those published for DSA (Table 40-7). When their interobserver data were categorized into four stenosis groups (0%, 1% to 49%, 50% to 99%, 100%), the κ value was only 0.654 $\pm$ 0.017 (our calculations)—again a figure resembling those found for DSA (Table 40-7). Therefore it is probable that at least some of the errors attributed to DSA may, in fact, relate to difficulties inherent in reading any angiographic study.

ARCH STUDIES

The ability to visualize the aortic arch and its branches with a less invasive test than conventional arteriography is one of the commonly mentioned advantages of intravenous DSA. These vessels are difficult to examine noninvasively. A report by Hesselink et al.[25] indicates that 90% of the vertebral images were of good or fair quality in patients referred for suspected vertebrobasilar disease. Moderate or severe disease was detected in 8% and total vertebral occlusion in 4%. Interestingly, these findings had little influence on therapeutic decisions, which were more often dictated by concomitant disease at the carotid bifurcation.

The importance of arch aortography in patients without vertebrobasilar disease has, however, been questioned. In a prospective study using conventional arteriographic techniques, Goldstein et al.[23] found that 41% of the arch aortograms were entirely normal; 28% revealed nonulcerated minor lesions of no clinical significance; 29% demonstrated nonsurgical lesions (for example, asymptomatic subclavian steal); and only 2% showed lesions of surgical importance (such as occlusion of the proximal common carotid or vertebral arteries). In our experience and in that of others, DSA is quite helpful in confirming the diagnosis of subclavian steal.

INTRACRANIAL STUDIES

The large intracranial vessels can usually be visualized with intravenous DSA. Problems related to resolution, vessel overlap, motion artifact, poor contrast, and scatter from the bony structures of the skull tend to degrade the image, making it difficult to obtain the fine detail necessary for accurate diagnosis.[14] Modic et al.[35] reported that 65% of the intracranial images were diagnostic but that the overall quality was inferior to conventional arteriography. An additional 22% were diagnostic but were susceptible to misinterpretation, and 13% were nondiagnostic or uninterpretable. In their study, 70% of the meningiomas, arteriovenous malformations, and aneurysms were recognized. At the Mayo Clinic, 8% of the DSA images overlooked significant intracranial lesions that were subsequently detected by conventional arteriography.[14] Among the lesions that were missed were severe stenoses or occlusions of the distal internal

carotid artery, carotid siphon, middle cerebral artery, and basilar artery.

Hesselink et al.[25] found that 24% of the basilar artery images and 58% of the posterior cerebral artery images were poor. They concluded that DSA does not adequately visualize the posterior cerebral or cerebellar arteries and that it overlooks minor disease and underestimates major disease of the basilar artery.

A positive DSA, therefore, may be helpful; but a negative study cannot be relied on to rule out arteriovenous malformations, small aneurysms, or occlusive disease of the intracranial arteries.[35]

ACCURACY COMPARED WITH NONINVASIVE TESTS

Few reports have been published comparing the accuracy of noninvasive tests and DSA to conventional arteriography in the same groups of patients.[8,17,28,50] Table 40-8 summarizes the noninvasive test results from three such studies. The DSA results are included in Tables 40-5 and 40-6. In general, the accuracies of the two tests appeared to be similar, but there were appreciable differences in a few isolated areas. For example, Turnipseed et al.[50], who used a continuous-wave Doppler flow-mapping device, found that DSA was more specific than the noninvasive test both for identifying the absence of any disease and for identifying stenoses with diameter reductions less than 50%. Eikelboom et al.[17], using a combination real-time B-mode scanner and a pulsed Doppler flow detector (Duplex scan), noted a very low NPV for DSA (55%) compared with that of the noninvasive test (100%) when both modalities were called on to rule out the presence of any stenosis. In their study the Duplex scan was more sensitive than the DSA but

Table 40-8. Accuracy of noninvasive tests in patients also undergoing DSA: correlation with conventional arteriography

Reference (method used)	Positive criterion (%stenosis)	Sensitivity (%)	Specificity (%)	PPV (%)	NPV (%)	Accuracy (%)
Turnipseed et al., 1982[50] (Doppler scan)	0*	57/59 (97)	11/13 (85)	57/59 (97)	11/13 (85)	68/72 (94)
	50	42/45 (93)	24/27 (89)	42/45 (93)	24/27 (89)	66/72 (92)
Eikelboom et al., 1983[17] (Duplex scan)	0*	94/94 (100)	3/14 (21)	94/105 (90)	3/3 (100)	97/108 (90)
	50	57/60 (95)	47/48 (98)	57/58 (98)	47/50 (94)	104/108 (96)
Kempczinski et al., 1983[28] (OPG-Gee)	50	22/27 (81)	36/38 (95)	22/24 (92)	36/41 (88)	58/65 (89)

*Any detectable disease considered positive.

far less specific (high false positive rate). For differentiating hemodynamically significant from non-hemodynamically significant disease, DSA and noninvasive tests had practically identical accuracies in both Eikelboom's and Kempczinski's reports.[17,28]

Perfect agreement between the noninvasive tests and conventional arteriography occurred in 81% of the studies by Turnipseed et al. and in 71% of those by Eikelboom et al.[17,50] The κ value was 0.756 ± 0.058 for the noninvasive data of Turnipseed et al. and 0.610 ± 0.059 for that of Eikelboom et al. Comparing the agreement figures and the κ statistics for the noninvasive tests with the data in Table 40-7 suggests that noninvasive tests and conventional arteriography are somewhat less well correlated than DSA and conventional arteriography.

When the DSA results in Tables 40-5 and 40-6 are compared with results of noninvasive tests reported in the literature and elsewhere in this book, it is evident that the accuracy of DSA exceeds that of many noninvasive tests and approaches that of the best.[46] DSA seems to be better than most of the noninvasive imaging techniques for distinguishing total occlusion of the internal carotid artery from severe stenosis. (The remote physiologic tests, oculoplethysmography, supraorbital sonography, etc. are unable to make this distinction.) As discussed earlier in this chapter, DSA has a reported sensitivity of 96% and PPV of 100% for total occlusion. Combining the data of Eikelboom et al.[17] and Roederer et al.,[42] Duplex scanning had a sensitivity of 98% (54/55) and a PPV of 96% (54/56). Turnipseed et al.[50] reported that continuous-wave Doppler scanning identified 14 of 18 total occlusions (78% sensitivity) and correctly predicted 14 of 15 total occlusions (93% PPV). On the other hand, analysis of our earlier data with pulsed Doppler imaging revealed a sensitivity and PPV of only 64%.[47] Total occlusions can also be overlooked by echo scanning methods that do not incorporate Doppler flow studies, since fresh thrombi may have an acoustic density similar to that of blood.

Of the noninvasive tests, only the echo scanning methods are capable of detecting ulcers, but their accuracy in this regard is disputed. Although DSA and conventional arteriography are not particularly accurate either, they are better than most noninvasive tests for identifying ulcers or wall irregularity. The reported ability of echo scans to char-

acterize plaque morphology (in terms of soft vs. hard or the presence of intraplaque hemorrhage) is potentially an advantage that these noninvasive tests have over DSA.

Because of inadequate resolution, motion artifact, and orientation of the image, DSA has missed weblike stenoses that have been detected noninvasively.[2] Even in the assessment of the larger intracranial arteries, where the DSA usually excels, noninvasive tests may detect stenoses that have been overlooked by DSA. For example, Kempczinski et al.[28], in their comparative study of DSA and the Gee oculopneumoplethysmograph, found four hemodynamically significant lesions of the internal carotid siphon that were not identified by DSA but were detected by the noninvasive tests. If these four had been considered false negative results, the sensitivity of the DSA would have been reduced to 72%.

RISKS AND COMPLICATIONS

Although intravenous DSA is an invasive procedure, it is decidedly less risky than conventional cerebral arteriography. To our knowledge, no strokes have occurred as the result of DSA and local complications are relatively minor.[8,10,21]

At the University of Virginia, Faught et al. found that 6.8% of patients undergoing conventional arteriography for stroke or TIAs had transient cerebral complications, and another 5.4% had permanent neurologic deficits.[19] The risk was highest in those patients with severe stenosis and multiple TIAs, the very group that could benefit most from surgery. The statistics from other institutions have been less discouraging. Neurologic complications occurred in 4.2% of patients undergoing conventional arteriography for suspected cerebrovascular disease at the Mayo Clinic.[15] Only 0.6% were permanent, however. Hematomas developed in 4.4% of the patients, and other local complications (arterial thrombosis and infection) occurred in 0.5%. The incidence of serious local complications requiring surgery or prolonged hospitalization was only 0.3%. Systemic reactions were also rare, 1.9%. Since the risk of conventional arteriography varies from one hospital to the next, the deficits of DSA must be weighed carefully against the arteriographic stroke rate at each institution to determine which of the two radiologic procedures to employ.

Patients undergoing DSA for cerebrovascular diagnosis appear to be subjected to less radiation than those undergoing conventional arteriography. At

ical decisions using DSA or ultrasound?'' and then suggested an answer, ''Is it that we are accustomed to seeing a picture?''

Among others, Earnest et al.[14] feel that the additional information gained by obtaining conventional arteriography in patients being considered for carotid endarterectomy justifies the small additional risk. Detection of intracranial lesions, previously unrecognized on DSA, modified their therapeutic approach in 4 of 78 patients (5%). Folcarelli et al.[20] reviewed four patients on whom carotid endarterectomies had been performed on the basis of DSA alone in which overlooked lesions seriously threatened the outcome of the surgery. The lesions included a severely stenotic vertebral artery in a patient with occlusion of the opposite vertebral, a total occlusion of the internal carotid artery distal to the bifurcation, a 90% stenosis of the carotid siphon distal to the endarterectomy site, and a markedly narrowed common carotid artery. The latter complicated the insertion of a shunt, leading to a stroke. Since no denominator was provided in Folcarelli's study, it is impossible to determine the incidence of these problems.

Another concern is the possibility that DSA may fail to detect clinically significant lesions at the carotid bifurcation. We reviewed 70 internal carotid arteries that underwent endarterectomy after having been evaluated with DSA,[44] of which 24 (34%) were operated on solely on the basis of the DSA findings with no evident adverse effects. The remaining 46 arteries were also studied with conventional arteriography. In 2 of these (4%) the DSA proved to be falsely negative, and in 8 (17%) the DSA was uninterpretable. In other words, if DSA had been the only radiologic procedure used to select patients for operation, 10 (22%) of the endarterectomies would not have been performed.

Thus it is incumbent on those who would use DSA as the definitive diagnostic procedure to ensure that *important* lesions are not being missed at the carotid bifurcation or in other vital components of the cerebral circulation. Clouding the picture, however, are the issues of cost-effectiveness and what constitutes an important lesion. Despite the fact that DSA may miss a few lesions at the aortic arch, in the vertebrobasilar system, and in the intracranial carotid arteries, many would argue that the great majority of these lesions are inconsequential. While few surgeons would knowingly neglect low-grade lesions at the carotid bifurcation in patients with hemispheric symptoms, a large

number are less convinced of the importance of stenotic lesions in asymptomatic patients or in those with nonhemispheric symptoms.

Because false positive DSA images are relatively infrequent, they are numerically of less concern in a population with a high prevalence of disease. They do, of course, assume more importance when DSA is used as a screening procedure.

In view of these considerations, it is not surprising that no consensus has emerged regarding the appropriate use of DSA. Perhaps the only point on which all investigators agree is the necessity for obtaining conventional arteriograms when the DSA is incomplete, ambiguous, or not clear.

An interesting development is the emphasis that some authors are placing on the complementary roles of DSA and noninvasive testing.[1,4,28,40] For example, Kempczinski et al.[28] advocate the initial use of noninvasive testing on patients with asymptomatic bruits or nonhemispheric symptoms. Since the risk of stroke in these patients is generally assumed to be appreciable only when the carotid lesion is hemodynamically significant, noninvasive tests are quite likely to be accurate. Patients with negative noninvasive tests can be safely followed, and those that have positive tests may be referred for DSA as a definitive procedure. Because the NPV of DSA for hemodynamically significant lesions is high (Table 40-6), few potentially dangerous lesions are apt to be overlooked. This approach, therefore, has the dual virtues of being both rational and cost-effective. Both tests can be performed on an outpatient basis, and the patient need be hospitalized only if endarterectomy is planned. Of course, DSA could be employed as the initial procedure, but a large number of unnecessary DSAs would be required and the overall cost would increase.

Several approaches to hemispheric symptoms have been advocated by those who wish to avoid going directly to conventional arteriography. In patients with typical TIAs or reversible ischemic deficits, Kempczinski et al.[28] suggest using DSA as the initial procedure. If the study is adequate and the findings agree with the symptoms, it can function as the definitive diagnostic procedure and endarterectomy can be performed without further x-ray studies. Demonstration of an occlusion or other inoperable lesion would also obviate the need for conventional arteriography. In all other cases, including those in which the DSA appears normal, conventional arteriography is required. Thiele[49] supports the initial use of Duplex imaging in patients with hemispheric symptoms. Because of the high NPV of Duplex imaging (Table 40-8), there is little chance that DSA would detect a lesion missed by this technique. Consequently, when the Duplex scan is negative or indicates a low-grade lesion, the patient is referred directly for a conventional arteriogram. To avoid another potentially inconclusive study, a similar approach is taken when the Duplex scan suggests total occlusion of the internal carotid artery. If, however, the Duplex scan shows a high-grade lesion, DSA may be performed with reasonable confidence as the definitive diagnostic procedure. Any disagreement between the two studies requires resolution by conventional arteriography. For like reasons, Raines[40] and Bendick et al.,[4] who use real-time echo imaging, favor DSA in those patients in whom the tests are strongly positive and conventional arteriography in those in whom the tests indicate low-grade disease.

As a less hazardous procedure than conventional arteriography, intravenous DSA may be used early after a stroke to rule out thrombi or critical stenosis that may require anticoagulation therapy or emergent surgery.[28] It may be the only possible radiographic procedure, short of direct carotid puncture, in patients with no arterial access. Finally, it usually provides sufficiently adequate visualization of the arch structures to detect subclavian steal and often to detect vertebral disease—diagnoses that are difficult to confirm noninvasively.

Our preference, at present, is to use noninvasive tests for the initial evaluation of patients with suspected cerebrovascular disease and conventional arteriography when a surgical procedure is contemplated.[44] From time to time arteriography has revealed unexpected intracranial lesions—such as aneurysms or tumors—that have altered our therapeutic approach. Moreover, we appreciate the fine detail provided by conventional arteriography, we are uncomfortable with the fuzzy images of DSA, and—based on our assessment of DSA vs. conventional arteriography—we are skeptical of its accuracy. Only when the patient has no ready arterial access or when a previously unsatisfactory conventional arteriogram has been obtained do we order DSA as the definitive diagnostic procedure.[21] However, when we are referred a patient who has already had a good quality DSA that demonstrates findings compatible with the patient's symptoms, and when the computed tomographic scan is negative (a constellation that is occurring with increasing frequently), we will proceed with surgery with-

out conventional arteriography. To date, we have recognized no adverse effects of this approach.

Postoperative follow-up

DSA has been used in the immediate postoperative period to rule out thrombosis occurring at the endarterectomy site in patients who awake with neurologic deficits or who develop deficits in the first 12 to 24 hours.[24] Noninvasive imaging methods are difficult to apply to the fresh wound because of sutures, swelling, hematomas, and disrupted tissue planes that produce multiple acoustic interfaces. Supraorbital Doppler sonography and oculopneumoplethysmography can be used, but these tests lack sensitivity. Hertzer et al.[24] report that normal DSA findings avoided unnecessary reoperations in four of six patients with postoperative strokes. Blaisdell,[5] in his discussion of Hertzer's paper, questioned the use of DSA in this setting, pointing out that obtaining DSA necessitates a delay that could compromise the ability of the surgeon to reverse the neurologic deficit. He favored immediate return to the operating room rather than expending time on diagnostic tests. Responding to Blaisdell's comments, Hertzer proposed a selective approach.[24] Patients with small internal carotid arteries and those in whom the arteriotomy closure had been difficult should be returned immediately to the operating room, since the likelihood of thrombosis is high. On the other hand, when no technical problems were encountered during the operation and when the chance of intraoperative embolization was high, DSA should be performed. The likelihood of thrombosis in these patients is low; the outcomes of relatively few would be compromised by the delay; and most would be spared the trauma and expense of another surgical procedure.

Hertzer's group[24] has also used DSA to assess the early technical results of carotid endarterectomy. Studies performed before hospital discharge revealed that 1.9% of the internal carotid arteries and 4.7% of the external carotid arteries had occluded. Postoperative stenoses were found in 4.3% of the internal carotid arteries (all of which were mild) and in 2.0% of the external carotid arteries. Again, the use of noninvasive tests during this period is fraught with many of the same problems just outlined.

For long-term follow-up, noninvasive tests have the advantage of being less expensive and sufficiently accurate to detect recurrence or progression of disease. Archer et al.,[2] using both DSA and continuous-wave Doppler scanning, identified recurrent stenoses in 9% of internal carotid arteries that had been subjected to operation and in 18% of the surgically untreated arteries. They concluded that DSA should be performed when the noninvasive tests demonstrated hemodynamically significant progression or when there were recurrent symptoms of cerebral ischemia.

Screening

It has been suggested that DSA be used to screen patients at high risk for cerebrovascular disease, including those with poorly controlled hypertension, diabetes, hyperlipidemia, or arteriosclerosis at other sites and those scheduled for coronary artery bypass.[21] Again, it would seem more appropriate to employ the less expensive, less traumatic, and less time-consuming noninvasive tests for this purpose.

The proposal that DSA be employed when arteriography is only ''marginally indicated'' lacks intellectual appeal and encourages indiscriminant use of the modality.[21] By and large the results of such ill-conceived studies do not contribute to the patient's well-being and are disproportionately expensive. Unfortunately, our experience with DSA in a community hospital setting suggested that this is exactly the way it was being used in a large proportion of the cases.[44]

Estimation of cerebral blood flow

Because intravenous DSA simultaneously delivers contrast material to all arteries feeding the intracerebral circulation, the patterns of cortical opacification could theoretically provide a method for assessing cerebral blood flow.[29] To test this hypothesis, Awad et al.[3] correlated DSA findings with regional cerebral blood flow measured by the ^{133}Xe inhalation technique in a series of patients with unilateral internal carotid occlusion. Symmetric hemispheric opacification confirmed the presence of adequate interhemispheric collateral vessels but did not rule out reduced blood flow. On the other hand, delayed cortical opacification on the side of the carotid occlusion did not necessarily imply reduced blood flow or inadequate collateral vessels. This application of DSA, therefore, appears to have limited value.

COST-EFFECTIVENESS

DSA is less expensive than conventional arteriography. Part of this reduction is in film costs, which average less than $15 (including magnetic

tape) for DSA compared with $65 to $150 or more with the conventional procedure.[10,22,35] But the major cost saving relates to the fact that DSA can be done as an outpatient procedure, thereby avoiding the expense and inconvenience associated with hospitalization. Although conventional arteriography can also be performed as an outpatient procedure in selected patients, currently most patients are admitted for at least 24 hours.

Freedman[22] has calculated that the cost per lesion identified by inpatient carotid arteriography would be $1500, assuming that the cost of each study was $1200 and that 80% of the studies were positive. If DSA were performed before hospitalization at a cost of $500 and if conventional arteriograms were obtained on all 80% that were positive, the cost per lesion identified would rise to $2033. The cost per lesion would, however, fall to $1433 if conventional arteriograms were required to corroborate 50% of the positive DSAs and to $950 if they were required in only 10% of the positive DSAs. Therefore DSA would provide significant savings only if 90% of the studies could be accepted as definitive.

At our institution, total charges including professional fees average about $450 for DSA, $850 for conventional arteriography, and $150 for a noninvasive carotid screen.[44] The estimated cost of hospitalization for 2 nights including routine laboratory studies and attending physician's fees is $475. Based on these figures, noninvasive testing appears to be the most economical method for correctly diagnosing the presence or absence of internal carotid arterial disease (Table 40-11). Although DSA is much less expensive than conventional arteriography, this advantage is almost eliminated when hospitalization is required. If a screening test is required before conventional arteriography, noninvasive testing has the advantage of adding very little to the overall diagnostic cost.

This rather simplistic approach does not take into account the number of conventional arteriograms that might be avoided by DSA or the number of patients who could undergo endarterectomy without further radiographic study. To address these issues, the comparative costs of DSA and noninvasive testing in 1000 patients were calculated from the following data: of 1771 patients having noninvasive carotid testing in our laboratory, 328 (19%) subsequently underwent conventional arteriography and 112 (6%) underwent carotid endarterectomy.[47] Of 688 patients originally studied with DSA, 78 (11%) had conventional arteriography and

Table 40-11. Cost per correctly diagnosed internal carotid artery

	Any disease		50% diameter stenosis		Conventional arteriography
	UA*	DSA†	UA*	DSA†	
Accuracy	86%	88%	92%	93%	100%
Accurate and interpretable‡	78%	80%	84%	85%	100%
Outpatient cost	$96	$281	$89	$264	$425
Inpatient cost	$400	$578	$371	$555	$663

*UA, pulsed Doppler ultrasonic arteriography; data from our laboratory, 1982-1983.
†Data from Tables 40-5 and 40-6.
‡Assuming that 9% of the UA and DSA examinations were uninterpretable.

70 (10%), carotid endarterectomy (24 of the carotid endarterectomies were performed without conventional arteriography and 32 of those undergoing conventional arteriography were not operated on).[44] Based on these percentages and the average cost of these tests as mentioned earlier, the cost of the total diagnostic workup for 1000 patients screened initially by outpatient DSA would be 48% higher than that for an equivalent number screened by the noninvasive modality ($595,750 vs. $401,750). In fact, DSA would be slightly more expensive than noninvasive testing even if DSA totally obviated the need for conventional arteriography ($450,000 vs. $401,750). In terms of cost per endarterectomy, the difference would be less striking ($8511 vs. $6696), but DSA would still be 27% more costly. Obviously, if the diagnostic workup in all 1000 patients had been limited to conventional arteriography, the cost would have been two to three times as high; but it is unlikely that this would have occurred.[6] Our data indicate that 44% of the DSAs and 52% of the noninvasive tests were done for localizing symptoms (TIA, stroke, amaurosis fugax).[44,47] If 50% of the patients had localizing symptoms and only those with localizing symptoms were subjected to conventional arteriography, the total cost would have been $662,500, which is 65% higher than the cost for screening the entire group noninvasively but only 11% higher than that for screening with DSA.

The problem of cost-effectiveness is complex. These analyses have not considered the adverse effects of unnecessary or ill-advised conventional arteriography, nor have they considered the increased morbidity and mortality that might result from overlooking a significant lesion with noninvasive testing or DSA. Other variables, such as the prevalence of disease in the population, the clinical judgment, diagnostic ability, and prejudices of the attending physician; and the less tangible concerns of the patient (inconvenience, pain, apprehension) are all important parts of the overall picture that have not been included in these analyses. Nevertheless, they do suggest that intravenous DSA is less cost-effective than noninvasive testing and only moderately more so than conventional arteriography.

THE FUTURE

The early anecdotal reports of clinical success with intravenous DSA led some enthusiasts to predict that it would largely replace conventional arteriography; this promise remains unfulfilled.[41] Although some of the problems that plague DSA could be partially overcome by the routine use of central venous catheterization, a larger bolus of contrast medium, increased radiation dose per frame, a greater number of exposures, more views, and more sophisticated immobilization techniques, these measures would increase the cost, the amount of radiation, and the risk of renal damage, congestive heart failure, myocardial infarction, and local complications.[14,26] Artifacts caused by swallowing may not be eliminated even when nonionic contrast media are used; even if this approach were successful it would be prohibitively expensive.[29,51] Although remasking is now almost universally employed, it rarely salvages an image obscured by severe motion artifact. Investigative techniques, such as dual energy subtraction and hybrid subtraction (a combination of temporal subtraction and energy subtraction), hold some promise of eliminating swallowing artifacts.[6,34,41] These methods, however, provide no help with misregistration of bone.

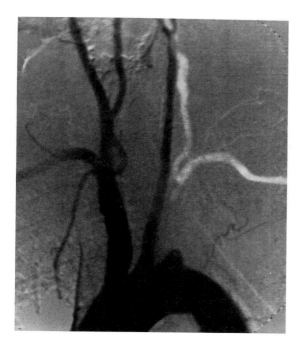

Fig. 40-6. Intraarterial DSA of aortic arch demonstrating occlusion of proximal left subclavian artery, retrograde flow in left vertebral artery, and reconstitution of distal left subclavian artery.

Because of the problems with intravenous DSA, there has been increasing interest in intraarterial DSA.[13,21,29,52] Although the intraarterial route is more invasive than the intravenous, it avoids motion artifact and can be used to obtain selective views of the extracranial and intracranial vessels, thereby eliminating vessel overlap. In addition, image quality is considerably better. Compared with conventional arteriography, intraarterial DSA requires less contrast material, decreases the need for selective catheterization, reduces film cost and examination time, and may be used to store an image to facilitate selective catheterization.[13] The disadvantages include reduced spatial resolution, limited field size, and inability to conduct simultaneous biplanar examinations. Our radiologists now commonly obtain an intraarterial DSA of the aortic arch and vertebrobasilar systems in conjunction with conventional selective carotid arteriography (Fig. 40-6).

SUMMARY

Intravenous DSA is less invasive, less hazardous, and less expensive than conventional cerebrovascular arteriography but is more invasive, haz-ardous, and expensive than noninvasive testing. Unlike noninvasive testing, to which there are few restrictions, DSA must be avoided in patients who are allergic to contrast media and should be used cautiously in those with renal insufficiency or unstable cardiac disease. It cannot be employed in agitated or uncooperative patients.

Image quality is usually inferior to that obtained with conventional arteriography. About 10% of the studies are uninterpretable because of misregistration artifacts, and a significant number are incomplete because of vessel overlap. Although positive studies are reliable predictors of disease, negative studies are less reliable. Web stenoses and thrombi may be overlooked, and low-grade lesions tend to be underestimated. Diagnostic quality images do, however, discriminate accurately between hemodynamically and nonhemodynamically significant disease. Moreover, DSA detects stenoses at the carotid bifurcation with an accuracy approximating that of the better noninvasive imaging methods; it excels in identifying the presence or absence of total occlusion. Another advantage, not shared by noninvasive methods, is the capacity to visualize the aortic arch and intracranial vessels; however, this advantage is of borderline significance, since lesions at the aortic arch seldom influence therapeutic decisions and DSA cannot be relied on to rule out intracranial lesions. The detection of ulcers by any diagnostic technique is an imprecise science, and for this purpose DSA is probably no better or no worse than conventional arteriography or noninvasive imaging. On the other hand, B-mode scans may provide unique (and possibly prognostically valuable) information regarding plaque morphology, but DSA, like other radiographic techniques, cannot.

Although good quality DSAs are being used by many surgeons as the definitive preoperative diagnostic examination in well-selected patients, this approach has not been universally accepted. A growing awareness of the limitations of DSA has prompted the development of protocols that use noninvasive testing to determine which patients should undergo DSA and which patients require conventional arteriography. Despite these well-considered efforts, there is evidence that many physicians continue to use little discretion in their selection of patients for DSA. Although the number of conventional arteriograms obtained has decreased, the total number of cerebrovascular radiologic examinations has expanded severalfold, thereby increasing overall diagnostic costs. For pre-operative screening, DSA is probably less cost-effective than noninvasive tests but is cheaper than routine conventional arteriography, provided that 50% or more of the conventional arteriograms can be avoided.

The exact role of intravenous DSA in the evaluation of extracranial carotid lesions remains to be clarified. It clearly has many advantages, but at present it is not sufficiently accurate to replace conventional arteriography, and it is too invasive and too expensive to replace noninvasive testing.

REFERENCES

1. Ackerman, R.H., et al.: Complementary roles of a noninvasive test battery and DSA in evaluating carotid artery disease, AJNR 4:757, 1983.
2. Archer, C.W., et al.: Digital subtraction angiography and continuous-wave Doppler studies. Their use in post-operative study of patients with carotid endarterectomy, Arch. Surg. 118:462, 1983.
3. Awad, I., et al.: Intravenous digital subtraction angiography: an index of collateral cerebral blood flow in internal carotid occlusion, Stroke 13:469, 1982.
4. Bendick, P.J., Jackson, V.P., and Becker, G.J.: Comparison of ultrasound scanning/Doppler with digital subtraction angiography in evaluating carotid occlusive disease, Med. Instrum. 17:220, 1983.
5. Blaisdell, F.W.: Discussion of Hertzer, N.R., et al.: Early patency of the carotid artery after endarterectomy: digital subtraction angiography after two hundred sixty-two operations, Surgery 92:1056, 1982.
6. Brody, W.R., et al.: Intravenous arteriography using digital subtraction techniques, JAMA 248:671, 1982.
7. Brown, P.M., and Johnston, K.W.: The difficulty of quantifying the severity of carotid stenosis, Surgery 92:468, 1982.
8. Celesia, G.G., et al.: Digital subtraction arteriography. A new method for evaluation of extracranial occlusive disease, Arch. Neurol. 40:70, 1983.
9. Chikos, P.M., et al.: Observer variability in evaluating extracranial carotid artery stenosis, Stroke 14:885, 1983.
10. Chilcote, W.A., et al.: Digital subtraction angiography of the carotid arteries: a comparative study in 100 patients, Radiology 139:287, 1981.
11. Cohen, J.: Weighted kappa: nominal scale agreement with provision for scaled disagreement or partial credit, Psychol. Bull. 70:213, 1968.
12. Croft, R.J., Ellam, L.D., and Harrison, M.J.G.: Accuracy of carotid angiography in the assessment of atheroma of the internal carotid artery, Lancet 1:997, 1980.
13. Crummy, A.B., et al.: Digital subtraction angiography: current status and use of intraarterial injection, Radiology 145:303, 1982.
14. Earnest, F. IV, et al.: The accuracy and limitations of intravenous digital subtraction angiography in the evaluation of atherosclerotic cerebrovascular disease: an angiographic and surgical correlation, Mayo Clin. Proc. 58:735, 1983.
15. Earnest, F. IV, et al.: Complications of cerebral angiography: a prospective assessment of risk, AJNR 4:1191, 1983.
16. Edwards, J.H., et al.: Angiographically undetected ulceration of the carotid bifurcation as a cause of embolic stroke, Radiology 132:369, 1979.
17. Eikelboom, B.C., et al.: Digital video subtraction angiography and duplex scanning in assessment of carotid artery disease: comparison with conventional angiography, Surgery 94:821, 1983.
18. Eikelboom, B.C., et al.: Inaccuracy of angiography in the diagnosis of carotid ulceration, Stroke 14:882, 1983.
19. Faught, E., Trader, S.D., and Hanna, G.R.: Cerebral complications of angiography for transient ischemia and stroke: prediction of risk, Neurology 29:4, 1979.
20. Folcarelli, P., et al.: Pitfalls of carotid surgery based on digital subtraction angiography, Bruit 7:13, 1983.
21. Forbes, G.S., et al.: Digital angiography. Introducing digital techniques to clinical cerebral angiography practice, Mayo Clin. Proc. 57:683, 1982.
22. Freedman, G.S.: Economic analysis of outpatient digital angiography, Applied Radiology 11:29, (May/June) 1982.
23. Goldstein, S.J., et al.: Limited usefulness of aortic arch angiography in the evaluation of carotid occlusive disease, AJR 138:103, 1982.
24. Hertzer, N.R., et al.: Early patency of the carotid artery after endarterectomy: digital subtraction angiography after two hundred sixty-two operations, Surgery 92:1049, 1982.
25. Hesselink, J.R., et al.: Intravenous digital subtraction angiography of arteriosclerotic vertebrobasilar disease, AJR 142:255, 1984.
26. Hoffman, M.G., Gomes, A.S., and Pais, S.O.: Limitations in the interpretation of intravenous carotid digital subtraction angiography, AJR 142:261, 1984.
27. Kaseff, L.G.: Positional variations of the common carotid artery bifurcation: implications for digital subtraction angiography, Radiology 145:377, 1982.
28. Kempczinski, R.F., et al.: A comparison of digital subtraction angiography and noninvasive testing in the diagnosis of cerebrovascular disease, Am. J. Surg. 146:207, 1983.
29. Little, J.R., et al.: Digital subtraction angiography in cerebrovascular disease, Stroke 13:557, 1982.
30. Lusby, R.J., and Ehrenfeld, W.K.: Carotid artery surgery based on digital subtraction angiography, Am. J. Surg. 144:211, 1982.
31. Martin-Paredo, V., et al.: Risk of renal failure after major angiography, Arch. Surg. 118:1417, 1983.
32. Merren, M.D.: Defending DSA (letter), Vasc. Diagn. Ther. 4:11, March/April 1983.
33. Metz, C.E.: Basic principles of ROC analysis, Semin. Nucl. Med. 8:283, 1978.
34. Mistretta, C.A., et al.: Recent advances in digital radiography, Ann. Radiol. 26:537, 1983.
35. Modic, M.T., et al.: Digital subtraction angiography of the intracranial vascular system: comparative study in 55 patients, AJNR 2:527, 1981.
36. Passariello, R., et al.: Radiation exposure of the patient in conventional and digital intravenous angiography, Ann. Radiol. 26:548, 1983.
37. Pavlicek, W., et al.: Patient doses during digital subtraction angiography of the carotid arteries: comparison with conventional angiography, Radiology 145:683, 1982.
38. Persson, A.V.: Will intravenous digital angiography provide new clinical information (editorial), Vasc. Diagn. Ther. 3:5, October/November 1982.
39. Persson, A.V.: Reply to Merren, M.D.: Defending DSA (letter), Vasc. Diagn. Ther. 4:11, March/April 1983.
40. Raines, J.K.: Effect of DVI arteriography on the noninvasive vascular laboratory, Proceedings of the eighteenth meeting of AAMI, Arlington, Va., 1983.
41. Riederer, S.J., and Kruger, R.A.: Intravenous digital subtraction: a summary of recent developments, Radiology 147:633, 1983.

42. Roederer, G.O., et al.: Ultrasonic Duplex scanning of extracranial carotid arteries: improved accuracy using new features from the common carotid artery, J. Cardiovasc. Ultrasonography 1:373, 1982.

43. Robillard, P., et al.: Digital angiography: current status, J. Can. Assoc. Radiol. 34:95, 1983.

44. Russell, J.B., et al.: Digital subtraction angiography for evaluation of extracranial carotid occlusive disease: comparison with conventional arteriography, Surgery 94:604, 1983.

45. Shehadi, W.H., and Toniolo, G.: Adverse reactions to contrast media, Radiology 137:299, 1980.

46. Sumner, D.S.: Noninvasive method for preoperative assessment of carotid occlusive disease. I. Statistical interpretation of test results, Vasc. Diagn. Ther. 2:41, June/July 1981.

47. Sumner, D.S., Russell, J.B., and Miles, R.D.: Are noninvasive tests sufficiently accurate to identify patients in need of carotid arteriography? Surgery 91:700, 1982.

48. Sundberg, J.: Localization of atheromatosis and calcification in the carotid bifurcation: a post mortem radiographic investigation, Acta Radiol. 22:521, 1981.

49. Thiele, B.L.: Arteriography, applications and pitfalls. Extracranial arterial disease: pathophysiology, diagnosis, treatment, and natural history. Paper presented at symposium, Hilton Head, S.C., April 26, 1984.

50. Turnipseed, W.D., et al.: A comparison of standard cerebral arteriography with noninvasive Doppler imaging and intravenous angiography, Arch. Surg. 117:419, 1982.

51. Turski, P.A., et al.: Limitations of intravenous digital subtraction angiography, AJNR 4:271, 1983.

52. Wilms, G., et al.: Digital intravenous and intraarterial subtraction angiography. Applications to the intracranial vascular system, Fortschr. Röntgenstr. 138:140, 1983.

53. Wood, G.W., et al.: Digital subtraction angiography with intravenous injection: assessment of 1,000 carotid bifurcations, AJNR 4:125, 1983.

CHAPTER 41

Other noninvasive techniques in cerebrovascular disease

ROBERT W. BARNES

Currently the most frequently used noninvasive screening techniques in cerebrovascular disease include periorbital Doppler ultrasound; ocular plethysmography, with or without carotid phonangiography; and carotid ultrasonic arteriography, with or without flow analysis. Several other noninvasive techniques have been developed to detect cerebrovascular lesions, particularly in the extracranial carotid arteries. Although some of these techniques have limited accuracy and clinical application, others have proved to be as reliable as some of the more commonly employed methods. The techniques to be described can be classified as indirect or direct methods. Most *indirect* techniques assess alterations in pressure or flow in the ophthalmic artery or its periorbital branches; these techniques include supraorbital photoplethysmography, carotid compression tonography, ophthalmodynamometry, pneumatic tonometry, and facial thermography. In addition, measurement of regional cerebral blood flow has occasionally been used to infer extracranial carotid occlusive disease. The *direct* techniques assess carotid morphology and include radionuclide arteriography or carotid scanning and computerized tomography. In this chapter are reviewed the techniques and results of these indirect and direct carotid screening methods.

INDIRECT TECHNIQUES
Supraorbital photoplethysmography

Technique. The photoelectric plethysmograph was originally described by Hertzman.[16] The use of the photoplethysmograph (PPG) to screen for extracranial carotid occlusive disease was independently described by Howell,[18] Fuster et al.,[12] and Heck and Price.[15] Original photoelectric transduc-

ers contained an incandescent light source, which was beamed into the superficial layers of the skin. Light reflected from the skin was received by a photoelectric cell. The amount of backscattered light varied with the amount of blood in the superficial circulation of the skin. A voltage output of the photoelectric cell permitted recording of pulsatile fluctuations in microcirculation of the skin. The incandescent light absorption by blood was somewhat influenced by the saturation of hemoglobulin, and the light source potentially provided a heating effect on the superficial layers of the skin. Recent refinements in transducer design have led to an infrared light–emitting diode and adjacent phototransistor*; this device is not affected by hemoglobin saturation and does not result in heating of the skin. It was used in a prospective study of patients undergoing contrast arteriography for suspected cerebrovascular disease.[2,3]

Two PPG transducers are applied above the medial aspect of each eyebrow by using clear two-faced plastic tape. The transducers are connected to a two-channel recorder to permit continuous recording of supraorbital pulse amplitude. The supraorbital region of the forehead is normally supplied by the frontal and supraorbital arteries, which are terminal branches of the ophthalmic artery. While recording bilateral supraorbital pulsations, the technologist sequentially compresses the branches of each external carotid artery (superficial temporal, infraorbital, and facial arteries) and then each common carotid artery in turn. Carotid compression is carried out low in the neck to avoid stimulation of baroreceptors and to prevent dis-

*Medsonics, Mountain View, Calif.

lodgement of emboli from a diseased carotid bifurcation. Several thousand common carotid compressions have been carried out without a single instance of stroke or cardiac arrest.

Normally the supraorbital pulse amplitude is not significantly diminished by compression of external carotid artery branches. Occasionally a slight reduction in pulse amplitude occurs, but the diminution should be by no more than 33% below the resting pulse amplitude. Greater attenuation of supraorbital pulsation in response to compression of a branch of the external carotid artery suggests a possible significant stenosis (greater than 50% diameter reduction) or occlusion of the extracranial internal carotid artery. Normally supraorbital pulse amplitude is diminished only by compression of the ipsilateral common carotid artery. In the presence of significant carotid occlusive disease, intracranial collateral circulation may be inferred if ipsilateral common carotid compression fails to attentuate the supraorbital pulse. Collateral circulation from the contralateral carotid artery via the circle of Willis may be documented if contralateral carotid compression results in diminution of supraorbital pulsation. If sequential compression of each common carotid artery fails to alter supraorbital pulsation, intracranial collateral via the vertebrobasilar system is inferred.

Results. The accuracy of supraorbital PPG studies was established in a prospective screening of 78 consecutive patients undergoing contrast arteriography for suspected cerebrovascular disease. The PPG examination yielded abnormal results in all 20 occluded internal carotid arteries and all 16 vessels with significant (greater than 50%) stenosis. As expected, only 10 of 44 vessels with less than 50% stenosis were associated with abnormal PPG findings. Results were false positive in 8 (11%) of 76 arteries that were normal by contrast arteriography. When compared with the results of periorbital Doppler ultrasound in this group of patients,[2] the supraorbital PPG proved to be more sensitive (100% vs. 94%) but less specific (89% vs. 96%). When the two techniques were used in combination and the results were in agreement, the sensitivity was 100% in detecting significant carotid stenosis or occlusion and the specificity was 97% in arteries that were angiographically normal; however, the techniques rarely detected nonobstructive carotid stenosis (less than 50%).

Supraorbital PPG provides simple, rapid, and objective hard-copy data about both internal carotid

systems simultaneously. The technique is not influenced by the presence of bilateral carotid disease of balanced severity. The technique does not require ocular anesthesia. The greatest limitation of the method is the frequent false positive result; thus an abnormal study also should be investigated by some other noninvasive technique, such as periorbital Doppler ultrasound, to rule out a false positive result. However, the simplicity of the method and its high sensitivity to hemodynamically significant disease makes the method useful for screening large numbers of asymptomatic patients who may be at risk for harboring carotid occlusive disease. Currently such an application of this instrument is being used to screen all patients undergoing coronary artery bypass surgery or major peripheral vascular reconstruction at our institution. A normal study virtually excludes the risk of severe carotid occlusive disease, although abnormal results require clarification by another noninvasive method. Supraorbital PPG has also been useful for continual monitoring of ophthalmic artery flow dynamics during carotid endarterectomy.[13] The ratio of supraorbital pulse amplitude during and prior to carotid clamping correlates well with the carotid back (stump) pressure (r = 0.87, p < .001). The supraorbital PPG monitor permits assessment of adequacy of blood flow through the carotid shunt as well as the integrity of the carotid endarterectomy after closure of the arteriotomy.

Carotid compression tonography

Technique. Carotid compression tonography records volume adjustments within the eye in association with carotid compression. The technique was originally described by Barrios and Solis.[4] An electronic recording tonometer (Mueller*) permits recording of ocular pulse and pressure level on a standard recorder. Once the tracing is stabilized, sequential compression of the ipsilateral and the contralateral carotid artery is performed. The test is repeated while recording tracings from the opposite eye. The three parameters used to interpret the tests include comparison of the pulse amplitudes between each eye, determination of the slope of recovery of ocular pressure on release of carotid compression, and assessment of intraocular pressure responses to compression of the contralateral carotid artery. Normally, ipsilateral carotid compression results in a rapid fall in intraocular pres-

*V. Mueller and Co., Chicago, Ill.

sure, which recovers rapidly on release of carotid compression. Also normally, intraocular pressure is not affected by compression of the contralateral carotid artery. In the presence of hemodynamically significant obstruction of the extracranial internal carotid artery the ocular pulse amplitude may be diminished, the recovery time for return of intraocular pressure to the baseline is delayed, and the intraocular pressure may diminish on compression of the contralateral carotid artery.

Results. Cohen et al.[8] reported the results of carotid compression tonography in 122 patients who underwent contrast arteriography for suspected cerebrovascular disease. The sensitivity of the test in detecting hemodynamically significant stenosis or occlusion of the internal carotid artery was 92% in a group of 82 patients with greater than 50% stenosis or occlusion of the artery on arteriogram. In 40 patients with insignificant or no demonstrable abnormality on carotid arteriogram, carotid compression tomography was normal in 75%. This test seems to share many of the attributes of supraorbital PPG, particularly in being fairly sensitive but somewhat nonspecific. The technique is objective and relatively inexpensive. The method, like other noninvasive techniques, is insensitive to nonobstructive carotid occlusive disease of less than 50% diameter reduction.

Ophthalmodynamometry

Technique. As originally described by Bailliart,[1] ophthalmodynamometry (ODM) involves measurement of the gram force applied to the eye to obliterate arterial pulsations in the branches of the retinal artery (systolic pressure) or to create maximal pulsation in these vessels (diastolic pressure). The vessels are observed through an ophthalmoscope, and the gram force applied by the foot plate of the ophthalmodynamometer is read from the scale on the instrument.

Results. ODM has been widely used by ophthalmologists, but the results have been less accurate than with other newer noninvasive screening techniques. In a study of 45 patients by Kobayashi et al.,[22] a significant difference in retinal artery pressure between the two eyes was seen in only 74% of patients with at least one severely stenotic carotid artery. Even in the patients with minimal disease of the opposite vessel, only 80% showed significant asymmetry of the retinal artery pressure. The presence of severe bilateral carotid occlusive disease resulted in significant differences in retinal artery

pressure in only 55% of patients studied. From these data ODM would appear to be a less accurate screening technique than other periorbital or direct carotid methods.

Pneumatic tonometry

Technique. Pneumatic tonometry,[23] or oculocerebrovasculometry (OCVM), combines a pneumatic applanation tonometer with a vacuum system for increasing intraocular pressure to measure the ophthalmic artery pressure more directly than with oculopneumoplethysmography of Gee (OPG-Gee). The pressure at which ocular pulsations cease during progressive increase in intraocular pressure induced by incremental increases in vacuum applied to the sclera is graphically and digitally recorded as the intraocular pressure. The device also permits comparison of the amplitude of each ocular pulse.

Results. Langham et al.[23] determined that ophthalmic artery systolic pressures in normal control subjects averaged 89.0 ± 2.1 mm Hg, which was 66% ± 1% of the brachial arterial systolic pressure (a value similar to that measured by OPG-Gee). In 20 patients with ≥95% stenosis of the internal carotid artery documented by arteriography, mean ophthalmic artery pressure was 49.9 ± 4.1 mm Hg, which was 33% ± 3% of the brachial systolic pressure. Russell et al.[27] found that OCVM was 100% sensitive but only 36% specific in detecting or excluding ≥50% stenosis of the internal carotid artery in a small series of 19 arteries visualized arteriographically.

Thermography

Technique. Inasmuch as the supraorbital region of the forehead is normally supplied by blood from the internal carotid arteries by ophthalmic artery branches, this area of the face is normally at a slightly higher temperature than other areas. Asymmetric coolness of one supraorbital area may indicate significant obstruction of the ipsilateral internal carotid artery. Although direct temperature measurement using thermistor thermometry is possible,[26] most investigations of supraorbital temperature have involved the use of infrared thermography.[28] In this test the patient is permitted to accommodate to a constant temperature room. The thermograph interrogates the infrared energy emission from the skin of the face. Polaroid photographic recordings of the oscilloscope image represent heat energy as proportional shades of gray. Thermograms may be obtained with the subject at rest or with provocative maneuvers such as forehead cooling or compression of the superficial temporal arteries. Normally the thermal patterns on the forehead are symmetric. Abnormal thermograms are defined as those with temperature asymmetry in the supraorbital region of 0.7° C or greater.

Results. Capistrant and Gumnit[7] reported the accuracy of conventional facial thermography and their results with provocative tests of facial cooling and temporal artery compression in patients undergoing contrast arteriography. With routine thermography the sensitivity of the test was only 57% in 30 patients with carotid occlusive disease. Test results were abnormal in only 5 of 14 patients with carotid stenosis and 12 of 16 with internal carotid occlusion. The specificity was 92%, with five false positive results in 65 patients without significant carotid disease. With the provocative test of superficial temporal artery compression, the sensitivity was increased to 83% of the 30 patients with significant carotid occlusive disease. The specificity was 92% of the 59 patients without significant carotid disease. Addition of a forehead cooling provocative test resulted in a sensitivity of 81% and a specificity of 84%. These results suggest that facial thermography correlates with the presence of carotid occlusive disease, especially when provocative tests are performed, but it does not have the accuracy of some of the other indirect screening techniques and is not economically feasible in mass screening of healthy individuals.

DIRECT TECHNIQUES
Radionuclide arteriography
Technique. Radionuclide angiography provides rapid-sequence dynamic flow imaging of injected isotope before static brain imaging. The radionuclide sodium pertechnetate ^{99m}Tc is rapidly injected intravenously, and serial Polaroid photographs are obtained with a gamma camera positioned over the head and neck of the patient. Sequential dynamic flow images reveal the course of the isotope up the carotid and vertebral arteries and subsequently through the cerebral circulation. Although resolution of vascular defects is not possible with this technique, delay in cerebrovascular flow and maldistribution of flow are recorded.

Results. Radionuclide angiography is a useful adjunct to static brain imaging; however, the limited resolution and relatively low sensitivity make this technique less accurate than other noninvasive screening techniques. The reported sensitivity to

hemodynamically significant extracranial carotid disease averages 60%, with a specificity of approximately 90%.[10,19] With internal carotid occlusion the sensitivity of this test is only about 75%, and with carotid stenosis the sensitivity drops to about 50%. The technique is expensive and should only be considered as an adjunct to brain scanning if the later procedure is indicated in the symptomatic patient.

Radionuclide carotid scanning
Technique. In contrast to dynamic flow scanning, a static carotid scan involves the detection of localized accumulation of isotope-labeled particles, such as fibrinogen or platelets, at areas of thrombosis or ulceration of the cervical carotid artery. A variety of preparations have been employed, including technetium [^{99m}Tc]sulfur colloid albumin aggregates,[25] [^{123}I] or [^{131}I]fibrinogen,[20-24] and technetium [^{99m}Tc] or [^{111}In]-autologous platelets.[9,14] After injection of the radionuclide-labeled particles, the cervical area over the carotid arteries is scanned with a scintillation detector. Sites of increased radioactivity suggest localization of the labeled particles at sites of vascular injury, atherosclerotic ulceration, or carotid thrombosis.

Results. Most studies to date using static radionuclide carotid scanning have involved experimental animals in whom carotid trauma or ulceration has been created. A few clinical studies suggest the potential application of these techniques.[14,24] However, future prospective clinical trials with validation with contrast arteriography or operative carotid endarterectomy will be necessary before the true value of these techniques in humans is established.

Computed tomography
Technique. Computed tomography (CT) involves scanning of a portion of the body with a narrow beam of x rays from different multiple angles at equally spaced intervals. The attenuation of the x-ray beam is measured by photon detectors, and absorption values of tissues are calculated by computer. X-ray absorption coefficients, or densities, are calculated for blocks of tissue and are displayed as a matrix of numerous white, gray, or black picture points on a cathode ray tube.[17] The major impact of CT scanning in assessment of cerebrovascular disease is in its ability to detect intraparenchymal hemorrhage and intracranial lesions that may mimic stroke.[6] Recently the technique has

Table 41-1. Qualitative comparison of noninvasive cerebrovascular techniques

Technique	Simplicity	Portability	Cost	Sensitivity	Specificity
Supraorbital photoplethysmography	+ +	+ +	+	+ +	+
Carotid compression tonography	+ +	+ +	+	+ +	+
Ophthalmodynamometry	+ +	+ +	+ +	0	+ +
Thermography	0	0	0	0	+ +
Radionuclide angiography	0	0	0	0	+ +
Carotid static scans	0	0	0	+	?
Computed tomography	0	0	0	?	?

+ +, Good; +, fair; 0, poor.

been used for direct assessment of the cervical carotid arteries to define carotid calcification in patients with transient ischemic attacks.[11]

Results. Indirect application of CT scanning suggests that in most patients with transient ischemic attacks, study results will be normal and that in patients who have suffered stroke, scans will show abnormal findings in at least 48 hours.[21] In a small series all 17 patients with transient ischemic attack and angiographically abnormal arteries showed carotid calcification on CT scans of the neck.[11] Of three patients with normal arteries, the cervical tomograms showed normal findings; however, further clinical investigation, including the use of CT scans enhanced by injection of contrast medium, will be necessary before the clinical value of this technique is established.

SUMMARY

Most of the noninvasive cerebrovascular screening techniques described demonstrate less overall accuracy than the other indirect and direct carotid screening methods. Exceptions to this are supraorbital PPG and carotid compression tonography, which are quite sensitive to hemodynamically significant carotid occlusive disease. However, both of these techniques are somewhat less specific than other indirect periorbital screening tests. Nevertheless, the simplicity and rapidity of these tests make them useful for mass screening of patients at risk for harboring carotid occlusive lesions. The other techniques are either much less accurate or more expensive and time consuming and have not gained widespread acceptance in diagnosis of cerebrovascular disease. A summary of the qualitative attributes and limitations of these techniques is shown in Table 41-1.

All of these techniques share the same limitations of other noninvasive studies with respect to their role in evaluating patients with symptoms of hemispheric transient ischemic attack or stroke. Because at least 50% of patients with extracranial cerebrovascular disease have nonobstructive plaques or ulcerative lesions that are a source of cerebral emboli, none of the indirect techniques are sensitive to these lesions, which are only reliably assessed by contrast arteriography.[5] Although the direct carotid imaging and flow analysis techniques may eventually improve the detection of such lesions, any patient who has suffered symptoms of hemispheric ischemia deserves contrast arteriography if an operation for a carotid lesion is being considered.

On the other hand, many asymptomatic patients or those with atypical nonlateralizing symptoms are benefitted by a study with noninvasive cerebrovascular techniques. Most of the techniques mentioned are more cumbersome and less accurate than other methods discussed earlier; however, supraorbital PPG and carotid tonography share many of the attributes of more commonly used techniques and should be considered as alternate methods to screen patients with suspected asymptomatic cerebrovascular disease. The tests are also useful to monitor patients in the perioperative period and to longitudinally follow the natural history or the results of medical or surgical therapy of patients with carotid artery disease.

REFERENCES

1. Bailliart, P.: La pression artérielle dans les branches de l'artère centrale de la rétine: nouvelle technique pour la déterminer, Ann. Ocul. (Paris) 154:648, 1917.
2. Barnes, R.W., et al.: Doppler ultrasound and supraorbital photoplethysmography for noninvasive screening of carotid occlusive disease, Am. J. Surg. 134:183, 1977.
3. Barnes, R.W., et al.: Supraorbital photoplethysmography: simple accurate screening for carotid occlusive disease, J. Surg. Res. 22:319, 1977.

4. Barrios, R.R., and Solis, C.: Carotid-compression tono-graphic test: its application in the study of carotid-artery occlusions, Am. J. Ophthalmol 62:116, 1966.

5. Bone, G.E., and Barnes, R.W.: Limitations of the Doppler cerebrovascular examination in hemispheric cerebral ischemia, Surgery 79:577, 1976.

6. Campbell, J.K.: Use of computerized tomography and radionuclide scan in stroke, Stroke 3:11, 1977.

7. Capistrant, T.D., and Gumnit, R.J.: Detecting carotid occlusive disease by thermography, Stroke 4:57, 1973.

8. Cohen, D.N., et al.: Carotid compression tonography, Stroke 6:257, 1975.

9. Davis, H.H., et al.: Scintigraphic detection of atherosclerotic lesions and venous thrombi in man by indium-111-labelled autologous paltelets, Lancet 1(8075):1185, 1978.

10. Foo, D., and Henrickson, L.: Radionuclide cerebral blood flow and carotid angiogram: correlation in internal carotid artery disease, Stroke 8:39, 1977.

11. Frisén, L., et al.: Detection of extracranial carotid stenosis by computed tomography, Lancet 1:1319, 1979.

12. Fuster, B., et al.: Extracranial internal and external carotid territories as mapped by photoelectric plethysmography, Acta Neurol. Lat. Am. 15:1, 1969.

13. Garrett, W.V., Slaymaker, E.E., and Barnes, R.W.: Noninvasive perioperative monitoring of carotid endarterectomy, J. Surg. Res. 26:255, 1979.

14. Grossman, Z.D., et al.: Platelets labeled with oxine complexes of Tc-99m and In-111. II. Localization of experimentally induced vascular lesions, J. Nucl. Med. 19:488, 1978.

15. Heck, A.F., and Price, T.R.: Opacity pulse propagation measurements in humans: atraumatic screening for carotid artery occlusion, Stroke 1:411, 1970.

16. Hertzman, A.B.: Blood supply of various skin areas as estimated by the photoelectric plethysmography, Am. J. Physiol. 124:328, 1938.

17. Hounsfield, G.N.: Computerized transverse axial scanning (tomography). I. Description of system, Br. J. Radiol. 46:1016, 1973.

18. Howell, W.L.: Photosensor monitoring of supraorbital blood flow, Med. Ann. D.C. 36:730, 1967.

19. Jhingran, S.G., and Johnson, P.C.: Radionuclide angiography in the diagnosis of cerebrovascular disease, J. Nucl. Med. 14:265, 1973.

20. Kaufman, H.H., et al.: Radioiodinated fibrinogen for clot detection in a canine model of cervical carotid thrombosis, J. Nucl. Med. 19:370, 1978.

21. Kinkel, W.R., and Jacobs, L.: Computerized axial transverse tomography in cerebrovascular disease, Neurology 26:924, 1976.

22. Kobayashi, S., Hollenhorst, R.W., and Sundt, T.M.: Retinal arterial pressure before and after surgery for carotid artery stenosis, Stroke 2:569, 1971.

23. Langham, M.E., To'mey, K.F., and Preziosi, T.J.: Carotid occlusive disease: effect of complete occlusion of internal carotid artery on intraocular pulse/pressure relation and an ophthalamic arterial pressure, Stroke 12:759, 1981.

24. Mettinger, K.L., et al.: Detection of atherosclerotic plaques in carotid arteries by the use of ^{123}I-fibrinogen, Lancet 1:242, 1978.

25. Pollack, E.W., et al.: Arterial scan versus radiographic angiography in detection of shallow arterial ulcers, Am. Surg. 43:242, 1977.

26. Price, T.R., and Heck, A.F.: Correlation of thermometry and angiography in carotid arterial disease, Arch. Neurol. 26:450, 1972.

27. Russell, J.B., et al.: Oculocerebrovasculometry: a new procedure for the measurement of the ophthalamic artery pressure, Bruit 4:34, 1980.

28. Wood, E.H.: Thermography in the diagnosis of cerebrovascular disease, Radiology 83:540, 1964.

CHAPTER 42

Intraoperative assessment of carotid endarterectomy

RALPH B. DILLEY

Intraoperative assessment of the technical result of carotid endarterectomy is important, primarily because the outcome of the operation depends on a technically perfect procedure; if it is not achieved there is a high risk of a postoperative neurologic event. Although the correlation between a technical defect discovered at the time of operation and postoperative stroke is inferential, Blaisdell et al.[1] uncovered a 25% incidence of technical defects, or thrombosis, when they performed 100 successive operative angiograms after carotid endarterectomy. Although it is not certain that these 25 patients with technical defects would have gone on to have a postoperative stroke, clearly the presence of such an operative defect must be considered an indication for correction. It is also intuitively obvious that discovery of a technical surgical problem in the operating room before skin closure is far preferable to allowing the patient to awaken with a stroke or other neurologic deficit and then have to decide on a course of action. Although many investigators have ascribed most postoperative neurologic deficits to emboli released into the intracerebral circulation during mobilization, it seems likely that technical problems with the operative repair may play a more important role than previously thought.

The second main reason for intraoperative assessment relates to the development of early postoperative re-stenosis, which most often is caused by myointimal hyperplasia. Intraoperative assessment becomes important in ruling out persistent disease (incomplete removal of atheromatous plaque), as differentiated from recurrent disease, so that routine noninvasive follow-up examinations of the operative segment only reflect the development of recurrent stenosis. The incidence of such

recurrences and the problems posed by them are discussed in Chapter 46.

Unfortunately, it is not sufficient to palpate the common, external, and internal carotid arteries to determine whether a postoperative defect is present. Even in cases of significant obstruction, it is rare that a decrease in the amplitude of the pulse will allow this determination to be made. Moreover, it is generally uncommon to feel a thrill in postoperative obstructions.

Current techniques for evaluating the operative segment after closure of the vessel are primarily based on data obtained with intraoperative arteriography, a technique with which there has been considerable experience.[1,2,5] In addition, there is significant recent interest in B-mode real-time imaging at the time of operation, Doppler spectral analysis, or a combination of these techniques (Duplex scanning).

COMPLETION OPERATIVE ARTERIOGRAPHY

Although operative arteriography has been considered a standard technique for assessing the intraoperative result of carotid endarterectomy, it has not been universally accepted for a number of reasons. The technique is cumbersome and requires the presence of an x-ray technician and a portable x-ray unit at the conclusion of the arteriotomy closure. The technician must then return the cassette to a facility that develops the film and return the developed film to the operating room for interpretation by the surgeon. The surgeon must be skilled in timing the exposure to the injected contrast medium and must develop skill in assessing operative arteriograms with respect to intimal flaps, obstruction, and kinks, in both the internal and external carotid arteries. In centers where a significant number of these procedures are performed, there is the risk of exposure of operating room personnel to x rays, and adequate shielding must be provided. In addition, the resultant film views the operative segment in only one plane, and a significant lesion may be missed. Finally, there is always the potential risk of embolism, because contrast material must be injected through a syringe and catheter system into the carotid artery, and of contrast media toxicity, because concentrated dye is injected directly into the cerebral circulation. Despite these limitations, completion angiography remains the most useful in determining the technical adequacies of carotid endarterectomy and, if performed with care, the complications can be minimized.

After the patient has been placed on the operating table and before the operative procedure is started, a scout film should be taken to ensure that no extraneous radiopaque material will interfere with the angiogram and that the x-ray technique is adequate. After the arteriotomy incision has been closed, all clamps and retractors must be removed from the wound so these will not interfere with the subsequent arteriogram. In addition, this allows the artery to return to its normal position in the neck. A 20-gauge needle is attached to a length of intravenous tubing, and a syringe is filled with 60% iothalamate meglumine (Conray 60). Extreme caution must be taken to ensure that the entire system is free of air bubbles, which might be introduced into the artery. Once the injection syringe and associated tubing and needle have been prepared, the x-ray machine is positioned over the operating field and a sterilely draped x-ray shield is provided for the surgeon. An arterial clamp is placed across the common carotid artery at the lower end of the wound, and the needle is introduced into that vessel above the clamp. Again, great care must be taken that no air is present in the system. The volume of injected contrast medium should be approximately 5 to 7 ml, depending on the size of the artery. The x-ray exposure is made as the last bit of material is injected into the artery. The needle should be removed from the artery immediately and the arterial clamp removed. The resultant arteriogram provides detailed anatomic information about the endarterectomized segment and clearly defines obstructions, kinks, residual disease, or elevated intimal flaps at the distal end of the segment. Any such defects should be repaired promptly and the arteriogram repeated.

With careful technique and experience, consis-

tently high-quality arteriograms from which useful information can be derived can be produced. In our institution operative arteriograms have been performed routinely during the last 285 carotid operations, with no obvious complication attributable to the arteriogram. Technical defects, repaired before awakening the patient, occurred in 7% to 8% of the patients, and mild permanent postoperative neurologic deficits occurred in 1.2%. Only one patient has died after carotid endarterectomy, of myocardial infarction on the fourth postoperative day.

B-MODE REAL-TIME IMAGING

With the advance of ultrasonic imaging techniques, it appeared appropriate to apply these devices to intraoperative carotid assessment because it seemed likely they offered an answer to many of the problems inherent with operative arteriography. The experimental basis for this conclusion was developed by Coelho et al.,[3,4] who demonstrated that real-time ultrasonic scanning of exposed vessels in experimental animals could use the sensitive resolution potential of high-frequency scanners. Their studies suggested that flaps as small as 1 mm could be identified in these exposed vessels and that ultrasonography was more sensitive than intraoperative angiography in the detection of intravascular thrombi and diameter reduction.

The technique was extended to the clinical arena by Siegel et al.,[6] who examined 74 carotid arteries after endarterectomy using either a High Stoy 7.5 MHz or a Biosound 12 MHz transducer. Saline solution in the wound provided acoustic coupling, and multiple transverse and longitudinal sections through the vessel were obtained. They were able to demonstrate a 27% incidence of technical abnormalities with this technique. Many of these occurred in the proximal common carotid artery at the site where the obstructing plaque was divided and represented a transition from unendarterectomized to endarterectomized vessel. The significance of this finding is clearly not great, and if the common carotid lesions are excluded, the incidence of significant technical abnormality was 12%. Unfortunately, these studies were not always controlled with intraoperative angiography, so it is uncertain as to how many positive angiograms might have been obtained. In addition, criteria for arterial reexploration were not developed in this study.

Our own experience with B-mode real-time imaging in the operating room includes approximately 60 patients and seven different commercially available B-mode real-time imagers. In addition, a variety of transducers were used, and a significant amount of time was required to learn these techniques in the operating room. In only 26 patients was the quality of the study sufficiently good to allow detailed analysis in comparison with intraoperative angiography. Table 42-1 compares real-time postoperative imaging with postoperative angiography in assessing the upper end of the endarterectomy in the internal carotid artery. In 21 of 26 patients both postoperative angiography and

Table 42-1. Intraoperative assessment of internal carotid artery

	Postoperative real-time imaging		
	Normal	Abnormal	Total
Postoperative angiography			
Normal	21	1	22
Abnormal	1	3	4
TOTAL	22	4	26

postoperative real-time imaging yielded normal results. In one patient the angiogram showed normal findings and the imaging technique demonstrated a significant lesion, and in one patient the angiogram showed an abnormality and the imaging technique gave normal results. In three patients both techniques demonstrated significant technical problems. Fig. 42-1 demonstrates an abnormal obstruction of the internal carotid artery at at the upper end of the endarterectomy and the corresponding postoperative image in the transverse plane demonstrating the same lesion. The vessel above and below this obstruction was entirely normal by B-mode imaging (Fig. 42-2). Fig. 42-3 demonstrates an acceptable intraoperative arteriogram and an associated intraoperative B-mode image in the longitudinal plane, which clearly demonstrates an intimal flap. On the basis of this the artery was reexplored and the intimal flap was confirmed and corrected. Table 42-2 details our experience with 26 external carotid artery end points and demonstrates that all angiographic abnormalities were confirmed by real-time imaging. Fig. 42-4 dem-

A

B

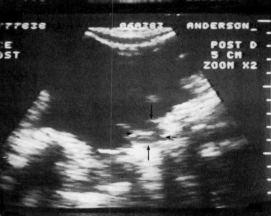

Fig. 42-1. A, Intraoperative arteriogram demonstrates high kink and obstruction at site where endarterectomy ends. **B,** B-mode real-time image of internal carotid artery at same site as in A. Arrows indicate obstructed artery.

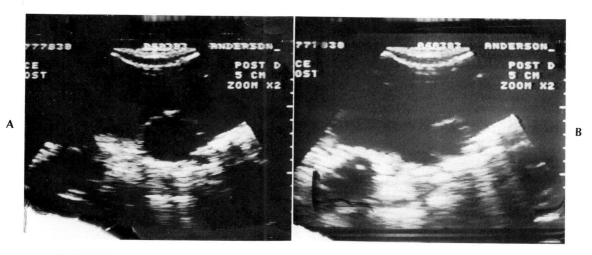

Fig. 42-2. In same patient as in Fig. 42-1, B-mode real-time image of internal carotid artery below *(A)* and above *(B)* site of obstruction.

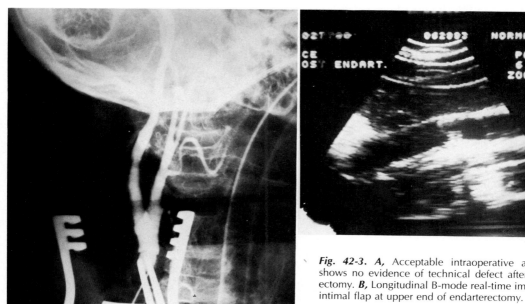

Fig. 42-3. *A,* Acceptable intraoperative arteriogram shows no evidence of technical defect after endarterectomy. *B,* Longitudinal B-mode real-time image shows intimal flap at upper end of endarterectomy.

Table 42-2. Intraoperative assessment of external carotid artery

	Postoperative real-time imaging		
	Normal	Abnormal	Total
Postoperative angiography			
Normal	22	0	22
Abnormal	0	4	4
TOTAL	22	4	26

onstrates an external carotid arteriogram (associated with a total chronic internal carotid artery occlusion) with an intimal flap at the upper end of the endarterectomy site. Fig. 42-5 demonstrates the external carotid artery in transverse section by real-time imaging just proximal to the intimal flap and then at the intimal flap.

Although the B-mode real-time images have been accurate in a small number of cases in picking up technical defects at the conclusion of carotid

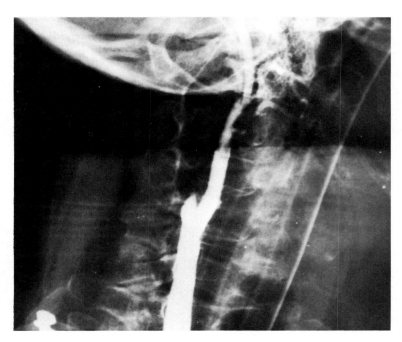

Fig. 42-4. Postendarterectomy intraoperative arteriogram shows nonobstructive high external carotid intimal flap.

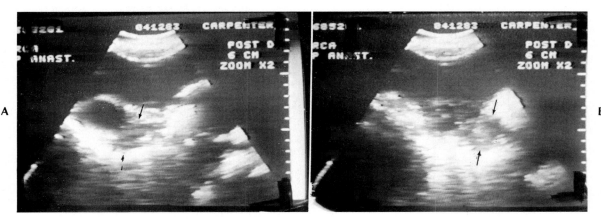

Fig. 42-5. B-mode real-time image of same external carotid artery shown in Fig. 42-4, after endarterectomy below *(A)* and at site of obstruction *(B)*. Arrows show adjacent totally occluded internal carotid artery.

endarterectomy, significant problems remain. Transducer configuration is a major problem in that many commercial products are large, bulky, and difficult to position over the carotid artery. Because many sites to be examined are high on the internal carotid artery, it can be difficult to direct the transducer because of the limited space between the styloid process and the ramus of the mandible. Unfortunately, this is the most difficult area to examine with currently available transducers. Further, many of the transducer systems cannot be sterilized and require cumbersome draping techniques at the time of operation, which is time consuming and increases the potential for contamination. This problem clearly needs to be addressed. In addition, a significant learning period is required to produce accurate images and to interpret the findings. The images obtained with some units have a significant number of artifacts and make it difficult to develop criteria on which to base the decision for reexploration. However, these problems appear solvable, and clearly, real-time B-mode imaging has the potential to replace angiography because there is no radiation exposure and no risk of air embolism, images are instantly available, and repeat studies may be performed without risk to the patient or the surgeon.

PULSED DOPPLER REAL-TIME SPECTRAL ANALYSIS

In addition to B-mode imaging, pulsed Doppler velocity tracings with spectral analysis have been used for intraoperative assessment of arterial reconstruction in the carotid area. Zierler et al.[7] have used a direction-sensitive 20 MHz pulse Doppler velocity meter with a sterilizable probe mounted on a 16-gauge needle. Fig. 42-6 illustrates the carotid artery bifurcation after endarterectomy and how the probe is positioned to sample velocity patterns at points within the arterial lumen (1.3 to 11.5 mm from the end of the probe). The criteria for flow disturbance include estimation of peak systolic frequency up to 16 KHz for mild or moderate flow disturbances, with the addition of minimal spectral broadening for mild flow disturbances and spectral broadening throughout systole for moderate flow disturbances. Severe flow disturbances are characterized by peak systolic frequencies above 16 KHz and spectral broadening throughout most of systole. Zierler studied 50 patients, all of whom underwent completion operative angiography to confirm the operative findings. A significant number of patients had mild flow disturbances after endarterectomy, even with normal findings on operative angiograms, which suggests that the oper-

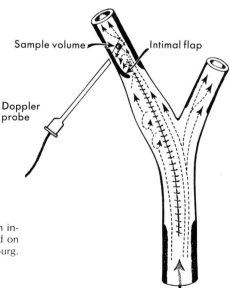

Fig. 42-6. Postendarterectomy carotid bifurcation with intimal flap in internal carotid artery. Small (20 MHz) ultrasonic transducer mounted on 16-gauge needle samples velocity patterns. (From Zierler, R.E.: Vasc. Surg. 1:73, 1984.)

ation itself produces these abnormal changes. Although the data obtained from such studies are objective and assess physiologic variables, the criteria between mild, moderate, and severe flow disturbances are close and appear to be useful only insofar as they suggest the need for an operative arteriogram. They do not appear to be specific enough to develop criteria for reexploration of the operative segment without additional anatomic information.

Consequently, to make decisions about reopening the vessel, one would have to add to pulsed Doppler ultrasound either real-time B-mode imaging or an operative arteriogram for anatomic information on which to base criteria for reexploration of the operative segment. The combination of these modalities might prove more cumbersome for the surgeon and more difficult to interpret in the short time available than operative arteriograms, and it is not yet clear that these multiple evaluations will be the simplest or most sensitive approach to the problem.

CONCLUSIONS

A need exists for a simple, direct method of evaluating the technical results of carotid endarterectomy. Although this classically has been done by completion operative arteriograms, vascular surgeons have not universally accepted this approach because of the inherent disadvantages of the tech-

nique. B-mode real-time imaging offers the prospect of a significant advance in this field. The technique should be simple, reproducible, and allow viewing of the reconstructed segment in several planes. Currently a number of commercial units are available for intraoperative B-mode imaging, but in most the probe design makes it difficult to apply the probe to the artery and record adequate images. Many of these problems should be resolved over the next few years so that a simple portable unit that will allow rapid confirmation of a technically perfect result will become available.

REFERENCES

1. Blaisdell, F.W., Lim. Jr., R., and Hall, A.D.: Technical result of carotid endarterectomy: arteriographic assessment, Am. J. Surg. 114:239, 1967.
2. Bowald, S., Eriksson, E., and Faberberg, S.: Intraoperative angiography in arterial surgery, Acta Chir. Scand. 144:463, 1978.
3. Coelho, J.C.U., et al.: Detection of arterial defects by real time ultrasound scanning during vascular surgery: an experimental study, J. Surg. Res. 30:535, 1981.
4. Coelho, J.C.U., et al.: An experimental evaluation of arteriography and imaging ultrasonography in detecting arterial defects at operation, J. Surg. Res. 32:130, 1982.
5. Collins Jr., G.J., et al.: Stroke associated with carotid endarterectomy, Am. J. Surg. 135:221, 1978.
6. Sigel B., et al.: Imaging ultrasound in the intraoperative diagnosis of vascular defects, J. Ultrasound Med. 2:337, 1983.
7. Zierler, R.E., Bandyk, D.F., and Thiele, B.L.: Intraoperative assessment of carotid endarterectomy, J. Vasc. Surg. 1:73, 1984.

CHAPTER 43

Cerebral blood flow measurements during carotid endarterectomy

THORALF M. SUNDT, Jr.

In collaboration with W. Richard Marsh, M.D., Robert E. Anderson, Joseph M. Messick, Jr., M.D., and Frank W. Sharbrough, M.D.*

From January 1972 through December 1983, 1772 carotid endarterectomies were performed in patients with carotid ulcerative-stenotic disease on the neurovascular surgical service at the Mayo Clinic. These patients were routinely monitored with intraoperative cerebral blood flow (CBF) measurements and continuous electroencephalograms (EEGs). The EEG was found to be a sensitive monitor of neurologic function. No patients awoke after the operative procedure with a new neurologic deficit not predicted by EEG. The critical CBF (flow required to maintain normal EEG findings) varied somewhat with the anesthetic agent but approximated 30% of normal CBF of 50 ml/100 g/min. Shunts were usually placed if flow fell below 18 to 20 ml/100 g/min during occlusion for endarterectomy in patients under enflurane or halothane anesthesia and below 15 ml/100 g/min for patients under combined forane-fentanyl anesthesia.

Patients were categorized into four groups before surgery according to medical, neurologic, and angiographically determined risk factors. Baseline and occlusion CBF values were significantly lower in the highest risk group in comparison to similar measurements in the lowest risk group. Occlusion flow rate <10 ml/100 g/min was recorded in 8% of patients with grade 1 risk, 15% with grade 2, 19% with grade 3, and 28% with grade 4. Shunts were used in approximately 41% of the patients. This varied slightly according to the anesthetic agent used: halothane in 41%, enflurane in 45%, and forane in 28%. Occlusion flow rate below the

*Mayo Clinic and Medical School, Rochester, Minn.

critical level was found in 24.9% of all patients (0 to 4 ml/100 g/min in 3%, 5 to 9 ml/100 g/min in 7%, and 10 to 14 ml/100 g/min in 14%). In an additional 15% of patients with borderline flow rates (15 to 20 ml/100 g/min) shunts often were used, some of these because of a preexisting EEG abnormality related to a preoperative infarct. Shunts were required in 54% of patients who were neurologically unstable before surgery but in only 29% of patients who were neurologically stable before the operation. Saphenous vein patch grafts were used in more than 90% of the operative procedures. In this chapter is described the use of intraoperative CBF measurements in carotid artery surgery.

Intraoperative monitoring techniques were adopted more than 12 years ago after the results of endarterectomy without monitoring were analyzed and found to be unacceptable. At that time our overall morbidity-mortality was less than 5% but was associated with a group of patients at lower risk than are currently undergoing surgery at this institution. Although the arterial procedure itself seldom took longer than 15 to 20 minutes, a number of patients awoke after surgery with either a major or minor neurologic deficit, some transient, others permanent. Although ever cognizant of the risk of intraoperative embolization, we did not feel that these deficits were attributable to that cause. Furthermore, a postoperative internal carotid artery occlusion rate approaching 3% was documented in more than 100 patients operated on without patch grafting (the identification of the occlusion in two patients by a reduction in the postoperative retinal artery pressure measurement led to prompt reconstruction of the endarterectomy with patch grafting before the development of a neurologic deficit). An agonizing reappraisal led to the decision to perform a more meticulous endarterectomy and to patch graft routinely. Coupled with this approach was the need to provide cerebral protection by indwelling shunts either routinely or selectively during the period of carotid occlusion, because the period of occlusion for patch grafting obviously would be longer.

We report the results of the intraoperative correlation of continuous EEGs with intermittent CBF measurements. Results and complications of the operative procedure have been previously reported in detail. Attention is focused on intraoperative complications and those complications following surgery specifically related to the phenomenon of cerebral hyperperfusion.

METHODS

This report includes all patients operated on for carotid stenosis by our neurovascular surgical service between January 1, 1972, and January 1, 1984. Surgery was performed by one of four staff surgeons or by a chief resident with one of those staff surgeons acting as first assistant. Approximately 65% of the operations were performed on the senior author's service. During the entire period of the report, patients were classified into one of four categories on the basis of preoperative risk factors.

Preoperative risk factors

Early in our experience certain preoperative risk factors were correlated with specific types of complications.[34,42] The following represent the major, but by no means the only, considerations in determining the patient's surgical risk:

1. Medical risk factors: presence of symptomatic coronary artery disease (angina pectoris) or myocardial infarction within 6 months of the date of surgery, severe hypertension (blood pressure greater than 180/110), chronic obstructive pulmonary disease, physiologic age more than 70 years, and severe obesity
2. Neurologic risk factors: progressive neurologic deficit, presence of a deficit for less than 24 hours before surgery, frequent daily transient ischemic attacks, or symptoms of generalized (as opposed to focal) cerebral ischemia

3. Angiographically determined risks: coexisting stenosis of the internal carotid artery in the siphon area, extensive involvement of the vessel to be operated on with the plaque extending more than 3 cm distally in the internal carotid artery or 5 cm proximally in the common carotid artery, bifurcation of the carotid artery at the level of the second cervical vertebra in conjunction with a short or thick neck, occlusion of the opposite internal carotid artery, evidence of a soft thrombus extending from the ulcerative lesion or small vessel occlusions from multiple emboli, and a slowed intracranial circulation time on angiography. The degree of stenosis per se was not considered a risk factor.

Classification of patients

On the basis of the foregoing general risk factors it is possible to create a system for grading a patient's potential risk for surgery.[42] Although a given patient does not always fit neatly into a particular group, this system does provide a framework for comparative purposes. The patients were categorized as follows:

Grade 1: neurologically stable (no neurologic risk factors) with no major medical or angiographically determined risks, with unilateral or bilateral ulcerative-stenotic disease.

Grade 2: neurologically stable with no major medical risks but with significant angiographically determined risks.

Grade 3: neurologically stable with major medical risks with or without significant angiographically determined risks.

Grade 4: major neurologic risks with or without associated major medical or angiographically determined risks. Angiograms in this group frequently showed both a slowed flow and multiple small vessel occlusions.

Preoperative evaluation

Before surgery all patients underwent detailed medical and neurologic examination, along with retinal artery pressure (RAP) measurements and oculoplethysmography (OPG). Both the intracranial and extracranial vessels were visualized on cerebral angiography. Digital subtraction angiograms (DSAs) were found useful for postoperative studies and, in fact, became routine, but were seldom accepted for the preoperative evaluation of the disease process.

Intraoperative monitoring

Anesthesia. The anesthetic technique used has been reported previously. The depth of anesthesia was carefully controlled to get a sensitive EEG tracing, and the arterial carbon dioxide tension ($Paco_2$) was held constant to have comparable conditions for the comparison of CBF measurements. There was considerable variation of CBF with the anesthetic agent. The mean ($\pm SD$) baseline $Paco_2$ values were 40 ± 5 torr with halothane, 40 ± 5 torr with enflurane, and 39 ± 3 torr with forane-fentanyl. The mean ($\pm SD$) baseline mean arterial pressure (MAP) determinations were 135 ± 21 torr with halothane, 126 ± 19 torr with enflurane, and 125 ± 35 torr with forane-fentanyl.

Cerebral blood flow measurements. Region CBF measurements were determined from clearance curves obtained from the extracranial detection of intraarterially injected ^{133}Xe. The technique has been described in detail previously.[45] All instruments for recording counts were located in an adjacent monitoring room (Fig. 43-1). No cumbersome equipment was present in the operating suite. The indicator was injected through a No. 27 needle into the common carotid artery with the external carotid artery temporarily occluded. Each injectate contained 200 to 300 μCi^{133} Xe diluted to 0.2 to 0.3 ml total volume with physiologic saline solution. Customarily three measurements were obtained: one before occlusion, one during occlusion, and one after restoration of flow. If a shunt was used, a fourth measurement, and sometimes a fifth, was obtained with the shunt in place.

Operative technique

A saphenous vein patch graft was used routinely except in patients with particularly large vessels. A shunt was always placed when both the EEG and the CBF indicated cerebral ischemia during the period of occlusion and frequently placed if the CBF was marginal, even if the EEG pattern remained unchanged. This latter indication for shunting was particularly important in patients with a preoperative cerebral infarction and abnormal EEG findings, because changes on the EEG are more difficult to identify and because these individuals appear to have a lower tolerance for ischemia. A shunt was never placed until the normal lumen of the vessel was visualized beyond the limits of the plaque. If a temporal artery pulse was not present after flow had been restored, the origin of the external carotid artery was temporarily occluded and

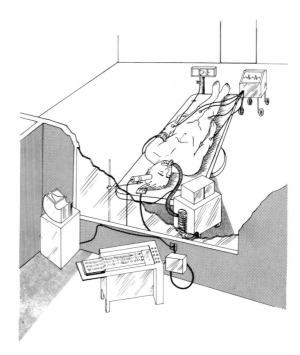

Fig. 43-1. Equipment arranged for simultaneous cerebral blood flow measurements and electroencephalograms during operative procedure. All cumbersome equipment and paraphernalia are housed in adjacent monitoring room so as not to encroach on working space of surgical or anesthesia teams.

the shelf of elevated plaque or intima invariably present at the distal limit of the resection excised through a separate short arteriotomy in that vessel. Routinely, 4000 to 5000 U heparin was given before occlusion of the vessels, and this heparin was not reversed.

Postoperative monitoring

All patients underwent detailed neurologic examination when they awakened from anesthesia. They remained in the intensive care unit for 24 hours, during which time postoperative RAPs and OPGs were obtained. Most patients had postoperative EEG studies, which were usually completed on the sixth or seventh day postoperatively. Currently, patients undergo routine DSA studies on the fifth or sixth day after the operation.

RESULTS
Cerebral blood flow vs. anesthetic agent and patient category

Table 43-1 summarized intraoperative CBF measurements in 1692 patients and correlates these measurements with the anesthetic agent used dur-

Table 43-1. Cerebral blood flow according to anesthetic used and grade of risk

Time of measurement	Grade 1		Grade 2		Grade 3		Grade 4	
	n	$\overline{X} \pm SD$	n	$\overline{X} \pm SD$	n	$\overline{X} \pm SD$	n	$\overline{X} \pm SD$
HALOTHANE								
Baseline	157	62 ± 26	88	57 ± 28	141	51 ± 21	82	48 ± 20
Occlusion	157	34 ± 18	86	31 ± 18	143	27 ± 15	80	24 ± 13
Shunt	43	44 ± 15	41	53 ± 18	65	43 ± 17	47	42 ± 12
Postocclusion	158	69 ± 27	89	68 ± 26	143	62 ± 23	84	61 ± 21
ENFLURANE								
Baseline	313	49 ± 18	189	45 ± 19	204	42 ± 18	145	37 ± 21
Occlusion	311	27 ± 13	188	23 ± 13	200	21 ± 11	143	18 ± 12
Shunt	105	39 ± 15	96	35 ± 11	109	36 ± 13	91	35 ± 14
Postocclusion	317	51 ± 18	192	50 ± 19	211	48 ± 19	155	50 ± 21
FORANE								
Baseline	99	37 ± 15	74	37 ± 17	94	32 ± 13	50	29 ± 17
Occlusion	98	23 ± 10	74	21 ± 12	95	19 ± 9	51	17 ± 9
Shunt	24	26 ± 6	22	33 ± 9	26	27 ± 10	25	31 ± 14
Postocclusion	104	41 ± 18	76	45 ± 18	100	37 ± 15	63	52 ± 16

Table 43-2. Cerebral blood flow vs. EEG during carotid endarterectomy: January 1, 1972, to December 31, 1983

Flow (ml/100 g/min)	No. of patients with change in EEG within 2 min of occlusion			No. of patients without change in EEG within 2 min of occlusion			
	Halothane	Enflurane	Forane	Halothane	Enflurane	Forane	Total
0-4	10	23	14	0	1	1	49
5-9	19	76	18	1	2	8	124
10-14	42	74	17	8	51	37	229
15-19	41	45	9	25	92	53	265
20-24	0	0	1	47	122	74	244
25-29	0	0	0	56	104	34	194
30-99	0	1	0	212	248	59	520
TOTAL	112	219	59	349	602	266	1625

ing the operation and the patient's preoperative risk category. Data in 80 patients are not included because an anesthetic agent other than halothane, enflurane, or forane-fentanyl was used. The discrepancy between the number of patients with postocclusion flow and those with baseline flow relates to technical problems in delivering the indicator to the brain in patients with a very high-grade stenosis (99.9%) or a physiologic occlusion.

There is a statistically significant difference among the baseline flow measurements in comparable grades of risk in patients operated on under these three anesthetic agents. There is also a significant difference between the baseline and occlusion flows in the patients of grade 4 risk compared with those of better risk (grades 1 and 2) operated on under the same anesthetic agent.

Correlation of EEG and CBF measurements

The severity of EEG changes observed with varying degrees of ischemia is illustrated in Fig. 43-2. Table 43-2 summarizes changes seen in the EEG with carotid occlusion according to the anesthetic agent used. It should be noted that in patients with a low CBF shunting often was performed before the development of an EEG change. In such cases the plaque was usually removed from the distal internal carotid artery before placing the shunt so that the period of occlusion before placement of a shunt approximated 2 to 4 minutes.

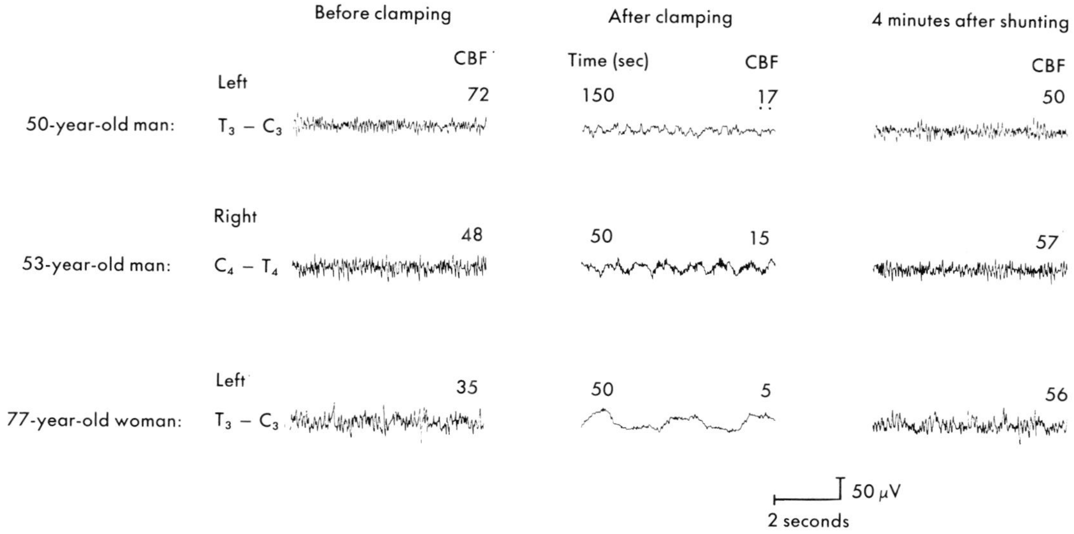

Fig. 43-2. Correlation between electroencephalograms and cerebral blood flow measurements during carotid endarterectomy. Severity of EEG change parallels reduction in cerebral blood flow.

Cerebral blood flow and stump pressure

Stump pressures were measured in 100 consecutive patients to correlate these measurements with the occlusion CBF. These data are summarized in Fig. 43-3.

Embolic complications

Embolic complications during the operation are easily identified by a very dramatic change in the EEG. There were 17 embolic complications during the surgery, for an incidence of about 1%. One half of these led to only a transient EEG change, but one half were associated with a major or minor neurologic deficit.

There were five cases of emboli through a functioning shunt during the operation in this series. Three of these were major events related to proximal atherosclerosis and, in retrospect, might possibly have been avoided with more experience. The other two embolic complications were minor, and the patients regained normal EEG findings before awakening from anesthesia and had normal neurologic function in the recovery room.

There were 12 embolic complications not related to shunts. Of these 11 occurred during the exposure of the vessel (1 with induction of anesthesia), and 1 developed as the patient was awakening from anesthesia. Six of these led to a transient EEG change and 6 to a neurologic complication.

DISCUSSION
Monitoring and shunting during surgery

Between January 1972 and January 1984 we performed 1772 endarterectomies for carotid stenosis using the intraoperative monitoring techniques described. The correlation of CBF measurements with EEGs in these cases has been excellent, as indicated in Table 43-2, which summarizes data from 1628 patients operated on under halothane, enflurane, or forane-fentanyl. Occlusion flow rate was between 0 and 4 ml/100 g/min in 45 patients, between 5 and 9 ml/100 g/min in 121, and between 10 and 14 ml/100 g/min in 235. Using the xenon washout technique, flow less than 5 ml/100 g/min is difficult to quantitate and can be equated with zero flow. Thus we believe that 3% of the patients in our group would definitely have sustained a cerebral infarction without shunting because of inadequate collateral flow. Another 7% to 8%, patients with flow rates between 5 and 9 ml/100 g/min, probably would have sustained an infarction with any prolonged period of occlusion. Patients with flow between 10 and 14 ml/100 g/min, representing 14% of the group, may or may not have withstood the period of ischemia, as discussed later. Shunts were also used in a large number of patients with flows between 15 and 20 ml/100 g/min for fear that the EEG would fail to reveal regions of focal ischemia in the deep white matter

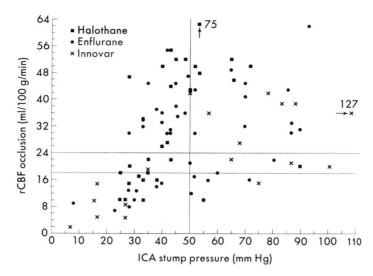

Fig. 43-3. Scattergram of occlusion regional cerebral blood flows *(rCBF)* plotted against internal carotid artery *(ICA)* stump pressures. Vertical line represents stump pressure of 50 torr (considered critical level). Two horizontal lines represent critical flow level (rCBF ≤ 18 ml/100 g/min) and margin zone (rCBF 18 to 24 ml/100 g/min). Regression lines for each anesthetic agent were calculated. Expressed for halothane, $rCBF_{occl} = 0.51$ (stump pressure) ± 9.94, r = 0.43. Expressed for enflurane, $rCBF_{occl} = 0.26$ (stump pressure) ± 16.51, r = 0.39. Expressed for forane = fentanyl $rCBF_{occl} = 0.27$ (stump pressure) ± 0.93, r = 0.68.

or basal ganglia with these borderline flow rates or because of a preoperative region of infarction or ischemia. Occasionally patients with flow rates greater than 20 ml/100 g/min also received shunts if they had a preexisting EEG abnormality related to preoperative infarct, because we have found, as have others, that these patients are particularly vulnerable to marginal flow.* Shunts are usually not inserted until the plaque has been removed from the distal internal carotid artery except in cases in which flow is less than 5 ml/100 g/min or in which there has been a dramatic and catastrophic change in EEG patterns (usually these are simultaneous events—one does not occur without the other).

In a total of 694 of the 1692 endarterectomies performed under these three anesthetic agents cerebral protection was provided by indwelling shunts during the operation. However, there was a statistically significant difference in the frequency of shunt usage according to both the grade of risk and the anesthetic agent used. Thus shunts were placed in 41% and 45% of patients operated on under halothane and enflurane, respectively, compared with only 28% of patients operated on under forane (often supplemented with fentanyl).

*References 9, 17, 18, 24, 34, 48.

There was also a statistically significant difference in blood flow among patients categorized according to the anesthetic agent used. The highest flow rates were seen with halothane and the lowest with forane (supplemented in many cases with fentanyl). An analysis of the data in Table 43-1 shows significant differences in baseline and postocclusion CBF in patients operated on under the three agents studied (p < .001). Halothane was associated with higher flow rates than enflurane, which in turn was associated with higher flow rates than forane. Halothane occlusion and shunt flow rates were also significantly higher when compared with enflurane and forane, but there were less striking differences between the latter agents. The use of fentanyl with forane skews these comparisons.

In comparing CBF according to the grade of patient risk, there were statistically significant differences in the baseline and occlusion flow rates in grade 4 compared with grade 1, with values in the grade 4 patients being lower (p < .001). There were no differences in the postocclusion flow values.

Shunts were required in only 29% of grade 1 candidates for surgery but were required in 54% of patients who were grade 4 candidates for surgery. Furthermore, both the baseline and occlusion flow rates were lower in the patients at higher risk. This leads to the conclusion that the microembolic and hemodynamic theories for transient ischemic attacks and infarctions are not mutually exclusive. Areas of brain functioning on a marginal flow of 40% to 50% of normal are particularly vulnerable to the effects of emboli.

Conversely, Whisnant et al.[51] performed a detailed multivariant analysis of a group of patients with transient ischemic attacks operated on between 1970 and 1974 and found that no patients with high occlusion flow rates had an intraoperative or postoperative stroke. Furthermore, this group had no stroke in 4.5 years of follow-up evaluation, indicating that the prognosis is good in individuals with high collateral flow.

Critical flow and ischemic tolerance

The critical flow rate required to maintain a normal EEG pattern may be higher than that required to maintain basic cell metabolism, so that even with a state of physiologic paralysis cell death is prevented and recovery is possible after a certain latency. We have found some biologic variation in the critical flow required to maintain cell viability. Data from both our studies[43,44] and the studies of Boysen et al.[5] show that the critical flow for the former ranges between 15 and 20 ml/100 g/min, and laboratory studies suggest that the critical flow for the latter in primates is between 10 and 15 ml/100 g/min.[2] It follows that the ischemic tolerance of neural tissue is proportional to both the duration and severity of flow reduction. The precise duration that these reduced flows can be tolerated before cellular injury occurs is unknown.[1,2]

Intraoperative cerebral blood flow measurements using intraarterially injected xenon are a great deal more reliable than blood flow measurements using the inhalation xenon technique in which the true severity of ischemic lesions are not identified. With the intraarterial injection technique a representative amount of indicator arrives in the area predestined for ischemia before occlusion of the vessel, and thus measurements are based on the clearance of indicator from the true region of ischemia.[15] With the systemic administration of xenon, intravenously or by inhalation, artifact in these measurements develops related to ''look-through,'' in which the blood flow probe measures from normally perfused tissue deep to the area of ischemia, because the obstructions to the arterial in-flow prevent the indicator from arriving in the ischemic zone.[15]

CBF measurements in the laboratory animal are difficult because of the small size of the brain studied and the even smaller areas of brain subjected to ischemia. Furthermore, the common laboratory animals—the dog, cat, and rat—have excellent collateral circulations over the cortex, so that areas of ischemia often lie remote from the area of measurement. The primate unfortunately remains the only animal in which CBF measurements comparable to those in the human can be acquired. In these animals it is very difficult to perform accurate measurements of CBF throughout a period of prolonged ischemia and salvage the particular animal for a long-term preparation to determine the ultimate areas of infarction. Thus it is necessary to extrapolate from one study to another and measure blood flow,[15] energy metabolites,[41] and zones of infarction in different preparations[40,49] and then cross correlate the results.

The squirrel monkey makes an excellent model for focal incomplete cerebral ischemia, and our early studies on this subject suggested that the animals could tolerate a 60% to 70% reduction in CBF for approximately 1 hour. This did not exclude microinfarctions, because nonuniform characteristics of flow in areas of incomplete ischemia were readily apparent in the microcirculation.[49] During this time of incomplete ischemia there was a steady decrease in adenosine triphosphate levels and a rise in lactate levels.[41] However, these animals were operated on under barbiturate anesthesia, and at that time we did not understand the protective effects of this agent. Thus this tolerable period of 1 hour might be a good bit shorter in the awake animal; studies by other investigators suggest that this is indeed the case.[11,22]

During the period of these investigations (1965 to 1972) it was our belief that seldom, if ever, would CBF fall below a critical level of cell viability during carotid endarterectomy, because collateral flow from one source or another would be able to sustain a flow of at least 10 to 15 ml/100 g/min, particularly if the patient were protected with an elevated blood pressure. With greater experience we found that this was not the case. In some patients hemispheric blood flow falls to essentially zero with carotid occlusion, approximating quite closely the situation of cardiac arrest or animal decapitation in which both clinical experience and laboratory data[28] suggest that within 4 to 9 minutes of zero flow irreparable brain damage begins to occur.

The laboratory confirmation of the clinical impressions had to await the elegant studies of Symon et al.[1,2,6,7,47] in the Rhesus monkey. This group established that blood flow less than 15 ml/100 g/min results in paralysis of neuronal activity and that flow less than 10 ml/100 g/min results in ionic shifts that may be irreversible if allowed to persist. The true level of tolerance for ischemia in patients with flow between 5 and 10 or 10 and 15 ml/100 g/min is unknown, but recent studies stress the variability and focality of histologic changes in these levels.[7,22] We prefer not to speculate as to how long a particular person can retain physiologic paralysis without developing neuronal damage. There is some recent evidence that incomplete ischemia, which is associated with a greater degree of acidosis than is complete ischemia, because of continued glycolysis, has complications uniquely related to its acidosis.[36]

Skillful general anesthesia

Possibly the most sensitive monitor of neurologic function is the awake patient, and some very experienced surgeons still use this method of monitoring.[20] We prefer general anesthesia, because it is safe in the hands of competent anesthesiologists, protects the patient's airway, facilitates high exposure of distal internal carotid artery lesions, and improves the comfort of both the patient and the surgeon. However, to date, barbiturates are the only anesthetic agents that have unequivocally been proved to protect the brain and improve tissue tolerance to ischemia.[19,25,27,29,30] Our recent experience suggests that the critical flow does seem to be lower with isoflurane but these are only preliminary data. Data from Michenfelder's[26] laboratory suggest that this may be a valid observation.

Short occlusion time

In our judgment, rapid performance of endarterectomy is fraught with hazard. The plaque must be removed meticulously from the vessel, with no lip of intima distally to serve as a source of dissection and no stump of the external carotid artery to serve as a source of emboli. In our experience the best reconstruction of the vessel is achieved with a saphenous vein patch graft, which extends the period of occlusion approximately 15 minutes. The only series of patients operated on without patch angioplasty routinely undergoing postoperative angiograms (by an experienced and respected group) is reported to demonstrate a 20% occlusion rate of the external carotid artery and a 4% occlusion rate of the internal carotid artery.[12]

Hyperperfusion syndromes

Our most common complication after endarterectomy is related to the group of high-risk patients, in which there has been a very marked increase in CBF during the operative procedure.[44] This usually occurs several days after surgery in patients with a low baseline CBF measurement before endarterectomy and a ≥200% increase in flow after endarterectomy. This paralysis of autoregulation leads to an ipsilateral hemispheric hyperperfusion and associated vascular headaches. Fortunately, in most patients this seems to be limited to unilateral headache. However, in some patients it has been associated with paroxysmal lateralizing epileptiform discharges, cerebral hemorrhage, and migraine variants. Most all of these patients, except those with headaches alone, have undergone angiography at the time of the complication, and in none of them have we identified major intracranial vessel occlusion. Hemorrhage into an area of previous infarction is a well-known complication of endarterectomy.[8,53] However, these hyperperfusion syndromes have occurred in patients without a major area of infarction. These complications have only been infrequently reported,[52] leading us to the concern that they might be uniquely related to our policy of not reversing the heparin given at surgery, a policy based on the protective effects of heparin on the thrombogenic surface of a freshly endarterectomized vessel.[13] Alternatively, lacking CBF monitoring, these complications might not be recognized as unique by other groups and attributed to a different mechanism.

Comments

Experience can be defined as a compilation of complications. Experience of most of the outstanding pioneers in this field led them to conclude that routine shunting[10,21,48] or some form of monitoring (awake patient or internal carotid artery back pressure)[17,31] with selective shunting was advisable. It was the experience of these individuals that a number of complications occurred that could not be attributed to embolic events. Those of us who are now second-generation surgeons and who shared the disappointments of their first-generation mentors vividly recall certain types of complications that were frequent enough that they were not anecdotal. One of these, in patients operated on under local anesthesia, was the onset of an acute and profound hemiplegia with carotid occlusion that was irreversible with restoration of flow 20 to 30 minutes thereafter.

There is no room for a cavalier attitude toward carotid endarterectomy. It can be a relatively easy operation or an extremely difficult procedure. In either case, it remains a dangerous operation with intraoperative risks of embolization or infarction from inadequate flow during the period of occlusion and postoperative risks of occlusion or embolization[14,31,32,48] from vessels inadequately reconstructed or from complications of cerebral hyperperfusion following the restoration of a normal perfusion pressure to a vascular bed with paralyzed autoregulation.[44]

Effects of endarterectomy

It is important to note that our measurements were of CBF, not flow through the artery, and were performed under static, controlled conditions. Even in cases in which there was not a major change in CBF,[5] using electromagnetic arterial flow probes along with simultaneous CBF measurements, we found an increase in arterial flow and the contribution to total CBF from the vessel operated on if a high-grade stenosis was present.

The cerebral hemispheric arterial circulation can be divided into two general types of arteries: (1) the conducting vessels, consisting of the internal carotid artery and its major trunks, which divide into a network of interlacing and anastomosing smaller branches on the brain's surface, and (2) the penetrating or nutrient arterioles, which arise on the surface of the brain from the conducting vessels and enter the brain parenchyma.[37] In normal humans there is only a 10% to 15% drop in perfusion pressure between the origin of the internal carotid artery and the penetrating vessels.[3] The conducting vessels can be regarded as a pressure equalization reservoir modulated by the sympathetic nervous system.[16,46] True cerebral autoregulation probably resides in the penetrating arterioles, which apparently are modulated by an intrinsic nervous system taking origin in the brainstem.[4,23,35,38] Those arterioles must be supplied with an adequate perfusion pressure to function normally. The normalization of RAPs after endarterectomy indicates the restoration of a normal perfusion pressure permits the parenchymal arterioles to return to a more normal tone, from one of maximal dilation, and thus the brain's autoregulatory ability is restored.

The microembolic[39,50] and hemodynamic theories[33] for transient ischemic attacks and infarcts are not mutually exclusive. Areas of brain functioning on a marginal flow of 40% to 50% of normal are particularly vulnerable to the effects of emboli. Furthermore, plaque deposits that cause a severe degree of stenosis, which therefore represent a significant hemodynamic lesion, are more likely to develop deep ulcer craters than those of lesser severity.

Thus endarterectomy in a patient with a high-grade stenosis and ulceration (1) removes a source of emboli,[39] (2) restores a normal distal perfusion pressure and the capability for normal autoregulation, (3) increases flow through the artery and, depending on collateral flow, increases CBF, and (4) prevents progression of the stenosis to occlusion.

REFERENCES

1. Astrup, J., Siesjo, B.K., and Symon, L.: Thresholds in cerebral ischemia: the ischemic penumbra, Stroke 12:723, 1981.
2. Astrup, J., et al.: Cortical evoked potential and extracellular K$^+$ and H$^+$ at critical levels of brain ischemia, Stroke 8:51, 1977.
3. Bakay, L., and Sweet, W.H.: Cervical and intracranial intra-arterial pressures with and without vascular occlusion, Surg. Gynecol. Obstet. 95:67, 1952.
4. Bates, D., et al.: The effect of lesions in the locus coeruleus on the physiological responses of the cerebral blood vessels in cats, Brain Res. 136:431, 1977.
5. Boysen, G.: Cerebral hemodynamics in carotid surgery, Acta Neurol. Scand. (suppl.) 52:1, 1973.
6. Branston, N.M., Hope, D.T., and Symon, L.: Barbiturates in focal ischemia of primate cortex: effects of blood flow distribution, evoked potential and extracellular potassium, Stroke 10:647, 1979.
7. Branston, N.M., Strong, A.J., and Symon, L.: Extracellular potassium activity, evoked potential and tissue blood flow: relationship during progressive ischaemia in baboon cerebral cortex, J. Neurol. Sci. 32:305, 1977.
8. Bruetman, M.E., et al.: Cerebral hemorrhage in carotid artery surgery, Arch. Neurol. 9:458, 1963.
9. Callow, A.D., and O'Donnell, T.F.: Electroencephalogram monitoring in cerebrovascular surgery. In Bergan, J.J., and Yao, J.S., editors: Cerebral vascular insufficiency, New York, 1983, Grune & Stratton, pp. 327-341.
10. Crawford, E.S., et al.: Surgical treatment of occlusive cerebrovascular disease, Surg. Clin. North Am. 46:873, 1966.
11. Crowell, R.M., et al.: Temporary occlusion of the middle cerebral artery in the monkey: clinical and pathological observations, Stroke 1:439, 1970.
12. Diaz, F.G., et al.: Early angiographic changes after carotid endarterectomy, Neurosurgery 10:151, 1982.
13. Dirrenberger, R.A., and Sundt, T.M., Jr.: Carotid endarterectomy: temporal profile of the healing process and effects of anticoagulation therapy, J. Neurosurg. 48:201, 1978.

14. Giannotta, S.L., Dicks, R.E., and Kindt, G.W.: Carotid endarterectomy: technical improvements, Neurosurgery 7:309, 1980.

15. Hanson, E.J., Jr., Anderson, R.E., and Sundt, T.M., Jr.: Comparison of [85]krypton and [133]xenon cerebral blood flow measurements before, during, and following focal incomplete ischemia in the squirrel monkey, Circ. Res. 36:18, 1975.

16. Harper, A.M., et al.: The influence of sympathetic nervous activity on cerebral blood flow, Arch. Neurol. 27:1, 1972.

17. Hays, R.J., Levinson, S.A., and Wylie, E.J.: Intraoperative measurement of carotid back pressure as a guide to operative management of carotid endarterectomy, Surgery 72:953, 1972.

18. Hertzer, N.R., et al.: Internal carotid back pressure, intraoperative shunting, ulcerated atheromata, and the incidence of stroke during carotid endarterectomy, Surgery 83:306, 1978.

19. Hoff, J.T., et al.: Barbiturate protection from cerebral infarction in primates, Stroke 6:28, 1975.

20. Imparato, A.M., et al.: Cerebral protection in carotid surgery, Arch. Surg. 117:1073, 1982.

21. Javid, H., et al.: Seventeen-year experience with routine shunting in carotid artery surgery, World J. Surg. 3:167, 1979.

22. Jones, T.H., et al.: Thresholds of focal cerebral ischemia in awake monkeys, J. Neurosurg. 54:773, 1981.

23. Langfitt, T.W., and Kassell, N.F.: Cerebral vasodilatation produced by brain-stem stimulation: neurogenic control vs. autoregulation, Am. J. Physiol. 215:90, 1968.

24. Matsumoto, G.H., et al.: EEG surveillance as a means of extending operability in high risk carotid endarterectomy, Stroke 7:554, 1976.

25. Michenfelder, J.D.: The interdependency of cerebral functional and metabolic effects following massive doses of thiopental in the dog, Anesthesiology 41:231, 1974.

26. Michenfelder, J.D.: Personal communication, 1982.

27. Michenfelder, J.D.: Cerebral protection by barbiturate anesthesia: use after middle cerebral artery occlusion in Java monkeys, Arch. Neurol. 33:345, 1976.

28. Michenfelder, J.D., and Theye, R.A.: The effects of anesthesia and hypothermia on canine cerebral ATP and lactate during anoxia produced by decapitation, Anesthesiology 33:430, 1970.

29. Michenfelder, J.D., and Theye, R.A.: Effects of fentanyl, droperidol, and innovar on canine cerebral metabolism and blood flow, Br. J. Anaesth. 43:603, 1971.

30. Michenfelder, J.D., and Theye, R.A.: Cerebral protection by thiopental during hypoxia, Anesthesiology 39:510, 1973.

31. Murphey, F., and Maccubbin, D.A.: Carotid endarterectomy: a long-term follow-up study, J. Neurosurg. 23:156, 1965.

32. Perdue, G.D.: Management of post-endarterectomy neurologic deficits, Arch. Surg. 117:1079, 1982.

33. Pessin, M.S., et al.: Mechanisms of acute carotid stroke, Ann. Neurol. 6:145, 1979.

34. Phillips, M.R., et al.: Carotid endarterectomy in the presence of contralateral carotid occlusion: the role of EEG and intraluminal shunting, Arch. Surg. 114:1232, 1979.

35. Raichle, M.E., et al.: Central noradrenergic regulation of cerebral blood flow and vascular permeability, Proc. Natl. Acad. Sci. USA 72:3726, 1975.

36. Rehncrona, S., Rosen, I., and Siesjö, B.K.: Brian lactic acidosis and ischemic cell damage: biochemistry and neurophysiology, J. Cereb. Blood Flow Metab. 1:297, 1981.

37. Saunders, R.L., and Bell, M.A.: X-ray microscopy and histochemistry of the human cerebral blood vessels, J. Neurosurg. 35:128, 1971.

38. Sahlit, N.M., et al.: Carbon dioxide and cerebral circulatory control. III. The effects of brainstem lesions, Arch. Neurol. 17:342, 1967.

39. Siekert, R.G., Whisnant, J.P., and Millikan, C.H.: Surgical and anticoagulant therapy of occlusive cerebral vascular disease, Ann. Intern. Med. 48:637, 1963.

40. Sundt, T.M., Jr., Grant, W.C., and Garcia, J.H.: Restoration of middle cerebral artery flow in experimental infarction, J. Neurosurg. 31:311, 1969.

41. Sundt, T.M., Jr., and Michenfelder, J.D.: Focal transient cerebral ischemia in the squirrel monkey: effect on brain adenosine triphosphate and lactate levels with electrocorticographic and pathologic correlation, Circ. Res. 30:703, 1972.

42. Sundt, T.M., Jr., Sandok, B.A., and Whisnant, J.P.: Carotid endarterectomy: complications and preoperative assessment of risk, Mayo Clin. Proc. 50:301, 1975.

43. Sundt, T.M., Jr.: Cerebral blood flow measurements and electroencephalograms during carotid endarterectomy, J. Neurosurg. 41:310, 1974.

44. Sundt, T.M., Jr., et al.: Correlation of cerebral blood flow and electroencephalographic changes during carotid endarterectomy, Mayo Clin. Proc. 56:533, 1981.

45. Sundt, T.M., Jr., et al.: Monitoring techniques for carotid endarterectomy, Clin. Neurosurg. 22:199, 1975.

46. Symon, L.: A comparative study of middle cerebral pressure in dogs and macaques, J. Physiol. (Lond.) 19:449, 1967.

47. Symon, L.: The relationship between CBF, evoked potentials and the clinical features in cerebral ischaemia. Proceedings of the twenty-third Scandinavian Neurological Congress Acta Neurol. Scand. (suppl. 78) 62:175, 1980.

48. Thompson, J.E.: Complications of carotid endarterectomy and their prevention, World J. Surg. 3:155, 1979.

49. Waltz, A.G., and Sundt, T.M., Jr.: The microvasculature and microcirculation of the cerebral cortex after arterial occlusion, Brain 90:681, 1967.

50. Whisnant, J.P., et al.: Effect of anticoagulants on experimental cerebral infarction, Circulation 20:56, 1959.

51. Whisnant, J.P., Sandok, B.A., and Sundt, T.M., Jr.: Carotid endarterectomy for unilateral carotid system transient cerebral ischemia, Mayo Clin. Proc. 58:171, 1983.

52. Wilkinson, J.T., Adams, H.P., Jr., and Wright, C.B.: Convulsions after carotid endarterectomy, JAMA 244:1827, 1980.

53. Wylie, E.J., Heim, M.F., and Adams, J.R.: Intracranial hemorrhage following surgical revascularization for treatment of acute stroke, J. Neurosurg. 21:212, 1964.

CHAPTER 44

Evolution of carotid arterial disease in asymptomatic patients with bruits

GHISLAINE O. ROEDERER, YVES E. LANGLOIS, and D. EUGENE STRANDNESS, Jr.

The link that exists between atherosclerotic lesions in the extracranial vessels and symptoms of cerebrovascular insufficiency is well known. In a previous report Hass et al.[9] stated that 74% of patients with cerebrovascular insufficiency have at least one significant lesion at a surgically accessible site in the neck. In patients with localized neurologic symptoms, surgical removal of the obstructing atheroma has proved to be very effective in relieving symptoms and reducing the incidence of subsequent stroke.[2,5,18,20,23] On the other hand, there is a lack of convincing evidence to support the role of prophylactic carotid endarterectomy in asymptomatic patients with a cervical bruit and an internal carotid artery lesion. With wider application of noninvasive testing, more carotid lesions are being discovered, creating a difficult dilemma for physicians confronted with this problem. Although there appears to be no doubt that some patients with carotid artery disease will benefit from carotid endarterectomy, much needs to be learned regarding the selection of such patients. The information concerning this issue remains incomplete.

Over the past several years a great deal of interest has been paid to the finding of a bruit over the middle portion of the neck as a possible indication of carotid artery disease. However, in the attempt to evaluate carotid bifurcation disease by the presence of a bruit alone, it must be remembered that all bruits are not necessarily associated with significant internal carotid atherosclerosis.[4,14,24] In our laboratory more than half of the internal carotid arteries on the side of a cervical bruit were reduced

by less than 50% of their original diameter. Similarly, very severe lesions or occlusions may not be associated with a cervical bruit. Despite these facts, auscultation of the neck in search of a carotid bruit remains an important aspect of the physical examination and should be done in all patients with symptoms of cerebrovascular insufficiency, all patients older than 40 years, those who show evidence of atherosclerotic disease elsewhere in the body.

The attention paid to the finding of a bruit over the midportion of the neck has become greater since a report by Thompson et al.,[19] who noted a significant incidence of transient ischemic attack (TIA) (27%) and stroke (17%) in 138 patients observed over an average of 46 months. Supported by their work and others,[3,7] Thompson et al. recommended prophylactic endarterectomy in selected asymptomatic patients, claiming a decline in the incidence of TIAs (4.5%) and stroke (4.6%) as a result of surgical procedure. The control population used in their study was not chosen randomly, however, and their report included all stroke events, without further reference to the type and location of the stroke. In contrast, other reports have presented differing viewpoints. Two studies based on epidemiologic data have documented the clinical outcome of asymptomatic patients with cervical bruits. Wolf et al.[22] reported a stroke rate of 12% in 171 asymptomatic patients with a neck bruit observed up to 8 years. Although this rate is almost twice the expected incidence, about half of the strokes were either nonischemic or were caused by emboli originating from the heart or not appropriate to the site of the bruit. From the rural Evans County, Georgia study, Heyman et al.[10] reported a stroke rate of 14% in asymptomatic patients with a cer-

☐ Supported by Grant HL-20898 from the National Institutes of Health.

465

vical bruit. Although the presence of a bruit signaled an increased risk of ischemic heart disease and death, a poor correlation was noted between the side of the bruit and the side of the stroke.

OUTCOME AFTER ENDARTERECTOMY

Operative mortality of 0% to 2% and perioperative stroke rates of 2% to 4% have been reported in asymptomatic patients undergoing carotid endarterectomy.[11,21,23] Although these results appear acceptable for a prophylactic procedure, the ensuing benefit of endarterectomy when compared with medical treatment or retreatment remains unproved in the asymptomatic patient. The risk of late stroke after endarterectomy ranges from 2% to 11% in reported series, 3% to 5% of these being fatal.[5,18,21] Also, recent evidence from our laboratory indicates that 2 years after carefully performed carotid endarterectomy the rate of recurrent high-grade stenoses is in the range of 19%[25]

Another aspect to consider when prophylactic endarterectomy is contemplated in asymptomatic patients is that, in general, these patients have a shortened life expectancy after surgery. Javid et al.[16] reported a death rate of 27% over a period of 3 years in their series of elderly patients who underwent an operation for an asymptomatic carotid stenosis. The majority of the deaths were of myocardial origin.

NATURAL HISTORY STUDIES

All of the natural history studies currently available have monitored the clinical outcome as the primary end point. Although clinical end points are the most important concerns, they are rarely specific enough to document the underlying basis of the event. Despite the obvious interest in detecting carotid arterial disease, it is surprising that so little information exists on the natural history of the lesions themselves. The only arteriographic data on the fate of carotid artery lesions was reported by Javid et al.[12] Repeat angiograms were performed in 93 patients at intervals of 1 to 9 years (mean, 3 years) after the initial angiograms. Only patients with lesions that reduced the arterial diameter by less than 60% were included in the study. When changes in the disease state were expressed in annual percent changes from the initial findings, disease progression of less than 25% per year was noted in at least one side in 22% of patients who did not undergo surgery. Although age, sex, and diabetes did not appear to influence the rate of

progression in their series, hypertension, the presence of a bruit, and the initial extent of the disease all appeared to be directly related to the likelihood of rapid changes in the carotid plaque. Up until recently only contrast angiography was available to monitor in vivo the extent of atherosclerotic disease.

In the last 15 years numerous noninvasive procedures have been developed to evaluate carotid disease. Despite the widespread availability of these tests, only two studies describe the natural outcome in asymptomatic patients with carotid lesions that were detected noninvasively. Kartchner and McRae[13] used oculoplethysmography (OPG) and phonoangiography (CPA) as noninvasive screening methods. With an average follow-up of 2 years, they reported a 3% stroke rate in asymptomatic patients with either a positive OPG or CPA findings. When both tests were found positive, the stroke rate rose to 12%. However, more than half of the patients with positive OPG or CPA results underwent a prophylactic endarterectomy, and 41% of the strokes in this group were nonischemic, caused by cardiac emboli, occurred during surgery, or were on the side not operated on. Also, it is not clear whether these strokes were preceded by TIAs. Although suggestions were given regarding the long-term surveillance of selected patients, no data were available on the pattern of changes at the bifurcation and their relevance to the clinical outcome. Barnes et al.[1] reported a 1.5% incidence of stroke without warning symptoms and a 14% incidence of hemispheric TIAs in patients with detectable carotid disease observed for an average of 11 months. Of the 254 patients with no detectable carotid lesions, none suffered a stroke and 2 (0.8%) reported symptoms suggestive of TIAs. They recommended careful follow-up of such patients, awaiting the development of TIAs rather than recommending endarterectomy. In the study by Barnes et al.,[1] patients with detectable carotid lesions underwent sequential continuous-wave Doppler studies, but no data were presented on the natural evolution of the detected plaques.

OUR EXPERIENCE

In January 1980 a prospective study was initiated to follow with ultrasonic Duplex scanning the course of carotid occlusive disease in a consecutive series of asymptomatic patients with a midcervical bruit.[15] The aim of the study was to determine (1) the stability of arterial lesions at the carotid bifur-

Duplex

	A	B	C	D	E	TOTAL
Normal	47	9				56
1% to 15%	4	49	8			61
16% to 49%		14	62	4		80
50% to 99%		1	7	91	1	100
100%				1	38	39
TOTAL	51	73	77	96	39	336

(% Diameter reduction)

Fig. 44-1. Accuracy of Duplex scanning vs. angiography.

cation, (2) the occurrence and type of neurologic symptoms developing during follow-up, and (3) the possible role of risk factors on disease progression.

Patient population

Between January 1980 and June 1982, 203 asymptomatic patients with a midcervical bruit on auscultation were referred to our laboratory for evaluation of carotid arterial occlusive disease and recruited for the study. None of these patients had undergone a previous carotid endarterectomy, and none had previous history of TIAs or stroke.

Of these 203 patients, 162 were available for follow-up and provide the data for this analysis. Of the remaining 41 patients, 2 died of myocardial infarction less than 1 year after their initial visit, 24 were still alive and asymptomatic but failed to comply with the follow-up protocol, 10 were lost to follow-up, 1 underwent bilateral prophylactic endarterectomy shortly after the initial visit, and 4 underwent a prophylactic operation of the side contralateral to an occlusion and their data were excluded from analysis.

Patients were seen at 6-month intervals for the first year and yearly thereafter. In addition to bilateral arm blood pressure measurements and neck auscultation, the patient's history was recorded using a standard questionnaire and Duplex scanning of the extracranial carotid arteries was performed. Additional data gathered on each subject included a review of the medical history, previous treatment, and potential risk factors, such as cigarette smoking and hypertension.

Duplex scanning

At each visit an ultrasonic Duplex scanner* was used to evaluate the extracranial portion of the carotid arteries. This method combines a B-mode image and a pulsed Doppler unit. The quadrature outputs of the Doppler signal are subjected to a real-time spectrum analysis that uses a digital fast Fourier transform (FFT) method with a mode normalized output.†

The assessment of carotid artery disease depends on the interpretation of spectral changes in the center-stream velocity patterns recorded from specific sites along the carotid arteries. The parameters used for classification of the spectra include peak systolic frequency, end diastolic frequency, amount of spectral broadening during systole, and overall shape of the waveforms. Using these features, disease at the carotid bifurcation is classified into six categories: normal; 1% to 15%, 16% to 49%, 50% to 79%, and 80% to 99% diameter reduction; and occlusion.

Validation of the methods has shown an overall agreement of 82% with contrast angiography.[16,17] The ability to recognize normal arteries (specificity) is 84%, and the sensitivity of the method for the detection of disease is 99%. For each category of disease the accuracy is about 80% when compared with angiography (Fig. 44-1).

*Mark V Duplex scanner, Advanced Technology Laboratory, Bellevue, Wash.
†Honeywell, Inc., Denver.

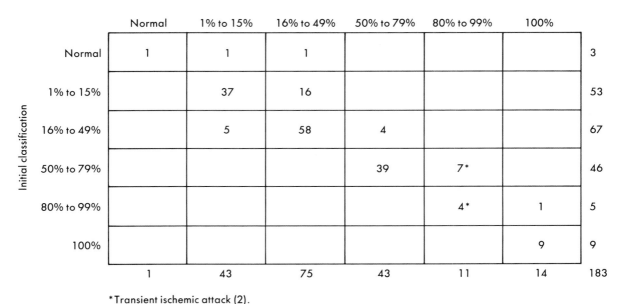

*Transient ischemic attack (2).

Fig. 44-2. Follow-up visit at 6 months.

Disease progression

Disease progression was defined as a change of disease classification by at least one category, from less severe to more severe, from the first visit to the last visit. Review of serial studies for the 162 patients revealed that findings in 101 (62%) patients remained unchanged on both sides, 50 (31%) showed disease progression on one side only, and 11 (7%) showed disease progression in both internal carotid arteries.

At 6 months, 103 patients were seen (Fig. 44-2). Of these, 23 had undergone a prophylactic endarterectomy on one side. Of the 183 nonoperated sides studied, 174 were patent initially, thus considered at risk for progression of disease. Of these, 80% (139 of 174) remained unchanged since the original visit, 17% (30 of 174) were classified as more severe, and 3% (5 of 174) were classified as a lesser degree of stenosis. None of the patients seen at 6 months suffered a stroke, but two experienced TIAs. In one instance the TIA occurred on the side with 80% to 99% stenosis that remained stable, and the other was associated with a 50% to 79% lesion that progressed to 80% to 99% stenosis. One lesion originally classified in 80% to 99% category had occluded at 6 months, without symptoms.

At 12 months, 95 patients were seen (Fig. 44-3). Twenty-four of these patients had undergone

unilateral endarterectomy. Of the 166 nonoperated sides studied, 157 were patent initially, thus considered at risk for progression. Of these, 26% (41 of 157) were classified as more severe and 3% (4 of 157) as less severe. Two new episodes of TIAs and two strokes were reported at the 12-month visit. TIAs occurred on the sides of a 50% to 79% lesion that had progressed to an 80% to 99% lesion at 6 months and was occluded at 12 months. One patient suffered a spontaneous stroke on the side of an internal carotid artery that was already occluded at the time of entry into the study. The contralateral side was narrowed by a less than 15% stenosis. The other stroke occurred during a contrast carotid arteriogram on the side of a stable 16% to 49% lesion defined on angiography as a 20% diameter-reducing stenosis.

At 24 months (Fig. 44-4), 64 patients were seen, and of the 110 patent sides at risk for progression, 27% (30 of 110) had progressed to a more severe category of disease and 4% (4 of 110) were classified as one category less severe. One patient experienced a TIA on the side of a 1% to 15% diameter reducing lesion in the internal carotid artery that remained stable. One patient suffered a stroke on the side of an internal carotid artery that had progressed from a 50% to 79% lesion to an 80% to 99% stenosis at 12 months and was found occluded at the time of the stroke. This patient had

Initial classification	Normal	1% to 15%	16% to 49%	50% to 79%	80% to 99%	100%	
Normal	3	2					5
1% to 15%		31	20			1	52
16% to 49%		4	41*	7		1	53
50% to 79%				36	7†	2†	45
80% to 99%			\		1	1	2
100%						9*	9
	3	37	61	43	8	18	166

*Stroke (2)—1 during angiography (the 16% to 49% lesion).

†Transient ischemic attack (2).

Fig. 44-3. Follow-up visit at 12 months.

Initial classification	Normal	1% to 15%	16% to 49%	50% to 79%	80% to 99%	100%	
Normal		4	1				5
1% to 15%		22*	10	2			34
16% to 49%		4	25	7	1	1	38
50% to 79%				29	2	2†	33
80% to 99%							0
100%						2	2
	0	30	36	38	3	6	112

*Transient ischemic attack (1).

†Stroke (1).

Fig. 44-4. Follow-up visit at 24 months.

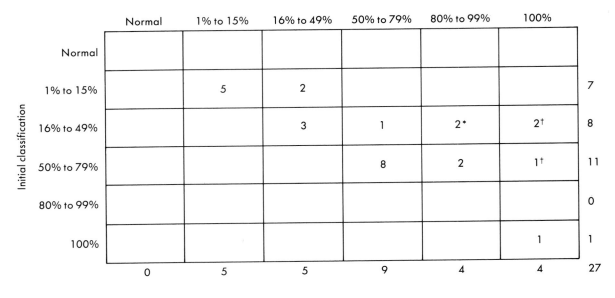

	Normal	1% to 15%	16% to 49%	50% to 79%	80% to 99%	100%	
Normal							
1% to 15%		5	2				7
16% to 49%			3	1	2*	2†	8
50% to 79%				8	2	1†	11
80% to 99%							0
100%						1	1
	0	5	5	9	4	4	27

Initial classification

*Transient ischemic attack (1).

†Stroke (2).

Fig. 44-5. Follow-up visit at 36 months.

reported previous episodes of TIAs on the side of the progression.

At 36 months (Fig. 44-5), 17 patients were seen, and of the 26 unoperated patent sides, 38% (10 of 26) had progressed to a more severe category. One patient reported new episodes of TIAs, and one patient suffered a stroke. Another patient developed a stroke 2 months after his 36-month visit. One patient suffered a stroke on the side of a 16% to 49% stenosis that progressed to an 80% to 99% lesion. One patient suffered a stroke on the side of a 16% to 49% lesion that had progressed to an 80% to 99% stenosis and was found occluded at the time of the stroke (Fig. 44-6). The other stroke occurred at 38 months on the side of a lesion that had progressed from a 50% to 79% lesion to an 80% to 99% stenosis at 36 months and was now occluded. Neither of these two patients experienced warning symptoms before the stroke.

To obviate the problem inherent to the structure of the study, an actuarial life table analysis was chosen to provide a more accurate means of estimating true rates of events. The absolute end points for the life table analysis shown in Fig. 44-7 were (1) symptoms (TIA or stroke), (2) disease progression in the internal carotid artery from a less than 50% to a more than 50% diameter-reducing lesion, and (3) evidence of progression in all cat-

egories of disease. The analysis showed an annual rate of occurrence of symptoms of 4%. At 3 years, 36% of the sides initially classified in the less than 50% category progressed to a more than 50% lesion. The average annual rate of progression to this category of disease was 8%. When progression in all categories are considered, 60% of the sides will have progressed after 3 years.

Symptoms, occlusions, and disease progression

Spontaneous appearance of symptoms occurred in 10 patients. Three suffered unheralded thromboembolic strokes, 1 had a TIA followed by a stroke, and 6 had TIAs only. In addition, 1 patient suffered a stroke during a contrast study on the side of a stable 16% to 49% lesion. That patient was asymptomatic before angiography.

Of the four spontaneous strokes, three occurred without warning TIAs, for an overall rate of unpredictable stroke of 1.8%. The annual rate of incidence of TIA is 3%. It is interesting to note that, although 90% of the spontaneous symptoms were associated with a more than 80% stenosis at the time of occurrence of the symptoms, 40% occurred on sides that were narrowed by less than 50% stenosis at the time of recruitment. Not considering the stroke that occurred on the side of an already occluded internal carotid artery, 89% of the symp-

Right internal carotid artery

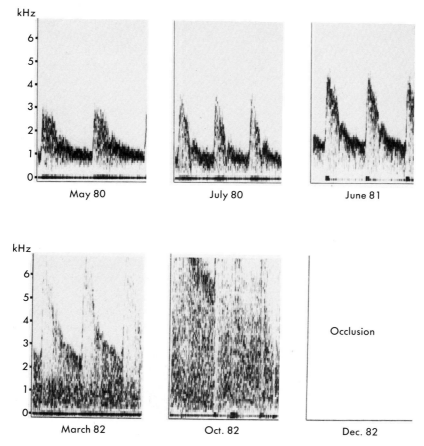

Fig. 44-6. Spectral changes in 59-year-old asymptomatic patient. On right side, lesion progressed from 16% to 49% lesion in May 1980 to 80% to 99% stenosis in December 1982. Two months later, patient suffered right hemispheric stroke and ipsilateral internal carotid artery was found occluded. Contralateral side remained stable in the 50% to 79% category. (From Roederer, G.O., et al.: The natural history of carotid arterial disease in asymptomatic patients with cervical bruits, Stroke. 15(4):566, 1984. By permission of the American Heart Association, Inc.)

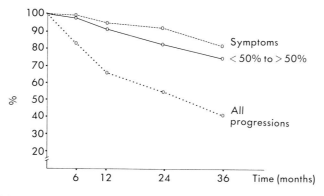

Fig. 44-7. Life table analysis. Annual rate of symptoms was 4%. Mean annual rate of progression from <50% to >50% lesion was 8%. When disease progression in all categories is considered, about 60% of sides will have progressed after 3 years of follow-up. (From Roederer, G.O., et al.: The natural history of carotid arterial disease in asymptomatic patients with cervical bruits, Stroke 15(4):566, 1984. By permission of the American Heart Association, Inc.)

toms (4 of 5 isolated TIAs and all three spontaneous strokes) were preceded by disease progression to a greater than 80% stenosis. Disease progression to beyond an 80% stenosis also preceded the occurrence of an occlusion in all cases where sequential studies were available. Progression of a lesion to more than 80% stenosis is an important finding in that it was found to carry a 35% risk of developing ischemic symptoms or ipsilateral occlusion within 6 months and a 46% risk at 12 months.

Conversely, only 1.5% of the lesions that remained in the less than 80% category produced a complication; one TIA occurred on the side of a stable 1% to 15% stenosis, and there was silent occlusion of three sides. These findings strongly suggest that it is safe to observe asymptomatic patients with a less than 80% diameter-reducing lesion of the carotid arteries and to delay angiography and surgery until the first appearance of TIA or the finding of a marked progression of the disease.

Risk factors for progression

Twelve potential risk indicators and second-order combinations were examined to evaluate their relationship with the occurrence of disease progression. These factors were (1) age, (2) sex, (3) history of high blood pressure, (4) treatment for high blood pressure, (5) measured systolic blood pressure, (6) measured diastolic blood pressure, (7) history of ischemic heart disease, (8) history of peripheral arterial occlusive disease, (9) history of diabetes mellitus, (10) smoking habits, (11) treatment with aspirin, and (12) treatment with dipyridamole.

No correlation was found between carotid artery disease progression and history of high blood pressure, treatment for high blood pressure, levels of systolic or diastolic pressure, sex, history of ischemic heart disease, and history of peripheral vascular disease. Also, the proportion of patients who showed progression during follow-up was the same whether taking aspirin and dipyridamole in combination (37%, 14 of 37), aspirin or dipyridamole alone (34%, 16 of 47), or neither of these drugs (40%, 31 of 78).

When the prevalence of carotid artery disease was examined in relation to age, an interesting observation was made. In the group of subjects older than 65 years at the time of entry into the study, the proportion of those in whom disease progressed was found to be lower (29%, 22 of 76) than in the younger group (45%, 39 of 86). The

difference was significant at p = .02 (Fisher exact test). This difference could not be explained by a difference in duration of follow-up but tends to disappear after accounting for the original state of disease.

A positive history of cigarette smoking emerged as an important risk factor for progression of carotid artery disease. Of those who had no history of smoking, 24% progressed as opposed to 42% for those who reported a positive history of cigarette smoking. Discontinuing smoking appeared to decrease the risk of progression. Although the difference did not reach statistical significance, the risk of progression decreased from 47% (36 of 77) for those who continued smoking during the study to 34% (15 of 44) for those who quit smoking before entering the study.

Occurrence of disease progression was also found higher in patients with diabetes (58%, 11 of 19) than in the nondiabetic group (35%, 50 of 143; p = 0.04).

To account for the contribution of the risk factors for disease progression, a multivariate stepwise discriminant analysis was performed. Age, diabetes, and smoking were found to be independent contributors to the risk of carotid artery disease progression.

Continued surveillance of asymptomatic patients with carotid artery disease is now feasible using accurate noninvasive tests that are safe and easily repeatable. A better understanding of the natural history of carotid artery disease will permit a more enlightened management of disease in these patients. It will be feasible to identify subsets of patients who will benefit from closer surveillance or prophylactic treatment. Our data suggest that it is safe to observe asymptomatic patients with noninvasive tests until disease has progressed beyond 80% diameter reduction or until the appearance of TIAs.

ACKNOWLEDGMENTS

We thank Marian Chinn and Lorraine Jenson for preparation of the manuscript, and ATL and Honeywell, Inc. for providing instrumentation used in this study.

REFERENCES

1. Barnes, R.W., et al.: The natural history of asymptomatic carotid disease in patients undergoing cardiovascular surgery, Surgery 90:1075, 1982.
2. Callow, A.D.: An overview of the stroke problem in the carotid territory, Am. J. Surg. 140:181, 1980.
3. Cooperman, M., Martin, E.W., and Evans, W.E.: Significance of asymptomatic carotid bruits, Arch. Surg. 113:1339, 1978.

4. David, T.E., et al.: A correlation of neck bruits and atherosclerotic arteries, Arch. Surg. 107:729, 1973.
5. DeWeese, J.A., et al.: Results of carotid endarterectomies for transient ischemic attacks: five years later, Ann. Surg. 178:258, 1973.
6. DeWeese, J.A., et al.:Endarterectomy for atherosclerotic lesions of the carotid artery, J. Cardiovasc. Surg. 12:299, 1971.
7. Dorazio, R.A., Esset, F., and Nesbit, N.J.: Long term follow-up of asymptomatic carotid bruit, Am. J. Surg. 140:212, 1980.
8. Fell, G., et al.: Importance of noninvasive ultrasonic Doppler testing in the evaluation of patients with asymptomatic carotid bruits, Am. Heart J. 102:221, 1981.
9. Hass, W.K., et al.: Joint study of extracranial arterial occlusion. II. Arteriography, techniques, sites and complications, JAMA 203:159, 1968.
10. Heyman, A., et al.: Risk of stroke in asymptomatic persons with cervical bruits: a population study in Evans County, Georgia, N. Engl. J. Med. 302:838, 1980.
11. Javid, H., et al.: Carotid endarterectomy for asymptomatic patients, Arch. Surg. 102:389, 1971.
12. Javid, H., et al.: Natural history of carotid bifurcation atheroma, Surgery 67:80, 1970.
13. Kartchner, N.M., and McRae L.P.: Noninvasive evaluation and management of asymptomatic carotid bruit, Surgery 6:840, 1977.
14. Riles, T.S., et al.: Symptoms, stenosis and bruit, Arch. Surg. 116:218, 1981.
15. Roederer, G.O., et al.: The natural history of carotid arterial disease in asymptomatic patients with cervical bruits, Stroke 15(4):566, 1984.
16. Roederer G.O., et al.: Ultrasonic Duplex scanning of extracranial carotid arteries: improved accuracy using new features from the common carotid artery, J. Cardiovasc. Ultrasonogr. 1:373, 1982.
17. Roederer, G.O., et al.: A simple spectral parameter for accurate classification of severe carotid disease, Bruit 8:174, 1984.
18. Stanford, J.R., Lubow, M., and Vasko, J.S.: Prevention of stroke by carotid endarterectomy, Surgery 83:259, 1978.
19. Thompson, J.E., Patman, R.D., and Talkington, C.M.: Asymptomatic carotid bruit:long-term outcome of patients having endarterectomy compared with unoperated controls, Ann. Surg. 188:308, 1978.
20. Thompson, J.E., Austin, D.J., and Patman, R.D.: Carotid endarterectomy for cerebrovascular insufficiency: long term results in 592 patients followed up to thirteen years, Ann. Surg. 172:663, 1970.
21. Thompson, J.E., Patman, K.D., and Persson, A.J.: Management of asymptomatic carotid bruits, Am. Surg. 42:77, 1976.
22. Wolf, P.A., et al.: Asymptomatic carotid bruit and the risk of stroke, JAMA 245:1442, 1981.
23. Wylie, E.J., and Ehrenfeld, W.K.: In Extracranial occlusive cerebrovascular disease: diagnosis and treatment, Philadelphia, 1970, W.B. Saunders Co.
24. Ziegler, D.K., et al.: Correlation of bruits over the carotid artery with angiographically demonstrated lesions, Neurology 21:860, 1971.
25. Zierler, R.E., et al.: Carotid artery stenosis following endarterectomy, Arch. Surg. 117:1408, 1982.

CHAPTER 45

Asymptomatic carotid disease in preoperative patients: perioperative and late stroke risk

ROBERT W. BARNES

Asymptomatic carotid disease occurs in one of the following circumstances: (1) as an incidental cervical bruit, (2) contralateral to symptomatic carotid disease, or (3) in a preoperative patient. Although controversy exists about the management of asymptomatic carotid disease, most physicians have recommended prophylactic endarterectomy of severe carotid stenosis in patients who are candidates for major operations, particularly before vascular or cardiac surgery. This philosophy reflects the feeling that patients undergoing major operations associated with potential hypotension or blood loss may suffer perioperative strokes in the presence of severe asymptomatic carotid occlusive disease. However, most previous studies are based on identification of patients at risk by the presence of asymptomatic carotid bruits. Recently asymptomatic carotid disease has been detected by noninvasive screening methods. Unfortunately, most previous studies have been retrospective and nonrandomized. Furthermore, previous studies have reported prophylactic endarterectomy that is carried out either as a staged procedure or simultaneous with the intended major operation. Recent prospective studies suggest that a nonoperative approach to asymptomatic disease in the preoperative patient may be associated with similar, if not reduced, risk of perioperative stroke when compared with retrospective studies in which prophylactic carotid endarterectomy was used. In this chapter are reviewed the previous retrospective and prospective studies with respect to the perioperative and late morbidity and mortality of patients with asymptomatic carotid disease associated with major cardiovascular operations.

DEFINITIONS
Asymptomatic carotid bruit

Asymptomatic carotid disease is most often identified in a patient with a midcervical bruit discovered incidentally on physical examination. Such bruits should be distinguished from bruits radiating from the aortic valve or aortic arch vessels, including the innominate, subclavian, or common carotid arteries. Innominate and subclavian artery bruits are detected in the supraclavicular fossa. Common carotid bruits have maximal intensity in the low anterior neck between the sternocleidomastoid muscle and the trachea. Carotid bifurcation bruits demonstrate maximal amplitude in the midcervical region near the angle of the mandible. Most carotid bifurcation bruits occur during systole and may represent stenosis of either the internal or external carotid arteries. A midcervical bruit that extends throughout systole and into diastole is pathognomonic of severe internal carotid stenosis.

Asymptomatic carotid disease

Significant obstruction of the carotid artery may exist in the absence of a cervical bruit. Examples of such disease include severe stenosis (greater than 85% diameter reduction) or occlusion of the internal carotid artery. On the other hand, a midcervical bruit may represent external carotid stenosis, which alone does not pose a risk for stroke. I prefer the term asymptomatic carotid *disease* to define lesions of the carotid artery, regardless of the presence or absence of a bruit. Such asymptomatic carotid disease is often detected by noninvasive diagnostic screening techniques.

DIAGNOSTIC METHODS
Clinical examination

The cerebrovascular evaluation includes a record of each radial, subclavian, and superficial temporal artery pulse. Significant obstruction of the internal carotid artery does not alter the amplitude of the common carotid artery pulse, which is diminished only in the presence of proximal common carotid (or innominate) artery disease. Diminution of the temporal pulse suggests external carotid artery obstruction. Bruits are elicited from the aortic ejection area, each supraclavicular fossa, low in the anterior neck, the midcervical region, the posterior cervical area (representing vertebral artery stenosis), and each orbit (a bruit representing carotid siphon stenosis).

Noninvasive diagnostic techniques

Indirect techniques include periorbital Doppler ultrasound and oculoplethysmography. These techniques are sensitive to severe stenosis (greater than 75% reduction in diameter) or occlusion of the internal carotid artery. In addition, the Doppler examination or oculopneumoplethysmography of Gee (OPG-Gee) during carotid compression permits estimation of collateral hemispheric perfusion pressure. These methods are insensitive to nonobstructive (ulcerative) carotid plaques and do not distinguish between operable carotid stenosis and inoperable occlusion of the internal carotid artery.

Direct carotid screening techniques include carotid phonoangiography for qualitative or quantitative analysis of bruits, Doppler ultrasonic evaluation of carotid flow disturbances using audible or spectral analysis techniques, and ultrasonic imaging of the carotid artery using continuous or pulsed Doppler flow visualization, real-time B-mode imaging, or combined (Duplex) scanning techniques. These methods are more sensitive to nonobstructive (ulcerative) and severe carotid lesions and are capable of distinguishing between operable carotid stenosis and inoperable carotid occlusion. The direct screening techniques are generally more complex and expensive than indirect methods.

Arteriography

Contrast arteriography remains the diagnostic standard for detection of carotid artery disease, particularly in patients who are candidates for operation. *Intravenous* angiography (digital subtraction angiography, [DSA or DIVA]) carries less risk and discomfort for the patient but provides less resolution and does not permit selective views of the extracranial or intracranial circulation. I recommend this procedure only in patients with evidence of severe internal carotid stenosis by direct noninvasive diagnostic techniques. *Intraarterial* angiography, including aortic arch and selective four-vessel views, provides optimal visualization of the extracranial and intracranial circulation but is associated with more patient discomfort and a small risk of stroke or arterial complications. I recommend selective intraarterial angiography for symptomatic patients with noninvasive evidence of minimal or no carotid disease or internal carotid artery occlusion.

MANAGEMENT
Prophylactic carotid endarterectomy

Table 45-1 depicts the results of both retrospective and prospective studies using prophylactic carotid endarterectomy as staged procedures or simultaneous with coronary artery bypass. In the 11 retrospective studies reported in the decade between 1972 and 1982,* the overall stroke rate in the 747 reported patients was 5.2% and incidence of myocardial infarction was 6.0%. The overall perioperative mortality was 10.2%. Of the 274 patients undergoing staged carotid endarterectomy followed by coronary artery bypass, the perioperative stroke rate was 3.6% and the incidence of myocardial infarction was 10.6%, with 11.0% mortality. Of the 473 patients undergoing simultaneous prophylactic carotid endarterectomy and coronary artery bypass grafting, the perioperative stroke rate was 6.1%, perioperative myocardial infarction rate was 3.4%, and mortality was 9.8%. These studies suggest that staged prophylactic endarterectomy results in a lower perioperative stroke rate but a significantly higher incidence of perioperative myocardial infarction than in patients undergoing simultaneous carotid endarterectomy and coronary artery bypass grafting.

In the single prospective study of prophylactic carotid endarterectomy in patients undergoing coronary artery bypass grafting screened with direct noninvasive carotid techniques,[3] the perioperative stroke rate associated with simultaneous prophylactic endarterectomy was 10%, with a 4% permanent stroke rate.

*References 2, 6-8, 10, 12-16, 20.

Table 45-1. Prophylactic carotid endarterectomy

Author	Technique	No. of patients	Stroke (%)	MI* (%)	Death (%)
RETROSPECTIVE STUDIES (CORONARY BYPASS)					
Bernard et al., 1972	Staged	15	7	27	33
	Simultaneous	16	7	0	0
Lefrak and Guinn, 1974	Staged	34	3	15	18
Urschel et al., 1976	Staged	24	4	4	0
	Simultaneous	8	0	0	0
Okies et al., 1977	Simultaneous	16	13	6	6
Mehigan et al., 1977	Staged	25	4	4	8
	Simultaneous	24	13	0	8
Hertzer et al., 1978	Staged	59	3	10	2
	Simultaneous	115	9	10	4
Ennix et al., 1979	Staged	77	5	13	18
	Simultaneous	51	1	3	3
Crawford et al., 1980	Staged	40	0	5	5
	Simultaneous	48	2	2	2
Rice et al., 1980	Simultaneous	54	4	0	0
Craver et al., 1982	Simultaneous	68	2	2	0
Schwartz et al., 1982	Simultaneous	73	10	0	10
PROSPECTIVE STUDY (CORONARY BYPASS)					
Brener et al., 1983	Simultaneous	29	10†		

*Mi, Myocardial infarction.
†Four percent permanent.

NONOPERATIVE THERAPY

Table 45-2 depicts the results of studies reported with a nonoperative approach to asymptomatic carotid disease in patients undergoing cardiac or peripheral vascular reconstructive surgery. Combining the early and late follow-up reports of Treiman et al.[5,9,17,18] of 1330 patients undergoing major vascular reconstructive surgery, the overall stroke rate was 1.1%. Of the 211 patients with asymptomatic bruit, the perioperative stroke rate was 0.5%. Of the 1119 patients without asymptomatic carotid bruit, the perioperative stroke rate was 1.2%. These studies suggest that the presence of asymptomatic carotid bruit does not increase the rate of perioperative stroke in patients undergoing major vascular reconstruction.

Kartchner and McRae[11] reported a retrospective study of the outcome of patients screened by oculoplethysmography and carotid phonoangiography who were undergoing major cardiovascular procedures. Of the 42 patients with significant carotid obstruction as defined by these noninvasive techniques, there was a 17% incidence of perioperative stroke. Of the 192 patients without asymptomatic carotid disease or in whom such disease had been prophylactically removed, the perioperative stroke rate was 1%.

Three independent prospective studies have used direct noninvasive screening techniques to identify patients with asymptomatic carotid disease before major peripheral arterial or coronary artery bypass grafting.[1,4,19] In these three recent studies the overall perioperative stroke rate in patients not undergoing prophylactic endarterectomy was 2.7% in the 627 patients screened. Of the 157 patients with noninvasive evidence of significant carotid obstruction, the perioperative stroke rate was 3.6%. Of the 470 patients with normal direct carotid noninvasive studies, the perioperative stroke rate was 2.4%. This difference is not statistically significant. These prospective studies suggest that noninvasive evidence of significant asymptomatic carotid occlusive disease does not significantly increase the risk of perioperative stroke in patients who do not undergo prophylactic carotid endarterectomy.

In our own study[1] there was a poor correlation between the presence of asymptomatic cervical

Table 45-2. Nonoperative therapy

Author	Carotid bruit	Carotid stenosis	Patients (n)	Stroke (%)
RETROSPECTIVE STUDIES (VASCULAR SURGERY)				
Treiman et al., 1973	Present	—	40	0
	Absent	—	156	1
Carney et al., 1977	Present	—	35	0
	Absent	—	213	2
Evans and Cooperman, 1978	Present	—	92	0
	Absent	—	496	1
Treiman et al., 1979	Present	—	84	1
	Absent	—	410	1
Kartchner and McRae, 1982	—	Present	42	17
	—	Absent	192	1

Author	Carotid stenosis	No. of patients	Perioperative problems		Late problems		
			Stroke (%)	Death (%)	TIA (%)	Stroke (%)	Death (%)
RETROSPECTIVE STUDIES (VASCULAR SURGERY)							
Turnipseed et al., 1980	Present	76	5	—	—	—	—
	Absent	254	4	—	—	—	—
Barnes et al., 1981	Present	63	3	11	14	3	9
	Absent	386	1	1	1	0	1
Breslau et al., 1981	Present	18	0	—	—	—	—
	Absent	84	1	—	—	—	—

bruit and the presence of significant obstruction by direct noninvasive carotid screening techniques. Of the 898 arteries screened, only 36.9% of the 65 arteries with bruit had noninvasive direct Doppler evidence of significant carotid obstruction. Conversely, of the 88 arteries with significant carotid occlusive disease by noninvasive techniques, bruits were present in only 27.3% of the vessels. There was a significant correlation of the presence of asymptomatic carotid bruit or disease with perioperative mortality, ranging from 18.2% of patients with both noninvasive evidence of carotid obstruction and cervical bruit to 0.3% mortality in patients without evidence of carotid obstruction or bruit. This increased mortality was present in the late follow-up of patients who suffered an 11.1% mortality in the presence of both carotid obstruction and bruit vs. 0.8% late mortality in patients without evidence of carotid obstruction or bruit. Of 69 patients with asymptomatic carotid disease who suffered no perioperative neurologic deficits, late follow-up revealed a 19% incidence of late neurologic deficits in follow-up ranging up to 4 years. However, in 15% the deficit was a transient ischemic attack and in only three (4%) patients did a stroke occur in the absence of antecedent transient ischemic attack. Only one of the strokes (1.5%) occurred on the side of original carotid disease. This study suggests that asymptomatic carotid disease in the preoperative patient does not pose a significant threat of perioperative stroke. However, such patients will frequently develop late postoperative neurologic deficits, which must be screened for and corrected with prophylactic endarterectomy before future stroke. Asymptomatic carotid disease is a marker of increased risk for perioperative or late postoperative mortality from myocardial infarction.

DISCUSSION

Although most physicians consider asymptomatic carotid disease a significant risk factor for perioperative stroke in patients undergoing major cardiovascular procedures, recent prospective studies using sensitive direct carotid noninvasive screening techniques fail to support this hypothesis. Indeed, the three prospective studies reported to date are associated with a lower incidence of perioperative stroke in patients not undergoing prophylactic endarterectomy than in the retrospective studies reported to date in which prophylactic endarterectomy is carried out before or at the time of major cardiovascular surgery. The reported studies, however, do point out two major risk factors of patients with asymptomatic carotid disease before cardiovascular operation. The presence of such carotid disease is an indication that the patient is at increased risk for perioperative or late coronary artery morbid events. A case could be made for performing coronary angiography in such patients to identify high-risk coronary lesions that might require prophylactic endarterectomy before major peripheral vascular reconstructions. A second major risk in patients with asymptomatic carotid disease is the significant incidence of late neurologic deficits in the postoperative follow-up period. However, most of these deficits are transient ischemic attacks, which may lead the physician to recommend prophylactic endarterectomy to prevent future stroke. Few patients suffer stroke in the absence of antecedent transient ischemic attack. In our own study less than 2% suffered stroke on the side of the original carotid lesion detected preoperatively.

Thus, all patients undergoing major cardiovascular procedures should be screened with noninvasive direct carotid diagnostic techniques to identify the presence of asymptomatic carotid disease. Such disease does not require correction before the major operation. However, the value of carotid screening is twofold. First, it identifies patients at risk of possible morbid coronary events in the perioperative and late postoperative period. Second, it permits careful follow-up and education of patients with asymptomatic carotid disease to detect subsequent transient ischemic attacks before the development of stroke. Such symptomatic patients in the follow-up period may undergo prophylactic carotid endarterectomy, yet avoid such surgical intervention in the vast majority (approximately 80%) who do not develop symptoms in the postoperative follow-up.

REFERENCES

1. Barnes, R.W., et al.: The natural history of asymptomatic carotid disease in patients undergoing cardiovascular surgery, Surgery 90:1075, 1981.
2. Bernhard, V.M., Johnson, W.D., and Peterson, J.J.: Carotid artery stenosis, Arch. Surg. 105:837, 1972.
3. Brener, B.J., et al.: A four year experience with preoperative noninvasive carotid evaluation of 2026 patients undergoing cardiac surgery, J. Vasc. Surg. 1:326, 1984.
4. Breslau, P.J., et al.: Carotid arterial disease in patients undergoing coronary artery bypass operations, J. Thorac. Cardiovasc. Surg. 82:765, 1981.
5. Carney, W.K., Jr., et al.: Carotid bruit as a risk factor in aortoiliac reconstruction, Surgery 81:567, 1977.
6. Craver, J.M., et al.: Concomitant carotid and coronary artery reconstruction, Ann. Surg. 195:712, 1982.
7. Crawford, E.S., Palamara, A.E., and Kasparian, A.S.: Carotid and noncoronary operations: simultaneous, staged, and delayed, Surgery 87:1, 1980.
8. Ennix, C.L., Jr., et al.: Improved results of carotid endarterectomy in patients with symptomatic coronary disease: an analysis of 1,546 consecutive carotid operations, Stroke 10:122, 1979.
9. Evans, W.E., and Cooperman, M.: The significance of asymptomatic unilateral carotid bruits in preoperative patients, Surgery 83:521, 1978.
10. Hertzer, N.R., et al.: Staged and combined surgical approach to simultaneous carotid and coronary vascular disease, Surgery 84:803, 1978.
11. Kartchner, M.M., and McRae, L.P.: Carotid occlusive disease as a risk factor in major cardiovascular surgery, Arch. Surg. 117:1086, 1982.
12. Lefrak, E.A., and Guinn, G.A.: Prophylactic carotid artery surgery in patients requiring a second operation, South. Med. J. 67:185, 1974.
13. Mehigan, J.T., et al.: A planned approach to coexistent cerebrovascular disease in coronary artery bypass candidates, Arch. Surg. 122:1403, 1977.
14. Okies, J.E., MacManus, O., and Starr, A.: Myocardial revascularization and carotid endarterectomy: a combined approach, Ann. Thorac. Surg. 23:560, 1977.
15. Rice, P.L., et al.: Experience with simultaneous myocardial revascularization and carotid endarterectomy, J. Thorac. Cardiovasc. Surg. 79:922, 1980.
16. Schwartz, R.L., et al.: Simultaneous myocardial revascularization and carotid endarterectomy, Circulation 66 (suppl. 1):97, 1982.
17. Treiman, R.L., et al.: Carotid bruit: significance in patients undergoing an abdominal aortic operation, Arch. Surg. 106:803, 1973.
18. Treiman, R.L., et al.: Carotid bruit: a follow-up report on its significance in patients undergoing an abdominal aortic operation, Arch. Surg. 114:1138, 1979.
19. Turnipseed, W.D., Berkoff, H.A., and Belzer, F.O.: Postoperative stroke in cardiac and peripheral vascular disease, Ann. Surg. 192:365, 1980.
20. Urschel, H.C., Razzuk, M.A., and Gardner, M.A.: Management of concomitant occlusive disease of the carotid and coronary arteries, J. Thorac. Cardiovasc. Surg. 72:829, 1976.

CHAPTER 46

Recurrent carotid artery stenosis

MARTIN H. THOMAS, RALPH B. DILLEY, and EUGENE F. BERNSTEIN

Extracranial carotid artery disease causes ischemic cerebral symptoms and stroke from microemboli and inadequate cerebral perfusion.[12] Carotid endarterectomy reduces morbidity and mortality in such patients, particularly after transient ischemic attacks (TIAs).[3,38] Also, in selected cases, these are reduced in patients with asymptomatic carotid bruits.[37] Although carotid endarterectomy was initially thought to provide permanent protection against occlusive and ulcerated lesions of the carotid bifurcation, several reports of recurrent stenosis following carotid surgery have appeared.* Initially, recurrent stenosis was detected only on the basis of clinical events with an incidence of 1% to 4% (Table 46-1). The first large series (1654 patients) reported showed only a 1.5% symptomatic recurrent stenosis rate,[34] whereas more recent rates up to 3.4% have been reported.[8] Two additional angiographic studies, although incomplete, suggest a recurrent carotid stenosis rate of about 7% after 5 years or more.[10,33]

The introduction of sensitive noninvasive methods for the assessment of carotid arteries has permitted a more routine and complete follow-up of patients after surgery. Such noninvasive methods have revealed recurrent stenosis rates from 9%[10,39] to as high as 19%[32,41] (Table 46-2). If such recurrent stenoses are associated with the development of clinically significant symptoms, then their detection would gain increasing importance.

At the Scripps Clinic, routine vascular laboratory follow-up with spectral analysis detected 38 recurrent carotid lesions in 257 carotid arteries after surgery (15.5%). Three were complete occlusions (1.2%), two of which occurred within 2 months. An additional 20 arteries were stenosed from 50%

to 99% for a total frequency of hemodynamically significant lesions of 9% (23 out of 257). Fifteen (6%) other stenoses were classified as 20% to 49% of the internal carotid artery (ICA) diameter, and a further 25 carotid arteries exhibited Doppler velocity patterns compatible with minor degrees of stenosis less than 20%. These latter spectra are of doubtful significance postoperatively and have not been included in the further analysis.

Table 46-1. Reported incidence of recurrent carotid stenosis based only on clinical symptoms

Author	Year	Incidence (%)
Stoney[34]	1976	1.5
French[11]	1977	0.6
Cossman[8]	1978	3.6
Hertzer[15]	1979	1.3
Cossman[9]	1980	3.4
Callow[3]	1982	1.7

Table 46-2. Reported incidence of recurrent carotid stenosis based on noninvasive laboratory examinations

Author	Year	Incidence (%) Symptomatic	Total
Kartchner[20]	1979	—	7.9
Kremen[22]	1979	1.7	9.8
Turnipseed[39]	1980	2.5	11.3
Cantelmo[5]	1981	4.5	12
Zierler[41]	1982	5.5	19
Salvian[32]	1983	4.8	11.4
Lynch[23]	1983	1.9	12.9
Thomas[36]	1984	1.7	14.8

*References 5, 8, 10, 33, 34, 39.

Fourteen recurrent lesions were documented in men and 24 in women; thus 9% of male and 25% of female carotid arteries had recurrent stenosis after surgery. Sixteen lesions developed within 3 months, 22 within 6 months, and 29 (76%) within 1 year. Only one of the remaining nine patients had been examined within a year, was found to be normal, and subsequently had recurrent stenosis. The other eight had not attended the clinic in the first 12 months and returned later with stenotic lesions. It is therefore possible that some or all of these eight also had a recurrent stenosis in the first year.

Regression of lesions was documented in three patients. Eight arteries were also examined by conventional or digital subtraction angiography, and the recurrent stenosis was confirmed in every case.

Other than the sex distribution, there did not appear to be any difference in preoperative status between the 219 patients with nonstenosed and the 38 patients with stenosed carotid arteries (Table 46-3). Clinical indications for surgery and preoperative degree of stenosis were proportionately similar among those patients who developed recurrent stenosis and those who did not. Neither was any difference noted between the two groups for diabetes mellitus, hypertension, or smoking habits.

Of the 38 patients with carotid recurrent stenosis, 6 underwent another operation within 4 years and 4 within a year. All 6 had developed lesions of greater than 50%, and clinical symptoms were present in 4: TIAs in three and a bruit audible to the patient in the fourth. Subocclusions of greater than 95% diameter reduction were seen in the other 2. Thus in the relatively short average follow-up period of 20 months, 16% of the patients with recurrent stenosis and 30% of those with a hemodynamically significant recurrent stenosis (greater than 50%) required another operation.

Our data confirm that recurrent stenosis of the carotid artery is a significant problem for the vascular surgeon. Noninvasive tests reveal a much larger number of postoperative recurrent stenoses than were suggested by clinical criteria alone. Spectral analysis has proved a reliable noninvasive method for assessing the carotid artery and can detect stenoses that do not limit flow, as well as those that narrow the lumen over 50%.[1,41] Spectral analysis is less invasive than digital subtraction angiography and probably as accurate.

Kremen[22] detected 9.8% hemodynamically significant stenoses using the ocular pneumoplethys-

mograph (OPPG), although the interval after surgery that the patients were studied is not clear. Using oculoplethysmography and carotid phonoangiography (OPG-CPA), supplemented in some later patients by Doppler imaging, Cantelmo[5] found 9% significant stenoses, whereas Turnipseed[39] found 8.9% using Doppler imaging alone.[10] These figures are remarkably consistent with our own 9% for stenoses equal to or greater than 50% diameter narrowing. Zierler[41] reported an initial incidence of 36% flow-limiting stenoses in the first year following operation, although only 19% persisted, a figure not confirmed by other studies. Available long-term studies[27] suggest that disease progression on the operated side occurs at the same rate as on the unoperated side. It should be emphasized that in very few of the prior studies was intraoperative angiography employed routinely.

The true incidence of non-flow-limiting recurrent stenosis is not known. Most studies have not reported stenoses of less than 50%, usually because the available instrumentation has not been sufficiently accurate. Several of the indirect and plethysmographic methods depend on changes in pressure and flow to detect a stenosis and are therefore of little use in diagnosing the more moderate lesions. Cantelmo[5] reported 3% non-flow-limiting stenoses, but since OPG-CPA was used, this figure is probably low. Our study demonstrated 15 (6%) stenoses from 20% to 50%. Another 25 patients' carotid arteries showed spectral changes consistent with stenoses less than 20%. Whereas the former group clearly represent true recurrent stenoses, the significance of the latter group remains less certain. Some degree of spectral broadening can be expected from arterial wall compliance changes after endarterectomy and probably does not represent pathologic recurrent stenosis in most cases. Since no other studies of minimal and moderate recurrent stenosis following carotid surgery have been reported, the precise frequency of these lesions remains unknown. The significance of the mild and moderate lesions is also uncertain, as is the likelihood that these lesser grades of stenosis progress to a tight stenosis or cause clinical problems.

Stenoses were recorded at the first postoperative examination at 1 month in 11 of our cases. Review of these patients' intraoperative angiograms did not reveal any significant surgically related narrowing. Progression of disease from apparently normal at 1 month to severely stenosed at 3 months was also documented. Twenty-nine of the lesions appeared within 1 year. These figures suggest that recurrent stenosis may occur remarkably quickly. The condition did not progress in every case, and three patients even showed regression of early stenotic lesions. The phenomenon of regression was also described by Zierler[41] and may be a result of remodeling, as has been demonstrated in animals[26] and humans.[33] Thus the early stenotic lesion occurring in the first few months has the potential to worsen or to improve.

The stenotic lesion that develops within 1 year is not a result of atheroma. This early lesion apparently is caused by myointimal hyperplasia[30,34] and seems to be platelet mediated. Platelets adhere rapidly to the exposed collagen surface of the endarterectomized segment of carotid artery (Fig. 46-1). Collagen-induced platelet aggregation mediated by platelet-dense granule nucleotides and other substances follows. These activated, adherent platelets release a mitogenic factor that promotes proliferation of arterial wall smooth muscle cells.* The resulting myointimal hyperplasia has been examined histologically in specimens obtained at the time of operation for recurrent stenosis and is different from atherosclerosis.[34] Stoney and String[34] described myointimal proliferation in 11 specimens removed from patients within 15 months of the initial endarterectomy and typical changes of atherosclerosis in a further 20 lesions removed 2 to 20 years later.[34] The late recurrent atherosclerotic lesion may be removed by standard techniques, whereas the early myointimal lesion does not separate easily and should be treated by widening the artery with a patch.[8]

Angiographically the stenosis secondary to myointimal hyperplasia is smooth and regular and occurs at the site of the endarterectomy, whereas the recurrent atherosclerotic lesion tends to be irregular, ulcerated, and worse beyond the end of the previous endarterectomy site. A similar phenomenon of smooth muscle proliferation has been reported after arterial reconstruction in the leg using vascular grafts.[41]

In our experience, no difference was found in the incidence of diabetes mellitus, hypertension, clinical indications for carotid endarterectomy, preoperative severity of disease, or smoking habits among the patients whose carotid arteries had recurrent stenosis compared to those whose arteries

*References 6, 13, 17, 24, 25, 28-31.

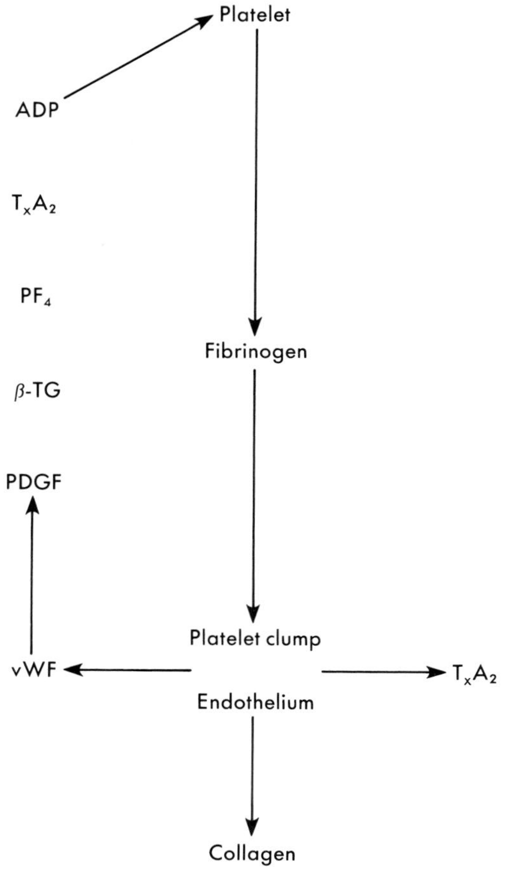

Fig. 46-1. Scheme of platelet-mediated myointimal hyperplasia. Rapid platelet adherence to exposed subendothelial collagen involves interaction of collagen with von Willebrand's factor and platelet membrane glycoprotein. Released ADP and T_xA_2 act synergistically to recruit and, with fibrinogen bridging, to aggregate more platelets. PDGF released into subendothelium promotes intimal migration and proliferation of smooth muscle cells. *ADP,* adenosine diphosphate; T_xA_2, thromboxane A_2; *PF₄,* platelet factor 4; *βTG,* β thromboglobulin; *PDGF,* platelet-derived growth factor; *vWF,* von Willebrand's factor.

stayed open (Tables 46-3 and 46-4). Clagett et al.[7] described a high incidence of continued smoking in the recurrent stenosis group, but was unable to demonstrate any difference in other factors. Neither the present study nor that of Clagett et al.[7] used objective means, such as carboxyhemoglobin or thiocyanate measurements, to monitor tobacco consumption. Since patient's witness as to their tobacco consumption is notoriously unreliable, no firm conclusions can be drawn on the role of cigarette smoking.[35]

Table 46-3. Incidence of recurrent stenosis following carotid endarterectomy at Scripps Clinic

	Total arteries (257)		Recurrent stenoses (38)	
	No.	%	No.	% of Total
Males	161	63	14	9
Females	96	37	24	25
Preoperative stenosis of hemodynamic significance (>50%)	169	66	23	9
Diabetes mellitus	28	11	4	36
Smoking history	208	81	25	12
Hypertension	136	53	16	12

Table 46-4. Relationship of carotid recurrent stenosis to indications for endarterectomy and operative factors

Operative factors	Total No.	Recurrent stenosis	
		No.	%
INDICATION FOR SURGERY			
Amaurosis fugax	39	8	21
Motor TIA	76	12	32
Prior stroke	69	7	18
Asymptomatic stenosis	70	11	29
Other indications	1	0	0
SURGERY PERFORMED			
Patch angioplasty	16	0	0
Bilateral operation	30	6	16

One outstanding feature of our results is the high frequency of recurrent stenosis among women. In another clinical study, Cossman[9] found 11 out of 14 patients with symptomatic carotid recurrent stenosis were female. This finding was also confirmed in a case control study in which the male/female ratio among patients with recurrent stenosis was 1.6:1 compared to 2.9:1 for the whole group. Women tend to have higher platelet counts than men, and the explanation for the predominance of recurrent stenosis among women could be sex differences in platelet behavior. Significant sex differences in platelet aggregation have been demonstrated in rats, guinea pigs,[19] and humans.[18] All our patients were given aspirin with dipyridamole postoperatively, although their compliance rate is unknown. Platelet response to aspirin also shows sex differences in animals and humans. Aspirin reduced the thrombosis rate and mortality of testosterone-treated rats with indwelling aortic cannulae[40] and also reduced thrombosis in male rabbits, but not in female rabbits.[21] Hirsch[16] showed a differential effect of aspirin on bleeding time between men and women. The Canadian Cooperative Study of aspirin and sulphinpyrazone in patients with threatened stroke reported a risk reduction in stroke or death of 48% for men, but none for women.[4] This evidence suggests that the difference between male and female recurrent stenosis rates is real and probably mediated through their platelet response to endarterectomy.

In summary, carotid recurrent stenosis after endarterectomy is more frequent than previously believed with hemodynamically significant lesions recurring in 9%, most within 1 year of surgery and more frequently in women. Some of these patients also develop cerebrovascular symptoms, which may be indications for further surgery. Whether these lesions have true clinical or prognostic significance in the absence of symptoms is not known. However, routine postoperative screening with noninvasive vascular laboratory techniques appears worthwhile in these patients and may permit identifying patients at high risk before other signs.

ACKNOWLEDGMENT

The clinical review described in this chapter was performed by Martin H. Thomas during a research fellowship at the Scripps Clinic and Research Foundation supported from grants from the Vascular Disease Foundation and a Welcome Traveling Fellowship.

REFERENCES

1. Blackshear, W.M., et al.: Detection of carotid occlusive disease by ultrasonic imaging and pulsed Doppler spectrum analysis, Surgery 86:298, 1979.
2. Breslau, P.J., et al.: Evaluation of carotid bifurcation disease, Arch. Surg. 117:58, 1982.
3. Callow, A.D.: An overview of the stroke problem in the carotid territory, Am. J. Surg. 140:181, 1980.
4. Canadian Cooperative Study Group: A randomized trial of aspirin and sulphinpyrazone in threatened stroke, N. Engl. J. Med. 299:53, 1978.
5. Cantelmo, N.L.: Non-invasive detection of carotid stenosis following endarterectomy, Arch. Surg. 116:1005, 1981.
6. Chesebro, J.H., et al.: A platelet inhibitor drug trial in coronary artery bypass operations, N. Engl. J. Med. 307:73, 1982.
7. Clagett, G.P., et al.: Etiologic factors for recurrent carotid artery stenosis, Surgery 93:313, 1983.

8. Cossman, D.V., et al.: Early restenosis after carotid endarterectomy, Arch. Surg. 113:275, 1978.
9. Cossman, D.V., et al.: Surgical approach to recurrent carotid stenosis, Am. J. Surg. 140:209, 1980.
10. Edwards, W.S., Wilson, T.A.S., and Bennett, A.: The long-term effectiveness of carotid endarterectomy in prevention of strokes, Ann. Surg. 168:756, 1965.
11. French, B.N., and Rewcastle, N.B.: Recurrent stenosis at site of carotid endarterectomy, Stroke 8:597, 1977.
12. Gunning, A.J., Pickering, G.W., and Robb-Smith, A.H.T.: Mural thrombosis of the internal carotid artery and subsequent embolism, Q. J. Med. 33:155, 1964.
13. Harker, L.A., Schwartz, S.M., and Ross, R.: Endothelium and arteriosclerosis, Clin. Haematol. 10:283, 1981.
14. Harker, L.A., Slichter, S.J., and Sauvage, L.R.: Platelet consumption by arterial prosthesis: the effects of endothelialization and pharmacologic inhibition of platelet function, Ann. Surg. 186:594, 1977.
15. Hertzer, N.R., Martinez, B.D., and Beven, E.G.: Recurrent stenosis after carotid endarterectomy, Surg. Gynecol. Obstet. 149:360, 1979.
16. Hirsch, J., Blajehman, M., and Kaegl A.: The bleeding time: platelet function testing, DHEW Pub. No. (NIH) 78-1087, Washington, D.C., 1978.
17. Imparato, A.M., et al.: Intimal and neointimal fibrous proliferation causing failure of arterial reconstructions, Surgery 72:1007, 1972.
18. Johnson, M., Ramey, E., and Ramwell, P.W.: Sex and age differences in human platelet aggregation, Nature 253:355, 1975.
19. Johnson, M., and Ramwell, P.W.: Androgen mediated sex differences in platelet aggregation, Physiologist 17:256, 1974.
20. Kartchner, M.M., and McRae, L.P.: Oculoplethysmography and carotid phonoangiography. In Bernstein, E.F., editor: Noninvasive diagnostic techniques in vascular disease, ed. 2, St. Louis, 1982, The C.V. Mosby Co.
21. Kelton, J.G., et al.: Sex differences in the antithrombotic effects of aspirin, Blood 52:1073, 1978.
22. Kremen, J.E., et al.: Restenosis or occlusion after carotid endarterectomy, Arch. Surg. 114:608, 1979.
23. Lynch, T.G., Hobson, R.W., II, and Berry, S.M.: The role of real-time B-mode ultrasonography and ocular pneumoplethysmography following carotid endarterectomy, Am. Surg. 49:31, 1983.
24. McCann, R.L., Hager, P.O., and Fuchs, J.C.A.: Aspirin and dipyridamole decrease intimal hyperplasia in experimental vein grafts, Ann. Surg. 191:238, 1980.
25. Metke, M.P., et al.: Reduction of intimal thickening in canine coronary bypass vein grafts with dipyridamole and aspirin, Am. J. Cardiol. 43:1144, 1979.
26. Moore, S., Friedman, R.J., and Gent, M.: Resolution of lipid containing atherosclerotic lesions induced by injury, Blood Vessels 14:193, 1977.
27. Norrving, B., Nilsson, B., and Olsson, J.E.: Progression of carotid disease after endarterectomy: a Doppler ultrasound study, Ann. Neurol. 12:548, 1982.
28. Pantely, G.A., et al.: Failure of antiplatelet and anticoagulant therapy to improve patency of grafts after coronary artery bypass: a controlled randomized trial, N. Engl. J. Med. 301:962, 1979.
29. Ross, R., and Vogel, A.: The platelet derived growth factor, Cell 14:203, 1978.
30. Ross, R., and Glomset, J.A.: The pathogenesis of atherosclerosis: part 1, N. Engl. J. Med. 295:369, 1976.
31. Rutherford, R.B., and Ross, R.: Platelet factors stimulate fibroblasts and smooth muscle cells quiescent in plasma serum to proliferate, J. Cell Biol. 69:196, 1976.
32. Salvian, A., et al.: Cause and noninvasive detection of restenosis after carotid endarterectomy, Am. J. Surg. 146:29, 1983.
33. Schultz, H., Fleming, J.F.R., and Awerbuck, B.: Arteriographic assessment of carotid endarterectomy, Ann. Surg. 171:509, 1970.
34. Stoney, R.J., and String, S.T.: Recurrent carotid stenosis, Surgery 80:705, 1976.
35. Thomas, M.H.: Smoking ans vascular surgery, Br. J. Surg. 68:601, 1981.
36. Thomas, M.H., et al.: Recurrent carotid artery stenosis following endarterectomy, Ann. Surg. 200:74, 1984.
37. Thompson, J.E., Patman, R.D., and Talkington, C.M.: Asymptomatic carotid bruit: long-term outcome of patients having endarterectomy compared with unoperated controls, Ann. Surg. 188:308, 1978.
38. Thompson, J.E., and Talkington, C.M.: Carotid endarterectomy, Ann. Surg. 184:1, 1976.
39. Turnipseed, W.D., Berkoff, H.A., and Crummy, A.: Postoperative occlusion after carotid endarterectomy, Arch. Surg. 115:573, 1980.
40. Uzunova, A.D., Ramey, E.R., and Ramwell, P.W.: Gonadal hormones and pathogenesis of occlusive arterial thrombosis, Am. J. Physiol. 234:H454, 1978.
41. Zierler, R.E., et al.: Carotid artery stenosis following endarterectomy, Arch. Surg. 117:1408, 1982.

CHAPTER 47

The natural outcome of carotid artery lesions on the side contralateral to endarterectomy

GHISLAINE O. ROEDERER, YVES E. LANGLOIS, and D. EUGENE STRANDNESS Jr.

Removal of the obstructing atheroma has proved effective in relieving symptoms and reducing the incidence of subsequent stroke in patients having focal neurologic symptoms.[2,3,16,17,20] On the other hand, the natural history of carotid artery disease on the contralateral side after endarterectomy remains uncertain, and management of these patients is a source of controversy. Some surgeons advocate a prophylactic operation for those vessels with significant lesions,[8,10,11] whereas other recommend a more conservative approach, intervening only when symptoms develop.[1,4,6,7] This debate will continue until data are available that put into perspective the natural history and clinical consequences of the disease, the long-term benefit of endarterectomy, and those factors that may influence therapeutic results.

SURGICAL RESULTS

To fulfill its goal, carotid endarterectomy should prevent recurrent transient ischemic attacks (TIAs) and a completed stroke. The key questions in the evaluation of this issue are as follows:

1. Which patients are at risk for stroke and would benefit from the operation?
2. Can the operation be performed with an acceptable risk of stroke?
3. Will the procedure protect the patient from further neurologic complications?

There is no doubt that patients with TIAs are prone to develop a stroke. Statistics vary from different reported series, but, in general, about 40% will develop a stroke within 5 years of the first

TIA.[19] These patients are prime candidates for endarterectomy. The same rationale also dictates surgical treatment in patients with either a mild or moderate neurologic deficit following a first stroke. However, the treatment of asymptomatic patients with carotid lesions and those having nonhemispheric symptoms is less clear.

If carotid endarterectomy is to be recommended for the treatment of both asymptomatic and symptomatic patients, the mortality and morbidity should be better than observed with nonoperative management. As estimated by Hass,[5] the combined mortality and morbidity of the operation should not exceed 3%, if it is to be the treatment of choice.

Most published surgical series would satisfy these criteria, reporting mortality of about 1% and morbidity of about 2% following carotid endarterectomy.[2,3,16,17,20] Although the operation can be performed with good immediate results, the risk of late stroke following a carotid endarterectomy ranged from 2% to 10% in reported series with 3% to 5% of these being fatal.[2,16,18]

To evaluate the benefit of prophylactic endarterectomy on the contralateral side, it is important to compare those surgical results with data on the outcome of nonsurgically treated patients.

LONG-TERM CLINICAL STUDIES

Several studies to date have attempted to clarify the natural history of carotid disease in the artery contralateral to the operated side. Clinical reports favoring a prophylactic surgical management of lesions found opposite an initial endarterectomy are based on high stroke rates that range from 4.5% to 36% when patients are conservatively followed. The occurrence of stroke as the initial symptom

□ This work was supported by NIH grant no. HL-20898.

further confirms these views.[8,10,11] Other reports have presented differing views.

Humphries et al.[6] retrospectively analyzed 168 patients (182 arteries) with angiographically confirmed stenoses of the internal carotid artery (ICA) equal to or greater than a 50% diameter reduction, but no symptoms referable to that vessel. Of the 168 patients, 111 had undergone carotid endarterectomy on one side. The patients were followed for an average of 32 months, and 26 of them developed TIAs, all of whom underwent a successful endarterectomy. Three patients developed symptoms that were ignored and subsequently went on to a completed stroke. Only 1 patient sustained a stroke without premonitory symptoms. Based on these data, they suggested withholding the surgery until the appearance of TIAs. The safety of following patients until the appearance of TIAs is corroborated by unheralded stroke rates ranging from 0% to 4% and by the frequent presence of warning symptoms before the stroke events.[1,4,6,7]

Given the uncertainties concerning the management of these patients, others have elected to follow noninvasively the contralateral carotid lesions and study the natural outcome of the lesions themselves and the relationship between changes in the disease states and the late occurrence of symptoms.

In a retrospective analysis, Norving et al.[9] used a continuous-wave (CW) Doppler device to evaluate patients 1 to 13 years (mean, 6 years) following a unilateral operation. These data suggest that there is a relationship between carotid disease progression and appearance of ipsilateral symptoms. The proportion of symptom-related sides in the group of patients with nonoperated arteries that progressed and those that did not was 18% and 4%, respectively.

OUR EXPERIENCE

A study was designed with an ultrasonic Duplex scanner to follow the natural course of atherosclerotic disease in patients with nonoperated carotid arteries contralateral to endarterectomy. The aim of the study was to determine the rate of disease progression and its relationship to the development of clinical events. A recent report addressed the outcome of 134 patients serially studied over a period extending to 48 months after a unilateral endarterectomy.[15] The patients were studied before the operation and at 3, 6, 9, 12, and 18 months, and then yearly. The results of the initial noninvasive study were compared to those of subsequent visits.

At each visit a standard interview was conducted relative to the presence and development of symptoms and their time of occurrence. Auscultation was routinely carried out over the upper chest, the supraclavicular areas and along the neck, and up to the angle of the jaw. Finally, an ultrasonic Duplex scan of the extracranial arteries was performed.

The extent of arterial narrowing was determined by spectral analysis of the pulsed Doppler signal. The spectral waveforms are displayed graphically on light-sensitive paper with time on the horizontal axis, frequency on the vertical axis, and amplitude expressed as shades of gray. The spectral criteria used to identify and grade disease in the ICA and the results comparing Duplex scanning with spectral analysis and cerebral contrast angiography have been reported previously.[12] The extent of disease at the carotid bifurcation is classified into six categories: (1) normal, (2) 1% to 15% diameter reduction, (3) 16% to 49%, (4) 50% to 79%, (5) 80% to 99%, and (6) occlusion.

A table was constructed for each of the five follow-up intervals after the initial noninvasive study, and the rates of disease change from one category to another were calculated.

DISEASE PROGRESSION

At 6 months, 101 patients were seen, and 94 of the 101 contralateral ICAs remained unchanged (92%). Of the remaining 8 vessels, 7 progressed from a 1% to 15% stenosis to a 16% to 49% lesion, and 1 from a 50% to 79% stenosis to a greater than 80% lesion. At this time, four TIAs were reported. Symptoms that occurred were related to the side of a greater than 80% lesion in 2 patients and on the side of a 50% to 79% lesion in 2 others. In all 4 instances, the state of disease had remained unchanged (Fig. 47-1).

At 12 months, 93 patients were seen and 80 of the 93 contralateral sides remained stable (86%). One side initially classified in the 16% to 49% category was now classified in the 1% to 15% category. Of the 12 sides that progressed (12%), 5 went from a mild to a 16% to 49% lesion, and 4 from a 16% to 49% to a 50% to 79% stenosis. Also, of the 3 arteries classified in the greater than 80% category at 12 months, 1 had a less than 50% stenosis initially, and 2 had progressed from a 50% to 79% lesion. One TIA occurred on the side of a stable 1% to 15% stenosis (Fig. 47-2).

At 24 months, a change in the state of disease

Initial visit	Normal	1% to 15%	16% to 49%	50% to 79%	80% to 99%	100%	
Normal	2						2
1% to 15%		28	7				35
16% to 49%			38				38
50% to 79%				23*	1		24
80% to 99%					2*		2
	2		45	23	3		101

*Transient ischemic attack.

Fig. 47-1. Carotid disease at 6 months.

Initial visit	Normal	1% to 15%	16% to 49%	50% to 79%	80% to 99%	100%	
Normal	1						1
1% to 15%		23*	5				28
16% to 49%		1	34	4	1		40
50% to 79%				22	2		24
80% to 99%							
	1	24	39	26	3		93

*Transient ischemic attack.

Fig. 47-2. Carotid disease at 12 months.

was observed in 12 of 61 arteries (19%). Of these, 5 initially classified as less than 50% lesions progressed to a 50% to 79% stenosis and 2 severe lesions progressed to a greater than 80% category. Finally, one side with a 16% to 49% stenosis on the initial examination occluded. At 12 months, 4 new TIAs were reported. One was associated with the development of an occlusion, and one occurred on the side of a 16% to 49% lesion that had progressed to a 50% to 79% stenosis. Two additional patients experienced symptoms, one with a 50%

to 79% lesion and the other with a 16% to 49% stenosis. Both lesions were stable (Fig. 47-3).

At 36 months, 9 of 27 sides studied showed evidence of progression (33%). The state of disease went from mild to 16% to 49% lesion in 3, moderate to a 50% to 79% stenosis in 3 and severe to a greater than 80% lesion in 2. One side with an initial 16% to 49% stenosis had occluded. The only TIA reported at 36 months occurred on the side of a 1% to 15% lesion that had progressed to a 16% to 49% stenosis (Fig. 47-4).

Initial visit	Normal	1% to 15%	16% to 49%	50% to 79%	80% to 99%	100%	
Normal		1					1
1% to 15%		13	2				15
16% to 49%		1	18*	5*		1*	25
50% to 79%				18*	2		20
80% to 99%							
		15	20	23	2	1	61

*Transient ischemic attack.

Fig. 47-3. Carotid disease at 24 months.

Initial visit	Normal	1% to 15%	16% to 49%	50% to 79%	80% to 99%	100%	
Normal							
1% to 15%		5	3*				8
16% to 49%			8	3		1	12
50% to 79%				5	2		7
80% to 99%							
		5	11	8	2	1	27

*Transient ischemic attack.

Fig. 47-4. Carotid disease at 36 months.

	Normal	1% to 15%	16% to 49%	50% to 79%	80% to 99%	100%	
Normal							
1% to 15%		4	1	1			6
16% to 49%	1	5*	1		1*	1	9
50% to 79%					2		2
		5	6	2	3	1	17

Initial visit (left axis label)

*Transient ischemic attack.

Fig. 47-5. Carotid disease at 48 months.

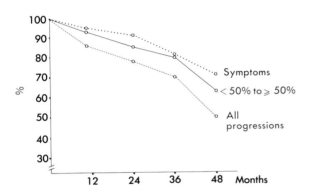

Fig. 47-6. Life table analysis. Endpoints examined were (1) occurrence of symptoms, (2) progression of disease beyond 50%, and (3) progression of disease in all categories. Mean annual rate of appearance of symptoms was calculated at 5% per year. At 4 years, approximately half of patients will show some progression of disease in unoperated ICA. About one-third will have progressed beyond 50% narrowing point.

At 48 months, 7 of 17 arteries had progressed (41%). Of these, 4 with less than 50% stenosis initially had become greater than 50% lesions or occlusions. At this time, 3 new TIAs were reported: one on the side of a stable 16% to 49% lesion and one on the side of a 16% to 49% stenosis that progressed to a greater than 80% lesion. The third episode occurred on the side of a stable 50% to 79% lesion (Fig. 47-5).

The absolute endpoints for the life table analysis are shown in Fig. 47-6. The mean annual rate of occurrence of symptoms was 5%. At 48 months, 37% of the sides progressed to a greater than 50% lesion for a mean annual rate of progression to this category of disease of 7%. When progression for all categories of disease was considered, the mean annual rate was 13%.

During the course of follow-up, a total of 22 out of 134 patients (16%) showed some progression of disease on the side opposite the operation. There were two occlusions. A total of 13 patients (10%) developed focal symptoms relative to the side without endarterectomy. All events were TIAs, and there were no strokes.

Interestingly, no difference in progression was found between patients with an initial bruit and those without. Of the 77 sides without a bruit, 13 (17%) progressed and of the 57 sides with a bruit, 9 (16%) progressed. Neither the appearance of a new bruit nor the disappearance of a previously noted bruit correlated with progression. Surprisingly, when progression of carotid artery disease was examined with respect to age at the time of entry in the study, disease change was found more rapid in patients under 65 years of age.

A strong relationship was also observed between

Table 47-1. Disease progression beyond 80% diameter reduction and symptoms

	Diameter reduction		
	<80%	≥80%	Totals
No symptoms	117	4	121
Symptoms	9	4	13
TOTALS	126	8	134

the development of symptoms and the finding of a greater than 80% stenosis either initially or during follow-up. The risk of subsequent symptoms was 7% for lesions not progressing beyond 80% and 50% for lesions progressing beyond 80% (Table 47-1). The relationship reached a strong statistical significance (p = .003). Despite the fact that there were no stroke events, we believe that the finding of a greater than 80% lesion may justify the performance of an angiographic contrast study and prophylactic endarterectomy. This belief is supported by recently reported findings on nonoperated asymptomatic patients with midcervical bruits followed over a period extending to 3 years.[20] It can be inferred from this study that it is appropriate to follow noninvasively the carotid artery without operation opposite the side of a previous endarterectomy. Surgical treatment can be delayed until the appearance of TIAs or progression of disease to a greater than 80% stenosis. Further follow-up studies should bring more thorough understanding of the natural history of atherosclerosis at the carotid bifurcation and assist in establishing optimal methods of patient management.

ACKNOWLEDGMENTS

The authors wish to thank Marian Chinn and Lorraine Jenson for preparation of this manuscript and ATL and Honeywell, Inc. for providing instrumentation used in this study.

REFERENCES

1. Bergan, J.J.: Carotid endarterectomy: a follow-up study of the contralateral nonoperated carotid artery, Ann. Surg. 188(6):748, 1978.
2. Callow, A.D.: An overview of the stroke problem in the carotid territory, Am. J. Surg. 140:181, 1980.
3. DeWeese, J.A., et al.: Results of carotid endartrectomies for transient ischemic attacks—five years later, Ann. Surg. 178:258, 1973.
4. Durward, Q.J., Ferguson, G.G., and Barr, H.W.K.: The natural history of asymptomatic carotid bifurcation plaques, Stroke 13:459, 1982.
5. Hass, W.K.: An approach to the maximal acceptance stroke complication rate after surgery for transient cerebral ischemia (TIA), Stroke 10:104, 1979.
6. Humphries, A.W., et al.: Unoperated, asymptomatic significant internal carotid artery stenosis: a review of 182 instances, Surgery 80(6):695, 1976.
7. Levin, S.M., Sondheimer, F.K., and Levin, J.M.: The contralateral diseased asymptomatic carotid artery: to operate or not? An update, Am. J. Surg. 140:203, 1980.
8. Moore, W.L., et al.: Asymptomatic carotid stenosis: immediate and long-term results after prophylactic endarterectomy, Am. J. Surg. 138:228, 1979.
9. Norrving, B., Nilsson, B., and Olsson, J.E.: Progression of carotid disease after endarterectomy: a Doppler ultrasound study, Ann. Neurol. 12:548, 1982.
10. Podore, P.C., et al.: Asymptomatic contralateral carotid artery stenosis: a five year followup study following carotid endarterectomy, Surgery 88(6):748, 1980.
11. Riles, T.S., et al.: Comparison of results of bilateral and unilateral carotid endarterectomy five years after surgery, Surgery 91(3):258, 1982.
12. Roederer, G.O., et al.: Ultrasonic Duplex scanning of extracranial carotid arteries: improved accuracy using new features from the common carotid artery, J. Cardiovasc. Ultrasonography 1(4):373, 1982.
13. Roederer, G.O., et al.: The natural history of carotid arterial disease in asymptomatic patients with cervical bruits, Stroke 15(4):566, 1984.
14. Roederer, G.O., et al.: A simple spectral parameter for accurate classification of severe carotid disease, Bruit 8:174, 1984.
15. Roederer, G.O., et al.: Natural history of carotid artery disease on the side contralateral to endarterectomy, J. Vasc. Surg. 1:62, 1984.
16. Stanford, J.R., Lubow, M., and Vasko, J.S.: Prevention of stroke by carotid endarterectomy, Surgery 83:259, 1978.
17. Thompson, J.E., Austin, D.J., and Patman, R.D.: Carotid endarterectomy for cerebrovascular insufficiency: long-term results in 592 patients followed up to thirteen years, Ann. Surg. 172:663, 1970.
18. Thompson, J.E., Patman, R.D., and Talkington, C.M.: Asymptomatic carotid bruit: long-term outcome of patients having endarterectomy compared with unoperated controls, Ann. Surg. 188(3):308, 1978.
19. Toole, J.F.: Management of transient ischemic attacks. In Scheinberg, P., editor: Cerebrovascular disease, New York, 1976, Raven Press.
20. Wylie, E.J., and Ehrenfeld, W.K.: Extracranial occlusive cerebrovascular disease: diagnosis and treatment, Philadelphia, 1970, W.B. Saunders Co.

CHAPTER 48

Controversies in the noninvasive evaluation of extracranial arterial disease

THE EDITORS

Since publication of the first two volumes of this book, considerable progress has been made in the development, testing, and application of a variety of diagnostic procedures. Some of these methods are relatively new, and we are beginning to see, possibly for the first time, some obsolete techniques disappear from the laboratory.

TESTS USED

The birth and maturation of this field has yielded the development and application of a variety of techniques. When the simple continuous-wave (CW) Doppler systems were first used to evaluate arterial and venous disorders, we felt evaluation of the carotid bifurcation would be a simple task. Direct ultrasonic scans across the carotid bifurcation were attempted as early as 1966 to assess the presence of a stenosis, but were rapidly discarded for the following reasons: (1) the location and angle of the bifurcation were unknown (2) only an audible interpretation was available, and (3) we failed to recognize the difference in flow patterns between the external carotid arteries (ECA) and internal carotid arteries (ICA). Thus we set this method aside, but it was later developed by others who had a better appreciation of the flow patterns in the two branches of the common carotid artery (CCA).[10]

The indirect tests (periorbital Doppler systems[3] and oculoplethysmography[6,9]) were introduced to detect disease in the ICA by making observations at the level of the eye—a point removed from the site of disease. In theory, and as now appreciated in practice, these tests are useful only to detect those lesions that reduce pressure and flow. The major problem with these approaches relates to their inability to differentiate a high-grade stenosis from a total occlusion. In addition, they are not suitable for long-term studies to follow the progression of a plaque through all stages of development. The OPG-GEE is the most quantitative indirect test, since it measures ophthalmic artery pressure. There appears to be little doubt that it is the best test of its kind currently in use. Although the OPG-GEE may be useful in predicting which asymptomatic patients are likely to subsequently develop transient ischemic attacks (TIA) and strokes, there have been no reports substantiating this claim.

The use of the Doppler effect to generate images of the artery where flow is occurring has produced encouraging results.[7] A stenosis can be differentiated from a total occlusion, and, with the aid of spectral analysis of velocity patterns recorded from suspicious areas, it is possible to detect degrees of narrowing that are not sufficient to reduce pressure and flow. These devices are cheaper than the more complex ultrasonic Duplex systems and will probably continue to be used by those laboratories that are working within a more limited budget.

Given the rapid improvements in B-mode imaging systems and the further sophistication of Doppler system methods and analysis of velocity patterns, it was only natural that these two diagnostic approaches would be combined into a single system.[1] Setting aside the issue of cost, the combined anatomic and physiologic approach is attractive. Although every diagnostic system currently marketed combined B-mode imaging with a Doppler device (usually pulsed), there is continuing disagreement about the relative value of these two modalities. On one hand, the proponents of high-resolution imaging stress the importance of the anatomic display and employ the Doppler system mainly to identify the branches of the bifurcation and to verify the presence of an occluded ICA. This argument would have merit if the image alone were sufficient to accurately detect and define the degree of stenosis for all degrees of involvement. Current experience suggests that B-mode imaging is best suited for the detection and classification of early lesions.[4] As the plaque becomes more complicated in terms of its constituents and the degree of stenosis becomes more severe, the accuracy of B-mode imaging in predicting the degree of narrowing becomes less.

The use of pulsed Doppler and spectral analysis is based on the premise that stenoses of the ICA will produce predictable degrees of a velocity increase and that spectral broadening will permit a classification of lesions into rather large categories of narrowing (that is, normal, 1% to 15%, 16% to 49%, 50% to 79%, 80% to 99%, and occlusion). This hypothesis has been validated by more than one study.[2]

Another important consideration relates to the application of the available tests for natural history studies. In theory the image of the artery as seen in the B-mode should be useful for detecting sequential changes in the plaque. To date the use of imaging for this purpose has not been demonstrated, and it is unlikely to be the case for some time to come. This is a result of the fact that the measurement of a dimension change becomes a problem even with high-resolution systems, particularly with lesions such as the atherosclerotic plaque. The plaque is not uniform in terms of constituents that may influence both the reflection and transmission of ultrasound. In addition, atherosclerosis rarely produces an axisymmetric lesion within the artery. Both of these considerations present a serious problem for the application of any ultrasonic imaging technique, particularly for such a complex bifurcation as that found in the neck.

Suprisingly, the use of a change in velocity patterns appears to be promising for long-term studies.[11] Any increase in the degree of narrowing must result in an increase in the velocity at the site of narrowing as long as two conditions have been met: (1) there has been no change in the flow in the prestenotic segment and (2) the site from which the velocity recordings are made corresponds to the point of maximal narrowing. The carotid circulation is rather unique in that flow does not appear to show the same changes commonly observed in

peripheral arteries under a wide variety of conditions that often occur, for example, a change in ambient temperature and marked variations in sympathetic activity. The results reported in Chapters 34 and 39 are encouraging and tend to support the use of changes in velocity patterns to follow the progress of carotid bifurcation disease.

What of the future? Whereas progress has now slowed to some degree, continued improvements in both the image quality and methods of signal processing will continue to occur. When the point is reached where both image quality and Doppler signal analysis have reached their optimal level of development, the two approaches will be happily joined. At this point, it is clear that both approaches can be used in a single instrument to derive the maximum amount of information.

PATIENT CLASSIFICATION

The classification of patients with symptoms remains fairly standard: (1) TIA, (2) completed stroke with partial or complete recovery, (3) completed stroke without recovery, (4) nonspecific symptoms that are neither focal nor lateralizing, (5) so-called subclavian steal syndrome, and (6) the asymptomatic patient with a bruit.

Traditionally, it has been accepted practice to perform arteriography for the first two categories, and possibly the third, and not use noninvasive testing procedures. This is particularly true for those patients who are considered potential candidates for endarterectomy. The use of noninvasive tests in this circumstance was considered unnecessary and wasteful. This view should no longer be considered true if we accept the following tenets: (1) patients with carotid bifurcation disease should be followed by noninvasive testing after endarterectomy; (2) with the increasing accuracy of the newer methods, some patients may not require angiography, for example those with total occlusions; and (3) the results of the noninvasive test may help decide which type of angiographic procedure is required, for example, selective standard methods or digital subtraction arteriography.

With regard to endarterectomy, the problem of early recurrent stenosis appears to be more common than earlier studies suggested.[13] We now know that this early recurrent stenosis is secondary to myointimal proliferation and not a result of technical error in most instances. This pathophysiology is poorly understood, but likely represents the response of the artery to injury. A properly performed endarterectomy leaves a large area of smooth muscle cells exposed to the flowing blood, which in some cases leads to rapid proliferation with the production of a smooth lesion that appears to have some characteristic features of the fibrous plaque. Because we know so little about this lesion and its natural history, it will be important to establish its incidence and clinical effects on those patients who undergo this common operation. In addition, it may be possible to test the usefulness of drugs that have been postulated as useful in the prevention of myointimal proliferation.

Asymptomatic patient with a cervical bruit

The asymptomatic patient with a cervical bruit continues to be a problem for the medical community both in determining the risk of a subsequent stroke and in deciding how the patient should be managed. These asymptomatic patients are usually seen because a bruit has been detected on a routine physical examination or because major surgery, such as aneurysm resection or aortocoronary bypass grafting has been scheduled.[5,8]

The asymptomatic patient constitutes somewhere between 10% and 20% of patients referred to a vascular laboratory.[5] If only patients with high-grade stenoses (greater than 50% diameter reduction) are of concern, prescreening would be useful and cost-effective. The latter is particularly true when compared to the costs of arteriography in studying this population. Although there will be some variability from one study to another, it appears that at least one-third of the sides with a bruit will have a high-grade stenosis. It is also recognized that whereas the prevalence of high-grade lesions is lower on the side free of the bruit, it is not insignificant and is in the range of 15% diameter reduction.

An important study of the natural history of these patients is to be found in Chapter 44. This study showed that a very high-grade lesion (greater than 80% diameter reduction) is associated with the development of symptoms or a total occlusion of the ICA. This was true irrespective of whether the lesion was found at the time of the initial screen or developed during follow-up. The same type of findings were noted for the side contralateral to an endarterectomy (Chapter 47).

Although there still remains some disagreement, the patient with high-grade carotid artery stenosis and coronary artery disease should not have concomitant operative procedures in most circumstances. It appears that prescreening has its greatest benefit in identifying those patients who are worthy of close follow-up after the aortocoronary bypass grafting has been carried out.

DIGITAL SUBTRACTION ARTERIOGRAPHY

The ability to obtain reasonable images with an intravenous injection or with small intraarterial amounts of contrast material has been an exciting prospect. The early reports of this method suggested that conventional arteriography and noninvasive methods would shortly become obsolete. This prophecy proved to be incorrect. Surprisingly, it has only been recently that many problems associated with the standard methods of arteriography have been appreciated.[12]

The major advantage of the digital subtraction method was touted to be the added safety provided by using a central venous injection site. Whereas this method can be used in outpatients, the total dye load is significant and, most important, resolution is often a problem. Although there was some variation in the reported incidence of unsatisfactory studies when the venous route was used, it was generally in the range of 10% to 20%. Even in the satisfactory studies, the views of the bulb were often limited and the image quality was not as good as that observed with the conventional studies.

Because of these problems, it is now accepted that the venous route for injection should be used selectively and that better results can be obtained with small volumes of dye delivered by a small catheter placed in the aortic arch. Using this approach it is feasible not only to visualize the arch and the bifurcation, but the intracranial arteries as well. This is an improvement, but it still may be necessary on occasion to use the selective multiplanar–view technique that is familiar to most of us. This is particularly true in patients with TIAs who are found to be either normal or to have minimal disease when prescreened using ultrasonic Duplex scanning.

Although surprising, the results of direct noninvasive tests can be helpful in selecting the type of arteriographic procedure to be used. If we assume that the noninvasive test is capable of documenting the state of the carotid bulb for all stages of disease, intelligent choices as to the arteriographic procedure can be made. For example, if a symptomatic patient has either a normal or minimally diseased carotid bulb, then the best possible contrast study is needed, which is the standard approach. On the other hand, a patient with a high-grade lesion may not require similar resolution for documentation, and either an intravenous route or the arterial route with a small catheter in the arch may be chosen. However, when it is important to visualize all components of the arterial contribution to the brain with the best possible resolution, then the standard arteriographic procedure must be used.

REFERENCES

1. Barber, F.E., et al.: Ultrasonic Duplex echo-Doppler scanner, IEEE Trans. Biomed. Eng. 21:109, 1979.
2. Breslau, P.J.: Ultrasonic duplex scanning in the evaluation of carotid artery disease, medical thesis, Maastricht, Holland, 1982, University of Limburg.
3. Brockenbrough, E.J.: Screening for the prevention of stroke: use of a Doppler flowmeter, 1970, Information and education research support unit of Washington/Alaska Regional Medical Program.
4. Comerota, A.J., et al.: Real-time B-mode carotid imaging. A three-year multicenter experience, J. Vasc. Surg. 1:84, 1984.
5. Fell, G., et al.: Importance of noninvasive ultrasonic Doppler testing in the evaluation of patients with asymptomatic carotid bruits, Am. Heart J. 102:21, 1981.
6. Gee, W., Oller, D.W., and Wylie, E.J.: Noninvasive diagnosis of carotid occlusion by ocular plethysmography, Stroke 7:18, 1976.
7. Hokanson, D.E., et al.: Ultrasonic arteriography: a noninvasive method for arterial visualization, Radiology 102:435, 1972.
8. Ivey, T.D., et al.: Management of patients with carotid bruits undergoing cardiopulmonary bypass, J. Thorac. Cardiovasc. Surg. 87:183, 1984.
9. Kartchner, M.M., McRae, L.P., and Morrison, F.D.: Noninvasive detection and validation of carotid occlusive disease, Arch. Surg. 106:528, 1973.
10. Planiol, T., and Pourcelot, L.: Doppler effect study of the carotid circulation. In deVlieger, M., White, D.N., and McCreedy, V.W., editors: Proceeding of the second world congress on Ultrasonics in Medicine, New York, 1974, American Elsevier Publishing Co., Inc.
11. Roederer, G.O., et al.: Natural history of carotid artery disease on the side contralateral to endarterectomy, J. Vasc. Surg. 1:62, 1984.
12. Thiele, B.L., and Strandness, D.E., Jr.: Accuracy of angiographic quantification of peripheral atherosclerosis, Prog. Cardiovasc. Dis. 3:223, 1983.
13. Zierler, R.E., et al.: Carotid artery stenosis following endarterectomy, Arch. Surg. 117:1408, 1982.

CHAPTER 49

Clinical problems in peripheral arterial disease: is the clinical diagnosis adequate?

STEFAN A. CARTER

The diagnosis of arterial obstruction should be made by clinical assessment backed by laboratory data. In the majority of patients with occlusion or narrowing of the arterial supply to the extremities, clinical assessment is adequate to detect even milder degrees of narrowing, to estimate the relative severity of the disease, and to decide on the general approach to management. In addition, the major site of obstruction frequently may be localized. This chapter reviews methods of clinical diagnosis of peripheral arterial disease and in the concluding section relates the roles of clinical diagnosis and laboratory investigation.

HISTORY

The history should be taken first; when carefully elicited it will often indicate to the physician the presence or absence of arterial obstruction and its severity even before beginning the physical examination. However, a negative history does not rule out the presence of arterial obstruction. Many patients with long-standing obstruction have no symptoms, particularly if they lead a sedentary existence or if their exercise tolerance is limited more by another condition, such as cardiac or pulmonary disease, or by other limb pathology.

Symptoms of peripheral arterial disease

The symptoms of peripheral arterial disease include pain, impotence, coldness, and Raynaud's phenomena. Raynaud's phenomena are discussed further in the section on peripheral arterial disease of the upper extremities and in Chapter 63.

Since the pain secondary to arterial disease has specific characteristics, the time taken by the physician to elicit these characteristics and the circum-

stances under which the pain occurs is worthwhile because it will usually allow determination of whether or not the symptom is caused by arterial disease.

Pain associated with exercise. Pain during exercise (walking), or intermittent claudication, occurs when blood flow to the skeletal muscle is insufficient to meet the metabolic demands of the exercising muscle; it is thought to be related to the accumulation of metabolites. The discomfort is variously described as cramps, tiredness, tightness, aching, or pain. The important characteristics are that the pain is absent during the first part of the walk, begins after a relatively constant distance has been traversed, and disappears within a few minutes after the patient stops walking. The distance the patient walks before the onset of the discomfort can vary from a fraction of one city block to half a mile or more, depending on the severity of the condition. Also, the distance may vary to some extent depending on the speed of walking, the type of terrain, and the presence or absence of an incline. It is of value to try to ascertain whether the discomfort disappears rapidly when the patient stops walking and stands still. However, many individuals do not like to stop in the middle of the street and will try to reach their destination and sit down, since it appears that relief is obtained faster when the patient sits down. This may be because of lower intramuscular pressure in the legs in the sitting position, which impedes arterial inflow to a lesser extent than does a standing position in which the muscles of the legs contract to some extent to maintain posture. Intermittent claudication practically never occurs solely from standing and should not be confused with pain in the feet caused by weight bearing, which may occur in various other disorders.

The usual site of claudication is in the muscles of the leg distal to the knee. This is frequently the case not only in patients with obstruction at the level of the thigh but also in those with aortoiliac disease. Other patients with aortoiliac obstruction may experience hip, thigh, or lower back claudication with or without more distal discomfort. In patients with very distal disease, for example, when only branches of the popliteal artery are involved, discomfort brought on by exercise tends to involve the foot and may have atypical features.

In some patients, spinal or other neuromuscular disorders mimic intermittent claudication. For example, compression of the cauda equina during walking may result in pain.[20,30,36,68] For this reason the term *pseudoclaudication* has been coined. The physician may obtain clues as to the presence of such conditions by inquiring whether or not similar pain occurs when the patient is sitting, lying, or standing, or whether it is brought on by certain movements such as bending. Also the nature of the discomfort may be different. An important point is that patients with pseudoclaudication often have to sit or even lie down to obtain relief, and a considerable period of time, for example, 15 minutes or much longer, may be necessary for the discomfort to disappear. Table 49-1 summarizes the features of intermittent claudication caused by arterial disease and of pseudoclaudication produced by spinal conditions. Characteristics of pain that are not typical of vascular disease should arouse suspicion that another cause may be present.

Neurologic examination, examination of the spine, electromyography, determination of nerve conduction velocity, noninvasive tests of arterial function, angiography, and myelography may be needed to distinguish the respective roles of the spinal and arterial pathologic conditions, especially if the two coexist.[30,42] However, it is relevant that in a study of 52 patients with diagnostic problems in whom various tests of spinal and vascular status were carried out, at least 70% could have been diagnosed by critical assessment of the patients' symptoms.[30]

Pain at rest. When arterial obstruction is more severe, patients may complain of pain in the limb at rest. This occurs when blood flow is insufficient to meet even the relatively low metabolic demands of the resting tissue. The characteristic features of ischemic rest pain are its distal distribution and relation to posture. The pain usually involves the toes and the foot. Pain proximal to the ankle also may be present if there is severe pain in the foot and toes. However, pain limited to the more proximal parts of the limb is not caused by arterial disease unless there is skin breakdown and ulceration that give rise to local pain. In the absence of ulceration, pain at rest in the upper parts of the legs, thighs, or hips is practically never caused by chronic ischemia.

Ischemic pain is increased or occurs only when the patient is supine, and it is frequently nocturnal. Relief is often obtained by putting the limb in a dependent position, probably because of the increased hydrostatic pressure in the collateral vessels, which results from the weight of the long column of blood. The increased hydrostatic pressure decreases resistance by distending the collateral vessels and thus leads to increased blood flow and relief of pain.[13,26,43] Some patients relate that the dependent position alone does not bring about relief but that walking around the room will alle-

Table 49-1. Features of the history in patients with intermittent claudication caused by arterial disease and patients with pseudoclaudication

History of discomfort	Arterial disease	Pseudoclaudication
Onset	Occurs after walking a distance	Produced by walking, prolonged standing, straightening or bending, or turning the back (even in bed)
Nature	Cramp, tiredness, ache, squeezing	Tingling, weakness, clumsiness
Relation to distance walked	Constant	Variable
Relief	Within minutes after cessation of walking (while standing)	May have to sit or lie down for 15 minutes or longer

viate the pain. This may be caused by the activation of the venous pump, which reduces venous pressure and thus increases the arteriovenous pressure gradient available to cause blood to flow through the foot, in addition to the distention of the collateral channels.[27]

A more severe form of pain at rest may be caused by ischemic neuropathy, which can result from damage to the nerves by ischemia. This intense pain may consist of paroxysms of sharp shooting pain superimposed on the more constant diffuse pain, and the relationship to posture may be lost.

Impotence. Patients with proximal arterial disease may experience impotence related to absent or decreased erection. A demonstration of decreased penile systolic pressure is of help in determining the presence of significant arterial obstruction in the blood supply of the penis and thus provides evidence that the symptom is related to an impairment of arterial circulation.[25]

Coldness. Patients with arterial obstruction may complain of coldness of the extremities, although coldness is not a specific symptom of organic arterial obstruction. History of asymmetric coldness in one of the limbs or in some of the digits is a more likely indication of the presence of arterial disease.

Other aspects of history

One should also inquire about evidence of arterial disease in other vascular beds, since arteriosclerosis obliterans—the most common cause of arterial obstruction in the limbs—is a diffuse disease and frequently involves coronary vessels, the arteries supplying the brain, and other organs at times. Therefore patients should be questioned about a history of myocardial infarction, angina, or cerebrovascular disease. The presence of risk factors that increase the likelihood of development of arteriosclerotic complications should be ascertained by determining the presence or absence of hypertension, diabetes mellitus, and smoking. The presence of arterial disease in other vascular beds is important to assess because it increases the surgical risk, which should be considered if reconstructive surgery is contemplated. The elimination or treatment of risk factors is important because it tends to improve prognosis to life and limbs.[34] Other less common causes of arterial obstruction should be kept in mind. For example, patients should be asked whether they suffer from migraine headaches, because medications used in the treat-

ment of migraine, such as ergot or methysergide, may result in arterial occlusion, which is reversible if discontinued early.[11,39,54] Moreover, intermittent claudication occasionally has been reported in patients with severe anemia,[51] pheochromocytoma,[60] or amyloidosis,[23] without organic obstruction in the main arterial pathways.

PHYSICAL EXAMINATION
Palpation of peripheral pulses

At rest. Palpation of pulses is the mainstay of physical examination, and its importance cannot be overemphasized. To acquire this simple skill, trainees must take time to practice palpation, time that will be richly rewarded. In feeling for a pulse, one must persist and try repeatedly after slightly altering the position of the palpating fingers, the pressure applied, and the position of the examined limb. If there is doubt as to the presence or absence of the patient's pulse, counting the pulse that one is feeling introduces an element of objectivity to an otherwise subjective examination. One should count the pulse aloud for 10 to 12 beats while an assistant who feels an easily palpable pulse such as the radial pulse reports whether the examiner is keeping in rhythm with the patient's pulse. If an assistant is not available, the patient may be asked to do Valsalva's maneuver to alter the heart rate to determine whether the change can be detected. Alternatively, the physician's own pulse rate may be altered by breath-holding or exercise. If the pulse cannot be counted in this manner, it is probably absent. Without these precautions one is liable to mistake the pulse in one's own finger, or at times repetitive movements of the patient's tendon, for the patient's pulse. If the pulse is palpable, one has to decide whether or not it is diminished, because a diminished pulse indicates the presence of a proximal occlusive or stenotic process. The pulse distal to an arterial obstruction has diminished amplitude and increased upstroke time. To decide whether or not the pulse is diminished, one may consider the quality of the pulse itself, but comparison with the contralateral pulse or with the corresponding pulse in the upper limb is more helpful. If the pulse is weaker than in the contralateral limb, there is strong evidence of the presence of a proximal occlusive or stenotic process. However, since the disease may be bilateral, the examiner should also compare the pulse in the lower limbs with an upper limb pulse. In normal subjects the arterial pressure wave becomes more peaked during distal propagation, its upstroke time shortens, and the amplitude increases, mainly because of the increase in the systolic pressure.[8,41] Therefore inappropriate conclusions might be drawn if proximal pulses in the lower limbs were compared with distal pulses in the upper limbs. One should compare the femoral and popliteal pulses with the brachial pulse, and the pedal pulses with the radial or ulnar pulses.

In examining a patient's arterial system, all the accessible arteries should be palpated. In the arterial supply to the brain, carotid pulses should be palpated carefully, preferably in the lower part of the neck, so as not to press over the area of carotid bifurcation and stimulate sensitive baroreceptors in the carotid sinus, which could result in bradycardia or asystole. Superficial temporal and facial pulses also should be felt. A decrease in these pulses may be caused by obstruction of the external carotid artery. However, asymmetry of the superficial temporal or facial arteries may be caused by an increase in the size of these vessels on the side of an internal carotid obstruction, when the flow in them tends to compensate for absent or diminished flow through the internal carotid system.

Unless the patient's abdomen is very large or there is guarding, the width of the abdominal aorta should be estimated to detect the presence of an abdominal aneurysm. The possibility of increased arterial width should also be considered when palpating the lower abdominal quadrants, the groins, and the popliteal fossae, because of the possibility of aneurysms of the iliac, femoral, and popliteal arteries. In a patient in whom both femoral arteries are absent or markedly diminished, deep palpation over the epigastrium to detect the presence of the aortic pulse may be of value, since absence of the epigastric pulsation suggests the presence of high obstruction of the abdominal aorta,[58] whereas in the more common obstruction in the region of the aortic bifurcation, the epigastric pulse is usually easily palpable.

In the lower extremities femoral, popliteal, dorsalis pedis, and posterior tibial pulses should be felt routinely. The femoral pulse often can be followed down the thigh along the course of the superficial femoral artery. Except in very large extremities, the pulse can be followed at least approximately 10 cm distal to the groin and often all the way to the region of the adductor canal. This is done by proceeding gradually along the course of the vessel, finger-breadth by finger-breadth, using deep palpation with both hands. If the pulse

stops short at the groin or high in the thigh, and especially if the finding is unilateral, an occlusion of the common femoral artery that tends to render the limb more ischemic or a high obstruction of the superficial femoral artery near the division of the common femoral artery may be suspected, rather than the more common site of occlusion in the adductor canal. It is my practice to feel all the pulses with the patient supine. In the case of the popliteal pulse I place the fingers of both my hands behind the patient's knee to palpate in the popliteal fossa while counterpressure is applied on the front of the knee with my thumbs and/or the thenar eminences of my hands. The pressure applied and the position of the fingers may have to be altered slightly. In some patients the pulse may be felt more readily if the knee is flexed to a slight extent while searching for the pulse. The best place to start palpation is below the level of the knee joint where there is less tissue between the skin and the bone and the vessel can be compressed against the flat posterior surface of the tibia.[29] However, in some patients who may have occlusion of the popliteal artery in the popliteal fossa, the pulse may be palpable only in the upper part of the popliteal space above the level of the joint.

The dorsalis pedis artery usually arises from the anterior tibial artery, but in some patients it may originate from the peroneal artery and in such cases takes a more lateral course on the dorsum of the foot. At times the dorsalis pedis pulse cannot be felt if the ankle is excessively plantar flexed[33] or if the patient's feet are very cold. Palpation in front of the ankle between the malleoli in patients in whom posterior tibial and dorsalis pedis pulses may be absent may reveal the presence of a good quality pulse, which indicates that at least the peroneal or the anterior tibial artery is patent down to that level. Since the dorsalis pedis artery is congenitally absent in 5% to 10% of normal individuals,[3,33,45] absence of the dorsalis pedis pulse does not by itself signify arterial disease. Absence of the posterior tibial pulse is more significant because these vessels are rarely absent as a result of congenital anomaly.[3,45]

In the upper limbs palpation should include the subclavian, axillary, brachial, radial, and ulnar pulses. The Allen test provides evidence as to the patency of the wrist arteries into the palms. It is important to avoid pitfalls that at times may lead to a false positive Allen test.[21] The ulnar artery, more often than the radial artery, may be compressed by stretching the skin over it with the examiner's fingers. Excessive dorsiflexion of the wrist when the patient makes a fist may compress the radial and ulnar vessels where they cross the wrist and may lead to a false positive test. Also, if the patient's hand is opened and the fingers extended forcibly, the skin may be stretched taut over the palm, which may lead to relative pallor because of interference with circulation through the compressed small vessels in the stretched skin.

The principle of the Allen test may also be used in assessing patency of the dorsalis pedis and posterior tibial arteries into the foot.[21] Elevation of the foot instead of clenching of the fist is used to produce pallor of the skin.

After exercise. If a patient has palpable pulses and the examiner is not sure whether or not they are diminished, it may be helpful to ask the patient to walk or do other exercise, and then repeat the palpation. If a proximal stenosis is responsible for the symptoms, distal pulses will usually disappear as a result of the exercise, and marked pallor of the foot may develop. This phenomenon is caused by pronounced vasodilatation in the vessels of the skeletal muscle, which leads to increased flow through the stenosis with resulting loss of pressure energy, fall in distal pressure, and disappearance of pulses.[15,19,38] Pallor of the foot develops because the flow is preferentially diverted from the skin to the proximal and vasodilated skeletal muscle.[19]

Maneuvers to detect arterial compression. Palpation of the radial artery, or if the radial pulse is absent or diminished, palpation of the ulnar or brachial pulse, is carried out during "shoulder girdle maneuvers" to detect compression by structures in the thoracic outlet. The maneuvers include palpation of the pulse during hyperabduction, during the costoclavicular maneuver (exaggerated military position), and during the Adson or scalene maneuver. Details of the various maneuvers are given in classic textbook descriptions.[22,72] Compression will be demonstrated by marked diminution or disappearance of the pulse. However, such a finding does not prove that symptoms are caused by compression in the thoracic outlet, since these tests show positive results in a significant proportion of asymptomatic normal subjects.[72] If the maneuver reproduces the patient's symptoms, it suggests that they are caused by the compression, but the diagnosis has to be based on an overall evaluation of the patient.

Disappearance of the pedal pulses during active plantar flexion or during forced passive dorsiflexion of the ankle may provide a clue to the presence of the popliteal artery entrapment.[14,49]

Estimation of skin temperature

Although it is difficult to estimate the absolute temperature of the skin, differences of 1° to 2° C between sites can easily be detected by palpation. Maintained asymmetric difference in the skin temperature of the corresponding sites of the distal parts of the limbs favors the presence of arterial obstruction. Also, lower temperature of individual digits suggests the presence of local interference with blood flow. However, since severe obstruction in the arterial tree is required before resting blood flow is significantly decreased, the absence of coldness does not rule out mild or moderate arterial disease.

Although skin temperature of the acral part of the limb (for example, the foot) may be lower distal to the site of the obstruction, at the level of the occlusion, collateral circulation tends to increase and may lead to a local increase in skin temperature. When the popliteal artery is occluded, collateral circulation develops around the knee by way of the geniculate system. This is frequently manifested by increased skin temperature of one or both sides of the knee on the involved side,[28] and at times the enlarged geniculate vessels may be palpable on the side of the knee joint. Therefore the finding of a cold foot with a warm knee strongly suggests an occlusion of the popliteal artery. Similarly the skin of the lower thigh, usually on the medial aspect, is often warmer in limbs with occlusion of the superficial femoral artery in the adductor canal.

Auscultation

At rest. Auscultation is an important part of the physical examination of the arterial system but tends to be neglected and underestimated. Murmurs or bruits may be produced by arteriovenous fistulae, aneurysms, or vascular tumors.[18,31,74] More frequently, a bruit indicates the presence of an arterial stenotic lesion and may allow localization of a lesion or lesions and distinction between a complete occlusion and a stenosis. Auscultation should be carried out over both sides of the neck and supraclavicular fossae, and if there are symptoms or suggestion of arterial disease in the arterial supply to the upper limbs, it should also be carried out in the axillary and upper brachial regions. Auscultation should also include listening over all quadrants of the abdomen, in some cases over the back, in the groins, along the length of the medial aspect of the thighs over the course of the superficial femoral arteries, and in the popliteal fossae. If the presence of an arteriovenous malformation is suspected, auscultation over more distal parts of the extremities should be included. Auscultation of the chest is important to reveal murmurs that might be transmitted to the neck, supraclavicular fossae, or epigastrium.

It is important not to exert excessive pressure with the diaphragm of the stethoscope because the vessel may be compressed, resulting in an artifactual bruit. This tends to occur over superficial vessels such as the common femoral arteries in the groin and the popliteal vessels. It is more difficult to create an artifactual bruit over the lower abdomen or the thigh, and one may apply a fair amount of pressure initially to be sure that good apposition is present so that a soft bruit will not be missed. If a bruit is heard, the pressure should be relaxed to ascertain whether it disappears.

The frequency of bruits will depend on the population studied. In over 300 patients with peripheral arteriosclerosis obliterans referred for assessment to the Vascular Laboratory at St. Boniface General Hospital in Winnipeg, Manitoba, abdominal bruits were found in 30% of the patients, a bruit in one or both groins in 48%, a bruit over the thigh distal to the groin in 26%, and a popliteal bruit in 11%.[9] Widmer et al.[71] used auscultation together with other tests to screen about 2000 factory workers for arterial disease. They found that the presence of bruits was a useful sign in detecting arterial pathology, indicating that it may provide an easy and valuable screening method for population studies. Although bruits over some sites, especially in the neck and supraclavicular regions, over the epigastrium, and at times in the region of the groins, may be found in apparently normal, usually young, subjects and in hyperkinetic states,[31,48,50,56,70] consideration of the clinical condition, the age of the subject, details of the physical findings, and the effect of exercise will usually suggest whether the bruit is functional or is likely to be caused by pathologic conditions. Pathologic bruits as compared to functional bruits are longer and may extend into diastole, particularly after exercise.[24,31,50,57] Bruits over the flanks, the lower abdominal quadrants, and the region of the adductor canal are rarely functional.[56,70] Also, bruits over the thigh in the region of

the adductor canal, likely a result of early atherosclerotic lesions, may be found not infrequently in limbs in which the ankle systolic pressure at rest is within normal limits.[9]

After exercise. Exercise of the extremity usually increases the intensity and duration of the bruit and thus is helpful in confirming the finding when the bruit is soft or difficult to hear at rest. Also, in the presence of a mild arterial narrowing there may be no bruit at rest when the blood flow is relatively low. Increased flow following exercise by increasing velocity through and distal to the stenosis results in increased turbulence and often in an audible bruit, thus unmasking the presence of a stenotic lesion.[6,24,53,63]

Distinction between a complete occlusion and a stenosis is of value in patients in whom emboli from aneurysms, ulcerated plaques, or areas of poststenotic dilation in the proximal part of the arterial tree may lead to localized small vessel occlusions in the distal part of the limb manifested by localized ischemic areas such as cyanotic digits[35] or irregular patches of discoloration with associated symptoms.[37] Demonstration of a bruit after exercise in such a case demonstrates the presence of a patent pathway through which embolization can occur.[9] Auscultation after exercise may also be of help in localizing the lesions, for example, when there are multiple stenoses, by allowing more precise localization of the maximum intensity of the bruits. A change in hemodynamics as a result of drug administration may also change the characteristics of the bruits and be of practical value.[65,66]

Maneuvers to detect arterial compression. In examining patients for the presence of compression in the thoracic outlet, it is helpful to auscultate in the paraclavicular region. During the maneuvers referred to earlier under palpation of pulses, systolic bruits may be heard as the subclavian artery is compressed. They usually disappear together with the distal pulse as the maneuver is completed.[22] The bruit can be heard transiently as the maneuver is reversed. Such examinations may be helpful in assessing patients with suspected thoracic outlet syndrome, but the presence of bruits during the maneuvers does not prove by itself that the symptoms are caused by outlet compression because these findings also occur in a significant number of asymptomatic subjects.

Other maneuvers to localize the site of bruits. Dowell and Sladen[17] recently drew attention to an interesting and valuable maneuver aimed at the localization of bruit-producing lesions. The "bruit-occlusion test" consists of manual compression of an artery distal to the bruit. If the bruit disappears, stenosis is likely to be present proximally in the compressed artery or in its parent vessel. Conversely, if the bruit is unchanged or increases, the site of the lesion is likely to be in an unoccluded branch of the parent vessel. A decrease in the bruit may be caused by stenosis of the parent vessel or may indicate a multiple origin. A change in the intensity of the bruit is usually most noticeable during the first few beats after compression and after release of the efferent vessel. For example, a bruit in the groin, if caused by the stenosis at the takeoff of the superficial femoral artery, will disappear when the superficial femoral artery is compressed a few inches distally, may decrease in intensity if it is in the common femoral or external iliac artery, and will remain unchanged or increase if located in the profunda femoris artery. The same procedure can be applied to the elucidation of bruits in other parts of the arterial tree.

In a patient who has a bruit in the right supraclavicular fossa and lower part of the neck and a murmur in the right second interspace, marked diminution of the bruit over the supraclavicular area and disappearance from the second interspace during compression of the upper brachial artery confirm the absence of aortic stenosis and the presence of a stenotic lesion in the subclavian or innominate artery. Disappearance of an abdominal bruit in the paraumbilical region on the compression of the right femoral artery in the groin, indicates that it originates in the abdominal aorta or the right common or external iliac vessels and not in a visceral aortic branch. Auscultation of the abdominal bruits can be carried out during bilateral femoral compression. A bruit that originates in the aortoiliac region may disappear or may only decrease because of flow continuing through patent internal iliac vessels. On the other hand, if the bruit does not change or becomes louder it is likely that it originates from a side branch of the abdominal aorta, such as a renal, celiac, or mesenteric artery. Accentuation of a carotid bruit may be produced by compression of the contralateral carotid artery.[31,57]

Significance of arterial auscultation in peripheral vascular disease was demonstrated by correlation of the auscultatory findings with systolic pressure measurements in 309 patients with arterial obstruction and 149 without arterial disease.[9] Examination for bruits after limb exercise and during compression maneuvers provided additional important information. The findings of the study confirmed that auscultation over the peripheral arteries should be an integral part of the physical examination of patients for arterial disease, since it often provides valuable information about the presence and site of arterial lesions. In a number of cases, bruits resulting from early arterial lesions may be found before the onset of symptoms and even in the presence of normal resting ankle pressures.[9]

Inspection

Trophic changes in the skin. Chronic severe impairment of blood flow leads to changes in the skin that can be noted by inspection. Since the flow is usually decreased to the greatest extent in the most distal part of the limb, such trophic changes are commonly found in the toes and feet. They include thinning of the skin, attenuation or disappearance of the skin ridges on the plantar aspects of the distal phalanges of the digits, thickening of the nails, dryness and scaliness, and loss of hair on the toes. Absence of hair on the more proximal parts of the limbs is of little significance, since it occurs frequently in patients without arterial disease. The presence of abnormal discoloration in the supine position may indicate local ischemia. Persistent cyanosis usually indicates severe ischemia or a preinfarction stage. Scattered, irregular cyanotic areas, at times resembling livedo reticularis, may be caused by multiple small emboli of thrombotic or atheromatous material from proximal ulcerated plaques, sites of poststenotic dilatation, or aneurysms.[35,37]

Chronic ulcers or gangrenous lesions are also most commonly found on the toes and feet but may occur more proximally as a result of injury in limbs with severe arterial obstruction. Skin cracking, which may lead to a chronic lesion, should be looked for in the skin of the heels and between the toes. Ulcers secondary to venous insufficiency are commonly found in the region of the ankle, most often on the medial aspect. They are usually associated with induration of the skin caused by fibrosis of subcutaneous tissue and with brown pigmentation of the skin of the ankle or lower leg. Painful hypertensive ischemic ulcers occur in the leg, often on the lateral aspect of the ankles.[62]

Positional color changes. Observation of changes in the color of the skin with changes in the position of the limb is useful in assessing the severity of arterial obstruction. With the patient supine, the examiner lifts the patient's legs with the knees straight as far above the bed as possible without causing discomfort to the patient. The soles of the feet and the toes are observed for the development of pallor. Deathly pallor develops in the presence of severe arterial obstruction, whereas lesser degrees of pallor signify milder disease. It is important to observe the elevated feet for about a minute or longer, since the pallor may not develop for some time. After observation for pallor is completed, the patient is asked to sit up with the feet over the side of the bed and to let them hang loosely. The feet are observed for the development of increased rubor. Relaxation of smooth muscle in the walls of the small vessels of the skin because of ischemia leads to the accumulation of a greater volume of blood in these small vessels when hydrostatic pressure is increased in the dependent position and thus results in a deeper color.

Venous filling time. It is convenient to combine observations for positional color changes with a determination of the venous filling time. When the patient sits up and hangs the legs over the side of the bed, the dorsum of the foot is observed for the time it takes for the veins to fill. This represents a rough index of blood flow to the foot and normally varies from less than 10 seconds to 20 seconds or more. Although several textbooks indicate 10 or 15 seconds as the upper limit of normal, in my experience this is true only if there is peripheral vasodilatation and a high blood flow. When the patient is vasoconstricted because of coldness or nervousness, the venous filling time in normal subjects may be 20 seconds or longer. The finding of a difference of 5 or more seconds between the filling time of the two feet provides strong evidence of the presence of obstruction or of more severe obstruction on the side with the longer filling time. In the presence of venous insufficiency, however, the veins of the foot may fill from above, and the test can be misleading.

Other aspects of the physical examination

Since symptoms in the lower limbs may be caused by a number of conditions other than arterial disease, it may be worthwhile to examine the extremities for the presence of several other conditions. Neurologic examination with testing of the tendon jerks and sensation may demonstrate abnormalities because of neuropathy, for example, in diabetics, or because of nerve root compression resulting from disease of the spine. Tenderness may suggest the presence of phlebitis or of a muscular abnormality, although calf muscle tenderness may be present in patients with intermittent claudication, especially if the arterial occlusion is relatively recent or sometimes if the patient has walked long distances despite claudication. Increased temperature in the joints may be caused by active arthritic condition. Edema may point to venous or lymphatic obstruction, although hydrostatic edema may be present in patients with severe arterial disease who may sleep over protracted periods of time with their limbs in a dependent position.

PERIPHERAL ARTERIAL DISEASE OF THE UPPER EXTREMITIES

Although arterial disease in the vessels supplying the upper limbs is less common than in the lower extremities, arterial obstruction from the subclavian to the digital arteries occurs as a result of atherosclerosis,[12] Takayasu's disease,[73] embolism,[73] thoracic outlet syndromes,[16,67,73] complications of diagnostic arterial catheterization,[16] thromboangiitis obliterans,[73] trauma,[16,67,73] and various conditions that affect more distal arteries of the hand or digits.[67,73] An obstruction of the subclavian arteries by arteriosclerosis obliterans is not uncommon in older subjects, and the left subclavian artery is affected more frequently than the right.[12] Such obstruction may be asymptomatic and manifested only by an unequal brachial pressure in the two upper limbs. However, since the involvement of the subclavian arteries may be bilateral, it may result in abnormally low blood pressure in both brachial regions; in such a case brachial blood pressure measurement may give an erroneous notion of the patient's central blood pressure. This consideration makes it mandatory to listen for the presence of bruits in the paraclavicular regions, which, if present, may provide clues as to the presence of stenotic lesions in the subclavian vessels and abnormally low brachial blood pressures. Patients with arterial obstruction in the upper extremities may have symptoms of claudication, pain at rest, and skin ulceration or gangrene. The characteristics of the symptoms and principles of physical examination discussed earlier in this chapter apply to the assessment of patients with the disease of the arterial supply of the upper limbs.

Raynaud's phenomena are symptoms of peripheral arterial disease that affect predominantly the acral parts of the extremities and especially the digits. They consist of episodes of white or cyanotic discoloration, usually of the fingers or toes, which may involve a part of the digit or the whole digit and at times, more proximal parts of the hands and feet. Raynaud's phenomena are thought to be a result of spasm or critical closure of digital arteries. The vasospastic episodes are precipitated by exposure of the extremities or of the body to cold and, at times, by emotional upsets. Although they may involve the toes, they occur more frequently in the fingers. They may be secondary to a variety of primary conditions that include connective tissue disorders, trauma, arteriosclerosis or thromboangiitis obliterans, exposure to drugs and toxic substances, use of vibratory tools, and other conditions. In some patients the symptoms are primary and not related to another disorder.

The diagnosis of Raynaud's phenomena is made by history of the characteristic episodic discoloration. Although a number of physiologic tests to objectively document Raynaud's phenomena have been described, varying proportions of false negative results occur with virtually all types of tests, which include assessment of responses of blood flow, skin temperature, and local systolic pressures to a cold challenge. Thus Raynaud's phenomena continue to be elusive in some patients in laboratory studies, and this parallels the clinical experience of the inability to consistently provoke the attacks in the physician's office by putting patients' limbs under cold water.

Although demonstration of a primary condition to which Raynaud's phenomena might be secondary is often made by a combination of careful clinical assessment and various laboratories studies, in some patients the vasospastic attacks may precede the development of other manifestations of the primary disorder by a number of years. Certain clues in the clinical assessment may suggest that Raynaud's phenomena are secondary. They include unilateral vasospastic attacks or episodes that consistently involve only some digits of an extremity, evidence of organic arterial obstruction, the presence of severe ischemia or necrosis, and the recent onset of severe symptoms.

ROLE OF CLINICAL ASSESSMENT IN MANAGEMENT AND FOLLOW-UP

Decisions concerning management of the patient are based on the results of the clinical findings and, as may be indicated, laboratory assessment of the individual patient in the context of the knowledge of the natural history of the disease. Patients with arteriosclerosis obliterans in the vessels supplying the extremities are more likely to have an underlying involvement of the vessels supplying other vascular beds. Many patients eventually die of cardiac or cerebral complications of atherosclerosis.[32,55,61,69] Therefore the search for underlying disease in other vascular beds and assessment for the presence of risk factors are of primary importance. The factors that adversely influence prognosis include diabetes, smoking, hypertension, and hyperlipidemia.

Despite frequent development of further obstructive lesions in the arterial tree of the same or contralateral limb,[4,64] the prognosis for the limbs is good in nondiabetic patients with intermittent claudication, and the amputation rate is between 1% and 2% per year or 10% to 12% at 10 years.[4,45a,61] The prognosis in patients with diabetes mellitus and claudication is not as good, and the rate of amputation has been estimated at two to three times that in nondiabetics.[32,61] In the majority of patients who have intermittent claudication, the symptoms improve.[4,47,61,69] Considerable improvement often occurs gradually after the occurrence of an occlusive process or its progression. The symptomatic improvement may be paralleled by a gradual increase in the ankle systolic pressure[7] and in maximal blood flow, which may continue for a year or longer.[5] Numerous studies also indicate that walking exercise training is frequently followed by a great improvement in the walking ability,[59] and about 75% of the patients with claudication may achieve remarkable walking ability despite moderately severe arterial obstruction.[10]

The relatively benign prognosis for limbs with intermittent claudication and the potential for good walking ability have to be taken into account in making decisions about the advisability of arterial reconstructive surgery, since these patients may have an increased surgical risk related to the underlying arteriosclerotic involvement of the vessels supplying the heart and brain. On the other hand, the presence of persistent pain at rest or unhealed ulceration and gangrene warrant a more aggressive surgical approach.

Patients with arterial occlusive disease to the extremities should be followed at regular intervals by clinical assessment and when indicated by noninvasive pressure measurements. An increase in the severity of the symptoms, such as intermittent claudication, suggests progression of the severity of the arterial obstruction. However, since severity of the claudication is also influenced by the amount of walking that the patients perform, it is not uncommon for patients, especially those who live in cold northern climates, to experience more severe symptoms when they resume walking in the spring after being inactive during the winter without any progression of the arterial disease. Absence of the progression may be ascertained by physical examination and confirmed by noninvasive pressure measurements. On the other hand, the severity of the arterial obstruction may increase before a change in clinical manifestations and may also be demonstrated by pressure measurements.[7,64]

SUMMARY

Previous sections of this chapter reviewed clinical assessment of patients for peripheral arterial disease. When carried out carefully by experienced clinicians, the clinical diagnosis is adequate in the majority of patients. The clinician's experience, ability, and willingness to take time to carry out the clinical assessment are important. Errors in diagnosis occur when assessment is carried out by less experienced personnel.[2] Comparisons of the results of clinical diagnosis and noninvasive testing of arterial disease have been published. Significant correlations exist between physical findings and the results of the physiologic studies,[40,44] but the latter provide more quantitative data. One study reported a significant percentage of false positive and false negative results obtained by clinical assessment when noninvasive hemodynamic testing was used as a criterion of the arterial disease.[46] In another study, in which angiographic findings were used as a criterion, clinical diagnosis by experienced vascular surgeons was as useful as the results of vascular laboratory testing.[2] It seems that it is not an important issue whether clinical diagnosis or laboratory studies are better, because most physicians will agree that the patient should be thoroughly evaluated clinically and laboratory studies should be carried out as needed to improve the assessment and assist in the diagnosis or management. The finding of false negative history is to be expected because many patients with complete occlusion of the main artery to the limb may be asymptomatic if they are limited in their ability to exercise by another condition. The sensitivity of the physical examination to detect an arterial lesion will depend on the thoroughness of the procedure, for example, whether arterial auscultation is carried

out over various sites, before and after exercise, and with compression maneuvers. Auscultation after exercise and auscultation during arterial compression are worthwhile methods for finding milder stenotic lesions and for localizing the origin of bruits. Bruits may occur at times at rest or after exercise in the presence of minor stenotic lesions and in limbs in which systolic pressures may be within normal limits.[9] Such bruits could be referred to as "clinically false positive" information. Yet this type of examination may be useful in screening for early atherosclerotic lesions and may be applied to population studies[71] for the purpose of preventive health measures, perhaps in combination with simple noninvasive testing.[52]

There is no doubt that laboratory investigations are needed in the evaluation of patients with arterial disease and might include both noninvasive testing and angiography. Angiography is most important in providing the surgeon with detailed information about the anatomy of the diseased arteries when planning surgery, but because it is associated with a small but significant incidence of complications, it should never be used just to make a diagnosis.

Noninvasive testing is useful and of great practical importance in the assessment and management of patients with peripheral arterial disease. It provides a quantitative, objective documentation of arterial obstruction and of its severity, against which the progress of the disease can be gauged in individual patients and in the determination of its natural history. Laboratory measurements are especially valuable in the assessment and diagnosis of patients with pseudoclaudication or with other conditions, such as diabetic neuropathy, especially when these conditions coexist with arterial obstruction. Systolic pressure measurement in the penis is of special value in the assessment of arterial obstruction that may cause impotence. Noninvasive testing is helpful in the management of patients by estimating the chances of healing of skin lesions and of elective surgical procedures in limbs with arterial obstruction and of amputation sites. The tests may assist in selecting patients for specific medical and surgical therapies. Physiologic measurements also will provide new data of value in research, which are necessary to gain a better understanding of the pathophysiology of disease and to develop improved diagnostic and therapeutic methods.

REFERENCES

1. Reference deleted in proofs.
2. Baker, W.H., et al.: Diagnosis of peripheral occlusive disease, Arch. Surg. 113:1308, 1978.
3. Barnhorst, D.A., and Barner, H.B.: Prevalence of congenitally absent pedal pulses, N. Engl. J. Med. 278:264, 1968.
4. Bloor, K.: Natural history of arteriosclerosis of the lower extremities, Ann. R. Coll. Surg. Engl. 28:36, 1961.
5. Bollinger, A.: Kollateraldurchblutung bei Verschlüssen der Gliedmassenarterien, Angiologica 3:293, 1966.
6. Bühler, F., Da Silva, A., and Widmer, L.K.: Die Arterienauskultation zur Früherfassung der Atherosklerose, Schweiz. Med. Wochenschr. 98:1932, 1968.
7. Carter, S.A.: Clinical measurement of systolic pressures in limbs with arterial occlusive disease, JAMA 207:1869, 1969.
8. Carter, S.A.: Effect of age, cardiovascular disease, and vasomotor changes on transmission of arterial pressure waves through the lower extremities, Angiology 29:601, 1978.
9. Carter, S.A.: Arterial auscultation in peripheral vascular disease, JAMA 261:1682, 1981.
10. Carter, S.A., et al.: Exercise program in intermittent claudication, Physiologist 23:184, 1980.
11. Conley, J.E., Boulanger, W.J., and Mendeloff, G.L.: Aortic obstruction associated with methysergide maleate therapy for headaches, JAMA 198:808, 1966.
12. Crawford, E.S., et al.: Surgical treatment of occlusion of the innominate, common carotid, and subclavian arteries: a 10 year experience, Surgery 65:17, 1969.
13. Dahn, I., et al.: On the conservative treatment of severe ischemia, Scand, J. Clin. Lab. Invest. 19(suppl. 99):160, 1966.
14. Darling, R.C., et al.: Intermittent claudication in young athletes: popliteal artery entrapment syndrome, J. Trauma 14:543, 1974.
15. DeWeese, J.A.: Pedal pulses disappearing with exercise, N. Engl. J. Med. 262:1214, 1960.
16. Dick, R.: Arteriography in neurovascular compression at the thoracic outlet, with special reference to embolic patterns, Am. J. Roentgenol. Radium Ther. Nucl. Med. 110:141, 1970.
17. Dowell, A.J., and Sladen, J.G.: The bruit-occlusion test: a clinical method for localizing arterial stenosis, Br. J. Surg. 65:201, 1978.
18. Edwards, E.A., and Levine, H.D.: Peripheral vascular murmurs, Arch. Intern. Med. 90:284, 1952.
19. Edwards, E.A., Cohen, N.R., and Kaplan, M.M.: Effect of exercise on the peripheral pulses, N. Engl. J. Med. 260:738, 1959.
20. Evans, J.G.: Neurogenic intermittent claudication, Br. Med. J. 2:985, 1964.
21. Fairbairn, J.F., II: Approach to the patient with peripheral vascular disease. In Fairbairn, J.F., II, Juergens, J.L., and Spittell, J.A., Jr.: Peripheral vascular diseases, ed. 4, Philadelphia, 1972, W.B. Saunders Co.
22. Fairbairn, J.F., II, and Clagett, O.T.: Neurovascular compression syndromes of the thoracic outlet. In Fairbairn, J.F., II, Juergens, J.L., and Spitell, J.A., Jr.: Peripheral vascular diseases, ed. 4, Philadelphia, 1972, W.B. Saunders Co.
23. Fairbairn, J.F., II, Juergens, J.L., and Spittell, J.A., Jr.: Clinical manifestations of peripheral vascular disease. In Fairbairn J.F., II, Juergens, J.L., and Spittell, J.A., Jr.: Peripheral vascular diseases, ed. 4, Philadelphia, 1972, W.B. Saunders Co.
24. Garrison, G.E., Floyd, W.L., and Orgain, E.S.: Exercise in the physical examination of peripheral arterial disease, Ann. Intern. Med. 66:587, 1967.
25. Gaskell, P.: The importance of penile blood pressure in cases of impotence, Can. Med. Assoc. J. 105:1047, 1971.
26. Gaskell, P., and Becker, W.J.: The erect posture as an aid to the circulation in the feet in the presence of arterial obstruction, Can. Med. Assoc. J. 105:930, 1971.
27. Gaskell, P., and Parrott, J.C.: The effect of a mechanical venous pump on the circulation of the feet in the presence of arterial obstruction, Surg. Gynecol. Obstet. 146:582, 1978.
28. Gaylis, H.: Warm knees and cold feet; a new sign in arterial occlusion, Lancet 1:792, 1966.
29. Ger, R.: Palpation of the popliteal pulse, Surgery 60:615, 1966.
30. Goodreau, J.J., et al.: Rational approach to the differentiation of vascular and neurogenic claudication, Surgery 84:749, 1978.
31. Harvey, W.P.: Some newer or poorly recognized findings on clinical auscultation. (I), Mod. Conc. Cardiovasc. Dis. 37:85, 1968.
32. Hughson, W.G., et al.: Intermittent claudication: factors determining outcome, Br. Med. J. 1:1377, 1978.
33. Ison, J.W.: Palpation of dorsalis pedis pulse, JAMA 206:2745, 1968.
34. Janzon, L., et al.: Intermittent claudication and hypertension. Ankle pressure and walking distance in patients with well-treated and nontreated hypertension, Angiology 32:175, 1981.
35. Karmody, A.M., et al.: ''Blue toe'' syndrome, Arch. Surg. 111:1263, 1976.
36. Kavanaugh, G.J., et al.: ''Pseudoclaudication'' syndrome produced by compression of the cauda equina, JAMA 206:2477, 1968.
37. Kazmier, F.J., et al.: Livedo reticularis and digital infarcts: a syndrome due to cholesterol emboli arising from atheromatous abdominal aortic aneurysms, Vasc. Dis. 3:12, 1966.
38. Keitzer, W.F., et al.: Hemodynamic mechanism for pulse changes seen in occlusive vascular disease, Surgery 57:163, 1965.
39. Kempczinski, R.F., Buckley, M.J., and Darling, R.C.: Vascular insufficiency secondary to ergotism, Surgery 79:597, 1976.
40. Krähenbuhl, B., and Rohr, J.: Artères périphériques: palpation manuelle et examen par la méthode de Doppler, Schweiz. Med. Wochenschr. 104:240, 1974.
41. Kroeker, E.J., and Wood, E.H.: Comparison of simultaneously recorded central and peripheral arterial pressure pulses during rest, exercise and tilted position in man, Circ. Res. 3:623, 1955.
42. Lamerton, A.J., et al.: ''Claudication'' of the sciatic nerve, Br. Med. J. 286:1785, 1983.
43. Lezack, J.D., and Carter, S.A.: Systolic pressures in arterial occlusive disease with special reference to the effect of posture, Clin. Res. 17:638, 1969.
44. Lorentsen, E.: The plantar ischemia test (contribution to the discussion about local blood pressure measurements in patients with peripheral arterial insufficiency), Scand. J. Clin. Lab. Invest. 31(suppl. 128): 149, 1973.
45. Ludbrook, J., Clarke, A.M., and McKenzie, J.K.: Significance of absent ankle pulse, Br. Med. J. 1:1724, 1962.
45a. Naji, A.: Femoropopliteal vein grafts for claudication analysis of 100 consecutive cases, Ann. Surg. 188:79, 1978.
46. Marinelli, M.R., et al.: Noninvasive testing vs. clinical evaluation of arterial disease, JAMA 241:2031, 1979.

47. McAllister, F.F.: The fate of patients with intermittent claudication managed nonoperatively, Am. J. Surg. 132:593, 1976.

48. McLoughlin, M.J., Colapinto, R.F., and Hobbs, B.B.: Abdominal bruits, JAMA 232:1238, 1975.

49. Miles, S., et al.: Doppler ultrasound in the diagnosis of the popliteal artery entrapment syndrome, Br. J. Surg. 64:883, 1977.

50. Pennetti, V., and Di Renzi, L.: On some phonoarteriographic aspects of peripheral arterial murmurs due to hyperactivity and to obliterating arteriopathies, Angiologica 7:8, 1970.

51. Pickering, G.W., and Wayne, E.J.: Observations on angina pectoris and intermittent claudication in anaemia, Clin. Sci. 1:305, 1934.

52. Prineas, R.J., et al.: Recommendations for use of noninvasive methods to detect atherosclerotic peripheral arterial disease—in population studies, Circulation 65:1561, 1982.

53. Provan, J.L., Moreau, P., and MacNab, I.: Pitfalls in the diagnosis of leg pain, Can. Med. Assoc. J. 121:167, 1979.

54. Rackley, C.E., et al.: Vascular complications with use of methysergide, Arch. Intern. Med. 117:265, 1966.

55. Reunanen, A., Takkunen, H., and Aromaa, A.: Prevalence of intermittent claudication and its effect on mortality, Acta Med. Scand. 211:249, 1982.

56. Rivin, A.U.: Abdominal vascular sounds, JAMA 221:688, 1972.

57. Royle, J.P.: Auscultation of peripheral arteries, Med. J. Aust. 2:488, 1969.

58. Sako, Y.: Arteriosclerotic occlusion of the midabdominal aorta, Surgery 59:709, 1966.

59. Saltin, B.: Physical training in patients with intermittent claudication. In Cohen, L.S., Mock, M.B., and Ringquist, I., editors: Physical conditioning and cardiovascular rehabilitation, New York, 1981, John Wiley & Sons, Inc.

60. Scharf, Y., et al.: Intermittent claudication with pheochromocytoma, JAMA 215:1323, 1971.

61. Schatz, I.J.: The natural history of peripheral arteriosclerosis. In Brest, A.N., and Moyer, J.H., editors: Atherosclerotic vascular disease: a Hahnemann symposium, New York, 1967, Appleton-Century-Crofts.

62. Schnier, B.R., Sheps, S.G., and Juergens, J.L.: Hypertensive ischemic ulcer. Am. J. Cardiol. 17:560, 1966.

63. Schoop, W.: Frühdiagnose stenosierender Arterienveränderungen, Dtsch. Med. Wochenschr. 92:1723, 1967.

64. Strandness, D.E., Jr., and Stahler, C.: Arteriosclerosis obliterans.: Manner and rate of progression, JAMA 196:1, 1966.

65. Strano, A., and Di Renzi, L.: Stethoacoustic findings on peripheral arteries and phonoarteriographic records in normal young subjects during the intravenous infusion of adrenalin, Angiology 21:678, 1970.

66. Ueda, H., et al.: Quantitative assessment of obstruction of the aorta and its branches in "Aortitis Syndrome," Jpn. Heart J. 7:3, 1966.

67. Velayos, E.D., et al.: Clinical correlation analysis of 137 patients with Raynaud's Phenomena, Am. J. Med. Sci. 262:347, 1970.

68. Verstraete, M.: Pseudo-intermittent claudication, Angiologia 7:212, 1970.

69. Verstraete, M.: Current therapy for intermittent claudication, Drugs 24:240, 1982.

70. Widmer, L.K., and Glaus, L.: Zur Epidemiologie des Verschlusses von Gliedmassenarterien, Schweiz. Med. Wochenschr. 100:761, 1970.

71. Widmer, L.K., et al.: Zur Häufigkeit des Gliedmassenarterienverschlusses bei 1864 berufstätigen Männern, Schweiz. Med. Wochenschr. 97:102, 1967.

72. Wright, I.S.: Neurovascular syndromes of the shoulder girdle. In Vascular diseases in clinical practice, ed. 2, Chicago, 1952, Year Book Publishers, Inc.

73. Yao, J.S.T., et al.: A method for assessing ischemia of the hand and fingers, Surg. Gynecol. Obstet. 135:373, 1972.

74. Zoneraich, S., and Zoneraich, O.: Diagnostic significance of abdominal arterial murmurs in liver and pancreatic disease, Angiology 22:197, 1971.

CHAPTER 50

The preoperative selection of patients: what must the surgeon know?

ANDREW N. NICOLAIDES

Symptoms such as pain on walking, cold feet, or blue toes are common complaints suggestive of ischemia. The internist or vascular surgeon must first exclude the presence of osteoarthritis, sciatica, or venous insufficiency. Although this may be easy in the majority of patients, it can be difficult when ischemia is mild, and especially when arthritis may coexist. Evidence of peripheral ischemia, such as nutritional changes, cold feet, and absent pulses, will confirm the suspicion of arterial disease noted in the history. Rest pain, especially at night, will make the diagnosis even easier, and an urgent admission to the hospital and arteriography will be arranged with the expectation of early revascularization. However, in some claudicants such clearcut evidence of ischemia may be absent because nutritional changes do not exist and all the peripheral pulses are present when the patient is examined at rest (Chapter 49).

Careful examination reveals four main groups of patients with the following conditions: (1) absent or weak femoral pulses suggesting that at least aortoiliac disease is present, (2) absent foot pulses but normal femoral pulses suggesting femoropopliteal disease, (3) normal foot and femoral pulses at rest that become weak or disappear on exercise with a variable number of minutes elapsing before their return, and (4) normal foot and femoral pulses at rest not altered by exercise. In the 1960s these were the basic observations to consider before a decision could be made that arterial disease was present or that it was of such severity that reconstruction would be justified, if judged to be feasible by the arteriogram. At that time arteriography was an invariable sequel to the clinical examination. However, the noninvasive investigations recently developed supplement the history and clinical examination and in many patients allow clinical decisions without resorting to angiography.

The purpose of this chapter is to analyze the surgeon's approach to the diagnosis of arterial disease, the decision to proceed to arteriography, vascular reconstruction, and the selection of the correct procedure in light of information obtained from noninvasive investigations. The discussion is developed through a series of questions a surgeon should consider regarding a patient with symptoms suggesting arterial disease.

IS THERE ARTERIAL DISEASE?

The value of the history and clinical examination and particularly the examination of pulses in determining the presence of arterial disease has been discussed in the previous chapter. If the pulses are absent, the clinical examination alone is enough to determine the presence of arterial disease; the noninvasive tests are not necessary to make a diagnosis, and their use is mainly to document the presence and degree of disease. In the presence of weak pulses the noninvasive tests are also unnecessary, but they can provide objective confirmation. The ankle pressure at rest will be enough for this and is useful in obese patients or in the presence of ankle edema when the pulses may not be easily palpable. However, in the presence of normal pulses and pain on walking the noninvasive tests are necessary to determine the presence or absence of disease. In such patients the ankle pressure should be measured both at rest and after exercise, because it is possible to have normal pulses and a normal ankle pressure at rest, with a fall in ankle pressure after exercise as the sole indicator of disease (Chapters 51, 52, and 55).

It is now well established that the fall in ankle pressure after a standardized exercise test on a treadmill (Chapter 55) and the disappearance of pulses and pulse reappearance time during reactive hyperemia (Chapter 56) are the most sensitive measures of the presence and severity of occlusive arterial disease. A recent study of 400 patients referred to our outpatient clinic with pain on walking has demonstrated the relative accuracy of the pulses, pressure index at rest, and ankle pressure after exercise in relation to the presence of significant arterial disease.[6] The presence of absence of foot pulses at rest, the pressure index at rest, and the ankle pressure after exercise were recorded in the most symptomatic of the two limbs of all 400 patients. A standard procedure was followed. The patient first rested on a couch for 30 minutes. The brachial and ankle pressures were measured, and the patient walked on a treadmill at 4 km/hr for a maximum of 5 minutes or until he was stopped by claudication. The brachial and ankle pressures were measured 1 minute after the end of exercise and then every 2 minutes until they returned to the preexericse level. Aortography was the objective arbiter of the presence of arterial disease; a lesion causing more than 40% stenosis in diameter was considered significant. It can be seen from Fig. 50-1 that the ankle pressure after exercise was the most sensitive index of the presence or absence of significant disease and that relying on the pulses alone would have resulted in the wrong diagnosis in 9% of patients. Whenever the exercise ankle pressure was increased or unchanged, the aorto-gram was normal and the symptoms were the result of other conditions such as osteoarthritis, sciatica, and venous insufficiency. Thus an *increase* in ankle pressure after exercise is a definite indicator of the absence of hemodynamically significant arterial disease, and patients can be saved from any further unnecessary vascular investigations.

Although the pressure index has been used in vascular surgery for many years, it is only recently that it has been realized that the relationship between brachial systolic and ankle systolic pressures is nonlinear.[2] Belcaro et al. have studied 200 patients having cardiac catheterization by measuring aortic or brachial pressure and ankle systolic pressure using Doppler ultrasound. These measurements were done during catheterization for cardiac investigation, during operations, and in the intensive care unit. None of the patients had peripheral arterial disease. A nonlinear relationship was found between the systemic pressure and the systolic ankle pressure. For systemic pressure of less than 100 mm Hg or greater than 200 mm Hg, the ankle pressure was on average 25% lower. For systemic pressure 100 mm Hg to 200 mm Hg, the ankle pressure was the same or slightly higher (Fig. 50-2). These data indicate that in normal limbs the pressure index at rest is 1.0 to 1.2 when the systolic brachial pressure is between 100 and 200 mm Hg, but in patients with hypotension or hypertension it may be less than 1.0. This is an important observation that will prevent vascular surgeons from making erroneous diagnoses of arterial disease in the presence of hypertension or hypotension.

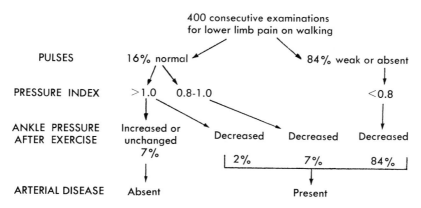

Fig. 50-1. The value of pulses, pressure index, and ankle pressure after exercise in determining the presence or absence of arterial disease.

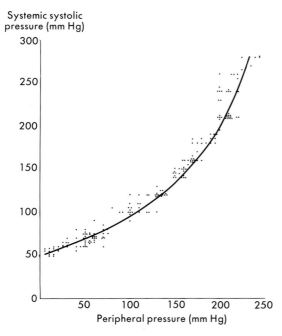

Fig. 50-2. Relationship between systemic and peripheral systolic pressures. Regression tends to be straight line through origin in normotensive patients only.

WHAT IS THE SEVERITY OF THE DISEASE?

From the history and clinical examination it is possible to classify patients into three groups: patients with mild disease and mild claudication, patients with moderate disease and severe claudication, and patients with severe disease with a limb in danger. A more precise classification is very difficult without objective quantitative assessment. The information provided by our vascular laboratory is essential because it provides such a quantitative measure of the severity of the disease.

The measurement of ankle pressure became simple in the late 1960s because of the development of instruments that could detect flow in small vessels distal to a pneumatic cuff[3,4,11,12] (Chapters 51 to 59). It is now realized that the grading of pulses as normal, weak, or absent by palpation lacks precision, however sensitive and trained the examiner's fingers may be.

The relationship of systolic ankle pressure to the presence or absence of foot pulses was determined in the following study.[9] Limbs of 82 patients in the ward were randomly selected and examined by two observers. They were classified as group A if any of the foot pulses were palpable and as group B if both foot pulses (posterior tibial and dorsalis pedis) were absent. The examiners were not aware of the angiographic findings or the operation proposed for these patients. The ankle pressure was subsequently determined by a third person who did not know the previous findings. Pulses were present in 52 limbs (group A) and absent in 30 limbs (group B). The distribution of the two groups in relation to ankle pressure is shown in Fig. 50-3. Pulses were palpable in 50 (96%) of 52 limbs with an ankle pressure greater than 100 mm Hg and only in 1 (4%) of 23 limbs with ankle pressures less than 70 mm Hg. They were palpable in 6 (50%) of 12 limbs with ankle pressures between 70 and 100 mm Hg. These results demonstrate that palpation is a very crude screening test with relatively little quantitative value. Thus when the ankle systolic pressure is 110 mm Hg, foot pulses may be graded as normal, though this pressure may be only 60% of the brachial systolic pressure (180 mm Hg) in a patient with claudication. At a pressure of 70 mm Hg the foot is not in immediate danger, but at a pressure of 30 mm Hg it is, yet palpation may reveal cold feet with absent pulses in both cases.

The decrease in ankle pressure after a standard exercise and the time taken for it to return to the preexercise level (recovery time) are good indicators of the severity of the disease, whereas the time of onset of claudication is an accurate measure of the patient's incapacity (Chapter 55).

WHERE IS THE DISEASE?

There are good reasons why one must determine whether the disease is in the aortoiliac or femoropopliteal segment, is distal to the popliteal artery, or is in more than one segment. In the case of aortoiliac reconstruction the results are good; endarterectomized iliac vessels or grafts remain patent for many years, and the patients remain symptom free. However, the results of femoropopliteal reconstruction are not as good; the primary failure rate is significant, and at least 30% to 50% of grafts become occluded in 5 years. Finally, lesions distal to the popliteal artery are usually not amenable to reconstruction. The surgeon knows that the patient will derive greater and longer lasting benefit from aortoiliac reconstruction than from femoropopliteal reconstruction and would recommend that the aortoiliac operation be performed for fewer symptoms than the femoropopliteal operation in patients with claudication. Often the surgeon cannot decide by clinical observation alone whether in a patient with

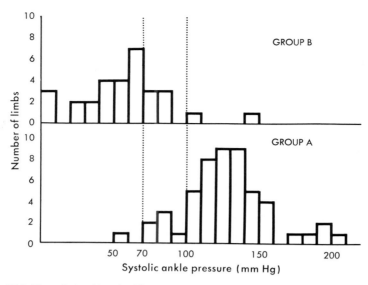

Fig. 50-3. The relationship of ankle pressure to the presence or absence of foot pulses.

obvious superficial femoral occlusion and femoral pulses, there is also an added element of aortoiliac disease. Simple auscultation may reveal a bruit at the common femoral artery, but its significance may not be certain.

A clue about the site and extent of disease can be obtained from the recovery time (that is, the time taken for the decreased ankle pressure after exercise to return to the preexercise level). A recovery time of less than 5 minutes means that there is a single lesion only and that this is most probably in the femoropopliteal segment.[12] A recovery time between 5 and 15 minutes suggests a single lesion also, but this is usually in the aortoiliac region. A recovery time that is longer than 15 minutes suggests multiple occlusions.

The recordings of Doppler velocity tracings from the common femoral artery together with velocity tracings from the ankle and the measurements made from them (Chapters 3, 7, and 53) will supplement the pressure measurements and recovery time and help to localize the disease. The principle involved is the fact that velocity tracings distal to a stenosis or occlusion are damped. In the majority of cases it is possible to localize disease by visual inspection of such tracings and to classify limbs into the following four groups: (1) no disease, (2) aortoiliac disease only, (3) femoropopliteal disease only, and (4) disease with combined aortoiliac and femoropopliteal lesions. The use of the pulsatility index, damping factor, or other measurements made on the velocity tracings and the use of segmental pressures (Chapters 10, 11, 51, and 52) will also document the severity of the disease at different sites. Although these measurements are useful for documentation and objective follow-up, in practice they are not necessary for diagnostic purposes and for clinical decisions. Visual inspection of the Doppler velocity tracings usually is adequate to classify the limbs into the four classes mentioned earlier and to answer the next question.

IS THE AORTOILIAC SEGMENT NORMAL?

The condition of the aortoiliac segment is a key question for the management of claudication. It determines the decision of whether to proceed to angiography and what type of angiogram to do, lumbar or femoral. After identifying the presence of occlusive arterial disease, the surgeon should determine whether the aortoiliac segment is normal (that is, whether the disease is confined to the superficial femoral artery), because disease confined to the superficial femoral artery is a very benign condition. In our vascular laboratory we have so far followed up 250 patients with superficial femoral artery occlusion and an aortoiliac segment that was either normal or had less than 30% stenosis in diameter.[7] There was a clinical improvement in 92% of patients with an increase in the mean pressure index from 0.4 to 0.6. Deterioration occurred in only 8%; four of these patients required operations and three were successful. Only one patient had amputation.

It has already been mentioned that the femoral pulse and presence or absence of bruits may offer clues about the presence of aortoiliac disease. However, if the Doppler velocity tracings from the common femoral artery are triphasic[8] they will confirm that the aortoiliac segment is normal. This will be sufficient to enable the surgeon to decide that the disease is distal to the inguinal ligament and that reconstruction is not indicated if the patient can cope with most daily activities and work. When this decision is made, angiography becomes unnecessary and the patient is saved from admission to the hospital and an expensive investigation. The patient is followed up in the vascular laboratory instead.

HOW SIGNIFICANT IS THE AORTOILIAC LESION IN PATIENTS WITH COMBINED AORTOILIAC AND FEMOROPOPLITEAL DISEASE?

The significance of the aortoiliac lesion in a patient with both aortoiliac and femoropopliteal disease is the most difficult question of all, but it is beyond the scope of this chapter. It is now recognized that even biplane angiograms cannot give the functional significance of borderline lesions. The pulsatility index[5] and other measurements made on the Doppler velocity tracings[8] (Chapters 3, 7, and 53) and the simultaneous measurement of changes in flow in the muscles of the thigh and calf in response to exercise[1] (Chapter 57) are attempts to grade aortoiliac lesions and to supplement the arteriogram with functional information.

THE FINAL DECISION

The final decision whether to recommend an operation or not is based on a weighing of the severity of symptoms, the incapacity experienced by the patient, and the danger to the limb if operation is not done, against the risk of reconstruction and both the long- and short-term results of reconstruction. One must be able to say how long the reconstruction will last, particularly if operating for mild or moderate claudication. Finally we must be able to say what the short-term results will be. A patient will not be grateful after a successful arterial reconstruction if he is still just as incapacitated by angina or pain from an osteoarthritic hip. The surgeon must assess the severity of these conditions and decide whether these symptoms can be relieved too, since these conditions coexist with arterial disease in many patients. For example, one may decide that a patient should have a coronary reconstruction first with subsequent arterial reconstruction. We had 50 such patients who had coronary artery bypass grafts followed by a peripheral arterial operation and who now have resumed responsible and demanding occupations.

Many patients with lower limb ischemia have occult myocardial ischemia. They give a history of one or more myocardial infarctions in the past or a history of angina that disappeared when the claudication distance decreased. In our practice, 56% of those with claudication have electrocardiographic evidence of myocardial ischemia on exercise, although only 3% develop angina.[13] We have found that although their walking ability may be limited, they are able to exercise on a bicycle ergometer and raise their heart rate to a level that will give meaningful electrocardiographic results. In addition, the ability to diagnose the presence of one-, two-, or three-vessel coronary disease noninvasively by electrocardiographic chest-wall mapping during bicycle ergometry[10] offers the chance to select the high-risk group that is responsible for the perioperative mortality (3% to 5%) and late mortality, which can be as high as 30% at 2 years in patients undergoing peripheral vascular reconstruction.

The presence of a carotid bruit will indicate the need for noninvasive carotid testing (Chapter 28); if a hemodynamically significant lesion is suggested, arteriography will be done with a view to performing carotid endarterectomy before peripheral reconstruction to minimize the risk of preoperative or postoperative stroke.

SUMMARY

The questions posed by the surgeon and the clinical decisions that are based on the answers presented are summarized in the dichotomous algorithm shown in Fig. 50-4. In our practice, 10% of patients who come to us because of pain on walking do not have arterial disease. Their symptoms are the results of other conditions. We also find that 60% of the patients have mild claudication with superficial femoral occlusion and a normal iliac segment (Fig. 50-4). They are treated conservatively. Thus 70% of patients are saved from any further investigation, and only 30% of our patients require an arteriogram.

The flow chart shown in Fig. 50-4 is an oversimplification of the surgeon's approach, and variations will occur from center to center. Every sur-

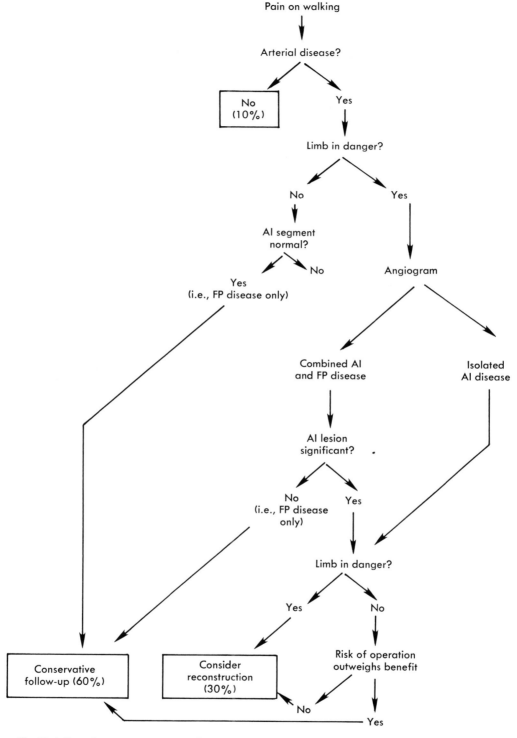

Fig. 50-4. Flow chart summarizing initial management of patients with suspected arterial disease, showing decisions based on history, clinical examination, and information obtained from noninvasive tests. *AI,* Aortoiliac; *FP,* femoropopliteal.

geon should construct a chart according to the information obtained from the noninvasive tests, provided the steps and decisions taken can be justified.

In summary, the noninvasive tests are valuable aids to the surgeon who must learn to use them to supplement the history and clinical examination to find out precisely what is wrong with the patient, where and how severe the disease is, why the patient is complaining, and when surgical intervention is necessary. Most important of all is knowing when not to intervene.

REFERENCES

1. Angelides, N.S., and Nicolaides, A.N.: Simultaneous isotope clearance from the muscles of the calf and thigh, Br. J. Surg. 67:220, 1980.
2. Belcaro, G., and Nicolaides, A.N.: The variation of pressure index in relation to systemic systolic blood pressure, Br. J. Surg. 70:693, 1983.
3. Carter, S.A.: Indirect systolic pressures and pulse waves in arterial occlusive disease of the lower extremities, Circulation 37:624, 1968.
4. Carter, S.A.: Clinical measurement of systolic pressures in limbs with arterial occlusive disease, JAMA 207:1869, 1969.
5. Johnston, K.W., and Tarashuk, I.: Validation of the role of pulsatility index in quantitation of the severity of peripheral arterial occlusive disease, Am. J. Surg. 131:295, 1976.
6. Koliopoulos, P.: The relationship of pressure measurements before and after exercise to the severity of arterial disease, master's thesis, Athens, Greece, 1981, Athens University.
7. Levien, L., et al.: The natural history of superficial femoral artery occlusion, abstract presented to the Vascular Society of Great Britain and Ireland, Oxford, England, Dec. 18, 1979.
8. Nicolaides, A.N., et al.: The value of Doppler blood velocity tracings in the detection of aortoiliac disease in patients with intermittent claudication, Surgery 80:774, 1976.
9. Poller, M., and Nicolaides, A.N.: Unpublished data, 1977.
10. Salmasi, A.M., et al.: Electrocardiographic chest wall mapping in the diagnosis of coronary artery disease, Br. Med. J. 287:9, 1983.
11. Strandness, D.E., Jr., and Bell, J.W.: An evaluation of the hemodynamic response of the claudicating extremity to exercise, Surg. Gynecol. Obstet. 119:1237, 1964.
12. Yao, J.S.T., Hobbs, J.T., and Irvine, W.T.: Ankle systolic pressure measurements in arterial disease affecting the lower extremities, Br. J. Surg. 56:675, 1969.
13. Vecht, R.J., et al.: Resting and treadmill electrocardiographic findings in patients with intermittent claudication, Int. Angiol. 1:119, 1982.

CHAPTER 51

Role of pressure measurements in vascular disease

STEFAN A. CARTER

In collaboration with Eugene R. Hamel*

Blood flow to an organ is determined by the difference in pressure between the large arteries and veins and by the resistance to flow of a given vascular bed. Under normal conditions the resistance to flow depends primarily on the degree of vasoconstriction in the microcirculation. Large and distributing arteries offer relatively little resistance to flow, and the mean pressure does not fall much between the aorta and small arteries of the limbs such as the radial or the dorsal artery of the foot.[115] Whereas the mean pressure falls slightly, the amplitude of the pressure wave and the systolic pressure actually increase as the wave travels distally because of the presence of increasing stiffness of the walls of the arteries toward the periphery and the presence of the reflected waves.[115,207]

Encroachment on the lumen of an artery by an atherosclerotic plaque or a stenosis may result in diminished pressure and flow distal to the lesion, but since arteries offer relatively little resistance to flow compared with the microcirculation, the encroachment on the lumen has to be relatively extensive before changes in hemodynamics become manifest. Studies in humans and in experimental animals indicate that about 90% of the cross-sectional areas of the aorta has to be encroached on before there is a change in the distal pressure and flow, whereas in smaller arteries such as the iliac, femoral, carotid, and renal the "critical stenosis" varies from 70% to 90%.[137,184] Experiments with graded stenoses in animals indicate that although the diastolic pressure does not fall until the

stenosis is severe, decrease in systolic pressure is a sensitive index of the fall in mean pressure and of the altered shape and amplitude of the pressure wave distal to the stenosis.[220] Studies in humans indicate that systolic pressure measured at rest is a far more sensitive index of the occlusive or stenotic process than a measurement of blood flow.[65,125]

The presence of occlusive arterial disease in the extremities may be demonstrated in the majority of patients by a careful history and physical examination as outlined elsewhere in this volume. Precise information about the site and severity of the lesions can be obtained by angiography. However, clinical assessment is subjective and provides only qualitative information, whereas angiography is invasive, may result in complications, and gives no information per se about the degree of functional impairment.[53,111,113] Measurement of systolic pressure, which can be performed by noninvasive methods easily and repeatedly, provides a quantitative, objective, and sensitive index of the occlusive process and complements the information obtained by clinical assessment and, where appropriate, by angiography.

This chapter reviews information that can be obtained from measurements of systolic pressures, examines their limitations, and surveys the application of the measurements to the diagnosis, follow-up, and management of patients with disease of the arterial supply to the extremities.

PRINCIPLES AND LIMITATIONS OF NONINVASIVE MEASUREMENTS
Principles

Technical details of the measurements of blood pressure are discussed elsewhere in this volume.

□ Supported by grants-in-aid from the Manitoba Heart, Manitoba Medical Service, and St. Boniface General Hospital Research Foundations.
*Vascular Laboratory, St. Boniface General Hospital, Winnipeg, Manitoba, Canada.

The method of noninvasive measurement uses pneumatic cuffs, which are applied around the extremity. Pressures may be measured anywhere the cuffs can be applied around the limb. Cuffs have to be of proper size because otherwise high or low readings may be obtained.[71,74] The cuffs are inflated to a pressure sufficient to stop blood flow into the distal part of the limb. During slow deflation of the cuff some method is used to detect the pressure in the cuff at which the flow into the distal part of the limb resumes. That pressure represents the systolic pressure at the level of the cuff. Various methods have been used to detect the resumption of blood flow. They include volume,[65] air,[186] photocell,[175,216] and strain-gauge plethysmography[196]; the appearance of oxyhemoglobin in the light reflected from the skin[67]; "visual flush" technique[24]; ultrasonic flow detectors[25,191]; capacitance pulse pickups[24]; and isotope clearance.[121] When carefully performed, all these techniques appear to give accurate estimations of the systolic pressures as judged by the results of intraarterial measurements,[16,79,148,191] they agree with one another,[24,25,71,121,225] and the reproducibility of the measurements is comparable to that of the routine measurements of brachial blood pressure by auscultation.[24] However, it cannot be overemphasized that to obtain valid measurements meticulous attention to detail is necessary. During measurements the patient should be comfortably warm. Pressures are measured routinely with the patient supine. Any deviation from 'his position, which could result in a difference ʾetween the level of the heart and the limb segment in which the pressure is measured, would require correction for the differences in the hydrostatic level.[142] Careful attention has to be given to the maintenance of the instruments that detect the resumption of blood flow and to the mercury manometers or other pressure transducers. Proper deflation rates of the cuff pressures during measurements, appropriate width and length of the cuffs, and the use of sufficient number of replicate measurements are necessary to obtain acceptable reproducibility.

We previously reported that single replicate determinations of systolic pressures could differ from the mean of three or more measurements by up to 11 mm Hg for the auscultatory brachial pressure and up to 14 mm Hg for the ankle and thigh pressures.[24] Expressed as ratios of the lower limb to brachial systolic pressure, these differences corresponded to 0.09 and 0.13 for the ankle and thigh

pressure measurements, respectively. Measurements in the lower limbs repeated on another day within 1 month varied by an average of 0.06 with maximal deviations up to 0.16 when expressed as fractions of the brachial systolic pressures. These data were obtained using capacitance pulse pickups to measure pressures in the lower limbs. However, similar results are obtained for ankle pressures using ultrasonic flow detectors[5] or digital pressures using various techniques.[32,119,146,156,216] Therefore when individual patients are followed or the effects of treatments are evaluated, small differences in the peripheral pressures should not be considered significant.

Limitations

Noninvasive measurements of pressures are influenced by a number of factors and have limitations. These factors and limitations must be kept in mind or the results may be interpreted incorrectly and lead to improper evaluation of the arterial status of the patient. Lack of awareness of such limitations may be partly responsible for conflicting reports on some of the practical applications of the pressure measurements.

Effect of the interruption of blood flow by the measuring cuff. Inflation of the cuff around the limb interrupts blood flow into the part of the limb under and distal to the cuff and therefore tends to decrease blood flow in the vessels proximal to the cuff. This decrease in flow leads to a smaller fall in pressure along the vessels proximal to the cuff and tends to increase the measured pressure, an effect especially important in the presence of proximal stenotic lesions. Such effects are more pronounced when measurements are carried out at the more proximal sites in the extremities and the flows to a relatively large tissue mass are interrupted.

Effect of the girth of the limb. When the girth of the limb is large in relation to the width of the cuff, the pressure in the cuff may not be transmitted completely to the vessels in the central part of the limb and the measured pressures may be greatly exaggerated. Such exaggerated pressures are commonly encountered in the measurements at the level of the thighs and are further referred to in the section on pressures proximal to the ankles.

Effect of the rigidity of the arterial walls. In a certain percentage of cases, rigidity of the arterial walls, usually caused by Mönckeberg's sclerosis, may interfere with pressure measurements. Calcification may lead to "incompressibility" of the arterial walls in the legs so that it may be impossible to stop the flow even with cuff pressures of 300 mm Hg or more.[24,196] In some instances the flow will be stopped, but the required pressure is greater than the blood pressure because additional force is needed to deform the stiff arterial walls, and falsely high pressure values may be obtained.[27,210] Theoretical considerations indicate that increased elastic stiffness modulus, increased wall thickness to radius ratio, and viscoelasticity contribute to this phenomenon.[56,178] Falsely high brachial pressure measurements as a result of arterial rigidity have also been reported.[189,205] The frequency with which arterial rigidity interferes with valid measurements of the systolic pressures using blood pressure cuffs has not been established. Earlier reports suggested that the frequency may be 1% or less,[24,90] whereas more recent publications report an incidence of about 3%,[122] 10%,[136] or higher.[62,213] An evaluation of the incidence of falsely high pressures is complicated by differences in the criteria for what is considered as normal pressure in various laboratories, by exaggerated values in limbs with large girth, and in some cases by difficulties in determining the presence of functionally significant arterial lesions from angiograms. Medial calcification occurs most frequently in patients with diabetes,[52,136] but has also been reported in those undergoing chronic corticosteroid therapy, in renal dialysis patients,[98] and after renal transplantation.[83] Neuropathy and surgical sympathectomy promote medial calcification in diabetic and nondiabetic patients.[52,76] We found it impossible to assess from x-ray films whether or not arterial calcification will interfere with the measurement of the systolic pressure.[27] Also, Bone and Pomajzl[19] found no correlation between the extent to which the noninvasive method overestimated the pressure obtained by intraarterial measurements and the extent of roentgenographic density of arterial calcification.

Certain clues may suggest that falsely high pressures are measured. Such clues may be noted by the technical personnel who perform the measurements and taken into account when reporting and interpreting the data. These clues include the following:

1. An unusually high ankle/brachial artery pressure ratio, that is, one exceeding 1.3 or 1.35, may be reported.

2. When ultrasonic flow detectors are used, a much higher pressure may be required to stop the flow during inflation of the cuffs (closing pressure)

than the pressure at which the flow resumes during deflation (opening pressure). We found in 80 patients with arterial occlusive disease that the closing ankle pressure was significantly higher than the opening pressure ($p < .001$) at times by 50 mm Hg or more. There was no significant difference in the case of brachial pressure measurements. Similar findings were recently reported by Thulesius and Länne.[211] Theoretical considerations indicate that in addition to wall rigidity, viscoelasticity may also contribute to this phenomenon.[56]

3. The progression of the segmental systolic pressures measured along the extremities may be abnormal. Noninvasive measurements show pressures that are higher in the more proximal parts of the limbs because of larger limb girth. The presence of an arterial obstruction will further contribute to the finding of lower pressures at the more distal sites. When this progression is altered and a considerably higher pressure is found distally, there is a fair likelihood that falsely high pressures are present.[62]

4. The arterial flow sounds heard, when using an ultrasonic flow detector to measure systolic pressure, may not appear to correspond to the pressure values. Ordinarily in limbs with normal or near-normal hemodynamics, triphasic or biphasic flow sounds are heard, whereas in the presence of a significant obstruction, single sounds are present and their volume varies inversely with the severity of the obstruction.[210]

5. When pressure measurements are repeated over a period of time in patients who are in a stable condition, the results vary little.[24,97] Finding a large increase during follow-up, without apparent reason, should alert the physician or technical personnel that development of increased arterial rigidity may be resulting in a falsely high pressure.

When it is suspected that ankle pressure may be overestimated because of the rigidity of the arterial walls or it cannot be measured at all, certain measures can be used in the assessment of the patient. Recording pressures at several levels proximal to the ankle may be helpful,[62] although finding a falsely high pressure at one level increases the chances that measurements at other levels may also be incorrect. Falsely high pressures are known to occur at the level of the forefoot[185] and proximally. On the other hand, calcification of the arteries of the toes is less extensive and less frequent and, in our experience and that of others,[19] does not appear to interfere with the measurements. Therefore measurement of the pressure in the toes is of special value in such cases. Also, externally recorded pressure pulse waves[24,122,136,161,174] or the flow waves obtained using the Doppler ultrasonic method[61,62,64,77,106] may be of practical value in correctly assessing the circulation of patients in whom arterial rigidity may interfere with the pressure measurements. The use of waveform analysis is based on reports that in the majority of patients with peripheral arterial disease, the measurements of pressures and arterial wave recordings appear to give comparable results and to correlate well.[24,104,136]

Obstruction in parallel vessels. Where two or more parallel vessels of comparable size are under the cuff, the measurement will usually reflect the pressure in the artery with the highest pressure and will not detect stenotic or occlusive lesions in the other vessels.[24] Therefore the measurements will not detect isolated obstruction in the internal iliac, profunda femoris, tibial, peroneal, ulnar, or individual digital arteries nor interruption of one of the palmar or plantar arches.

Effects of changes in the vasomotor tone. Changes in the vasomotor state affect arterial pressures. When blood flow is increased during peripheral vasodilation induced by body heating, exercise, or reactive hyperemia, more pressure energy is used in causing flow through stenotic lesions, collaterals, and small distal vessels, and therefore distal blood pressure is reduced. Conversely, when the flow is lower at rest, or when the patient is cool, the pressure tends to be higher. These considerations explain why pressures measured at rest are within normal limits in limbs with mild stenotic lesions and why digital pressures are altered significantly by changes in the vasomotor tone. In addition, a high tone of the smooth muscle in the wall of the smaller distal arteries of the limbs may result in an apparent reduction of the measured systolic pressure. Pressures measured in the digits are particularly affected by these phenomena, which are discussed further in the sections that deal with these measurements.

FINDINGS IN ARTERIAL DISEASE OF THE LOWER EXTREMITIES

To demonstrate the presence of arterial disease in the lower extremities, systolic pressure in the lower limb has to be compared with an index of the pressure proximal to the site of the occlusive or stenotic process. For that purpose brachial sys-

tolic pressure measured by the ausculatory technique is usually used, and the leg pressure is expressed as a percentage of the brachial systolic pressure[24,25] or as the ratio of the lower limb to the brachial pressure, a so-called systolic pressure index.[210,225] Since arterial disease may occur in the vessels supplying the upper limbs, it is important that pressures be measured in both arms and that clinical examination for the presence of supraclavicular bruits be carried out to identify patients who may have bilateral arterial disease in the upper limbs. Failure to identify such patients might lead to erroneous conclusions if the pressure in the lower limb is compared with an abnormally low brachial blood pressure.

Ankle pressures

Although, as will be discussed later, segmental measurements of blood pressure at various levels in the limbs proximal to the ankles may provide additional information of practical value and measurements of pressures in the toes are superior for the evaluation and practical applications in certain groups of patients, systolic pressure measured at the level of the ankles has been used most frequently for a routine assessment of the occlusive process in the lower extremities. Measurements using cuffs of the standard 12 cm width give values that agree well with intraarterial measurements.[16,148,191] Ankle pressures reflect the overall occlusive process in the main proximal arteries, which may be amenable to arterial reconstruction, except for disease of individual vessels distal to the division of the popliteal artery. In the absence of disease in more proximal arteries, ankle pressures may be normal when one or two of the popliteal branches are occluded.[24] For example, a normal pressure may be measured in the presence of the occlusion of the anterior and posterior tibial arteries when there is a large peroneal vessel free of disease.[24] However, when ankle pressures are measured using ultrasonic flow detectors, a clue may be obtained about disease in the individual tibial branches. A difference of more than 15 mm Hg between pressures measured by detecting flow over the dorsal artery of the foot and the posterior tibial artery suggests a lesion in the vessel that gives the lower pressure, although a smaller difference does not rule it out.[25] These considerations should also be kept in mind when interpreting pressure measurements at the level of the calf.

Blood flow measured at rest often is within normal limits in limbs with an arterial occlusive process.[65,125] In contrast to flow measurements, resting systolic pressures have been reported by Naumann,[144] Winsor,[222] and Gaskell[65] to be diminished, and this finding has since been confirmed by numerous reports. Strandness and co-workers,* in a series of publications, successfully applied pressure measurements to the assessment and follow-up of patients with peripheral vascular disease. Because of systolic amplification ankle pressure is almost always greater than brachial pressure in the absence of a significant narrowing. Although some reports give ankle pressures of 90% of the brachial pressure or less as the lower limit of normal,[210] it is likely that the presence of mild stenotic lesions in asymptomatic patients or the use of too wide a cuff[210] is responsible for the low readings, and therefore a more correct lower limit of normal is 97% of the brachial pressure.[24,25,225] Experience with a large number of cases suggests that the lower

*References, 9, 10, 187, 188, 192, 193, 195-199, 204.

limit of normal for the ankle pressures, measured using blood pressure cuffs, may increase with age. This is supported by the finding that the difference between the thigh or calf pressure and the brachial pressure is greater in older patients.[12] In subjects of the age usually encountered in patients with arteriosclerosis obliterans, ankle pressures that are equal to or even a few millimeters of mercury greater than brachial pressures may be associated with a mild arterial stenosis.[26,29] The apparent increase in the pressure in the legs as compared with that in the arm in older patients may be related to the greater increase in stiffness of the walls of the leg arteries with aging.[218] This could result in some overestimation of the pressure in the lower limbs.[12] Intraarterial measurements actually indicate that systolic amplification in the aortoiliac axis[163] and in the arteries of the lower limbs[28] does not increase with age.

Correlation with angiography. Carter[24,25] and Yao et al.[225] correlated measurements of ankle systolic pressures with angiographic documentation of the disease in large series of cases. Fig. 51-1 illustrates

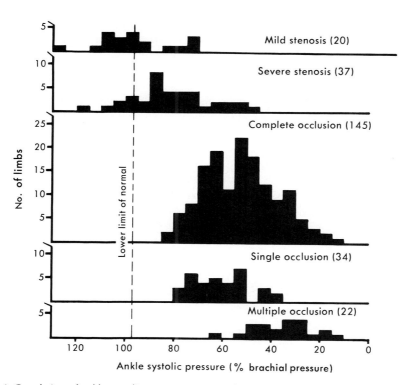

Fig. 51-1. Correlation of ankle systolic pressures measured at rest with angiographic findings. Numbers in parentheses indicate number of limbs. (From Carter, S.A.: JAMA 207:1869, 1969. Copyright 1969, American Medical Association.)

that ankle pressures are always abnormal in limbs with complete arterial occlusion. In most cases they do not exceed 80% of the brachial pressure, but in some limbs with well-developed collateral pathways pressures may range from 80% to 90%. In limbs with a single complete occlusion the pressure is usually 50% or more of the brachial pressure, whereas in those with two or more occlusions in series it is usually less than 50%. The presence of some overlap is not surprising because of differences in the length, diameter, and number of the collateral pathways. For example, it is often observed that soon after an acute arterial occlusion the ankle pressure may be quite low, often less than 50% of the brachial pressure. However, over a period of time as the collateral circulation and symptoms improve, the pressure increases to values greater than 50%.

In limbs with arterial stenosis, pressures range from about 50% of the brachial levels to values within normal limits. This is also not surprising, since the degree of narrowing varies and considerable encroachment on the lumen has to be present before there are appreciable effects on distal flow and pressure.[137,184] In the majority of patients with stenotic lesions and normal ankle pressures shown in Fig. 51-1 there were no symptoms.[25]

Effect of changes in blood flow. It is known that the decrease in pressure across an arterial narrowing or across collateral pathways, which bypass an arterial occlusion, depends on the rate of blood flow. This has been well documented by studies on the ''critical arterial stenosis'' in experimental animals and in humans.[137,179,184] The pressure drop increases with increased blood flow, which may be produced by vasodilation in the peripheral resistance vessels in the limb distal to the site of the arterial obstruction. An increase in blood flow may result in a pressure gradient in a case of a mild narrowing, when there is no pressure drop under resting or low-flow conditions. Since blood flow through the skin of the extremities increases manyfold when there is need to eliminate heat as part of the function of the regulation of the body temperature,[78,177] the question arose whether physiologic changes in cutaneous blood flow might influence pressure measurements in limbs with arterial disease. To study the effect of changes in skin blood flow, body heating and cooling were induced in 13 normal subjects by a modification of the procedure of Gibbon and Landis.[75,206] The presence of large changes in blood flow was con-

firmed by the finding of changes in digital skin temperatures that exceeded 10° C in all cases. There was a systematic increase in the ankle systolic pressure with body cooling that amounted to 20 mm Hg or more in 8 subjects ($p < .001$). However, body cooling was also associated with an increase in central blood pressure as shown by an increase in the brachial pressure. The systematic change in ankle pressure with body cooling was diminished or abolished when ankle pressure was expressed as percentage of the brachial systolic pressure, and the difference between heating and cooling became insignificant ($p > .05$). Ankle pressure expressed as percentage of brachial pressure was higher during cooling in eight and lower in five limbs. The differences were never greater than 15%, in most cases less than 10%. These findings indicate that smaller changes in cutaneous blood flow during routine measurements of ankle pressures in patients with peripheral arterial disease are not likely to affect the results appreciably when ankle pressure is expressed as percentage of the brachial pressure.

Changes in blood flow through the large muscle mass of a lower limb in response to various interventions can result in larger changes in blood flow and have profound effects on distal arterial pressure. Distal pressures have been measured after exercise and in response to reactive hyperemia. Types of exercise used include walking at a fixed rate in a corridor,[129] walking on a treadmill at various speeds and elevations,* toe stands[23] and step test,[36] and flexion-extension exercise of the ankle.[26] Cappelen and Hall[23] demonstrated a large decrease in the intraarterially recorded pressure from the dorsal artery of the foot in limbs with intermittent claudication during exercise. Strandness et al.[110,190,193,204] studied changes in ankle blood pressure and calf blood flow in response to exercise in normal limbs and in limbs of patients with arterial disease at various levels. Fig. 51-2 shows that in the presence of a severe arterial stenosis there is a profound drop in ankle pressure after exercise that takes several minutes to return to the preexercise level. The time course of the return of the pressure closely parallels the time course of the postexercise hyperemia shown by the calf blood flow. The extent of the postexercise pressure drop and the time required for it to return to the preexericse level depend on the number, severity, and level of the sten-

---

*References. 110, 125, 190, 193, 195, 204, 224.

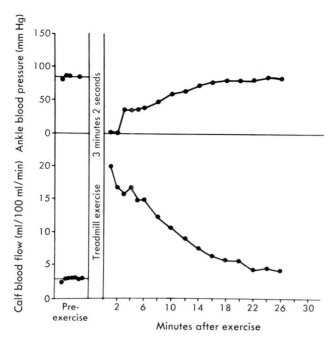

Fig. 51-2. Effect of exercise on ankle systolic pressure and calf blood flow in a limb with severe arterial stenosis. (From Sumner, D.S., and Strandness, D.E., Jr.: Surgery 65:763, 1969.)

otic or occlusive lesions.[36,125,193,204,224] Thus measurements of pressure after exercise provide more physiologic information about circulation in limbs with arterial disease than do measurements taken at rest. Similar changes in pressure in limbs with arterial disease occur during reactive hyperemia produced by a period of occlusion of blood flow to the limb using thigh cuffs inflated to suprasystolic pressures.[18,46,103] The degree of postexercise or reactive hyperemia depends also on the severity of the exercise or the period of ischemia. When ischemia is prolonged or the exercise severe, ankle systolic pressure will decrease to some extent even in normal limbs,[134,190] and a positive brachial-to-ankle pressure difference may develop.[26,134]

Demonstration of the presence of mild arterial disease. Fig. 51-1 showed that in some patients with an arterial stenosis ankle pressure may be within normal limits. Although the majority of such patients do not have symptoms, on occasion patients with symptoms consistent with intermittent claudication may have ankle pressures that, at rest, are greater than the brachial pressure.[26,192] Measurement of pressure after exercise is then of help in deciding whether the symptoms are a result of ar-

terial disease.[195] Fig. 51-3 shows changes in the ankle pressure and the brachial-ankle pressure difference in such a patient. The ankle pressure was higher than the brachial pressure at rest but fell profoundly after supine exercise, which consisted of flexion-extension of the ankle for 2½ minutes at a rate of one a second, and took several minutes to return to preexercise level. Although ankle pressure after exercise decreased in relation to the brachial pressure in 34 of 37 limbs of normal subjects, it remained higher than the brachial in 30 of these limbs.[26] The greatest brachial-ankle pressure difference after exercise in the normal group was 7 mm Hg. Statistical evaluation of the results in the normal limbs indicates that after this type of exercise the brachial-ankle difference should be less than 9 mm Hg. A difference of 9 to 16 mm Hg represents a borderline response, and more than 16 mm Hg is abnormal. Ankle pressures at rest were normal in 7 of 14 limbs with mild arterial disease and in 13 of 18 with questionable arterial disease.[26] All 14 limbs with mild arterial disease showed abnormal responses to exercise. Among the limbs with questionable disease 11 had an abnormal response, 4 responses were borderline, and 3 were within normal limits.

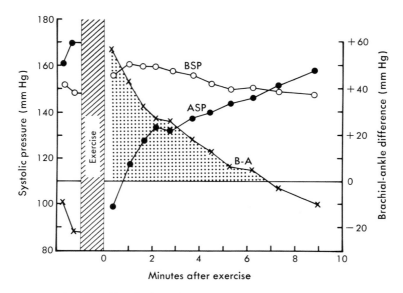

Fig. 51-3. Response of ankle and brachial systolic pressure to leg exercise in a patient with questionable arterial disease. Scale on left is for ankle systolic pressure (*ASP*, solid circles) and brachial systolic pressure (*BSP*, open circles); scale on right is for brachial minus ankle pressure difference. *B-A*, Crosses; dotted area indicates positive difference. (Reprinted by permission. From N. Engl. J. Med. 287:578, 1972.)

A correlation exists between the brachial-ankle difference at rest and after exercise. We often find in older patients that if ankle pressure at rest is less than 110% of the brachial, the response to exercise is abnormal; if it is 115% or more at rest, then the response is within normal limits. Measurements after supine exercise may have some advantage as compared with testing after walking, since the first measurement can usually be obtained within 10 to 20 seconds after cessation of exercise, and a longer time may be necessary to obtain the first measurement after walking. In some patients with mild stenotic lesions the drop in ankle pressure may be quite transient and difficult to demonstrate if the first measurements are not obtained quickly. Simultaneous measurement of brachial pressure increases the usefulness of the test because, on occasion, ankle pressure might show little change after exercise, but a simultaneous increase in the brachial pressure would indicate that an abnormal brachial-ankle pressure difference had developed.

There is considerable interest in the measurements of distal systolic pressures in response to exercise and reactive hyperemia. Large numbers of patients are tested by these methods in vascular laboratories,[123] and recent studies compare the results of pressure measurements following various forms and intensities of exercise and during reac-

tive hyperemia.[3,96,131,133] There are advantages and disadvantages in the various methods of testing. Measurements during reactive hyperemia do not require the patient to walk, can be carried out in laboratories that do not possess treadmills, and are generally less time consuming. However, measurement after exercise may separate more completely patients with mild disease from normal subjects and is preferable for the assessment of patients with "pseudoclaudication" and normal resting ankle pressures.[96] Also, in patients who had femoropopliteal bypass surgery, application of suprasystolic pressures over the graft for a considerable period of time may not be advisable at least in the early postoperative period.[96] There is no doubt that measurements after exercise or during reactive hyperemia are useful in making the diagnosis in patients with mild or questionable arterial disease. Disappearance of previously palpable pulses or development or increase in the intensity of arterial bruits is a clinical counterpart to the increased blood flow after exercise.[7,29] However, measurement of ankle pressure provides a more objective and quantitative method. A normal pressure response can rule out arterial disease as the cause of symptoms and is particularly useful in the diagnosis of patients with pseudoclaudication who may develop pain in the limbs on walking as a result of spinal or neuromuscular disorders.[55,96] Measurements after stress are of value in such cases and in other selected patients and provide physiologic information about the functional state of the circulation that may be of interest for research purposes and special applications. However, in the majority of patients with clinically significant arterial obstruction, measurements of pressure at rest are sufficient to demonstrate the presence and to assess the severity of the obstruction, and the measurements after stress are not needed for clinical purposes.[165] This is also corroborated by close correlation between the brachial-ankle pressure difference at rest and after exercise.[26,133]

Cholesterol crystal or atherothrombotic embolization from the sites of ulcerated atherosclerotic lesions in the proximal but patent arterial tree[2,108] can occlude small muscular arteries, as documented by muscle biopsies.[2,108] Although intermittent claudication primarily caused by occlusion of the small muscular arteries appears to be rare, measurement of blood flow after exercise might demonstrate an abnormality in such cases.[66]

Pressures proximal to the ankles

Winsor[222] reported in 1950 on segmental measurements at various levels in the upper and lower limbs in 10 young normal subjects and showed that the measurements were abnormal in patients with arterial disease. A large number of reports have since appeared. However, such measurements are affected by various artifacts more than ankle pressures. Also, differences in the techniques and width of cuffs used in the various studies can affect the results and further limit the practical usefulness of such studies.*

Thigh pressures. Relatively greater range of variation in the girth and shape of the thigh contributes to a fairly large range of values found in normal patients and patients with arterial disease. In the majority of studies systolic pressures at the level of the thigh were found to be higher than brachial systolic pressure. There is little doubt that thigh pressures tend to be overestimated because cuff pressure may not be transmitted completely to the vessels in the central part of this wide region of the limb. Intraarterial pressure measurements show that femoral pressure at the groin corresponds closely to the brachial systolic pressure,[167] but systolic pressure increases distally in the limb, with

pressures in the dorsal artery of the foot and the posterior tibial artery being consistently greater than femoral pressure.[28,115,120] Therefore "true" pressures in the upper part of the thigh should be only slightly greater than brachial pressure, but the difference would be expected to increase in the lower part of the thigh and distally.

A review of the published results suggests that cuffs of the standard width of 12 cm or narrower, even if the bladder is long, tend to overestimate thigh pressure considerably.[43,63] Cuffs 15 to 18 cm in width with a long bladder appear to give values that correspond reasonably well with the pressures that would be expected on the basis of intraarterial findings. Since considerable taper of the circumference of the thigh in some subjects makes it difficult to apply wider cuffs, the 15 cm cuff may give a better fit in such cases and therefore more consistent results, even though the values may be overestimated to some extent.[24,112] Bell et al.[11] reported that thigh pressure did not differ significantly from the brachial (range − 22 to + 28 mm Hg) in 30 normal subjects. They used an 18 cm wide cuff but did not state where along the thigh the cuff was applied. Using a 15 cm cuff at the lower thigh (above the knee), we found that the pressure averaged 116% of the brachial pressure in 24 subjects without peripheral vascular disease, with the lower limit of normal 107% of brachial pressure.[24] Although assessment of the vessels proximal to the groin is very important for practical decisions regarding surgical management, it cannot always be made reliably by noninvasive methods.

The pressure at the upper thigh is greatly influenced by the size of the limb and the width of the measuring cuffs, and normal standards have to be determined by each laboratory. It is helpful to measure the circumference of the limb at the site of the measurement and to take it into account in the interpretation of the results. In our laboratory 12 cm wide cuffs are used at the upper thigh, and, from experience, the pressure at the upper thigh has to exceed the brachial pressure by 30 mm Hg if it is to be considered normal. It appears that the main value of the measurements at the upper thigh is to exclude hemodynamically significant aortoiliac occlusive disease at rest when the pressure is clearly normal.[57] However, such pressures measured at rest do not rule out mild proximal lesions. Measurements during reactive hyperemia or following intraarterial injection of vasodilating agents are needed for that purpose.[21,35]

*References 11, 24, 43, 63, 130, 186.

If the pressure at the upper thigh is lower than that of the arm or significantly lower than that of the opposite limb, significant obstruction is present at or proximal to the upper thigh. The obstruction might be proximal to the groin or in the upper part of the thigh, especially in limbs with obstruction of the superficial femoral artery and a poorly developed or diseased profunda artery. If the pressure at the upper thigh is equal or only slightly higher than the arm pressure and there is little difference between the two lower limbs, the presence of an obstruction at or proximal to the upper thigh cannot be ruled out.[194] Consideration of all information including clinical findings, pressure at the upper thigh, pressure gradients distally along the limb, and angiography results may help elucidate the problem. If it is important to assess more precisely the arteries proximal to the groin to make therapeutic decisions, other methods may have to be resorted to in individual patients. The techniques that may be useful include comparison of intraarterial pressures measured in the femoral and brachial arteries,[21,35,82,217] and recording of blood flow velocity waves from over the femoral arteries.[61,104] An abnormally low thigh pressure usually indicates the presence of disease at or proximal to that level, but normal pressure may not rule out disease of the superficial femoral artery, depending on the placement of the cuffs and the site of the occlusion. When the superficial femoral artery is occluded near its origin and the deep femoral artery enlarges to provide collateral circulation to the distal part of the limb, a cuff at the thigh that overlies the superficial femoral occlusion may give pressure values within normal limits because the measurement gives the high pressure in the enlarged deep femoral artery.[24]

Calf pressures. In 30 normal subjects, with the cuffs applied just below the knees, Bell et al.[11] found pressures to average 5 mm Hg above the brachial (range − 16 to + 28 mm Hg) using an 18 cm wide cuff and digital plethysmography. Cutajar et al.[43] used a standard 12 cm cuff and Doppler ultrasonic flow detector in another group of 30 normal subjects and found the pressure to average 117% of the brachial with a range of 100% to 140%. Similar results were reported by Fronek et al.[63]

Pressure gradients. Abnormal differences between pressures measured at the upper thigh, above the knee (low thigh), at the calf, and at the ankle

may provide information about the number and site of the occlusive or stenotic lesions. Findings to date have been correlated with angiographic documentation of the disease.* Despite the differences in the size of the cuffs and the techniques used in different studies, most workers agree that a gradient of less than 20 mm Hg between contiguous sites along the extremity is normal. Usually, gradients of 20 to 30 mm Hg would be considered borderline and greater than 30 mm Hg abnormal.[6,196] Cuff artifacts are probably responsible for the apparently ''normal'' gradients without an arterial lesion. In the presence of an obstruction these and other measurement artifacts can at times seriously affect segmental pressure measurements and the apparent pressure gradients. When there is a proximal lesion, the level at which the cuff is applied to measure pressure in the extremity distal to the lesion could affect the measurements and contribute to an apparent gradient.[120] For example, blood flow through collaterals bypassing an iliac occlusion would be lower when a thigh cuff is inflated than during inflation of an ankle cuff, since flow through a large part of the limb would be cut off during the measurement of thigh pressure. This would tend to increase the pressure measured at the thigh and increase the thigh-ankle difference. Also, falsely low pressures may at times be measured in the presence of arterial obstruction distal to the cuffs,[13] and the measurements can be affected by the type of flow-sensing device and the site at which it is applied.[59] Below the knee the presence of three branches of the popliteal artery in parallel and the capacity for extensive collateral interconnections in this part of the limb may result in normal gradients from the calf to the ankle in the presence of an extensive occlusive process.[192] It is desirable to measure brachial pressure by ausculation simultaneously with the lower limb pressures and to make corrections for changes in the brachial pressure.[63] At times, when the patient's thigh is large, inflation of the cuff to a high pressure may cause considerable discomfort and result in an increase in the central and peripheral blood pressures.[11,24] Differences of more than 15 to 20 mm Hg between pressures in the two lower limbs measured at the same level are also indicative of arterial disease.[63]

---

*References 12, 24, 63, 81, 84, 196.

Pressures distal to the ankles

Since ankle pressures may not provide information about disease in the individual branches of the popliteal artery, do not reflect arterial disease that may be present in the small vessels distal to the ankle, and can give falsely high values in the presence of medial calcification, there is considerable interest in the measurement of the more distal pressures.

Foot pressures. Winsor[222] reported on the measurements using 13 cm wide cuffs applied to the ankle and the foot in 10 young normal individuals and found that the average difference between the ankle and foot pressures was 17 mm Hg, although the range of values was not given. He found that the difference was increased in some patients with peripheral arterial disease. Hirai and Shionoya[88] studied 50 limbs of patients with thromboangiitis obliterans with angiographic documentation of occlusion of the arteries distal to the popliteal bifurcation and without evidence of more proximal disease. They measured foot pressures using 6 cm wide cuffs and photoelectric plethysmography and found that the pressures averaged between 50 and 60 mm Hg lower than brachial systolic pressure, although they did not report data in subjects without arterial obstruction. In all limbs the difference exceeded 20 mm Hg with a range of more than 20 to about 100 mm Hg. The average difference between ankle and foot systolic pressures averaged approximately 40 mm Hg, although individual values of the differences were not given. The difference between foot and toe pressure in the same study was significantly greater in those patients who had foot claudication and averaged 40 to 50 mm Hg, although it appears that there was considerable overlap between limbs with and without foot claudication.

Gaskell[69] studied foot pressures in the limbs of 59 normal subjects 19 to 59 years of age and in 43 patients with arterial disease and angiographic visualization of limb arteries, including the vessels down to and including the foot. A spectroscopic method was used to determine systolic endpoint during deflation of contoured 9 cm wide cuffs wrapped around the forefoot. Foot pressures were compared with ankle systolic pressures. On the basis of this study the difference between the ankle and foot pressures in normal subjects should be less than 30 mm Hg. A larger difference is abnormal. Since pressure differences along the distal

parts of the lower and upper limbs may be increased in hypertension even in the absence of arterial obstruction, abnormally high ankle-to-foot pressure differences could be present in hypertensive patients, although further data to establish this point are needed. In patients with additional significant obstruction in the proximal arteries, low ankle pressures, and low blood flows in the feet, differences between ankle and foot pressures of less than 30 mm Hg may be associated with obstruction of the foot arteries. Also, foot pressures have been reported to give falsely high values in some cases with medial calcification.[185] Measurements of foot pressures may be of special value in the assessment of distal arterial obstruction when pressures cannot be measured in the toes because of previous amputations or the presence of skin lesions.

Toe pressures. There are many reports on the pressures measured in the toes. Measurements in patients with arterial disease were reported as early as 1934.[58] Conrad and Green[42] found that systolic pressures in the second toe were decreased in patients with severe arterial disease and that the brachial-toe pressure difference was increased. They reported that in normal subjects there was no significant difference between the brachial and toe pressures. However, they used a 1 cm wide cuff, which is too narrow and which probably gave values too high for the pressures in the digits. Pressures measured using pneumatic cuffs will be overestimated if the cuff is too narrow and may be underestimated if it is too wide.[71,74,127] There appears to be a range of cuff widths in which the measured pressure does not change much. This was shown for the toes,[127] fingers,[71] and the brachial region[74]; in the latter case the findings were compared with intraarterial recordings. In the second toe, systolic pressures show little change with cuffs between 2 and 3 cm in width.[127] Since a certain length of the digit is needed to apply the sensing device distal to the cuff, the 2 cm cuff was used in our studies.[32,127,128] We also found that a 3 cm cuff on the big toe gave values comparable to those from the 2 cm cuff on the second toe.[32]

Since cuffs are usually applied at the base of the toe, the measurements cannot detect disease in the vessels situated more distally near the tip of the digit. Also, since digits have two main lateral arteries, occlusion of only one of these vessels would not be detected.[50] Comparison of measurements in the toes with the cuff applied at the base and 1 cm distally along the digit showed no significant differences in normal subjects, indicating that there is no steep fall in the pressure along the toe and that small differences in the exact positioning of the cuff are not important as long as the proximal edge of the cuff is not more than 1 cm from the base of the digit.[127]

Measurements are carried out with the patients in a supine position, and the toes are then higher relative to the level of the heart than the sites where pressures are measured proximally in the lower and in the upper limbs. This difference in level corresponds to an average difference of 9 mm Hg in hydrostatic pressure.[127] We do not correct for the difference in level because the uncorrected values reflect the transmural pressure that exists when the patients are in bed in the supine position. The very low values recorded in some patients with severe occlusive disease emphasize the importance of treatment by having the limbs in the dependent position, which results in increase in hydrostatic pressure.[32,127] The near zero or unmeasurable toe pressures in some patients indicate that there may be little or no blood flow in their toes in the supine position.[32]

In normal subjects toe pressures are always found to be lower than ankle pressures and usually lower than brachial systolic pressures.[127] Validity of these findings would require comparison with direct pressure measurements, which are not available. However, our data on the relation of the toe pressures to proximal pressures are similar to those obtained by intraarterial studies in vessels of comparable size in dogs.[202] Also, a single report on measurement of intraarterial pressure in a finger artery showed that finger pressure was lower than the brachial pressure.[148] The decrease in systolic pressure between the ankle and the toe must be a result of smaller diameter of the arteries of the feet, which results in damping of the pressure wave, and greater resistance, which leads to a loss of some of the pressure energy during flow through the foot.

Since the arteries of the feet offer a greater resistance to flow than do the more proximal conduit vessels, the change in pressure along the foot is affected by changes in blood flow to a greater extent than are the more proximal pressures. We found in normal subjects that systolic pressure in the second toe decreased during body heating as compared to body cooling, and the ankle-toe and brachial-toe pressure differences showed opposite changes, that is, they increased during body heating and

decreased during body cooling.[127] Other researchers reported similar changes in pressures with changes in the vasomotor tone in the digits of the lower[42,155] and upper extremities.[49,72] Measurements in patients with arterial disease are usually carried out under normal resting conditions. We determined normal values by studying pressures in 45 subjects without peripheral vascular disease whose ages ranged from 18 to 70 years.[32] Measurements were carried out with the subjects supine at a room temperature of about 21° C, with the trunk covered by an electric blanket to prevent excessive body cooling. The lower limit of normal for the toe pressure was found to be 50 mm Hg, and 64% of the brachial systolic pressure. For the ankle-toe gradient the upper limit of normal was 70 mm Hg.

In patients with hypertension but without peripheral vascular disease the systolic pressures in the toes are higher, as are the ankle-toe pressure gradients.[32] Therefore an ankle-toe gradient of more than 70 mm Hg may not signify arterial obstruction in the presence of systemic hypertension. However, toe pressures expressed as a percentage of the brachial pressure are not different in hypertensive patients, and therefore this parameter, if abnormal, indicates the presence of proximal arterial disease whether or not hypertension exists.[32]

Correlation of measurements of toe pressures with angiographic findings in 102 limbs showed that the pressures were abnormal in 97% of limbs with arterial occlusion and in 74% of limbs with stenotic lesions,[32] indicating that these pressures represent a valid index of the occlusive process. Since they reflect disease in the smaller distal vessels of the limb, which is not the case with the pressures measured more proximally, they are of special value in assessing the overall extent and severity of disease whether or not there is concomitant involvement of the larger proximal arteries.[32,94,128] Measurement of toe pressures may also allow assessment of the occlusive process in those cases in which arterial calcification interferes with the measurement of the more proximal pressures.[94] In addition to the measurements in patients with arteriosclerosis obliterans, toe pressures have been successfully applied to the assessment of the occlusive process in thromboangiitis obliterans and Raynaud's phenomenon.[32,88] In these conditions arterial lesions are usually situated in the smaller distal vessels,[50,132,181] and ankle pressures may be normal.[32] It is important to carry out the measurements with the patients comfortably warm[32] because, in the presence of vasospasm or high tone in the smooth muscle of the digital arteries, values too low, which do not represent an organic occlusive process, may be recorded.[81,120]

Systolic pressures in the toes have also been studied by Gundersen[80,81] and numerous other investigators.* Their results are similar to those presented earlier.

Skin pressures

Nielsen et al.[152] and Holstein and Lassen[92] reported on measurements of "skin" blood pressures. The method consists of detecting the pressure in the cuff at which blood flow in the skin directly under the cuff begins. A photoelectric probe or clearance of an isotope can be used for that purpose. Skin pressures are lower than the ordinarily measured systolic pressures except in some patients with a severe occlusive process. Although they correlate well with the diastolic pressure in normotensive subjects,[92] they are higher in the presence of hypertension.[152] The measurements probably represent systolic pressure in small vessels of the skin. As will be discussed later, they may be of value in predicting prognosis for healing.

Table 51-1 shows guidelines for interpretation of pressures at various levels in the lower limbs. However, the values will depend on the size of the cuffs used and the girth of the limbs.

Relation to symptoms

Intermittent claudication. The absolute levels of ankle systolic pressure show wide variation in pa-

*References 93, 94, 101, 121, 146, 149, 155, 166, 175, 185, 213, 216.

tients with claudication. It has been reported that claudication can occur in normotensive patients with ankle pressures as high as 100 mm Hg.[66] Raines et al.[174] found that average ankle systolic pressures at rest in patients with "limiting claudication" was 77 mm Hg with a large range of values. Fig. 51-4 shows distribution of ankle pressures in 160 patients with claudication studied in our laboratory. There is no significant difference between patients with and without diabetes. The presence of hypertension among the group accounts for some of the high pressures and the mean of 95 mm Hg. Since ankle pressure falls markedly with exercise in the presence of a proximal stenosis or occlusion, absolute ankle pressures at rest do not reflect the hemodynamic situation during exercise when claudication occurs. The relationship of the ankle pressure to brachial blood pressure is a better index of the occlusive process. Yao[223] reported in 1970 that in 213 limbs with claudication ankle systolic pressure averaged 59% of the brachial pressure, with a range of 20% to 100%. Similar average ankle pressures between 57% and 65% of the brachial pressure and wide ranges were reported by Cutajar et al.,[43] Lennihan and Mackereth,[123] and others,[6,208] and agree with our experience, which is illustrated in Fig. 51-5. As was discussed earlier, in an occasional patient with claudication and a normal ankle pressure at rest, the response to exercise is necessary to demonstrate the hemodynamic abnormality. The wide range of pressure values found in patients with claudication is related in part to the variations in the site, length, and number of the occlusive or stenotic lesions and the development of collateral circulation. However, other factors are likely to contribute as well.

Table 51-1. Systolic pressure values in the lower extremities at rest

Pressure (mm Hg)	Normal	Borderline	Abnormal
Difference between right and left limbs at same level	Below 15	15-20	Above 20
Upper thigh-brachial difference	Above 30	Below 30	Below 30
Gradients along lower limbs proximal to ankle	Below 20	20-30	Above 30
Ankle (% of brachial)	Above 103*	97-103	Below 97
Ankle-foot difference†	Below 30	30	Above 30 (? less than 30)‡
Ankle-toe difference†	Below 65	65-70	Above 70 (? 60)‡
Toe	Above 50	50	Below 50
Toe (% of brachial)	Above 70	64-70	Below 64

*In the presence of a mild stenosis, response to exercise may be needed to demonstrate abnormality.
†May be above normal in patients with hypertension without arterial obstruction.
‡With severe proximal disease and low flows.

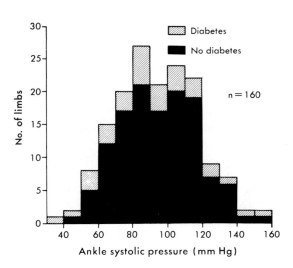

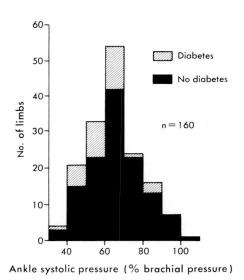

Fig. 51-4. Absolute values of ankle systolic pressure measured at rest in limbs with intermittent claudication. *n*, Number of limbs.

Fig. 51-5. Ankle systolic pressure expressed as percentage of brachial systolic pressure in limbs with intermittent claudication. *n*, Number of limbs.

Lorentsen[130] and Yao et al.[226] found correlation coefficients of less than 0.5 between ankle pressures and the maximal walking distance, even though the correlation with resting ankle pressure was as good as or better than with hyperemic muscle blood flow. To investigate further the relationship of the pressures to the walking ability, brachial and ankle systolic pressures were measured at rest and after a standard walk on a treadmill at 2 mph on a 7% grade in 28 patients with claudication. The maximal walking time correlated significantly with ankle systolic pressure and brachial-ankle pressure difference at rest and after exercise as well as with the return time of the ankle systolic pressure (p < .01). Figs. 51-6 and 51-7 show brachial-ankle pressure differences at rest and after the standard walk plotted against the maximal walking distance. Eight patients with occlusive disease who were able to walk half a mile or more without having to stop had resting ankle systolic pressure that ranged from 72 to 112 mm Hg or 61% to 93% of the brachial pressure. Their brachial-ankle pressure difference at rest varied from 10 to 58 mm Hg, and 3 minutes after exercise, from 41 to 122 mm Hg. The highest correlation of −0.72 was with brachial-ankle pressure difference after exercise, but the correlation coefficients with this difference at rest (−0.69) and with ankle systolic pressure at rest expressed as percentage of brachial pressure (0.66) were nearly as high. These findings indicate

that severity of the occlusive process as determined by the measurements of the ankle and brachial systolic pressures at rest and after walking is an important determinant of the walking ability of patients with intermittent claudication. The remaining variability is probably caused by other factors such as differences in motivation, in the distribution of the available blood flow to the more ischemic muscle groups, or in the ability of the muscle to extract oxygen and nutrients from the available blood flow.[1,44] Some of these factors may in turn be influenced by the amount of exercise the patients perform in their daily lives.

Because ankle pressures do not reflect arterial obstruction in the distal part of the extremity and may be falsely exaggerated by arterial rigidity, measurements of systolic pressures in the toes have been gaining a more prominent role in the assessment of patients. In similarity to the ankle pressures, there is a wide variation of the digital pressures in patients with intermittent claudication. Carter and Lezack[32] reported in 1971 that systolic pressure in the toes averaged 62 mm Hg and 43% of brachial systolic pressure in patients with intermittent claudication secondary to arteriosclerosis obliterans. There was no significant difference between patients with and without diabetes. However, in patients with claudication resulting from thromboangiitis obliterans the pressures were lower and averaged 30 mm Hg and 24% of the brachial pres-

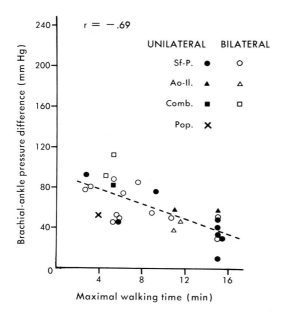

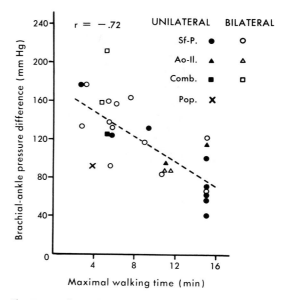

Fig. 51-6. Relationship of maximal walking time to brachial minus ankle pressure difference measured at rest in limbs with intermittent claudication. Maximal walking time was determined on treadmill at 2 mph and on a 7% elevation. Calculated regression line and correlation coefficient (r) are shown. *Sf-P.*, Superficial femoropopliteal; *Ao-Il.*, aortoiliac; *Comb.*, combined aortoiliac and superficial femoropopliteal; *Pop.*, popliteal.

Fig. 51-7. Relationship of maximal walking time to brachial and ankle pressure difference 3 minutes after a standard 5-minute walk on the treadmill at 2 mph and on a 7% elevation. Calculated regression line and correlation coefficient (r) are shown. *Sf-P.*, Superficial femoropopliteal; *Ao-Il.*, aortoiliac; *Comb.*, combined aortoiliac and superficial femoropopliteal; *Pop.*, popliteal.

sure. This finding may be a result of more severe distal arterial obstruction in this group of patients. Our findings have recently been confirmed by other researchers.[175,213,216] Figs. 51-8 and 51-9 show distribution of the systolic pressure in the toes in limbs with intermittent claudication studied in our laboratory.

Rest pain and skin lesions. Patients with a more advanced occlusive process manifested by pain at rest or lesions of the skin have lower pressures. Yao[223] found an average ankle systolic pressure of 26% of the brachial pressure in 77 patients with pain at rest, with a range from values near 0% to 65%, and similar findings have been reported by others.[6,43,123,208] Raines et al.[174] found that absolute ankle systolic pressure averaged 36 mm Hg in limbs with pain at rest and 52 mm Hg in those with lesions of the skin, again with a wide range of values.

The wide range of values in patients with symptoms and signs of severe ischemia is related to the following considerations. As indicated previously, ankle pressures may not reflect disease in the branches of the popliteal artery below the knee nor

in the smaller vessels distal to the ankles. Such distal disease may be present because of the basic disease process, as a result of thrombosis secondary to local trauma, infection, or stasis,[41] and, in some cases, thromboembolism or atheroembolism from complicated atherosclerotic plaques located proximally in the arterial tree.[2,108] Also, ankle systolic pressures could be overestimated in some patients with arterial calcification, and this is more likely to happen in the presence of diabetes.[24,174,196] Figs. 51-10 and 51-11 show our findings of the ankle systolic pressure given in millimeters of mercury and expressed as percentage of the brachial pressure, respectively. In limbs with rest pain but without skin breakdown, pressure is usually less than 40% of the brachial pressure and less than 60 mm Hg. Patients with diabetes do not differ from those without diabetes (p > .2). In the limbs with skin lesions the range of values is greater, and some limbs have ankle pressures that are nearly normal. Although there is considerable overlap, pressures are significantly higher in the limbs of patients with diabetes (p < .01 for absolute values and p < .02 for percentage of brachial pressure).

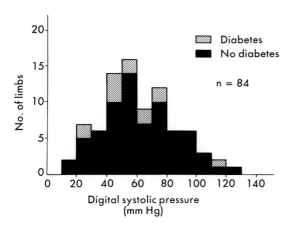

Fig. 51-8. Absolute values of systolic pressure measured in second toe in limbs with intermittent claudication. *n,* Number of limbs.

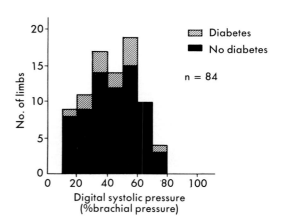

Fig. 51-9. Systolic pressure measured in second toe expressed as percentage of brachial systolic pressure in limbs with intermittent claudication. *n,* Number of limbs.

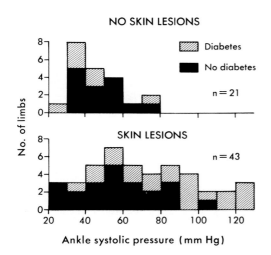

Fig. 51-10. Absolute values of ankle systolic pressure in limbs with severe rest pain, without and with skin lesions. *n,* Number of limbs.

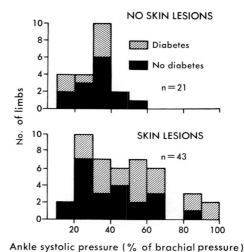

Fig. 51-11. Ankle systolic pressure expressed as percentage of brachial systolic pressure in limbs with severe rest pain, without and with skin lesions. *n,* Number of limbs.

Systolic pressures measured in the toes correlate better with the presence of severe ischemia.[31] We reported previously that in patients with rest pain, with or without ischemic skin lesions, systolic pressures in the toes averaged 33 mm Hg and 21% of the brachial systolic pressure.[32] There was no significant difference between diabetic and nondiabetic patients. Fig. 51-12 shows that in 96% of limbs with severe rest pain with or without skin lesions the pressures were less than 30 mm Hg. The two high digital pressures in the group with

skin lesions were in patients with lesions involving a single toe and not the one in which the pressure was measured. Similar results were reported by other researchers.[80,175,213,216] The findings demonstrate that systolic pressures measured in the toes correlate better than do ankle pressures with clinical evidence of severe ischemia, and they seem to provide a better index of the overall occlusive process, which may include obstruction in the more distal vessels of the extremity. The somewhat higher average pressures in limbs with skin lesions may

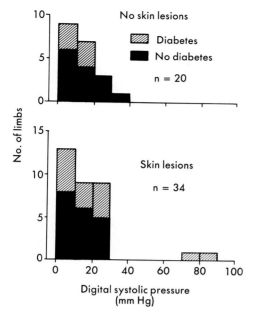

Fig. 51-12. Absolute values of systolic pressure in toes in limbs with severe rest pain, without and with skin lesions. *n,* Number of limbs.

be because of the lesions developing as a result of a precipitating cause, such as trauma in some limbs with relatively less severe disease. Higher ankle pressure found in some patients with diabetes and ischemia may be a result of the overestimation of the systolic pressure because of arterial calcification, but it can also be caused, at least in part, by the presence of more extensive distal disease in the diabetic patients.[40,200] The finding of higher ankle-toe pressure differences in some diabetic patients and in the majority of symptomatic patients with thromboangiitis obliterans,[32] whose disease is primarily in the small distal vessels of the extremities[182] but who are not known to have calcified arteries, also supports this contention.

APPLICATION TO THE ASSESSMENT AND MANAGEMENT OF DISEASE OF THE LOWER EXTREMITIES
Diagnosis and follow-up of patients

Previous parts of the chapter demonstrated that measurements of pressures provide a quantitative, reproducible, and sensitive method for determination of the presence and severity of the occlusive process in limbs with arterial disease. Since the measurements are noninvasive and can be performed easily and repeatedly, they lend themselves

well to the follow-up of individual patients and to the documentation of the natural history of the disease.

Although in the majority of patients the diagnosis can be made on the basis of history and physical examination, several reports indicate that changes in pressures frequently occur before there are clear changes in the clinical findings.* For example, development of obstruction in the arterial tree following diagnostic catheterization has been documented by pressure measurements even in the absence of symptoms.[8,14] Measurement of pressure is of special value in those patients who may have symptoms in the extremities caused by a spinal, arthritic, or muscular disorder that may mimic arterial disease or coexist with it[55,96] and in those with mild disease.[26] Measurement of ankle pressure at rest will document the presence or absence of proximal disease in most cases, but in some patients with mild stenotic lesions the response of pressure to exercise may have to be determined. The finding of normal or nearly normal pressure will usually eliminate the need for angiography. Addition of pressure measurements in the toes is necessary when more proximal pressures are incorrect because of medial calcification. Toe pressures are also of special value in the assessment of the presence and severity of the distal disease and useful in patients with a severe or primarily distal occlusive process associated with diabetes, thromboangiitis obliterans, or Raynaud's phenomenon.[32]

Even when disease is obvious by clinical assessment, measurement of pressure provides a baseline against which future changes in the disease process can be monitored. Studies of reproducibility of the measurements indicate that changes in ankle and toe pressure expressed as a percentage of the brachial pressure are significant if they are 15% or more, whereas differences of 10% to 15% are of borderline significance.[24,166] If a patient with known arterial disease develops a change in symptoms, measurement of pressure can be of help in deciding whether the change or new symptom is caused by the progression of the disease.

Natural history of disease

Progression of the occlusive process. Pressure measurements have been applied to the study of the progression of the occlusive process.[124,197] Development of disease in the second limb in patients

_____

*References 25, 124, 143, 193, 197, 198.

with unilateral occlusive process is frequent.[197] Patients often show objective improvement during the first year after the onset of symptoms, and then there are no significant changes in many cases over periods of up to 4 years[124] or longer.[143] These reports provide objective evidence that supports the findings of previous clinical studies that prognosis in limbs with arteriosclerosis obliterans is generally good.[15,20,181] Patients with disease involving the femoral and popliteal arteries showed a more variable clinical course than did those with localized superficial femoral block.[124] There was little or no deterioration in limbs with good runoff on angiography, whereas significant deterioration occurred over 3 years in the group with poorest runoff. Limbs with poor runoff that came to amputation had significantly lower ankle pressures expressed as percentage of the brachial pressure than did those with poor runoff that did not require amputation. Serial pressure measurements often showed deterioration without an obvious clinical change, suggesting that surgical intervention in such cases might improve limb salvage.[124] A low incidence of progression of disease in patients with isolated lesions above the inguinal ligament and in those with combined proximal and distal disease was found in the majority of patients followed with pressure measurements.[124,143,197]

Measurements of systolic pressure in the toes have also been applied to the study of the progression of the arterial obstruction and are especially useful in the study of severe ischemia when ankle pressures are unreliable because of medial calcification. Paaske and Tønnesen[166] showed that prognosis for limb salvage was poor when toe systolic pressure was less than 8% of the brachial pressure and improved at higher pressures. The study also showed the importance of the follow-up of patients with repeated measurements, since some patients with initially low pressures showed an increase in the measurements over a 2-year period and did not develop rest pain or skin breakdown. Such studies provide information that is of help in making decisions about the management of individual patients on a more rational basis.

Population studies. Since pressure measurements provide a sensitive index of arterial obstruction and can be performed easily and repeatedly, their value in the study of the prevalence of arterial disease in population studies was recognized by the American Heart Association[171] and used by a number of researchers. The brachial-ankle pressure difference

was found to correlate significantly with smoking, hypertension, and hyperlipedemia in patients with intermittent claudication.[99] The researchers suggested that such measurements could be used to quantitate the severity of the arteriosclerotic process and to evaluate the relationship to the factors that influence its progression. Ankle pressure measurements were used to estimate prevalence of peripheral arteriosclerotic disease in a 60-year-old population in Denmark.[183] Both ankle and toe pressure measurements were applied to the study of the prevalence of arteriosclerosis obliterans in patients with diabetes mellitus.[9,10,164] These and similar studies provide important epidemiologic information on the prevalence of arterial disease in various patient subgroups, the relationship to smoking, and the results of various therapeutic interventions.

It is important to realize that the sensitivity of the pressure measurements to detect an early arteriosclerotic process will depend on the criteria used. The evidence discussed earlier in this chapter indicates that mild stenotic lesions may be present in limbs with a resting ankle pressure that lies between 100% and 115% of the brachial systolic pressure. Assessment of the response of the ankle pressure to exercise would be required to demonstrate such mild stenotic lesions. Also, as emphasized by the American Heart Association,[171] the noninvasive studies should be combined with clinical assessment. There is evidence that auscultation for bruits, especially over the superficial artery in the region of the adductor canal in the thigh at rest and after exercise, is a sensitive index of mild arterial lesions. Such bruits may be present in limbs with normal systolic pressures.[29]

Medical therapy

Measurements of pressure can be used to guide and evaluate medical therapy. Segmental pressure measurements have been reported to be of help in the management of a patient with arterial occlusion secondary to ergotism that may regress spontaneously[109] and to assist in the treatment of severe ischemia with drug-induced systemic hypertension by monitoring distal systolic pressure.[81,117] The use of dependent position in the treatment of severe ischemia of the limbs is supported by the findings that in the presence of severe occlusion the increase in the ankle[70] and digital[126] pressures with dependency is greater than the increase in hydrostatic level, presumably because of the distention of the collateral vessels. Combination of the upright posture with intermittent venous compression may increase blood flow in the presence of arterial obstruction by increasing the arteriovenous pressure gradient across the foot. Significant increases in skin blood flow measured using the xenon clearance method occurred when a mechanical venous pump was used in patients with arterial obstruction in the sitting position, but only when arterial obstruction was severe, as indicated by the ankle pressure of 60 mm Hg or less.[73]

Vasodilators have been shown to decrease digital blood pressure distal to occlusion and are probably not indicated, particularly in the presence of severe ischemia.[81] Walking on a raised heel did not change the response of ankle systolic pressure to exercise nor the walking time of patients with claudication.[37] On the other hand, treatment with clofibrate resulted in a significant improvement in the response of ankle pressure to exercise in a group of patients with intermittent claudication and high plasma fibrinogen level.[170] Similarily, defibrination by subcutaneous injections of ancrod for 5 weeks was followed by improvement of the symptoms and statistically significant increases in resting ankle pressure and its response to exercise, which improved by 25% or more.[48] In a study of patients with intermittent claudication, cessation of smoking was followed by significant improvement of the walking distance, resting ankle pressures, and ankle pressures after exercise, whereas patients who continued to smoke showed no significant changes.[172]

Numerous reports indicate that exercise improves walking ability of patients with intermittent claudication. The mechanism of improvement is not clear, but it is likely that several factors may contribute to the remarkable walking ability that many patients achieve in the exercise programs.[34,180] Some studies reported increases in blood flow in response to training,[1,117] whereas others did not.[228] Similarly, early clinical studies reported increases in the ankle systolic pressure at rest and in response to exercise after training,[187,188] whereas more recent studies showed only modest increases.[34,38] We found that remarkable walking ability may be achieved in about 75% of patients with intermittent claudication.[34] Good walking ability may be achieved in patients with obstruction either proximal or distal to the inguinal ligament, in patients with combined disease, in patients with and without ischemic heart disease and diabetes, and in patients taking beta blocking drugs. Similar degrees of improvement were also observed in patients with widely varying severity of obstruction as assessed by systolic pressure measurements. Good walking ability was achieved by patients whose ankle systolic pressures were as low as 55 mm Hg and 40% of brachial systolic pressure and toe systolic pressures as low as 30 mm Hg.[34]

Prognosis for healing

The use of pressure measurements to determine prognosis for healing is one of its most important practical applications. Patients with severe ischemia and skin lesions in whom arterial reconstruction may be associated with a significant risk because of the associated cardiovascular disease present a common clinical problem. If the lesion were to heal without surgery, the risk to life could be avoided. In other patients arterial reconstruction may not be feasible because disease is too extensive. In such cases one often persists with conservative management in the hope that the lesion will heal. In many patients, however, the conservative approach fails and amputation is carried out, often after a long period of suffering and hospitalization. In 1973 we demonstrated that measurements of distal systolic pressures can be helpful in making decisions in such cases.[27] If ankle pressure was less than 55 mm Hg, healing did not take place and major amputation had to be carried out in diabetic and nondiabetic patients. The chances for healing were good in nondiabetic patients when the ankle pressure was greater than 55 mm Hg, whereas in the diabetic patients the chances for healing were uncertain even with high ankle pressures. This finding is not surprising because of the frequency of severe obstruction in the small distal vessels of the limbs in the diabetic patients and higher incidence of medial calcification that may render ankle pressure unreliable. On the other hand, toe pressures correlated well with healing in the limbs of both diabetic and nondiabetic patients. Chances of healing were uncertain when the pressure was less than 30 mm Hg and good when it was higher. Slightly lower chances of healing in the diabetic patients are probably related to the impairment of the tissue reparative processes by the metabolic disorder, increased susceptibility to infection, and neuropathy. These early results have since been confirmed by numerous studies. Raines et al.[174] reported that healing was unlikely when ankle pressure was less than 55 mm Hg and that higher pressures were required for healing to occur in diabetic patients.

Table 51-2. Relationship of systolic pressure to prognosis for healing of skin lesions of the toes or feet

Pressure (mm Hg)	Probability of healing (%)	
	No diabetes	Diabetes
Ankle		
Below 55	0	0
55 to 90	85	45
Above 90	100	85
Toe		
Below 20	25	29
20 to 30	73	40
30 to 55	100	85
Above 55	100	97
Skin		
Below 20	0	0

Scandinavian researchers[93,118,120,160] applied measurements of toe and skin blood pressures extensively to the assessment of prognosis for healing with similar results. Table 51-2 summarizes the relationship of the pressure measurements to the prognosis for healing of skin lesions of the toes or feet based on a large combined experience in Copenhagen and in our laboratory.

The finding that a distal arterial pressure of about 30 mm Hg is necessary to achieve healing of skin lesions is in agreement with recent findings[19,175,184] on the relationship of the toe systolic pressures to the healing of distal amputations of the feet and toes. Another situation in which systolic pressures may be used to estimate the chances of healing is elective surgery in the feet of patients with arterial obstruction, for the purpose of correcting bunions, hammer toes, or other pathologic conditions, for example, excising neuromas. When there is clinically evident arterial obstruction, there may be reluctance to consider surgery, and patients may be left at times with significant disability. We reviewed our experience in 16 orthopedic procedures in the feet of patients with various degrees of arterial disease. Healing occurred without difficulties in all cases. Although the degree of arterial obstruction estimated by distal systolic pressure measurements was mild in many cases, the ankle pressure was decreased in some to 60 to 70 mm Hg and in four cases the digital systolic pressures were 40 to 60 mm Hg. This experience and the other data on the relationship of pressures to healing sug-

gest that when systolic pressure exceeds 30 mm Hg in the toes of nondiabetic subjects and 55 mm Hg in diabetic patients, elective surgery can probably be safely done, although there is a need for the study of a larger number of cases.

It seems reasonable that a pressure of about 30 mm Hg in the small arteries is usually needed to maintain an effective arteriovenous pressure difference and to provide adequate nutritional blood flow and thus promote healing. Although adequate blood flow and oxygen delivery to the tissues are the important parameters necessary for healing, they depend on the available driving pressure and peripheral resistance in the microcirculation. There is evidence that when the ability of the small vessels to vasoconstrict is abolished by local heating or ischemia, the flow and oxygen delivery depend primarily on the available arterial pressure, which is reflected in the distal systolic pressure measurements. This concept is supported by the finding of a good correlation between transcutaneous measurements of oxygen tension in limbs with arterial obstruction and distal systolic pressures[39,54,219] and by corresponding correlations between ischemia, pressures, and other measurements of digital circulation.[101] The question remains why healing occurs in some limbs in which the measured pressures are even lower[27,93,166] and why some patients with very low pressures may have no symptoms.[32,93] Several considerations may be relevant. Technical factors, for example, too tight application of the measuring cuffs, might result in falsely low pressures, since the digital arteries with low pressures might be compressed or even closed more easily by a tightly applied cuff. Theoretically, vasospasm resulting from local cooling or sympathetic vasoconstriction can decrease apparent digital systolic pressures,[156] but this seems unlikely in ischemic feet in which a high concentration of metabolites would be expected to lead to the relaxation of the vascular smooth muscle. During measurements, usually carried out with the patient in the supine position, the toes are higher than the level of the heart, which results in an average decrease in the measured pressure of 9 mm Hg.[127] Therefore it is likely that when patients lie in a different position the digital pressure is slightly higher. Also, it has been shown that when limbs with severe arterial obstruction are in a dependent position the increase in digital pressure is greater than expected from the difference in hydrostatic level,[126] which should result in an increased arteriovenous pressure gradient. The digital pressures will also vary with the changes in the hemodynamic state of the patient. If a patient's central blood pressure is relatively low during the measurements and high at other times, lower systolic pressure measured in the toes during the test would not represent higher pressures that may otherwise exist. Digital pressures are known to vary with changes in blood flow and vasomotor tone;[49,86,127] they are lower if blood flow is higher and conversely increase when there is peripheral vasoconstriction and blood flow decreases. Therefore it is important to measure pressures with the patients comfortably warm and avoid pronounced vasoconstriction or vasodilation. For example, following a strong vasodilating stimulus, higher blood flow proximal to the toe could result in a relatively low digital pressure, which would suggest a worse prognosis than actually might be present. It is possible that in some limbs with lesions and arterial obstruction pronounced vasodilation and relatively high flows might be present as a result of inflammation, ischemia,[138,139] or neuropathy[51] in the presence of toe pressures below 30 mm Hg. If it is suspected that such a situation may be present, the use of some index of distal blood flow, such as the recording of digital pulse volume changes using strain-gauge or photocell plethysmography,[161] or measurement of skin blood flow,[135] may provide important information. Also, repetition of the pressure measurements during follow-up is important, because in some patients subsequent testing may show an increase in pressure and suggest a better prognosis.[93,166]

APPLICATION TO THE ASSESSMENT AND MANAGEMENT OF DISEASE OF THE UPPER EXTREMITIES

Disease in the arteries supplying the upper limbs is less common than in the lower extremities, but the occlusive process in the arterial tree from the subclavian to the digital vessels occurs as a result of atherosclerosis,[22,102] Takayasu's disease,[227] embolism,[227] thoracic outlet syndromes,[47,215,227] complications of diagnostic arterial catheterization,[47,100] thromboangiitis obliterans,[181] trauma,[47,215,227] and various conditions that affect small distal arteries of the hand or digits.[132,215,227] As in the case of the lower limbs, measurements of systolic pressures in the upper limbs provide information about the presence, site, and severity of the stenotic or occlusive process and thus aid in the diagnosis and management of patients.

Obstruction in the main arterial pathways

An occlusive or stenotic process in the subclavian or axillary artery will result in a decrease of the brachial blood pressure. There are many publications that deal with obstruction of the subclavian arteries, including those about patients with subclavian steal syndrome.[168] Results of pressure measurements in 15 limbs with subclavian stenosis or occlusion studied in our laboratory, combined with the data from five published reports,[22,102,169,173,214] show that the difference in the brachial systolic pressures between the two arms averaged 41 ± SD 14 mm Hg (range 20 to 70) in 21 cases of subclavian stenosis and 64 ± SD 25 (range 24 to 130) in 29 cases with a complete occlusion. The difference exceeded 50 mm Hg in 23 cases with occlusion and only in 3 with a stenosis. Although it has been stated that differences in pressure of more than 30 mm Hg between the two arms are indicative of the disease,[102] studies of blood pressure differences between the two arms in large series of subjects[176,201] suggest that differences greater than 15 mm Hg should arouse suspicion. At times the difference in the blood pressure between the two arms may underestimate the severity of the disease, since the disease may be bilateral and a milder lesion may exist in the limb with the higher pressure. A comparison with pressure measurement in the lower limbs may provide a more accurate assessment of the significance of the occlusive process to the upper extremities in such cases.[227] Arm exercise will result in the drop of pressure distal to a hemodynamically significant lesion, and this procedure may be of additional help in the assessment of patients.[214,227] Lamis et al.[116] reported that distal segmental pressure measurements after hyperemia were of help in the evaluation of the donor subclavian or innominate vessels before axillo-axillary bypass graft for occlusion of the contralateral subclavian artery.

Among six cases of obstruction in the axillary region we found differences in blood pressure between the two arms that ranged from 40 to 68 mm Hg in four patients, whereas in two who sustained an injury to the axillary region at a relatively young age and had few or no symptoms, the difference was only 20 mm Hg and was not increased by exercise. This finding might be explained by the potential for the development of abundant collateral circulation in the shoulder region.[227]

With increased use of arterial catheterization for diagnostic purposes, complications that result in the obstruction of the brachial artery are becoming one of the more common causes of the occlusive process of the arteries of the upper limbs.[100] Among 10 patients with obstruction in the brachial region referred to our laboratory, in 8 the obstruction was secondary to a diagnostic catheterization. The mean difference between brachial pressures was only $11 \pm$ SD 12 mm Hg (range -2 to 36), and it exceeded 20 mm Hg in only two patients. On the other hand, the difference in forearm pressure averaged $44 \pm$ SD 15 mm Hg (range 30 to 79). The difference between brachial pressures did not reflect the severity of the occlusive process. The situation here is similar to that in the thigh, where high pressures may be measured in the presence of the obstruction of the superficial femoral artery because of the enlargement of the deep femoral artery. In the upper limb an enlarged deep brachial artery was probably responsible for relatively high pressures recorded in the arms of these patients. Determination of forearm or wrist pressures using a Doppler ultrasonic flow detector over the radial and ulnar vessels may at times give different readings over the two vessels. This was the case in one patient in this series in whom a much lower pressure recorded with the Doppler flow detector over the radial artery was caused by thrombotic occlusion of this vessel in addition to the brachial occlusion. All patients whose obstruction was secondary to arterial catheterization had symptoms consistent with intermittent claudication and associated coldness of the hand. The pressures in the fingers were also reduced. An abnormally large difference between the blood pressures in the two upper limbs that is not associated with an obstructive arterial lesion may occur in patients with supravalvular aortic stenosis. It has been suggested that asymmetric jet effects lead to the observed pressure difference.[60]

Finger pressures in the assessment of distal diseases including Raynaud's phenomenon

Systolic pressures in the fingers have been measured for at least 80 years, and earlier studies were reviewed by others.[58,71] After correction for the difference in level between fingers and toes in the supine position, pressures in the fingers were found to be, on the average, 13 mm Hg higher than in the toes.[127] In general, pressures in the fingers behave in a similar way to those measured in the toes. In an elegant study in 1939, Doupe et al.[49] demonstrated that finger pressures increased during pe-

ripheral vasoconstriction and decreased during vasodilation and that the difference between the brachial and finger pressures showed opposite changes. Similar results were reported by Gaskell and Krisman,[72] and Lezack and Carter.[127] Gaskell and Krisman[71] also studied the effect of various cuff widths and found that cuffs 3 to 4 cm wide appeared to give consistent results.

Although there are differences in the results of various studies related, at least in part, to differences in the techniques and possibly to differences in the vasomotor state of the subjects,[49,72,127,149] finger pressures are generally lower than brachial pressures except at times under the condition of pronounced peripheral vasoconstriction.[49,50,72,127] Intra-arterial measurements indicate that there is also amplification of the systolic pressure along the arteries of the upper limbs,[115] although it may not be as pronounced as in the lower limbs. The report of a direct measurement from a finger artery indicates that a decrease in pressure occurs between the wrist and the finger.[148] Similar to the findings in the lower limbs, increased brachial-to-digit pressure differences may be found in patients with hypertension without an occlusive arterial process.[72]

Organic obstruction. Downs et al.[50] carried out a careful study of pressure measurements in the fingers of normal subjects and patients with angiographically demonstrated occlusive process in the arteries of the hands and fingers using 38 mm wide cuffs applied around the proximal phalanx. Their findings were that systolic finger pressures of less than 70 mm Hg, wrist-digit gradients of more than 30 mm Hg, and brachial-finger differences of more than 35 to 40 mm Hg strongly suggest the presence of an occlusive process at or proximal to the digit. Also, differences between simultaneously measured pressures in the corresponding fingers should not exceed 15 mm Hg.

Measurements of finger pressures in normal subjects and in patients with arterial obstruction were also reported by Gundersen[80,81] and others.[86,149,153] Their results are similar, but some differences are related to the use of a narrower 24 mm wide cuff[81,153,155] as compared with the 38 mm cuffs used in the study of Downs et al.[50] Hirai[86] studied a large number of normal subjects and patients with arterial disease using a 24 mm wide cuff to measure pressures at both the proximal and intermediate phalanges of the fingers. He did not find significant differences between the measurements at the proximal and middle phalanges despite a previous report, which indicated that the pressure at the middle phalanges is about 5 mm Hg lower than at the base of the digit.[85] He also reported that brachial-finger differences should not exceed 20 mm Hg in normal subjects less than 50 years of age and 25 mm Hg in older subjects without arterial disease. The differences between the findings of Hirai[86] and Downs et al.[50] might be a result of the use of different widths of the cuffs, but also of the different vasomotor state of the subjects, since Hirai did not specify the conditions under which the measurements were carried out, whereas Downs et al. studied subjects who were kept warm by means of an electric blanket. It is necessary for each laboratory to apply and develop appropriate normal standards according to the techniques and procedures that are used, although to assess the presence and severity of the organic arterial obstruction, the measurements in the limbs and particularly in the digits should be carried out with the patients and extremities at least comfortably warm.

Measurements of systolic pressures in the fingers to assess arterial obstruction have limitations similar to those discussed with respect to the assessment of the obstruction in the lower limbs and the more proximal disease in the upper limbs. If only one of the two digital arteries is occluded, the measured pressure will be normal.[50,86] Also, if obstruction is present in the digital arteries in the distal part of the finger, the obstruction may be detected only if the cuff is placed at the intermediate phalanx and normal values obtained at the proximal phalanx. In cases of very distal disease even measurements at the intermediate phalanx may be normal, and the evidence of obstruction may only be obtained by assessment of distal blood flow or skin temperature.[30]

Hirai found normal finger pressure in all 184 fingers with at least one normal arterial pathway to the digit as assessed by angiographic findings.[86] Among 203 fingers with occlusion of both digital arteries or more proximal vessels supplying the digit, abnormal pressures were recorded in 173 digits. In 30 fingers with ''falsely negative'' results there were no symptoms in the majority. Such normal results are a result of the occasional development of very large collateral channels that may form connections between two occluded digital arteries,[50] the presence of other large collateral pathways within the palm, very distal obstructions in the digit, and the uncertainty of the evaluation of the angiographic findings in relatively small arteries

of the hands and fingers.[86] These considerations, however, do not detract from the value of pressure measurements in the digits in the assessment of the arterial obstruction to the fingers. Such false negative results are relatively infrequent, usually not associated with severe impairment of blood flow, and may be taken into account in the interpretation of the results.

Prognosis for healing. Pressure measurements in the fingers may be of value in assessing prognosis for healing. In a study of 23 patients, we found that chances for early healing were high when finger systolic pressure exceeded 55 mm Hg, the brachial-finger pressure difference was less than 50 mm Hg, and the maximal difference among the fingers was less than 30 mm Hg.[30] Early healing was also likely when finger temperature of 10° C or more above room temperature was achieved during body heating. However, slow healing over a period of up to a year or more occurred in all digits in which the pressure exceeded 25 mm Hg.[30]

Cold sensitivity. Although digital pressures usually increase during peripheral vasoconstriction, in patients with cold sensitivity abnormally low digital pressures may be recorded when the patient or the extremities are cold, because excessive force is exerted by the smooth muscle in the digital arteries in such cases.[120] This phenomenon has been applied to the study of patients with cold sensitivity in the elegant studies of Krähenbuhl et al.[114] and Nielsen and Lassen.[157]

The method, which is described in greater detail in Chapter 63, uses measurement of systolic pressure in locally cooled fingers. In normal subjects the pressure in the locally cooled digits was reported to fall by an average of only 15% when the local temperature was lowered to 10° or 5° C, whereas in patients with Raynaud's phenomena it fell precipitously, often to unobtainable values, indicating closure of the digital arteries.[156,209] The frequency of the occurrence of digital artery closure with local cooling was increased by the addition of body cooling.[156] This interesting technique gave an early promise of providing a sensitive and specific test for the diagnosis of Raynaud's phenomena, and some studies reported good separation between normal subjects and patients.[89,156] However, other reports indicate that subjects without Raynaud's phenomena may at times exhibit abnormal decrease in the finger pressure with local cooling at times even to zero,[114,154] and in other studies more than 20% of patients with Raynaud's phenomena did not show an abnormal response.[33,209] Also, in patients with Raynaud's phenomena, abnormal responses and closure may occur during body cooling without local cooling of the fingers.[33] The method appears to provide an interesting approach to the evaluation of the digital arteries and has been used to assess these vessels in patients with arterial obstruction,[87,158] hypertension, and diabetes,[212] and to evaluate the effect of various therapeutic interventions.[150,151,159] However, further research is needed before the role and limitations of this method in the diagnosis and management of patients with vasospastic disorders can be established.

OTHER APPLICATIONS
Assessment of procedures to eliminate arterial obstruction

Organic arterial occlusion or stenosis may be eliminated by surgery or by percutaneous transluminal dilation. Pressure measurements have been used in the assessment of the results of these procedures and attempts made to apply the measurements to help select patients for treatment. The use of pressures in relation to the surgical treatment is dealt with in detail in Chapter 52. There are reports of successful use of the measurements to assess the results of transluminal dilation,[105,107,162] but these and numerous other studies on this subject are not reviewed in detail. It is clear, however, that the measurements are useful in the assessment of patients before surgery or angioplasty, in the immediate and long-term follow-up after the procedures, and in the objective evaluation of the results. The methods, criteria, and use of the measurements are essentially similar to those discussed in earlier sections of this chapter. The role of the measurements in predicting the chances of success of specific procedures is also discussed in other chapters. Pressure measurements by themselves may not be able to predict with complete accuracy the chances of success of treatment, which may also be influenced by the nature and extent of the obstruction, the techniques and materials used, and other factors; therefore such expectations may be unrealistic.[189]

Healing of major amputations

Healing of major amputations is discussed in detail in Chapter 58. Although pressure measurements at the ankles and at more proximal sites in the lower limbs have been used to try and predict healing of below-knee and above-knee amputations, the results are not as consistent as in the case of healing of lesions in the feet and toes, distal amputations, and elective surgery of the toes and feet discussed earlier in this chapter. These findings should not be surprising. Toe pressures are a good index of perfusion pressure close to the level of the lesion or surgery in the feet. On the other hand, ankle and proximal pressures may not reflect the perfusion pressure in the small skin vessels in the areas where healing after major amputations has to occur, and those pressures may also be unreliable in the presence of medial calcification. It appears that measurements of skin perfusion pressures at the sites of amputation may represent a more appropriate index for prediction of healing of these more proximal procedures. Good results using this method have been reported.[91,95]

Penile pressure in the assessment of impotence

Gaskell[68] was the first to report on the use of measurements of systolic blood pressure in the penis in normal young men, patients with occlusive arterial disease in the extremities but without impotence, and impotent patients. He found that in the absence of arterial obstruction, systolic pressure in the penis should not be less than the mean brachial blood pressure taken as the diastolic plus one third of the pulse pressure. Using this criterion, there were only two patients who had abnormally low penile pressures and claimed to be potent and only one patient with a normal pressure and impotence. Numerous studies of penile pressure measurements in the assessment of impotence have appeared since. In most studies the ratio of the penile systolic to the brachial systolic pressure has been reported and not the difference between mean brachial and penile systolic pressure used by Gaskell. In a study of 97 patients at the Vascular Laboratory at St. Boniface General Hospital in Winnipeg we found that there is a good correlation between penile/brachial systolic pressure ratio and the difference between the penile systolic and brachial mean pressures, with the correlation coefficient of 0.93 ($p < .001$). A zero difference between penile systolic and brachial mean pressures corresponded to the penile systolic pressure of 72% of the brachial pressure. Therefore lower pressures suggest the presence of arterial obstruction in the arterial supply of the penis, and this agrees with other reports.[140,141] The relationship of penile blood pressure to the occurrence of impotence is complex, since there are a number of other factors that may affect the erectile function. This subject is discussed in detail in Chapter 67.

Popliteal artery entrapment

Popliteal artery entrapment may be responsible for a history of intermittent claudication in young patients, although routine physical examination may show normal peripheral pulses before complications occur. The diagnosis should be suspected if pedal pulses disappear or diminish markedly with sustained active plantar flexion or with passive dorsiflexion at the ankle. Recording of abnormal pulse waves and of diminished ankle systolic pressure will corroborate the diagnosis.[45]

Coarctation

Comparison of the ankle and brachial systolic pressures can be used to assess patients with coarctation and to evaluate the efficacy of surgical treatment. Bollinger et al.[17] found that the difference between the brachial and ankle systolic pressures at rest averaged 70 mm Hg in 12 patients. Patients with coarctation of the thoracic aorta did not have intermittent claudication, despite the significant difference in pressures between the upper and lower limbs. The peak calf blood flow after 3 minutes of ischemia was normal in patients with coarctation,[17] suggesting that extensive collateral circulation that develops early in life is able to provide adequate blood flow to the exercising muscles of the lower extremities. In four patients with coarctation we found that, after exercise of the lower limbs, the ankle systolic pressure showed little or no change.

Peripheral arteriovenous fistula

Systolic pressure measurements have been applied to the study of the circulation in limbs distal to arteriovenous fistulas. Distal to a large fistula, ankle pressures are decreased at rest and show an abnormal fall in response to exercise that resembles the response in limbs with occlusive arterial process.[192,199] Compression of the fistula results in an increase of the ankle pressure.

SUMMARY AND CURRENT STATUS

As is well known, noninvasive measurements of brachial blood pressure using pneumatic cuffs were introduced during the nineteenth century and have been an essential tool in the clinical assessment and management of patients. Noninvasive measurements of systolic pressure in the fingers and in the lower limbs including the toes were carried out beginning early in this century. These early reports are referred to in the 1934 paper by Formijne.[58] In 1950 Winsor[222] reported on the segmental pressure measurements in the upper and lower limbs in normal subjects and patients with arterial obstruction, and in 1956 Gaskell[65] demonstrated that ankle systolic pressures measured at rest were a better index of the arterial obstruction than measurements of blood flow at rest and as good as measurements of blood flow in response to reactive hyperemia. The advent of extensive use of arterial surgery led to increased interest in the development of noninvasive methods for assessment of patients with peripheral arterial disease. The pioneering work of Strandness, which began in the early 1960s and has continued since, provided a major stimulus for the interest and further development of noninvasive pressure measurements by other researchers. As a result, pressure measurements have become an accepted method of evaluation of patients with arterial disease in diagnostic laboratories throughout the world. We became interested in the measurements of pressures in the toes in mid-1960s[126,127] and applied them to the assessment of arterial obstruction and estimation of the chances of healing of skin lesions.[32,128] These studies, those by Gundersen,[80,81] and those by others* lead to the documentation of the value of such distal measurements in the assessment and management of patients. In 1971 Gaskell[68] reported on the use of penile systolic pressure in the assessment of impotence, and other similar studies followed. The increasing interest in the use of pressure measurements to assess peripheral arterial disease is illustrated by the large number of papers, symposia, and courses on this subject during the past 10 to 15 years. Extensive work of numerous researchers has allowed a better assessment of the value and specific applications of the measurements as well as their limitations.

The ankle systolic pressure measured at rest probably provides the best single index of the presence and severity of the arterial obstruction in the main arterial channels proximal to the division of the popliteal artery. Ankle pressure equal to the brachial systolic pressure should be used as a practical rule of thumb for the lower limit of normal.

*References 93, 94, 101, 121, 146, 149, 155, 166, 175, 185, 213, 216.

However, mild stenotic lesions may be present in the limbs, in which ankle pressure exceeds brachial pressure by up to about 15%, and at times there may be associated symptoms of intermittent claudication. Measurements of pressures after exercise or during reactive hyperemia are useful in the demonstration of such mild stenotic lesions and in the differentiation of the causes of symptoms in patients who may have pseudoclaudication associated with neurospinal disorders, especially when arterial disease coexists. However, measurements after stress do not usually add practical information to the resting ankle pressure measurements if these are clearly abnormal. Measurements after stress should not be a part of a routine assessment of all patients with arterial disease. Measurements of segmental pressures at different levels have not fulfilled the promise of early enthusiastic reports. The results of these more proximal measurements are affected severely by various artifacts. The most useful information they may provide is evidence for the absence of significant obstruction proximal to the groin when the pressure at the upper thigh is considerably higher than brachial systolic pressure (by at least 30 mm Hg), in the presence of a strong femoral pulse, and in the absence of bruits. When the upper thigh pressure is lower, the presence of significant proximal lesions cannot be ruled out without resorting to other methods, including invasive pressure measurements. Segmental measurements frequently do not provide reliable information about the site of the obstruction and the number of lesions along the arterial tree of the extremity. The value of the ankle pressure by itself can give a reasonably good idea as to whether there is a single lesion or multiple sites of obstruction.

Since ankle and more proximal pressures may be falsely high in limbs with medial calcification and do not provide evidence about obstruction in the more distal vessels of the limbs, measurements of systolic pressures in the toes that appear not to be subject to these limitations have been shown clearly to be of great value and should be available in diagnostic vascular laboratories. In the absence of extensive or deep-seated infection, such as osteomyelitis, systolic pressures in the toes are an excellent index of healing of skin lesions, amputations, and elective surgical procedures in the toes and feet of patients with arterial disease. Pressures of 30 mm Hg or greater indicate excellent prognosis for healing in nondiabetic patients and good prognosis in diabetic patients, with a pressure of 55 mm Hg assuring healing in nearly 100% of cases—even in the diabetic patients. These findings fit well with physiologic concepts, since pressure of 30 mm Hg probably approaches the value of arterial pressure necessary to provide a minimum pressure gradient for an effective tissue blood flow. Together with other techniques, measurements of penile systolic pressures are of value in the assessment of impotence.

Measurements of pressures provide an objective and quantitative method for the assessment of the presence and severity of the arterial obstruction in the extremities and are of value in following individual patients, in population studies to assess the natural history and prevalence of arterial disease, and in the evaluation of results of specific therapeutic interventions. It appears that noninvasive pressure measurements may not be able to reliably predict the success of various therapies, although their role in conjunction with other methods remains to be fully elucidated. Such a finding should not be surprising, since pressure in the main arterial channels is not the only factor affecting the success of therapeutic procedures. This consideration also applies to the healing of major amputations, although measurements of skin pressure, which probably reflects pressure in the small arteries supplying the areas in question, appear to be a good predictor in similarity to the pressure measurements in the toes in the case of healing in the distal parts of the extremities.

There is abundant evidence that noninvasive pressure measurements are extremely useful in the assessment, follow-up, and management of patients with arterial disease and provide an objective method for the evaluation of results of therapeutic procedures. Judicious use of the measurements for routine assessment of patients is not only justified but necessary. Careful attention to the techniques and the use of the appropriate normal standards is of critical importance, since the normal range of values may be different when different techniques, and particularly when cuffs of different widths, are used in the measurements. Also, care has to be exercised in evaluating benefits of therapy when the resulting changes in pressure are relatively small and may be within the range of variability of the measurements. Various limitations of specific measurements must be kept in mind when interpreting the results and applying them to the assessment and management of patients. It must also be emphasized that the measurements should not be used as a substitute for careful clinical assessment but only in conjunction with it.

ACKNOWLEDGMENT

I wish to thank all members of the technical, nursing, and secretarial staff of the Vascular Laboratory of St. Boniface General Hospital for their excellent help over the past 25 years, to students who participated in our research, and numerous colleagues in our and other medical centers for the stimulation and motivation of my interest in the role of pressure measurements.

REFERENCES

1. Alpert, J.S., Larsen, O.A., and Lassen, N.A.: Exercise and intermittent claudication, Circulation 39:353, 1969.
2. Anderson, W.R.: Necrotizing angiitis associated with embolization of cholesterol, Am. J. Clin. Pathol. 43:65, 1965.
3. Baker, J.D.: Poststress Doppler ankle pressures, Arch. Surg. 113:1171, 1978.
4. Baker, R.J., Chunprapaph, B., and Nyhus, L.M.: Severe ischemia of the hand following radial artery catheterization, Surgery 80:449, 1976.
5. Baker, J.D., and Dix, D.: Variability of Doppler ankle pressures with arterial occlusive disease: an evaluation of ankle index and brachial-ankle pressure gradient, Surgery 89:134, 1981.
6. Baker, W.H., and Barnes, R.W.: Revitalizing the ischemic limb, Geriatrics 28:56, 1973.
7. Barner, H.B., et al.: Intermittent claudication with pedal pulses, JAMA 204:958, 1968.
8. Barnes, R.W., et al.: Complications of percutaneous femoral arterial catheterization, Am. J. Cardiol. 33:259, 1974.
9. Beach, K.W., Brunzell, J.D., and Strandness, D.E., Jr.: Prevalence of severe arteriosclerosis obliterans in patients with diabetes mellitus, Arteriosclerosis 2:275, 1982.
10. Beach, K.W., and Strandness, D.E., Jr.: Arteriosclerosis obliterans and associated risk factors in insulin-dependent and non-insulin-dependent diabetes, Diabetes 29:882, 1980.
11. Bell, G., et al.: Indirect measurement of systolic blood pressure in the lower limb using a mercury-in-rubber strain gauge, Cardiovasc. Res. 7:282, 1973.
12. Bell, G., et al.: Measurements of systolic pressure in the limbs of patients with arterial occlusive disease, Surg. Gynecol. Obstet. 136:177, 1973.
13. Bernstein, E.F., et al.: Thigh pressure artifacts with noninvasive techniques in an experimental model, Surgery 89:319, 1981.
14. Bloom, J.D., et al.: Defective limb growth as a complication of catheterization of the femoral artery, Surg. Gynecol. Obstet. 138:524, 1974.
15. Bloor, K.: Natural history of arteriosclerosis of the lower extremities, Ann. R. Coll. Surg. Engl. 28:36, 1961.
16. Bollinger, A., Barras, J.P., and Mahler, F.: Measurement of foot artery blood pressure by micromanometry in normal subjects and in patients with arterial occlusive disease, Circulation 53:506, 1976.
17. Bollinger, A., Mahler, F., and Gruentzig, A.: Peripheral hemodynamics in patients with coarctation, normotensive and hypertensive arteriosclerosis obliterans of the lower limbs, Angiology 22:354, 1971.
18. Bollinger, A., Mahler, F., and Zehender, O.: Kombinierte Druck- und Durchflussmessungen in der Beurteilung arterieller Durchblutungsstörungen, Dtsch. Med. Wochenschr. 95:1039, 1970.
19. Bone, G.E., and Pomajzl, M.J.: Toe blood pressure by photoplethysmography: an index of healing in forefoot amputation, Surgery 89:569, 1981.
20. Boyd, A.M.: The natural course of arteriosclerosis of the lower extremities, Proc. R. Soc. Med. 55:591, 1962.
21. Brener, B.J., et al.: Measurement of systolic femoral arterial pressure during reactive hyperemia: an estimate of aortoiliac disease, Circulation 50(suppl.):259, 1974.
22. Bryant, L.R., and Spencer, F.C.: Occlusive disease of subclavian artery, JAMA 196:109, 1966.
23. Cappelen, C., Jr., and Hall, K.V.: The effect of obstructive arterial disease on the peripheral arterial blood pressure, Surgery 48:888, 1960.
24. Carter, S.A.: Indirect systolic pressures and pulse waves in arterial occlusive disease of the lower extremities, Circulation 37:624, 1968.
25. Carter, S.A.: Clinical measurement of systolic pressures in limbs with arterial occlusive disease, JAMA 207:1869, 1969.
26. Carter, S.A.: Response of ankle systolic pressure to leg exercise in mild or questionable arterial disease, N. Engl. J. Med. 287:578, 1972.
27. Carter, S.A.: The relationship of distal systolic pressures to healing of skin lesions in limbs with arterial occlusive disease, with special reference to diabetes mellitus, Scand. J. Clin. Lab. Invest. 31(suppl. 128):239, 1973.
28. Carter, S.A.: Effect of age, cardiovascular disease, and vasomotor changes on transmission of arterial pressure waves through the lower extremities, Angiology 29:601, 1978.
29. Carter, S.A.: Arterial auscultation in peripheral vascular disease, JAMA 261:1682, 1981.
30. Carter, S.A.: Finger systolic pressures and skin temperatures in severe Raynaud's syndrome: the relationship to healing of skin lesions and the use of oral phenoxybenzamine, Angiology 32:298, 1981.
31. Carter, S.A.: The definition of critical ischaemia of the lower limb and distal systolic pressures, Br. J. Surg. 70:188, 1983.
32. Carter, S.A., and Lezack, J.D.: Digital systolic pressures in the lower limb in arterial disease, Circulation 43:905, 1971.
33. Carter, S.A., and Perlman, E.: The effect of vasomotor state on finger systolic pressures during local cooling in Raynaud's syndrome, Paper presented at the thirteenth World Congress International Union of Angiology, Rochester, Minn., 1983.
34. Carter, S.A., et al.: Exercise program in intermittent claudication, Physiologist 23:184, 1980.
35. Castaneda-Zuniga, W., et al.: Hemodynamic assessment of obstructive aortoiliac disease, Am. J. Roentgenol. 127:559, 1976.
36. Chamberlain, J., Housley, E., and Macpherson, A.I.S.: The relationship between ultrasound assessment and angiography in occlusive arterial disease of the lower limb, Br. J. Surg. 62:64, 1975.
37. Chavatzas, D., and Jamieson, C.W.: The doubtful place of the raised heel in patients with intermittent claudication of the leg, Br. J. Surg. 61:299, 1974.
38. Clifford, P.C., et al.: Intermittent claudication: is a supervised exercise class worthwhile? Br. Med. J. 280:1503, 1980.
39. Clyne, C.A.C., et al.: Oxygen tension on the skin of ischemic legs, Am. J. Surg. 143:315, 1982.

40. Conrad, M.C.: Large and small artery occlusion in diabetics and nondiabetics with severe vascular disease, Circulation 36:83, 1967.

41. Conrad, M.C.: Abnormalities of the digital vasculature as related to ulceration and gangrene, Circulation 38:568, 1968.

42. Conrad, M.C., and Green, H.D.: Hemodynamics of large and small vessels in peripheral vascular disease, Circulation 29:847, 1964.

43. Cutajar, C.L., Marston, A., and Newcombe, J.F.: Value of cuff occlusion pressures in assessment of peripheral vascular disease, Br. Med. J. 2:392, 1973.

44. Dahllöf, A.-G., et al.: Metabolic activity of skeletal muscle in patients with peripheral arterial insufficiency, Eur. J. Clin. Invest. 4:9, 1974.

45. Darling, R.C., et al.: Intermittent claudication in young athletes: popliteal artery entrapment syndrome, J. Trauma 14:543, 1974.

46. Delius, W.: Hämodynamische Untersuchungen über den systolischen Blutdruck und die arterielle Durchblutung distal von arteriellen Gefässverschlüssen an den unteren Extremitäten, Z. Kreislaufforsch. 58:319, 1969.

47. Dick, R.: Arteriography in neurovascular compression at the thoracic outlet, with special reference to embolic patterns, Am. J. Roentgenol. Radium Ther. Nucl. Med. 110:141, 1970.

48. Dormandy, J.A., Goyle, K.B., and Reid, H.L.: Treatment of severe intermittent claudication by controlled defibrination, Lancet 1:625, 1977.

49. Doupe, J., Newman, H.W., and Wilkins, R.W.: The effect of peripheral vasomotor activity on systolic arterial pressure in the extremities of man, J. Physiol. 95:244, 1939.

50. Downs, A.R., et al.: Assessment of arterial obstruction in vessels supplying the fingers by measurement of local blood pressures and the skin temperature response test—correlation with angiographic evidence, Surgery 77:530, 1975.

51. Edmonds, M.E., Roberts, V.C., and Watkins, P.J.: Blood flow in the diabetic neuropathic foot, Diabetologia 22:9, 1982.

52. Edmonds, M.E., et al.: Medial arterial calcification and diabetic neuropathy, Br. Med. J. 284:928, 1982.

53. Edwards, W.S., and Carmichael, J.D.: Aorto-iliac reconstruction without preoperative aortogram, Ann. Surg. 165:853, 1967.

54. Eickhoff, J.H., and Engell, H.C.: Transcutaneous oxygen tension (tcPO$_2$) measurements on the foot in normal subjects and in patients with peripheral arterial disease admitted for vascular surgery, Scand. J. Clin. Lab. Invest. 41:743, 1981.

55. Evans, J.G.: Neurogenic intermittent claudication, Br. Med. J. 2:985, 1964.

56. Fenton, T.R., Carter, S.A., and Vaishnav, R.N.: Collapse and viscoelasticity of diseased human arteries, J. Biomech., 1984. (In press.)

57. Flanigan, D.P., et al.: Utility of wide and narrow blood pressure cuffs in the hemodynamic assessment of aorto-iliac occlusive disease, Surgery 92:16, 1982.

58. Formijne, P.: Investigation of the patency of peripheral arteries, Am. Heart. J. 10:1, 1934.

59. Franzeck, U.K., Bernstein, E.F., and Fronek, A.: The effect of sensing site on the limb segmental blood pressure determination, Arch. Surg. 116:912, 1981.

60. French, J.W., and Guntheroth, W.G.: An explanation of asymmetric upper extremity blood pressures in supravalvular aortic stenosis, Circulation 42:31, 1970.

61. Fronek, A., Coel, M., and Bernstein, E.F.: Quantitative ultrasonographic studies of lower extremity flow velocities in health and disease, Circulation 53:957, 1976.

62. Fronek, A., Coel, M., and Bernstein, E.F.: The importance of combined multisegmental pressure and Doppler flow velocity studies in the diagnosis of peripheral arterial occlusive disease, Surgery 84:840, 1978.

63. Fronek, A., et al.: Noninvasive physiologic tests in the diagnosis and characterization of peripheral arterial occlusive disease, Am. J. Surg. 126:205, 1973.

64. Fronek, A., et al.: Ultrasonographically monitored postocclusive reactive hyperemia in the diagnosis of peripheral arterial occlusive disease, Circulation 48:149, 1973.

65. Gaskell, P.: The rate of blood flow in the foot and calf before and after reconstruction by arterial grafting of an occluded main artery to the lower limb, Clin. Sci. 15:259, 1956.

66. Gaskell, P.: Laboratory tests of circulation in the limbs, Manitoba Med. Rev. 45:540, 1965.

67. Gaskell, P.: The measurement of blood pressure, the critical opening pressure, and the critical closing pressure of digital vessels under various circumstances, Can. J. Physiol. Pharmacol. 43:979, 1965.

68. Gaskell, P.: The importance of penile blood pressure in cases of impotence, Can. Med. Assoc. J. 105:1047, 1971.

69. Gaskell, P.: Personal communication, 1979.

70. Gaskell, P., and Becker, W.J.: The erect posture as an aid to the circulation in the presence of arterial obstruction, Can. Med. Assoc. J. 105:930, 1971.

71. Gaskell, P., and Krisman, A.M.: An auscultatory technique for measuring the digital blood pressure, Can. J. Biochem. Physiol. 36:883, 1958.

72. Gaskell, P., and Krisman, A.M.: The brachial to digital blood pressure gradient in normal subjects and in patients with high blood pressure, Can. J. Biochem. Physiol. 36:889, 1958.

73. Gaskell, P., and Parrott, J.C.W.: The effect of a mechanical venous pump on the circulation of the feet in the presence of arterial obstruction, Surg. Gynecol. Obstet. 146:583, 1978.

74. Geddes, L.A., and Tivey, R.: The importance of cuff width in measurement of blood pressure indirectly, Cardiovasc. Res. Cent. Bull. 14:69, 1976.

75. Gibbon, J.H., and Landis, E.M.: Vasodilatation in lower extremities in response to immersing forearms in warm water, J. Clin. Invest. 11:1019, 1932.

76. Goebel, F.-D., and Füessl, H.S.: Mönckeberg's sclerosis after sympathetic denervation in diabetic and non-diabetic subjects, Diabetologia 24:347, 1983.

77. Gosling, R.G., and King, D.H.: Arterial assessment by Doppler-shift ultrasound, Proc. R. Soc. Med. 67:447, 1974.

78. Greenfield, A.D.M., Shepherd, J.T., and Whelan, R.F.: The proportion of the total hand blood flow passing through the digits, J. Physiol. 113:63, 1951.

79. Grüntzig, A., Schlumpf, M., and Bollinger, A.: Direkt und indirekt gemessner Druckgradient bei Stenosen der Becken- und Oberschenkelarterien. In Kriessmann, A., and Bollinger, A., editors: Ultraschall-Doppler-Diagnostik in der Angiologie, Stuttgart, 1978, Georg Thieme Verlag.

80. Gundersen, J.: Diagnosis of arterial insufficiency with measurement of blood pressure in fingers and toes, Angiology 22:191, 1971.

81. Gundersen, J.: Segmental measurements of systolic blood pressure in the extremities including the thumb and the great toe, Acta Chir. Scand. 426(suppl.):1, 1972.

82. Haimovici, H., and Escher, D.J.: Aortoiliac stenosis, Arch. Surg. 72:107, 1956.

83. Hällgren, R., et al.: Arterial calcification and progressive peripheral gangrene after renal transplantation, Acta Med. Scand. 198:331, 1975.

84. Heintz, S.E., et al.: Value of arterial pressure measurements in the proximal and distal part of the thigh in arterial occlusive disease, Surg. Gynecol. Obstet. 146:337, 1978.

85. Hirai, M., Nielsen, S.L., and Lassen, N.A.: Blood pressure measurement of all five fingers by strain gauge plethysmography, Scand. J. Clin. Lab. Invest. 36:627, 1976.

86. Hirai, M.: Arterial insufficiency of the hand evaluated by digital blood pressure and arteriographic findings, Circulation 58:902, 1978.

87. Hirai, M.: Cold sensitivity of the hand in arterial occlusive disease, Surgery 85:140, 1979.

88. Hirai, M., and Shionoya, S.: Intermittent claudication in the foot and Buerger's disease, Br. J. Surg. 65:210, 1978.

89. Hoare, M., et al.: The effect of local cooling on digital systolic pressure in patients with Raynaud's syndrome, Br. J. Surg. 69(suppl.):S27, 1982.

90. Hobbs, J.T., et al.: A limitation of the Doppler ultrasound method of measuring ankle systolic pressure, Vasa 3:160, 1974.

91. Holstein, P., Dovey, H., and Lassen, N.A.: Wound healing in above-knee amputations in relation to skin perfusion pressure, Acta Orthop. Scand. 50:59, 1979.

92. Holstein, P., and Lassen, N.A.: Radioisotope clearance technique for measurement of distal blood pressure in skin and muscles, Scand. J. Clin. Lab. Invest. 31(suppl. 128):143, 1973.

93. Holstein, P., and Lassen, N.A.: Healing of ulcers on the feet correlated with distal blood pressure measurements in occlusive arterial disease, Acta Orthop. Scand. 51:995, 1980.

94. Holstein, P., and Sager, P.: Toe blood pressure in peripheral arterial disease, Acta Orthop. Scand. 44:564, 1973.

95. Holstein, P., Sager, P., and Lassen, N.A.: Wound healing in below-knee amputations in relation to skin perfusion pressure, Acta Orthop. Scand. 50:49, 1979.

96. Hummel, B.W., et al.: Reactive hyperemia vs. treadmill exercise testing in arterial disease, Arch. Surg. 113:95, 1978.

97. Hutchison, K.J., and Williams, H.T.: Calf blood flow and ankle systolic blood pressure in intermittent claudication monitored over five years, Angiology 29:719, 1978.

98. Ibels, L.S., et al.: Arterial Calcification and pathology in uremic patients undergoing dialysis, Am. J. Med. 66:790, 1979.

99. Janzon, L., et al.: The arm-ankle pressure gradient in relation to cardiovascular risk factors in intermittent claudication, Circulation 63:1339, 1981.

100. Jeresaty, R.M., and Liss, J.P.: Effects of brachial artery catheterization on arterial pulse and blood pressure in 203 patients, Am. Heart J. 76:481, 1968.

101. Jogestrand, T., and Berglund, B.: Estimation of digital circulation and its correlation to clinical signs of ischaemia—a comparative methodological study, Clin. Physiol. 3:307, 1983.

102. Johnson, C.D., Zirkle, T.J., and Smith, L.L.: Occlusive disease of the vessels of the aortic arch, Calif. Med. 108:20, 1968.

103. Johnson, W.C.: Doppler ankle pressure and reactive hyperemia in the diagnosis of arterial insufficiency, J. Surg. Res. 18:177, 1975.

104. Johnston, K.W.: Role of Doppler ultrasonography in determining the hemodynamic significance of aortoiliac disease, Can. J. Surg. 21:319, 1978.

105. Johnston, K.W., Colapinto, R.F., and Baird, R.J.: Transluminal dilation, Arch. Surg. 117:1604, 1982.

106. Johnston, K.W., and Taraschuk, I.: Validation of the role of pulsatility index in quantitation of the severity of peripheral arterial occlusive disease, Am. J. Surg. 131:295, 1976.

107. Kaufman, S.L., et al.: Hemodynamic measurements in the evaluation and follow-up of transluminal angioplasty of the iliac and femoral arteries, Radiology 142:329, 1982.

108. Kazmier, F.J., et al.: Livedo reticularis and digital infarcts: a syndrome due to cholesterol emboli arising from atheromatous abdominal aortic aneurysms, Vasc. Dis. 3:12, 1966.

109. Kempczinski, R.F., Buckley, C.J., and Darling, R.C.: Vascular insufficiency secondary to ergotism, Surgery 79:597, 1976.

110. King, L.T., Strandness, D.E., Jr., and Bell, J.W.: The hemodynamic response of the lower extremities to exercise, J. Surg. Res. 5:167, 1965.

111. Knox, W.G., Finby, N., and Moscarella, A.A.: Limitations of arteriography in determining operability for femoropopliteal occlusive disease, Ann. Surg. 161:509, 1965.

112. Kotte, J.H., Iglaner, A., and McGuire, J.: Measurements of arterial blood pressure in arm and leg: comparison of sphygmomanometric and direct intra-arterial pressures with special attention to their relationship in aortic regurgitation. Am. Heart J. 28:476, 1944.

113. Kottke, B.A., Fairbairn, J.H., II, and Davis, G.D.: Complications of aortography, Circulation 30:843, 1964.

114. Krähenbühl, B., Nielsen, S.L., and Lassen, N.A.: Closure of digital arteries in high vascular tone states as demonstrated by measurement of systolic blood pressure in the fingers, Scand. J. Clin. Lab. Invest. 37:71, 1977.

115. Kroeker, E.J., and Wood, E.H.: Beat-to-beat alterations in relationship of simultaneously recorded central and peripheral arterial pressure pulses during Valsalva maneuver and prolonged expiration in man, J. Appl. Physiol. 8:483, 1956.

116. Lamis, P.A., Stanton, P.E., Jr., and Hyland, L.: The axillo-axillary bypass graft, Arch. Surg. 111:1353, 1976.

117. Larsen, O.A., and Lassen, N.A.: Medical treatment of occlusive arterial disease of the legs, Angiologia 6:288, 1969.

118. Lassen, N.A., and Holstein, P.: Use of radioisotopes in assessment of distal blood flow and distal blood pressure in arterial insufficiency, Surg. Clin. North Am. 54:39, 1974.

119. Lassen, N.A., Krähenbühl, B., and Hirai, M.: Occlusion cuff for routine measurement of digital blood pressure and blood flow, Am. J. Physiol. 232:H338, 1977.

120. Lassen, N.A., Tönnesen, K.H., and Holstein, P.: Distal blood pressure (editorial), Scand. J. Clin. Lab. Invest. 36:705, 1976.

121. Lassen, N.A., et al.: Distal blood pressure measurements in occlusive arterial disease, strain gauge compared to xenon-133, Angiology 23:211, 1972.

122. Lazarus, H.M., et al.: Doppler ankle pressures and stiff arteries. In Diethrich, E.B., editor: Noninvasive cardiovascular diagnosis: current concepts, Baltimore, 1978, University Park Press.

123. Lennihan, R., Jr., and Mackereth, M.A.: Ankle blood pressures as a practical aid in vascular practice, Angiology 26:211, 1975.

124. Lewis, J.D.: Pressure measurements in the long-term follow up of peripheral vascular disease, Proc. R. Soc. Med. 67:443, 1974.

125. Lewis, J.D., et al.: Simultaneous flow and pressure measurements in intermittent claudication, Br. J. Surg. 59:418, 1972.

126. Lezack, J.D., and Carter, S.A.: Systolic pressures in arterial occlusive disease with special reference to the effect of posture, Clin. Res. 17:638, 1969.

127. Lezack, J.D., and Carter, S.A.: Systolic pressures in the extremities of man with special reference to the toes, Can. J. Physiol. Pharmacol. 48:469, 1970.

128. Lezack, J.D., and Carter, S.A.: The relationship of distal systolic pressures to the clinical and angiographic findings in limbs with arterial occlusive disease, Scand. J. Clin. Lab. Invest. 31(suppl. 128):97, 1973.

129. Lorentsen, E.: Blood pressure and flow in the calf in relation to claudication distance, Scand. J. Clin. Lab. Invest. 31:141, 1973.

130. Lorentsen, E.: Calf blood pressure measurements. The applicability of a plethysmographic method and the results of measurements during reactive hyperaemia, Scand. J. Clin. Lab. Invest. 31:69, 1973.

131. Lorentsen, E.: The vascular resistance in the arteries of the lower leg in normal subjects and in patients with different degrees of atherosclerotic disease, Scand. J. Clin. Lab. Invest. 31:147, 1973.

132. Lynn, R.B., Steiner, R.E., and Van Wyk, F.A.K.: Arteriographic appearance of the digital arteries of the hands in Raynaud's disease, Lancet 1:471, 1955.

133. Mahler, F., Schlumpf, M., and Bollinger, A.: Knöchel-arteriendruck nach standardisierter Gehbelastung bei Gesunden und bei Patienten mit arterieller Verschlusskrankheit. In Kriessman, A., and Bollinger, A., editors: Ultraschall-Doppler-Diagnostik in der Angiologie, Stuttgart, 1978, Georg Thieme Verlag.

134. Mahler, F., et al.: Postocclusion and postexercise flow velocity and ankle pressures in normals and marathon runners, Angiology 27:721, 1976.

135. Malone, J.M., et al.: The "Gold Standard" for amputation level selection: xenon-133 clearance, J. Surg. Res. 30:449, 1981.

136. Matesanz, J.M., Patwardhan, N., and Herrmann, J.B.: A simplified method for evaluating peripheral arterial occlusive disease in a clinical vascular laboratory, Angiology 29:791, 1978.

137. May, A.G., Van de Berg, L., DeWeese, J.A., and Rob, C.G.: Critical arterial stenosis, Surgery 54:250, 1963.

138. McEwan, A.J., and Ledingham, I.M.: Blood flow characteristics and tissue nutrition in apparently ischaemic feet, Br. Med. J. 3:220, 1971.

139. McEwan, A.J., Stalker, C.G., and Ledingham, I.M.: Foot skin ischaemia in atherosclerotic peripheral vascular disease, Br. Med. J. 3:612, 1970.

140. Metz, P.: Erectile function in men with occlusive arterial disease in the legs, Dan. Med. Bull. 30:185, 1983.

141. Metz, P., and Bengtsson, J.: Penile blood pressure, Scand. J. Urol. Nephrol. 15:161, 1981.

142. Mitchell, P.L., Parlin, R.W., and Blackburn, H.: Effect of vertical displacement of the arm on indirect blood-pressure measurement, N. Engl. J. Med. 271:72, 1964.

143. Mozersky, D.J., Sumner, D.S., and Strandness, D.E., Jr.: Long-term results of reconstructive aortoiliac surgery, Am. J. Surg. 123:503, 1972.

144. Naumann, M.: Der Blutdruck in der Arteria dorsalis pedis in der Norm und bei Kreislaufstörungen, Z. Kreislaufforsch. 31:36, 1939.

145. Nicolaides, A.N., Fernandes e Fernandes, J., and Angelides, N.A.: The effect of profundaplasty on ankle pressure and walking distance: an objective assessment using Doppler ultrasound and a treadmill. In Diethrich, E.B., editor: Noninvasive cardiovascular diagnosis: current concepts, Baltimore, 1978, University Park Press.

146. Nielsen, P.E.: Digital blood pressure in patients with peripheral arterial disease, Scand. J. Clin. Lab. Invest. 36:731, 1976.

147. Nielsen, P.E.: Digital blood pressure in normal subjects and patients with peripheral arterial disease, Scand. J. Clin. Lab. Invest. 36:725, 1976.

148. Nielsen, P.E., Barras, J.-P., and Holstein, P.: Systolic pressure amplification in the arteries of normal subjects, Scand. J. Clin. Lab. Invest. 33:371, 1974.

149. Nielsen, P.E., Bell, G., and Lassen, N.A.: The measurement of digital systolic blood pressure by strain gauge technique, Scand. J. Clin. Lab. Invest. 29:371, 1972.

150. Nielsen, P.E., and Nielsen, S.L.: Digital arterial tone in hypertensive subjects treated with cardioselective and non-selective beta-adrenoreceptor blocking agents, Dan. Med. Bull. 28:76, 1981.

151. Nielsen, S.L., Olsen, N., and Henriksen, O.: Cold hypersensitivity after sympathectomy for Raynaud's disease, Scand. J. Thor. Cardiovasc. Surg. 14:109, 1980.

152. Nielsen, P.E., Poulsen, H.L., and Gyntelberg, F.: Skin blood pressure measured by a photoelectric probe and external counterpressure, Scand. J. Clin. Lab. Invest. 31(suppl. 128):137, 1973.

153. Nielsen, P.E., and Rasmussen, S.M.: Indirect measurement of systolic blood pressure by strain gauge technique at finger, ankle and toe in diabetic patients without symptoms of occlusive arterial disease, Diabetologia 9:25, 1973.

154. Nielsen, S.L., Sørensen, C.J., and Olsen, N.: Thermostatted measurement of systolic blood pressure on cooled fingers, Scand. J. Clin. Lab. Invest. 40:683, 1980.

155. Nielsen, P.E., et al.: Reduction in distal blood pressure by sympathetic nerve block in patients with occlusive arterial disease, Cardiovasc. Res. 7:577, 1973.

156. Nielsen, S.L.: Raynaud phenomena and finger systolic pressure during cooling, Scand. J. Clin. Lab. Invest. 38:765, 1978.

157. Nielsen, S.L., and Lassen, N.A.: Measurement of digital blood pressure after local cooling, J. Appl. Physiol. 43:907, 1977.

158. Nielsen, S.L., et al.: Raynaud's phenomenon in arterial obstructive disease of the hand demonstrated by locally provoked cooling, Scand. J. Thor. Cardiovasc. Surg. 12:105, 1978.

159. Nobin, B.A., et al.: Reserpine treatment of Raynaud's disease, Ann. Surg. 187:12, 1978.

160. Noer, I., Tønnesen, K.H., and Sager, P.: Preoperative estimation of run off in patients with multiple level arterial obstructions as a guide to partial reconstructive surgery, Ann. Surg. 188:663, 1978.

161. Oliva, I., and Roztočil, K.: Toe pulse wave analysis in obliterating atherosclerosis, Angiology 34:610, 1983.

162. O'Mara, C.S., et al.: Hemodynamic assessment of transluminal angioplasty for lower extremity ischemia, Surgery 89:106, 1981.

163. O'Rourke, M.F., et al.: Pressure wave transmission along the human aorta, Circ. Res. 23:567, 1968.

164. Osmundson, P.J.: A prospective study of peripheral occlusive arterial disease in diabetes. II. Vascular laboratory assessment, Mayo Clin. Proc. 56:223, 1981.

165. Ouriel, K., et al.: A critical evaluation of stress testing in the diagnosis of peripheral vascular disease, Surgery 91:686, 1982.

166. Paaske, W.P., and Tønnesen, K.H.: Prognostic significance of distal blood pressure measurements in patients with severe ischaemia, Scand. J. Thor. Cardiovasc. Surg. 14:105, 1980.

167. Pascarelli, E.F., and Bertrand, C.A.: Comparison of blood pressures in the arms and legs, N. Engl. J. Med. 270:693, 1964.

168. Patel, A., and Toole, J.F.: Subclavian steal syndrome—reversal of cephalic blood flow, Medicine (Baltimore) 44:289, 1965.

169. Piccone, V.A., Jr., Karvounis, P., and LeVeen, H.H.: The subclavian steal syndrome, Angiology 21:240, 1970.

170. Postlethwaite, J.C., and Dormandy, J.A.: Results of ankle systolic pressure measurements in patients with intermittent claudication being treated with clofibrate, Ann. Surg. 181:799, 1975.

171. Prineas, R.J., et al.: Recommendations for use of noninvasive methods to detect atherosclerotic peripheral arterial disease—in population studies, Circulation 65:1561A, 1982.

172. Quick, C.R., and Cotton, L.T.: The measured effect of stopping smoking on intermittent claudication, Br. J. Surg. 69(suppl.):S24, 1982.

173. Rahman, A., and Rodbard, S.: Timing of the arterial sounds in the subclavian steal syndrome, Arch. Intern. Med. 125:1027, 1970.

174. Raines, J.K., et al.: Vascular laboratory criteria for the management of peripheral vascular disease of the lower extremities, Surgery 79:21, 1976.

175. Ramsey, D.E., Manke, D.A., and Sumner, D.S.: Toe blood pressure a valuable adjunct to ankle pressure measurement for assessing peripheral arterial disease, J. Cardiovasc. Surg. 24:43, 1983.

176. Reinle, E.: Über Blutdruckdifferenzen zwischen rechtem und linkem Arm, Schweiz. Med. Wochenschr. 93:1616, 1963.

177. Roddie, I.C., Shepherd, J.T., and Whelan, R.F.: The contribution of constrictor and dilator nerves to the skin vasodilatation during body heating, J. Physiol. 136:489, 1957.

178. Sacks, A.H.: Indirect blood pressure measurements: a matter of interpretation, Angiology 30:683, 1979.

179. Sako, Y.: Value of flowmeter and pressure measurements during vascular surgery: clinical and experimental, Surg. Clin. North Am. 47:1383, 1967.

180. Saltin, B.: Physical training in patients with intermittent claudication. In Cohen, L.S., Mock, I., and Ringquist, M.B., editors: Physical conditioning and cardiovascular rehabilitation, New York, 1981, John Wiley & Sons, Inc.

181. Schatz, I.J.: The natural history of peripheral arteriosclerosis. In Brest, A.N., and Moyer, J.H., editors: Atherosclerotic vascular disease: a Hahnemann symposium, New York, 1967, Appleton-Century-Crofts.

182. Schatz, I.J., Fine, G., and Eyler, W.R.: Thromboangiitis obliterans, Br. Heart J. 28:84, 1966.

183. Schroll, M., and Munck, O.: Estimation of peripheral arteriosclerotic disease by ankle blood pressure measurements in a population study of 60-year-old men and women, J. Chronic Dis. 34:261, 1981.

184. Schultz, R.D., Hokanson, D.F., and Strandness, D.F., Jr.: Pressure-flow and stress-strain measurements of normal and diseased aortoiliac segments, Surg. Gynecol. Obstet. 124:1267, 1967.

185. Schwartz, J.A., et al.: Predictive value of distal perfusion pressure in the healing of amputation of the digits and the forefoot, Surg. Gynecol. Obstet. 154:865, 1982.

186. Siggaard-Andersen, J., et al.: Blood pressure measurements of the lower limb. Arterial occlusions in the calf determined by plethysmographic blood pressure measurements in the thigh and at the ankle, Angiology 23:350, 1972.

187. Skinner, J.S., and Strandness, D.E., Jr.: Exercise and intermittent claudication. I. Effect of repetition and intensity of exercise, Circulation 36:15, 1967.

188. Skinner, J.S., and Strandness, D.E., Jr.: Exercise and intermittent claudication. II. Effect of physical training, Circulation 36:23, 1967.

189. Sprague, D.H., and Kim, D.I.: Pseudohypertension due to Mönckeberg's arteriosclerosis, Anesth. Analg. 57:588, 1978.

190. Stahler, C., and Strandness, D.E., Jr.: Ankle blood pressure response to graded treadmill exercise, Angiology 18:237, 1967.

191. Stegall, H.F., Kardon, M.B., and Kemmerer, W.T.: Indirect measurement of arterial blood pressure by Doppler ultrasonic sphygmomanometry, J. Appl. Physiol. 25:793, 1968.

192. Strandness, D.E., Jr.: Peripheral arterial disease. A physiologic approach, Boston, 1969, Little, Brown & Co.

193. Strandness, D.E., Jr.: Exercise testing in the evaluation of patients undergoing direct arterial surgery, J. Cardiovasc. Surg. 11:192, 1970.

194. Strandness, D.E., Jr.: Common pitfalls in the noninvasive evaluation of lower extremity arterial insufficiency. In Diethrich, E.B., editor: Noninvasive cardiovascular diagnosis: current concepts, Baltimore, 1978, University Park Press.

195. Strandness, D.E., Jr., and Bell, J.W.: An evaluation of the hemodynamic response of the claudicating extremity to exercise, Surg. Gynecol. Obstet. 119:1237, 1964.

196. Strandness, D.E., Jr., and Bell, J.W.: Peripheral vascular disease: diagnosis and objective evaluation using a mercury strain gauge, Ann. Surg. 161(suppl.4):1, 1965.

197. Strandness, D.E., Jr., and Stahler, C.: Arteriosclerosis obliterans. Manner and rate of progression, J.A.M.A. 196:1, 1966.

198. Strandness, D.E., Jr., and Sumner, D.S.: Applications of ultrasound to the study of arteriosclerosis obliterans, Angiology 26:187, 1975.

199. Strandness, D.E., Jr., Gibbons, G.E., and Bell, J.W.: Mercury strain gauge plethysmography. Evaluation of patients with acquired arteriovenous fistula, Arch. Surg. 85:215, 1962.

200. Strandness, D.E., Jr., Priest, R.E., and Gibbons, G.E.: Combined clinical and pathologic study of diabetic and nondiabetic peripheral arterial disease, Diabetes 13:366, 1964.

201. Sturm, A., Jr., Puentes, F., and Scheja, H.W.: Ursachen der Blutdruckdifferenzen zwischen dem rechten und linken Arm, Dtsch. Med. Wochenschr. 95:1914, 1970.

202. Sugiura, T., and Freis, E.D.: Pressure pulse in small arteries, Circ. Res. 11:838, 1962.

203. Sumner, D.S.: Presidential address: Noninvasive testing of vascular disease—fact, fancy, and future, Surgery 93:664, 1983.

204. Sumner, D.S., and Strandness, D.E., Jr.: The relationship between calf blood flow and ankle blood pressure in patients with intermittent claudication, Surgery 65:763, 1969.

205. Taguchi, J.T., and Suwangool, P.: "Pipestem" brachial arteries. A cause of pseudohypertension, JAMA 228:733, 1974.

206. Tanner, J.: Studies on medium-sized arteries in man. B.Sc. (Med.) thesis, University of Manitoba, no. 22947, September, 1964.

207. Taylor, M.G.: Wave travel in arteries and the design of the cardiovascular system. In Attinger, E.O., editor: Pulsatile blood flow, New York, 1964, McGraw-Hill Book Co.

208. Thulesius, O.: Beurteilung des Schweregrades arterieller Durchblutungsstörungen mit dem Doppler-Ultraschallgerät. In Bollinger, A., and Brunner, U., editors: Aktuelle Probleme in der Angiologie, Bern, 1971, Hans Huber Publishers.

209. Thulesius, O., Brubakk, A., and Berlin, E.: Response of digital blood pressure to cold provocation in cases with Raynaud's Phenomena, Angiology 32:113, 1981.

210. Thulesius, O., and Gjöres, J.E.: Use of Doppler shift detection for determining peripheral arterial blood pressure, Angiology 22:594, 1971.

211. Thulesius, O., and Länne, T.: The importance of arterial compliance and tone for the determination of ankle systolic pressure, Paper presented at the thirteenth World Congress of the International Union of Angiology, Rochester, Minn., 1983.

212. Thulesius, O., Valmin, K., and Todoreskov, R.: Response of finger systolic blood pressure to cold provocation in cases with hypertension and diabetes, Clin. Physiol. 2:513, 1982.

213. Tønnesen, K.H., et al.: Classification of peripheral occlusive arterial diseases based on symptoms, signs, and distal blood pressure measurements, Acta Chir. Scand. 146:101, 1980.

214. Toole, J.F., and Tulloch, E.F.: Bilateral simultaneous sphygmomanometry. A new diagnostic test for subclavian steal syndrome, Circulation 33:952, 1966.

215. Velayos, E.D., Robinson, H., Porciuncula, F.U., and Masi, A.T.: Clinical correlation analysis of 137 patients with Raynaud's phenomenon, Am. J. Med. Sci. 262:347, 1970.

216. Vincent, D.G., et al.: Noninvasive assessment of toe systolic pressures with special reference to diabetes mellitus, J. Cardiovasc. Surg. 24:22, 1983.

217. Weismann, R.E., and Upson, J.F.: Intra-arterial pressure studies in patients with arterial insufficiency of lower extremities, Ann. Surg. 157:501, 1963.

218. Wezler, K., and Standl, R.: Die normalen Alterskurven der Pulswellengeschwindigkeit in elastischen und muskulären Arterien des Menschen, Z. Biol. 97:265, 1936.

219. White, R.A., et al.: Noninvasive evaluation of peripheral vascular disease using transcutaneous oxygen tension, Am. J. Surg. 144:68, 1982.

220. Widmer, L.K., and Staub, H.: Blutdruck in stenosierten Arterien, Z. Kreislaufforsch. 51:975, 1962.

221. Wilbur, B.G., and Olcott, C., IV: A comparison of three modes of stress on Doppler ankle pressures. In Diethrich, E.B., editor: Noninvasive cardiovascular diagnosis: current concepts, Baltimore, 1978, University Park Press.

222. Winsor, T.: Influence of arterial disease on the systolic blood pressure gradients of the extremity, Am. J. Med. Sci. 220:117, 1950.

223. Yao, J.S.T.: Haemodynamic studies in peripheral arterial disease, Br. J. Surg. 57:761, 1970.

224. Yao, J.S.T.: Exercise testing using Doppler ultrasound and xenon clearance techniques, Angiology 26:528, 1975.

225. Yao, J.S.T., Hobbs, J.T., and Irvine, W.T.: Ankle systolic pressure measurements in arterial disease affecting the lower extremities, Br. J. Surg. 56:676, 1969.

226. Yao, J.S.T., et al.: A comparative study of strain-gauge plethysmography and Doppler ultrasound in the assessment of occlusive arterial disease of the lower extremities, Surgery 71:4, 1972.

227. Yao, J.S.T., et al.: A method for assessing ischemia of the hand and fingers, Surg. Gynecol. Obstet. 135:373, 1972.

228. Zetterquist, S.: The effect of active training on the nutritive blood flow in exercising ischemic legs, Scand. J. Clin. Lab. Invest. 25:101, 1970.

CHAPTER 52

Surgical use of pressure studies in peripheral arterial disease

JAMES S.T. YAO

Of the various techniques for recording systolic pressure in the lower limb, the Doppler ultrasound flow velocity detector technique[49,53,58] is the most versatile method and has been shown to provide an objective approach in the evaluation of patients with occlusive arterial disease. At present, segmental systolic pressure measurement is a standard routine in most medical centers dealing with reconstructive vascular surgical procedures. The use of Doppler ultrasound provides useful information in the preoperative and postoperative phases of management of patients undergoing reconstructive procedures.

Applications of ankle systolic pressure measurement in *clinical practice* are multiple. The accompanying outline summarizes surgical applications of ankle systolic pressure in occlusive peripheral arterial disease affecting the lower extremity. In upper extremity ischemia the use of pressure measurement of the forearm or digital arteries is helpful to elucidate Raynaud's phenomenon and various forms of hand ischemia.

Segmental pressure measurement of the lower extremity includes high and low thigh, calf, and ankle levels. Also, toe pressure recorded by either Doppler ultrasound or photoplethysmography may offer further hemodynamic information. Table 52-1 shows the normal values of systolic pressures commonly used in many vascular laboratories.

CONFIRMATION OF THE PRESENCE AND LOCATION OF ACUTE AND CHRONIC ARTERIAL OCCLUSIONS

Confirmation of the clinical diagnosis of occlusive arterial disease constitutes the first step in the treatment of these patients. The absence of a palpable pedal pulse often leads to the diagnosis of occlusive arterial disease. In borderline situations such as the presence of ankle edema and obesity, which make assessment of the pedal pulse difficult, the level of ankle pressure recorded by the ultrasound technique often refutes or confirms the diagnosis instantly. In patients with occlusive arterial disease in whom the pedal pulses are not palpable, the Doppler ultrasound flow velocity detector is able to detect flow signals from either the posterior tibial or dorsal artery of the foot. These flow signals represent the supply by collateral flow pathways, which could be used for registration of systolic pressure endpoint by the indirect cuff technique.

Pressures measured at the thigh, calf, and ankle may aid in establishing the site of occlusion. In the presence of iliac artery or common femoral artery occlusion, pressure recorded at these sites gives similar information, that is, the absence of a pressure gradient. In contrast, a pressure gradient is noted between thigh and ankle levels when there is occlusion affecting the femoropopliteal segment. In multiple occlusions affecting the aortoiliac and femoropopliteal segments different pressure gradients in the thigh and ankle are also seen, with the ankle pressure being much lower than in patients with single occlusions.

Ankle systolic pressure, when compared with the brachial systolic pressure, gives the index of isch-

□ Supported in part by the Dr. Scholl Foundation and the Northwestern University Vascular Research Fund.

Table 52-1. Normal values for Doppler arterial examination

Pressure area	Pressure values
Ankle systolic pressure	>Brachial systolic pressure (<40 mm Hg = limb-threatening ischemia)
Ankle pressure index (ankle/brachial ratio)	>1.0
Thigh systolic pressure	
Upper (narrow cuff)	30-40 mm Hg > brachial systolic pressure
Lower (wide cuff)	20-30 mm Hg > brachial systolic pressure
Thigh pressure index	>1.1
Pressure gradients	<30 mm Hg between adjacent sites
Toe systolic pressure index	0.7 ± 0.19 (0.35 ± 0.15 = claudication; 0.11 ± 0.10 = rest pain)
Finger systolic pressure index	>0.95
Treadmill exercise test (2 mph, 12% grade)	Elevated or no decrease of ankle pressure after 5 minutes' walking time

Reproduced with permission from Pearce, W.H., Yao, J.S.T., and Bergan, J.J.: Noninvasive vascular diagnostic testing in Ravitch, M.M., et al. (eds): CURRENT PROBLEMS IN SURGERY Vol. 20, No. 8, Copyright © 1983 by Year Book Medical Publishers, Inc., Chicago.

emia. Such a pressure index, as suggested by Winsor,[53] has been shown to correlate significantly with initial clinical symptoms[58] and the angiographic findings.

The absolute level of ankle systolic pressure and the pressure index are useful to express hemodynamic data. The pressure index helps distinguish normal from abnormal limbs, whereas the absolute pressure level helps in determining limb viability. Fig. 52-1 illustrates the receiver operating characteristic (ROC) curves reported by Ouriel and Zarins[38] for these two parameters in the diagnosis of arterial occlusive disease. The specificity was 99% for presence of disease and 100% for absence of disease. Ankle systolic pressure, however, is more useful to determine limb viability (Fig. 52-1, *B*). Ankle systolic pressure less than 40 mm Hg is always associated with limb-threatening ischemia, and such a level has been recommended as an objective hemodynamic criterion for defining critical ischemia.[27] When arterial occlusion involves more distal arteries, the toe pressure recording may be a better index to establish the presence of severe ischemia. Toe pressure measurement may be subject to wide variations, and duplicate measurements may be needed for a reliable study.[47]

Similar to all physiologic measurements, ankle pressure is subject to variability, and this variation must be considered when evaluating the results of a longitudinal study. In our study,[55] as well as others,[2] a change in ankle pressure index of 0.15 was considered to be significant, but any change less than 0.15 was considered a result of measurement variation.

EVALUATION OF INTERMITTENT CLAUDICATION

Intermittent claudication may be arterial, venous, or neurogenic in origin. In the majority of patients, careful history taking and physical examination should establish the diagnosis. Measurement of ankle pressure and observation of its change after a standard treadmill exercise provide a simple test in the diagnosis of claudication of vascular origin. This is particularly true in patients initially having intermittent claudication who are found to have pedal pulses. These pulses, derived from collateral flow, often are associated with a decrease of ankle pressure and often disappear after exercise. The so-called pulse-disappearing phenomenon can be verified simply by recording the ankle pressure after treadmill exercise. When there is a significant drop of ankle pressure after exercise, disability as a result of neurogenic origin can be ruled out and vice versa.

After treadmill exercise, the degree of ankle pressure drop and the time for the pressure to return to preexercise level are the two important components that offer hemodynamic information. The degree of ankle pressure drop immediately after termination of exercise reflects the degree of inflow obstruction, whereas the recovery time denotes the adequacy of collateral pathways. In the presence of superficial femoral or femoropopliteal artery occlusion the pressure drop is often to 50% of the preexercise level. In contrast, patients with iliac artery occlusion will have a greater drop in ankle pressure (70% to 90%) immediately following exercise because of shunting of blood to the thigh

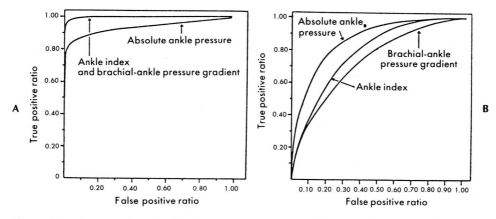

Fig. 52-1. ROC curves illustrating absolute ankle pressure and ankle index to discriminate between **A,** normal and arteriographically diseased limbs and, **B,** viable and nonviable limbs. (From Ouriel, K., and Zarins, C.K.: Arch. Surg. 117:1297, Copyright 1982, American Medical Association.

muscle groups. The return of pressure to the preexercise level is often within 5 to 7 minutes because of the adequacy of collateral pathways in these patients. When there are two levels of occlusion, the picture becomes more complex. Following exercise, blood flow must traverse two collateral networks. A profound drop of ankle systolic pressure, often to an unrecordable level, results. Likewise, the recovery time is prolonged because of multiple levels of occlusion. An understanding of these hemodynamic changes helps determine the type of surgical corrective procedure to be used in these patients.

Different types of postexercise pressure curves have been reported by Chamberlain et al.[11] Their findings correlated well with the angiographic appearance. Of great interest is the finding that associated deep femoral artery disease often is found with a severe depression of ankle pressure after exercise. Such information is useful to supplement the angiographic findings before reconstructive procedures, and it may help in the selection of patients for deep femoral artery reconstruction. The postexercise pressure response is also useful in planning a logical approach to patients who have coexistent neurogenic and vascular claudication.[22]

In addition to detection of atherosclerotic occlusive disease, the Doppler examination can detect popliteal artery entrapment. If entrapment is present, the ankle pressure will decrease when the leg is placed in passive hyperextension with the foot dorsiflexed.[39]

Following is an outline of the surgical application of ankle systolic pressure in occlusive peripheral arterial disease.

1. Confirmation of clinical diagnosis
2. Ischemic index (ankle/brachial pressure ratio)
   a. Degree of ischemia
   b. Status of runoff
   c. Patency of reconstructed artery
   d. Long-term follow-up
3. Level of amputation
4. Response to sympathetic ablation
5. Prognosis for healing of skin lesions
6. Exercise test
   a. Differential diagnosis for neurogenic claudication
   b. Functional assessment of angiographic stenosis
   c. Functional assessment of result of reconstructive surgery

SELECTION OF OPERATION AND OPERATIVE CANDIDATES

Hemodynamic study of inflow arteries. The importance of recognizing iliac artery stenosis before superficial femoral artery reconstruction has been stressed by many authors. Failure to correct a significant inflow defect often results in failure of a femorodistal bypass. When there is angiographic evidence of stenotic lesions affecting both the iliac and superficial femoral arteries, the lesion giving rise to the ischemic symptoms must be identified.

Using the ankle pressure measurement and flow waveform recordings from the common femoral artery, the hemodynamic consequences of anatomic disease in the iliac artery can be assessed to identify significant lesions.[54] A segmental pressure measurement that shows a significant pressure gradient (greater than 50 mm Hg) between thigh and ankle levels signifies that the occlusion of the femoropopliteal segment is of hemodynamic significance. The degree of ankle pressure drop following treadmill exercise is also helpful in the evaluation of proximal arterial lesions. Since there is only minor shunting of blood to thigh muscles, patients with femoropopliteal disease alone have only moderate reduction in postexercise ankle pressure. Conversely, inflow disease of the aortoiliac segment produces more profound drops in ankle pressure. When functionally significant disease is present in both segments, ankle pressures often fall to zero following exercise and remain depressed for a prolonged period. Correction of the aortoiliac arterial occlusion often reverts the postexercise pattern to that of a single anatomic occlusion.

By identifying which angiographically demonstrated lesion of the iliac artery has hemodynamic significance, one can more intelligently select the most appropriate operation. When the anatomic iliac disease is not functionally significant, femoropopliteal reconstruction can be expected to provide gratifying results. Likewise, if the previous information suggests that the iliac occlusion is limiting inflow, it must be corrected before femoropopliteal bypass is considered. The common femoral flow pattern, the segmental pressure, and its change after exercise should be taken into consideration in planning reconstructive procedures in patients with combined occlusions.

To identify iliac artery stenosis, Bone et al.[7] have recommended the use of a narrow cuff to record upper thigh pressure. In our laboratory, as well as others,[15-17] it has been found that the upper thigh pressure measurement added little information on the status of inflow. The presence of a superficial femoral artery occlusion alters the result of upper thigh pressure recordings. Whereas a normal upper thigh pressure is generally reliable in ruling out hemodynamically significant aortoiliac occlusive disease, an abnormal pressure does not differentiate between aortoiliac and superficial femoral artery disease. In the study by Flanigan et al.,[17] it was found that the upper thigh pressure could not identify a significant iliac lesion when there was an associated femoropopliteal artery occlusion. Also, the upper thigh pressure was not as accurate as intraoperative femoral artery pressure measurement.[17] If there is difficulty in determining which lesion is hemodynamically significant, intraoperative pressure measurement with pharmacologic vasodilation appears to be a more reliable technique.[19]

The use of ankle pressure and its response to treadmill exercise is also helpful in planning inflow procedures for patients with claudication. When a femoro-femoral graft is considered and the adequacy of the donor artery inflow needs to be determined, a decrease in ankle pressure in the donor limb after exercise is ominous. In our analysis of 44 patients who underwent femorofemoral grafting for claudication, 50% of the patients had deterioration of donor limb hemodynamics after surgery. All of these patients had a decrease in ankle pressure after treadmill exercise.[24] Four of the patients had a normal triphasic waveform recorded at the donor common femoral artery. It would appear that resting flow velocity recording is not sufficient when the presenting symptom is claudication, and that evaluation by treadmill exercise is needed to assess the adequacy of inflow.

Pressure index as a prognostic indication in femoropopliteal reconstruction.

Traditionally, adequacy of distal runoff is determined by angiographic appearance. As described in the previous sections, there is a highly significant correlation between the severity of ischemia and the degree of ankle systolic pressure reduction. It would appear, then, that the level of ankle pressure may further supplement information on the success of the reconstructive surgery. Isolated lesions of the femoropopliteal segment produce only modest reduction in ankle pressure and are usually associated with intermittent claudication. Extensive occlusive disease of the femoropopliteal segment and distal vessels produces severe ischemia and demonstrates severe depression in the ankle systolic pressure. Since distal pressure is inversely related to the proximal resistance, markedly reduced ankle pressures connote extremely high resistance to blood flow through the collateral bed or the popliteal and distal arteries. Ankle systolic pressure level represents the status of collateral flow, and it should bear an inverse relation to the extent of arterial occlusion.

Although the ankle pressure index may affect the prognosis of a femoropopliteal bypass,[13] the ankle pressure index alone has little value as a prognosticator of a bypass graft to the tibial or peroneal vessels. In patients with femoropopliteal occlusion, a low or unrecordable ankle pressure should not be interpreted as an indication for amputation. Such a finding merely suggests the presence of severe occlusive disease distal to the popliteal trifurcation and that a bypass graft to the popliteal artery proximal to the diseased tibial artery is frequently associated with thrombosis. In our recent analysis,[57] the level of ankle pressure or the pressure index correlated well with the status of popliteal artery run-off in patients with normal aortoiliac inflow. In the presence of severe popliteal occlusive disease with involvement of the tibial or peroneal artery, the pressure index is often much lower (0.22 ± 0.13) than in patients with patent vessels distal to the popliteal trifurcation (0.55 ± 0.09). Also, the pressure gradient between the thigh and ankle helps to determine the severity of popliteal disease with tibial vessel involvement. When severe trifurcation disease is present, a large pressure gradient may develop between the lower thigh and ankle levels. A femoral graft with anastomosis onto the popliteal artery without correction of the pressure gradient is often associated with a high rate of failure. In this situation, a bypass with the anastomosis placed onto a tibial vessel that bypasses the pressure gradient is desirable. Therefore the use of the thigh-ankle pressure gradient together with visual inspection of the degree of damping of the flow waveforms helps to select the type of bypass procedure. The pressure level alone should not determine the operability of patients with tibial artery disease. Also, the level of pressure has no prognostic value in tibial bypasses.[12]

Determination of response to sympathetic ablation. Obviously, different factors influence the outcome in any given patient. A calcified artery may give a falsely high pressure reading and invalidate the results. Moreover, there have been reports that diabetic patients seem to benefit less from sympathectomy.[35,52] Autosympathectomy has been cited as the reason for failure in some of these patients. Nevertheless, the importance of pressure measurements in relation to sympathectomy lies in the selection of patients who will not respond to sympathectomy. Unless there is adequate distal perfusion, lumbar sympathectomy is seldom effective. These patients, when identified preoperatively, will be spared an unnecessary operation.

Recently Walker and Johnston[52] have found that patients with an ankle pressure less than 30 mm Hg did not respond to sympathetic blockade. The 30 mm Hg level as an indicator for a positive response to sympathetic ablation has also been suggested by Nielsen et al.[35] They found that a drop in toe pressure after sympathetic blockade to a level less than 30 mm Hg was accompanied by a decrease in subcutaneous blood flow measured adjacent to the ischemic area. In a report by Pistolese et al.,[40] 38 of 143 patients with a low pressure index had symptoms worsen after sympathectomy. Although an upper thigh pressure has been suggested by Plecha et al.[41] as being useful to predict the response to lumbar ablation, we have found that the ankle systolic pressure remains a better indicator.

Selection of amputation level. Determining the level of amputation for severe, uncorrectable ischemia remains a challenging problem, particularly after failed femoropopliteal or femorotibial grafting. A major objective of noninvasive technology has been to predict the most distal amputation that would heal primarily. Several techniques are now currently available for this determination. These include ^{133}Xe clearance, thermography, and transcutaneous O_2 recording.[25,33,45]

Unlike the xenon technique, Doppler segmental pressure measurement is a simple technique. In a series of 66 patients who had major amputations, we used the ankle systolic pressure; the waveforms recorded from the posterior tibial, anterior tibial, and dorsalis pedis arteries; and the pressure in the lower thigh to determine the level of amputation.[14] Our data suggest that, when there is no detectable flow in the popliteal artery, an above-knee amputation is advisable. On the other hand, detectable flow in the popliteal artery allows the recording of thigh pressure, and, if the thigh pressure exceeds 50 mm Hg, a below-knee amputation should be attempted because the chance for success is high. This has also been suggested by others.[4,30,34] All patients who had audible signals at the posterior tibial or dorsalis pedis artery had a successful below-knee amputation. The use of pressure level alone may be fallacious, since the presence of infection and the operative technique strongly influence the surgical result. Nicholas,[34] using a calf systolic pressure of 70 torr and an ankle pressure greater than 30 torr, found a high false negative rate with negative predictive values of 32% and 40%.

Minor amputation includes digit or forefoot amputation. It has been reported that an ankle systolic pressure over 35 mm Hg is sufficient for wound healing,[10] although others rely on a higher level.[21] The use of ankle systolic pressure alone should be interpreted with caution. A high ankle pressure does not necessarily guarantee the success of a toe or forefoot amputation because the pressure level may not reflect the status of perfusion of the toes or forefoot. This is particularly true in diabetics, in whom the ankle pressure is unreliable.[26,46] The use of toe pressure may prove a better way to assess the level of minor amputations.[5]

Photoplethysmography (PPG) may be used instead of Doppler ultrasound or strain-gauge recording. Using a PPG endpoint of 20 mm Hg, Schwartz et al.[46] and Barnes et al.[5] observed uniform healing in all minor forefoot and digital amputations.

DETERMINATION OF GRAFT PATENCY FOLLOWING RECONSTRUCTIVE SURGERY

Arterial reconstruction for occlusive disease is now an established procedure. There is, however, no single convenient, objective, bedside method of monitoring the blood flow and patency of the vessel after operation. The return of a pedal pulse usually indicates successful surgery, but the variability in palpation of pulses by different observers, especially in borderline cases and in the presence of postoperative edema, often makes this method unreliable. Doppler ankle sphygmomanometry offers a simple and reliable method of assessing the patency of arterial reconstructions. Determination of ankle systolic pressure can be made as often as required and is of particular value in patients in whom a residual lesion is present, making the return of a palpable pedal pulse unlikely. This situation is often encountered in patients with occlusions affecting both the aortoiliac and superficial femoral arteries, where reconstruction is done at the aortoiliac level. It may also be seen in patients with occlusion of the femoropopliteal artery with severe disease below the trifurcation of the popliteal artery. In deep femoral artery reconstruction, where there is a concomitant occlusion of the femoropopliteal segment, ankle systolic pressure recording is probably the only reliable, objective method to ascertain the result of operation.

In more than 500 cases analyzed in our laboratory successful arterial reconstruction in single segment disease (aortoiliac or superficial femoral) was followed by an immediate increase of ankle pressure to a level close to a pressure index of 1.0 at the termination of the surgical procedure or within 6 hours postoperatively. On occasion despite the absence of palpable pedal pulses immediately fol-

lowing the procedure, a delayed return of ankle pressure may be observed. Under this circumstance ankle pressure normally would rise within 6 hours after the completion of the procedure. Infrequently, the return of ankle pressure is delayed in aortoiliac reconstructions because of prolonged clamping of the aorta or excessive blood loss. In these cases, however, flow signals at the popliteal artery level are often detectable despite the absence of flow signals in the posterior tibial or dorsal arteries of the foot. After the elapse of anesthetics, 6 to 12 hours after surgery, ankle pressure often returns to a higher level than before surgery.

Reconstructions undertaken in the presence of residual distal disease (deep femoral artery reconstruction with disease involving the popliteal artery or aortoiliac reconstruction in patients with combined occlusions of the aortoiliac and femoral arteries) usually do not have an associated return of pedal pulses by palpation. Success of the reconstruction in this instance is best documented by ankle pressure measurement, and the level of ankle pressure is often double the preoperative level.

Ankle pressure recording is a simple method of monitoring patency of arterial reconstructions. Perhaps the greatest value of this technique is in detection of failure when success has been assumed. Failure of a reconstruction is indicated by a steady drop in ankle pressure or pressure index during the immediate postoperative period or by failure to improve ankle pressure higher than the preoperative level in a 6- to 12-hour observation period. Early return to the operating room for correction of technical error often converts failure to success. The simplicity of ankle pressure measurement has allowed nursing personnel to perform hourly ankle pressure measurements in the recovery room and intensive care unit. Such measurements should be made routinely in addition to palpation of pedal pulses in all hospitals dealing with vascular reconstructive procedures.

EVALUATION OF NEW TREATMENT MODALITIES AND FOLLOW-UP OF BYPASS GRAFTS

The use of noninvasive tests is essential in epidemiologic settings for diagnosis of atherosclerotic peripheral arterial disease and for recording the progress of the disease process. In an epidemiologic study, Marinelli et al.[31] have found clinical examination of pulses to be totally unreliable. One fifth of the patients with normal physical examination results were found to have abnormal results by ankle pressure determination. Recently the American Heart Association Council on Epidemiology has recommended the use of Doppler ultrasound to record the ankle-arm pressure index before and after standard treadmill exercise as a diagnostic tool for field studies.[43] The ankle pressure index can serve as baseline data to follow the natural history of the disease.

New therapeutic procedures are always being introduced as alternative treatments to surgery, and Doppler ultrasound examination provides an objective means to evaluate these procedures. The efficacy of transluminal balloon dilation or thrombolytic therapy, for example, needs to be verified objectively. Several studies[18,23,37] have demonstrated that the results of balloon dilation, when assessed by hemodynamic measurement, are inferior to those obtained by assessment of symptomatic improvement alone. The role of vasodilating agents in the treatment of claudication remains unclear. Evaluation of such vasodilator treatment can be obtained, since resting and exercise ankle systolic pressures provide objective tests to determine the efficacy of this pharmacologic approach.[28,32,42] More important, assessment of the result of any type of reconstructive surgery by an objective technique is essential to establish the effectiveness of the procedure. For instance, we have found that the femorofemoral graft is effective in limb salvage situations; however, the procedure gives less than optimal results in patients with claudication.[24] There has been concern about the effect of knee flexion on limb hemodynamics when prosthetic grafts are used, but ankle pressure measurement has demonstrated no ill effect during knee flexion.[9]

In later follow-up, ankle pressure measurement is the single most useful method to detect graft stenosis[6,60] and confirm graft occlusion. A steady decrease in ankle pressure is indicative of progression of the disease distal to the bypass or graft stenosis. The latter is frequently observed in patients with saphenous vein grafts.

A patent bypass graft by arteriography has been considered the hallmark of success of reconstructive surgery. In contrast to this belief, a bypass graft may be patent by arteriography yet provide no functional improvement. This patent but hemodynamically failed graft can be detected by serial Doppler ultrasound examinations. A change in ankle pressure of 0.15 is considered to be hemodynamically significant and indicates the need for repeat arteriography. A hemodynamically failed graft, if recognized early, may be corrected by surgery before graft failure by complete thrombosis.[36] The frequent use of Doppler ankle pressure recording during the follow-up period should be routine in the assessment of the results of reconstructive surgery.

Finally, postoperative or follow-up study by noninvasive techniques can determine whether an additional reconstructive procedure is necessary to achieve the desired result.[7,50] The need for a further bypass procedure is commonly seen in patients who have multiple-level disease and in whom a proximal reconstruction is performed in the presence of a distal occlusion. If there is no improvement in the ankle pressure after aortoiliac or profunda femoris reconstruction, a distal bypass graft to relieve symptoms is often warranted.[1,8,44]

REFERENCES

1. Archie, J.P.: Objective improvement after aortofemoral bypass for exercise ischemia, Surg. Gynecol. Obstet. 149: 374, 1979.
2. Baker, J.D., and Dix, D.: Variability of Doppler ankle pressure with arterial occlusive disease: an evaluation of ankle index and brachial-ankle pressure gradient, Surgery 89:134, 1981.
3. Baker, W.H., and Barnes, R.W.: Minor forefoot amputation in patients with low ankle pressure, Am. J. Surg. 133:331, 1977.
4. Barnes, R.W., Shanik, G.D., and Slaymaker, E.E.: An index of healing below the knee amputations using leg blood pressure by Doppler ultrasound, Surgery 79:13, 1976.
5. Barnes, R.W., et al.: Prediction of amputation wound healing: the roles of Doppler ultrasound and digit photoplethysmography, Arch. Surg. 116:80, 1981.
6. Berkowitz, H.D., et al.: Value of routine vascular laboratory studies to identify vein graft stenosis, Surgery 90:971, 1981.
7. Bone, G.E., et al.: Value of segmental limb blood pressure in predicting results of aortofemoral bypass, Am. J. Surg. 132:733, 1976.
8. Brewster, D.C., et al.: Aortofemoral graft for multilevel occlusive disease: predictors of success and need for distal bypass, Arch. Surg. 117:1593, 1982.
9. Burnham, S.J., et al.: Nonvein bypass in below-knee reoperation for lower limb ischemia, Surgery 84:417, 1978.
10. Carter, S.A.: The relationship of distal systolic pressure to healing of skin lesions in limbs with arterial occlusive disease, with special reference to diabetes mellitus, Scand. J. Clin. Lab. Invest. 31(suppl. 128):239, 1973.
11. Chamberlain, J., Housley, E., and MacPherson, A.I.S.: The relationship between ultrasound assessment and angiography in occlusive arterial disease of the lower limb, Br. J. Surg. 62:64, 1975.

12. Corson, J.D., et al.: Doppler ankle systolic blood pressure: prognostic value in vein bypass grafts of the lower extremity, Arch. Surg. 113:932, 1976.

13. Dean, R.H., et al.: Prognostic indicators in femoro-popliteal reconstructions, Arch. Surg. 110:1287, 1975.

14. Dean, R.H., et al.: Predictive value of ultrasonically derived arterial pressure in determination of amputation level, Am. Surg. 41:731, 1975.

15. Faris, I.B., and Jamieson, C.W.: The diagnosis of aorto-iliac stenosis: a comparison of thigh pressure measurement and femoral artery flow velocity profile, J. Cardiovasc. Surg. 16:597, 1975.

16. Flanigan, D.P., et al.: Correlation of Doppler-derived high thigh pressure and intra-arterial pressure in the assessment of aorto-iliac occlusive disease, Br. J. Surg. 68:423, 1981.

17. Flanigan, D.P., et al.: Utility of wide and narrow blood pressure cuffs in the hemodynamic assessment of aortoiliac occlusive disease, Surgery 92:16, 1982.

18. Flanigan, D.P., et al.: Anatomic and hemodynamic evaluation of percutaneous transluminal angioplasty, Surg. Gynecol. Obstet. 154:181, 1982.

19. Flanigan, D.P., et al.: Aortofemoral or femoropopliteal revascularization? A prospective evaluation of the papaverine test, J. Vasc. Surg. 1:215, 1984.

20. Garrett, W.V., et al.: Intraoperative prediction of symptomatic result of aortofemoral bypass from changes in ankle pressure index, Surgery 82:504, 1977.

21. Gibbons, G.W., et al.: Noninvasive prediction of amputation level in diabetic patients, Arch. Surg. 114:1034, 1979.

22. Goddreau, J.J., et al.: Rational approach to the differentiation of vascular and neurogenic claudication, Surgery 84:749, 1978.

23. Gunn, I.G., et al.: Haemodynamic assessment following iliac artery dilatation, Br. J. Surg. 68:858, 1981.

24. Harris, J.P., et al.: Assessment of donor limb hemodynamics in femorofemoral bypass for claudication, Surgery 90:764, 1981.

25. Holloway, G.A., Jr., and Burgess, E.M.: Cutaneous blood flow and its relation to healing of below-knee amputation, Surg. Gynecol. Obstet. 146:750, 1978.

26. Holstein, P., et al.: Distal blood pressure in severe arterial insufficiency: strain-gauge, radioisotopes, and other methods. In Bergan, J.J., and Yao, J.S.T., editors: Gangrene and severe ischemia of the lower extremities, New York, 1978, Grune & Stratton, Inc.

27. Jamieson, C.W.: The definition of critical ischaemia of a limb (editorial), Br. J. Surg. 69(suppl.):S-2, 1982.

28. Jones, N.A.G., et al.: A double-blind trial of suloctidil v. placebo in intermittent claudication, Br. J. Surg. 69:38, 1982.

29. Lassen, N.A., and Holstein, P.: Use of radioisotopes in assessment of distal blood flow and distal blood pressure in arterial insufficiency, Surg. Clin. North Am. 54:39, 1974.

30. Lee, B.Y., Trainer, F.S., and Kavner, D.: Noninvasive hemodynamic evaluation in selection of amputation level, Surg. Gynecol. Obstet. 149:241, 1979.

31. Marinelli, M.R., et al.: Noninvasive testing vs. clinical evaluation of arterial disease, a prospective study, JAMA 241:2031, 1979.

32. Mashiah, A., et al.: Drug therapy in intermittent claudication: an objective assessment of the effects of three drugs on patients with intermittent claudication, Br. J. Surg. 65:342, 1978.

33. Moore, W.S., et al.: Prospective use of Xenon Xe[133] clearance for amputation level selection, Arch. Surg. 116:80, 1981.

34. Nicholas, G.G., Myers, J.L., and DeMuth, W.: The role of the vascular laboratory: criteria in the selection of patients for lower extremity amputation, Ann. Surg. 195:469, 1982.

35. Nielsen, P.E., et al.: Reduction in distal pressure by sympathetic nerve block in patients with occlusive arterial disease, Cardiovasc. Res. 7:577, 1973.

36. O'Mara, C.S., et al.: Recognition and surgical management of patent but hemodynamically failed arterial grafts, Ann. Surg. 193:467, 1981.

37. O'Mara, C.S., et al.: Hemodynamic assessment of transluminal angioplasty for lower extremity ischemia, Surgery 89:106, 1981.

38. Ouriel, K., and Zarins, C.K.: Doppler ankle pressure: an evaluation of three methods of expression, Arch. Surg. 117:1297, 1982.

39. Pearce, W.H., Yao, J.S.T., and Bergan, J.J.: Noninvasive vascular diagnostic testing, Curr. Probl. Surg. 20(8):460, 1983.

40. Pistolese, G.R., et al.: Criteria for prognostic evaluation of the results of lumbar sympathectomy: clinical, hemodynamic, and angiographic findings, J. Cardiovasc. Surg. 23:411, 1982.

41. Plecha, F.R., et al.: A new criterion for predicting response to lumbar sympathectomy in patients with severe arteriosclerotic occlusive disease, Surgery 88:375, 1980.

42. Porter, J.M., and Baur, G.M.: Pharmacologic treatment of intermittent claudication, Surgery 92:966, 1982.

43. Prineas, R.J., et al.: Recommendations for use of noninvasive methods to detect atherosclerotic peripheral arterial disease—in population studies. Am. Heart Assoc. Council on Epidemiology, Circulation 65:1561A, 1982.

44. Queral, L.A., et al.: Selection of reconstructive surgery for lower-limb ischemia by noninvasive testing. In Diethrich, E.B., editor: Noninvasive cardiovascular diagnosis, ed. 2, Littleton, Mass., 1981, PSG Publishing Co.

45. Roon, A.J., Moore, W.S., and Goldstone, J.: Below-knee amputation: a modern approach, Am. J. Surg. 134:153, 1977.

46. Schwartz, J.A., et al.: Predictive value of distal perfusion pressure in the healing of the digits and the forefoot, Surg. Gynecol. Obstet. 154:865, 1982.

47. Sondergroth, T.R., et al.: Variability of toe pressure measurements, Bruit 6:14, 1982.

48. Stoney, R.J., James, D.R., and Wylie, E.J.: Surgery for femoropopliteal artherosclerosis: a reappraisal, Arch. Surg. 103:548, 1971.

49. Strandness, D.E., Jr., and Bell, J.W.: Peripheral vascular disease: diagnosis and objective evaluation using a mercury straingauge, Ann. Surg. 161(suppl. 1):35, 1965.

50. Sumner, D.S., and Strandness, D.E.: Aortoiliac reconstruction in patients with combined iliac and superficial femoral artery occlusion, Surgery 84:348, 1978.

51. Verta, M.J., Jr., et al.: Forefoot perfusion pressure and minor amputation for gangrene, Surgery 80:729, 1976.

52. Walker, P.M., and Johnston, K.W.: Predicting success of a sympathectomy: a prospective study using discriminant function and multiple regression analysis, Surgery 87:216, 1980.

53. Winsor, T.: Influence of arterial disease on the systolic blood pressure gradients of the extremity, Am. J. Med. Sci. 220:117, 1950.

54. Yao, J.S.T.: Haemodynamic studies in peripheral arterial disease, Br. J. Surg. 57:761, 1970.

55. Yao, J.S.T.: Discussion of Baker, J.D., and Dix, D., Surgery 89:137, 1981.

56. Yao, J.S.T., and Bergan, J.J.: Predictability of vascular reactivity to sympathetic ablation, Arch. Surg. 106:676, 1973.
57. Yao, J.S.T., and Nicolaides, A.N.: Transcutaneous Doppler ultrasound in the management of lower limb ischemia. In Nicolaides, A.N., and Yao, J.S.T., editors: Investigation of vascular disorders, New York, 1981, Churchill Livingstone.
58. Yao, J.S.T., Hobbs, J.T., and Irvine, W.T.: Ankle systolic pressure measurement in arterial disease affecting the lower extremities, Br. J. Surg. 56:676, 1969.
59. Yao, J.S.T., et al.: A comparative study of strain-gauge plethysmography and Doppler ultrasound in the assessment of occlusive arterial disease of the lower extremities, Surgery 71:4, 1972.
60. Yao, J.S.T., et al.: Postoperative evaluation of graft failure. In Bernhard, V.M., and Towne, J.B., editors: Complications in vascular surgery, New York, 1980, Grune & Stratton, Inc.

CHAPTER 53

Quantitative velocity measurements in arterial disease of the lower extremity

ARNOST FRONEK

The application of the Doppler principle to ultrasonic examination of the arterial system represents the single most important stimulus in the development of the vascular laboratory. Early publications[14,47,48] were quickly followed by additional reports that recognized the potential of the Doppler ultrasonic velocity meter (Doppler meter) for the objective analysis of arterial occlusive disease.[46,52,53,54] In addition to a simple auscultatory analysis of the Doppler signals, the advantages of recorded output were immediately used. The limitations of the early nondirectional Doppler instruments were eliminated when McLeod[36,37] described an approach to determine the direction of blood flow. When the limitations of McLeod's original recommendation to detect flow direction were recognized, a number of alternative technical solutions were subsequently reported (Chapter 7).

The first reports demonstrating the usefulness of Doppler examination of the arterial system interpreted the recorded signals on a qualitative basis using pattern recognition. Even today this type of interpretation is the most widely used for a number of reasons. First, the differences between normal and pathologic tracings of advanced stages of arterial occlusive disease are so clear that additional signal analysis seems unnecessary and time-consuming. However, qualitative evaluation only uses a fraction of the information contained in the recorded Doppler signal, especially in less advanced or borderline cases.

The biggest obstacle to quantitating Doppler signals is that the Doppler frequency shift depends on the angle between the ultrasonic beam and the main velocity vector (Chapter 3). As will be described, two recent developments, the introduction of spe-

cial probes that determine the angle of the ultrasonic beam[17,21,42] and the application of the Duplex principle (Chapter 60), have opened new avenues for Doppler quantitation.

SEMIQUANTITATIVE DOPPLER SIGNAL EVALUATION

Gosling et al.[18,19] and Woodcock et al.[57] described a pulsatility index (PI) that is insensitive to the angle of the probe. The PI is a ratio of the peak-to-peak Doppler velocity amplitude to the mean Doppler velocity value:

$$PI = \frac{Peak\text{-}to\text{-}peak}{Mean}$$

The range of PI values given are abdominal aorta 2 to 6, common femoral artery 5 to 10, popliteal artery 6 to 12, and posterior tibial artery 7 to 15. The PI is essentially not influenced by variations of the Doppler beam angle.[20] Originally the values used for the calculation of the PI were obtained on the basis of a Fourier analysis with the expectation that this approach, although more complex, would be sensitive even to minute changes in hemodynamics.[58] However, the Fourier analysis added little to the accuracy of the method.[57] Since then the PI has been calculated on the basis of simple Doppler system tracings without Fourier analysis.

In addition to the PI, Gosling et al. described two other indices to increase the overall sensitivity and specificity of the examination. The damping factor (DF) measures the degree of attenuation of the Doppler signal, which is expressed as a ratio of two adjacent PIs as follows:

$$DF = \frac{PI \text{ (proximal site)}}{PI \text{ (distal site)}}$$

The normal range of DF measured from the femoral artery to the popliteal artery is 0.79 ± 0.30 and measured from the popliteal artery to the posterior tibial artery is 0.94 ± 0.35.

The transit time (T) is defined as the time it takes for the Doppler signal to travel from one measurement site to another. Since the velocity signal is a function of the driving pressure, which is practically synchronous with the arterial wall displacement, the results are inversely related to the pulse wave velocity (PWV) as the following:

$$PWV = \frac{l}{T}$$

where l is the distance between two measurement sites and T is the time for the pulse to travel from the proximal to the distal sensing site. The published values of t measured from the femoral artery to the popliteal artery are 42.2 ± 4.8 msec and measured from the popliteal artery to the posterior tibial artery are 40.1 ± 4.6 msec. The T and mean blood pressure relationship confirms this assumption. A classification based on these three indices to identify the approximate topography and severity of the disease has been developed.

These results have been confirmed by a number of other researchers who found the PI as informative as the Fourier pulsatility index[27,28] and who also found a good correlation of PI with angiographic findings.[22,26,28] On the other hand, there are several reports[3,8,56] concluding that there is a poor relationship between the PI and the severity of the disease, although it is generally accepted that a low PI is a confirmation of very severe arterial occlusive disease. Demorais and Johnston[10] found a good correlation of the PI with intraoperative femoral artery pressure values. On the other hand, most researchers concluded that the diagnostic value of the transit time is limited.

Humphries et al.[24] found a good correlation of Gosling's indices with angiographic findings, although their accuracy in detecting moderate stenoses was unsatisfactory. They found, however, that a rise-time ratio (distal-proximal rise time) yields results at least as accurate as the PI and is easier to obtain.

The clinical need to determine the hemodynamic significance of aortoiliac obstruction stimulated a number of researchers to search for other helpful indices. Archie and Feldman[1,2] used a minimum-maximum ratio referring to the recorded Doppler signals, whereas Nicolaides et al.[39] used a slightly

modified PI labeled waveform index (RI) and found little correlation with the severity of disease. Flanigan et al.[13] in a carefully designed experimental study, demonstrated that although femoral artery PI tends to decrease with increasing degrees of stenosis, it only occurs after similar changes in pressure are demonstrated. Most important these results were seriously influenced by concomitant changes in the superficial femoral artery, which is a factor neglected in previous studies. This circumstance reduces the accuracy of the velocity-based conclusions under clinical conditions. In a recent study, Segard et al.[49] found that the diagnosis of aortoiliac artery obstruction can be determined accurately on the basis of the Doppler velocity signal. Accuracy, however, decreased in the presence of a concomitant superficial artery obstruction.

Fitzgerald et al.[11,12] developed a classification of lower extremity arterial occlusive disease using a combination of PI, DF, and T. Although his results were compared grossly with angiography, there is no information on the influence of distal obstruction on the monitored values.

The influence of superficial femoral artery obstruction on common femoral velocity data can be explained by the effect of distal resistance on the reverse velocity component of the femoral artery velocity pulse. It has been shown in a number of experimental[43,52] and clinical studies[31,34] that increased resistance leads to an increase in the reverse velocity component, whereas peripheral vasodilation, whether pharmacologic or physiologic (postocclusive reactive hyperemia), leads to its reduction or even complete disappearance. It is therefore understandable that a combination of proximal and distal resistance changes (for example, iliac and superficial femoral artery stenosis) may produce challenging diagnostic problems.

QUANTITATIVE FLOW VELOCITY DETERMINATION

As previously pointed out, one of the prerequisites for the quantitative assessment of flow velocities in the arteries of the lower extremities is the simultaneous recording of the Doppler-shifted signals and the beam velocity angle. In the future this will be possible either by using multiple crystal probes[7,17,21,41,42] or by using Duplex systems[7] (Chapter 60). At the present time these systems, with the exception of the Duplex scanner, are not commercially available, although the need for some degree of quantification is urgent in the daily diagnostic routine. Fronek et al.[15] reported absolute flow velocity values from the femoral, posterior tibial, and dorsalis pedis arteries using a precalibrated Doppler velocity metering system[55] (Fig. 53-1). A calibration curve was first obtained with a 0.5% Sephadex suspension (substituting blood) circulating in polyethylene tubing. The probe position was adjusted to yield the maximum deflection for a given flow velocity (scanning the tubing and then changing the angle until maximum output was obtained). Under these conditions, excellent linearity was obtained up to about 60 cm/sec with most commercially available Doppler meters[50] (Fig. 53-2). Under clinical conditions, highly reproducible results have been obtained with the same approach (maximum amplitude search by scanning the artery horizontally, and after a maximum signal obtained, varying the angle of the probe again until a maximum signal was recorded). The probe was then fixed in position with a magnetic clamp. It is possible to introduce artifacts (by careless positioning, probe movement, etc.), but reproducible tracings can be obtained routinely by a skilled vascular technician (Fig. 53-3).

Table 53-1 summarizes the data obtained under these conditions in 39 normal subjects.[15] These values are close to those obtained by Risøe and Wille.[44] Nimura et al.,[40] however, obtained far higher values, which would also imply unacceptably high blood flow values.[44]

In addition to peak flow, reversed, and mean velocity, a number of calculated indices proved to be useful, that is deceleration and peak-mean velocity ratio (Table 53-2 and Fig. 53-4). These velocity measurements are especially valuable in combination with other findings or are suggestive of disease where other measurements (for example, segmental pressure) may be falsely negative, as when vessel compliance is reduced and upper thigh pressure is erroneously normal or even elevated.[16]

QUALITATIVE EVALUATION OF DOPPLER VELOCITY SIGNALS

The Doppler-shifted signal obtained from the main arteries (femoral, popliteal, posterior tibial, and dorsalis pedis) of the lower extremity can be useful even without quantitative evaluation.[4,5,30,52] Generally accepted criteria of disease are reduction of amplitude, absence of reversed velocity component (especially in the femoral artery), rounded peak velocity, and a shallow, descending portion of the velocity tracing.

Two special qualitative signs specific for two different lesions have been described. Fitzgerald et al.[12] described a high-frequency signal with a specific ripple that could be recognized by Doppler auscultation or that produced a doublehump on the Doppler tracing in patients with abdominal aneurysm. On the other hand, Nicolaides et al.[39] described a special disturbance in the femoral artery velocity tracing after exercise in cases of significant aortoiliac disease. Unfortunately, statistics on the accuracy of both of these findings are not available.

In addition to this pattern recognition, auscultatory evaluation of the Doppler signal is important especially where recording facilities are not available. Under these circumstances, special attention must be given to any significant changes in the normal audio spectrum, and particularly to signals with an unusually high pitch, coarse or rough sounds, monotonous sounds, and weak signals.[4] Much like cardiologic auscultation, this type of Doppler signal evaluation requires considerable training and experience.

Profunda femoris artery Doppler examination. Becker et al.[6] described a set of maneuvers to identify the course and patency of the profunda femoris artery, using a 4 MHz Doppler velocity meter. These results were recently confirmed by Luizy et al.[30] Because this artery is important as a supply route to the distal part of the leg in cases of superficial femoral artery obstruction,[35,38] this test may help in planning both angiography and surgery.

Popliteal artery Doppler examination. Although the assessment of the popliteal artery velocity signal is considered an important part of the complete arterial evaluation, there are few reports describing normal and pathologic values of popliteal artery flow velocity. This is probably because examination of the popliteal artery is somewhat more difficult than examination of the other limb arteries, but it is not beyond the standard training capacity of a good technician. It is helpful to examine the patient lying on one side with the knees slightly bent, using the same maneuver described for all other arteries (for example, scanning for maximum amplitude). Under those conditions the normal values summarized in Table 53-3 can be expected.

The determination of popliteal artery flow velocity has also been reported under dynamic conditions after exercise.[32] The reproducibility was good and correlation with venous occlusion plethysmography yielded a straight line up to about 20

Table 53-1. Normal velocity values

	Peak forward velocity (cm/sec)	Peak reverse velocity (cm/sec)	Mean velocity (cm/sec)	Acceleration (cm/sec^2)	Deceleration (cm/sec^2)	Peak velocity/ mean velocity	Acceleration/ deceleration
Femoral artery n = 78 extremities	40.7 ± 10.9*	6.5 ± 3.6	9.8 ± 5.3	353.0 ± 113.1	250.9 ± 60.0	4.8 ± 1.6	1.4 ± 0.2
Posterior tibial artery n = 78	16.0 ± 10.0	2.0 ± 2.3	4.0 ± 3.5	145.0 ± 73.3	129.8 ± 75.7	4.8 ± 2.5	1.2 ± 0.1
Dorsalis pedis artery n = 73	16.8 ± 5.7	1.3 ± 2.2	3.4 ± 1.6	160.5 ± 55.3	137.9 ± 54.5	6.0 ± 4.1	1.3 ± 0.5

*Mean ± standard deviation.

Table 53-2. Velocity measurement in patients with angiographic evidence of arterial disease

	Peak forward velocity (cm/sec)	Peak reverse velocity (cm/sec)	Mean velocity (cm/sec)	Acceleration (cm/sec^2)	Deceleration (cm/sec^2)	Peak velocity/ mean velocity	Acceleration/ deceleration
Femoral artery							
Normal (n = 78)	40.7 ± 10.9	6.5 ± 3.6	9.8 ± 5.3	353.0 ± 113.1	250.0 ± 60.0	4.8 ± 1.6	1.4 ± 0.2
Group I (n = 14)	25.8 ± 9.4*	3.5 ± 3.5	8.9 ± 2.9	260.7 ± 176.6	122.9 ± 75.6*	3.1 ± 1.1*	2.0 ± 1.1
Group II (n = 27)	30.3 ± 15.4*	4.2 ± 4.4	8.9 ± 4.2	352.5 ± 193.8	181.0 ± 117.0*	3.6 ± 0.8*	2.2 ± 1.1
Group III (n = 70)	20.9 ± 11.2*	0.8 ± 1.9*†	7.9 ± 4.2	208.5 ± 166.2*	91.0 ± 70.7*†	2.7 ± 0.8*	2.7 ± 1.6*
Posterior tibial artery							
Normal (n = 78)	16.0 ± 10.0	2.0 ± 2.3	4.0 ± 3.5	145.0 ± 73.7	129.8 ± 75.7	4.8 ± 2.5	1.2 ± 0.1
Group I (n = 14)	13.4 ± 11.5	2.2 ± 2.9	4.4 ± 3.3	165.7 ± 191.8	79.2 ± 62.4	3.0 ± 0.76	1.9 ± 0.9
Group II (n = 25)	13.3 ± 6.6	1.2 ± 1.5	7.4 ± 7.0*	121.7 ± 59.5	77.2 ± 82.9*	2.8 ± 1.1*	1.8 ± 0.7*
Group III (n = 66)	11.7 ± 8.2*	0.4 ± 1.1*†	5.2 ± 4.2	89.6 ± 64.7*	43.0 ± 40.2*†	2.1 ± 0.8*	2.5 ± 1.5*
Dorsalis pedis artery							
Normal (n = 73)	16.8 ± 5.7	1.3 ± 2.2	3.4 ± 1.6	160.5 ± 55.3	137.9 ± 54.5	6.0 ± 4.1	1.3 ± 0.5
Group I (n = 13)	14.7 ± 6.4	2.0 ± 2.4	4.7 ± 2.4	168.2 ± 121.4	79.9 ± 50.8*	3.4 ± 1.5	2.0 ± 0.8
Group II (n = 27)	11.4 ± 9.2*	0.9 ± 1.9*	4.3 ± 3.2	116.9 ± 93.4*	71.8 ± 55.0*	2.6 ± 0.9*	2.0 ± 1.1
Group III (n = 60)	6.9 ± 6.5*	0.2 ± 0.5*	3.6 ± 3.4	68.9 ± 65.9*	28.9 ± 20.8*†	2.0 ± 0.7*	2.6 ± 1.4*

*Control group vs. I, II, or III. Significant at $p < .01$.
†Group III vs. I and II. Significant at $p < .01$.

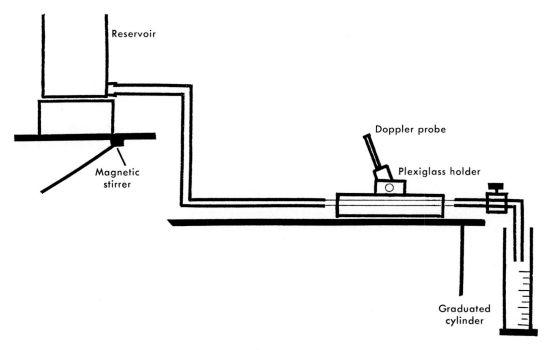

Fig. 53-1. Apparatus for in vitro calibration of Doppler flow probe (Parks 806).

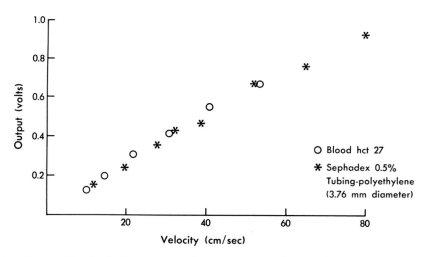

Fig. 53-2. Relationship of velocity to output voltage as determined with Parks 806 Doppler Directional Velocity Meter. Note excellent linearity when either blood or Sephadex is used.

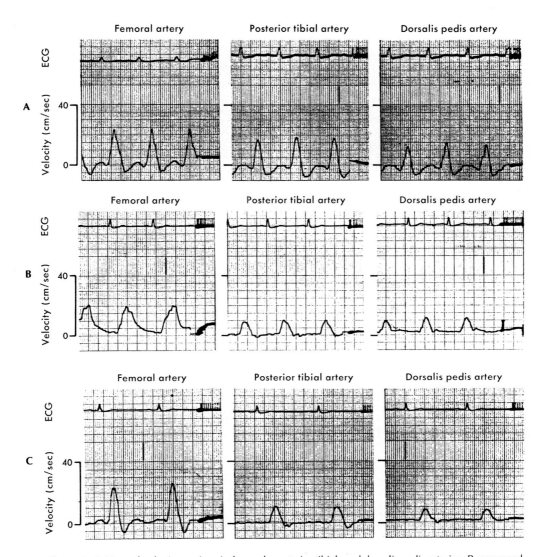

Fig. 53-3. A, Normal velocity tracings in femoral, posterior tibial, and dorsalis pedis arteries. Paper speed is 25 mm/sec, and at end of each tracing it is reduced to 1 mm/sec for recording mean velocity. Note sharp upslope, downslope, and prominent reverse component in all three vessels. Peak forward velocity is less in posterior tibial and dorsalis pedis arteries when compared with femoral artery. **B,** Velocity tracings from femoral, posterior tibial, and dorsalis pedis arteries in patient with aortoiliac stenosis. Paper speed is 25 mm/sec, and at end of each tracing it is reduced to 1 mm/sec for recording mean velocity. Note prolonged upslope, downslope, and absence of reverse component in all three vessels. In femoral artery tracing signal also does not return to zero baseline. Presence of changes in all three vessels is indicative of disease above femoral artery level. **C,** Velocity tracings from femoral, posterior tibial, and dorsalis pedis arteries in patient with femoropopliteal stenosis. Paper speed is 25 mm/sec, and at end of each tracing it is reduced to 1 mm/sec for recording mean velocity. Upslope, downslope, peak forward, and reverse velocities are normal in femoral artery tracing but abnormal or absent in posterior tibial and dorsalis pedis arteries. Changes are consistent with disease in superficial femoral artery.

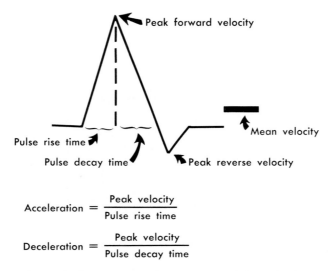

$$\text{Acceleration} = \frac{\text{Peak velocity}}{\text{Pulse rise time}}$$

$$\text{Deceleration} = \frac{\text{Peak velocity}}{\text{Pulse decay time}}$$

Fig. 53-4. Diagram of normal velocity signal. Pulse rise time, peak forward velocity, pulse delay time, peak reverse velocity, and mean velocity are measured directly from tracing. Acceleration, deceleration, and peak velocity/mean velocity are then calculated from measured variables.

Table 53-3. Popliteal artery flow velocity values

Parameter	Normal value	Standard deviation
Peak (cm/sec)	29.3	±5.9
Decay time (msec)	117.3	±18.3
Deceleration (cm/sec)	253.2	±47.0
Peak/mean	8.6	±6.3
Reversal (cm/sec)	10.2	±2.9
Mean velocity (cm/sec)	4.4	±2.3

ml/min/ 100 ml (the Doppler output was expressed in frequency).

Pedal arch Doppler examination. Patency of tibial artery grafts primarily depends on patency of the pedal arch.[9,25] In view of the difficulties in adequately visualizing the pedal arch angiographically,[23,29,51] Roedersheimer et al.[45] began to systematically examine the feasibility of a functional Doppler evaluation of the pedal arch. They identified three Doppler examination sites—dorsalis pedis artery, posterior tibial artery, and deep plantar artery (in the first metatarsal space). To determine which tibial vessel was communicating with the pedal arch, an Allen type of test was used. While listening to or recording the pedal arch signal in the first metatarsal space, the inflow arteries at the malleolar level were alternately compressed. Compression of the remaining tibial artery, which is analogous to the Allen test, resulted in the disap-

pearance of the pedal arch signal. On the other hand, if more than one tibial artery communicated with the pedal arch, compression of one tibial vessel resulted in attenuation, but not in disappearance of the pedal arch signal. In addition, greater attenuation after one tibial artery is compressed suggests that it is the preferred artery to receive the bypass graft.

Aneurysm. Fitzgerald et al.[12] described typical changes at the level of and below aortic and femoral aneurysms. They observed a special rippling effect that could also be identified acoustically. Unfortunately, the tracings presented in the original publications were obtained with a nondirectional Doppler velocity meter, so that evaluation is difficult. Additional information from other investigators is not currently available.

SUMMARY

Application of the Doppler principle to flow velocity determination represents one of the most important contributions to angiology in the last two decades. It has developed from simple pattern recognition to more quantitative evaluation criteria. We can expect that the application of frequency analysis and the future commercial availability of double crystal probes will reduce the difficulty of probe/velocity angle determination and permit more reliable quantitation of flow velocity determination in the arterial system of the lower extremities.

REFERENCES

1. Archie, J.P., and Feldman, R.W.: Intraoperative assessment of the hemodynamic significance of iliac and profunda femoris artery stenosis, Surgery 90:76, 1981.
2. Archie, J.P., and Feldman, R.W.: Determination of the hemodynamic significance of iliac artery stenosis by noninvasive Doppler ultrasonography, Surgery 91:419, 1982.
3. Baird, R.N., et al.: Upstream stenosis: its diagnosis by Doppler signals from the femoral artery, Arch. Surg. 115:1316, 1980.
4. Barnes, R.W., Russell, H.E., and Wilson, M.R.: Doppler ultrasonic evaluation of arterial disease, Audiovisual instruction, Iowa City, Iowa, 1975, University of Iowa Press.
5. Barsotti, J., et al.: L'effet Doppler, son utilisation en pathologie et chirurgie vasculaire peripherique, Nouv. Presse Med. 2677, 1972.
6. Becker, F., Demercière, and Perrin, M.: Examen de l'artère fémorale profonde par vélocimétrie ultrasonique, Doppler Ultrason. 1:63, 1980.
7. Blackshear, W.M., Jr., et al.: Detection of carotid occlusive disease by ultrasonic imaging and pulsed Doppler spectrum analysis, Surgery 86:698, 1979.
8. Bone, G.E.: The relationship between aortoiliac hemodynamics and femoral pulsatility index, J. Surg. Res. 32:228, 1982.
9. Dardik, H., Ibrahim, I.M., Dardik, I.: Evaluation of glutaraldehyde tanned human umbilical cord vein as a vascular prosthesis for bypass to the popliteal, tibian and peroneal arteries, Surgery 83:577, 1979.
10. Demorais, D., and Johnston, K.W.: Assessment of aortoiliac disease by noninvasive quantitative Doppler waveform analysis, Br. J. Surg. 68:789, 1981.
11. Fitzgerald, D.E., and Carr, J.: Doppler ultrasound diagnosis and classification as an alternative to arteriography, Angiology 26:183, 1975.
12. Fitzgerald, D.E., et al.: Detection of arterial aneurysms with Doppler ultrasound, J. Irish Coll. Phys. Surg. 5:11, 1975.
13. Flanigan, D.P., et al.: Femoral pulsatility index in the evaluation of aortoiliac occlusive disease, J. Surg. Res. 31:392, 1981.
14. Franklin, D., Schlegel, W.M., and Rushmer, R.F.: Blood flow measured by Doppler frequency shift of back-scattered ultrasound, Science 134:564, 1961.
15. Fronek, A., Coel, M. and Bernstein, E.F.: Quantitative ultrasonographic studies of lower extremity flow velocities in health and in disease, Circulation 53:953, 1976.
16. Fronek, A., Coel, M., and Bernstein, E.F.: The importance of combined multi-segmental pressure and Doppler flow velocity studies in the diagnosis of peripheral arterial occlusive disease, Surgery 84:840, 1978.
17. Furuhata, H., et al.: An ultrasonic Doppler method designed for the measurement of absolute blood velocity values, Jpn. J. Med. Elec. Bioeng. 16:264, 1978.
18. Gosling, R.G., and King, D.H.: Continuous wave ultrasound as an alternative and complement to X-rays in vascular examinations. In Reneman, R.S., editor: Cardiovascular applications of ultrasound, Amsterdam 1974, North Holland Publishing Co.
19. Gosling, R.G., and King, D.H.: Ultrasonic angiology, In Harcus, A.W., and Addenson, L., editors: Arteries and veins, Edinburgh, 1975, Churchill Livingstone.
20. Gosling, R.G., et al.: The quantitative analysis of occlusive peripheral arterial disease by a noninstrusive ultrasonic technique, Angiology 22:52, 1971.
21. Hansen, L.P., Cross, G., and Light, L.H.: Beam-angle independent Doppler velocity measurement. In Woodcock, Y., editor: Clinical blood flow measurement, New York, 1976, Pitman Medical.
22. Harris, P.L., et al.: The relationship between Doppler ultrasound assessment and angiography in occlusive arterial disease of the lower limbs, Surg. Gynecol. Obstet. 138:911, 1974.
23. Hishida, Y.: Peripheral arteriography using reactive hyperemia, Jpn. Circ. J. 27:349, 1963.
24. Humphries, K.N., et al.: Quantitative assessment of the common femoral to popliteal arterial segment using continuous wave Doppler ultrasound, Ultrasound Med. Biol. 6:99, 1980.
25. Imparato, A.M., et al: The results of tibial artery reconstruction procedures, Surg. Gynecol. Obstet. 138:33, 1974.
26. Johnston, K.W., Maruzzo, B.C., and Cobbold, R.S.C.: Doppler methods for quantitative measurement and localization of peripheral arterial disease by analysis of the blood flow velocity waveform, Ultrasound Med. Biol. 4:209, 1978.
27. Johnston, K.W., Maruzzo, B.C., and Taraschuk, I.C.: Fourier and peak-to-peak pulsatility indices: quantitation of arterial occlusive disease. In Taylor, D.E.M., and Whamond, J., editors: Non-invasive clinical measurement, Baltimore, 1977, University Park Press.
28. Johnston, K.W., and Taraschuk, I.: Validation of the role of pulsatility index in quantitation of the severity of peripheral arterial occlusive disease, Am. J. Surg. 131:295, 1976.
29. Kahn, P.C., et al.: Reactive hyperemia in lower extremity arteriography: an evaluation, Radiology 90:975, 1968.
30. Kriessmann, A., and Bollinger, A.: Ultraschall Doppler-Diagnostik in der Angiologie, Stuttgart, 1979, Georg Thieme.
31. Lee, B.Y., Castillo, H.T., and Madden, J.L.: Quantification of the arterial pulsatile blood flow wave form in peripheral vascular disease, Angiology 21:595, 1970.
32. Lubbers, J., et al.: A continuous wave Doppler velocimeter for monitoring blood flow in the popliteal artery, compared with venous occlusion plethysmograph of the calf, Pflugers Arch. 382:241, 1979.
33. Luizy, L., et al.: Exploration de l'artere femorale profonde par U.S. Doppler continue en 4MHz, J. d'Echo. et de Méd. Ultrasonore 2:37, 1981.
34. Mahler, F., et al.: Postocclusion and post-exercise flow velocity and ankle pressures in normals and marathon runners, Angiology 27:721, 1976.
35. Martin, P., et al.: On the surgery of atherosclerosis of the produnda femoris artery, Surgery 71:182, 1972.
36. McLeod, F.D.: Directional Doppler demodulation, Proc. Conf. Med. Biol. 27:1, 1967.
37. McLeod, F.D.: Calibration of CW and pulsed Doppler flowmeters, Proc. Conf. Engr. Med. Biol. 12:271, 1970.
38. Morris, G.C., et al.: Surgical importance of the profunda femoris artery, Arch. Surg. 82:52, 1961.
39. Nicolaides, A.N., et al.: The value of Doppler blood velocity tracings in the detection of aortoiliac disease in patients with intermittent claudication, Surgery 80:774, 1976.
40. Nimura, Y., et al.: Studies on arterial flow pattern instantaneous velocity spectrums and their phasic changes with directional ultrasonic Doppler technique, Br. Heart J. 36:899, 1974.
41. Peronneau, P.P., et al.: Debitmetrie sanguine par ultrasons. Developpement et applications experimentales, Europ. Surg. Res. 1:147, 1969.
42. Peronneau, P.P., et al.: Theoretical and practical aspects of pulsed Doppler flowmetry: real-time application to the measure of instantaneous velocity profiles in vitro and in vivo. In Reneman, R.S., editor: Cardiovascular applications of ultrasound, Amsterdam, 1974, North Holland Publishing Co.

43. Pritchard, W.H., et al.: A study of flow pattern responses in peripheral arteries to the injection of vasomotor drugs, Am. J. Physiol. 138:731, 1943.

44. Risøe, C., and Wille, S.Ø.: Blood velocity in human arteries measured by a bidirectional ultrasonic Doppler flowmeter, Acta Physiol. Scand. 103:370, 1978.

45. Roedersheimer, R.L., Feins, R., and Gree, R.M.: Doppler evaluation of the pedal arch, Am. J. Surg. 142:601, 1981.

46. Rushmer, R.F., Baker, D.W., and Stegall, H.F.: Transcutaneous Doppler flow detection as a nondestructive technique. J. Appl. Physiol. 21:554, 1966.

47. Satomura, S.: Study of the flow patterns in peripheral arteries by ultrasonics, J. Acoust. Soc. Jpn. 15:151, 1959.

48. Satomura, S., Kanako, Z.: Ultrasonic blood rheograph, Proceedings of the Third International Conference on Medical Electronics, London, 1960.

49. Segard, M., Carey, P., and Fronek, A.: Doppler velocity indices and topographic diagnosis of peripheral arterial occlusive disease, Proceedings of the Symposium on Noninvasive Diagnostic Techniques in Vascular Disease, San Diego, 1982.

50. Shoor, P.M., Fronek, A., and Bernstein, E.F.: Quantitative transcutaneous arterial velocity measurements with Doppler flowmeters, Arch. Surg. 114:911, 1979.

51. Soulen, R.L., et al.: Angiographic criteria for small-vessel bypass, Radiology 107:513, 1973.

52. Strandness, D.E., and Sumner, D.S.: Ultrasonic techniques in angiology, Berne, Switzerland, 1975, Hans Huber.

53. Strandness, D.E. Jr., et al.: Ultrasonic flow detection: a useful technique in the evaluation of peripheral vascular disease, Am. J. Surg. 113:311, 1967.

54. Strandness, D.E., Jr., et al.: Transcutaneous directional flow detection: a preliminary report, Am. Heart J. 78:65, 1969.

55. Thangavelu, M., Fronek, A., Morgan, R.: Simple calibration of Doppler velocity metering, Proc. San Diego Biomed. Symp. 16:1, 1977.

56. Ward, A.S., and Martin, T.P.: Some aspects of ultrasound in the diagnosis and assessment of aortoiliac disease, Am. J. Surg. 140:200, 1980.

57. Woodcock, J.P., Gosling, R.G., and Fitzgerald, D.E.: A new noninvasive technique for assessment of superficial femoral arterial obstruction, Br. J. Surg. 59:226, 1972.

58. Woodcock, J.P., et al.: Physical aspects of blood-velocity measurement by Doppler-shifted ultrasound. In Roberts, C., editor: Blood flow measurement, London, 1972, Sector Publisher, Ltd.

CHAPTER 54

The pulse volume recorder in peripheral arterial disease

JEFFREY K. RAINES

Recent advances in electronics, a more complete understanding of peripheral hemodynamics, and the vigorous development of clinical criteria have made the use of quantitative segmental plethysmography an important component in the routine evaluation of peripheral vascular disease.

After years of instrumentation development in the Fluid Mechanics Laboratory at the Massachusetts Institute of Technology[10-12] and clinical trials in the Vascular Laboratory, Massachusetts General Hospital,[2,5,13] the pulse volume recorder (PVR)* has emerged. The PVR is basically a quantitative segmental plethysmograph that has been designed for high sensitivity and oriented toward clinical use (Fig. 54-1).

To use the PVR, appropriate blood pressure cuffs are placed on the extremity or digit, and a measured quantity of air is injected until a preset pressure is reached. This procedure ensures that at a given pressure the cuff volume surrounding the limb is constant from reading to reading. The PVR electronic package measures and records instantaneous pressure changes in the segmental monitoring cuff. Cuff pressure change reflects alteration in cuff volume, which in turn reflects momentary changes in limb volume. PVR units are calibrated so that 1 mm Hg pressure change in the cuff provides a 20 mm chart deflection.

During the design phase, frequency response of the complete device (cuff/electronic system) was tested. The system has a flat response to 20 Hz, which is sufficient to evaluate the higher frequency components of the human arterial pressure pulse contour. Additional experiments were performed

*Life Sciences, Inc., Greenwich, Conn.

to verify that linearity is maintained over the full range of clinical interest. For arterial studies the output of the PVR electronics is AC coupled with a 1-second time constant.

To determine how closely the volume pulse contour resembles the pressure pulse contour, simultaneous PVR traces were compared with direct intraarterial pressure recordings taken at the same location. Fig. 54-2 shows a typical comparison in which mean cuff pressures were adjusted between 30 and 80 mm Hg in 10 mm Hg increments. The cuff pressure must be sufficiently high to allow adequate contact between the cuff bladder and the limb segment. Since the cuff pressure will by necessity reduce the transmural pressure in the underlying arteries, distortion of the recorded pulse contour will result at higher cuff pressures. In clinical practice a cuff pressure of 65 mm Hg has been found to give excellent pneumatic gain and surface contact as well as to maintain the important contour characteristics.

PVR INDICES

PVR amplitude. In clinical trials extending over 8 years, PVR amplitudes were found to remain highly reproducible in the same patient if constant cuff volumes and pressures were used.[5] Significant changes were consistently correlated with alterations in the underlying vasculature. There were variations in amplitudes from patient to patient. Amplitude can be affected by ventricular stroke volume, blood pressure, vasomotor tone, and volume. Despite this impressive list, consistency has been the rule in clinical practice, with patients in some cases returning every 3 or 4 months for repeat examinations. In our vascular laboratory alone we

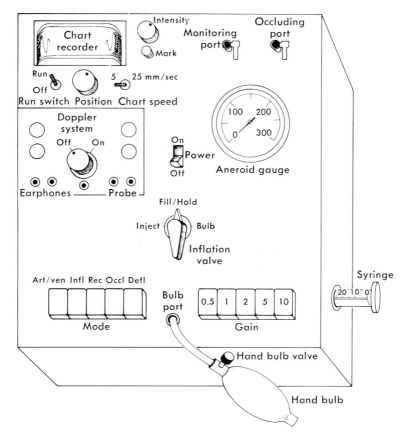

Fig. 54-1. Pulse volume recorder (PVR).

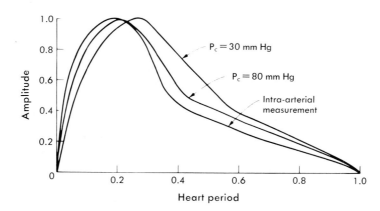

Fig. 54-2. PVR contours at different cuff pressures (P_c) compared with intraarterial measurement in femoral artery.

have performed over 15,000 lower extremity studies. Similarly, the presence of limb edema has not influenced the height or contour of the PVR recording.

Pulse volume amplitudes, however, are universally affected by exercise. In normal subjects the amplitude increases following standard exercise tests. On the other hand, patients with occlusive arterial disease uniformly show a diminution in pulse volume at the ankle following exercise. In addition, there is a definite relationship between the degree of ischemia as determined by the maximum walking time and the relative fall in pulse volume amplitude. In some cases the recovery time required to establish preexercise pulse amplitudes is useful.

PVR contour. Indications of occlusive arterial disease as demonstrated by the PVR contour include (1) decrease in the rise of the anacrotic limb, (2) rounding and delay in the pulse crest, (3) decreased rate of fall of the catacrotic limb, and (4) absence of the reflected diastolic wave.

In our experience the reflected diastolic wave is of particular diagnostic significance, since we have not seen it in the presence of demonstrable occlusive disease. The hemodynamic principles of this phenomenon at rest and after exercise are described in detail by Raines.[10] Examples of normal and abnormal PVR contours are given in Fig. 54-3.

Limb pressures. In most cases the Doppler velocity detector can be used to measure limb systolic pressures. Also, the PVR can be used to measure limb or digit systolic and diastolic pressures by placing the occlusion cuff proximal to the monitoring cuff. Pressures are determined at the site of the occlusion cuff when its pressure obliterates the PVR recording in the distal monitoring cuff. As pressure is lowered in the occluding cuff, oscilla-

tions in the monitoring device increase in amplitude, the maximum excursions occurring at the diastolic level. This method is reliable even at low pressures and does not require specific positioning over an artery, as does the Doppler ultrasonic velocity detector. This method may be the only applicable procedure to obtain a limb pressure when no Doppler signals are obtainable. The systolic and diastolic pressures obtained by the PVR have been compared with intraarterial pressures obtained by radial and femoral artery cannulation. The agreement is excellent for systolic pressure and always within 10 mm Hg for diastolic pressure determinations.

It has been shown that arterial occlusions or high-grade stenoses produce pressure differences in the limb at rest.[5,10,14,16] However, less significant degrees of stenosis, particularly at the aortoiliac level, may not. The hemodynamic significance of such minor degrees of arterial narrowing and the functional capacity of the collateral circulation are best evaluated by resting PVR tracings and the response of PVR amplitudes and pressures after measured exercise.

The remainder of this chapter deals with procedures, techniques, and clinical criteria used in conjunction with the PVR.

EVALUATING ARTERIAL HEMODYNAMICS IN THE LOWER EXTREMITIES

Lower limb vascular laboratory examinations may be performed both before and after exercise and in the resting state. Examples of such examinations in the lower limbs at rest are PVR recordings and systolic pressure measurements at the thighs, calves, and ankles of both legs, Doppler velocity detection in the feet, documentation of pulses and bruits, and brachial blood pressure. Ex-

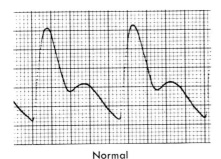

Normal

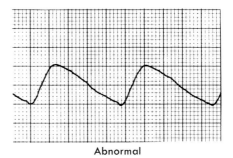

Abnormal

Fig. 54-3. Normal and abnormal pulse volume recordings taken at ankle level. Cuff pressure, 65 mm Hg; cuff volume, 75 cc.

ercise testing is performed when history, clinical examination, and symptoms indicate.

PVR cuffs are placed snugly around both thighs, calves, and ankles (six cuffs in all). The thigh cuff bladders are 36×18 cm, whereas the bladders in the cuffs for the calves and ankles are 22×12 cm.

Each recording is taken separately. The thigh cuff may be inflated using the hand bulb to a pressure of 65 mm Hg (air volume ≈ 400 cc). For the calf and ankle level the cuff pressure should also be 65 mm Hg with an injected volume of 75 ± 10 cc using the syringe. If this criterion is not met, the cuff must be reapplied at a slightly different tension. With practice, reapplication is rarely necessary.

To obtain systolic pressure at the thigh, calf, and ankle of a lower extremity, the PVR or the Doppler velocity detector may be used.

After completion of resting studies, exercise testing is performed and maximum walking time determined. If minimal or no symptoms occur, a 5-minute standard walking time is selected. Immediately after exercise, PVR recordings and pressures are measured at the ankle level and compared with resting values. In addition, postexercise brachial blood pressure is recorded.

When it is desirable to evaluate perfusion at the transmetatarsal or digital level, PVR recordings can be obtained at these levels. For transmetatarsal tracings a pediatric cuff (12×7 cm bladder) is used. The bladder is placed in contact with the anterior portion of the foot; 65 mm Hg is the desired cuff pressure, with an injected volume of 50 ± 10 cc.

For digital tracings, specifically designed cuffs[9] are used (7×2 cm and 9×3 cm bladders); 40 mm Hg is the recommended cuff pressure, with an injected volume of approximately 5 cc.

PVR recordings are classified into five categories, as listed in Table 54-1, and are combined with pressure data to define various clinical states.

The information given in Tables 54-1 to 54-6 has been developed at the Vascular Laboratory of the Massachusetts General Hospital and represents experience gained from 4500 examinations.[13] These tables establish objective criteria useful for the clinical management of peripheral vascular disease.

Rest pain. Table 54-2 summarizes data gathered to provide objective criteria for evaluation of patients with a complaint of rest pain.

Diabetics have significantly elevated ankle pres-

Table 54-1. Definition of PVR categories

PVR category	Chart deflection (mm)	
	Thigh and ankle	Calf
1	>15*	>20*
2	>15†	>20†
3	5 to 15	5 to 20
4	<5	<5
5	Flat	Flat

From Raines, J.K., et al.: Surgery 79:21, 1976.
*With reflected wave.
†No reflected wave.

Table 54-2. Vascular laboratory criteria for evaluation of rest pain

	Unlikely	Probable	Likely
Ankle pressure (mm Hg)			
Nondiabetic	>55	35 to 55	<35
Diabetic	>80	55 to 80	<55
Ankle PVR category			
Nondiabetic and diabetic	1,2,3	3,4	4,5

From Raines, J.K., et al.: Surgery 79:21, 1976.

Table 54-3. Vascular laboratory criteria for the prediction of lesion healing

	Unlikely	Probable	Likely
Ankle pressure (mm Hg)			
Nondiabetic	<55	55 to 65	>65
Diabetic	<80	80 to 90	>90
Ankle PVR category			
Nondiabetic and diabetic	4,5	3	1,2,3

From Raines, J.K., et al.: Surgery 79:21, 1976.

sure, since they often have medical calcinosis of peripheral vessels. This has the effect of artificially elevating the measured ankle pressure.[15] In fact, in at least 5% to 10% of diabetic patients, ankle pressures cannot be determined at all because of incompressible vessels. In these patients the PVR tracings are the only measurable parameter. It is especially important in the diabetic patient to be able to differentiate between primary neuropathic pain and primary ischemic pain.

Foot lesions. Table 54-3 provides objective criteria for the evaluation of patients with foot lesions.

In a recent study diabetic patients represented only 15% of patients in the rest pain group; 54%

of those with necrosis were diabetic. This emphasizes the clinically recognized fact that diabetics are far more prone to develop traumatic lesions, perhaps because of the frequent incidence of peripheral neuropathy. Diabetic patients frequently have artifically elevated pressures as a result of calcified vessels; this pressure difference is approximately 25 mm Hg. Furthermore, because of more distal small vessel involvement in the diabetic patient, a digital or forefoot lesion may develop or progress at a higher ankle pressure than in the nondiabetic patient.

In predicting healing of foot lesions, determination of ankle pressure and PVR recordings at the ankle, transmetatarsal, and digital levels are again and most important measurements.

Below-knee amputation healing. In the patient with advanced arteriosclerotic peripheral vascular disease in whom arterial reconstruction is not possible and who comes to amputation, it is generally agreed that a below-knee amputation is preferable from the standpoint of rehabilitation. However, it is also recognized that significant morbidity and mortality are present in this group of patients, particularly those in whom a more distal amputation fails and who therefore require a second procedure. Since the prediction of successful healing of a below-knee amputation on the basis of clinical or arteriographic information is often a difficult task requiring considerable experience, easily obtained and objective vascular laboratory measurements that prove helpful in this regard have been sought.

Table 54-4 summarizes current criteria developed to predict the chances of successful below-knee amputation. We are currently in the process of deriving similar criteria for transmetatarsal and digital amputations. In these instances distal PVR recordings play an important role. In fact, it has been our experience that in the absence of sepsis and osteomyelitis a toe amputation will heal if a pulsatile PVR tracing is found at the base of the digit in question. In addition, for the same clinical presentation a transmetatarsal amputation will heal if a pulsatile PVR tracing is present at the transmetatarsal level.

Evaluation of claudication. In the patient with lower extremity pain on exertion it is of utmost importance to distinguish symptoms caused by neurologic or orthopedic processes from those produced by vascular insufficiency. In fact, both entities may coexist. If true claudication is present, it is also important to determine accurately the pa-

Table 54-4. Vascular laboratory criteria for primary healing or below-knee amputation

	Unlikely	Probable	Likely
Pressure (mm Hg)			
Calf	>65	>65	>65
Ankle	>30	>30	>30
PVR category			
Calf	4,5	4	1,2,3
Ankle	5	4	1,2,3,4

From Raines, J.K., et al: Surgery 79:21, 1976.

Table 54-5. Vascular laboratory criteria for limiting claudication

	Unlikely	Probable	Likely
Postexercise ankle pressure (mm Hg)	>50	>50	>50
Postexercise ankle PVR category	2,3	4	4,5

From Raines, J.K., et al.: Surgery 79:21, 1976.

tient's degree of disability and to establish a quantitative baseline with which medical or surgical therapy can be compared. However, it is often difficult to accomplish this by history and physical examination alone; a vascular laboratory examination including treadmill exercise should be routine in the workup of such patients.

In evaluating the presence or absence of true claudication the most important parameters are ankle pressure and ankle PVR recording after measured treadmill exercise. Patients are exercised until significant symptoms are produced. The treadmill time at which this level of pain is reached, as previously mentioned, is called the maximum walking time and occurs sometime between the onset of symptoms and the point at which the patient developes disabling pain. The endpoint of the maximum walking time has been shown to be the most reliable.

Table 54-5 provides simple criteria for the laboratory evaluation of limiting claudication.

It should be pointed out that for maximum use of these tables, PVR and pressure measurements *must complement* each other; pressures are not always obtainable and, taken alone, may be misleading. PVR recordings are rarely misleading and are enhanced by pressure measurements. However, when pressures cannot be measured accurately,

PVR recordings may be used alone to form sound impressions.

Anatomic localization. Anatomic localization of hemodynamically significant peripheral vascular lesions by noninvasive means is another important contribution to patient management. Table 54-6 is given here as a simple guide for localization. It is important to note that laboratory findings and physical findings must be combined to produce accurate localization. Looking at one parameter is generally not sufficient. The case of combined disease is by far the most challenging; in 5% to 10% of patients with combined disease, noninvasive analysis, although it may define the hemodynamics, cannot accurately localize the major contributing lesion. In these cases an invasive femoral artery pressure study may be indicated.[1] A study is currently in progress at the Miami Heart Institute to define the accuracy and limitations of noninvasive testing in anatomic localization.

EVALUATING ARTERIAL HEMODYNAMICS IN THE UPPER EXTREMITIES

Occlusive arterial disease of the arteries supplying the upper extremities is rare when compared with the frequency of the disease in the lower extremities. However, arterial trauma and thrombosis following cardiac catheterization result in patients requiring evaluation of upper extremity arterial hemodynamics.

PVR cuffs (22 × 12 cm bladder) are placed snugly around the upper arm and forearm, and 100 ± 15 cc of air is injected with the syringe system into the upper cuff to produce a pressure of 65 mm Hg. This procedure is repeated for the forearm.

When the PVR is used to measure pressures, distal monitoring is obtained at the digital level using a digital cuff.

The upper extremity workup is completed by evaluating digital perfusion. This is done by taking PVR recordings at the base and tip of each digit, as well as digital systolic pressures. The larger digital cuff (9 × 3 cm bladder) is placed at the base of the digit and the smaller digital cuff (7 × 2 cm bladder) at the tip. PVR recordings are taken at these locations at a cuff pressure of 40 mm Hg; approximately 5 cc of atmospheric air is injected.

Systolic pressure at the base of the digits may be measured by using the PVR occlusion technique previously described.

EVALUATING VASOSPASTIC DISEASE

It is often important to differentiate digital small vessel disease from vasospastic disease. Vasospasm is characterized by loss of reflected wave, blunting, and reduced amplitude in the PVR recordings. When vasospasm first occurs, digital hemodynamics may be abnormal only when the patient is stressed, such as with cold or tension. Therefore such a patient should be studied at room temperature (a constant temperature room is not required) and also after digital immersion in iced water for 2 minutes. If the patient does not have nearly normal digital tip PVR recordings after 5 minutes at room temperature, vasospasm is probable.

In patients with more advanced vasospastic phenomena, abnormal PVR recordings will be present at room temperature at the digit tip level with near normal digital bases. With disease progression, the digit bases show abnormal recordings and systolic pressures.

In the further differentiation of vasospastic disease from occlusive disease and in predicting the effect of dorsal or lumbar sympathectomy, the study of digital perfusion with the PVR before and after nerve block has proved useful. If studies remain unchanged, sympathectomy may be of little help, and occlusive disease is suggested as a prime factor in the process. If perfusion is improved after block, the contribution resulting from vasospasm may be estimated and a basis for continued therapy established. Serial digital PVR studies also serve as a monitor for medical therapy.[8] We believe the chances of lesion healing are good if pulsatile PVR recordings can be determined at the tip level under normal conditions. This, of course, is modified if sepsis is present.

EVALUATING COMPRESSION SYNDROMES

The PVR can be helpful in thoracic outlet syndromes and popliteal artery entrapment.[3,6]

Most researchers believe the pain associated with thoracic outlet syndromes is neurologic, secondary to nerve compression at the lowest trunk of the brachial plexus by a cervical of first rib. Since the subclavian artery and the lower trunk of the brachial plexus are in close proximity, the artery also undergoes compression that may be monitored by the PVR.

The patient is first asked to sit erect off the side of the examining table. A PVR monitoring cuff is

Table 54-6. Anatomic localization

	ΔP_s			PVR			Postexercise		Exercise symptoms
	Arm-thigh	Thigh-calf	Calf-ankle	Thigh	Calf	Ankle	P_s, ankle† (mm Hg)	PVR category	
AI stenosis ODS	Yes	No	No	Abn	Abn	Abn	<50	5 (quick recovery)	Calf, thigh, buttocks
AI occlusion ODS	Yes	No	No	Abn	Abn	Abn	<20	5	Calf, thigh, buttocks
SFA occlusion (low) No AI disease*	No	Yes	Yes	Nor	Abn	Abn	20 to 50	4	Calf
SFA occlusion (high) No AI disease*	Yes	Yes	Yes	Abn	Abn	Abn	20 to 50	4	Calf, lower thigh
Combined disease AI + SFA	Yes	Yes	Yes	Abn	Abn	Abn	<10	5	Calf, thigh, buttocks
Tibial vessel disease	No	No	Yes	Nor	Nor	Abn	30 to 70	4	Foot, ankle, calf
Small vessel disease	No	No	No	Nor	Nor	Nor‡	—	—	—

AI, Aortoiliac; ODS, open distal system; SFA, superficial femoral artery; ΔP_s, systolic pressure difference; Abn, abnormal; Nor, normal; P_s, systolic pressure.
*No hemodynamically significant AI disease present.
†Values quoted are not absolute and are given as a guide.
‡PVR recordings at transmetatarsal region and/or digits reduced.

placed on the upper arm to be evaluated and is inflated to 65 mm Hg. Recordings are taken in the following positions:

1. Erect, with hands in lap
2. Erect, with arm at a 90-degree angle in the same plane as the torso
3. Erect, with arm at a 120-degree angle in the same plane as the torso
4. Erect, with arm at a 90-degree angle in the same plane as the torso and with shoulders in extended military-type brace
5. Same position as in 4 but with head turned sharply toward the monitored arm
6. Same position as in 4 but with head turned sharply away from the monitored arm

In general, PVR amplitudes increase as the arm is elevated. Arterial compression is present if the PVR amplitude goes flat in any of the standard positions. Since the syndrome is often bilateral, the other arm should always be studied. It should be noted that many asymptomatic individuals (25% is a good estimate) compress arteries supplying the arm in some of the positions outlined. Therefore it is important to base therapy on symptoms, physical findings, history, and ulnar nerve conduction in addition to vascular laboratory data.

Ischemic pain with exercise may occur because of intermittent compression or entrapment of the popliteal artery by the medial head of the gastrocnemius muscle. In such instances the popliteal artery passes medial to or through the fibers of the medial head of the gastrocnemius muscle, which may have an anomalous origin on the femur either cephalad or lateral to its normal position on the posterior face of the medial femoral condyle. Regardless of the anatomic or embryologic anomaly, however, the result is an episodic and functional occlusion of the popliteal artery that occurs with each plantar flexion. The significance of early detection and treatment of this abnormality is related to observations that progressive structural changes may occur in the arterial wall as a result of chronic and recurring trauma ultimately resulting in aneurysm formation, thrombosis, and loss of limb vitality. Less than 30 documented cases of the popliteal entrapment syndrome have been noted. Current review suggests that the syndrome may be characterized by (1) history of unilateral intermittent claudication in young men, (2) laboratory findings of diminution of ankle PVR recordings with sustained plantar flexion and/or passive dorsiflexion of the foot, and (3) angiographic findings of medial deviation of the popliteal artery.

In cases of suspected popliteal artery entrapment it is extremely important to perform a standard lower extremity examination as well as PVR re-

Table 54-7. Malformations

Malformation	Local PVR		Doppler abnormal superficial signals
	Amplitude	Reflected wave	
Venous	Normal	Present	Absent
Arteriovenous	Increased	Absent	Present

cordings at the ankle with sustained active plantar flexion and with passive dorsiflexion of the foot. Compression during any of these maneuvers is easily recognized.

With regard to entrapment in other clinical situations, the finding of normal PVR recordings in response to acute hip flexion and knee bending has been of help in advising patients who have had extraordinary, makeshift bypass grafts carried out for the treatment of sepsis or related problems. In many of these patients the grafts have been implanted lateral to the inguinal ligament, across the pubis, deep or superficial to muscle bellies and fascial bands, or around bony prominences at the knee. In such patients it is reassuring to know that the graft does not kink or become entrapped in varying limb positions.[5]

EVALUATING VASCULAR MALFORMATIONS

Pulse volume recordings taken on an extremity or digit over an area of suspected vascular malformation are helpful in differentiating the type of malformation and its extent. Doppler velocity detection over areas of suspected vascular malformation is also useful. Table 54-7 is presented as a simple guide.

In venous malformations arterial hemodynamics are not significantly affected. Therefore venous pressure remains within normal limits, and pulse volume is not increased. Also, peripheral resistance is normal, and arterial reflected waves recorded by the PVR are present. In arteriovenous malformation the compliant venous conduits undergo abnormal pulsatile pressure transmitted through the malformation from the arterial system. This results in increased pulse volume. Decreased local peripheral resistance results in loss of reflected wave.

INTRAOPERATIVE MONITORING

The PVR has been used extensively to monitor the results of reconstructive arterial surgery.[5] It is

acknowledged that experienced surgeons performing proximal arterial reconstructions in the presence of patent distal vessels can get a qualitative estimate of the excellence of revascularization by restoration of pedal pulses. However, pulses are not always restored and may be very difficult to appreciate in the operating room. The time to appreciate any operative misadventure is while in the operating room with the vessels exposed and not following a few hours of observation in the recovery room. Intraoperative monitoring is particularly valuable in the teaching setting and provides immediate objective evidence of technical success.

Intraoperative monitoring is essential in patients undergoing proximal arterial reconstruction in the presence of distal occlusive disease. This group of patients includes those with combined aortoiliac and femoropopliteal disease or those with femoropopliteal disease and associated tibial involvement. Absence of definable PVR amplitude in the limb segment immediately distal to the arterial reconstruction has led invariably to a successful search for a cause, whether an anastomotic stenosis, clamp injury, thrombosis, or embolus.

It is to be acknowledged that the PVR recording measured immediately following revascularization may be somewhat decreased. This ia particularly true if the ankle is monitored following aortoiliac reconstruction in patients with known femoropopliteal occlusive disease. This may reflect several factors, including vasoconstriction, hypotension, and hypovolemia. Therefore, with such patients, limb monitoring should be carried out as proximally as possible; the calf is ideal. In no recorded instance has there been a flat trace at the calf if the proximal reconstruction has been adequate. In cases where the pulse amplitude has not returned to more than 50% of its preoperative level, measurement of calf and ankle pressures has been used to complement the PVR measurements and verify the adequacy of the reconstruction. In patients with patent distal vessels the initial response following clamp removal has been immediate return of the PVR amplitude, usually to normal.

Technical errors during femoropopliteal bypass procedures may account for 6% to 15% of early and 15% to 30% of late failures.[4] Improperly constructed distal anastomoses with obstruction of the outflow tract, valvular or torsion defects with the vein graft, and distal thrombosis caused by intraoperative emboli are the principal causes of graft failure. Intraoperative arteriography has been suggested as a means of detection of these abnormalities. However, intraoperative arteriography is time-consuming, usually visualizes only one plane, and provides no physiologic information about the graft and distal runoff. In addition, the various angiographic techniques employed may lead to complications in themselves. The PVR provides physiologic information on (1) the distal runoff before insertion of the graft, (2) the condition and function of the distal and proximal anastomoses, and (3) the alignment of the saphenous vein.

Simulated pulse volume as monitored by the PVR has allowed correction of technical errors in the operating room, thus avoiding a repeat procedure. In this technique the PVR is connected to a monitoring cuff placed at the ankle; heparinized saline solution is "pulsed" by hand at the rate of ≈5 ml/sec at two stages: (1) through the popliteal arteriotomy by means of a Marx needle and (2) through the upper end of the graft following completion of distal anastomosis. After the proximal anastomosis is complete, the initial pulsatile blood flow propelled by the heart is also monitored. If abnormalities are found at any stage, reasons for hemodynamic defects are investigated.

RECOVERY ROOM MONITORING

Following peripheral arterial reconstruction in the presence of known distal occlusive disease, peripheral pulses may not be easily discernible, particularly in the early postoperative course. In addition, palpable pulses may disappear because of lower extremity edema later in the postoperative course. Noninvasive studies using the PVR have been of considerable value in following patients during this period.[5] Nursing personnel are able to monitor arterial reconstructions in the recovery area effectively despite the absence of palpable pulses. By detecting failure early, the surgeon is often able to correct problems, thus salvaging the reconstruction.

In practice the recovery room nurses take PVR recordings at set intervals. PVR amplitudes invariably remain stable or increase during the early postoperative period in the presence of a successful reconstruction. Failing PVR amplitudes, often but not always associated with diminution of the ankle/brachial systolic pressure ratio, invariably mean a failing arterial reconstruction in our experience. These findings should prompt early reexploration of the arterial reconstruction.

SUMMARY

Function is the most important consideration in evaluating lower extremity occlusive arterial disease. Evaluation such as described in this chapter can be done by means of noninvasive hemodynamic studies more precisely than by clinical examination or angiography. The overall functional accuracy of Tables 54-2 through 54-5 is greater than 95% when the clinical course is used as the standard. If disease is confined to a single level, these studies can anatomically localize (Table 54-6) the lesion in virtually 100% of cases. With bilevel disease, accuracy drops into a range of 90% to 95%.

The PVR (venous mode) in combination with its built-in Doppler system can perform lower and upper extremity noninvasive deep venous tree evaluations. This technique produces approximately 5% false positive and 2% false negative results.

Because of the flexibility of the transducer system in the PVR, it has been possible to build a simple attachment to the PVR for the measurement of ophthalmic artery pressure (ocular pneumoplethysmography—OPG*) The attachment is available in both unilateral and bilateral models. This measurement in combination with carotid audiofrequency analysis and cerebral Doppler evaluation has an overall accuracy of 94% in our hands.

Newest instrumentation

Recently a small group of vascular laboratory directors, vascular surgeons, electrical engineers, mechanical design engineers, and computer software and hardware engineers combined their skills to produce the automated procedures laboratory (PVR/APL).* The overall system is best described when its two major components are considered.

Measurement unit. The measurement unit (MU) (Fig. 54-4) provides the interface between the op-

*Life Sciences, Inc., Greenwich, Conn.

erator and the patient. In keeping with basic and validated systems, the MU contains menu-driven automated versions of the PVR, an advanced zero-crossing continuous-wave Doppler system (3.5 to 9.2 MHz), a dual-channel OPG (OPG II/500), and a digital carotid phonoangiograph (CPA II). The probes and cuffs are conveniently stored in the MU for use in the vascular laboratory, the operating room, or at the bedside. The unit has a minimum of buttons and controls, has the same floor space requirement as the current PVR, and is slightly taller. Its mobility also compares favorably.

The operator is prompted by a menu that appears on the cathod-ray tube (CRT) screen. Protocols for all standard vascular laboratory procedures are built in. The operator has control over the various steps in the protocols and may repeat any sequence as desired, such as the data stored (PVR tracings, limb pressures, ophthalmic artery pressures, or carotid phonoangiographic [CPA] data) and cuff inflation/deflation. To perform these functions the operator uses a controller that fits in the palm of one hand and has one button and two rocker switches. Patient data are stored on a floppy disk in the MU. At the completion of the tests the patient disk is removed for use in the analysis unit (AU), which is described later.

Besides being able to perform the standard lower extremity arterial, extracranial arterial, and lower extremity venous evaluations in combination with the AU, the MU can perform these studies independently. It also has a built-in strip-chart recorder for independent hard copy. Capacilities for digital studies, penile studies, femoral artery studies, lesion healing prediction, and amputation healing predictions are also included.

The MU used with the AU also has a built-in teaching program that outlines step by step all the required procedures. Actual patient data are displayed for immediate comparison by the student.

Analysis unit. The AU (Fig. 54-5) is a combination of the most advanced, supported microcomputer, specially designed software (an interface that allows the operator to communicate with the computer), and an advanced dot-matrix printer.

Patient data taken from the MU in disk form are displayed by the AU for analysis and final report printing. Reports may be generated after each patient examination or at another convenient time. The patient data are displayed on the CRT, and a menu-driven AU protocol guides the operator in entering the data. Final verification of the data is

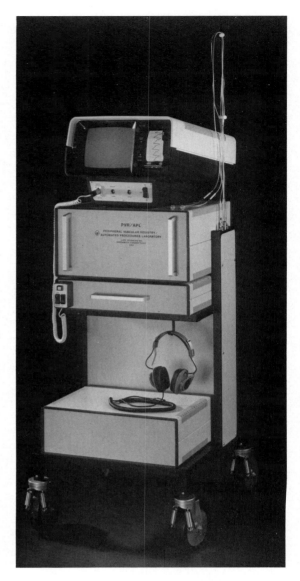

Fig. 54-4. Measurement unit (MU). (From Raines, J.: Vasc. Lab. Rev. 1:10, 1983.)

prepared by the operator with the help of the computer. When the patient data are complete, a quantitative interpretation is presented on the screen. This provides a firm diagnosis based on thousands of cases. The word processing capability of the system allows the operator or laboratory director to alter this interpretation. The operator then can instruct the AU to print the final clinical report. This report includes the history and physical examination information, the data that was measured including all tracings (PVR, OPG, and CPA), in-

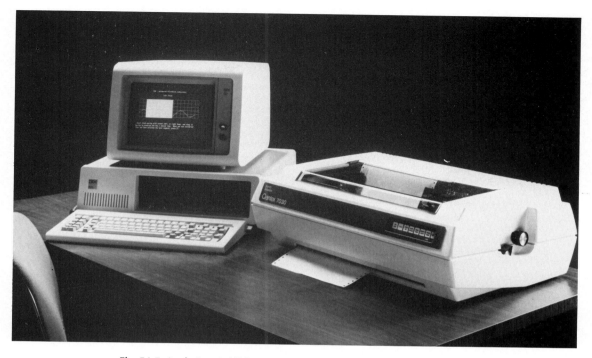

Fig. 54-5. Analysis unit (AU). (From Raines, J.: Vasc. Lab. Rev. 1:10, 1983.)

terepretation of the data, and a graphic display indicating the anatomic lesions of interest. Patient data are automatically stored on floppy disks in laboratory archives and entered into the peripheral vascular registry, which will be described.

Since the AU is also a powerful computer, a comprehensive office management system has been written for this equipment. The system generates patient logs, has complete office accounting files, includes automated billing, and prints insurance forms. In addition, IBM software for wordprocessing, electronic spread sheet analysis, statistical analysis, and BASIC language is compatible. There are also more than 2000 software packages written for this system by independent programming firms.

Peripheral vascular registry. A peripheral vascular registry is desirable for a number of reasons. The registry can improve patient management by reviewing previous experiences, new certification requirements, regional vascular societies, and surgical/medical results and generate interest in more automated research. This component has been built into the automated peripheral laboratory. It has been carefully designed to answer the maximum number of potential questions with the minimum amount of data entry and storage. In addition, most of the data obtained from the vascular laboratory studies are automatically placed in the registry. Extensive sorting, classification, and retrieval routines have been programmed into this system. This allows rapid clinical research on large patient populations. The hard disk in the IBM PC/XT can easily store more than 12,000 registry records for review. Since the registry is completely in software form, changes can be made easily at minimal cost. Nine files can be accessed by this registry as follows:

1. Census data, history, and physical findings
2. Lower extremity arterial laboratory data
3. Cerebral laboratory data
4. Lower extremity venous data
5. Lower extremity arteriography
6. Cerebral arteriography
7. Lower extremity venography
8. Compact surgical record
9. Complete follow-up record

The peripheral vascular registry allows the maximum use of measured noninvasive data in temporal management of patients, as well as in clinic research and natural history studies.

REFERENCES

1. Brener, B.J., et al.: Measurement of systolic femoral arterial pressure during reactive hyperemia, Circulation 50(suppl.):259, 1974.
2. Buckley, C.J., Darling, R.C., and Raines, J.K.: Instrumentation and examination procedures for a clinical vascular laboratory, Med. Instrum. 9:181, 1975.
3. Dale, W.A., and Lewis, M.R.: Management of thoracic outlet syndrome, Ann. Surg. 181:575, 1975.
4. Darling, R.C., and Linton, R.R.: Durability of femoropopliteal reconstructions, Am. J. Surg. 123:472, 1972.
5. Darling, R.C., et al.: Quantitative segmental pulse volume recorder: a clinical tool, Surgery 72:873, 1972.
6. Darling, R.C., et al.: Intermittent claudication in young athletes: popliteal artery entrapment syndrome, J. Trauma 14:543, 1974.
7. Gee, W., et al.: Ocular pneumoplethysmography in carotid artery disease, Med. Instrum. 8:244, 1974.
8. Gifford, R.W.: The arteriospastic diseases: clinical significance and management. In Brest, A.N., editor: Peripheral vascular disease: cardiovascular clinics, Philadelphia, 1971, F.A. Davis Co.
9. Gundersen, J.: Segmental measurements of systolic blood pressure in the extremities including the thumb and the great toe, Acta Chir. Scand. 462(suppl.):1, 1972.
10. Raines, J.K.: Diagnosis and analysis of arteriosclerosis in the lower limbs from the arterial pressure pulse, doctoral thesis, Massachusetts Institute of Technology, 1972, Cambridge, Mass.
11. Raines, J.K., Jaffrin, M.Y., and Rao, S.: A noninvasive pressure pulse recorder: development and rationale, Med. Instrum. 7:245, 1973.
12. Raines, J.K., Jaffrin, M.Y., and Shapiro, A.H.: A computer simulation of arterial dynamics in the human leg, J. Biochem. 7:77, 1974.
13. Raines, J.K., et al.: Vascular laboratory criteria for the management of peripheral vascular disease of the lower extremities, Surgery 79:21, 1976.
14. Strandness, D.E., Jr.: Peripheral arterial disease, Boston, 1969, Little, Brown & Co.
15. Taguchi, J.T., and Suwangool, P.: Pipe-stem brachial arteries: a cause of pseudohypertension, JAMA 228:733, 1974.
16. Yao, J.S.T.: Haemodynamic studies in peripheral arterial disease, Br. J. Surg. 57:761, 1970.

CHAPTER 55

Exercise ankle pressure measurements in arterial disease

D. EUGENE STRANDNESS, Jr., and R. EUGENE ZIERLER

The most common complaint of patients with chronic arterial occlusion is intermittent claudication. It is secondary to the inadequacy of the collateral circulation in fulfilling the metabolic requirements of the exercising muscle. Interestingly, numerous studies have confirmed that even with extensive multilevel occlusive disease, resting blood flows are maintained in the normal range because of the relatively low blood flow requirements at rest and the compensatory decrease in resistance that occurs distal to the areas of occlusion.

Exercise as a method of assessing the degree of disability associated with atherosclerosis is useful for the following reasons: (1) exercise is the specific activity that produces the symptoms; (2) the severity of pain, its localization, and the walking pattern can be simply assessed; (3) it is possible to determine the degree to which the collateral circulation can maintain distal perfusion pressure in response to a near maximal ischemic stimulus; (4) the recovery time that is, the period of postexercise hyperemia, can be accurately determined; (5) exercise can be valuable in distinguishing true claudication from the neurospinal conditions that mimic the pain of muscular ischemia; and (6) exercise may be the most sensitive method of assessing both disease progression and improvement.

Before considering the clinical application and usefulness of this type of testing, it is necessary to briefly review our current understanding of the normal physiologic response to exercise.

NORMAL PHYSIOLOGY
Limb blood flow

Blood flow is primarily distributed to the two major components of the limb: skin and muscle.

Because of its important role in thermal regulation, skin blood flow does, of course, vary widely depending on the ambient conditions. The proportion of skin to muscle in the limbs varies greatly by location, with progressively less muscle mass as one proceeds distally. The total blood flow to the leg is distributed to the major components: skin, muscle, bone, and fat. The level of resting flow to bone is dependent on the relative proportions of cancellous and noncancellous bone and is difficult to assess, particularly in terms of the redistribution that may occur in response to exercise.

Under resting conditions the average blood flow in the normal leg is in the range of 300 to 500 ml/min.[23] Grimby et al.[8] and Lassen and Kampp[13] measured resting flows in muscle by the xenon clearance method and found that, in general, flows vary between 1.8 and 2.5 ml/100 g/min in the muscle groups tested. At moderate levels of exercise, total leg blood flow increases by a factor of 5 to 10, while muscle blood flow rises to approximately 30 ml/100 g/min (Fig. 55-1). Muscle blood flow may reach 70 ml/100 g/min during strenuous exercise. After cessation of exercise, limb blood flow returns to resting values within 1 to 5 minutes.

Skin blood flow is extremely sensitive to changes in ambient temperature, and any value expressed must take this into account. Flows to the skin of the hand are much more variable than those to the foot, even with similar changes in temperature. Allwood and Burry,[1] for example, found foot blood flow to range from 0.2 ml/100 ml/min at 15° C to 16.5 ml/100 ml/min at 44° C. Corresponding temperature increases would produce much higher blood flows to the hand. Although there is no doubt that muscle flow can also respond to changes in

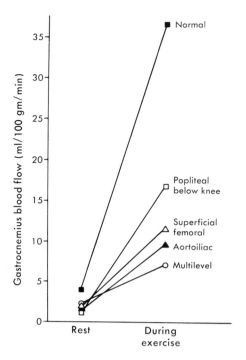

Fig. 55-1. Magnitude of increase in blood flow to muscle that occurs in normal subjects and in patients with varying degrees of occlusive arterial disease.

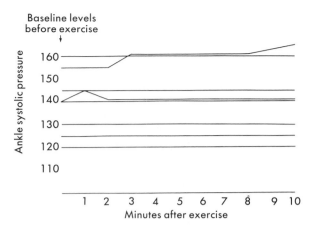

Fig. 55-2. Ankle systolic pressure values of eight normal subjects after walking on treadmill for 5 minutes at 2 mph on 12% grade. In every case pressure either remained at preexercise level or increased slightly. (From Strandness, D.E., Jr.: Surgery 59:325, 1966. By permission of The C.V. Mosby Co., St. Louis.)

temperature, it is much less variable than blood flow to skin and subcutaneous tissue.

Reactive hyperemia. One of the remarkable features of limb blood flow is the phenomenon commonly referred to as reactive hyperemia. A poorly understood aspect of this change is the fact that even a few seconds of arterial occlusion will produce an increase in flow even though the duration of occlusion is not sufficient to produce significant ischemia. The actual flow changes that are defined as reactive hyperemia are confined to those situations in which arterial flow has been occluded by a pneumatic tourniquet, whereas the changes that accompany walking will be referred to as the period of postexercise hyperemia.

Because flows to skin and muscle have not been measured simultaneously to assess the exact partition that occurs between these tissues, the exact distribution of reactive hyperemic flow is unclear. However, with reactive hyperemia the early marked increase in flow is largely confined to skin. During exercise, the great demands for blood are in muscle, and there may be a transient reduction in blood flow to skin and, in particular, to the distal foot. Thus with arterial occlusion there may be a tran-

sient but dramatic reduction in foot blood flow, the magnitude of which is related to the severity of the arterial disease.

Limb blood pressure

The limb blood pressure response to stress has been studied most frequently by indirect measurements of ankle systolic blood pressure. This information is must useful when expressed as the ratio of ankle systolic pressure to brachial systolic pressure. The ankle-to-arm pressure index has a mean value of 1.11 ± 0.10 in normal individuals at rest.[28] The following simple analogy to Ohm's law can be made:

$$P_1 - P_2 = RQ$$

where

$P_1 - P_2$ = Pressure drop across segment being evaluated
R = Resistance to flow
Q = Volume flow

As predicted by this analogy, there should be an increased pressure drop across an arterial segment as flow is increased either with exercise or with reactive hyperemia. However, Strandness and Bell[22] demonstrated little or no fall in systolic pressure at the ankle after exercise in normal subjects walking at 2 mph on a 12% grade. Stahler and Strandness[18] were also able to show that as the work load increased above this level there was a slight decrease in the ankle pressure immediately after exercise with some delay in recovery related to the

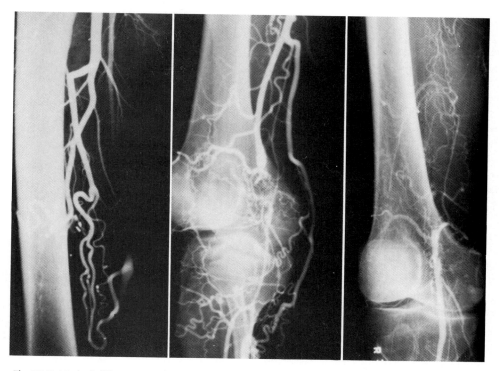

Fig. 55-3. Marked differences in degree of collateralization that can be observed in patients with disease of femoropopliteal segment.

level of the work load. Nevertheless, the work loads required to bring out this pressure fall were much more strenuous than those used in evaluating patients with intermittent claudication. Thus for practical purposes, the response of a normal leg to moderate exercise consists of little or no drop in ankle systolic pressure (Fig. 55-2).

EXERCISE PHYSIOLOGY WITH CHRONIC ARTERIAL OCCLUSION

The development of arterial stenoses or occlusions results in diversion of flow through the collateral channels, which, because of the very small size of the midzone components, are high-resistance conduits. Thus even under resting conditions there is an abnormal pressure drop across the collateral bed that reduces the perfusion pressure both to the muscle and skin distal to the site of involvement.

Although collateral resistance is relatively high and fixed, the resistance of a peripheral runoff bed such as the calf is quite variable. The muscular arterioles are primarily responsible for regulating peripheral resistance and controlling the distribution of flow to various capillary beds. Consider the common example of a limb with an occluded su-

perficial femoral artery. In this situation, the resistance offered by the profunda-geniculate collateral system is high, but a compensatory decrease in the peripheral calf resistance permits resting blood flow to remain in the normal range.[25] During exercise, the resistance of the proximal collateral bed remains high while the peripheral resistance continues to decrease. Since the ability of the peripheral vessels to compensate for the high proximal resistance is limited, exercise blood flow will be less than normal, and there will be a further pressure drop across the diseased arterial segment. The clinical result of this physiologic response is calf muscle ischemia with claudication.

In a normal patient, exercise even at moderate work loads produces a large increase in the blood flow to muscle. Although resting limb blood flow in patients with claudication is not significantly different from that in normal subjects, the same degree of exercise in patients with chronic arterial occlusion results in a much smaller increase in flow (Fig. 55-1). Thus the normal patient can dramatically increase limb blood flow immediately with stress in contrast to patients whose maximal limb blood flow is limited by the high-resistance collateral channels. This abnormal response is most easily demonstrated by recording the changes in ankle systolic pressure that follow treadmill exercise to the point of claudication.

As a patient walks, the pressures generated by the contracting muscles in the limb are in opposition to the intraarterial pressure. Therefore depending on the extent of the pressure drop accross the collateral bed, the pressure produced by each contraction may exceed that available for perfusion of the muscle. The situation is further complicated by the fact that the resistance vessels in skeletal muscle rapidly dilate in response to the ischemic stimulus. This marked vasodilation results in a further increase in pressure available to maintain flow. Thus a vicious cycle is created that can only be reversed by cessation of the exercise.

From a clinical standpoint it is clear that there is no single pressure-flow response that can be applied to every patient. The reasons for this are the wide variability of the following: (1) the anatomic patterns of arterial occlusion; (2) the availability and response of the collateral circulation, which also depends on the location of occlusions, duration of disease, degree of exercise maintained by the patient, and age (Fig. 55-3); (3) body weight; (4) systemic blood pressure; and (5) myocardial per-

formance. Thus all of these factors contribute to the degree of disability and the physiologic changes that accompany the disease. However, the advantage of exercise testing is that each patient can in a sense serve as their own control. The physiologic changes can then be measured and used for long-term studies of the natural history of the disease with or without therapy.[17,19,20]

Observed clinical patterns

As already discussed, the patterns that occur in normal patients are well characterized and when observed are adequate indices of normality, particularly if the level of stress is well documented. There are three general patterns of ankle pressure–calf blood flow responses that reflect the level and extent of disease and thus indirectly the collateral potential. These are best discussed in terms of single-segment and multisegment occlusive disease. Single-segment refers to isolated occlusions in either the aortoiliac area or superficial femoropopliteal segment. When both segments are occluded, the term multisegment is applied.

A brief mention should be made of the medium-sized arteries distal to the popliteal artery, that is, the tibial and peroneal vessels. Disease confined solely to these arteries will usually not produce

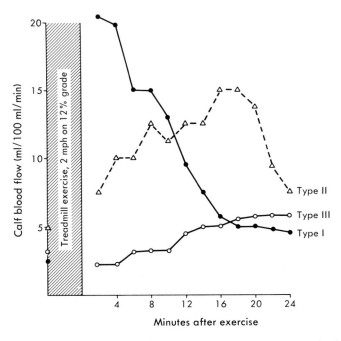

Fig. 55-4. Three patterns of calf blood flow observed in patients with intermittent claudication. See text for explanation. (From Strandness, D.E., Jr.: Cardiovasc. Clin. 3:53, 1971. By permission of F.A. Davis Co., Philadelphia.)

claudication but can produce problems involving perfusion of the foot. This is particularly true when distal occlusions are combined with disease at more proximal levels.

Before discussing the patterns observed, it must be emphasized that the resistance to flow offered by collateral arteries becomes greater as successive collateral channels are added, that is, serial resistances are additive. This will in large part explain why patients with multisegment disease and multiple collateral pathways always have the most severe symptoms.

Exercise testing for patients with vascular disease is generally carried out on a treadmill set for 2 mph on a 12% grade. This work load is easy for most patients, even elderly ones, and is sufficient to characterize the pressure-flow response that accompanies their disability. Sumner and Strandness[24] in a study of patients with claudication found the following three basic pressure-flow patterns (Fig. 55-4):

1. The calf blood flow increased immediately after exercise as the ankle pressure fell. The period of postexercise hyperemia was characterized by a lower than normal peak flow and a prolonged recovery time.

2. There was a marked delay in the calf blood flow reaching its lower than normal peak value.

3. The calf blood flow fell below even resting levels immediately after exercise, requiring prolonged periods of time for recovery.

An important observation resulting from these studies was that when simultaneous measurements were made of the ankle systolic pressure changes, there was an excellent correlation with the flow measurements (Fig. 55-5).

Some other important clinical observations regarding the response to exercise were as follows: (1) there is an inverse relationship between calf blood flow and ankle systolic pressure; (2) the ankle systolic pressure response can be used alone as an index of the ischemia that occurs rather than calf blood flow, which is much more difficult to measure; and (3) the degree of fall in pressure and its recovery time can be used as indicators of the severity of the hemodynamic abnormality.

CLINICAL APPLICATIONS OF EXERCISE TESTING

There is little doubt that resting systolic ankle pressures and ankle-to-arm indices are usually sufficient to establish the diagnosis of occlusive disease and its severity. For example, it is known that

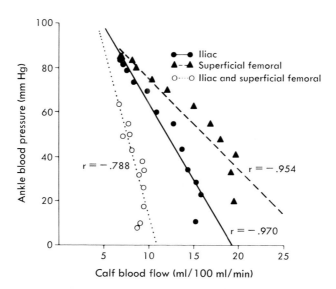

Fig. 55-5. Relationship between ankle blood pressure and calf blood flow in patients with varying degrees of arterial occlusion. (From Sumner, D.S., and Strandness, D.E., Jr.: Surgery 65:783, 1969. By permission of The C.V. Mosby Co., St. Louis.)

if the ankle-to-arm pressure index is greater than 0.5, single-segment disease is likely, whereas a lower pressure index is observed most commonly with multisegment disease. Furthermore, both the amount of improvement and the progression of disease can be documented in most cases by the resting pressures. It must therefore be determined what other factors justify the added testing.

Carter[4] has shown that patients with mild arterial occlusive disease and normal ankle systolic pressures at rest may have their lesions ''unmasked'' by exercise testing. In these cases, the collateral circulation provides adequate resting flow with little or no reduction in ankle pressure. However, since the capacity to increase flow is limited, pressure gradients may be accentuated when flow rates are increased by exercise. Thus exercise testing provides a method for detecting less severe degrees of arterial occlusive disease.

Patient testimony is highly subjective and is only sufficient for documenting the qualitative changes that have occurred. These pitfalls must be recognized by all clinicians who evaluate patients with claudication. The treadmill exercise test provides the following objective information: (1) the walking time at a constant work load; (2) the location, time of onset, and severity of pain; (3) the walking pattern as symptoms appear; (4) the critically important relationship between the ankle pressure response and walking time; (5) the degree of improvement following arterial surgery; and (6) the changes in the capacity of the collateral circulation.[17] In addition, walking on a treadmill simulates the activity that produces the patient's symptoms and determines the degree of disability under strictly controlled conditions. A variety of nonvascular factors may affect performance and can also be evaluated during treadmill exercise. These include musculoskeletal or cardiopulmonary disease, level of effort, patient motivation, and pain tolerance.

Walking on the treadmill is continued for 5 minutes or until symptoms force the patient to stop. The two most significant components of the response to exercise are: (1) the magnitude of the immediate drop in ankle systolic pressure; and (2) the time required for recovery to resting pressure. Changes in both of these parameters are proportional to the severity of arterial occlusive disease. Extended treadmill testing beyond the onset of claudication does not provide any additional diagnostic information.[14]

In general, the postexercise pressure changes in patients with arterial occlusive disease can be divided into three groups.[24] Ankle pressures that fall to low or unrecordable levels immediately after exercise and then return to resting values in 2 to 6 minutes suggest single-segment occlusive disease. Multisegment occlusive disease is usually associated with ankle pressures that remain low or unrecordable for up to 12 minutes. In patients with severe ischemia and rest pain, postexercise ankle pressures may be unrecordable for 15 minutes or more.

The obvious goal of any form of therapy is to improve the ability of the patient to walk. If the treadmill test is used in the same manner each time, the increase in walking time alone is one index of improvement. However, those not familiar with treadmill exercise must understand that walking time can be increased on the treadmill even when the disease is unchanged or occasionally is worse. Patients can accomplish this in several ways. First, they may grab the support bar of the treadmill, thus taking some of the weight off their legs. Second, they may walk with one leg slightly externally rotated to minimize the work required by the calf muscles. Both of these problems can be avoided by careful instruction and observation of the patient during walking. It is also possible to detect the patient who wants to give the impression of improvement by pushing himself beyond the point at which he would usually stop.

Differential diagnosis of leg pain

In recent years it has been recognized that there are patients with neurospinal disorders and degenerative joint disease who develop pain with walking that may mimic intermittent claudication. Although it is true that a carefully taken history will differentiate most of these patients, a normal treadmill test is further confirmation. A patient who develops leg pain on the basis of ischemia will *always* experience a drop in ankle pressure to an abnormal degree when exercised to the point of pain. If a normal exercise response is noted, some other cause for the symptoms must be sought.

Documenting results of treatment

It is important to recognize that the natural course of intermittent claudication is relatively benign, with only 1% to 2% of patients requiring amputation per year of follow-up.[2,10] Thus in the majority of patients, the degree of disability either remains stable or improves spontaneously. This improvement probably results from an increase in collateral flow occurring in response to the large pressure gradients produced in the leg during walking.[27] It is also possible that muscle cells are able to improve their function by undergoing some metabolic adaptation to chronic ischemia.[5] These observations provide the rationale for exercise therapy in patients with intermittent claudication.[12,16,17] Although an exercise program does increase the walking distance of many patients, the degree of clinical improvement that can be documented by treadmill testing is usually modest. The capacity of the collateral circulation to compensate for a major arterial occlusion is clearly limited, even during a maximal ischemic and hemodynamic stress.

The response of the ankle systolic pressure to treadmill exercise provides an ideal method for assessing the results of direct arterial surgery.[19,26] The patient who is improved by surgery but still not normal can easily have his condition documented. For example, a patient who walks on the treadmill for only 2 minutes before an operation and after the procedure doubles the walking time but still has the same abnormal hemodynamic response is definitely improved; the difference is that because of the increase in flow, it has simply taken longer to reach the same level of ischemia. Thus one of the great advantages of exercise testing is that it is possible to document the actual degree of improvement in physiologic terms (Fig. 55-6).

In patients with single-segment disease who undergo operation, the ankle pressure response to exercise should return to normal. If it does, then the exercise response indicates that all disease that is hemodynamically significant under the degree of stress applied has been corrected. When the response is improved but remains abnormal, there is either residual uncorrected disease or problems related to the reconstruction itself that continue to offer an abnormal amount of resistance to flow. Thus it is possible to use the response to exercise as an objective indicator of the degree of improvement, the extent of residual disease, and most importantly, the changes that may occur over time.[18,22,26]

Exercise testing has also been used to assess the results of pharmacologic therapy for occlusive arterial disease.[15,21] Clinical studies of vasodilator drugs have failed to show any objective benefit in patients with intermittent claudication or ischemic rest pain.[6,21] Furthermore, there is no evidence that vasodilators can increase flow through either collateral vessels or exercising muscle. Treadmill exercise testing was used to evaluate the rheologic agent pentoxifylline in a multicenter clinical trial.[15] Pentoxifylline inhibits platelet aggregation and reduces blood viscosity by altering the membrane flexibility of red blood cells. In this double-blind, placebo-controlled study the distance walked before onset of claudication increased in both the pentoxifylline and placebo groups; however, a significantly greater degree of improvement was ob-

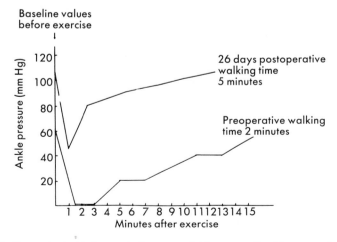

Fig. 55-6. Treadmill exercise test before and after successful femoropopliteal bypass graft with saphenous vein. Although walking time was increased to 5 minutes without symptoms, ankle pressure response remains abnormal. (From Strandness, D.E., Jr.: Surgery 59:325, 1966. By permission of The C.V. Mosby Co., St. Louis.)

served in the patients receiving pentoxifylline. The effect of this drug on the natural course of arterial occlusive disease is not known.

Exercise vs. reactive hyperemia testing

As previously mentioned, reactive hyperemia is an alternative to treadmill exercise for stressing the peripheral circulation. Inflating a pneumatic thigh cuff to suprasystolic pressure for 3 to 5 minutes will produce ischemia and vasodilation in the distal tissues. When cuff occlusion is released, the changes in ankle systolic pressure are qualitatively similar to those following exercise. However, there are several important differences between reactive hyperemia and postexercise hyperemia. Although normal subjects do not show a drop in ankle systolic pressure after treadmill exercise, a transient but definite drop is observed with reactive hyperemia.[9,11] This mean drop in ankle pressure is in the range of 17% to 34%. In patients with arterial occlusive disease, the response to reactive hyperemia is usually more prominent, and there is a good correlation between the maximal pressure drop with reactive hyperemia and the maximal pressure drop after treadmill exercise. There may be considerable overlap, however, in the ankle pressure response to reactive hyperemia among normal subjects and patients with arterial disease.[11] Furthermore, there is no correlation between reactive hyperemia and treadmill exercise with regard to the time for recovery to resting pressure. In general, patients with single-segment arterial disease show less than a 50% drop in ankle pressure with reactive hyperemia, whereas patients with multisegment arterial disease show a pressure drop greater than 50%.[9]

The reactive hyperemia test is simple and rapid to perform, and it is particularly useful for those patients who are unable to walk on the treadmill because of amputations or other physical disabilities. Although the use of cuff arterial occlusion has not been associated with thrombotic or embolic complications, it is not currently recommended for evaluation of patients after arterial reconstructions of the leg. The primary advantage of the treadmill exercise test is that it stresses the peripheral circulation in a physiologic manner and reproduces a patient's ischemic symptoms. Which type of stress test to use in a specific clinical situation will depend on individual patient characteristics, the time allotted for testing, and the equipment available.

CONCLUSIONS

One of the major limitations of treadmill exercise testing is the fact that when the patient has bilateral disease, the degree of disability is rarely the same for both limbs, so the exercise response will reflect functional impairment in the worse limb. Furthermore, it is not possible to predict on the basis of the test results alone the degree of disability that will remain when the flow to the most symptomatic limb has been corrected. For example, if a patient is stopped at 2 minutes with claudication involving one limb, correction of this side will increase the walking distance only to the extent that the other leg is involved.

The level of exercise used in most centers to evaluate peripheral arterial insufficiency involves a much lower work load than is commonly used to detect myocardial ischemia. There is increasing evidence that concomitant ECG monitoring may also provide useful data concerning the presence of coronary artery disease. Cutler et al.[7] in a series of 100 consecutive patients with peripheral arterial disease identified 46 patients who developed ventricular dysrhythmias, ischemia, or both, usually unassociated with symptoms. In this study, the unmasking of coexisting cardiac disease was a useful predictor of postoperative complications. There were 16 patients with abnormal ECGs who were subjected to direct arterial surgery; 6 of this group had postoperative myocardial infarctions, 2 of which were fatal. Carroll et al.[3] presented similar findings: of 46 consecutive patients, 23% demonstrated serious ECG abnormalities at this minimal work load.

We have not used concomitant ECG monitoring over the past 19 years. None of our subjects have died, but we have on occasion stopped the test because of angina or shortness of breath. Thus in terms of patient protection, ECG monitoring has not been necessary. Nonetheless, the studies just cited clearly indicate that if such surveillance is used, a significant number of patients with myocardial ischemia will be discovered. As noted in the series by Cutler et al.,[7] the tests also were useful in predicting the potential for postoperative myocardial infarction.

It is our feeling that all patients who are being considered for major arterial reconstructions should have a comprehensive cardiology evaluation. It is not clear that concomitant ECG monitoring would in fact modify our approach, since these patients are routinely evaluated by a cardiologist. Another factor to consider is the medico-legal issue of whether exercise testing at this low work load requires simultaneous ECG monitoring as the standard of practice. If this requirement is added to the usual testing for peripheral arterial disease, the procedure would have to be monitored by a physician familiar with those ECG changes associated with myocardial ischemia. Avoiding the need for ECG monitoring is one of the potential advantages of reactive hyperemia testing.

REFERENCES

1. Allwood, M.J., and Burry, H.S.: The effect of local temperature of blood flow in the human foot, J. Physiol. (Lond.) 124:345, 1954.
2. Boyd, A.M.: The natural course of arteriosclerosis of the lower extremities, Proc. R. Soc. Med. 55:591, 1962.
3. Carroll, R., et al.: Cardiac arrhythmias associated with standard 5-minute treadmill claudication testing, Proceedings of the Symposium on Noninvasive Diagnostic Techniques in Vascular Disease, San Diego, Sept. 10-14, 1979, University of California at San Diego, p. 69.
4. Carter, S.A.: Response to ankle systolic pressure to leg exercise in mild or questionable arterial disease, N. Engl. J. Med. 287:578, 1972.
5. Clyne, C.A.C., et al.: Ultrastructural and capillary adaption of gastrocnemius muscle to occlusive vascular disease, Surgery 92:434, 1982.
6. Coffman, J.D.: Vasodilator drugs in peripheral vascular disease, N. Engl. J. Med. 300:713, 1979.
7. Cutler, B.S., et al.: Assessment of operative risk with electrocardiographic exercise testing in patients with peripheral arterial disease, Am. J. Surg. 137:484, 1979.
8. Grimby, G., Haggendac, E., and Saltin, B.: Local xenon-133 clearance from the quadriceps muscle during exercise in man, J. Appl. Physiol. 22:305, 1967.
9. Hummell, B.W., et al.: Reactive hyperemia vs. treadmill exercise testing in arterial disease, Arch. Surg. 113:95, 1978.
10. Imparato, A.M., et al.: Intermittent claudication—its natural course, Surgery 78:795, 1975.
11. Keagy, B.A., et al.: Comparison of reactive hyperemia and treadmill tests in the evaluation of peripheral vascular disease, Am. J. Surg. 142:158, 1981.
12. Larsen, O.A., and Lassen, N.A.: Effect of daily muscular exercise on patients with intermittent claudication, Lancet 2:1093, 1966.
13. Lassen, N.A., and Kampp, M.: Calf muscle blood flow during walking studied by the Xe 133 method in normals and in patients with intermittent claudication, Scand. J. Clin. Lab. Invest. 17:447, 1965.
14. Mahler, D.K., et al.: Treadmill testing in peripheral arterial disease—what can be learned from extended testing? Bruit 6:21, 1982.
15. Porter, J.M., et al.: Pentoxifylline efficacy in the treatment of intermittent claudication—multicenter controlled double-blind trial with objective assessment of chronic occlusive arterial disease patients, Am. Heart. J. 104:66, 1982.
16. Skinner, J.S., and Strandness, D.E. Jr.: Exercise and intermittent claudication. I. Effect of repetition and intensity of exercise, Circulation 36:15, 1967.
17. Skinner, J.S., and Strandness, D.E., Jr.: Exercise and intermittent claudication. II. Effect of physical training, Circulation 36:23, 1967.
18. Stahler, C., and Strandness, D.E., Jr.: Ankle blood pressure response to graded treadmill exercise, Angiology 18:237, 1967.
19. Strandness, D.E., Jr.: Abnormal exercise responses after successful reconstructive arterial surgery, Surgery 59:325, 1966.
20. Strandness, D.E., Jr.: Exercise testing in the evaluation of patients undergoing direct arterial surgery, J. Cardiovasc. Surg. 11:192, 1970.
21. Strandness, D.E., Jr.: Ineffectiveness of isoxsuprine on intermittent claudication, JAMA 213:86, 1970.
22. Strandness, D.E., Jr., and Bell, J.W.: Peripheral vascular disease: diagnosis and objective evaluation using a mercury strain gauge, Ann. Surg. 161(suppl):1, 1965.
23. Strandness, D.E., Jr., and Sumner, D.S.: Hemodynamics for surgeons, New York, 1975, Grune and Stratton Inc.
24. Sumner, D.S., and Strandness, D.E., Jr.: The relationship between calf blood flow and ankle blood pressure in patients with intermittent claudication, Surgery 65:763, 1969.
25. Sumner, D.S., and Strandness, D.E. Jr.: The effect of exercise on resistance to blood flow in limbs with an occluded superficial femoral artery, Vasc. Surg. 4:229, 1970.
26. Sumner, D.S., and Strandness, D.E., Jr.: Hemodynamic studies before and after extended bypass grafts to the tibial and peroneal arteries, Surgery 86:442, 1979.
27. Winblad, J.N., et al.: Etiologic mechanisms in the development of collateral circulation, Surgery 45:105, 1959.
28. Yao, J.S.T.: Hemodynamic studies in peripheral arterial disease, Br. J. Surg. 57:761, 1970.

CHAPTER 56

Postocclusive reactive hyperemia in the testing of the peripheral arterial system: pressure, velocity, and pulse reappearance time

ARNOST FRONEK and EUGENE F. BERNSTEIN

The importance of pressure and velocity determinations in the diagnosis of peripheral arterial occlusive disease (PAOD) was discussed in Chapters 49 and 51 to 53. We are fully aware of the limitations of these techniques under resting conditions, especially in cases of borderline results. A logical step to increase the sensitivity of these tests is to stress the peripheral circulation in the hope that an increased blood flow induced by standardized local ischemia will (1) help to quantitate the vasodilatory response and (2) exaggerate the pressure drop across the stenotic lesion. Such stress testing is particularly important in those cases in which resting pressure and velocity results do not establish the diagnosis of PAOD unequivocally.

As Strandness has pointed out (Chapter 55), exercise has been one of the most widely used types of stress for this purpose because it is so clearly related to intermittent claudication. There are, however, several circumstances that limit the application of this otherwise highly sensitive and specific diagnostic technique: (1) the activity of the exercising subject precludes using some of the existing continuous monitoring techniques (velocity, pulse volume, etc.); (2) varying pain thresholds in different patients[20,40] may lower the standardization value of the test; (3) although the risk is small, a large percentage of patients with PAOD suffer also from coronary disease (in a clinical or subclinical form) and therefore ECG monitoring throughout the test may be advisable[9,39]; (4) there are a number of patients who are unable to undergo treadmill exercise (amputees, arthritics, patients with severe ischemia of the contralateral limb, cardiopulmonary limitation, neurologic disorders, etc.); and (5)

the expense and bulkiness of the treadmill may limit its application, especially if bedside use is considered. For all of these reasons postocclusive reactive hyperemia (PORH) has been considered by a number of investigators as an alternative stress procedure to increase the sensitivity and specificity of their respective tests.

Blood flow in the examined limb has been studied using venous occlusion plethysmography either with water or air as the communicating medium or with the mercury-in-rubber (Whitney) gauge.* The introduction of a simple electric calibration[8,22] may lead to wider use of the technique. Despite the well-established reliability of this approach, it has not found wide acceptance for routine clinical diagnostic studies, probably since (1) venous occlusion must be performed intermittently, so no continuous readout is possible and therefore the detection of the peak response may be missed, and (2) the evaluation is rather time-consuming, since the volume increase must be calculated separately for each run (although this last step can be automated).[16]

There are, however, three additional ways to use the transient increase in blood flow induced by temporary inflow compression: (1) the PORH ankle pressure response, (2) the ultrasonically monitored PORH flow velocity response, and (3) the peripherally monitored pulse reappearance time (PRT).

PORH ANKLE PRESSURE RESPONSE

Dornhorst and Sharpey-Schafer[14] described the significance of PORH as a standardized form of stress with ankle pressure measurements, and their

*References 1, 2, 4-6, 13, 16, 21, 24, 26, 29, 32-35, 38, 41.

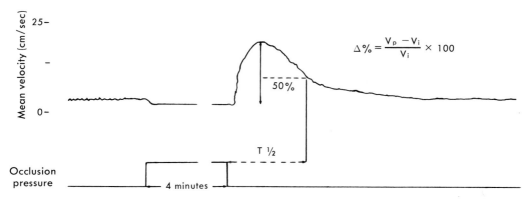

Fig. 56-1. Normal PORH femoral velocity response. Upper tracing is mean femoral artery flow velocity; lower tracing is occlusion pressure.

results were confirmed by a number of additional investigators.[11,25,31] Johnson[25] observed full pressure recovery in normal subjects within 1 minute, whereas patients with various degrees of arterial occlusive disease showed a significant delay in pressure recovery, with the pressure drop and delay related to the severity of the disease.

Several groups recently compared the efficiency of PORH with that of different exercise tests[3,23,39] and concluded that the drop in blood pressure is very similar when the 30-second PORH pressure response is compared with the 1-minute treadmill exercise response. The ankle flexion stress,[10] although very convenient and simple, led to a significantly smaller drop than the treadmill and PORH stress tests.[3,39]

ULTRASONOGRAPHICALLY MONITORED PORH VELOCITY RESPONSE

The PORH response following a transient flow obstruction can be recorded ultrasonographically.[18] To perform the procedure, the patient is placed in the supine position, and a standard pressure cuff is placed *below* the knee. (Suprasystolic inflation of a cuff placed *above* the knee may sometimes be unpleasant and may cause artifacts by exerting a pull on the ultrasonic probe.) A transcutaneous ultrasonic velocity meter is used, and the probe is placed at the level of the femoral artery with the tip aimed cephalad after the suitable angle and position (maximum output) have been identified. The probe is then held in position by a self-locking magnetic clamp.* A resisitance-capacitance filter with a time constant of 1 second may be added to

*Flex-O-Post Indicator Holder with Magnetic Base, Starrett Co., Athol, Mass.

the output stage of the original instrument (if not already built in) to obtain the mean flow velocity.

After a steady-state period has been reached, the cuff is inflated to the suprasystolic pressure. After 4 minutes the cuff is suddenly deflated, and the PORH response is continuously recorded until the velocity value returns to the control level. The response is evaluated in the following two ways (Fig. 56-1):

1. The percentage increase:

$$\frac{(\text{Peak velocity} - \text{Initial velocity})}{\text{Initial velocity}} \times 100$$

2. The recovery half-time ($T_{1/2}$), the time for the mean velocity to return to 50% of its peak response.

Control studies performed on 50 lower extremities in 25 healthy subjects helped establish the normal response: a 226% increase in femoral artery flow velocity (± 16.2 SEM) above the preocclusion value and a 25-second (± 1.5 SEM) $T_{1/2}$.

In contrast, patients with angiographically documented PAOD in the aortoiliac or femoropopliteal segments had a significantly lower peak response (55% $\pm$ 6.2 SEM) and a significantly longer recovery half-time (47.1 seconds $\pm$ 1.5 SEM). To date, more than 3000 patients have been studied with this technique, and for 400 of them, careful correlations have been made with their angiographic patterns. Based on this experience, we consider a peak velocity response of less than an 80% increase over control mean velocity and a $T_{1/2}$ longer than 35 seconds to be indicative of a pathologic condition. Fig. 56-2 shows a PORH velocity response before and after successful vascular reconstruction, as also recently reported by Myhre.[30]

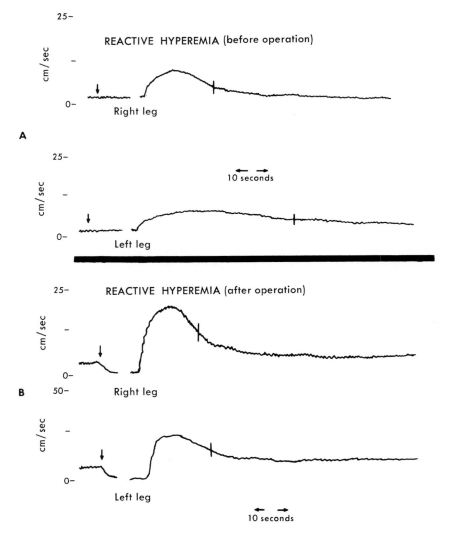

Fig. 56-2. PORH femoral artery velocity response. **A,** Right and left leg before operation. **B,** Right and left leg after operation.

PERIPHERALLY MONITORED PRT[17]

The technique of monitoring the PRT is based on clinical experience with the postexercise[12] disappearance of pedal pulses[15,27] and the significant decrease in distal arterial blood pressure seen in the presence of PAOD.[7,36,37] Since we established a qualitative similarity between the PORH and the postexercise reactive hyperemia response,[28] we extended the PORH test to include measuring the change in toe pulse volume induced by a 4-minute calf occlusion. The toe pulse volume can be recorded with a variety of suitable transducers. In the original study[17] a closed-loop mercury-in-rubber (Whitney) gauge was connected to a low-resistance bridge amplifier* with the output fed into an AC amplifier (band width 1 to 10 Hz) and recorded simultaneously with the PORH femoral arterial velocity response. After the 4-minute occlusion the cuff pressure was suddenly released, and the reappearance of the toe pulse was continuously recorded (Fig. 56-3).

Control values were established in 22 healthy subjects (44 limbs), in whom the average time for the toe pulse volume to return to 50% of its control amplitude (PRT/2) was 3.4 seconds ± 0.8 SEM.

*Model 270 plethysmograph, Parks Electronics, Beaverton, Ore., or SPG-16 Strain Gauge Plethysmograph, Medsonics, Mountain View, Calif., or EC-4 Plethysmograph, Hokanson, Issaquah, Wash.

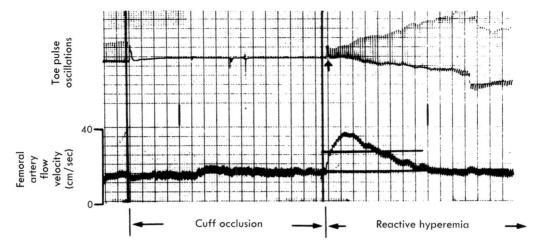

Fig. 56-3. Combined normal PORH femoral artery velocity and PRT/2 response.

Fig. 56-3 depicts a normal toe pulse reappearance time response recorded simultaneously with the ultrasonographically monitored PORH femoral artery velocity response. The very first volume pulse after cuff release is already higher than 50% of the preocclusion control amplitude. In addition, a typical overshoot response is demonstrated.

The PRT/2 has been correlated with angiographically documented disease in 58 patients (110 limbs). The average PRT/2 in patients with multilevel occlusive disease was 71.2 seconds (± 5.5 SEM), whereas the average PRT/2 in three other groups (isolated aortoiliac, femoropopliteal, and trifurcation occlusion) was around 25 seconds. Based on our overall experience with this technique, we consider a PRT/2 longer than 6 seconds to indicate a pathologic condition. These results were recently confirmed by Gutierrez and Gage[19] using a photoplethysmographic sensor.

DIAGNOSTIC VALUE OF THE PORH ANKLE PRESSURE, VELOCITY, AND PRT/2 RESPONSE

The three tests are closely related and represent three different indices of a common denominator—the hemodynamic response to transient tissue ischemia. Each test, however, documents a different aspect of the response.

The PORH ankle pressure and PRT/2 response are closest as to their genesis. As depicted schematically in Fig. 56-4, the peak PORH response is associated with a transient pressure drop of 80 mm Hg compared to a previous resting pressure drop of only 20 mm Hg. This increased pressure drop was induced by the transient increase in blood flow (from 100 to 400 ml/min) and therefore

$$\Delta P = \underset{R}{0.2} \times \underset{F}{400} = 80 \text{ mm Hg}$$

where

ΔP = Pressure drop across the stenosis
R = Resistance (expressed in relative units)
F = Flow at peak PORH response

With a declining flow response, the pressure drop decreases proportionally while the pressure increases by the same amount.

The same mechanism is also responsible for the PRT/2 response, but only the oscillatory component is recorded. The advantage of the PRT/2, however, is the ability to continuously monitor the pulse volume changes. It can be assumed that the PRT/2 value represents an index of overall perfusion, especially when monitored at the toe. Studies currently under way will demonstrate whether the two techniques (PORH ankle pressure and PRT/2 monitoring) yield results of comparable importance.

In contrast to these two methods, PORH velocity monitoring predominantly reflects the response at the femoral artery level and is highly sensitive to stenoses in the superficial femoral artery. The combination of these tests therefore has substantial advantage. For instance, a reduced PORH velocity response combined with a normal PRT/2 response suggests the presence of significant femoral artery occlusive disease with a well-developed collateral circulation. Similarly, in a patient who has under-

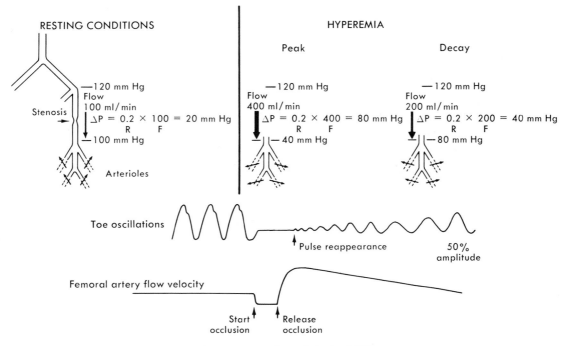

RESTING CONDITIONS

Stenosis

—120 mm Hg
Flow
100 ml/min
$\Delta P = 0.2 \times 100 = 20$ mm Hg
R   F
—100 mm Hg

Arterioles

HYPEREMIA

Peak

—120 mm Hg
Flow
400 ml/min
$\Delta P = 0.2 \times 400 = 80$ mm Hg
R   F
—40 mm Hg

Decay

—120 mm Hg
Flow
200 ml/min
$\Delta P = 0.2 \times 200 = 40$ mm Hg
R   F
—80 mm Hg

Toe oscillations

Pulse reappearance

50%
amplitude

Femoral artery flow velocity

Start
occlusion

Release
occlusion

Fig. 56-4. Hemodynamic basis of PRT.

gone a bypass operation without improvement of his femoral artery velocity PORH response, but with significant improvement of the PRT/2, benefit from the operation is based on an increase in the overall perfusion of the limb. In such cases the low PORH velocity response can be attributed to the topography of the bypassing vessel, or prosthesis, or to a local increase in vessel diameter at the site of suture, or from endarterectomy if the velocity probe incidentally monitored this site. Fig. 56-5 depicts changes in PORH and PRT/2 before and after vascular reconstruction.

All three techniques (PORH ankle pressure, PORH velocity response, and PRT/2) are useful adjunct diagnostic procedures, especially in cases when other noninvasive laboratory tests are equivocal. Depression and delay of PORH velocity response, as well as delay in PRT/2 response, indicate the presence of femoral artery occlusive disease and impairment of overall leg blood supply, respectively. Dissociation of these results, low PORH and normal PRT/2, generally indicates good collateral circulation, reducing the sequelae of arterial stenosis. On the other hand, normal segmental pressures (not only ankle pressures) in the presence of borderline symptomatology represent a strong indication to perform a stress test measuring the PORH response.

POSTEXERCISE VS. POSTOCCLUSIVE REACTIVE HYPEREMIA STRESS
Comparison of diagnostic value

As described in the preceding paragraphs and in Chapter 55, both methods have advantages and disadvantages that are complex. In view of currently available information and experience, the following conclusions can be drawn:

1. The postexercise reactive hyperemia (PERH) induces the most profound hemodynamic changes, reflected mainly in pressure drop and recovery time.

2. There are some limitations specific for the exercise test, especially when the treadmill is used. As mentioned earlier, constant ECG monitoring may be advisable in view of frequent concomitant coronary disease.[9,39] There are cases of limited mobility (amputees, or other cases of skeletomuscular or neurologic origin) that may distort the results because of difficulty in performing the study.

3. On the other hand, the PORH response leads to smaller hemodynamic changes, but these are standardized and applicable to every patient. The disadvantage of the shorter recovery time may be outweighed by the ease of recording the earliest poststress hemodynamic changes because the patient remains in the

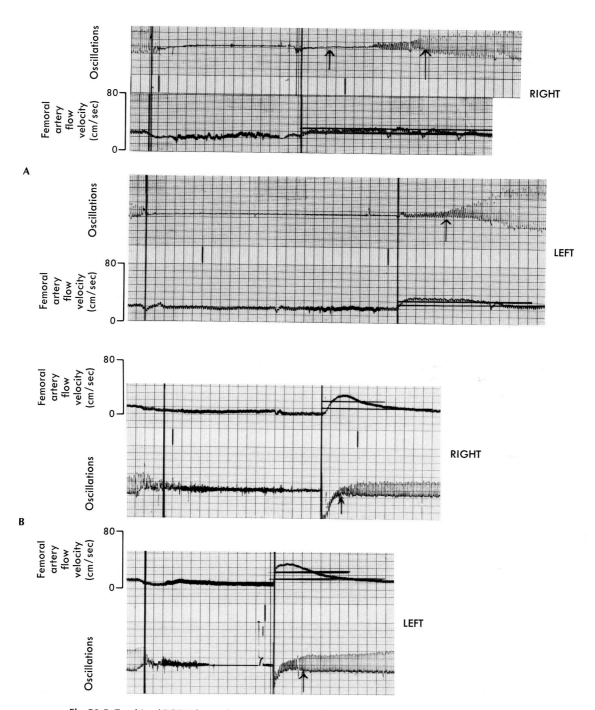

Fig. 56-5. Combined PORH femoral artery velocity and PRT/2 response. *A,* Before vascular reconstruction. First arrow is reappearance of the first pulse; second arrow is reappearance of 50% amplitude. *B,* After vascular reconstruction.

supine position and no time is lost in readjusting the instrumentation.

More investigations and experience with different types of stressors are needed for a definitive answer. The ideal dynamic test will have to be highly sensitive and specific and, at the same time, have a negligible effect on the overall cardiovascular system and be applicable to every patient, disregarding concomitant cardiopulmonary, neurologic, or musculoskeletal handicaps.

SUMMARY

Additional noninvasive diagnostic tests are desirable in cases with equivocal results based on resting peripheral circulatory hemodynamics. PORH measurement has some advantages when compared with that of PERH, since it permits continuous monitoring of the femoral artery velocity and the pulse volume response. It shows practically the same pressure drop as is seen during the postexercise response, although of shorter duration. The simplicity, absence of risk to the patient, and very good overall patient acceptance represent additional favorable factors.

Generally, a 4-minute period of ischemia is normally followed (1) by a return of ankle blood pressure to the control value within 60 seconds, (2) by an increase in femoral artery velocity by at least 100% above control levels, and (3) by a PRT/2 of 6 seconds or less. Conversely, a delayed return of ankle blood pressure of more than 120 seconds, an increase in femoral artery flow velocity less than 80% above control, and a delay of PRT/2 longer than 10 seconds indicate the presence of hemodynamically significant obstruction of the arterial system in the lower extremity.

Diagnostic implications of the described tests are discussed in light of their common hemodynamic basis: (1) a decrease in PORH velocity response with a normal PRT/2 response suggests the presence of significant femoral artery occlusive disease with a well-developed collateral circulation, (2) a decrease in PORH velocity response combined with a delayed PRT/2 response indicates the presence of femoral artery occlusive disease with an inadequate collateral circulation, and (3) a borderline segmental pressure can be conveniently clarified by repeating the pressure measurement during the PORH response.

REFERENCES

1. Abramson, D.J.: Circulation in the extremities, New York, 1967, Academic Press, Inc.
2. Abramson, D.J., Katzenstein, K.H., and Ferris, E.G., Jr.: Observations on reactive hyperaemia in various portions of the extremities, Am. J. Surg. 22:329, 1941.
3. Baker, J.D.: Post stress Doppler ankle pressures, Arch. Surg. 113:1171, 1978.
4. Bentley, T.H.: Muscle blood flow in patients with arteriosclerosis obliterans, Am. J. Surg. 96:193, 1958.
5. Bollinger, A.: Bedeutung der Venenverschlussplethysmographie in der angiologischen Diagnostik, Schweiz. Med. Wochenschr. 95:1357, 1969.
6. Bollinger, A.: Durchblutungsmessungen in der klinischen Angiologie, Bern, Switzerland, 1969, Hans Huber Medical Publisher.
7. Bollinger, A., et al.: Measurement of systolic ankle blood pressure with Doppler ultrasound at rest and after exercise in patients with leg artery occlusions, Scand. J. Clin. Lab. Invest. 31(suppl. 128):123, 1973.
8. Brakkee, A.J., and Vendrik, A.J.: Strain gauge plethysmography: theoretical and practical notes on a new design, J. Appl. Physiol. 21:701, 1966.
9. Carroll, R., et al.: Cardiac arrhythmias associated with standard 5-minute treadmill claudication testing, Paper presented at the Symposium on Noninvasive Diagnostic Techniques in Vascular Disease, San Diego, Sept. 10-14, 1979.
10. Carter, S.A.: Response of ankle systolic pressure to leg exercise in mild or questionable arterial disease, N. Engl. J. Med. 287:578, 1972.
11. Delius, W.: Hämodynamische Untersuchungen über den systolischen Blutdruck und die arterielle Durchblutung distal von arteriellen Gefässeverschlussen an den unteren Extremitäten, Z. Kreis. 58:319, 1969.
12. DeWeese, J.A.: Pedal pulses disappearing with exercise: a test for intermittent claudication, N. Engl. J. Med. 262:1214, 1960.
13. Dohn, K.: On clinical use of venous occlusion plethysmography of calf. II. Results in patients with arterial disease, Acta Med. Scand. 130:61, 1965.
14. Dornhorst, A.C., and Sharpey-Schafer, E.P.: Collateral resistance in limbs with arterial obstruction: spontaneous changes and effects of sympathectomy, Clin. Sci. 10:371, 1951.
15. Edwards, E.A., Cohen, N.R., and Kaplan, M.M.: Effect of exercise on peripheral pulses, N. Engl. J. Med. 160:738, 1959.
16. Ehringer, H.: Die reaktive Hyperämie nach arterieller Sperre. In Bollinger, A., and Brunner, U., editors: Messmethoden bei arteriellen Durchblutungsstorungen, Bern, Switzerland, 1971, Hans Huber Medical Publisher.
17. Fronek, A., Coel, M., and Bernstein, E.F.: The pulse-reappearance time: an index of over-all blood flow impairment in the ischemic extremity, Surgery 81:376, 1977.
18. Fronek, A., et al.: Ultrasonographically monitored postocclusive reactive hyperemia in the diagnosis of peripheral arterial occlusive disease, Circulation 43:149, 1973.
19. Gutierrez, J.Z., and Gage, A.A.: Toe pulse study (using the photopulse photoplethysmograph) in the diagnosis and evaluation of the severity of ischemic arterial disease of the lower extremities, Paper presented at Symposium on Noninvasive Diagnostic Techniques in Vascular Disease, San Diego, Sept. 10-14, 1979.
20. Hillestad, L.K.: The peripheral blood flow in intermittent claudication. IV. The significance of the claudication distance, Acta Med. Scand. 173:467, 1963.
21. Hillestad, L.K.: The peripheral blood flow in intermittent claudication. V. Plethysmographic studies, Acta Med. Scand. 174:23, 1963.

22. Hokanson, D.E., Sumner, D.S., and Strandness, D.E., Jr.: An electrically calibrated plethysmograph for direct measurement of limb blood flow, IEEE Trans. Biomed. Eng. 22:25, 1975.

23. Hummel, B.W., et al.: Reactive hyperemia vs. treadmill exercise testing in arterial disease, Arch. Surg. 113:95, 1978.

24. Hyman, C., and Winsor, T.: Blood flow redistribution in the human extremity, Am. J. Cardiol. 4:566, 1959.

25. Johnson, W.C.: Doppler ankle pressure and reactive hyperemia in the diagnosis of arterial insufficiency, J. Surg. Res. 18:177, 1975.

26. Lewis, T., and Grant, R.: Observations upon reactive hyperemia in man, Heart 12:73, 1925.

27. Mackereth, M., and Lennihan, R.: Ultrasound as an aid in the diagnosis and management of intermittent claudication, Angiology 21:704, 1970.

28. Mahler, F., et al.: Postocclusion and postexercise flow velocity and ankle pressures in normals and marathon runners, Angiology 27:721, 1976.

29. Myers, K.: The investigation of peripheral arterial disease by strain gauge plethysmography, Angiology 15:293, 1964.

30. Myhre, H.O.: Reactive hyperemia of the human lower limb. Measurement of postischaemic blood flow velocity in controls and in patients with lower limb artherosclerosis, VASA 2:145, 1975.

31. Myhre, H.O.: Reactive hyperemia of the human lower limb. A comparison between systolic pressure at the ankle after timed circulatory arrest and after exercise in controls and in patients with arthersclerosis, VASA 4:227, 1975.

32. Siggaard-Anderson, J.: Obliterative vascular disease, classification by means of the Dohn plethysmograph, Acta Chir. Scand. 130:190, 1965.

33. Snell, E.S., Eastcott, H.H., and Hamilton, M.: Circulation in lower limb before and after reconstruction of obstructed main artery, Lancet 1:242, 1960.

34. Storen, G.: Post-ischemic calf volume recording in functional evaluation of patients with intermittent claudication, Scand. J. Clin. Lab. Invest. 23:339, 1969.

35. Strandell, T., and Wahren, J.: Circulation in the calf at rest, after arterial occlusion, and after exercise in normal subjects and in patients with intermittent claudication, Acta Med. Scand. 173:99, 1963.

36. Strandness, D.E., Jr., and Bell, J.W.: An evaluation of the hemodynamic response of the claudicating extremity to exercise, Surg. Gyn. Obstet. 119:1237, 1964.

37. Sumner, D.S., and Strandness, D.E., Jr.: The relationship between calf blood flow and ankle blood pressure in patients with intermittent claudication, Surgery 65:763, 1971.

38. Whitney, R.J.: The measurement of volume changes in human limbs, J. Physiol. (Lond.) 121:1, 1953.

39. Wilbur, B.G., and Olcott, C.: A comparison of three modes of stress on Doppler ankle pressures. In Diethrich, E.B., editor: Noninvasive Cardiovascular Diagnosis, Baltimore, 1977, University Park Press.

40. Yao, S.T., et al.: A comparative study of strain-gauge plethysmography and Doppler ultrasound in the assessment of occlusive arterial disease of the lower extremities, Surgery 71:4, 1972.

41. Zelis, R., et al.: Effects of hyperlipoproteinemias and their treatment of the peripheral circulation, J. Clin. Invest. 49:1007, 1970.

CHAPTER 57

Applications of isotope technology to the clinical study of arterial disease

ANDREW N. NICOLAIDES and NICOS S. ANGELIDES

MEASUREMENTS AT REST

The principles and clinical applications of measurement of blood flow from the clearance of an isotope injected in a tissue have been described in Chapter 19. A new application has been the simultaneous measurement of changes in blood flow in the muscles of the thigh and calf using ^{99m}Tc.[1,2,3] This has led (1) to better understanding of the hemodynamics of the circulation in the lower limb and (2) to the development of a method of grading the degree of functional stenosis. The latter is particularly useful in limbs with both aortoiliac and superficial femoral stenoses.

Method

^{99m}Tc muscle clearance. A preparation of 40 μCi of ^{99m}Tc in 0.2 ml of saline solution is injected into the thickest part of the gastrocnemius and quadriceps muscles. The probes of two scintillation counters are placed on the skin at the site of injection. The position is marked to enable accurate replacement of the probes after exercise. Output from the detectors is recorded continuously as exponential curves by a two-channel pen recorder.

All subjects rest for 20 minutes before starting the test. Clearance curves are obtained for 10 minutes at rest; the patients then walk on a horizontal treadmill at 4.5 km per hour for 3 minutes or until they are forced to stop by claudication, following which, clearance curves are recorded for 20 minutes. At any time the percentage clearance per minute (T), which is proportional to muscle blood flow, can be obtained from the equation

$$T = \frac{f(t) - f(t + 1)}{f(t) + f(t + 1)} \times 200 \qquad (1)$$

where f(t) is the radioactivity measured at time t and f(t + 1) is the radioactivity measured 1 minute

later. The radioactivity cleared during 1 minute is f(t) − f(t + 1). The mean radioactivity during the same minute is [f(t) + f(t + 1)]/2, and therefore the percentage radioactivity cleared per minute is given by equation 1.

T is calculated at minute intervals and is plotted against time (Fig. 57-1).

Hyperemic index. The total excess of T, which is proportional to the total excess of blood, is calculated from the area A, representing the postexercise hyperemia (Fig. 57-1). This area can be calculated by measuring the height of the curve at minute intervals from the vertical line representing the end of exercise (Fig. 57-1) and taking the mean. The hyperemic index (HI), which represents time, was defined as the ratio of the total excess of T (area A) over the maximum value of T (height M) during the postexercise period (Fig. 57-1).

The two hyperemic indices obtained (one from the thigh and one from the calf) from the limbs studied are plotted against each other in a form of bivariate analysis.

Results

A number of clinical studies have been undertaken involving a total of 30 normal limbs from healthy volunteers and 216 limbs from patients with intermittent claudication who were also investigated with translumbar aortography. Characteristic patterns of changes in muscle blood flow have been found, depending on the site and severity of lesions.

Normal limbs. The changes of mean T in the thigh and calf of 30 normal limbs are shown in Fig. 57-2. Thigh and calf T are stable and comparable at rest. They show a fivefold increase immediately after exercise and both return to the

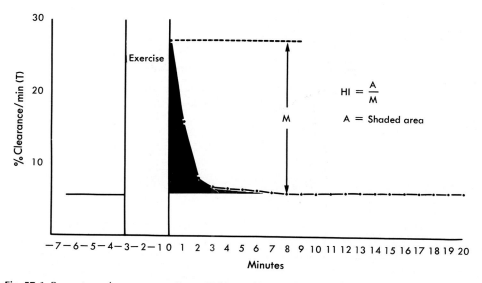

Fig. 57-1. Percentage clearance per minute (T) from calf of normal limb before and after exercise plotted against time. Method of calculation of hyperemic index (HI) is illustrated. (From Angelides, N., et al.: Br. J. Surg. 65:204, 1979.)

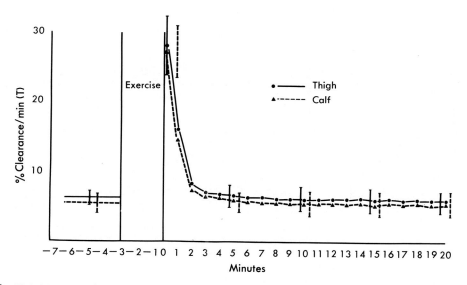

Fig. 57-2. Mean T and standard deviation in group of 30 normal limbs. (From Angelides, N., et al.: Br. J. Surg. 65:204, 1979.)

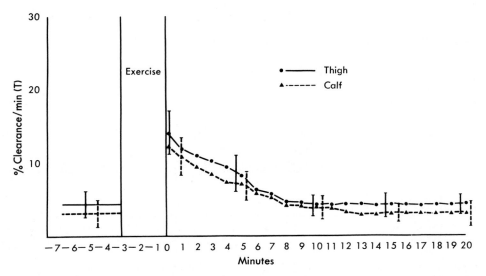

Fig. 57-3. Mean T and standard deviation in group of 35 limbs with iliac occlusion. (From Angelides, N., et al.: Br. J. Surg. 65:204, 1979.)

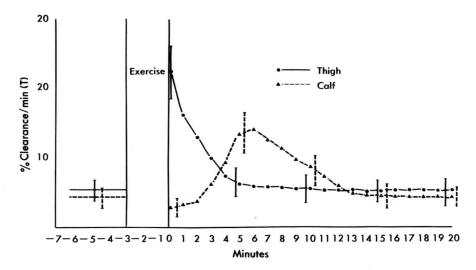

Fig. 57-4. Mean T and standard deviation in group of 46 limbs with superficial femoral artery occlusion. (From Angelides, N., et al.: Br. J. Surg. 65:204, 1979.)

preexercise level within 3 minutes. The maximum increase in T is observed during the first postexercise minute.

Limbs with aortoiliac occlusion. In limbs with aortoiliac occlusion (Fig. 57-3) the pattern is much the same, but the degree of hyperemia is less and the time to return to resting levels is prolonged (9 to 12 minutes). This means the flow changes are the same as in normal limbs, but flow is "throttled" by the occlusion, and blood flow via the collateral circulation is insufficient to permit normal postexercise hyperemia.

Limbs with femoropopliteal occlusion. In limbs with femoropopliteal occlusion (Fig. 57-4), there are differences between the pattern of clearance in the thigh and in the calf: the former behaves normally, while the latter shows a slightly diminished mean T immediately after exercise, rising to a peak at 6 minutes and thereafter returning to normal in a further 10 minutes. The only conceivable explanation of the delayed hyperemia in the calf is that because of the maximum vasodilation, there is too much blood shunted from the collateral circulation to the veins of the thigh, so that relatively little blood is available to the calf immediately after exercise. As the hyperemia in the thigh decreases, there is an increase in the pressure in the proximal part of the collateral circulation, thus restoring the pressure gradient across the collateral vessels. This then permits hyperemia in the calf where maximum dilation is still present.

Limbs with combined aortoiliac and femoropopliteal occlusions. In limbs with combined aortoiliac and femoropopliteal occlusions (Fig. 57-5), the thigh behaves much as in the group with aortoiliac occlusion (Fig. 57-3), but the calf shows near zero clearance immediately after exercise, rising to a peak at 10 minutes and then returning to normal in a further 10 minutes. These changes can be explained along lines similar to those used in the group of patients with superficial femoral occlusion only. The aortoiliac lesion is responsible for an aortofemoral gradient, which becomes even more pronounced immediately after exercise, producing a lower pressure in the profunda artery, a more prolonged reactive hyperemia in the thigh, and a more delayed onset of calf hyperemia.

Limbs with single or double stenoses. Limbs with a single iliac or superficial femoral stenosis show patterns that are intermediate between those described for normal limbs and those described for limbs with the corresponding single occlusions. Limbs with combined aortoiliac and femoropopliteal stenoses also show intermediate patterns depending on the severity of the lesions.

Plotting the hyperemic index of the calf against the hyperemic index of the thigh, the points representing limbs with similar lesions defined characteristic areas (Fig. 57-6). The results are reproducible so that these areas can be of diagnostic value (see key of areas *a-h* and *p-s* in Fig. 57-6).

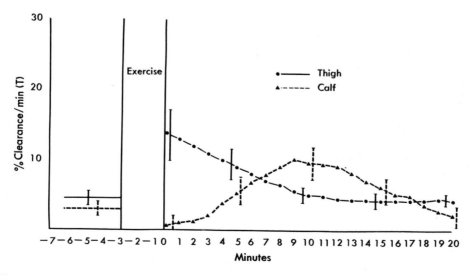

Fig. 57-5. Mean T and standard deviation in group of 25 limbs with combined aortoiliac and femoropopliteal lesions. (From Angelides, N., et al.: Br. J. Surg. 65:204, 1979.)

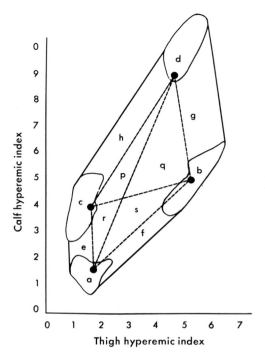

Fig. 57-6. Diagnostic chart based on calf and thigh hyperemic indices. *a*, Normal arterial tree; *b*, aortoiliac occlusion only; *c*, femoropopliteal occlusion only; *d*, aortoiliac and femoropopliteal occlusion; *e*, superficial femoral or popliteal stenosis only; *f*, aortoiliac stenosis only; *g*, aortoiliac occlusion and superficial femoral steonosis; *h*, superficial femoral occlusion and aortoiliac stenosis; *p*, aortoiliac and superficial femoral stenosis—SF stenosis > 70% > AI stenosis; *q*, aortoiliac and superficial femoral stenosis—AI stenosis > SF stenosis; *r*, aortoiliac and superficial femoral stenosis—AI stenosis < SF stenosis < 70%; *s*, aortoiliac and superficial femoral stenosis—SF stenosis < AI stenosis < 70%. (From Angelides, N., et al.: Br. J. Surg. 65:204, 1979.)

MEASUREMENTS DURING EXERCISE

The measurements in the studies just reported were made before and after exercise with the patient lying horizontal because of the heavy probes of the scintillation counters. The availability of lighter probes (80 g each) made measurements during exercise possible.

Method

The light scintillation probes (Model 45-25, Pallimedica) were strapped on the thigh and calf over the site of the injection. The same resting and exercise procedure described previously was used, but it became possible to obtain a clearance curve during exercise and from it calculate T using equation 1. This was done every 0.5 minutes during the 3-minute exercise period.

Five healthy volunteers (5 limbs) and 23 patients (25 limbs) with peripheral arterial disease were studied. All patients had aortography as part of their routine management.

Results

Characteristic patterns of changes in muscle blood flow during exercise have been found, depending on the site and severity of lesions. The changes of T in the thigh and in the calf of a normal limb, a limb with iliac occlusion only, a limb with superficial femoral artery occlusion only, and a limb with combined severe aortoiliac and femoropopliteal lesions, before, during, and after exercise are shown in Figs. 57-7 to 57-10. The mean values of thigh T and calf T and their standard deviations before, during, and after exercise are shown in Fig. 57-11 for normal limbs, in Fig. 57-12 for limbs with iliac occlusion only, in Fig. 57-13 for limbs with superficial femoral artery occlusion only, and in Fig. 57-14 for limbs with combined severe aortoiliac and femoropopliteal lesions (>70% stenosis or occlusion).

Before and after exercise the changes of T (or muscle blood flow) in the thigh and in the calf were similar to those described in earlier studies. During exercise, they were as follows:

In normal limbs there was a marked hyperemic response both in the thigh and calf. The maximum value of T was reached 30 seconds after the onset of walking and remained unchanged thereafter (Figs. 57-7 and 57-11). The decrease in flow during the first few seconds after the end of exercise is probably the result of the increase in venous pressure producing a decrease in arteriovenous gradient.

In limbs with iliac occlusion only, the pattern

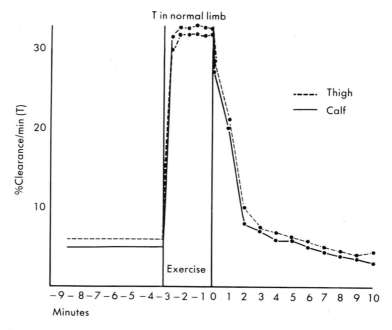

T in normal limb

Fig. 57-7. Changes of T in thigh and calf of normal limb before, during, and after exercise. (From Angelides, N.: Hemodynamic changes in the arterial circulation of the lower limb in patients with claudication, doctoral dissertation, London, 1980, London University.)

T in limb with proximal disease

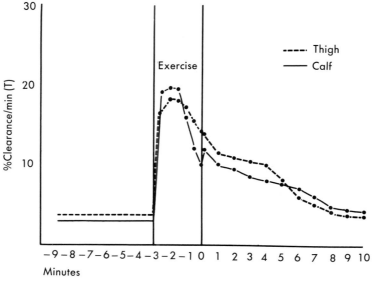

Fig. 57-8. Changes of T in thigh and calf of limb with iliac occlusion only, before, during, and after exercise. (From Angelides, N.: Hemodynamic changes in the arterial circulation of the lower limb in patients with claudication, doctoral dissertation, London, 1980, London University.)

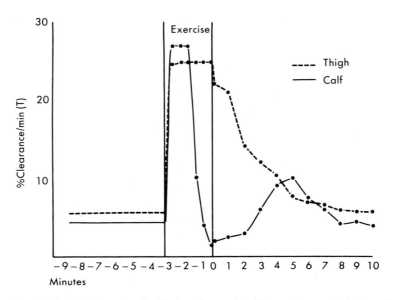

Fig. 57-9. Changes of T in thigh and calf of limb with superficial femoral artery occlusion only, before, during, and after exercise. (From Angelides, N.: Hemodynamic changes in the arterial circulation of the lower limb in patients with claudication, doctoral dissertation, London, 1980, London University.)

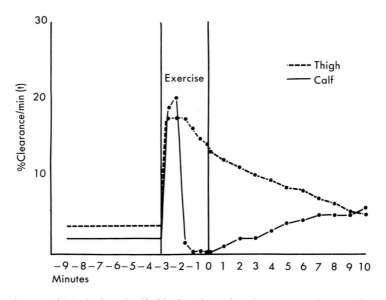

Fig. 57-10. Changes of T in thigh and calf of limb with combined severe aortoiliac and femoropopliteal lesions, before, during, and after exercise. (From Angelides, N.: Hemodynamic changes in the arterial circulation of the lower limb in patients with claudication, doctoral dissertation, London, 1980, London University.)

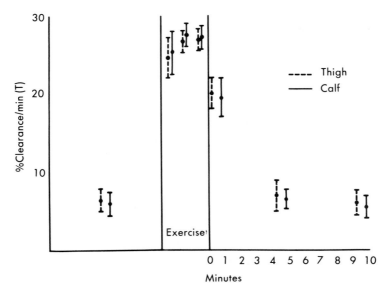

Fig. 57-11. Mean values of thigh T and calf T in normal limbs. (From Angelides, N.: Hemodynamic changes in the arterial circulation of the lower limb in patients with claudication, doctoral dissertation, London, 1980, London University.)

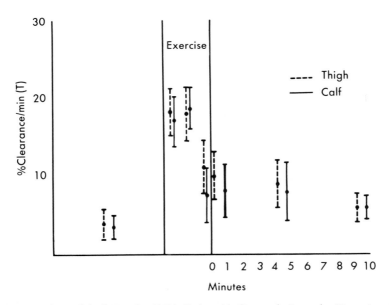

Fig. 57-12. Mean values of thigh T and calf T in limbs with iliac occlusion only. (From Angelides, N.: Hemodynamic changes in the arterial circulation of the lower limb in patients with claudication, doctoral dissertation, London, 1980, London University.)

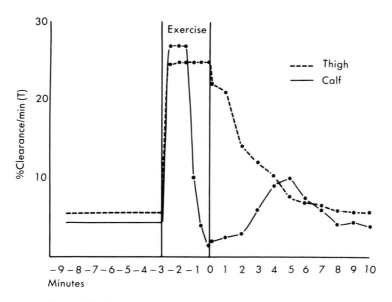

Fig. 57-13. Mean values of thigh T and calf T in limbs with superficial femoral artery occlusion only. (From Angelides, N.: Hemodynamic changes in the arterial circulation of the lower limb in patients with claudication, doctoral dissertation, London, 1980, London University.)

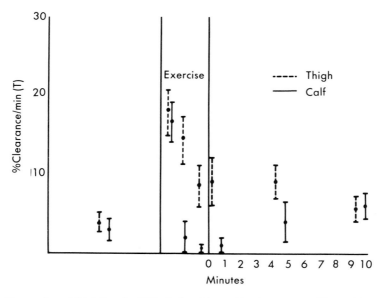

Fig. 57-14. Mean values of thigh T and calf T in limbs with combined severe aortoiliac and femoropopliteal lesions. (From Angelides, N.: Hemodynamic changes in the arterial circulation of the lower limb in patients with claudication, doctoral dissertation, London, 1980, London University.)

was diminished but equal in the thigh and calf. A hyperemic response was established 30 seconds after the onset of walking; it started to diminish but did not disappear at the end of exercise (Figs. 57-8 and 57-12).

In limbs with superficial femoral artery occlusion only, there was a different pattern of flow in the thigh from that in the calf. The former showed a flow pattern similar to that in normal limbs; the latter showed an initial hyperemic response, which disappeared by the third minute of walking; at the end of walking, little flow was present in the calf (Figs. 57-9 and 57-13).

Finally, in limbs with combined aortoiliac and femoropopliteal lesions the flow pattern in the thigh was similar to that in limbs with iliac occlusion only, while the flow pattern in the calf was less than the resting level by the second minute of walking; during the third minute of exercise, when claudication occurred, very little flow was found in the calf (Figs. 57-10 and 57-14).

These findings indicate that the maximum vasodilation in the muscles is reached during the first 30 seconds of exercise, and that in the presence of superficial femoral occlusion, the shunting of blood from the collateral circulation to the veins of the thigh, minimizing the blood available to the calf, occurs during the second minute of exercise. In the presence of an additional hemodynamically significant iliac lesion, this shunting occurs earlier and abolishes the flow in the calf. In these patients, this occurrence coincides with the clinical observation of the foot becoming white, with an unrecordable ankle pulse and pressure indicating absence of any detectable circulation.

SUMMARY

The use of ^{99m}Tc does not permit the determination of muscle blood flow in absolute values (that is, ml/100 ml of muscle/min) because its partition coefficient is not known. However, it will allow the measurement of changes in flow in arbitrary units (T). Five patients (five limbs) have been stud-

ied on 5 consecutive days in our laboratory to determine the reproducibility of the method. The coefficient of variation was 12% immediately after exercise when T was high (20%/min) and 30% at rest when T was low (3% to 5%/min).[1,2,3] The validity of ^{99m}Tc as a local radioactive tracer for the measurement of the flow of blood was tested by comparing it to the results obtained by ^{133}Xe clearance at rest and after exercise in five healthy volunteers. They were studied (five limbs) by both isotopes on 2 consecutive days. Similar changes in flow were demonstrated by both isotopes for increases in T up to 15% per minute. For higher flows, which occurred during the first minute after exercise, the ^{99m}Tc clearance was lower than ^{133}Xe by 20%.[1]

Although the original aim of these isotope studies was to understand the hemodynamic changes that occur with exercise, the simultaneous clearance of ^{99m}Tc from the thigh and calf developed into a diagnostic test. However, this is a complicated test, and it is unnecessary in patients with arterial occlusions, because the diagnosis can be made clinically. Single stenoses can be assessed by the reactive hyperemic response and pulse reappearance time (Chapter 56). The main value of the method may be in supplementing arteriography in patients with combined aortoiliac and femoropopliteal stenoses. The diagnostic chart shown in Fig. 57-6 indicates that the aortoiliac and femoropopliteal segments can each be graded as normal, having less than 70% stenosis and occlusion, without any error even in the presence of double segment disease.

REFERENCES

1. Angelides, N.: Hemodynamic changes in the arterial circulation of the lower limb in patients with claudication, doctoral dissertation, London, 1980, London University.
2. Angelides, N., and Nicolaides, A.N.: Simultaneous isotope clearance from the muscles of the calf and thigh, Br. J. Surg. 67:220, 1980.
3. Angelides, N., et al.: The mechanism of calf claudication: studies of simultaneous clearance of ^{99m}Tc from the calf and thigh, Br. J. Surg. 65:204, 1979.

CHAPTER 58

Amputation level determination using isotope clearance techniques

WESLEY S. MOORE and JAMES M. MALONE

The patient with vascular occlusive disease to the extent that lower extremity amputation is required presents the surgeon with a challenging problem. Correct judgment in amputation level selection combined with expert care can spell the difference between life and death and between successful rehabilitation with a prosthesis and a bed-and-wheelchair existence. This chapter will focus on the value of quantitative amputation level selection using isotope clearance techniques. These quantitative data can provide the surgeon with precise information as to the lowest level at which amputation can be carried out and expected to heal primarily. With this information the surgeon can perform an amputation at a level that spares maximum length for optimum prosthetic rehabilitation with a high degree of security that blood flow will be sufficient for healing.

MAGNITUDE OF THE AMPUTATION PROBLEM

There are between 30,000 and 50,000 lower extremity amputations performed each year in the United States. The vast majority are a result of either end-stage vascular occlusive disease or diabetic necrotizing infection. The amputation level that the surgeon selects has far-reaching implications for the patient, with respect to morbidity, mortality, and the likelihood for prosthetic rehabilitation. For example, amputation performed at the above-knee level in geriatric patients with vascular occlusive disease has been reported to carry a mortality as high as 50%, with a mean mortality of about 22%. In contrast, below-knee amputation carries an average mortality of 7%, with several series that employ immediate postoperative prostheses reporting mortality of less than 2%. Fur-

thermore, the patient who was ambulatory before the need for amputation can virtually be assured of ambulating on a prosthesis following unilateral amputation that spares the knee joint, in contrast to a mere 30% prosthetic rehabilitation rate following successful unilateral above-knee amputation. Finally, patients who can be accurately identified as having sufficient blood supply to heal a limited forefoot amputation not only will have a negligible morbidity and mortality, but also will have no need for a prosthetic appliance for ambulation. The problem with the vascularly impaired patient who requires amputation is that the amputation level that adequately encompasses the gangrenous or infectious process may or may not have sufficient blood flow to heal. The presence of viable, intact skin at the proposed amputation level is no assurance that blood flow is sufficient to heal a surgical incision, since healing requires a considerably greater blood flow than does the maintenance of viability in intact skin. The ideal test for amputation level selection is one that identifies the most distal level that successfully emcompasses the gangrenous or infectious process and possesses adequate blood flow to permit primary healing of the skin. The method for amputation level selection must be quantitative and have a sufficiently sharp endpoint to prevent an undue number of healing failures in those patients with flow rates that fall near the lower end of the "safe" scale. A sharp endpoint will encourage the surgeon not to proceed to the next higher amputation level in those patients with blood flow that falls near the low end of the "safe" scale, since that approach would deny many patients with healing potential at the lower level the benefits of a successful, conservative amputation.

CONVENTIONAL METHODS OF AMPUTATION LEVEL DETERMINATION
Level of distal palpable pulse

Older textbooks of surgery advocate the use of the level of most distal palpable pulse as the index for amputation level selection. For example, for a below-knee amputation to be recommended, it was stated that a popliteal pulse must be present and for a toe or transmetatarsal amputation, a pedal pulse. This very conservative method of level selection resulted in a high healing success rate, but it denied many patients who had healing potential at a conservative level the benefits of optimum amputation because of the absence of a palpable pulse. This fallacy was dramatically challenged by Lim et al.,[15] who reported a series of amputations for vascular occlusive disease empirically performed at the below-knee level regardless of pulse status. Despite the absence of a palpable popliteal pulse and, in some cases, absence of a femoral pulse, more than 70% of those amputations healed, indicating that nutritional skin blood flow was sufficient despite pulse deficit.

Trial and error

Some surgeons, frustrated by the lack of reliable criteria for level selection and wishing to save as much limb length as possible, would simply amputate at the most distal level that encompassed the gangrenous process, then repeat amputations at higher levels until healing ultimately took place. This approach was tempered somewhat by observing the amount of skin bleeding that occurred following incision. The disadvantages of this technique included multiple operations with increased morbidity, mortality, and prolonged hospitalization; also, a healing complication at one level might jeopardize healing at the next higher level, which might have had healing potential had it been selected initially.

Empiric "favorite" amputation level

A number of surgeons, concerned by the compromised healing and prolonged hospitalization seen in the vascularly impaired amputee, advocated the routine performance of amputation at the above-knee level. This approach was predicated on the hypothesis that healing would inevitably take place at this level. If the single objective were a healed amputation stump to facilitate early hospital discharge, this approach would have been quite satisfactory. Unfortunately, routine above-knee amputation led to a high mortality and an extremely poor record of prosthetic rehabilitation. Thus the advantage gained in early hospital discharge was rapidly lost in a permanently disabled patient.

A modification of the favorite level approach was the routine use of a below-knee amputation without application of any specific preoperative criteria for the likelihood of primary healing. This new clinical concept resulted in a decreased mortality and a significantly higher rehabilitation rate associated with preservation of the knee joint, but led to a 20% to 30% nonhealing rate, requiring second operation with revision at a higher level. Thus this method takes on some of the disadvantages of the trial and error technique.

Angiographic patterns of disease

There have been many attempts to review the angiographic patterns of occlusive arterial disease and to assess visible collateral pathways to determine the adequacy of blood flow to the skin. These have been uniformly unsuccessful in that static angiographic images provide no data on the dynamics of blood flow through collateral pathways.

NONINVASIVE METHODS OF AMPUTATION LEVEL SELECTION
Skin temperature

One of the earliest methods of noninvasive evaluation of blood flow was the use of skin temperature. A surface thermometer could be placed on the skin at the proposed level of an amputation site, and skin temperature could be recorded in tenths of a degree. Unfortunately, the temperature spread between skin with good blood flow and that with poor blood flow was not wide enough to identify a clear endpoint at the lower end of the skin temperature scale. Many patients with low temperatures, in fact, had adequate capillary skin blood flow to heal an amputation at the level measured. Thus the skin-temperature technique (using a surface thermometer) failed one of the critical criteria for the test to be of value.

However, the availability of new instrumentation has led to a renewed interest in the use of skin temperature for amputation level selection. Using a telethermometer,* Golbranson et al. found a significant correlation between skin-temperature readings and amputation stump healing.[7] Of 14 am-

*USI Series 400, Model 46 PVC, Yellow Springs Instrument Co., Yellow Springs, Ohio.

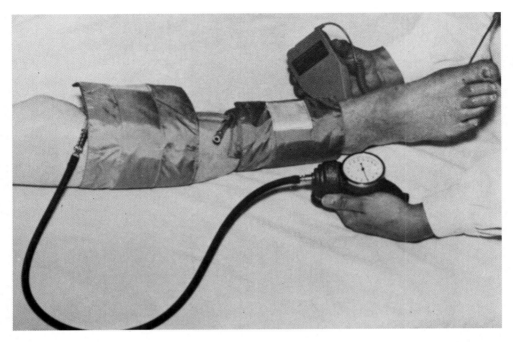

Fig. 58-1. Technique of measuring below-knee systolic blood pressure by Doppler ultrasound. (From Barnes, R.W., et al.: Surgery 79:13, 1976.)

putation stumps with skin temperatures above 32° C, 14 healed primarily (2 ray, 1 transmetatarsal, and 11 below-knee amputations). Of 14 amputations with skin temperatures between 30.5° and 32° C, 11 (78%) healed primarily (1 toe, 2 Syme's amputations, 8 below-knee amputations); however, only 3 of 6 (50%) distal amputations healed, whereas 8 of 8 below-knee amputations healed. Finally, neither of the 2 amputations healed in which the skin temperatures were below 30.5° C.

The ultimate role of skin temperature for amputation level selection, especially for Syme's, transmetatarsal, ray, and toe amputations, is unclear; however, further evaluation with new electronic temperature equipment seems warranted.

Hemodynamic indices

Several hemodynamic indices have been used recently to determine the optimal amputation level.[13] Raines et al.[24] reported their criteria based on pulse volume recordings, whereas Carter's experience[3] is based on ankle pressure measurements.

In 1976 Barnes et al.[1] reported their experience in 50 patients undergoing 53 amputations at the below-knee level in which retrospective correlation between segmental blood pressures and healing outcome were carried out. Segmental blood pressure measurements were obtained using wide cuffs at the upper and lower thigh, below-knee, and ankle levels. Evidence of flow as monitored by a Doppler flowmeter was sampled over the popliteal artery (Figs. 58-1 and 58-2). Of the 53 amputations, 31 (58%) went on to primary healing; 13 (25%) ultimately healed by secondary intention; and 9 amputations (17%) failed to heal and required revision at a higher level. All but one patient with undetectable audible flow in the popliteal artery failed to heal at the below-knee level. For all patients with popliteal pressures above 70 mm Hg the below-knee amputations healed. Those patients with a detectable signal at the popliteal artery but with pressures below 70 mm Hg had mixed results; 75% went on to either primary or secondary healing, but 25% of this group failed to heal. Thus those patients at the very low end of the spectrum (without audible flow at the popliteal artery) could have been clearly predicted to fail at the below-knee level, and this information could be used prospectively to recommend a higher amputation level. All patients with pressures at the high end of the scale (above 70 mm Hg) could be assured of healing at the below-knee level. The problem occurs in those patients who fall in the midrange between 70 mm Hg and no detectable flow. Of these, 75%

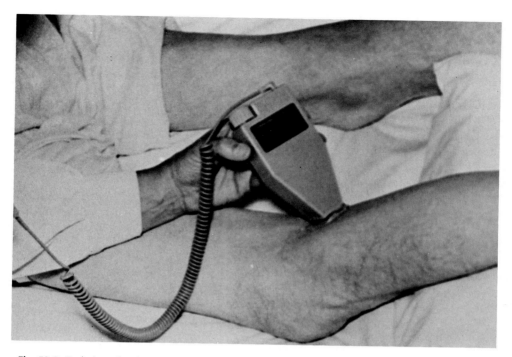

Fig. 58-2. Technique for detection of distal popliteal artery velocity signal. (From Barnes, R.W., et al.: Surgery 79:13, 1976.)

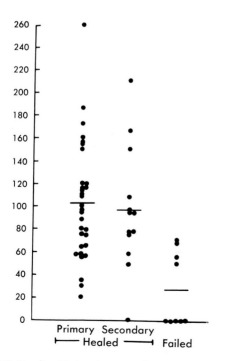

Fig. 58-3. Results of below-knee systolic pressure measurement according to healing status of below-knee amputation. (From Barnes, R.W., et al.: Surgery 79:13, 1976.)

healed and 25% failed to heal, once more approaching a trial and error technique for this indeterminate group and highlighting the fact that there is no sharp pressure endpoint between healing success and failure (Fig. 58-3).

Gibbons et al.,[6] reporting the experience from the Joslin Clinic, attempted to correlate pressure data with amputation experience in 66 diabetic patients who underwent forefoot amputation, this level having been selected on clinical grounds. Preoperative noninvasive testing, using segmental systolic ankle pressure and pulse volume recordings carried out at the thigh, calf, ankle, and forefoot, was used for a retrospective analysis. These authors noted that segmental blood pressure levels were erroneously high (greater than 200 mm Hg) because of arterial calcification and therefore were of no use in 56% of the patients studied. Ankle systolic blood pressure levels were low (suggesting healing failure had the data been used prospectively) in 36% of the patients who ultimately went on to healing success. Ankle blood pressure levels were high and suggested healing success in 64% of patients who ultimately failed to heal. Analysis of pulse volume recordings predicted healing failure in 50% of patients whose amputations went on to heal. These authors concluded that no patient should be denied a forefoot amputation based on segmental blood pressure or pulse volume recording data.

Bone and Pomajzl[2] reported healing data in 22 amputations at the digit or transmetatarsal level in which preoperative digital blood pressures were correlated. Infrared photoplethysmography combined with digit- and ankle-occluding blood pressure cuffs was used to determine toe and ankle systolic blood pressures. Out of these patients 18 (82%) were diabetic, 12 amputations (55%) went on to primary healing, and 10 (45%) required either postamputation revascularization to provide healing at the indicated level or reamputation at the below-knee level. The mean ankle blood pressure of limbs that went on to primary healing was 128 ± 49 mm Hg and did not differ significantly from the pressures in those amputations that failed to heal, of which the mean was 122 ± 71 mm Hg. Healing failures occurred with ankle blood pressures that ranged from 60 to more than 300 mm Hg. The mean value of toe blood pressure associated with healing was 89 ± 44 mm Hg, in contrast to the mean value of toe pressures in the healing failure group, which was 29 ± 6 mm Hg. Failure of forefoot amputation occurred in all 8 limbs with toe pressures less than 45 mm Hg and in 2 of 7 (29%) with toe pressures ranging from 45 to 55 mm Hg. Primary healing occurred in all 7 limbs with toe pressures greater than 55 mm Hg. These data suggest a reasonably sharp endpoint when toe blood pressure is used to monitor the likelihood of a forefoot amputation to heal.

Isotope clearance studies for blood flow measurement

In 1964 Lassen and colleagues[13] demonstrated that isotope clearance could be used to measure capillary blood flow in muscle tissue. ^{133}Xe, injected into muscle and monitored with a scintillation counter, could be used to calculate flow[12] at rest and following exercise. ^{133}Xe is a lipophilic, chemically inert, rare gas isotope whose only route for removal is to cross capillary cell membrane through a mass action or differential concentration effect. Therefore the rate of removal or clearance from an injection site is directly proportional to the capillary blood flow rate (Fig. 58-4). If one measures the partition coefficient between the tissue being studied and blood, the clearance information

can be put into the Ketty-Schmidt equation, which will yield numerical blood flow in milliliters per 100 grams of tissue per minute, as follows:

$$F = \frac{\log_e 2 \times \lambda}{T_{1/2}}$$

where

F = Flow in milliliters per 100 grams of tissue per minute
λ = Partition coefficient (0.7 for muscle and probably for skin)
T = Time for a complete decay of radioactivity at injection site

Other investigators have demonstrated that this technique could also be applied in the measurement of skin blood flow.[4,26] In reviewing the problem of amputation level selection and the need to establish a quantitative basis for precise preoperative level determination, Moore[13] reasoned that success or failure of amputation healing in patients with vascular occlusive disease should be a function of the nutritional (capillary) skin blood flow at the level selected. Since success in amputation surgery is dependent on skin healing, it seemed reasonable to apply Lassen's technique of capillary blood flow determination to measure skin blood flow at proposed levels of amputation and then retrospectively correlate healing data with preoperative flow rates. In 1973 Moore[18,19,20] reported his experience with 31 patients undergoing 33 below-knee amputations in which the level had been selected empirically on clinical criteria but in whom preoperative skin blood flow determinations were made, thus providing an opportunity for retrospective correlation. The technique of flow measurement was carried out in the following manner: 50 μCi of ^{133}Xe dissolved in 0.05 ml of sterile saline solution was drawn anaerobically into a syringe. Using a 26-guage needle, this was injected intradermally into the anterior midline skin, corresponding to a line ultimately to be used for the anterior incision for amputation (Fig. 58-5). The injection site raised a skin weal much like that of a tuberculin skin test. The needle was left in place for 30 seconds to permit equilibration and to prevent leaking of isotope along the needle track on removal. This injection site was chosen because we had observed that the most common site for a failure caused by ischemic necrosis was on the anterior midline skin. This suggested that the area of critical blood flow was at this anatomic site, and it therefore seemed reasonable to monitor this most sensitive area.

A scintillation probe was lightly taped to the leg

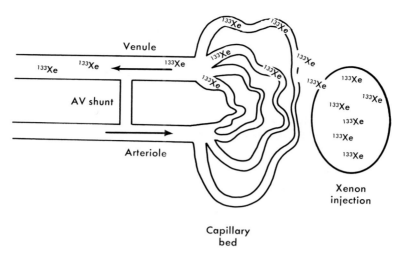

Fig. 58-4. Artist's concept of bolus of ^{133}Xe atoms in contact with capillary. Rate of diffusion of ^{133}Xe atoms across capillary cell membrane is function of differential concentration, and therefore of blood flow rate through capillary. Since ^{133}Xe is only removed by crossing capillary cell membrane, flow that takes place through arteriovenous fistulas will not affect measurement of ^{133}Xe clearance. (From Moore, W.S.: Arch. Surg. 107:798, 1973. Copyright 1973, American Medical Association.)

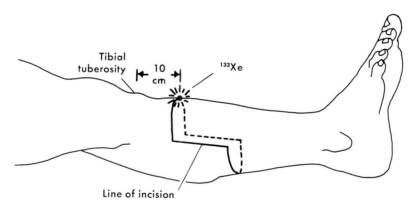

Fig. 58-5. Outline of proposed incision used for below-knee amputation. Intradermal injection of ^{133}Xe is made in midanterior portion of proposed skin incision so nutritional blood flow can be measured in this critical location. (From Moore, W.S.: Arch. Surg. 107:798, 1973. Copyright 1973, American Medical Association.)

adjacent to the point of injection. The probe was connected to a rate meter, which permitted the recording of the log of the counts per minute on a strip-chart recorder (Fig. 58-6). Recording was carried on for approximately 10 minutes. At that point the paper was removed, and a line tangent to the initial or steepest part of the curve was constructed and extrapolated to the point of zero activity. This line was used to calculate the $T_{1/2}$ (Fig. 58-7). Flow rates in the 33 cases studied ranged from a low of 2.2 ml/100 g of tissue/min to a high

of 17 ml/100 g of tissue/min, with a mean flow of 5.6 ml/100 g of tissue/min. All amputations were performed using a long posterior flap, and all patients were treated with immediate postoperative prostheses and ambulation beginning the day after amputation. The first cast changes were made 10 days after amputation, at which time the stump was inspected for healing. If healing was satisfactory, a second cast was applied and the patient was continued in ambulatory status for another 10 days, at which time the process was repeated. The third

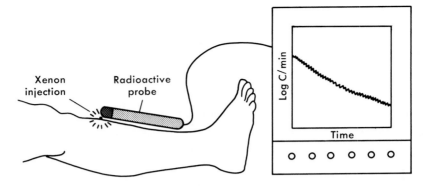

Fig. 58-6. Diagrammatic representation of method for measuring radioactive counts per minute and recording data on strip-chart recorder. (From Moore, W.S.: Arch. Surg. 107:798, 1973. Copyright 1973, American Medical Association.)

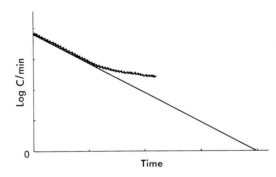

Fig. 58-7. Log of counts per minute plotted as function of time in order to convert exponential function to linear function. Only initial part of this curve measures skin blood flow; later part has admixture of subcutaneous flow. Line is drawn tangent to initial part of curve and extrapolated to zero time so theoretic time required for complete decay of radioactivity may be measured. (From Moore, W.S.: Arch. Surg. 107:798, 1973. Copyright 1973, American Medical Association.)

cast was usually left in place from 5 to 10 days, and then the patient was advanced to a permanent prosthesis.[21,22]

Using this approach, 3 (9%) of 33 amputations failed to heal because of ischemic necrosis at the suture line. Review of the preoperative flow studies revealed that these three amputations had the three lowest flow rates, corresponding to 2.2, 2.24, and 2.36 ml/100 g of tissue/min. All amputations with flow rates in excess of 2.6 ml/100 g of tissue/min went on to primary healing. These data suggest that the ^{133}Xe clearance technique would provide a sharp endpoint indicative of blood flow sufficient to heal at the below-knee level.

In 1977 Roon et al.[25] updated their experience with this technique and reported 62 extremities in which preamputation ^{133}Xe flow determinations were carried out. They noted that there were 10 extremities with flows less than 2.7 ml/100 g of tissue/min; 5 of these amputations healed, 3 primarily and 2 by prolonged secondary intention. The other 5 amputations failed to heal and required amputation at a higher level. It was our practice during that phase of the study to carry out a single determination of blood flow before amputation. We subsequently noted that there were several instances in which the preoperative blood flow seemed to be lower than we would have predicted on the basis of clinical observation. Because of this observation, we began to carry out a repeat measurement on each patient who demonstrated an initial flow of less than 2.6 ml/100 g of tissue/min. In the next 30 consecutive patients studied in this manner with flows in excess of 2.7 ml/100 g tissue/min, all went on to primary healing. Several of those patients had flows below the critical level on the initial examination but on repeat examination were found to have flows above the critical level and were offered the option of below-knee amputation. Patients whose flows repeatedly remained below the 2.6 level were not offered the below-knee amputation option.

Having established a critical flow threshold for healing, it seemed reasonable to apply these flow criteria to amputation levels other than the below-knee site. In collaboration with our colleagues in nuclear medicine, the technology of the gamma camera was introduced.[5] This permitted the simultaneous measurement of multiple levels of potential amputation with ^{133}Xe injection sites to select the most distal level encompassing the gangrenous process that had flow rates adequate to heal. Sites selected on the basis of ^{133}Xe studies included amputation of a single toe, transmetatarsal amputation, Syme's amputation, below-knee amputation, knee disarticulation, and above-knee amputation. The amputation level selected represented the most distal level, uninvolved with gangrene or infection, that had a flow rate of at least 2.6 ml/100 g of tissue/min. The healing data continued to validate the ^{133}Xe test results.

In 1981 Malone et al.[16] reported the results of ^{133}Xe skin blood flow studies in 45 patients using the gamma camera measurement technique. The range in ^{133}Xe skin blood flow rates was 2.1 to 22.0 ml/100 g of tissue/min and the mean blood flow was 5.9 ml/100 g of tissue/min. All amputations with ^{133}Xe skin blood flow rates in excess of 2.6 ml/100 g of tissue/min healed primarily. In addition, ^{133}Xe skin blood flow determinations were equally valid for diabetic and nondiabetic patients. These preliminary data on ^{133}Xe skin blood flow studies, using the gamma camera technique, were further validated in a subsequent report on 76 patients in late 1981.[17] Amputation levels included 6 toe amputations, 9 transmetatarsal amputations, 13 Syme's operations, 36 below-knee amputations, 7 knee disarticulations, 4 above-knee amputations, and 1 hip disarticulation. These data again showed that ^{133}Xe skin blood flow studies provided accurate objective information for amputation level selection at all levels of lower extremity amputation, although the cutoff point for healing was 2.2 rather than 2.6 ml/100 g of tissue/min. Once again, diabetes mellitus did not appear to affect the incidence of primary amputation wound healing. In addition, the second report[17] emphasized that ^{133}Xe skin blood flow studies could not be used in the presence of cellulitis or infection at the proposed level of blood flow determination.

Our ^{133}Xe skin blood data may be in contrast to a report by Holloway and Burgess.[8] Using a similar technique for measuring skin blood flow with ^{133}Xe, they found no difference between skin blood flow measurements of healing and nonhealing lower extremity amputations, although mean skin blood flow values were different. However, analysis of their data shows that all but two amputations with skin blood flows in excess of 2.6 ml/100 g of tissue/min healed primarily. In addition, the two healing failures occurred in patients who achieved primary wound healing but underwent secondary wound dehiscence caused by necrotic muscle.

Silberstein et al.[27] recently reported their data on the predictive value of intracutaneous ^{133}Xe clearance for amputation level determination using a measurement technique essentially identical to that used by Malone et al.[16,17] When skin blood flow measurements were greater than 2.4 ml/100 g of tissue/min, 38 of 39 amputations healed (97%), whereas only 4 of 7 amputations (57%) healed if skin blood flow was less than 2.4 ml/100 g of tissue/min ($p < .01$).

Based on data published to date on the use of ^{133}Xe for skin blood flow measurements, we would suggest that ^{133}Xe skin blood flows greater than 2.6 ml/100 g of tissue/min can reliably predict primary healing in the absence of infection at all levels of lower extremity amputation. The predictive accuracy of ^{133}Xe skin blood flows between 2.2 and 2.5 ml/100 g of tissue/min is not yet clear; however, it has been our practice to offer below-knee amputation to all patients with skin blood flows greater than 2.0 ml/100 g of tissue/min at the below-knee level.

It is of interest that attempts to correlate levels of distal palpable pulse or angiographic patterns of disease with healing and flow data have been uniformly unsuccessful. Many patients with extensive arterial occlusive disease, obliterating even the femoral pulse, turned out to have collateral blood flows sufficient to heal a transmetatarsal amputation. This indicated that only studies of capillary blood flow dynamics are adequate to select an appropriate amputation level.

Skin blood pressure determination using isotope clearance

In 1967 Nilsen et al.[23] reported their experience measuring arterial perfusion pressure in muscle by injecting a depot of [133]Xe (dissolved in saline solution and containing histamine) into the anterior tibial muscle. A small blood pressure cuff was placed over the injection site, and a scintillation counter was used to monitor the slope of clearance from the muscle injection site. The blood pressure cuff was slowly inflated until the slope of the clearance curve became flat, which was interpreted as being systolic perfusion pressure. In 1973, Holstein,[9] using a modification of this technique to retrospectively determine skin blood pressure in a group of patients having undergone lower extremity amputation, carried out a correlation between skin blood pressure and success or failure of healing. Holstein used a mixture of ^{133}Xe dissolved in saline solution with histamine and injected it intradermally in an area adjacent to the skin incision in a group of 24 patients who had undergone 29 amputations. This included 9 amputations at the above-knee level, 14 below the knee, and 6 distal amputations. The injections were performed postoperatively, and, following the injection, a blood pressure cuff was applied over the injection site with an air-filled bag connected to a mercury manometer interposed between the blood pressure cuff and the injection site. As the blood pressure cuff was inflated, pressure was generated within the air-filled bag and could be read off the mercury manometer (Fig. 58-8). The cuff was inflated in 5 mm increments until the clearance curve became flat, indicating that there was no flow to clear the radioisotope. This was interpreted as being systolic skin perfusion pressure (Fig. 58-9). Holstein noted

that no amputation stump healed when the pressure was below 20 mm Hg. He also noted that there were no failures when pressures were above 40 mm Hg, but between the range of 20 and 40 mm Hg there was a mixture of healing success and failure (Fig. 58-10).

In 1974 Lassen and Holstein[12] updated their experience using a further modification of this technique. They employed the 131 or 125 isotope of iodoantipyrine with histamine in saline solution to carry out the clearance study. Iodoantipyrine was used because this material is lipophobic and will remain confined to skin until removed. [133]Xe turned out to be unacceptable for this technique because it is lipophilic, and since the technique takes a half hour or more to perform, the isotope would diffuse into subcutaneous tissues and remain there, leading to an erroneous flow rate because of the slower flow in fat compared to skin. Retrospective blood pressures were determined following 51 amputations. There were 22 at the above-knee level and 29 at the below-knee level. Lassen and Holstein once again noted that there were no amputation successes when pressures were below 20 mm Hg (5 cases). When the skin blood pressure was be-

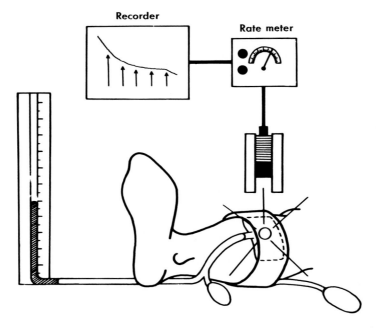

Fig. 58-8. Measurement of skin blood pressure on calf by flow cessation counterpressure. Local clearance from intradermal depot of [^{131}I]antipyrine mixed with histamine is registered by scintillation detector coupled to rate meter, output of which is recorded on penwriter. Counterpressure to depot is applied with ordinary blood pressure cuff. Plastic bag containing small amount of air is interposed between cuff and depot, and pressure directly to depot is measured by manometer connected to this bag. (From Lassen, N.A., and Holstein, P.: Surg. Clin. North Am. 54(1):45, 1974.)

tween 20 and 40 mm Hg, 3 of 12 amputations failed to heal because of ischemic necrosis, but 4 of 12 healed primarily and another 5 of 12 healed by secondary intention. When skin blood pressure was above 40 mm Hg, no amputation failed to heal because of ischemic necrosis (Fig. 58-11).

In 1979 Holstein et al.[10,11] expanded their series to 60 below-knee amputations in which skin blood flow measurement was carried out both preoperatively and again 4 to 9 weeks after operation. The technique once again employed the intradermal injection of 0.1 ml of a sterile solution containing 10 to 20 µCi of [^{131}I]antipyrene or 30 to 40 µCi

of [^{125}I]antipyrene mixed with 50 mg of histamine diphosphate. There were 8 amputation stumps with pressures below 20 mm Hg; 6 of 8 (75%) failed to heal, but 2 of the 8 (25%) went on to subsequent healing. There were 12 patients with pressures between 20 to 30 mm Hg; 4 (33%) failed to heal, but 8 (67%) did heal and were functional. There were 40 patients with pressures above 30 mm Hg; 4 (10%) failed to heal, and 36 (90%) went on to heal (Fig. 58-12).

The results of the skin blood pressure determination using isotope clearance studies provide only relative information concerning healing potential

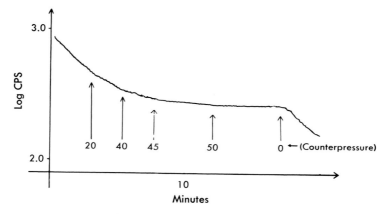

Fig. 58-9. Local clearance from intradermal depot of [^{131}I]antipyrine mixed with histamine. Stepwise increasing counterpressure results in stepwise decrease in clearance until flow cessation occurs (flat curve). (Skin blood pressure: 48 mm Hg. *CPS,* Counts per second.) (From Lassen, N.A., and Holstein, P.: Surg. Clin. North Am. 54[1]:46, 1974.)

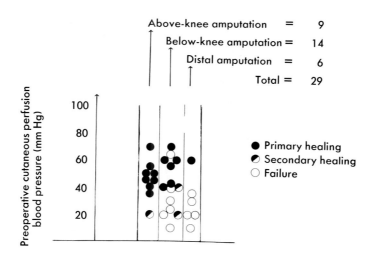

Fig. 58-10. Twenty-nine amputations performed in 24 patients. Results related to preoperative local cutaneous perfusion blood pressure measured at level of amputation with isotope clearance technique. (From Holstein, P.: Scand. J. Clin. Lab. Invest. 31(suppl. 128):246, 1973.)

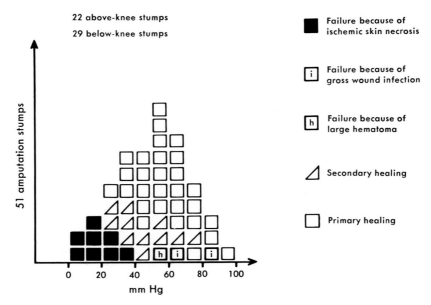

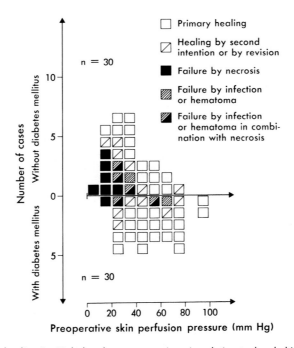

Fig. 58-11. Skin blood pressure values measured 2 to 8 weeks postoperatively in 51 amputation stumps (29 below-knee and 22 above-knee). Ischemic skin necrosis invariably caused reamputation when skin blood pressure was below 20 mm Hg. Between 20 and 39 mm Hg skin necrosis results in failure or slow secondary wound healing in most cases. Among 34 stumps with skin blood pressure of 40 mm Hg or more, there were 3 failures caused by wound infection or hematoma but no failures because of skin necrosis. (From Lassen, N.A., and Holstein, P.: Surg. Clin. North Am. 54(1):48, 1974.)

Fig. 58-12. Wound healing in 60 below-knee amputations in relation to local skin perfusion pressure measured preoperatively. (*Failure* indicates reamputation at above-knee level.) (From Holstein, P., et al.: Acta Orthop. Scand. 50:51, 1979.)

and have failed to provide a sharp endpoint that would delineate those patients who would heal from those who would not. Since blood pressure is only an indirect index of flow, it would appear more logical to use the same technique to directly provide flow data. This can be accomplished during a shorter time for measurement and can provide more accurate healing data than can a similar technique used to infer pressure data resulting in a less well-defined endpoint. Thus the isotope pressure studies have some of the same limitations found in the segmental limb pressure determinations using a blood pressure cuff with the Doppler flowmeter.

REFERENCES

1. Barnes, R.W., Shanik, G.D., and Slaymaker, E.E.: An index of healing in below-knee amputation: leg blood pressure by Doppler ultrasound, Surgery 79:13, 1976.
2. Bone, G.E., and Pomajzl, M.J.: Toe blood pressure by photopletysmography: an index of healing in forefoot amputation, Paper presented at the Symposium on Noninvasive Diagnostic Techniques in Vascular Disease, San Diego, Sept. 10-14, 1979.
3. Carter, S.A.: The relationship of distal systolic pressures to healing of skin lesions in limbs with arterial occlusive disease, with special reference to diabetes mellitus, Scand. J. Clin. Lab. Invest. 31(suppl. 128):239, 1973.
4. Chimoskey, J.E.: Skin blood flow by ^{133}Xe disappearance validated by venous occlusion plethysmograph, J. Appl. Physiol. 32:432, 1972.
5. Daly, M.J., and Henry, R.E.: Quantitative measurement of skin perfusion with xenon-133, J. Nucl. Med. 21:156, 1980.
6. Gibbons, G.W., et al.: Predicting success of forefoot amputations in diabetics by noninvasive testing, Arch. Surg. 114:1034, 1979.
7. Golbranson, F.L., Yu, E.C., and Gelberman, R.H.: The use of skin temperature determinations in lower extremity amputation level selection, Foot Ankle 3:170, 1982.
8. Holloway, G.A., Jr., and Burgess, E.M.: Cutaneous blood flow and its relation to healing of below knee amputation, Surg. Gynecol. Obstet. 146:750, 1978.
9. Holstein, P.: Distal blood pressure as guidance in choice of amputation level, Scand. J. Clin. Lab. Invest. 31(suppl. 128):245, 1973.
10. Holstein, P., Dovey, H., and Lassen, N.A.: Wound healing in above-knee amputations in relation to skin perfusion pressure, Acta Orthop. Scand. 50:59, 1979.
11. Holstein, P., Sager, P., and Lassen, N.A.: Wound healing in below-knee amputations in relation to skin perfusion pressure, Acta Orthop. Scand. 50:49, 1979.
12. Lassen, N.A., and Holstein, P.: Use of radioisotopes in assessment of distal blood flow and distal blood pressure in arterial insufficiency, Surg. Clin. North Am. 54(1):39, 1974.
13. Lassen, N.A., Lindjurg, J., and Munck, O.: Measurement of blood flow through skeletal muscle by intramuscular injection of Xenon-133, Lancet 1:686, 1964.
14. Lee, B.Y., et al.: Noninvasive hemodynamic evaluation in selecting of amputation level, Surg. Gynecol. Obstet. 149:241, 1979.
15. Lim, R.C., Jr., et al.: Below-knee amputation for ischemic gangrene, Surg. Gynecol. Obstet. 125:493, 1967.
16. Malone, J.M., Moore, W.S., and Leal, J.M.: Rehabilitation for lower extremity amputation, Arch. Surg. 116:93-98, 1981.
17. Malone, J.M., et al.: The "gold standard" for amputation level selection: xenon-133 clearance, J. Surg. Res. 30:449, 1981.
18. Moore, W.S.: Determination of amputation level: measurement of skin blood flow with xenon XE 133, Arch. Surg. 107:798, 1973.
19. Moore, W.S.: Determination of amputation level by measurement of skin blood flow (letter to the editor), Arch. Surg. 109:127, 1974.
20. Moore, W.S.: Skin blood flow and healing, Bull. Prosthet. Res. p. 105, Fall, 1974.
21. Moore, W.S., Hall, A.D., and Lim, R.C., Jr.: Below the knee amputation for ischemic gangrene. Comparative results of conventional operation and immediate postoperative fitting technic, Am. J. Surg. 124:127, 1972.
22. Moore, W.S., Hall, A.D., and Wylie, E.J.: Below knee amputation for vascular insufficiency, Arch. Surg. 97:886, 1968.
23. Nilsen, R., et al.: On the estimation of local effective perfusion pressure in patients with obliterative arterial disease by means of external compression over a xenon-133 depot, Scand. J. Clin. Lab. Invest. 19(suppl. 99):29, 1967.
24. Raines, J.K., et al.: Vascular laboratory criteria for the management of peripheral vascular disease of the lower extremities, Surgery 79:21, 1976.
25. Roon, A.J., Moore, W.S., and Goldstone, J.: Below-knee amputation: A modern approach, Am. J. Surg. 134:153, 1977.
26. Sejrsen, P.: Cutaneous blood flow in man studied by freely diffusible radioactive indicators, Scand. J. Clin. Lab. Invest. 19(suppl. 99):52, 1967.
27. Silberstein, E.B., et al.: Predictive value of intracutaneous xenon clearance for healing of amputation and cutaneous ulcer sites, Radiology 147:227, 1983.

CHAPTER 59

The predictive value of noninvasive testing in peripheral vascular disease

EUGENE F. BERNSTEIN

The early goals of noninvasive vascular diagnostic laboratories were the detection and definition of peripheral arterial occlusive disease.[11] Additional applications included screening for disease in asymptomatic patients, localizing the anatomic segment involved with greater precision, and intraoperative monitoring to ascertain the immediate outcome of arterial reconstruction. However, the greatest potential value of the vascular laboratory lies in its predictive capability. If more accurate estimates of the likelihood of success or failure of a given patient management procedure, such as an operative intervention, are available, then the laboratory will assume an essential role in the clinical management of patients with peripheral arterial occlusive disease. Since 1975, vascular laboratory data obtained before surgery have been correlated with the eventual success of reconstructive arterial operations, and these data are beginning to provide powerful predictors of the potential benefit of specific surgical reconstructive procedures in individual cases. This information may eventually represent an important contribution of the vascular laboratory to patient management.

PREOPERATIVE INDICES

Aortofemoral bypass represents the single most common and effective operation for dealing with peripheral arterial insufficiency, with a long-term patency rate exceeding 90%. Nevertheless, 10% to 30% of patients subjected to this procedure continue to have disabling symptoms.* To some degree this failure of symptomatic control represents the misapplication of aortofemoral bypass to patients with pseudoclaudication from neuro-or-

*References 2, 3, 5, 8, 14-16, 18, 20-22.

thopedic causes, which should be ruled out by a careful evaluation of the symptom complex and a standard preoperative vascular laboratory screening test. However, in addition, there is the difficult problem of multisegmental occlusive disease in which the decision to perform proximal or distal arterial reconstruction may be contingent on the constellation of angiographic and vascular laboratory data.

The earliest correlation of preoperative vascular laboratory information with the results of aortofemoral bypass was published by Bone et al.[3] in 1976 and included angiographic and hemodynamic data from 42 patients. The value of the thigh pressure index (TPI) was emphasized as critical in predicting the success of surgery. All 22 limbs with a TPI of 0.85 or less were improved following aortofemoral bypass (Table 59-1). In contrast, only 63% of patients with a TPI greater than 0.85 were clinically improved. Thus the authors emphasized that the development of a pressure gradient between the measurements taken at the brachial artery and those at the proximal thigh demonstrated significant aortofemoral occlusive disease and a high likelihood of successful surgery.

Unfortunately, when similar data were analyzed by Sumner and Strandness[21] the original conclusions of Bone et al. were not confirmed. In the Sumner series, 36% of the patients with poor results had preoperative TPI of less than 0.85. Sumner suggested that the upper TPI failed primarily because such pressures are subject to significant measurement artifacts, a finding confirmed by the clinical studies of Franzeck et al.[9] and experimental studies of Bernstein et al.[1] Additional data attempting to use thigh pressure measurements in the prediction of success following aortofemoral graft for

Table 59-1. Comparative data for predictive indices of the success of aortofemoral bypass

ALL LIMBS STUDIED

Test	Cutoff index	No. of limbs	Ability to predict (%)		Author
			Predicted success (%)	Predicted failure (%)	
TPI	0.85	52	100	37	Bone et al.[3]
IRR	0.2	129	91	26	Bernstein et al.[2]
TPRT	< 20	143	98	—	Bernstein et al.[2]
FPI	4	120	92	55 (all patients)	Thiele et al.[22]
	4	64	95	88 Aorto-iliac alone	Thiele et al.[22]
ΔFemoral-brachial index (pressure) (after papaverine)	0.15	20	100	100	Flanigan et al.[8]

MULTILEVEL DISEASE ONLY

Test	Cutoff index	No. of limbs	Predicted success (%)	Predicted failure (%)	Author
TPI	0.6	136	83	35	Brewster et al.[5]
API; TPRT	0.5; 0 to 20	74	100	43	Bernstein et al.[2]
TPRT	< 20	143	98	—	Bernstein et al.[2]
IRR	0.2	136	89	38	Brewster et al.[5]
FPI	4	81	88	60	Thiele et al.[22]
FP omega	0.2	40	81	92	O'Donnell et al.[16]
ΔFAP (after papaverine)	0.1	66	91	60	Brewster et al.[5]

multilevel occlusive disease have recently been presented by Brewster et al.[5] using a cutoff index of 0.6. In this more difficult group of patients, a TPI of 0.6 or less was associated with a good outcome in 83% of patients, whereas an index of greater than 0.6 was associated with a good outcome in only 65%.

Another pressure index was developed by Sumner and Strandness,[21] using the thigh-to-ankle pressure gradient to identify those patients with significant disease distal to the groin. This test, the index of runoff resistance (IRR), is calculated as thigh pressure minus ankle pressure divided by brachial pressure. In their study, essentially all patients with monosegmental aortoiliac disease and a low IRR (less than 0.2) improved after surgery. However, none of the indices measured by these researchers were reliable in predicting the results of aortofemoral bypass in patients with multilevel disease. Confirmation of these data was subsequently reported by Bernstein et al.[2] An IRR of less than 0.2 predicted success correctly in 91% of the patients. However, an index greater than 0.2

was associated with failure in only 26%. Thus a large number of patients with significant distal obstructive disease benefited from aortofemoral bypass. The IRR was also evaluated by Brewster et al.[5] in patients with multilevel disease where it also appeared to have significant predictive value, with a low index predicting success in 89% and a high index indicating failure correctly in 38%.

An alternative approach to the assessment of aortoiliac disease was investigated by Thiele et al.,[22] who analyzed the ability of the femoral pulsatility index (FPI), based on the femoral velocity waveform, to evaluate the hemodynamics of the aortoiliac segment. The FPI was calculated from the waveform by digitizing the envelope to obtain the mean amplitude and the peak-to-peak range. An FPI of 4 was determined to be critical. In comparison with the direct measurement of femoral artery pressures (FAP) before and after an injection of papaverine, the FPI correctly identified aortoiliac disease in 92% of 64 limbs studied, as well as in 92% of 36 limbs with combined aortoiliac and distal disease. However, a negative FPI (less than 4) was not as good in identifying the absence of aortoiliac disease in the face of occlusive disease of vessels distal to the inguinal ligament. Of 26 limbs with multisegmental disease studied in which the FPI was greater than 4, 25 limbs were hemodynamically normal for a sensitivity of 92%. However, of 55 limbs with an FPI value of less than 4 and combined aortoiliac and distal disease, only 33 were abnormal. Therefore the specificity of the FPI in combined disease was only 51%. In addition, these studies only confirmed the ability of the FPI to identify hemodynamically significant aortoiliac disease, but did not attempt to correlate the preoperative laboratory findings with eventual clinical symptom relief.

A plethysmographic correlation to the IRR was developed by O'Donnell et al.[16] and named the *FP omega*. This measurement represents the difference between the femoral and popliteal pulse volumes as measured by the pulse volume recorder (PVR). Using a cutoff criterion of 0.2, the technique was capable of predicting success in 81% of patients, and failure was predicted accurately in 92% of a selected group of patients with multilevel disease. Although the series is small (40 limbs), the data suggest that this is the most impressive preoperative noninvasive predictive index correlated with eventual symptomatic success published.

Finally, Bernstein et al.[2] have reported the value of the toe pulse reappearance time (TPRT/2)[10] in identifying those patients in whom aortofemoral bypass is most likely to be a clinical success. With a TPRT/2 less than 10, every patient was significantly improved by surgery, and with a TPRT of less than 20, 98% of the patients were improved. However, the ability of the test to predict future failures was not adequately described.

Because of the difficulties in identifying a single noninvasive measurement with significant predictive capability,[5,13,21] Bernstein et al. also evaluated the combination of the ankle pressure index (API) and the TPRT/2 in 74 limbs with multilevel disease. These criteria identified a group of patients in whom clinical success could be predicted with 100% accuracy and another group in which failure was predicted with a 43% likelihood.

Another effort at using multiple test data to discriminate between potential success and potential failure was published by Brewster et al.,[5] who identified five variables that were independent predictors of clinical outcome after aortofemoral bypass as follows:

1. Femoral pulse ($p = .002$)
2. Inflow disease on arteriogram ($p = .00001$)
3. Angiographic outflow tract ($p = .0003$)
4. IRR ($p = .003$)
5. Intraoperative PVR amplitude results ($p = .00001$)

The overall X^2/p value was $< .00001$. Using this model, 86% of outcomes were predicted correctly. This assessment, although identifying a variety of key predictive factors, was not much more accurate than several of the independent indices that have been discussed previously. In addition, only one vascular laboratory index, the IRR, was among the important indices.

Frustration with the noninvasive approaches has led to the use of semiinvasive techniques that generally involve femoral artery pressure measurements before and after the intraarterial injection of papaverine, as originally developed by Sako[19] and Brener.[4] Brewster et al.[5] confirmed the value of FAP measurements, using a cutoff index of a 10% change in pressure following femoral artery injection of papaverine as an indicator of significant proximal disease. Based on these criteria, in 66 limbs with multilevel disease the test was 91% accurate in predicting success and 60% accurate in predicting failure. Flanigan et al.,[8] using a similar test but relying on a 15% femoral pressure drop after papaverine, reported 100% success in separating eventual clinical symptomatic relief from clinical failure in 20 limbs.[8] Use of these semiinvasive techniques during angiography does not significantly add to the cost or morbidity of the preoperative patient workup. However, femoral puncture techniques are not as useful as a completely noninvasive approach that could be applied to evaluate patients who may not need simultaneous angiography and could be repeated following interventions such as balloon angioplasty or with symptom persistence or recurrence after surgery.

In addition to the value of individual pressure measurements, Bone emphasized the importance of the number of segmental pressure gradients distal to the groin. In extremities in which no abnormal preoperative pressure gradients were measured distal to the femoral artery, all extremities were symptomatically improved by aortofemoral bypass.[3] Of those limbs with a single gradient greater than 30 mm Hg of mercury, 76% obtained symptomatic relief. However, with two abnormal preoperative pressure gradients, the likelihood of success was only 29%, and all of these differences were statistically significant. These findings were confirmed in an additional review by Garrett et al.[12] in which the series was enlarged with essentially identical results. However, Sumner and Strandness[21] were unable to confirm the selectivity of this pressure classification. Bernstein et al.[2] evaluated a similar classification, dividing patients into those with pure aortoiliac disease, one additional distal pressure gradient, and two additional gradients. The data indicated a stepwise decreasing likelihood of symptom relief from aortofemoral bypass that reached a statistically significant level only in those patients with two gradients below the groin. Thus this classification was not more successful in identifying potential surgical failures than other efforts based on pressure measurements.

In summary, pressure-based noninvasive indices identify individuals in whom a high likelihood of surgical success can be predicted. However, they are not as capable of isolating future failures. Velocity-based information is essentially equal. PVR and TPRT data appear to offer greater accuracy, but the initial reports of success await future confirmation from other researchers.

INTRAOPERATIVE MONITORING

Garrett et al.[12] measured the API in 72 symptomatic extremities undergoing aortofemoral bypass as an indicator of eventual symptomatic relief. In this report, if the intraoperative API increased more than 0.1 during surgery, the eventual likelihood of clinical relief of symptoms was 100%. Patients with increases in the intraoperative API ranging from 0 to 0.1 generally had significant improvement in symptoms. All patients who failed to have any increase in their API during surgery reported no significant symptomatic improvement from the procedure. Similar results were reported by O'Donnell et al.,[15] using both Doppler systolic ankle pressure and segmental plethysmography. Whereas a significant increase in either the API or PVR amplitude suggests technical success of the procedure and its absence indicates that a search for technical misadventure should be undertaken, the surgeon's inability to detect a significant increase in either of these indices after a technically satisfactory procedure does not necessarily harbor failure. Kozloff et al.[13] have documented the fallibility of postoperative Doppler ankle pressures in a group of patients with limb-threatening ischemia. An increase in the ankle-to-arm pressure index was a reliable predictor of success, but its absence in

the early postoperative period, particularly in patients with occluded superficial femoral arteries, did not necessarily signify eventual clinical failure. Twenty limbs with occluded superficial femoral arteries did not demonstrate a significant increase until 3-hours postoperatively. However, within 24 hours, the ankle-to-arm pressure ratio should significantly exceed the preoperative value if the procedure has provided adequate revascularization.

Brewster et al.[5] have also commented on the value of intraoperative monitoring with PVR cuffs. In their experience, in patients with multilevel occlusive disease, an improved intraoperative PVR amplitude was associated with eventual clinical and hemodynamic success in 63 out of 65 limbs (97%). However, a lack of improvement was also associated with eventual clinical success in 48% of these patients. Thus the conclusions of Kozloff et al. using the ankle measure were confirmed by Brewster et al. for the PVR amplitude. Satiani et al.[20] also compared the postoperative ankle pressure measurement within the first 5 days after surgery with the eventual clinical result. In their experience the absence of an improvement of the ankle-to-brachial artery index of at least 0.1 within the first 5 postoperative days did predict a clinical failure in seven of eight limbs. O'Hara et al.[17] also reported the value of the PVR amplitude intraoperatively in detecting 15 instances of technical problems in approximately 400 arterial reconstructive procedures.

FEMOROPOPLITEAL BYPASS

In 1975 Dean et al.[7] correlated the late results of femoropopliteal reconstruction with the API in 115 patients. Intraoperative blood flow and angiographic runoff patterns were also correlated with graft patency. An 83% success rate was associated with patients in whom the preoperative API exceeded 0.4, and the success rate successively declined with decreasing API. If the API was less than 0.2, the success rate was only 9%. In a later review of this index by Corson,[6] all but one of the early failures were in limbs with a preoperative API greater than 0.5. However, late failures occurred in patients throughout the range of ankle pressures, and the ankle pressure measurement was not as well correlated with eventual success as in the Dean et al. study.

No additional data dealing with the clinical results of femoropopliteal or femorotibial bypass have been published. However, several groups are currently evaluating a number of preoperative vascular laboratory indices with eventual clinical success in these patient groups, and new data should become available in the near future.

SUMMARY

The discovery of valid and statistically significant predictors of the eventual success of major vascular reconstructive procedures for lower extremity ischemia is still in an early stage. Relatively few analyses of such data have been published, and the information is based on small series of patients, brief follow-up periods, and only a few standardized measurements. However, use of pressure, pulse volume, velocity, and reactive hyperemia modalities have been undertaken with promising results. Information regarding pressure measurement artifacts appears to explain some of the discrepancies with these measurements and emphasizes the potential importance of additional studies using velocity or plethysmographic techniques. Clearly the angiographic demonstration of localized aortoiliac disease is correlated with a high clinical success rate, and the noninvasive laboratory is unlikely to improve on this information. More difficult, but more important, is the problem of multilevel disease with an important aortoiliac component. A variety of researchers have now addressed this subgroup, and promising vascular laboratory data appear to increase the physician's ability to determine which segment is most important and which operative procedure should be recommended first. Combinations of measurements, including pressure, velocity, and reactive hyperemia data, remain to be fully explored and may increase the sensitivity of the assessment. Discriminate analysis of the application of derived-weighting factors may permit more selective characterization of patients preoperatively. However, even with the present limited information, the predictive power of these preoperative factors is impressive.

REFERENCES

1. Bernstein, E.F., et al.: Thigh pressure artifacts with noninvasive techniques in an experimental model, Surgery 89:319, 1981.
2. Bernstein, E.F., et al.: Toe pulse reappearance time in prediction of aortofemoral bypass success, Ann. Surg. 193:201, 1981.
3. Bone, G.E., et al.: Value of segmental limb blood pressures in predicting results of aorto-femoral bypass, Am. J. Surg. 132:733, 1976.
4. Brener, B.J., et al.: Measurement of systolic femoral arterial pressure during reactive hyperemia, Circulation 50(suppl):259, 1974.
5. Brewster, D.C., et al.: Aortofemoral graft for multilevel occlusive disease, Arch. Surg. 117:1593, 1982.
6. Corson, J.D., et al.: Doppler ankle systolic blood pressure: prognostic value in vein bypass grafts of the lower extremity, Arch. Surg. 113:932, 1978.
7. Dean, R.H., et al.: Prognostic indicators in femoropopliteal reconstruction, Arch. Surg. 110:1287, 1975.
8. Flanigan, D.P., et al.: Hemodynamic evaluation of the aortoiliac system based on pharmacologic vasodilatation, Surgery 93:709, 1983.
9. Franzeck, U., Bernstein, E.F., and Fronek, A.: The effect of sensing site on segmental limb pressure measurements, Arch. Surg. 116:912, 1981.
10. Fronek, A., Coel, M., and Bernstein, E.F.: The pulse-reappearance time: an index of over-all blood flow impairment in the ischemic extremity, Surgery 81:376, 1977.
11. Fronek, A., et al.: Non-invasive physiological tests in the diagnosis and characterization of peripheral arterial occlusive disease, Am. J. Surg. 126:205, 1973.
12. Garrett, W.V., et al.: Intraoperative prediction of symptomatic result of aortofemoral bypass from changes in ankle pressure index, Surgery 82:504, 1977.
13. Kozloff, L., et al.: Fallibility of postoperative Doppler ankle pressures in determining the adequacy of proximal arterial revascularization, Am. J. Surg. 139:326, 1980.
14. Martinez, B.D., Hertzer, N.R., and Beven, E.G.: Influence of distal arterial occlusive disease on prognosis following aortofemoral bypass, Surgery 88:795, 1980.
15. O'Donnell, T.F., Jr., et al.: A prospective study of Doppler pressures and segmental plethysmography before and following aortofemoral bypass, Surgery 86:120, 1979.
16. O'Donnell, T.F., Jr., et al.: Management of combined segment disease, Am. J. Surg. 141:452, 1981.
17. O'Hara, P.J., et al.: The value of intraoperative monitoring using the pulse volume recorder during peripheral vascular reconstructive operations, Surg. Gynecol. Obstet. 152:275, 1981.
18. O'Mara, C.S., et al.: Recognition and surgical management of patent but surgically failed arterial grafts, Ann. Surg. 193:467, 1981.
19. Sako, Y.: Papaverine test in peripheral arterial disease, Surg. Forum 17:141, 1966.
20. Satiani, B., Hayes, J.P., and Evans, W.E.: Prediction of distal reconstruction following aortofemoral bypass for limb salvage, Surg. Gynecol. Obstet. 151:500, 1980.
21. Sumner, D.S., and Strandness, D.E., Jr.: Aortoiliac reconstruction in patients with combined iliac and superficial femoral arterial occlusion, Surgery 84:348, 1978.
22. Thiele, B.L., et al.: A systemic approach to the assessment of aortoiliac disease, Arch. Surg. 118:477, 1983.

CHAPTER 60

Duplex scanning for the evaluation of lower limb arterial disease

KURT A. JÄGER, H.J. RICKETTS, and D. EUGENE STRANDNESS, Jr.

In collaboration with R.L. Martin, B.S.,* and C. Hanson, M.D.**

During the past 20 years there have been dramatic advances in the development of ultrasonic techniques to study vascular disorders.[1,12,21,22,27] With regard to the peripheral circulation, Doppler techniques have been widely applied.[10,15] The complexity of the systems varies from the pocket-sized continuous-wave (CW) systems to the sophisticated Duplex devices, which employ both B-mode imaging and Doppler ultrasound.[19] The simpler, directional CW systems are suitable for screening peripheral arteries and the measurement of limb blood pressures, but they also have serious limitations.[4,17,18,26,32] It is nearly impossible to obtain precise information on the angle of the sound beam, and this seriously limits the method in terms of quantitating the velocity changes that are observed.

The development of the Duplex system has revolutionized the area of noninvasive vascular studies.[1,2,8,19,20] For the first time it is possible to obtain a combination of anatomic, geometric, and velocity data from any desired location within the vascular system. Thus it is now feasible to scan the peripheral arteries from the level of the abdominal aorta to below the knee, making it possible to precisely locate the site(s) of involvement and quantitatively express the velocity patterns and changes across such segments.

INSTRUMENTATION

The Duplex scanner used in our laboratory (Ultra Imager)† combines a real-time B-mode imaging system with a pulsed Doppler unit. A single transducer (5 MHz) with a diameter of 13 mm is mechanically oscillated to generate both the fan-shaped sector image and the Doppler signal. The two-dimensional image can be stored electronically on the monitor and updated by request while the transducer is used in the pulsed Doppler mode. The position of the incident Doppler beam with respect to the vessel axis is displayed on the B-mode imager as a superimposed white line. The computed angle of the sound beam is provided as a numeric display. The discrete region in space where flow is measured is referred to as the *sample volume*. Its position along the line representing the incident Doppler beam is indicated by a small bar (Fig. 60-1). The B-mode and Doppler data are stored on videotape for review and evaluation at a later time. The hard copy recorder provides permanent visual records as strip-chart recordings or page prints.

B-mode imaging

The B-mode image is an ultrasonic topographic slice that allows visualization of the spatial relationships of the body structures in a two-dimensional presentation.[7,14,16] It is used to identify the artery of interest and to recognize anatomic variations (Fig. 60-1). Calcified plaques and obvious narrowings of the displayed artery on the B-mode imaging system are important guides to the examiner for correct placement of the sample volume in detecting disturbed flow patterns with the Doppler unit. Moreover, the B-mode image is a prerequisite for accurate placement of the sample volume to centerstream sites and to ensure a constant

*Research technologist, Department of Surgery, University of Washington School of Medicine, Seattle.
**Fellow in Interventional Radiology, University of Washington School of Medicine, Seattle.
†Honeywell, Inc., Denver.

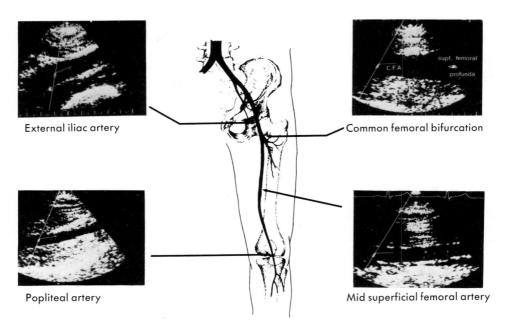

External iliac artery

Common femoral bifurcation

Popliteal artery

Mid superficial femoral artery

Fig. 60-1. B-mode image of distal external iliac artery, common femoral artery bifurcation *(CFA)*, superficial femoral artery, and popliteal artery of healthy volunteer. Axis of Doppler beam, angle of incidence, and sample volume placement are displayed.

angle of the Doppler beam with respect to the vessel axis. For standardization purposes we always use an angle of 60 degrees. It is obvious from the Doppler formula that the displayed velocity is greatly affected by the angle (cos Θ) of the incident sound beam. The importance of the angle can be demonstrated in its dramatic effect on the recorded blood velocity by simply tilting the Doppler probe (Fig. 60-2). It will be shown in subsequent sections how the accurate measurement of blood flow velocities allows classification of the degree of arterial stenosis.

A major disadvantage of the B-mode image is based on the fact that soft plaques and thrombi have an acoustic impedance similar to that of blood and may not be detected when B-mode techniques are employed alone.[19] Duplex systems minimize this deficiency.

Analysis of Doppler signals

The directional Doppler signals are analyzed both audibly and by spectral analysis. The spectral analysis is accomplished with the built-in digital real-time fast Fourier transform (FFT) spectrum analyzer. The analyzer generates 200 normalized spectra per second with a frequency resolution of 100 Hz. The graphic display shows time on the horizontal axis, velocity (cm/sec) on the vertical

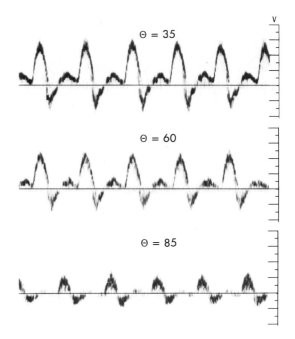

Fig. 60-2. Doppler velocity signals obtained from superficial femoral artery of normal subject. Waveforms were recorded within less than 1 minute at same recording site without moving scan head. Angle of incident Doppler beam was tilted by ± 25 degrees from 60 degrees (cos 60 = 0.5) to 35 degrees (cos 35 = 0.8) and 85 degrees (cos 85 = 0.1). Whereas peak systolic velocity of erythrocytes is assumed not to be affected, displayed peak systolic velocity changes dramatically when Doppler axis changes.

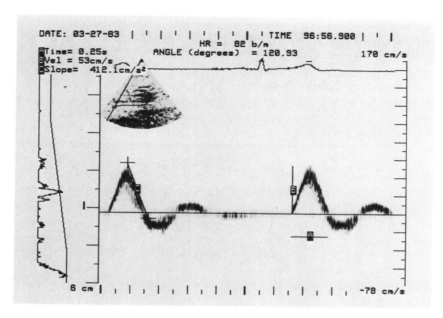

Fig. 60-3. Doppler signal is analyzed by real-time FFT spectrum analyzer and displayed with time on horizontal axis, velocity (cm/sec) on vertical axis and amplitude as shades of gray. Figure illustrates measurement of time (*A*, time of systolic forward flow, 0.25 sec) and velocity parameters (*B*, systolic peak velocity, 53 cm/sec). *C*, Slope: Deceleration = Peak systolic velocity divided by pulse decay time = 412.1 cm².

axis, and amplitude as shades of gray (Fig. 60-3). For any instant in time (of the heart cycle) the spectral width represents the entire range of velocity vectors within the sample volume. Thus the spectrum becomes broadened when turbulence is present.

SCANNING TECHNIQUE

The Duplex study is performed with the patient in a supine position. To get the best delineation of the femoral bifurcation, the leg may be slightly externally rotated. The popliteal artery is normally studied with the patient in a prone position and the feet elevated 20 to 30 degrees on a pillow. A generous amount of a water-soluble acoustic gel is used to couple the sound waves from the membrane of the scan head to the skin surface. The sites where flow velocities are routinely sampled include the iliac, the popliteal, the common femoral, and the deep femoral arteries and the proximal, mid, and distal parts of the superficial femoral artery. In addition, recordings are made from any site along the vessel axis from the aortic bifurcation to the popliteal trifurcation where flow disturbances are present.

The study is usually started in the groin by visualizing the common femoral artery. The examiner places the sample volume of the pulsed Doppler ultrasound in the centerstream of the vessel. The angle of the Doppler beam relative to the vessel axis is displayed on the screen. We maintain a Doppler angle of 60 degrees, which provides a standard signal for quantitative comparisons of peak velocities from different sites. Initial assessment of the common femoral artery flow signal permits a clue to the status of the aortoiliac and the femoropopliteal circulation. The scan head is then moved about to rapidly survey the vascular anatomy and the spatial relationships with other tissues and to depict anatomic landmarks. The vein is located alongside the artery and is usually easy to detect. The vein can be distinguished from the artery by exerting gentle pressure on the scan head, which will easily compress a nonthrombosed vein. The degree of pressure required to compress the vein can be used as a gauge of the correct placement of the scan head on the skin and ensures that the pressure exerted on the probe will not result in enough external compression to create an artificial stenosis. The deep and superficial femoral arteries are then visualized at their origin. The sample volume is moved along the displayed vessel axis to establish patency of the artery and to detect flow disturbances. After scanning the common femoral artery and the bifurcation, the scan head is moved up to the external iliac artery and then in a distal direction down to the adductor canal and popliteal artery. If the flow velocity pattern is normal, it is possible to scan the standard recording sites in a rapid sequence. However, if the stepwise examination shows an abnormality in the velocity waveform, a complete scan of the segment between the standard recording sites is needed to locate and precisely quantify the location and extent of the diseased segment.

Normal velocity patterns

Using this technique, 55 normal subjects were studied to establish the normal range of the flow velocity components for the defined arterial segments and to evaluate their alterations by age. There were 30 men and 25 women. The mean age was 51.9 years $\pm$ 14.3 years (standard deviation) with 16 subjects in the age group 21 to 40 years, 20 subjects in the age group 41 to 60 years and 19 subjects in the age group 61 to 80 years. None of the subjects had a history of peripheral vascular disease. All had a normal physical examination, normal resting ankle pressures, and a normal exercise test.

First, the diameter of the artery was measured from the B-mode image. Using the implemented software, two cross-hair cursors may be positioned by a joystick at the anterior and posterior walls of the artery and the distance between the two points is displayed on the screen. In this study, the mean diameter of the common femoral artery was 0.82 $\pm$ 0.14 cm and was 0.52 $\pm$ 0.11 cm at the popliteal artery (Table 60-1). On the average, women had a 0.15 cm smaller diameter than men), which was statistically significant (p > .001).

In the healthy individual, the velocity wave is oscillatory and has an initial systolic forward flow component followed by negative reverse flow and a second forward flow component during diastole.[2,9,24] Fig. 60-3 shows an original tracing as it is displayed on the screen at the time of the study. The figure also illustrates the measurement of the different time and velocity parameters of the waveform, which were performed on the frozen image by the computer in the Duplex unit. The means of the peak systolic and diastolic forward flow velocity and of the reverse flow velocity are listed in Table 60-1. At the femoral bifurcation the mean of the peak systolic velocity drops between the common femoral and superficial femoral arteries an average of 14 cm/sec. A marked drop of the peak velocity (25 cm/sec) can usually be measured across the adductor canal between the distal superficial femoral and the popliteal arteries.

Peak systolic and reverse flow velocity in normal arteries are only minimally affected by age or sex. The mean values of the diastolic forward flow velocity are stable in people 20 to 40 years and 40 to 60 years old. In the age group 60 to 80 years, however, a dramatic reduction in peak diastolic velocity was found. Comparison of men with women demonstrated a significant difference with lower values in women. Thus a biphasic waveform with forward and reverse flow components may be found in elderly healthy subjects. On the other hand, a quadriphasic waveform with an additional reverse flow component (Fig. 60-3) may be recorded in young subjects with a high elasticity of the arterial wall. A normal flow pattern shows a narrow spectral band. The spectral width is greater at the bifurcations because of flow disturbances and boundary layer separation. The reverse flow component in the deep femoral artery is shorter and lower than in the other segments. This can be explained by the relatively lower resistance in the arterial bed supplied by the deep femoral artery.

Table 60-1. Mean values and standard deviation measured at five different arterial segments in 55 healthy subjects

Artery studied	Diameter ± SD (cm)	V sys ± SD (cm/sec)	V rev ± SD (cm/sec)	V dias ± SD (cm/sec)
External iliac	0.79 ± 0.13	119.3 ± 21.7	41.5 ± 10.7	18.2 ± 7.5
Common femoral	0.82 ± 0.14	114.1 ± 24.9	40.6 ± 9.2	16.4 ± 8.3
Superficial femoral (proximal)	0.60 ± 0.12	90.8 ± 13.6	35.8 ± 8.2	14.5 ± 7.2
Superficial femoral (distal)	0.54 ± 0.11	93.6 ± 14.1	35.0 ± 9.8	14.6 ± 6.7
Popliteal	0.52 ± 0.11	68.8 ± 13.5	27.8 ± 9.2	9.8 ± 6.0

V sys, Peak systolic flow velocity; V rev, peak flow velocity of reverse flow component; V dias, peak flow velocity of diastolic forward flow; SD, standard deviation.

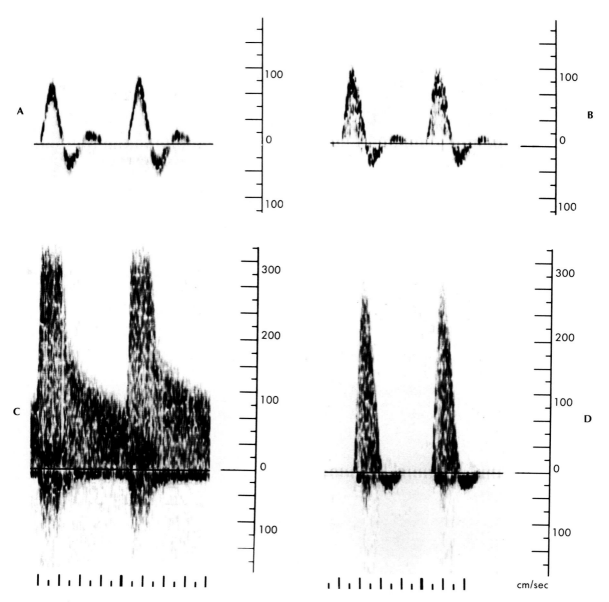

Fig. 60-4. Classification of spectra into arteriographic categories. *A,* Normal; *B,* 1% to 19% diameter reduction; *C,* 20% to 48% diameter reduction; *D,* 50% to 99% diameter reduction.

Velocity patterns in arterial disease

In patients with peripheral arterial disease, the degree of involvement can be classified using the pulsed Doppler signal. The three major criteria for disease classification are all derived from the Doppler spectral data and are based on the following:

1. The overall waveform contour
2. Peak systolic velocity
3. The spectral width referred to as spectral broadening

As compared with arteriography, the noninvasive findings are classified in five categories from A to E.

A   Normal, 0% diameter reduction. The criterion for normalcy is described in the preceding section. Figs. 60-2 to 60-4, *A* show normal waveforms.

B   Wall irregularities, 1% to 19% diameter reduction. Both the shape of the waveform and the peak systolic velocity are within normal range, but the spectrum is broadened (Fig. 60-4, *B*).

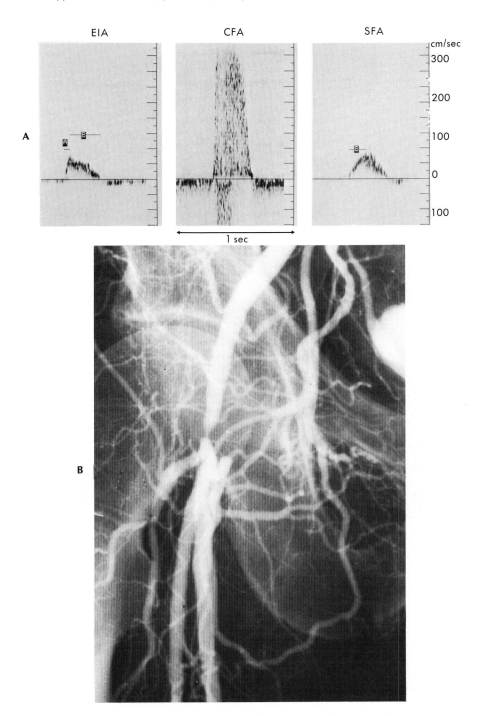

Fig. 60-5. Blood flow velocity tracings and arteriography of 61-year-old patient with high-grade stenosis of common femoral artery. *A, EIA,* External iliac artery; *CFA,* common femoral artery; *SFA,* superficial femoral artery. Peak systolic velocity at *EIA* is below normal values; pulse rise time *(A)* is reduced to 40 msec (90 to 100 msec is normal). Pulse decay time *(B)* is 260 msec, which is larger than normal (140 msec). Just distal to stenosis of *CFA,* a high increase in peak systolic velocity (wraparound) and marked spectral broadening are recorded. Distal to stenosis at *SFA,* peak velocity decreases rapidly and pulse rise time increases from 40 to 140 msec *(B).* Pulse decay time is 160 msec. *B,* Arteriogram demonstrates high-grade stenosis of right *CFA.*

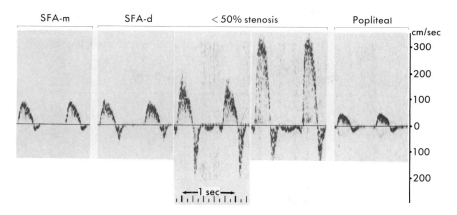

Fig. 60-6. Influence of peripheral resistance on displayed reverse flow component across stenosis. Peak forward flow velocity at mid-superficial femoral artery *(SFA-m)* and first recording at distal superficial femoral artery *(SFA-d)* is almost identical. First of three recordings at SFA-d, however, shows an arrow-shaped reverse flow component, which is indicating a marked increase in vascular impedance in front of stenosis. Following tracing was recorded just at beginning of stenosis. Systolic velocity is increasing and reverse flow velocity is becoming more pronounced. Third waveform of SFA-d was obtained at distal part of stenosis. At popliteal *(POPL)* artery peak systolic velocity and reverse flow component are normalized.

C 20% to 49% diameter reduction. The most striking finding is an increase in peak systolic velocity. This implies an increase by more than 30% with respect to the proximal recording site (Fig. 60-4, *C)*. The reverse flow component is maintained. The spectral broadening is marked. The flow patterns proximal and distal to the involved area are unchanged.

D 50% to 99% diameter reduction. A D lesion is characterized by the loss of reverse flow with only forward flow during the entire heart cycle. Thus the waveform becomes monophasic. The increase in systolic peak velocity is even more pronounced than in a 20% to 49% stenosis and the spectral broadening is extensive (Fig. 60-4, *D)*. The waveform proximal to the stenosis is affected only by a very tight stenosis. The distal waveform is abnormal, and the velocity is reduced with respect to the recording site proximal to the stenosis.

E Total occlusion. An occluded artery can be visualized on the sector image, but no flow is detected within the artery. The flow patterns proximal and distal to the occlusion are disturbed.

Using these criteria, a single stenosis along the arterial axis between the aortic bifurcation and popliteal trifurcation can be located and the degree of obstruction exactly determined. If multisegmental disease is present, the examiner must judge the actual waveform with respect to the shape of the spectra obtained at the next proximal segment. Changes in flow velocity and spectral width, how-ever, may be interpreted the same way as previously described for single stenoses. Since a high-grade stenosis and an occlusion affect both the proximal and the distal waveform, it is important to know whether the scan head should be moved proximally or distally to exactly locate the lesion and find the site of maximal flow disturbances. An important guide to the examiner for correct placement of the sample volume is the steepness of the systolic upslope or pulse rise time. The pulse rise time is short proximal to the obstruction and prolonged distal to the lesion (Fig. 60-5). The pulse delay time, or the duration of the downstroke period of the systolic curve, is longer in diseased vessels and can be considered a sensitive indicator for disturbed flow. The reverse flow component reflecting the peripheral vascular resistance shows a characteristic change in front of an obstruction. The peak of the reverse flow component is usually rounded. An increase in peripheral resistance, however, results in a symmetric tapered contour and a high peak reverse velocity (Fig. 60-6).

ANALYSIS OF RESULTS

Our first experiences are based on the results of the noninvasive Duplex scanning of 30 patients. The anatomic pattern of disease showed the following distribution: Combined aortoiliac and femoropopliteal disease was present in 22 legs. Of the 26 legs with only inflow or outflow disease, 12 involved the aortoiliac segment, whereas 14 in-

Table 60-2. Comparison of Duplex scanning results with conventional arteriography

Results of Duplex scan		Distribution according to conventional arteriography				
%Stenosis	No. of arteries	Normal	1%-19%	20%-49%	50%-99%	Total occlusion
Normal	97	**88**	7	1	1	
1-19	124	19	**80**	15	9	1
20-49	39	1	6	**21**	11	
50-99	41		3	1-	**36**	1
Total occlusion	37			1	3	**33**

volved the femoropopliteal segment. The asymptomatic contralateral leg without hemodynamically significant disease was studied 6 times. The results of the noninvasive Duplex study were compared with the arteriographic findings of a single radiologist. The arteriograms were also independently reviewed by a second radiologist who was also unaware of the results of the noninvasive study. Both the Duplex data and the arteriographic readings were available for final comparison in 54 legs involving 338 arterial segments.

The findings of the Duplex study as compared with conventional arteriography are cross tabulated in Table 60-2. Data with perfect agreement between arteriography and Duplex study are located on the diagonal line (in bold type) from the upper left to the lower right corner; overestimations may be found to the left and underestimations to the right of this line. Using the Duplex scanner, the degree of disease was overestimated by two categories 1.5% of the time (5/338), underestimated by two categories in 3% of the arteries studied (10/338), and underestimated by three categories in only 0.6% of the arteries studied (2/338).

Duplex scanning allows classification of the degree of involvement into the five categories mentioned earlier and categorization of disease to one of the seven levels of the arterial axis with an overall accuracy of 76.3% (258/338). The sensitivity of the test is 96%, the specificity 81%. The positive predictive value (PPV) reaches 92% while the negative predictive value (NPV) comes to 91% (Table 60-3).

The arteriograms of 257 arterial segments were also read by a second radiologist. The results of the arteriographic readings independently reported by radiologist 1 and radiologist 2 are cross tabulated in Table 60-4. Compared with the findings of radiologist 1, radiologist 2 overestimated the lesions by two categories in 1.9% of the cases (5/257), or

Table 60-3. Accuracy of Duplex scanning compared with conventional arteriography and of two independent arteriographic readings of the same films

	Arteriography vs. Duplex scanning	Arteriographic reading 1 vs. 2
Overall accuracy (%)	76	70
Sensitivity (%)	96	97
Specificity (%)	81	68
PPV (%)	92	88
NPV (%)	91	92

by more than two categories in 0.8% of the cases (2/257), and underestimated the lesions by two categories in 0.8% (2/257). Of the 257 segments, 181 were classified in the same category, resulting in a perfect agreement of 70% (Table 60-3). The sensitivity, specificity, PPV, and NPV of the two radiologists in classifying and localizing disease are also summarized in Table 60-5. Comparing the results of the noninvasive Duplex study with the arteriographic findings (radiologist 1) resulted in a better overall agreement and a higher specificity than comparing the readings of the two radiologists.

The following summary analyzes the accuracy of the technique in classifying disease as compared with arteriography (Table 60-5):

A. *Normal segment:* Of the 338 arterial segments studied with the Duplex scanner, 108 were classified by arteriography as normal. The ultrasonic data were in agreement with the arteriographic classification in 81.5% of the cases (88/108). The two radiologists were in agreement only 68% of the time.

B. *1% to 19% diameter reduction:* Spectral analysis of the pulsed Doppler signal provides nec-

Table 60-4. Comparison of two radiologists' readings of the same arteriograms

% Stenosis	No. of arteries	Normal	1%-19%	20%-49%	50%-99%	Total occlusion
Normal	72	49	21	1	1	
1-19	59	4	34	18	2	1
20-49	36		7	23	4	2
50-99	51		2	9	36	4
Total occlusion	39					39

The table header spans: **Results of first arteriographic reading** (% Stenosis, No. of arteries) and **Distribution according to second arteriographic reading** (Normal, 1%-19%, 20%-49%, 50%-99%, Total occlusion).

Table 60-5. Accuracy of Duplex scanning compared with conventional arteriography and of two independent arteriographic readings in classifying disease

Disease grade (%stenosis)	Arteriography vs. Duplex scanning (% agreement)	Arteriographic reading 1 vs. 2 (% agreement)
Normal	81	68
1-19	83	58
20-49	83	57
50-99	60	70
Total occlusion	94	100

essary physiologic information regarding the nature of the blood flow within the vessel. Spectral width is used to classify wall irregularities. The spectrum becomes broadened when turbulence is present or differences in blood flow velocity are detected within the sample volume. When the sample volume is placed close to the wall or at a bifurcation, there will be velocity gradients even in normal arteries.[19,28] Thus placement of the sample volume in the centerstream of the vessel is essential. Identification of spectral broadening by Duplex scanning resulted in a correct classification of wall irregularities in 83% (80/96). The interobserver agreement of the two radiologists for a 1% to 19% diameter reduction was only 58%.

C. *20% to 49% diameter reduction:* Blood flow velocities are known to increase across a stenosis. The results of experimental studies document a significant increase in peak systolic velocity when the diameter of the aorta is reduced by only 20%.[30] This is in contrast to the findings at the carotid bifurcation where a significant increase in peak systolic velocity is found only at the site of a greater than 50% diameter reduction.[8] The increase in velocity of the jet stream is in proportion to the degree of stenosis and to the pressure drop across the stenotic lesion. The conversion of pressure energy into kinetic energy can be detected by the rapidly changing nonlaminar flow vectors or turbulence that causes a marked spectral broadening. The distal propagation of poststenotic turbulence is proportional to the degree of the stenosis but is generally limited to a few centimeters.

Using the criteria of peak systolic velocity, spectral broadening, and the waveform contour, a perfect agreement with the arteriographic results was found in 54% of the lesions classified as a 20% to 49% diameter reduction by arteriography. Of the 39 segments considered on the basis of arteriography to be the site of a 20% to 49% stenosis, 15 (38%) were classified by Duplex scanning as having 1% to 19% stenosis. On the other hand, only 2 segments (5%) of this category were misclassified as having a greater than 50% diameter reduction. In judging a 20% to 49% stenosis the two radiologists agreed in 64% of the segments.

D. *50% to 99% diameter reduction:* The blood flow pattern is affected by the reduced peripheral resistance distal to a hemodynamically significant lesion. The reverse flow component of pulsatile flow is lost, and the Doppler waveform becomes monophasic. Various publications have reported that the absence of the reverse flow component under basic resting conditions may be considered an unambiguous sign of significant disease in the extremity arteries.[9,13,24] In the 50% to 99% diameter reduction group the described criteria resulted in an agreement between noninvasive study and arteriography in 60%, whereas the agreement between the two arteriographic reports was 70%.

E. *Total occlusion:* Complete occlusions were correctly classified by Duplex scanning in 94% (33/35) of the segments considered on the basis of arteriography to be occluded. All 39 segments reported by radiologist 1 to be totally occluded were classified the same by radiologist 2. Radiologist 2, however, reported 7 additional occlusions that were classified by radiologist 1 as 1% to 19% (1), 20% to 49% (2), or 50% to 99% (4) diameter reductions.

CLINICAL APPLICATIONS

Duplex scanning appears to have a high sensitivity (96%) and a fair specificity (81%) in identifying and localizing peripheral arterial disease. The results with scanning of the leg arteries may be compared with the recently reported results of ultrasonic Duplex studies in patients with carotid arterial disease.[20] The ability to identify extracranial carotid disease (sensitivity) is reported to be 99%, and the specificity, or ability to recognize normal arteries, is 84%. As in the carotid studies, we used five categories to classify the degree of involvement. Unlike the carotid artery, where the disease is mainly located at the bifurcation involving the orifice of the internal carotid artery, the arterial circulation of the lower extremity may be affected by atherosclerotic plaques at any segment between the aortic bifurcation and tibial arteries. Therefore the arterial system of the lower limb was divided into seven segments, and the results reflect the accuracy of the technique in attributing disease to the proper level as compared with arteriography.

Our results may not be compared with any other method of noninvasive assessment of lower extremity ischemia. At the present state of the art of noninvasive diagnosis of arterial obstruction using conventional methods, one can only distinguish to some extent between hemodynamically significant and nonsignificant obstructions.[3,13,23] Thus the binary decision, that is, more or less than 50% diameter reduction, is now expanded to the identification of five different degrees of obstruction. In addition, the traditional functional tests usually fail to establish the exact anatomic location of the obstruction.[11] Whether disease is proximal or distal to the inguinal ligaments is a key question for the management of patients with lower extremity ischemia.[6] Besides the difficulty involved in discriminating between aortoiliac and femoropopliteal involvement, presently available tests allow only crude estimations of whether disease is affecting the arteries proximal or distal to the knee.

Because of its great practical importance in vascular therapy, the diagnosis of iliac obstruction demonstrates the limitations of any diagnostic test. Using the Duplex scanner, disease of the iliac segment was always detected (100% sensitivity, with

conventional arteriography as the definitive test) when it was present, whereas normal arteries were recognized in 81% (specificity) of the cases studied. If only more than 50% diameter reduction by arteriography was considered to be a significant lesion, the specificity of the test reached 100%. Comparable results were obtained for the deep femoral artery. The only other test that permits an assessment of the circulation of the deep femoral artery is Doppler ultrasonic arteriography. Evaluation of this artery in patients with severe femorocrural obstructions is of particular importance in screening candidates for selective deep femoral revascularization.

Care was taken to analyze the accuracy of Duplex scanning in patients with only aortoiliac disease or femoropopliteal disease, as well as in patients with combined inflow and outflow disease. The results were not affected by the site of involvement or by multisegmental disease. The level and extent of the involvement should be established when either transluminal angioplasty or vascular surgery is being considered. The degree of obstruction will influence the manner in which the patient is managed. There is no doubt that the distinction between a high-grade stenosis and a total occlusion is of paramount clinical importance. A stenosis of the iliac artery, for example, is amenable to percutaneous transluminal angioplasty (PTA) with a good primary success rate, and favorable long-term results can be expected. Patients with iliac occlusion, on the other hand, usually are not considered good candidates for PTA. For the first time, normal arterial segments can be separated from those with wall irregularities and minimal disease. The information provided by the noninvasive Duplex technique allows assessment of the success rate of different treatment modalities and quantification of minor changes in diseases involving the arterial system. Epidemiologic studies designed to evaluate the true prevalence and incidence of atherosclerotic lesions are now feasible.

Contrast arteriography is considered the definitive diagnostic tool providing a road map for the surgeon. Besides the costs, discomfort, and complications of this invasive examination, the information provided is strictly anatomic, and it is often impossible to estimate the hemodynamic significance of a stenosis, even with films taken in two planes.[5,29] Despite all the objections to arteriography as a poor method to determine the state of the arterial circulation, we selected arteriography as the

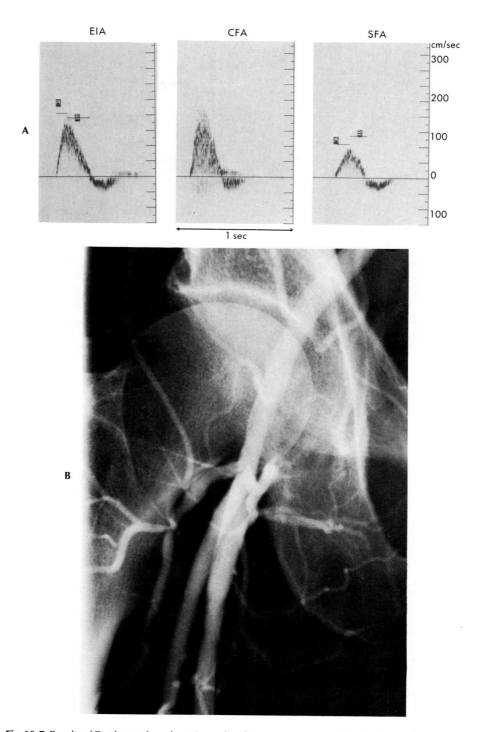

Fig. 60-7. Results of Duplex study and arteriography after percutaneous transluminal angioplasty (crossover PTA, Dr. E. Schneider) in patient demonstrated in Fig. 60-5. ***A,*** At *EIA,* peak systolic velocity, pulse rise time (***A*** = 90 msec), and decay time (***B*** = 190 msec) are improved. At *CFA,* peak velocity is almost normalized. Marked spectral broadening indicates that surface of dilated segment is rougher than expected from the arteriogram ***(B).*** At the *SFA,* the waveform, peak velocity of forward and reverse flow, pulse rise time (*A* = 100 msec), and pulse decay time (*B* = 140 msec) are normal. ***B,*** Arteriogram shows that stenosis at *CFA* was dilated and only minimal residual wall irregularities can be seen.

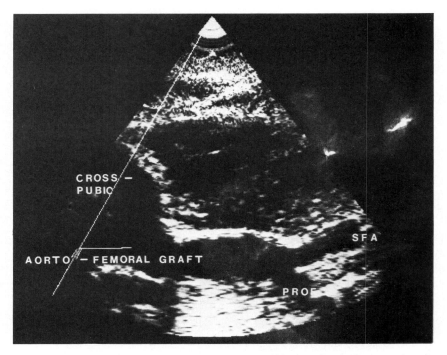

Fig. 60-8. After vascular surgery, operated arterial segment can be visualized. Then sample volume is moved along bypass and across anastomoses to establish patency and detect stenoses.

standard to which the results of the noninvasive Duplex scans were compared. In daily clinical practice no better method has been available. In our study, when two radiologists independently read the same films, they agreed on only 70% of the segments. In 97% they were in agreement that disease was present (sensitivity). The agreement in judging normal segments (specificity), however, was only 68%. The score obtained by Duplex scanning easily equals the score of two radiologists analyzing and assessing the lesions from the arteriograms. This not only demonstrates the deficiencies of the arteriography but also shows that the Duplex technique is as accurate as arteriography. The purpose of the study is not to replace the invasive radiologic test but to limit the number being done and to apply arteriography more selectively. Accurate functional assessment of disease combined with intraarterial pressure measurements should make it possible to select the proper patient population for either PTA or vascular surgery.[31] Thus candidates for a PTA may undergo this treatment without previous arteriography. After PTA the physiologic improvement can be recorded and the patency rate can easily be established in prospec-

tive studies (Fig. 60-7). The primary hemodynamic success rate seems to be not as impressive as assumed from the strictly anatomic arteriogram. In the same way, the primary success rate after vascular surgery and the frequency of reocclusions can be evaluated in follow-up studies.

During the early postoperative period, the proximal and distal anastomoses must be checked very carefully, since they are especially prone to recurrent stenosis (Fig. 60-8). In a short graft with good runoff, the peak velocity is expected to be equal at both sites. The degree to which blood flow velocity in the graft is affected by the runoff vessels is not known. It can be assumed that the waveform contour in itself is modified by the graft material (vein vs. synthetic graft), the length of the bypass, and the distal arteries. A minimal level of blood flow velocity or blood volume flowing through a graft may be a useful indicator for the prediction of graft failure.

Finally, a better understanding of the normal circulation is a prerequisite for an intelligent interpretation of disease. Attention must be focused on the most likely sites for atherosclerosis, such as bifurcations and the adductor canal.

SUMMARY

With the development of Duplex scanning, a method is now available that combines anatomic information with physiologic data. The technique permits a quantitative evaluation of the velocity changes at all levels of the limb from the aorta to below the knee. This makes it possible to detect both stenoses and occlusions. The application of this technique to the peripheral arterial system gave an overall accuracy of 76% in classifying the state of the artery in five categories and in localizing the exact sites of involvement. The ability of the technique to detect disease when it is present (sensitivity) is 96%; the ability of the technique to recognize normal arterial segments (specificity) is 81%. We found an overall agreement of only 70% between two radiologists independently analyzing and measuring the same films of our study. Their sensitivity was 97% with a specificity of 68%. By using the Duplex scanning method, the number of diagnostic arteriograms can be reduced. The technique allows a better selection of patients who can benefit from PTA or vascular surgery. Another important feature of the technique is that it can be used in follow-up to evaluate the changes that occur in bypass grafts and dilated segments.

REFERENCES

1. Baker, D.W.: Pulsed ultrasonic Doppler flow sensing, IEEE Trans. Sonics Ultrasonics 17:117, 1970.
2. Blackshear, W.M., Jr., Phillips, D.J., and Strandness, D.E., Jr.: Pulsed Doppler assessment of normal human femoral artery velocity patterns, J. Surg. Res. 27:73, 1979.
3. Campbell, W.B., et al.: Physiological interpretation of Doppler shift waveforms: the femorodistal segment in combined disease, Ultrasound Med. Biol. 9(3):265, 1983.
4. Carter, S.A.: Clinical measurements of systolic pressures in limbs with arterial occlusive disease, JAMA 207:1869, 1969.
5. Castaneda-Zuniga, Q., et al.: Hemodynamic assessment of obstructive aortoiliac disease, Am. J. Roentgenol. 127:559, 1976.
6. Charlesworth, D., et al.: Undetected aortoiliac insufficiency: a reason for early failure of saphenous vein bypass grafts for obstruction of the superficial femoral artery, Br. J. Surg. 62:567, 1975.
7. Davis, R.P., Neiman, H.L., and Yao, J.S.T.: Ultrasound scan in diagnosis of peripheral aneurysms, Arch. Surg. 112:55, 1977.
8. Fell, G., et al.: Ultrasonic duplex scanning for disease of the carotid artery, Circulation 64:1191, 1981.
9. Fronek, A., Coel, M., and Bernstein, E.F.: Quantitative ultrasonographic studies of lower extremity flow velocities in health and disease, Circulation 53:957, 1976.
10. Gosling, R.G., and King, D.H.: Continuous wave ultrasound as an alternative and complement to x-rays in vascular examinations. In Reneman, R., editor: Cardiovascular applications of ultrasound, New York, 1974, American Elsevier Publishers, Inc.
11. Heintz, S.E., et al.: Value of arterial pressure measurements in the proximal and distal part of the thigh in arterial occlusive disease, Surg. Gynecol. Obstet. 146:337, 1978.
12. Hokanson, D.E., et al.: Ultrasonic arteriography: a new approach to arterial visualisation, Biomed. Eng. 6:420, 1971.
13. Johnston, K.W., Maruzzo, B.C., and Cobbold, R.S.C.: Errors and artifacts of Doppler flowmeters and their solution, Arch. Surg. 112:135, 1977.
14. Leopold, G.R., Goldberger, L.E., and Bernstein, E.F.: Ultrasonic detection and evaluation of abdominal aortic aneurysms, Surgery 72:939, 1972.
15. Marinelli, M.R., et al.: Noninvasive testing vs. clinical evaluation of arterial disease. A prospective study, JAMA 241:2031, 1979.
16. Neiman, H.L., Lane, R.J., and Woods, C.W.: Ultrasound imaging of peripheral arteries. In Nicolaides, A.N., and Yao, J.S.T., editors: Investigation of vascular disorders, New York, 1981, Churchill Livingstone, Inc.
17. Nimura, Y., et al.: Studies on arterial flow patterns—instantaneous velocity spectrums and their phasic changes—with directional ultrasonic Doppler technique, Br. Heart J. 36:899, 1974.
18. Nippa, J.H., et al.: Phase rotation for separating forward and reverse blood velocity signals, IEEE Trans. Sonics Ultrasonics 22:340, 1975.
19. Phillips, D.J., et al.: Detection of peripheral vascular disease using the Duplex Scanner III, Ultrasound Med. Biol. 63:205, 1980.
20. Roederer, G.O., et al.: The natural history of carotid arterial disease in asymptomatic patients with cervical bruits, Stroke 15:605, 1984.
21. Rushmer, R.F., Baker, D.W., and Stegall, H.F.: Transcutaneous Doppler flow detection as a nondestructive technique, J. Appl. Physiol. 21:554, 1966.
22. Satumora, S.: Study of flow patterns in peripheral arteries by ultrasonics, J. Acoust. Soc. Jpn. 15:151, 1959.
23. Skidmore, R., et al.: Physiological interpretation of Doppler-shift waveforms. III. Clinical results, Ultrasound Med. Biol. 6:227, 1980.
24. Strandness, D.E., Jr.: Waveform analysis in the diagnosis of arteriosclerosis obliterans. In Strandness, D.E., Jr.: Peripheral arterial disease. A physiologic approach, Boston, 1969, Little, Brown & Co.
25. Strandness, D.E., Jr.: Noninvasive arteriography: a new approach for arterial visualization, Am. Surg. 38:494, 1972.
26. Strandness, D.E., Jr.: Noninvasive evaluation of arteriosclerosis: comparison of methods, Arteriosclerosis 3:103, 1983.
27. Strandness, D.E., Jr., McCutcheon, E.P., and Rushmer, R.F.: Application of a transcutaneous Doppler flowmeter in the evaluation of occlusive arterial disease, Surg. Gynecol. Obstet. 122:1039, 1966.
28. Strandness, D.E., Jr., and Sumner, D.S.: Hemodynamics for surgeons, New York, 1975, Grune & Stratton, Inc.
29. Thiele, B.L., et al.: Correlation of arteriographic findings with symptoms in patients with cerebrovascular disease, Neurology 30:1041, 1980.
30. Thiele, B.L., et al.: Pulsed Doppler waveform patterns produced by smooth stenosis in the dog thoracic aorta. In Taylor, D.E.M., and Stevens, A.L., editors: Blood flow. Theory and practice, London, 1983, Academic Press, Inc.
31. Thiele, B.L., et al.: A systematic approach to the assessment of aortoiliac disease, Arch. Surg. 118:477, 1983.
32. Yao, J.S.T., Hobbs, J.T., and Irvine, W.T.: Ankle systolic pressure measurements in arterial disease affecting the lower extremities, Br. J. Surg. 56:676, 1969.

CHAPTER 61

Postoperative screening in peripheral arterial disease

HENRY D. BERKOWITZ

There are multiple causes of femoropopliteal and femorotibial graft failures that occur at specific intervals in the postoperative period. The magnitude of this problem is indicated by the reported incidence of graft failure, which ranges from 3% to 18% during the early (30-day) postoperative period and 24% to 44% in the late (5-year) postoperative period.[5] In a recent summary of 555 femoropopliteal grafts, which reported a 34% overall failure rate, an analysis based on time showed that 15% of the failures occurred early, 65% developed by 1 year, and 79% appeared by the second postoperative year (Fig. 61-1).

Early failures are related to technical factors, including errors in constructing the anastomoses, an inadequate vein, or an inadequate distal vessel. Late failures appear to be more related to intrinsic hyperplastic lesions that develop within grafts near proximal and distal anastomoses and at the site of venous valves (Table 61-1) (Fig. 61-2 to 61-6). These lesions have been found in 11% to 33% of vein grafts[1,7,9,12,13] and approximately 75% appeared within the first postoperative year and 85% by the second postoperative year[1,6,8,12] (Table 61-2).

Progressive arteriosclerotic lesions, proximal and distal to graft anastomoses, are another source of graft failure. These lesions appear after the first year and account for an additional 15% of graft occlusions (Fig. 61-7).[13] Therefore it is essential to monitor the patients carefully during the first 2 postoperative years to diagnose stenotic lesions before they precipitate graft thrombosis. Although long-term graft patency following correction of stenotic lesions in the failing graft is excellent (>80%), poor long-term patency (19% to 37%) is a result of thrombectomy and repair of the failed (occluded) graft except in the immediate postoperative period.[1,3,7,13] Even with the addition of direct intraarterial thrombolytic therapy, immediate salvage rates of occluded grafts are still only 59%, and long-term patency rates are not yet available.[2] Szilagyi[9] showed that graft lesions are progressive and the untreated failing graft will ultimately occlude. Therefore close follow-up and aggressive treatment of these grafts should produce superior long-term patency rates. Sladen[7] demonstrated a 16% increase in overall 5-year patency of 173 femoropopliteal vein grafts after diagnosing and correcting stenotic lesions in 20% of the grafts. Since graft stenosis is more common in femorotibial bypasses, an even greater long-term benefit is to be expected from close surveillance of these grafts.[1]

In contrast to vein grafts, polytetrafluoroethylene (PTFE) grafts occlude precipitously with little advance warning and stenotic lesions are rarely diagnosed before graft thrombosis.[6] The most significant cause of failure is progression of distal arteriosclerotic disease, which has been found in 42% to 64% of occluded PTFE grafts.[6,10] This incidence is much higher than that found with vein grafts and suggests that PTFE may promote accelerated progression of down-stream atherosclerosis.[6] Graft thrombectomy and repair of stenotic lesions by patch graft angioplasty or distal extension grafts results in a 56% late (4-year) patency.[11] This is better than the patency obtained after treating occluded vein grafts, but worse than results achieved with stenotic vein grafts.

Recommended follow-up

"Clinical sensitivity on the part of the patient and surgeon is the key to diagnosis of graft stenosis."[7] Since 85% of graft lesions occur within 2 years of surgery, close surveillance is most important during this time. Follow-up examination

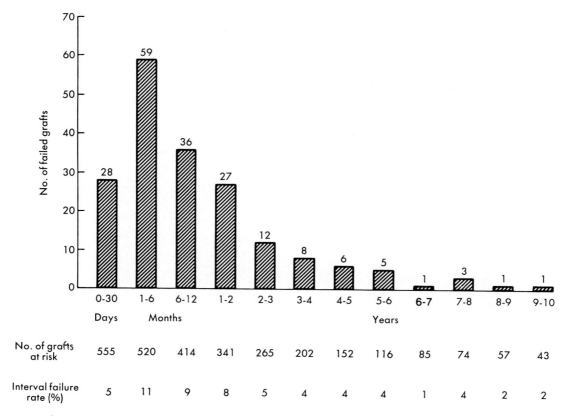

Fig. 61-1. Frequency of graft failure and interval failure rate in follow-up period after femoropopliteal bypass graft procedures. During study 188 grafts failed: 65% within 1 year and 79% by 2 years. (From Brewster, D.C., et al.: Arch. Surg. 118:1044, 1983. Copyright 1983, American Medical Association.)

Table 61-1. Arteriographic localization of vein graft stenosis

Location	No.
Proximal anastomosis	17
Vein	13
Artery	4
Midgraft	10
Fibrotic valve	10
Distal anastomosis	6
Vein	2
Artery	4
TOTAL LESIONS	33
TOTAL GRAFTS	30

From Berkowitz, H.D., et al.: Surgery 90:975, 1981.

should be performed every 3 months during the first 2 years and then at 6-month intervals thereafter. If clinical symptoms, physical examination, or vascular laboratory studies suggest a compromise in graft flow, immediate angiography is indicated. If the suspicion of graft stenosis is weak, repeat follow-up visits should be done at monthly intervals until the possibility of graft stenosis is verified or rejected by repeat noninvasive studies or arteriography.

Patients' responsibility. Patients must be impressed with the need to share in the responsibility for the outcome of their surgery. They are specifically instructed to note changes in walking ability, healing rate of ulcers, or development of new skin lesions, which are all signs of a potentially failing graft and are indications for a prompt reexamination. While it is difficult for patients to monitor their own peripheral pulse, they can usually be taught to feel pulsations in a subcutaneously implanted graft and are instructed to monitor the strength of the pulse at least twice a day and to report any significant decrease in pulse strength.

FAILURE OF CLINICAL SYMPTOMS TO DIAGNOSE ALL GRAFT STENOSES

Although an occluded graft with a return of preoperative symptoms of claudication or rest pain or

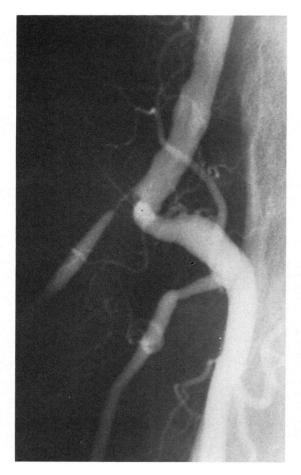

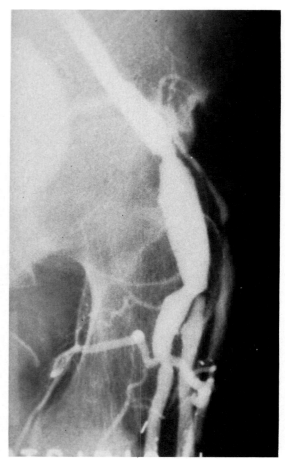

Fig. 61-2. Most common vein graft lesion located just distal to proximal anastomosis of femoropopliteal bypass graft. (From Berkowitz, H.D. et al.: Surgery 90:973, 1981.)

Fig. 61-3. Long irregular proximal vein graft stenosis in femorotibial graft. (From Berkowitz, H.D., et al.: Surgery 90:973, 1981.)

Table 61-2. Interval from surgery to appearance of vein graft lesion

Interval	No.
3 months	2
3-6 months	13
6-12 months*	8
12-24 months†	2
3 years	1
4 years	1
5 years	1
8 years‡	2
TOTAL	30

From Berkowitz, H.D., et al.: Surgery 90:975, 1981.
*77% appeared before 12 months.
†83% appeared before 24 months.
‡17% appeared within 3 to 8 years.

a cold, mottled, pulseless extremity is readily apparent, these symptoms and signs may be subtle or totally absent in the failing graft. A significant graft stenosis may be missed when the opposite extremity limits the patient's activity or a patient's general infirmity prevents sufficient exercise to induce symptoms. This is especially true if the opposite leg has been amputated or has severe peripheral vascular disease. Also, symptoms may not appear early in the leg initially revascularized for claudication because of difficulty in appreciating subtle decreases in walking ability that may come on slowly. Symptoms may even be absent after limb salvage operations when an ischemic lesion has already healed and the limb remains intact and pain free, despite significant graft stenosis or oc-

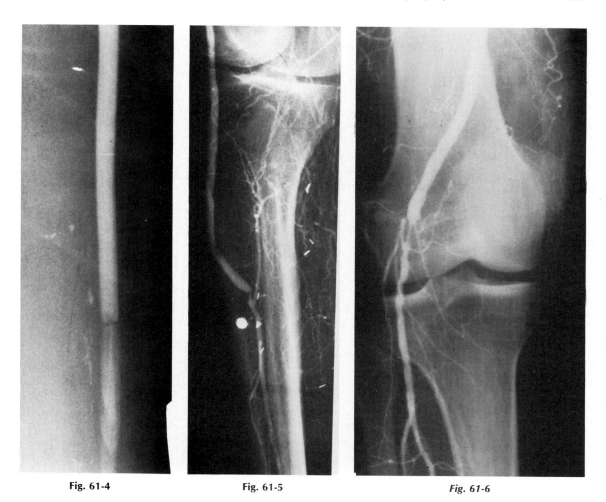

Fig. 61-4   **Fig. 61-5**   *Fig. 61-6*

Fig. 61-4. Stenosis produced by hyperplastic valve in midposition of femoropopliteal graft. (From Berkowitz, H.D., et al.: Surgery 90:974, 1981.)

Fig. 61-5. Stenosis just proximal to distal anastomosis of femoro-anterior tibial graft. (From Berkowitz, H.D., et al.: Surgery 90:975, 1981.)

Fig. 61-6. Stenosis at distal anastomosis involving artery and vein in femoropopliteal graft. (From Berkowitz, H.D., et al.: Surgery 90:975, 1981.)

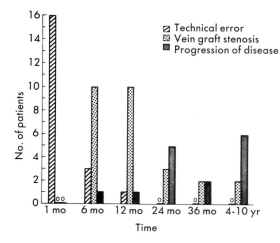

Fig. 61-7. Temporal distribution of three most frequent causes of failure in femoropopliteal graft. During first month 80% of technical errors occurred. Vein graft stenoses developed most often during first year; progression of artherosclerotic lesions was mainly responsible for failure after 1 year. (From Whittemore, A.D., et al.: Ann. Surg. 193:35, 1981.)

clusion. The most important part of the follow-up physical examination is to determine the presence or absence of graft or distal pulses. This can often be difficult if the leg is edematous or the patient is obese. While total absence of a previously strong peripheral pulse is often apparent, it may be difficult to appreciate a gradual decrease in pulse strength from one follow-up examination to another. Even in a subcutaneous graft, excellent pulses are often noted in grafts with significant graft stenoses because short stenotic lesions do not produce a significant pressure drop until at least 75% of the cross-sectional area is occluded. The graft pulse will also remain strong if a distal stenosis is present that may even accentuate the proximal pulse with a *water hammer* quality up to the point of total occlusion. A valuable examination for graft stenosis was described by Dowell and Sladen.[4] Temporary occlusion of the graft by manual palpation (easiest in a subcutaneously implanted graft) in the thigh or popliteal fossa will make the bruit associated with the graft stenosis disappear, whereas a bruit involving a native vessel will either diminish or be unchanged (Fig. 61-8). Since proximal anastomotic areas are the most common sites for graft stenosis, this is a valuable finding on physical examination, although it is not accurate enough to estimate the degree of stenosis and has been less valuable in diagnosing distal lesions.

Vascular laboratory studies in diagnosis

Vascular laboratory measurements consisting of segmental thigh, calf, and ankle segmental pressures, as well as pulse volume recorder (PVR) contour and amplitude, give excellent objective measurements that can readily be compared from one follow-up examination to another and may be the most valuable use of these studies. Baseline values are recorded in the postoperative period. The most reliable measurements are obtained approximately 7 to 10 days postoperatively. Earlier measurements are often inaccurate because of residual spasm, incisional pain, or the presence of edema. Even at 1 week, artifacts may make some measurements questionable. In these cases, repeat studies obtained after the first postoperative month invariably show higher values than those obtained earlier and are used for baseline values. Exercise measurements have not been used routinely in our postoperative follow-up, although they have the theoretic advantage of picking up milder degrees of stenosis.[7] A fall in ankle pressure index ≥ 0.2 from

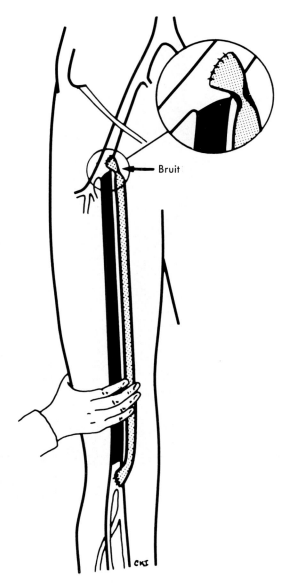

Fig. 61-8. Temporary occlusion of vein graft in thigh or popliteal fossa silences bruit of vein graft stenosis. (From Sladen, V.G., and Gilmore, J.C.: Am. J. Surg. 141:552, 1981.)

the postoperative value or previous follow-up examination is considered significant and suggests graft stenosis or occlusion.

PVR amplitude and curve contour are qualitatively graded according to predetermined standards (Fig. 61-9). Graft stenosis is diagnosed when the calf PVR amplitude is not at least 1 unit greater than the peak height of the thigh tracing or when the PVR curve contour changes from an "A" or "B" waveform to a "C" or "D" type. Although

Waveform analysis

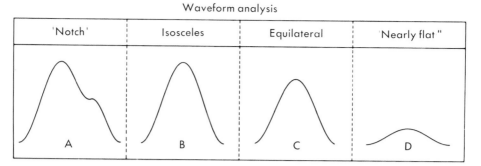

Fig. 61-9. Characterization of PVR amplitude and curve contour. **A,** Good amplitude (>10 mm) with the presence of a dicrotic notch. **B,** Good amplitude (>10 mm) with loss of dicrotic notch but general configuration of isosceles triangle (both side limbs equal and greater than base). **C,** Loss of amplitude and flattening of waveforms approaching configuration of equilateral triangle (all three sides equal). **D,** Poor amplitude (< 10 mm) with distinctly rounded (versus peaked) waveforms that may approach straight line.

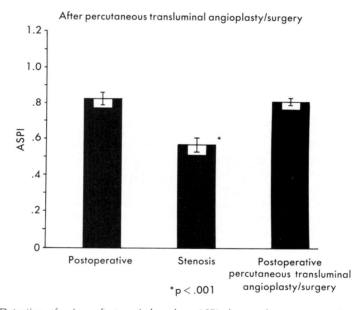

Fig. 61-10. Detection of vein graft stenosis based on ASPI changes from postoperative values. (From Berkowitz, H.D., et al.: Surgery 90:972, 1981.)

most stenoses will be diagnosed by changes in ankle systolic pressure indices (ASPI), PVR amplitude and contour are confirmatory and diagnostic when calcified vessels make segmental pressure measurements invalid or the pressure measurements are equivocal.

Comparison of vascular laboratory studies with clinical examination. Fig. 61-10 shows ankle systolic pressure indices (ASPI) obtained in 30 femoropopliteal and femorotibial grafts that developed graft stenosis. The mean postoperative ASPI was 0.83 ± 0.02 (SEM) and fell to 0.57 ± 0.04 when

graft stenosis was diagnosed (p < .001 paired comparison t-test). The mean decrement in ankle pressures from the postoperative values was 0.25 ± 0.03. ASPI fell ≤ 0.1 in only three limbs, and graft stenosis was diagnosed on the basis of clinical symptoms and PVR in these cases.

Patients' symptoms and clinical examinations were also analyzed and graded according to whether the patients were asymptomatic or had return of claudication or rest pain and whether distal or graft pulses were present or absent (Table 61-3). It is noteworthy that 57% of limbs had normal distal

Table 61-3. Diagnosis of vein graft stenosis based on clinical evaluation of distal pulses in 30 vein graft stenoses

	Distal pulse	
Symptoms	Normal (%)	Decrement/absent (%)
None	40	17
Claudication or rest pain	17	26
TOTAL	57	43

From Berkowitz, H.D., et al.: Surgery 90:972, 1981.

pulses and 57% were also asymptomatic. Forty percent were both asymptomatic and had normal distal pulses. Graft stenosis would not have been detected in this group without the vascular laboratory data. It is also probable that the vascular laboratory studies contributed to the diagnosis by reinforcing the need for repeat arteriography in the 17% of patients with symptoms but normal distal pulses and the 17% who were asymptomatic but had decreased distal pulses.

Management of graft stenosis

Once graft stenosis is suspected, arteriography should be performed promptly. Often it will be necessary to use extreme oblique views to visualize stenoses in and around the proximal anastomoses. Digital subtraction angiography (DSA) does not yet have the resolution to consistently show the discrete stenotic lesions that characterize many graft lesions.

Repair of graft stenosis can usually be accomplished by patch angioplasty or short-segment interposition graft.[7,13] Many of these lesions can also be treated nonoperatively with percutaneous transluminal angioplasty. This has allowed us to treat 24 of 30 graft stenoses without surgery.[1] Since most stenoses can be treated either with a simple operation or nonoperatively by using percutaneous transluminal angioplasty, the effort expended to detect the failing graft by frequent, meticulous follow-up examinations will be rewarded by improved late graft patency rates.

SUMMARY

Graft stenosis in femoropopliteal and femorotibial grafts occurs with a frequency of 11% to 33% and is probably most responsible for the late (5-year) failure rates of 24% to 44%. Within 2 years 85% of these lesions occur and are amenable to diagnosis before graft occlusion if careful monitoring of symptoms, pulses, and segmental limb pressures are obtained by patient, physician, and vascular laboratory. Correction of stenotic lesions before graft occlusion can be expected to give late patency rates of >80% and to improve overall graft patency rates significantly.

REFERENCES

1. Berkowitz, H.D., et al.: Value of routine vascular laboratory studies to identify vein graft stenosis, Surgery 90:971, 1981.
2. Berkowitz, H.D., Hargrove, W.C.III, and Roberts, B.R.: Thrombolytic therapy. In Kempczinski, R.F., editor: Management of the ischemic lower extremity, Chicago, Year Book Medical Publisher. (In press.)
3. Brewster, D.C., et al.: Femoropopliteal graft failures: clinical consequences and success of secondary reconstructions, Arch. Surg. 118:1043, 1983.
4. Dowell, A.J., and Sladen, J.G.: The bruit-occlusion test: a clinical method for localizing arterial stenosis, Br. J. Surg. 65:201, 1978.
5. Mehta, S.: A statistical summary of the results of femoropopliteal bypass surgery. Technical Note 175, Newark, 1980, W.L. Gore & Associates, Inc.
6. O'Donnell, T.F., et al.: Correlation of operative findings with angiographic and noninvasive hemodynamic factors associated with failure of polytetrafluoroethylene grafts, J. Vasc. Surg. 1:136, 1984.
7. Sladen, J.G., and Gilmore, J.L.: Vein graft stenosis: characteristics and effect of treatment, Am. J. Surg. 141:549, 1981.
8. Strandness, E.D.: Exercise ankle pressure measurements in arterial disease. In Bernstein, E.F., editor: Noninvasive diagnostic techniques in vascular disease, ed. 2, St. Louis, 1982, The C. V. Mosby Co.
9. Szilagyi, D.E., et al.: Biologic fate of autogenous vein implants as arterial substitutes, Ann. Surg. 178:232, 1973.
10. Veith, F.J., Gupta, S., and Daly, V.: Management of early and late thrombosis of expanded polytetrafluoroethylene (PTFE) femoropopliteal bypass grafts: favorable prognosis with appropriate reoperation, Surgery 87:581, 1980.
11. Veith, F.J., et al.: Progress in limb salvage by reconstructive arterial surgery combined with new or improved adjunctive procedures, Ann. Surg. 194:386, 1981.
12. Whitney, D.G., Kahn, E.M., and Estes, J.W.: Valvular occlusion of the arterialized saphenous vein, Ann. Surg. 42:879, 1976.
13. Whittemore, A.D., et al.: Secondary femoropopliteal reconstruction, Ann. Surg. 193:35, 1981.

CHAPTER 62

Problems in the evaluation of hand ischemia

OLAV THULESIUS

Hand ischemia may be the result of a variety of pathologic disturbances, among which—in contrast to the situation in the lower extremities—obliterative arteriosclerosis is not the main one. The most common type of digital ischemia is called *Raynaud's phenomenon* and consists of periods of reduced or totally obliterated digital circulation. The characteristic features of this disturbance are skin color changes, critical closing, and changes in sensory function.

Skin color changes. Raynaud's phenomenon is characterized by episodic color changes of the cutaneous circulation, involving three colors: blue, white, and red. Thomas Lewis[17] in 1929 was the first to devote much time to exploring the meaning of these color changes, which he correlated with levels of blood flow and local temperature. He actually introduced a color scale from V to VX, coding bright red to cyanotic violet. Color changes indicative of arterial closure occur after a certain minimal time (approximately 5 minutes); then cyanosis appears. Therefore shorter attacks may pass unrecognized. Cyanosis at low temperature (low tissue oxygen consumption) is an indication of stagnent or totally occluded flow. White skin color indicates a loss of blood from the subcutaneous venous plexus, which occurs after movements of digits "milk out" blood from the veins, with valves preventing backflow and arterial closure preventing refilling from the arterial side.

Critical closing. During Raynaud's attack there is a complete cessation of digital blood flow, which has been observed with the aid of capillary microscopy with direct visualization of blood flow in the nailfold capillaries.[2] Closure of the large digital arteries and not the arterioles seems quite reasonable, since reversible spastic closure of digital arteries can be demonstrated with arteriography be-

fore and after vasodilating procedures. Closure of subcapillary veins is an indication of decreased inflow and low capillary pressure together with passive emptying (the result of movement). There is no evidence of venous spasm, since there is a slow rise of capillary pressure when venous congestion is artificially imposed during the period of spasm and a rapid fall at the release of such congestion.[15]

The existence of a "critical closing phenomenon" as proposed by Burton[3] and Burton and Yamada[4] in 1951 has been debated.[1] Raynaud's phenomenon, however, with spastic closure of digital arteries seems to be an example of this phenomenon, which may also occur in normal individuals in conditions of high vasomotor tone.[14] The closing and, more specifically, the opening pressures (that is, the blood pressure at which blood starts flowing again after a fall in perfusion pressure) depend on such variables as vasomotor tone and the rheologic parameter to "yield stress" ratio (the pressure required to induce motion of blood) (Fig. 62-1).

Sensory functions. A characteristic aspect of Raynaud's attack is the appearance of paresthesias (numbness) and loss of tactile perception. As already shown by Lewis and Pochin[19] in 1938, asphyxia of an extremity leads to almost simultaneous defects of touch, temperature sense, and rapidly conducted pain. The loss of slowly conducted pain comes later and is preceeded by an exaggerated pain response. Recognition of position resulting from passive movement fails early and at the same time as touch and deep pressure.

CAUSES OF RAYNAUD'S ATTACK

There are essentially five different mechanisms that may be involved in the pathogenesis of Raynaud's phenomenon: (1) vasoconstrictor tone, (2)

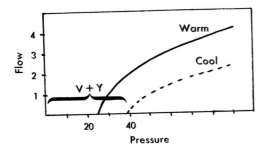

Fig. 62-1. Pressure-flow relationship in human forearm. Intercept on pressure axis is result of critical vascular closing (V) and yield stress (Y). (From Burton, A., and Yamada, S.: J. Appl. Physiol. 4:329, 1951.)

vascular abnormality, (3) blood pressure, (4) viscosity, and (5) immunologic factors.

Vasoconstrictor tone. The importance of an increased neurogenic vasoconstrictor tone was the original concept of Maurice Raynaud in 1862 when he described the disease that bears his name. This viewpoint can be explained by the fact that knowledge of small vessel disease such as obliterative arteriosclerosis was nonexistent at that time, and Raynaud found it sufficient to state that he could not find emboli in major arteries. The concept of an increased vasomotor tone as causative goes back to the enormous impact of Claude Bernard's description of vasomotor nerves in 1850. Since that time it was mainly the school of Thomas Lewis that questioned the importance of an augmented vasomotor tone. Their experiments with nerve blockade and sympathectomy showed that the elimination of vasomotor tone has only marginal effects on Raynaud's phenomenon and does not support the original hypothesis of an abnormally enhanced sympathetic tone as being causative.[17]

Recent studies on the adrenergic innervation of digital arteries using catecholamine fluorescence marking demonstrated that sympathetic innervation is confined to the medial-adventitial border just external to the smooth muscle layer. The specific fluorescence was, however, only found in young individuals, presumably an indication that sympathetic innervation is reduced with advancing age.[9]

Vascular abnormality. The heritage of Thomas Lewis' extensive studies on Raynaud's disease is the *local fault theory,* a concept that still stands but has not been clarified as yet. The simplest cause of such a vascular abnormality could be the special geometric features of the digital arteries, which are characterized by a prominent medial coat, giving a wall/lumen ratio of nearly 2:1, a feature other-

wise characteristic of sphincter vessels elsewhere in the body. This means that a small increase in vasoconstrictor tone is associated with a more pronounced luminal narrowing and markedly reduced blood flow, in comparison to thin-walled vessels, a situation first encountered in essential hypertension associated with medial hypertrophy.[8] Lewis himself thought of the possibility of undue wall hypertrophy or arterial occlusions in patients with Raynaud's phenomenon. His study to find such changes was equivocal, however.[18] Only in advanced cases with trophic changes of the fingertips was it possible to demonstrate marked thickening of the intima and complete closure; otherwise a thick tunica media and a slight intimal hyperplasia were present both in patients with Raynaud's disease and in normal individuals of similar age. The importance of wall abnormality has recently been documented by a delayed opening of digital arteries subsequent to tourniquet compression in patients with diabetes in which there is evidence of excessive accumulation of glycoproteins. These cases, however, did not have Raynaud's phenomenon, presumably because of a deficient vasomotor innervation.[30] In addition to vascular changes of the media and adventitia, the integrity of the endothelium is of critical importance, since it modulates smooth muscle tone through the generation of prostacyclin and other as yet undefined vasodilator substances.[34]

Blood pressure. Blood pressure must be an important factor in the critical closure of digital arteries, and it is surprising that this variable has been neglected for a considerable time. It is, however, reasonable to assume that arterial blood pressure plays an important role in the development of Raynaud's phenomenon. Evidence for this assumption are the following observations: Raynaud's phenomenon is seldom encountered in the toes, which can be because the vascular distending pressure usually is much higher in the lower extremities as a result of their added hydrostatic pressure. The natural history of primary Raynaud's phenomenon is characterized by a high percentage of spontaneous cures as shown by the follow-up study of Gifford and Hines[10] from the Mayo Clinic. This may be the result of the age-related increase in blood pressure. Moreover, primary Raynaud's phenomenon usually develops at an early age, at which time arterial blood pressure is much lower. Vasospastic phenomena with cyanosis seem to be frequent in cases with primary arterial hypotension and idiopathic hypokinetic circulation, such as *an-*

orexia nervosa.[7] I was able to show that arterial blood pressure in a population of patients with primary Raynaud's phenomenon is lower than in a comparable population of similar age.[28] Low blood pressure also plays a definite role in patients with secondary Raynaud's phenomenon caused by proximal occlusion of the supplying arteries, since this creates a territory of local hypotension distal to the arterial block.

Viscosity. During recent years several clinical studies have appeared reporting a slightly increased viscosity at low shear rates and low temperature.[11,32] The reason for the increased viscosity in some patients with idiopathic Raynaud's phenomenon has been reported to be an increased fibrinogen concentration,[13] whereas in others it may be the presence of cold agglutinins or cryoglobulins.[26] The importance of an increased viscosity is, however, not yet settled, and a recent publication did not show any significant elevation of whole blood viscosity in patients with cold-induced Raynaud's phenomenon.[12] Our experience points in the same direction. It cannot be denied that an increased blood viscosity must be an important *additional* factor in the production of vasospastic attacks, although enhanced viscosity is not the answer to the whole problem.

Immunologic factors. Immunologic factors, as encountered in collagen disease, play an important part in the development of secondary Raynaud's phenomenon. Many collagen disorders are associated with a variety of proliferative intimal lesions. The best known definitive association between a collagen disease and Raynaud's phenomenon is scleroderma, a disease mostly affecting women, a feature in common also with idiopathic Raynaud's phenomenon. The importance of immunologic factors in the pathogenesis of Raynaud's phenomenon is still most controversial, and the incidence of autoimmune disease varies between 4% and 81%.[10,24]

Cold provocation

Of the many pathogenetic factors discussed during the past 100 years there is only one that has never been challenged: the importance of cold as a decisive factor in the provocation of a typical Raynaud's attack. Cold can act in many ways to induce a slowing and ultimate stoppage of the digital circulation.

Blood flow in patients with Raynaud's phenomenon tends to be slightly lower than normal. This has been shown frequently both in patients with primary Raynaud's phenomenon[6,23] and in patients with scleroderma.[5] This means that local temperature in the digits is reduced and the fingers are more easily chilled. A chain of events is started at a critical temperature of 20° C[20] with increased viscosity, increased local vascular tone, and finally closure or subclosure of the main digital arteries.

The increased vascular tone resulting from cooling has been difficult to explain, since the contractile response of aortic smooth muscle is attenuated at lower temperatures, but the *duration* of the process, and hence relaxation, is prolonged.[31] On exposure to cold there is a marked increase in the affinity of the postjunctional α-adrenoreceptors for norepinephrine. This results in a constriction of the blood vessels and cessation of blood flow to the distal tissue. As the temperature of the tissues rapidly falls, sympathetic nerve conduction is interrupted and vasodilation occurs as a result of the cessation of norepinephrine release and the depressor action of cold on the contractile machinery. The resultant return of blood flow rewarms the tissue; nerve conduction is reestablished; and this, combined with the increased affinity of the α-adrenoreceptors for norepinephrine, leads to renewed vasoconstriction. Repetition of this cycle could result in the hunting reaction.[25]

The "catch" phenomenon. Experiments in our laboratory with gradual ischemic cooling of digits and measurements of reopening pressure with the technique of the Copenhagen group[14] have shown that closure is often preceded by a decreased opening pressure, and in patients with hypertension and diabetes (that is, two vascular diseases with medial hypertrophy), opening pressure is reduced.[30] I would explain this mechanism by the decrease of wall compliance (increased stiffness) caused by cold. This change in the wall property creates resistance to further deformation once the vessel has been closed by contraction or mechanical compression. Therefore I observed a retarded opening by intravascular forces (blood pressure) and hence a delayed recurrence of pulse. Evidence for this explanation is the fact that the closing phenomenon seen with the finger tourniquet is not observed with a proximal occlusion cuff at the hand.

The locally prolonged contraction process can be called a "catch" process (although the mechanism is not similar to the one seen in mollusks). Such a catch process should occur more easily in hypertrophied muscle and muscle with an abnormal content of viscous substances (such as probably seen in scleroderma and uremia).[16] Local compression, such as that connected with clutching of the hand, may be an additional factor setting forth the "catch" process in the cold stiff artery with increased tone.

EVALUATION OF DIGITAL ISCHEMIA

The main problem in the evaluation of digital ischemia without trophic changes of the finger-tips is related to the episodic nature of vascular spasm that must be provoked in the laboratory situation. Moreover, the excellent collateral circulation to the fingers with dual digital arteries makes it difficult to diagnose complete occlusions of one artery if the other is still patent.[35]

Our diagnostic evaluation includes the following steps:

1. Questionnaire
2. Digital plethysmography
3. Digital cold provocation
4. Doppler sonography

Questionnaire

The questionnaire essentially contains most of the relevant risk factors and gives a quantitative evaluation of the symptoms using a finger chart that can be applied to outline the extent of digital involvement. This information has been used to construct scores related to the severity of the disease. It could be shown that the "Raynaud score"

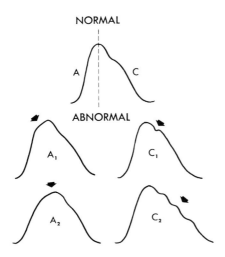

Fig. 62-2. Different types of pulse-wave abnormalities. Pulse curve can be divided into anacrotic *(A)* and catacrotic parts *(C)*. Vasospastic abnormalities are A_1 (slanting type), C_1 (high dicrotic notch), and C_2 (fragmented downstroke and low amplitude). Type A_2 is most commonly seen abnormality in occlusive arterial disease. (From Thulesius, O.: Acta Chir. Scand. Suppl. 465:53, 1976.)

is significantly correlated with the parameter derived from the cold provocation test.[29] The questionnaire has been adapted from Taylor and Pelmear.[27]

Digital plethysmography

Digital plethysmography is used to record volume pulses of the most distal parts of the finger pulp circulation. Either volumetric or photoelectric systems can be applied.[31] The diagnosis is based on the presence of abnormalities of the pulse waves and gross amplitude differences between individual fingers or hands before and after cooling and local heating. The degree of abnormality on cooling reflects vasospastic disorders (types A_1, C_1, and C_2); a delayed upstroke and crest time greater than 0.12 seconds after heating indicates obstructive vascular lesions as seen in secondary Raynaud's phenomenon (Fig. 62-2).

Digital cold provocation

The best reproducible technique of cold provocation is the test introduced by Nielsen and Lassen.[21] The principle is based on the determination of the reopening pressure (RP) of digital arteries locally cooled and subjected to arterial occlusion by a miniature cuff. Cooling and occlusion are performed using a plastic cuff (24 × 80 mm) with a double inlet for perfusion with water of different temperatures. Systolic digital blood pressure is determined indirectly using a mercury-in-Silastic strain gauge applied to the fingertip. Strain gauge signals (fingertip volume) and cuff pressure are recorded simultaneously on a six-channel Siemens-Elema Mingograph. Arterial occluding pressure is maintained at 240 mm Hg, and subsequent deflation is programmed in a standardized fashion, with a pressure drop of 5 mm/second. To ensure thorough cooling, the circulation to the finger is temporarily occluded by a cuff applied to the proximal phalanx of the same finger. Control pressures of an uncooled finger are recorded simultaneously from the contralateral, noncooled hand. The temperatures on both the cooled and the control finger are measured by thermocouples. Moreover, the blood pressure on the control arm is recorded (Fig. 62-3).

The cooled finger is measured at 35°, 30°, 25°, 20°, 15°, 10°, and 5° C. Normally, digital pressure after successive cooling does not fall more than 5% of the control level. The method is quite sensitive and has good reproducibility in patients with established Raynaud's phenomenon (Fig. 62-4).

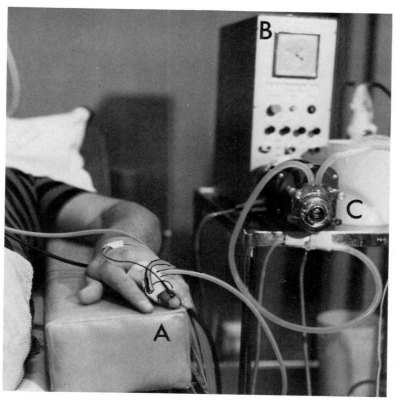

Fig. 62-3. Digital cooling test, Strain gauge at fingertip. *A,* Two proximal tourniquets are for arterial occlusion and perfusion with cold water from roller pump *(C). B,* Pressure source.

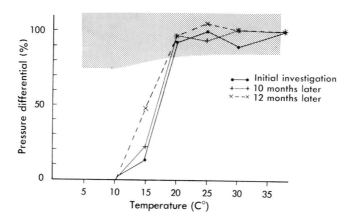

Fig. 62-4. Example of critical closing at 10° C in patient with Raynaud's phenomenon. Repeat measurements were performed 10 and 12 months later. Stippled area is normal range (mean value ± 2 standard deviations).

Doppler sonography

To test the patency of the digital arteries, the flow profile can be traced out to the fingertips after local direct heating in a water bath at 42° C. A finger chart is used to outline the patent arteries.[22]

REFERENCES

1. Ashton, H.: Critical closing pressure in human peripheral vascular beds, Clin. Sci. Mol. Med. 22:79, 1962.
2. Bollinger, A., Mahler, F., and Meyer, B.: Velocity patterns in nailfold capillaries in normal men and cases with Raynaud's disease and acrocyanosis, Bibl. Anat. 16:142, 1977.
3. Burton, A.: On the physical equilibrium of small blood vessels, Am. J. Physiol. 164:319, 1951.
4. Burton, A., and Yamada, S.: Relation between blood pressure and flow in the human forearm, J. Appl. Physiol. 4:329, 1951.
5. Coffman, J.D., and Cohen, A.: Total and capillary fingertip blood flow in Raynaud's phenomenon, N. Engl. J. Med. 285:259, 1971.
6. Downey, J.A., and Frewin, D.B.: The effect of cold on blood flow in the hand of patients with Raynaud's phenomenon, Clin. Sci. Mol. Med. 44:279, 1973.
7. Fohlin, L.: Body composition, cardiovascular and renal function in adolescent patients with anorexia nervosa, Acta Paediatr. Scand. Suppl. 268:1, 1977.
8. Folkow, B., Grimby, G., and Thulesius, O.: Adaptive structural changes of the vascular walls in hypertension and their relation to the control of peripheral resistance, Acta Physiol. Scand. 44:255, 1958.
9. Frewin, D.B., Waterson, J.G., and Whelan, R.F.: Catecholamine fluorescence in primate digital arteries, Aust. J. Exp. Biol. Med. Sci. 49:421, 1971.
10. Gifford, R.W., and Hines, E.A.: Raynaud's disease among women and girls, Circulation 16:1012, 1957.
11. Goyle, K.B., and Dormandy, J.A.: Abnormal blood viscosity in Raynaud's phenomenon, Lancet 1:1317, 1976.
12. Jahnsen, T., Skovborg, F., and Nielsen, S.L.: Blood viscosity and local response to cold in primary Raynaud's phenomenon, Lancet 2:1001, 1977.
13. Jarrett, P.E.M., Morland, M., and Browse, N.L.: Treatment of Raynaud's phenomenon by fibrinolytic enhancement, Br. Med. J. 2:523, 1978.
14. Krähenbühl, B., Nielsen, S.L., and Lassen, N.A.: Closure of digital arteries in high vascular tone states as demonstrated by measurement of systolic blood pressure in the fingers, Scand. J. Clin. Lab. Invest. 37:71, 1977.
15. Landis, E.: Micro-injection studies of capillary blood pressure in Raynaud's disease, Heart 15:247, 1930.
16. Läppchen, J., et al.: Raynaud-Phänomen bei Dialysepatienten, Dtsch. Med. Wochenschr. 102:521, 1977.
17. Lewis, T.: Experiments relating to the peripheral mechanism involved in spasmodic arrest of the circulation in the fingers, a variety of Raynaud's disease, Heart 15:7, 1929.
18. Lewis, T.: The pathological changes in the arteries supplying the fingers in warm-handed people and in cases of so-called Raynaud's disease, Clin. Sci. Mol. Med. 3:287, 1938.
19. Lewis, T., and Pochin, E.E.: Effects of asphyxia and pressure on sensory nerves, Clin. Sci. Mol. Med. 3:141, 1938.
20. Lottenbach, K.: Vasomotor tone and vascular response to local cold in primary Raynaud's disease, Angiology 22:4, 1971.
21. Nielsen, S.L., and Lassen, N.A.: Measurement of digital blood pressure after local cooling, J. Appl. Physiol. 43:907, 1977.
22. O'Reilly, M.J.G., et al.: Controlled trial of plasma exchange in treatment of Raynaud's syndrome, Br. Med. J. 1:1113, 1979.
23. Peacock, J.H.: The effect of changes in local temperature on the blood flows of the normal hand, primary Raynaud's disease and primary acrocyanosis, Clin. Sci. Mol. Med. 19:505, 1960.
24. Porter, J.M., et al.: The clinical significance of Raynaud's syndrome, Surgery 80:756, 1976.
25. Shepherd, J.T., Rusch, N.J., and Vanhoutte, P.M.: Effect of cold on the blood vessel wall, Gen. Pharmacol. 14:61, 1983.
26. Strandness, D.E., Jr.: Peripheral arterial disease, London, 1969, J. & A. Churchill, Ltd.
27. Taylor, W., and Pelmear, P.L.: Raynaud's phenomenon of occupational origin, Acta Chir. Scand. Suppl. 465:27, 1976.
28. Thulesius, O.: Methods for the evaluation of peripheral vascular function in the upper extremities, Acta Chir. Scand. Suppl. 465:53, 1976.
29. Thulesius, O., and Nielsen, S.L.: Digital circulation in cases with Raynaud-phenomena and treatment with Hydergin, proceedings of the eleventh International Congress on Angiology, Prague, 1978. (Abstract.)
30. Thulesius, O., Valmin, K., and Todoreskov, R.: Response of finger systolic blood pressure to cold provocation in cases with hypertension and diabetes, Clin. Physiol. 2:513, 1982.
31. Thulesius, O., Borgnis, F., and Dvorak, T.: Analysis of photoplethysmographic pulse curves with electronic derivation, Scand. J. Clin. Lab. Invest. Suppl. 128:159, 1973.
32. Tietjen, G.W., et al.: Blood viscosity, plasma proteins and Raynaud syndrome, Arch. Surg. 110:1343, 1975.
33. Todo, N., Hojo, M., and Sakae, K.: Modification by temperature of the response of isolated aorta to stimulatory agents and transmural stimulation, Blood Vessels 13:210, 1976.
34. Vanhoutte, P., and De Mey, J.: Control of vascular smooth muscle function by the endothelial cells, Gen. Pharmacol. 14:39, 1983.
35. Zweifler, A.: Detection of occlusive arterial disease in the hand in patients with Raynaud's phenomenon, Acta Chir. Scand. Suppl. 465:48, 1976.

CHAPTER 63

Finger systolic pressures in upper extremity testing for cold sensitivity (Raynaud's phenomenon)

STEEN L. NIELSEN and NIELS A. LASSEN

Digital vasoconstriction occurs during exposure to cold to preserve body temperature. This physiologic response is governed by the sympathetic nervous system and possibly by local effects of cold. Shortly after Bernard described the sympathetic nervous system, an exaggerated response of the digital circulation to cold or emotional stress was described by Raynaud in 1862.[19] The appearance of demarcated pallor or cyanosis of the digits on exposure to cold, with numbness and sometimes followed by hyperemic throbbing during rewarming,[1] has therefore been named Raynaud's phenomenon. The conditions provoking Raynaud's phenomenon were thoroughly investigated by Lewis and Pickering,[10] who concluded that the pallor was caused by complete *closure* of the digital arteries combined with venular constriction.

In recent reviews the phenomenon has been described in many different diseases.[2] Pathophysiologically the abnormal reaction of the digital arteries can be the result of exaggerated, cold-induced constriction of the smooth muscle cells in an otherwise normal artery (primary Raynaud's phenomenon). The closure can also be caused by stenotic processes in normally constricting digital arteries, or the impairment of the digital circulation can be association with an abnormally high blood viscosity (secondary Raynaud's phenomenon). This chapter summarizes an effective diagnostic test revealing the existence of digital arterial occlusive disease and cold hypersensitivity. The test is based on measurements of digital arterial blood pressure at normal hand and body temperature, respectively, after local digital cooling combined with body cooling. Our goal has been to find a reproducible test not only to detect Raynaud's phe-

nomenon, but also to quantitate the severity of the symptoms.

DETECTION OF ARTERIAL OBLITERATION IN DIGITS

For many years arteriography has been considered the best method to demonstrate arterial stenoses or occlusions. Elaborate techniques have been developed for hand arteriography.[17] Noninvasive determination of the hemodynamic importance of arterial stenoses in warm and cold hands is, however, more desirable.[20] Because measurements of digital blood flow and pulse amplitudes vary greatly in normal individuals and are difficult to standardize, we have developed methods to measure finger systolic pressure with a cuff technique. The detectors used are strain gauges, photocells, and Doppler ultrasound probes.

Techniques

All our subjects are investigated while they are supine with the hands at heart level after 15 minutes of rest at room temperature (22° to 24° C). The blood pressure cuffs for digits are made of plastic encircled by an easily attachable Velcro band.[6] The cuffs are routinely placed on the proximal phalanx of the thumb and on the intermediate phalanx of the other digits after powdering the skin with talc. Arm blood pressure measurements are taken via auscultation on both upper arms, and the finger cuffs are inflated to a suprasystolic pressure. During continuous deflation of the cuffs the appearance of the systolic signal is recorded by a mercury-in-Silastic strain gauge or a photocell placed on the pulp. Since the DC signal is used, the pulp must be squeezed for venous blood before cuff inflation.

Results

Cuff width. The intraarterial pressure in digits at thermoneutral conditions is very close to the brachial arterial pressure. This has been established by direct puncture of digital arteries and using "bladderfree" cuffs on the digits.[7] We therefore decided to adjust the width of the digit cuffs to give an indirectly recorded pressure in the digits of normal subjects as close as possible to the brachial pressure and with the smallest possible variation in repeated measurements. This was accomplished with a 24 mm wide cuff on digits I through IV, but on the fifth finger a 20 mm wide cuff was necessary.[6]

Reproducibility. The variation of indirectly recorded finger systolic blood pressures is small under the standard conditions just defined. The difference between recordings on different days shows a coefficient of variation of 5% and 10% for the arm and finger systolic pressures, respectively.[11]

Arm to finger and interphalangeal pressure gradients. The difference between arm and finger systolic pressures was small in three studies using the same technique, varying from slightly positive to slightly negative values.[4,6,11] This is attributable to differences in hand blood flow in the normal subjects investigated. Vasodilation of the hand with a high blood flow in the arteries of the forearm can increase the arm to finger pressure gradient by 20 mm Hg.[7] This is also the case with arteriovenous fistulas for hemodialysis on the forearm (proximal steal).

In each patient the expected finger systolic pressure can be calculated from the measured arm blood pressure, using the lower 95% limit of arm-to-finger systolic pressure gradient for normal subjects. The arm-to-finger pressure gradient is normally below 25 mm Hg, highest in older subjects.[4]

It should be noticed that there is a small but significant pressure gradient from the proximal to the intermediate phalanx on digits II through V using the same cuff at both sites.

Comparison with arteriographic findings. Table 63-1 summarizes a comparison between finger systolic pressure measurements and arteriographic findings.[4] Because of the rich collateral supply on the digits, ischemic signs first appear only with severe occlusive disease, that is, both volar digital arteries have to be occluded. Therefore a decreased finger systolic pressure in a patient indicates severe occlusive arterial disease on that finger. Because of the high reproducibility of the method, measurements can be repeated to follow the development of arterial occlusions. However, it cannot detect less severe obliterative disease if one digital artery is patent. Such cases might be traced by Doppler measurements, but controlled comparisons with arteriographic findings have not been made.

Pressure measurement during arterial compression. Finger systolic pressure can be measured during compression of the arteries at the wrist.[5] This can provide information regarding arterial dominance in the hand and constitutes a quantitation of Allen's compression test. On the thumb, for instance, the pressure declines less than 22% (95% confidence limit) after compression of the radial artery at the wrist. A greater reduction in pressure indicates an insufficient collateral supply in the hand.

Blood pressure in single arteries can be recorded with Doppler ultrasound, placing the cuff at the wrist or on the proximal phalanx. This method can provide the systolic pressure in the radial, ulnar, and volar digital arteries. Recordings on the digits might, however, be difficult, especially during va-

Table 63-1. Finger systolic pressures predicting arteriographic findings or finger ischemia

Disorder	Finger systolic pressure		Sensitivity* (%)	Specificity† (%)
	Decreased	**Normal**		
Arteriographic occlusion of digital arteries				
2	173	30	85	
0 or 1	0	184		100
Chronic ischemic skin lesions of fingers				
Yes	132	3	98	
No	41	211		84

*Positivity in disease.
†Negativity in health.

soconstriction, and pressures below 50 mm Hg cannot be measured.

Conclusion

Measurement of finger systolic pressure on the intermediate phalanx is easy to perform for suspected arterial obstruction of the digits. All digits should be investigated. The method has a good reproducibility, and with regard to severe obstructive disease on the digits, the specificity is high. The method is not capable of finding minor stenotic processes in the digital arteries. Whether these can be traced with Doppler ultrasound remains to be determined.

FINGER SYSTOLIC PRESSURE DURING COOLING

Measuring capillary pressure in the skin of patients with Raynaud's phenomenon, Landis[9] found that the pressure decreased almost to zero during an attack. This finding was taken to support the concept that complete closure of digital arteries during cold-provoked constriction causes Raynaud's phenomenon. However, capillary pressure is not recordable in clinical practice, and a measurement of zero pressure in the capillaries at the nailfold might be caused by arteriolar constriction alone. Lewis[10] proposed to detect digital arterial constriction by recording the pulse volume of the fingers. However, the pulse volume decreases both with arteriolar and with arterial constriction, and the pulse amplitude disappears at pressures below 30 to 50 mm Hg. For these reasons, pulse volume recordings are unable to distinguish arterial from arteriolar constriction on the digit or arterial closure from severe vasoconstriction.

We measure finger systolic pressure at the intermediate phalanx after cooling to detect arterial constriction.[7] A prerequisite for recording systolic blood pressure with a cuff technique is that the artery compressed by the cuff is a perfectly collapsible tube, that is, a tube that collapses when the transmural pressure is zero. It will then reopen when the pressure in the cuff during deflation reaches the intra-arterial pressure just proximal to the cuff. If, however, the artery compressed by the cuff is constricted (by cooling, for instance), then a transmural pressure gradient is necessary to overcome the increase in arterial tone and to reopen the vessel. The pressure gradient will therefore be observable as a decrease in the finger systolic pressure recording. The difference between the indirectly

recorded pressure before and after cooling therefore is the reopening pressure of the artery on the midphalanx that opens first. If Raynaud's phenomenon with closure of the arteries is provoked by the cooling procedure, the intraarterial pressure cannot reopen the artery compressed by the cuff and no pressure signal will be recordable until the constriction is released.

Techniques

Finger systolic pressure measurement and finger cooling can be performed with the same cuff (Fig. 63-1). It is necessary to cool the intermediate phalanx for 5 minutes with a suprasystolic pressure in the cuff to obtain a well-defined arterial temperature.[12] This time allows the temperature in the tissue around the artery to equilibrate with the skin temperature, which can be controlled by the water perfusing the cuff. The finger systolic pressure is measured after thermoequilibration. A decrease in pressure indicated that the digital artery has a positive reopening pressure. The degree of arterial constriction either can be expressed as the pressure decrease in millimeters of mercury, or the pressure in the cooled finger can be taken in percent of the pressure at 30° C.[11] A correction for changes in the perfusion pressure of the hand is based on simultaneous measurement of the systolic pressure in a reference finger on the same hand.

To provoke Raynaud's phenomenon, wherein a zero pressure should be recorded after finger cooling, it may be necessary to increase the sympathetic discharge to the digits by total body cooling.[11] This

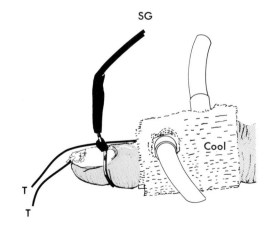

Fig. 63-1. Double-inlet plastic cuff encircled by Velcro band is placed on middle phalanx for both cooling and pressure recording. Strain gauge (SG) records pulse volume on outer phalanx, and thermistors (T) record temperature.

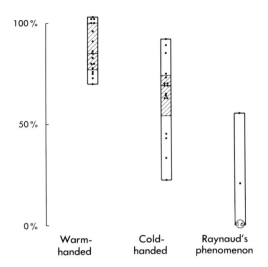

Fig. 63-2. Finger systolic pressure *(FSP)* measured after 5 minutes of cooling with water at 15° C is expressed as percentage of pressure at 30° C. Three groups of young women were investigated after 10 minutes of body cooling. Median and quartiles are presented.

can easily be performed with a cooling blanket with water perfusion capabilities covering the body. Our standard procedure is to perfuse the blanket with cold tap water (10° to 15° C) for 10 to 20 minutes. Finger cooling is started when the subject has a sensation of chilling (Fig. 63-2). It is also possible to study the local effect of finger cooling during body warming but this principle has not yet gained general acceptance.

Results

Cuff width. The reopening pressure of the digital arteries is calculated as the difference between pressures (Fig. 63-3) or as percent (Fig. 63-4) of the control normothermic value. It is therefore not as important to standardize the cuff width for this as it is for the systolic pressure measurements. The double inlet cuff for finger cooling was manufactured to be broader than that used for finger pressure measurements (30 as opposed to 24 mm Hg) to provide a greater contact surface for cooling. No significant difference in finger systolic pressures was noted when these two cuffs were compared on the same hand simultaneously.[11]

Reproducibility. The variation in pressure measurement at finger temperatures of 30° and 15° C in normal subjects is about the same as for measurements with conventional cuffs. The coefficient of variation is about 10%.[11]

Normal reaction to cooling. Three different groups of people were investigated: 17 young, indoor-working women; 20 young, indoor-working men; and 20 young to middle-aged, outdoor-working men.[14] When the body had been cooled for about 15 minutes, finger systolic pressure at a finger temperature of 15° C was found to be above 68% of the finger pressure at 30° C (given as the 95% lower limit). If the body was not cooled, a somewhat higher pressure was found in the finger cooled to 15° C, which indicates that the sympathetic discharge to the digits influences the arterial tone in normal individuals. Cooling of the digits to lower temperatures (10° and 5° C) decreased the finger systolic pressure; thus the digital arterial reaction to cooling is a graded response.

Abnormal reaction to cooling. In women complaining of cold hands, but without Raynaud's phenomenon, the finger arteries showed a more pronounced reaction than in women with warm hands (Fig. 63-2). The women were investigated after body cooling at a finger temperature of 15° C. Surprisingly, we found a completely normal reaction to finger cooling in women with acrocyanosis. In women with primary Raynaud's phenomenon, the pressure in the finger cooled to 15° C dropped from normal values to zero in nearly all subjects (Fig. 63-2). This indicates that closure of the digital arteries does occur during finger cooling in these patients and that the arteries have a prolonged reopening time during rewarming. Finger cooling can be continued to 10° or 5° C in patients not showing closure at 15° C. Repetition of the procedure may obviate release of an attack.

A well-defined group of patients with secondary Raynaud's phenomenon can be found among workers using vibrating hand tools. In both stone cutters and forest workers complaining of white, dead fingers in the cold, an abnormality in the digital arteries could be demonstrated by a pressure drop to zero at a temperature of 15° or 6° C after 20 minutes of body cooling.[16] Even more interesting was the finding of an abnormal reaction to cooling in workers without complaints, but using vibrating hand tools. This indicates that the method may be used not only to diagnose the disease, but also to follow the development of this occupational hazard. Vibration damage of the arteries in the hand occurs at different sites depending on the tool and its application. Therefore proximal stenotic arteries may be overlooked by cooling and pressure recording on a finger.

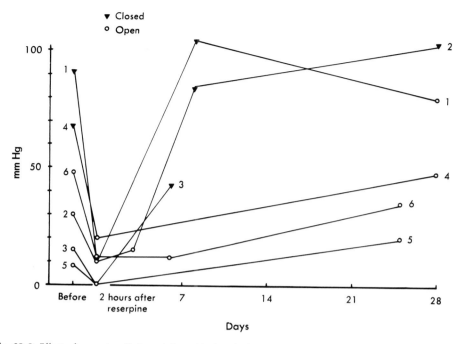

Fig. 63-3. Effect of reserpine (0.5 mg injected in brachial artery) on arterial constriction elicited by finger cooling to 20° C in six young women with severe Raynaud's phenomenon in their digits. Decreased constriction shortly after treatment correlated closely with clinical benefit.

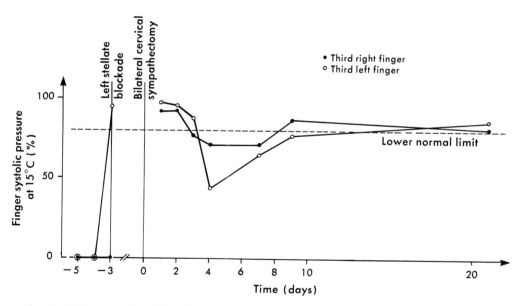

Fig. 63-4. Effect of stellate blockade and cervical sympathectomy in young woman with Raynaud's phenomenon. Finger systolic pressure at 15° C is expressed as percentage of control value at 30° C and measured after 10 minutes of total body cooling. Note normalization after blockade and hyperreactivity in degranulation period after sympathectomy.

Control of treatment. It is well known that most of the therapeutic attempts to relieve patients with Raynaud's phenomenon are directed at blocking the sympathetic nervous discharge and local effects of catecholamines on the digital arteries. Such attempts can be monitored by the method presented. Examples are given in Figs. 63-3 and 63-4.[13] Reserpine given intraarterially depletes the sympathetic vesicles of norepinephrine. For a few days after an injection of 0.5 mg reserpine in the brachial artery the abnormal reaction to cooling was prevented in the six young women with severe Raynaud's phenomenon (Fig. 63-3).

SUMMARY

Measurement of finger systolic pressure during combined finger and body cooling is a reliable method to record Raynaud's phenomenon. Some of the other methods listed in Table 63-2 do not have these advantages. The methods all differ in their provocation procedures, and detection of Raynaud's phenomenon is either indirect or qualitative in all. Because of the small groups investigated, there is only a minor difference in the efficiency of the different tests, which is calculated assuming a prevalence of Raynaud's phenomenon of 25%. The advantages of the finger systolic recording to detect vasoconstriction of the digital arteries are the precision of the method and the ability to record pressures down to zero. There is a need for standardization in provoking and detecting Raynaud's phenomenon. The method described in this chapter fulfills all the demands of precision and reproducibility and is efficient in routine clinical application. However, it may be difficult to detect an increased cold sensitivity caused by stenotic arteries in the palm or by neurologic disorders.

Table 63-2. Comparison of cold provocation tests to diagnose Raynaud's phenomenon

Cooling procedure											
Local		Room		Body					Predictive value if positive‡	Efficiency	Reference
°C	min	°C	min	°C	min	Detection	Sensitivity* (%)	Specificity† (%)			
Hand 4	1	6	—	—	—	Raynaud's phenomenon	78	100	62	85	15
Hand 15	10	15	—	—	—	Raynaud's phenomenon	50	100	40	62	8
Hand 15	10	15	—	—	—	Temperature delay	64	94	44	72	8
Hand 15	20	10	40	—	—	Raynaud's phenomenon	100	100	100	100	3
Arm 15	15	20	Shoulder —	15	15	Raynaud's phenomenon	44	100	40	58	18
Finger 0	1	24	30	—	—	Temperature delay	91	97	91	95	17
Finger 30-10	5	22	—	15	10	Finger systolic pressure	86	100	70	90	16
Finger 30-5	3	22	—	—	—	Pulse amplitude	50	100	40	62	21

*Positivity with Raynaud's phenomenon.
†Negativity without Raynaud's phenomenon.
‡Based on assumption of 25% prevalence of Raynaud's phenomenon.

REFERENCES

1. Allen, E.A., and Brown, G.E.: Raynaud's disease: a critical review of minimal requisites for diagnosis, Am. J. Med. Sci. 183:187, 1932.
2. Coffman, J.D., and Davies, W.T.: Vasospastic diseases: a review, Prog. Cardiovasc. Dis. 18:123, 1975.
3. Hellstrøm, B., and Myhre, K.: A comparison of some methods of diagnosing Raynaud phenomena of occupational origin, Br. J. Ind. Med. 28:272, 1971.
4. Hirai, M.: Arterial insufficiency of the hand evaluated by digital blood pressure and arteriographic findings, Circulation 58:902, 1978.
5. Hirai, M.: Digital blood pressure and arteriographic findings under selective compression of the radial and ulnar arteries, Angiology 31:21, 1980.
6. Hirai, M., Nielsen, S.L., and Lassen, N.A.: Blood pressure measurements of all five fingers by strain-gauge plethysmography, Scand. J. Clin. Lab. Invest. 36:627, 1976.
7. Krähenbühl, B., Nielsen, S.L., and Lassen, N.A.: Closure of digital arteries in high vascular tone states as demonstrated by measurement of systolic blood pressure in the fingers, Scand. J. Clin. Lab. Invest. 37:71, 1977.
8. Kylin, B., et al.: Hälso- och miljö undersökning bland skogsarbetere. A I rapport 5, Stockholm, 1968, Arbejdsmedicinska institutet.
9. Landis, E.M.: Micro-injection studies of capillary blood pressure in Raynaud's disease, Heart 15:247, 1928.
10. Lewis, T., and Pickering, G.W.: Observations upon maladies in which the blood supply to the digits ceases intermittently or permanently, and upon bilateral gangrene of digits. Observations relevant to so-called Raynaud's disease, Clin. Sci. Mol. Med. 1:327, 1934.
11. Nielsen, S.L.: Raynaud phenomena and finger systolic pressure during cooling, Scand. J. Clin. Lab. Invest. 38:765, 1978.
12. Nielsen, S.L., and Lassen, N.A.: Measurement of digital blood pressure after local cooling, J. Appl. Physiol. 43:907, 1977.
13. Nielsen, S.L., Olsen, N., and Henriksen, O.: Cold hypersensitivity after sympathectomy for Raynaud's disease, Scand. J. Thorac. Cardiovasc. Surg. 14:109, 1980.
14. Nielsen, S.L., Sørensen, C.L., and Olsen, L.N.: Thermostated measurement of systolic blood pressure on cooled fingers, Scand. J. Clin. Lab. Invest. 40:683, 1980.
15. Okada, A., et al.: Studies on the diagnosis and pathogenesis of Raynaud's phenomenon of occupational origin, Br. J. Ind. Med. 28:353, 1971.
16. Olsen, N., Nielsen, S.L., and Voss, P.: Cold response of digital arteries in chain saw operators, Br. J. Ind. Med. 39:82, 1982.
17. Porter, J.M., et al.: The diagnosis and treatment of Raynaud's phenomenon, Surgery 77:11, 1975.
18. Pyykkö, I.: The prevalence and symptoms of traumatic vasospastic disease among lumberjacks in Finland. A field study, Work Environ. Health 11:118, 1974.
19. Raynaud, M.: De l'asphyxie locale et de la gangréne symmetrique des extremités, Paris, 1862, Leclerc.
20. Sumner, D.S.: Raynaud's disease and Raynaud's phenomenon. In Strandness, D.E., and Sumner, D.S., editors: Hemodynamics for surgeons, New York, 1975, Grune & Stratton, Inc.
21. Wouda, A.A.: Raynaud's phenomenon, Acta Med. Scand. 201:519, 1977.

CHAPTER 64

Noninvasive evaluation of abdominal aortic aneurysms by ultrasonic imaging and computed tomography scanning

EUGENE F. BERNSTEIN, RONALD D. HARRIS, and GEORGE R. LEOPOLD

Aneurysm of the abdominal aorta is a common and dangerous manifestation of diffuse atherosclerosis, which increases in frequency after the sixth decade of life. The presence of an abdominal aortic aneurysm is most commonly first identified by the patient, who discovers a palpable pulsatile abdominal mass or mild abdominal discomfort. In about one fourth of the cases, however, the lesion is entirely asymptomatic and detected on routine physical examination; by abdominal x-ray, ultrasound, or computed tomography (CT) examination; at laparotomy for some other indication; or at postmortem examination.

Accurate confirmation of a clinical diagnosis of aneurysm made on the basis of physical examination or plain x-ray films alone is important, since a few patients have other lesions responsible for these findings, including overlying retroperitoneal or other visceral masses. For these reasons, to avoid unnecessary surgery, independent objective confirmation of the diagnosis is appropriate.

More detailed information concerning the size and configuration of the aneurysm increases the data base from which a decision for operation must be made. Both ultrasonic imaging and CT scanning have proven extremely useful in this regard.

Conventional contrast, digital subtraction, and isotope angiography have also been advocated in the diagnosis and characterization of abdominal aortic aneurysms. All angiographic studies define only the inner lumen of the aneurysm, which may provide grossly inaccurate data regarding size. Conventional contrast angiography is clearly invasive, requires hospitalization, has a small but definite complication rate, and is quite expensive. For this reason, it is our feeling that aortography should not be performed as a *diagnostic* procedure for abdominal aneurysms, but rather as a *preoperative* investigation, once surgery has been definitely decided on.[34,44] The purpose of the angiogram is to further delineate the anatomy of the paraaneurysmal structures, with particular emphasis on renal artery involvement or stenosis, multiple renal arteries, visceral artery lesions, and other vascular anomalies. In our view, therefore, angiography is a complementary procedure to ultrasound or CT scanning. Digital subtraction angiography (DSA) may well prove to be the ideal method for obtaining the additional information desired.[52]

THE PLAIN X-RAY FILM

Both anteroposterior (AP) and lateral views of the abdomen may demonstrate calcification in the wall of an abdominal aneurysm and therefore be diagnostic of its presence and indicative of its size. However, only 55% to 85% of patients with abdominal aneurysms have such calcification.[23] Further, in the AP view, the right wall of the aneurysm generally overlies the vertebral column and therefore does not always permit an accurate estimate of the transverse diameter of the lesion. In addition, such films may not reveal that the calcified left aortic wall is simply a portion of a tortuous aorta and not an aneurysmal one. In contrast, the lateral abdominal x-ray film is clearly diagnostic when positive and does provide a reasonably accurate estimate of aneurysm size. Unfortunately, particularly in the smaller aneurysms where size is more critical in evaluating the need for surgery, calcification is often absent.

ROLE OF ULTRASOUND AND CT SCANNING

In view of the limitations of the physical examination and conventional radiographs and the fact that both aortography and radionuclide aortic scans document only the lumen size and do not indicate the thickness of laminated clot and atheromatous material or other wall dimensions, other noninvasive and accurate means of diagnosis and sizing of abdominal aneurysms are important. Both ultrasound and CT scanning fulfill these requirements and permit routine documentation of the presence or absence of an abdominal aneurysm, an accurate depiction of its configuration and location, and good estimates of aneurysm size.

Until 1977 gray-scale echography was the most reliable tool for the evaluation and detection of abdominal aortic aneurysms. However, with the introduction of CT body scanning, it also has been recognized as a valuable radiographic diagnostic tool.

Applications of CT scanning and echography in the investigation of the aorta in both normal and pathologic states are quite similar. The two methods are equally accurate in identifying those patients with an aneurysm and properly diagnosing conditions wherein clinical suspicion of aneurysm is raised but aortic ectasia and tortuosity, an overlying abdominal mass, or a normal aorta in an asthenic person is found. Both techniques are safe, fast, noninvasive, and easily performed on an outpatient basis, and their fine detail also provides added information about other structures important to the surgeon at the time of operation. Details of the technical requirements for obtaining high-quality studies with both of these modalities and of the relative differences in information obtained by the two techniques form the basis of this chapter.

Ultrasound techniques

The use of a reflected beam of ultrasound to identify and characterize clinical pathologic conditions has been developed during the past two decades. In 1961 Donald and Brown first demonstrated an intraabdominal aortic aneurysm with ultrasound.[14] Further development of this methodology has involved the use of the A-mode scan, B-mode scan, B-mode real time, and M-mode ultrasound modalities. In each of these techniques a crystal is oscillated by electrical energy, producing

sound at frequencies exceeding 2 million cycles/sec, with each burst of ultrasound lasting approximately 1 microsecond. This ultrasonic beam is directed at the tissues to be studied and is reflected when it contacts any change in tissue density or tissue interface with a different acoustic impedance. The reflected waves then may be displayed on an oscilloscopic screen in a variety of ways.

In the A-mode presentation the reflected echoes are demonstrated as vertical deflections from a horizontal baseline. The spaces between the deflections represent the time for the echo to travel to the target and return to the receiver (Fig. 64-1). Knowing the velocity of sound in human tissues permits accurately converting this time delay into a depth scale in the direction of the sound beam. However, the A-mode scan is rarely used today in aneurysm studies.

By moving the transducer in a plane of section and representing echoes on the oscilloscope in accordance with the transducer position, a two-dimensional impression of the interior of the body may be obtained by what is referred to as B-mode scanning, or ultrasonic scanning (Fig. 64-2). This

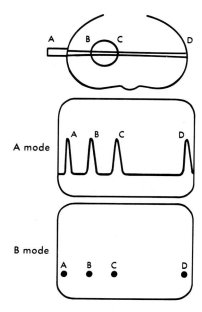

Fig. 64-1. Scheme of A-mode echography, which represents each reflecting surface as spike on oscilloscope, height of which is proportional to acoustic density difference between two materials at interface. In B-mode each such interface between different layers is represented as dot, brightness of which is proportional to density difference. It is comparable to looking down onto top of A-mode spikes. Each of these techniques provides one-dimensional output of distance between layers traversed by sound beam.

procedure usually involves the manual movement of a single transducer to fill in the picture of a particular body section.[17,18,33,35,43]

Early efforts with ultrasound in the diagnosis of abdominal aortic aneurysms involved the use of both A and B modes by Goldberg et al.[19] and Segal et al.[51] in 1966. In a subsequent study Evans et al.[5] first used B-mode scanning to demonstrate a three-dimensional picture of the aneurysm. In 1970 Leopold[36] pointed out the advantages of combining the A-mode and B-mode scan techniques, using

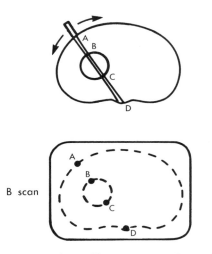

Fig. 64-2. B-scan is obtained by rotating B-mode transducer to obtain many B-mode reflections and storing them on oscilloscope screen. This permits building up detailed two-dimensional image in any plane or section.

the B-mode scan to identify and characterize the shape of the aneurysm, particularly in the longitudinal echogram, with follow-up identification of the maximum diameters in both anteroposterior (AP) and transverse planes with the A-mode technique (Figs. 64-3 to 64-7). Accuracy in sizing aneurysms using the combined technique approached 3 mm. Our current experience with this approach exceeds 700 cases at the University of California, San Diego, and we have increasingly more confidence in the sensitivity and accuracy of the method.[2,4,5,34,38]

Accuracy of B-mode ultrasound. Earlier studies of abdominal aneurysms with ultrasound, involving both A-mode and B-mode investigations to obtain three-dimensional data and accurate sizing, demonstrated the ability of the technique to adequately visualize such lesions in a routine manner. The first published correlation of the diagnostic capability of ultrasound with surgery, in 1971, indicated that B-mode scanning accurately diagnosed 79 of 80 cases of abdominal aneurysms, with one false positive in a patient with a paraaortic lymph node enlargement.[45] More recently, Maloney et al.[39] compared AP and lateral x-ray films with B-mode ultrasound images and found B-mode ultrasound accurately made the diagnosis and permitted size measurements in each instance. Further, the ultrasonic estimates of size averaged within 4 mm of the surgical measurement, far closer than the plain x-ray films. In addition, a study from the

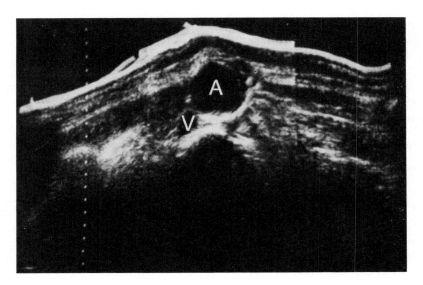

Fig. 64-3. B-scan echogram in transverse plane demonstrating abdominal aortic aneurysm *(A)* and inferior vena cava *(V).* Row of dots represents 1 cm scale.

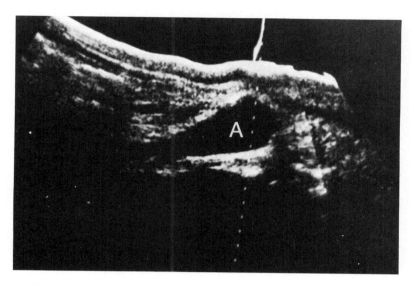

Fig. 64-4. Sagittal plane B-scan echo through abdominal aortic aneurysm *(A)* with sizing scale.

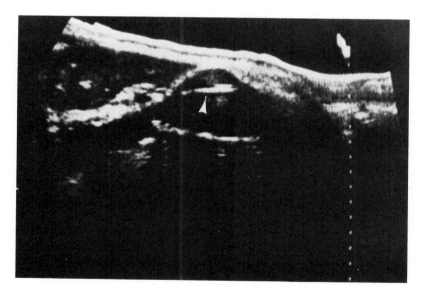

Fig. 64-5. Sagittal plane demonstration of large abdominal aortic aneurysm with thrombus (arrow) within lumen.

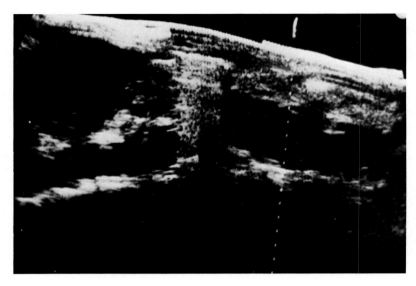

Fig. 64-6. Sagittal plane through large and tortuous abdominal aortic aneurysm, which leaves plane of echogram in center of study as it extends to patient's left beyond plane of examination.

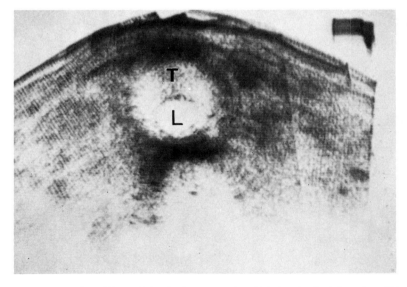

Fig. 64-7. Transverse section of large abdominal aneurysm in which intraluminal thrombus *(T)* is circumferential and lumen *(L)* is of normal size. Such lesion might well appear normal on aortography.

Cleveland Clinic demonstrated that B-mode ultrasound measurements were identical with operative measurements in 34% of the patients and within 0.5 cm in 75%.[31]

Finally, the reproducibility of B-mode ultrasound measurements has been demonstrated in our own experience, in which over 100 patients have been followed with repeated studies for up to 10 years, rather than operated on, because they represented poor-risk patients with small asymptomatic lesions.[2,3,5] Studies performed at 3-month intervals rarely vary by more than 2 or 3 mm and produce such consistent data that aneurysm growth rates can be accurately defined.

Other important advantages of ultrasound imaging include the ability to perform longitudinal reconstructions, which are helpful in differentiating tortuous aortas from those with small aneurysms and in measuring the AP diameter. In addition, the ability of real-time B-mode scanning to identify areas of aortic pulsation that are particularly prominent may permit selecting those lesions with an area of localized weakness prone to early rupture. However, data regarding this possibility are not available yet.

CT operating principles

The patient is placed on a couch that passes through an aperture in the scanner gantry. Around the aperture is either an array of highly sensitive x-ray detectors that are in precise alignment with the x-ray tube or single detectors that rotate. The x-ray beam is tightly collimated into a shape that matches the configuration of the detectors. As the beam passes through the anatomic structures, the intensity of the beam is altered by tissue absorption in the beam's path. The detectors convert this information into electric signals, which are precisely digitized for each sampling interval or until the scan is completed. The patient is then repositioned and another scan begun. A complex series of computer calculations defines the precise x-ray absorption value for each specific pixel point within the scanned section. These digital values are stored on a magnetic tape and represent a mathematic picture of the patient's anatomy. The data are then available for video display and can be manipulated for optimal evaluation and reproduction. The newest generation of scanners complete a scan in 2 to 5 seconds and have a skin surface radiation dose as low as 0.1 to 0.45 rad/section, depending on the manufacturer.

CT techniques. The approach may be tailored to each individual patient. One standard method is to palpate the maximal part of the abdominal mass and then scan from 3 cm above to 3 cm below this point[1,50] at 1 cm intervals. The patient is then given intravenous radiographic contrast material either by a bolus injection of 50 to 100 ml of a high iodine content substance (Renografin 76) or by an infusion of 300 ml of 25% to 30% of a meglumine diatrizoate solution (Reno-N-Dip 30%). Scans are then repeated following the contrast medium injection[28-30]

Another technique involves scanning from the xyphoid to below the umbilicus at 1 cm intervals to gain information about other intraabdominal organs, the proximal aorta, and the iliac arteries. Contrast material is then administered and the scans repeated, occasionally overlapping at 1 cm intervals to gain information about the patency of renal and visceral vessels. The renal status can also be determined after the administration of contrast material, particularly to identify problems of excretion and possible obstruction. If necessary, a primary contrast examination may be performed, especially in an emergency situation. After the contrast material is injected, the aorta itself, the aortic lumen, and thrombus within the aneurysm are clearly defined. The procedure without, and then with, contrast material takes about 60 minutes. A contrast scan alone takes 30 to 40 minutes to complete.

Evaluation of aneurysms by CT. In the early experience with CT, scans were done without IV contrast material, and although aneurysms could be recognized, the wall of the aorta was indistinguishable from the lumen unless the wall was calcified. Thrombi were indistinguishable from the blood in the lumen. The time involved in obtaining these early scans was 4 minutes, and the radiation dose approximated 8 rad to the skin.[1]

With newer scanners, especially with the 2-second scan time, the aortic diameter is easily measured even if not calcified, and the measurements correlate well with those obtained at surgery.[10,20,26] Vertebral body erosions associated with aneurysms are easily identified, and aneurysms may be distinguished from other intraabdominal masses or hematomas. CT is also helpful in distinguishing an aneurysm from tortuosity when an aneurysm is suspected by other radiographic or clinical examinations. Additional information gained by CT includes the variation in aortic position from its usual location anterior to and slightly to the left of the

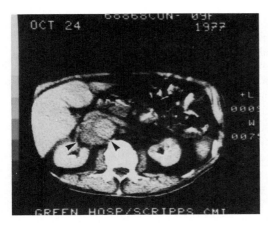

Fig. 64-8. This contrast-enhanced CT scan demonstrates amount of tortuosity that can occur in dilated aorta. Here aorta is seen far to right (arrowheads). Inferior vena cava is sitting on top of aorta, with renal veins stretched to gain access to it. CT scans are read with patient's right on viewer's left, as if looking up at section from patient's feet.

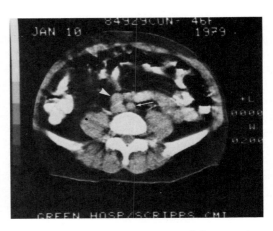

Fig. 64-9. This scan obtained below aortic bifurcation shows aneurysm of right common iliac artery (arrowhead) next to normal left side (small arrow).

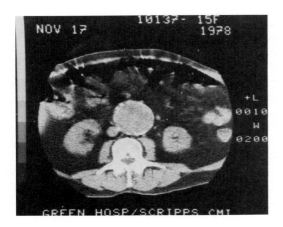

Fig. 64-10. Scan from patient with large amount of body fat shows how fat acts as contrast substance against which organs stand out. Here aneurysm dwarfs inferior vena cava.

vertebral bodies. With increasing tortuosity or dilation, it frequently swings considerably to the right (Fig. 64-8). Commonly, aneurysms of the iliac arteries are also encountered (Fig. 64-9), as well as dilation of the proximal aorta.

CT scanning may be of diagnostic use when ultrasound is not effective because of patient obesity, barium retention, or excessive intestinal gas. Obese patients are easily scanned because the fat acts as a contrast material against which the soft tissues stand out (Fig. 64-10). Gas also does not interfere with the CT scans, especially if the patient

is given an intravenous injection of 1 mg glucagon to inhibit bowel motility. Barium may produce some artifacts and can significantly degrade the scans. One very important source of CT artifacts is the presence of metallic surgical clips, since small detailed areas are obscured by streaks from the metal.

Size estimates of the aneurysms have been within 4 mm of findings at surgery. In a series of 23 patients the measurements were identical in 17 cases.[22,23]

One of the great advances in CT scanning involves the use of intravenous radiographic contrast material (RCM). Examinations with RCM have allowed detailed evaluation of lumen size and the position and amount of thrombus present. Phases of clot formation can be sharply defined regardless of the degree of organization.[10,22] Newer clot close to the lumen is less dense than the older clot close to the outer wall, as confirmed by serial sectioning of pathologic specimens.[22] In most cases the majority of thrombus lies anterior to the lumen, which is in turn located symmetrically somewhat posterior to the center (Fig. 64-11). The clot can also be further evaluated after contrast enhancement. Clot liquefaction or clot dissection can be identified by the presence of an eccentric lumen, often with a tail of contrast material seen close to the lateral wall (Fig. 64-12), indicating dehiscence of the clot.[22] A clot dissection can also be recognized by contrast material appearing around the edge of the clot[50] (Fig. 64-13).

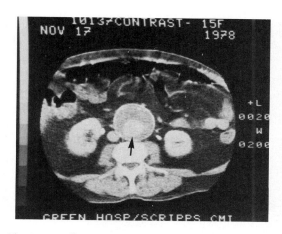

Fig. 64-11. Following intravenous administration of contrast material, lumen of aorta is enhanced by flowing blood (arrow). Thrombus is easily differentiated and is typically located anterior and lateral to lumen.

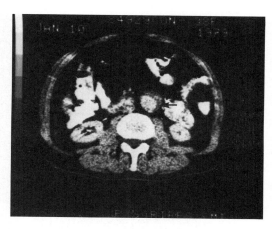

Fig. 64-12. In this contrast-enhanced scan lumen is eccentric (arrow), suggesting clot dissection.

Preoperative visualization of the inferior vena cava position in relation to the aorta and the state of the visceral vessels also can be ascertained. Aneurysmal dilation of the iliac arteries is easily determined, especially following contrast enhancement (Fig. 64-9), and is better seen by CT scanning than by echography. This is important preoperative information when assessing surgical risk and potential technical operative difficulties.[21,22,47] The presence of an inflammatory aneurysm can also be diagnosed with certainty[48] (Fig. 64-14).

Retroperitoneal hematomas secondary to leaking or rupturing aneurysms can be quickly assessed by CT, especially with contrast-enhanced scans. Extravascular blood is a high-density substance that disrupts the normal anatomic configurations in the retroperitoneum on the scans (Fig. 64-15, *A*). After RCM, the clot takes a characteristic lower density than surrounding structures, which normally "blush" with the contrast material (Fig. 64-15, *B*). The hematoma may also have some rim enhancement (Fig. 64-15, *B*) because of an inflammatory response around the hematoma.[10]

A new and important role for CT scanning has been the postoperative evaluation of patients undergoing aneurysmectomy. Repeat scans can follow the resolution of periprosthetic hematomas. Both aortoprosthesis disruption and false aneurysm formation have been diagnosed. There is no need to prepare the bowel in these patients, who often have an attendant paralytic ileus, which would render echo less effective. It also may be possible to

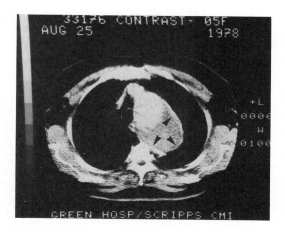

Fig. 64-13. In this patient contrast material is seen around edge of thrombus just beneath wall of aorta (arrowheads). This is sign of clot liquefaction and dehiscence.

distinguish early postoperative changes from those changes resulting from infection, where one of the early signs is the loss of periaortic fat.[6] An exceptional diagnostic finding, however, has been the identification of pockets of gas caused by pyogenic organisms (Fig. 64-16). These gas pockets are usually multiple and characteristically located posterior to the lumen. RCM enhancement demonstrates that these gas pockets are indeed extraluminal.[27,32] In distinction, gas can be found in normal patients up to 10 days after surgery, but the gas is seen anteriorly and is usually a single collection com-

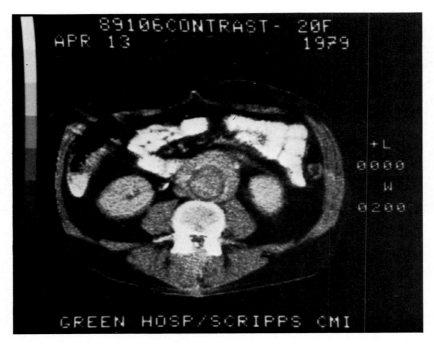

Fig. 64-14. Inflammatory aneurysm is clearly demonstrated with thick mantle of tissue anterior and lateral to aneurysm.

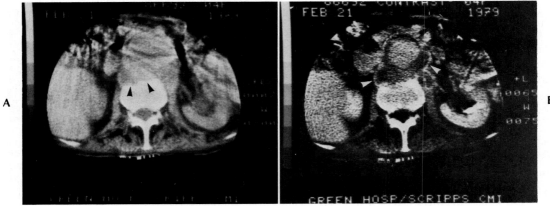

Fig. 64-15. Retroperitoneal hematoma surrounds leaking aortic prosthesis. **A,** High-density blood obscures normal anatomic configurations of aorta and anterior psoas muscle margins. Vertebral body erosions are also noted (arrowheads). Bleeding was a result of aortoprosthetic graft disruption. **B,** Contrast enhancement clearly delineates aortic lumen and limits of periprosthetic hematoma (arrowheads).

pared to the posteriorly located multiple gas bubbles of an abscess.[11,27,32] Inflammatory rim enhancement around a postgraft abscess after contrast injection is also a sign of infection (Fig. 64-17). Aspiration of periaortic fluid under CT guidance may be useful to confirm the diagnosis.[11]

Abdominal aneurysm expansion rates. Serial ultrasound studies have been obtained in 110 poor-risk patients with asymptomatic abdominal aortic aneurysms initially measuring 3.0 cm or greater in the largest transverse diameter. The expansion rates of these patients averaged 0.4 cm/year and are a useful general guideline in predicting the potential of any patient to develop increased aneurysm size and thus aneurysm rupture (Fig. 64-18). Although individual abdominal aneurysms may vary sub-

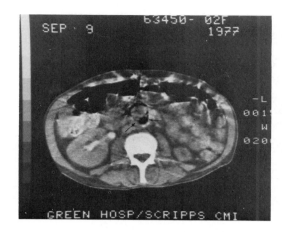

Fig. 64-16. This patient became febrile after aortic graft surgery. Scan shows collections of gas, which appear as black areas posterior to lumen of aorta (arrows). These gas pockets are felt to be pathognomonic for pyogenic infection.

A 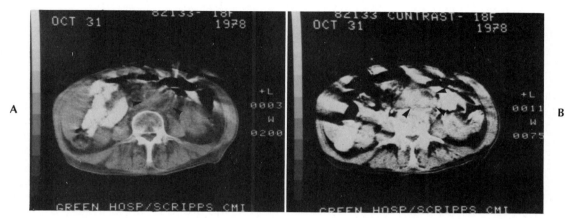 B

Fig. 64-17. This patient became febrile shortly after his aneurysm was resected and aortic wall wrapped over graft. **A,** Scan done without contrast material shows inhomogenous soft tissue densities below graft bifurcation (arrowheads). **B,** Scan after contrast material was injected in this patient demonstrates rim enhancement of wrapped aortic graft (arrowheads). Rim enhancement is also seen with infection, and abscess was found at this site.

stantially from this mean expansion rate and sudden expansion and rupture are always possible, these data have permitted a group of poor-risk patients with small, asymptomatic abdominal aneurysms and a low overall mortality to be followed.

The subsequent outcome of the 110 patients was ascertained with a mean follow-up of almost 4 years. Forty-six patients underwent elective resection because the aneurysm size increased to 6 cm or more or because of the development of symptoms. Thirty-six died from causes unrelated to their unoperated aneurysms, and 22 were still alive at the time of the most recent follow-up. Only 6 patients suffered aneurysm rupture, and, of these, 3 were not operated on electively because of severe incapacitating contraindications, such as hemiplegia and aphasia after cerebral vascular accident (CVA), even though their aneurysms were larger

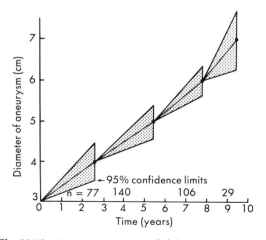

Fig. 64-18. Mean expansion rate of abdominal aortic aneurysm (±95% confidence limit) based on ultrasound data obtained from poor-risk patients observed at least 1 year after diagnosis.

than 6 cm. Two of these 6 patients had failed to continue the serial 3-month examinations and had not been studied for 18 months before rupture. Therefore only 3 of the 110 patients' aneurysms ruptured without warning while under this surveillance. The total mortality of the 110 patients as a result of aneurysm rupture or surgery was 7.5%. It appears that evaluating and following poor-risk patients with small and asymptomatic abdominal aneurysms by serial ultrasonic examinations permits identifying those in whom rupture is likely to occur, by either symptom development or increase in aneurysm size. Thus elective surgery can be done selectively in those patients. On the other hand, over half of the patients can be managed without surgery if they remain symptom free and the aneurysm remains less than 6 cm in size.

Comparative analysis of ultrasound and CT scanning

Echography has been shown to be quite accurate in diagnosing 98.8% to 100% of abdominal aneurysms[9,45,54] and generally correlates within 3 mm of the findings at surgery (Table 64-1).[38] However, in some hands the results have not been as reliable. One study found a consistent underestimation of size in up to 20% of patients by B-mode scans,[9] and another series[41,42] found that the size underestimation ranged from 1.3 to 3.0 cm. These errors may be caused by an increased wall thickness with old organized thrombus, leading to difficulty in acoustically separating the aortic wall from surrounding tissue. Wider discrepancies are present where there was heavy thrombus deposited in the walls of the aneurysm and in obese patients.[16,22] Whether such variations in data are a result of differences in equipment, its application, or skill in interpretation remains unknown at this time.

Ultrasound frequently can detect the presence of thrombus within an aneurysm, although the various phases of clot organization may not be as accurately distinguished as with CT scanning. The clinical importance of these distinctions remains uncertain at this time, however.

The presence of large amounts of interfering intestinal gas is a problem for ultrasound, particularly with paralytic bowel ileus. However, the abdominal aneurysm may push aside overlapping bowel in patients, so that the diagnosis can still be made in these instances. Radiodense contrast material such as barium in the bowel serves as an obstacle to both ultrasound and CT scans. Finally, in some obese patients, body size is too great to permit adequate penetration of the sound beam for an accurate anatomic examination.[46]

Ultrasound is extremely fast, simple, cheap, and usually effective in making the diagnosis. In addition, echography has at least two major advantages over CT scanning in being able to scan in a longitudinal plane and in using energy that is nonionizing. In a comparison between the two techniques in 20 patients, Raskin and Cunningham[49] felt that ultrasound was indeed superior because it was less expensive, was nonionizing, and provided longitudinal scans. Echography was as accurate as CT in determining aneurysm size and in revealing intraluminal thrombus. The limitation of CT to transverse scanning increases the likelihood of falsely diagnosing an aneurysm as an ectatic aorta swings transversely. However, whether such errors are common is still not known.

Table 64-1. Comparison of ultrasound and CT scan in the diagnosis and assessment of abdominal aortic aneurysms

Area compared	Ultrasound	CT scan
Examining modality	High-frequency sound (1-20 mHz)	X rays
Radiation dose (skin surface)/slice	None	0.1-2 rad
Time for examination	10-60 minutes	30-60 minutes
Cost of examination	$75-$150	$75-$300
Dependence on technician skill	Great	Modest
Dependence on interpretive skill	Great	Straightforward
Limitations	Intestinal gas, obesity; cannot distinguish clot from flowing blood	Motion; only cross-sectional images generally available now; metallic clips distort image
Accuracy in aneurysm diagnosis	Excellent	Excellent
Accuracy in aneurysm size estimates	± 3 mm	Not fully documented, but probably ± 3 mm

Finally, *real-time* ultrasonography represents an additional modality for the study of aortic wall motion that eliminated the need for highly skilled technical specialists and permits the recognition of aortic dissection. Further, this opportunity to study aortic wall motion may permit identifying localized areas of weakness that represent prerupture sites.

One of the problems with older CT scanners was the time required for each study. However, with the newer machines, the entire procedure can be accomplished in 30 to 60 minutes, which compares with 10 to 60 minutes for ultrasound examinations.

Radiation dosage has also been a CT drawback, particularly for serial studies, but with the newer scanners, the skin dose has been significantly reduced to 0.1 to 2 rads per slice,[40,55] and the patient dosage is no greater than that received from an upper gastrointestinal series.

The earlier advantage of ultrasound in performing longitudinal scans is rapidly being equalized by newer CT software packages that allow both longitudinal and coronal reconstruction images of the abdomen. However, these are available in less than 1% of the installations in this country at the present time.

Metallic hemostatic surgical clips produce serious CT image artifacts, especially when they are located adjacent to moving structures such as a pulsatile aorta. Because of their dependence on postoperative CT scans, most neurosurgeons have ceased using such clips for hemostasis, and vascular surgeons may find a similar tactic useful if the frequent postoperative use of CT scanning becomes progressively more valuable.

Improving ultrasonic and CT scanning technology should permit the risk-free, accurate diagnosis of abdominal aneurysms on a routine basis in an outpatient setting. The identification of patients without aneurysmal disease but with aortic ectasia or tortuosity will save such patients from needless angiography and laparotomy. The clear detection of unsuspected aneurysms and their differentiation from other intraabdominal masses will permit early elective aneurysm resection in other patients and should decrease the eventual mortality from this disease. In addition, the improved delineation of smaller anatomic details, which appears to be possible with the newer techniques, may permit localizing paraaneurysmal structures such as the renal arteries, anomalous venous conditions, and other items of importance to the vascular surgeon. Finally, the increasing trend toward mass screening

centers for the diagnosis of asymptomatic cardiovascular disease may well provide an opportunity for the use of ultrasound or CT screening of large numbers of patients for the presence of aneurysmal and other intraabdominal pathology. In the long run, availability, reproducibility, cost, and technical proficiency will be the final determinants in the choice of which of these two diagnostic modalities is best for examining patients with abdominal aortic aneurysms.

Thoracic aortic aneurysms. In the thoracic area, ultrasound is rarely of value because of its attenuation by the air-containing lungs. Thus CT scanning and DSA have become the only noninvasive modalities capable of identifying thoracic aortic aneurysms.[7] However, in this area preoperative angiography is considered mandatory to define the lesion and its relationship to other critical vessels. Since there are few or no data regarding the relationship of thoracic aneurysm size and likelihood of rupture, sizing thoracic aneurysms has not achieved the widespread clinical significance that such measurements obtain in the abdomen.

Femoral and popiteal arterial aneurysms. Both ultrasound and CT scanning are equally effective diagnostic tools for the femoral and popiteal areas.[12,13,25,52] However, echography has achieved far greater popularity in these areas because of the ease of such scanning and because the images are usually of high quality, since higher frequency probes that yield finer sensitivity can be used in these relatively superficial applications. Since the presence of aneurysms in these locations is an adequate indication for surgical therapy, details regarding size, shape, and neighboring structures are relatively unimportant in these locations.

SUMMARY

Both ultrasound and CT scanning are safe noninvasive methods with high reliability in making the diagnosis of abdominal aortic aneurysms. Both approaches also are capable of determining aneurysm size, probably within 3 to 4 mm. Limitations of echography include difficulty in imaging in the presence of large amounts of intestinal gas, retained abdominal barium, and marked obesity, but this is offset by the ease of obtaining longitudinal as well as transverse scans and the lack of patient exposure to ionizing radiation. CT scans are limited by metallic objects, the radiation dose, and cost, but provide excellent intraluminal delineation with the aid of radiographic contrast material and require less operator skill. Both techniques are now in widespread clinical use and are the preferred methods for diagnosing abdominal aortic aneurysms. Technical improvements are also beginning to provide additional useful anatomic details of paraaneurysmal structures. Long-term reductions in cost may permit the application of one or both methods for asymptomatic patient screening, as well as for following the patient who does not undergo early surgery. The second choice as to which technique to favor in the elective preoperative evaluation will depend on such factors as cost, availability, and local expertise in test result interpretation.

REFERENCES

1. Axelbaum, S.P., et al.: Computed tomographic evaluation of aortic aneurysms, AJR 127:75, 1976.
2. Bernstein, E.F.: Considerations in the management of poor-risk patients with small asymptomatic abdominal aortic aneurysms. In Varco, R.L., and Delaney, J.P.: Controversy in surgery. Philadelphia, 1976, W.B. Saunders Co.
3. Bernstein, E.F.: The natural history of abdominal aortic aneurysms. In Najarian, J.S., and Delaney, J.B., editors: Vascular surgery, Miami, 1978, Symposia Specialists.
4. Bernstein, E.F.: Ultrasound techniques in the diagnosis and evaluation of abdominal aortic aneurysms. In Bernstein, E.F., editor: Noninvasive diagnostic techniques in vascular disease, St. Louis, 1978, The C.V. Mosby Co.
5. Bernstein, E.F., et al.: Growth rates of small abdominal aortic aneurysms, Surgery 80:765, 1976.
6. Birnholtz, J.C.: Alternatives in the diagnosis of abdominal aortic aneurysm: combined use of isotope aortography and ultrasonography, AJR 118:809, 1973.
7. Bresnihan, E.R., and Keates, P.G.: Ultrasound and dissection of the abdominal aorta, Clin. Radiol. 31:105, 1980.
8. Brewster, D.C. et al.: Angiography in the management of aneurysms of the abdominal aorta, N. Engl. J. Med. 292:822, 1975.
9. Brewster, D.C., et al.: Assessment of abdominal aortic aneurysm size, Circulation 56(suppl. II):164, 1977.
10. Carter, B.L., and Wechsler, R.J.: Computed tomography of the retroperitoneum and abdominal wall, Semin. Roentgenol. 13:201, 1978.
11. Cunat, J.S., et al.: Periaortic fluid aspiration for recognition of infected graft: pulmonary report, AJR 139:251, 1982.
12. Davis, R.P., et al.: Ultrasound scan in diagnosis of peripheral aneurysms, Arch. Surg. 1112:55, 1977.
13. Dent, T.L., et al.: Multiple arteriosclerotic arterial aneurysms, Arch. Surg. 105:338, 1972.
14. Donald, L., and Brown, T.G.: Demonstration of tissue interfaces within the body by ultrasonic echo sounding, Br. J. Radiol. 34:539, 1961.
15. Evans, G.C., et al.: Echo-aortography, Am. J. Cardiol. 19:91, 1967.
16. Glaeve, A.H., et al.: Discordance in the sizing of abdominal aortic aneurysm and its significance, Am. J. Surg. 144:627, 1982.
17. Goldberg, B.B.: Suprasternal aortosonography, JAMA 215:245, 1971.
18. Goldberg, B.B., and Lehman, J.S.: Aortosonography: ultrasound measurement of the abdominal and thoracic aorta, Arch. Surg. 100:652, 1970.
19. Goldberg, B.B., Ostrum, B.J., and Isard, H.J.: Ultrasonic aortography, JAMA 198:119, 1966.
20. Gomes, M.N.: ACTA scanning in the diagnosis of abdominal aortic aneurysms, Comput. Tomogr. 1:51, 1977.
21. Gomes, M.N., and Hufnagel, C.A.: The use of CT scanning in the evaluation of aneurysms of the abdominal aorta, International Cardiovascular Society, Los Angeles, June, 1978.
22. Gomes, M.N., Hakkal, H.G., and Schellinger, D.: Ultrasonography and CT scanning: a comparative study of abdominal aortic aneurysms, Comput. Tomogr. 2:99, 1978.
23. Gomes, M.N., Schellinger, D., and Hufnagel, C.A.: Abdominal aortic aneurysms and CT scanning. Symposium on Total Body Computerized Tomography, Heidelberg, Germany, Sept. 29-Oct. 1, 1977.
24. Gore, I., and Hirst, A.J.: Arteriosclerotic aneurysms of the abdominal aorta: a review, Prog. Cardiovasc. Dis. 16:113, 1973.
25. Graham, L.M., et al.: Clinical significance of arteriosclerotic femoral artery aneurysms, Arch. Surg. 115:502, 1980.
26. Haaga, J., and Reich, N.E.: Computed tomography of abdominal abnormalities, The C.V. Mosby Co., St. Louis, 1978.
27. Haaga, J.R., et al.: CT detection of infected synthetic grafts: preliminary report of a new sign, AJR 131:317, 1978.
28. Harris, R.D., and Hougen, M.L.: Early diagnosis of tuberculous thoracic aortic aneurysm by computerized axial tomography, Comput. Tomogr. 2:49, 1978.
29. Harris, R.D., and Seat, S.G.: Value of computerized tomography in evaluation of kidney, Urology 12:729, 1978.
30. Harris, R.D., et al.: Computerized tomography of an aneurysm of the thoracic aorta, Comput. Tomogr. 3:81, 1979.
31. Hertzer, N.R., and Beven, E.G.: Ultrasound measurement and elective aneurysmectomy, JAMA 240:1966, 1978.
32. Hilton, S., et al.: Computed tomography of the postoperative abdominal aorta, Radiology 145:403, 1982.
33. Holm, H.H., et al.: Ultrasonic diagnosis of arterial aneurysms, Scand, J. Thorac. Cardiovasc. Surg. 2:140, 1968.
34. Karp, W., and Eklof, B.: Ultrasonography and angiography in the diagnosis of abdominal aortic aneurysm, Acta Radiol. (Diagn.) 19:955, 1978.
35. Lautela, E., and Tahti, E.: Echoaortography in abdominal aortic aneurysm, Ann. Chir. Gynaecol. 57:506, 1968.
36. Leopold, G.R.: Ultrasonic abdominal aortography, Radiology 96:9, 1970.
37. Leopold, G.R.: Gray scale ultrasonic angiography of the upper abdomen, Radiology 117:665, 1975.
38. Leopold, G.R., Goldberger, L.E., and Bernstein, E.F.: Ultrasonic detection and evaluation of abdominal aortic aneurysms, Surgery 72:939, 1972.
39. Moloney, J.D., et al.: Ultrasound evaluation of abdominal aortic aneurysms. Circulation 56(suppl. II): 1180, 1977.
40. Margulis, A.R., Boyd, D.P., and Korobkin, M.T.: Advantages and disadvantages of rotary body CT scanners. Symposium on Total Body Computerized Tomography, Heidelberg, Germany, Sept. 29-Oct. 1, 1977.
41. McGregor, J.C., Pollock, J.G., and Anton, H.C.: The value of ultrasonography in the diagnosis of abdominal aortic aneurysm, Scott. Med. J. 20:133, 1975.
42. McGregor, J.C., Pollock, J.G., and Anton, H.C.: The diagnosis and assessment of abdominal aortic aneurysms by ultrasonography, Ann. R. Coll. Surg. Engl. 58:388, 1976.
43. Mulder, D.S., et al.: Ultrasonic "B" scanning of abdominal aneurysms, Ann. Thorac. Surg. 16:361, 1973.
44. Nuno, I.N., et al.: Should aortography be used routinely in the elective management of abdominal aortic aneurysm? Am. J. Surg. 144:54, 1982.

45. Nusbaum, J.W., Freimanis, A.K., and Thomford, N.R.: Echography in the diagnosis of abdominal aortic aneurysm, Arch. Surg. 102:385, 1971.
46. Pederson, R., et al.: CT in the evaluation of abdominal aortic aneurysms. International Symposium and Course on Computed Tomography, Miami Beach, March, 1978.
47. Pond, G.D., and Hillman, B.: Evaluation of aneurysms by computerized tomography, Surgery 89:216-23, 1981.
48. Ramirez, A.A., et al.: CAT scans of inflammatory aneurysms: a new technique for preoperative diagnosis, Surgery 91:390, 1982.
49. Raskin, M.M., and Cunningham, J.B.: Comparison of computed tomography and ultrasound for abdominal aortic aneurysms: preliminary study, J. Comput. Assist. Tomogr. 2:21, 1978.
50. Schellinger, D.: CT of abdominal aortic aneurysms. Society of Computerized Tomography postgraduate course, San Diego, Feb. 24-Mar. 1, 1979.
51. Segal B.L., et al.: Ultrasound diagnosis of an abdominal aortic aneurysm, Am. J. Cardiol. 17:101, 1966.
52. Turnipseed, W.D., et al.: Digital subtraction angiography and B-mode ultrasonography for abdominal and peripheral aneurysms, Surgery 92:619, 1982.
53. Wheeler, W.E., Beachley, M.C., and Ranniger, K.: Angiography and ultrasonography. AJR 126:95, 1976.
54. Winsberg, F., Cole-Beuglet, C., and Mulder, D.S.: Continuous ultrasound "B"-scanning of abdominal aortic aneurysms, AJR 121:626, 1974.
55. Zaklad, H.: Low dose in computerized tomography.
55. Symposium on Total Body Computerized Tomography, Heidelberg, Germany, Sept. 29-Oct. 1, 1977. (Abstracts.)

CHAPTER 65

Noninvasive testing in the diagnosis and assessment of arteriovenous fistula

ROBERT B. RUTHERFORD

The diagnosis of an arteriovenous (AV) fistula may be obvious on physical examination by (1) the auscultation of a characteristic bruit, (2) the obliteration of a thrill producing a bradycardiac response, (3) the observation of secondary varicosities and cutaneous signs of chronic venous hypertension, or (4) in congenital AV fistulas, the association of a "birthmark" and limb overgrowth. Unfortunately such classic findings often are absent, and the diagnosis may only be suspected. Thus there is a need for noninvasive screening tests that confirm or refute such suspicions, as well as for simple and innocuous methods of estimating the magnitude of AV shunt flow in an extremity and practical means of serially monitoring naturally occurring AV fistulas or those created for angioaccess purposes. In addition to a number of invasive diagnostic techniques identifying the presence or absence of hemodynamically significant AV communications,* several noninvasive diagnostic approaches have recently been published. Changes in blood flow, detected by venous occlusive plethysmography,[22] pulse volume,[2,19] and segmental pressure[2,8] have been described, as well as changes in flow velocities determined by Doppler velocity measurements.[2,7,12,15] This chapter summarizes my experience with some of these techniques.

HEMODYNAMIC BACKGROUND

An understanding of the hemodynamics and pathophysiology of AV fistulas provides the necessary background for their noninvasive diagnosis. Sumner[20] recently has written a comprehensive and

detailed review on this subject.[20] Although increased arterial flow leading into the fistula, decreased resistance and mean arterial pressure in the involved extremity, and increased venous volume and pressure are common and well-recognized features, other hemodynamic changes are variable, depending on the size of the fistula and the degree of collateral circulation development. With small fistulas or good collateral development, effects distal to the fistula may be so minor as to be undetectable by current physiologic testing. With large fistulas or poor collateral development, a number of readily detectable hemodynamic disturbances occur that often are described collectively under the term *distal steal*. Systolic as well as mean arterial pressure is decreased distal to the fistula, as is pulsatility, as gauged by volume or pressure measurements. Reversal of flow in the artery distal to the fistula marks the turning point in fistula development. These changes, along with the secondary effect of obstructing flow through the fistula or its afferent or efferent arteries and veins, are the basis for many of the following tests.

SCREENING TESTS FOR EXTREMITY AV FISTULAS

Three noninvasive diagnostic tests that were primarily developed for the detection and localization of peripheral arterial occlusive lesions also constitute an effective screening battery for extremity AV fistulas: (1) segmental limb systolic pressure determinations (SLPs), (2) segmental limb plethysmography or pulse-volume recordings (PVRs), and (3) the analysis of arterial velocity tracings or waveforms (VWFs). The techniques of performing

*References 1, 6, 9-11, 13, and 14.

these tests are well established and are described elsewhere in this text (Chapters 51 to 54). These techniques are not elaborated on further here. Rather the focus is on the specific application of the SLP, PVR, and VWF to the diagnosis of extremity AV fistulas, a potential that has not been widely realized. Directional Doppler scans are discussed elsewhere.

Segmental limb systolic pressures

The SLP test is performed exactly as described for the detection and localization of peripheral arterial occlusive lesions. I prefer the four-cuff to the three-cuff method, with two standard-size rather than one large thigh cuff because although the second gives a more accurate estimate of true systolic pressure in the thigh arteries, the first provides better localization of arterial lesions.[8] The reduced peripheral resistance associated with AV fistulas *decreases* mean arterial pressure in the arterial tree but *increases* pulse pressure. Therefore, proximal to an AV fistula, SLPs will usually be increased[9] in comparison to those of the contralateral (normal) extremity, whereas distal to the fistula, SLPs may be normal or, if the fistula is "stealing" significantly from distal arterial flow, they may be *decreased*. This description applies primarily to the situation in which there is a *localized* and hemodynamically significant AV fistula, whether it be acquired or a congenital macrofistula. However, even in AV fistulas that are so diffusely located that segmental localization is not possible, the systolic pressure determinations in the involved extremity may be higher than those in the contralateral normal extremity, as long as fistula flow is significantly great.

Segmental limb plethysmography or pulse-volume recording

An AV fistula increases the volume changes normally produced by pulsatile arterial flow. These can be monitored by segmental strain-gauge, impedance, or volume plethysmography. Characteristically, proximal to the fistula these PVRs are greater than in the normal contralateral extremity, and they have a sharper systolic peak and a decreased or absent anacrotic notch. Distal to the fistula PVRs often are not changed until the digital level, where they may be decreased. However, this decrease is usually relatively less than the decrease in systolic pressure. As previously observed for SLPs, the magnitude of these plethysmographic

changes and their ability to localize an extremity AV fistula depend on the type of fistula and the volume of fistula flow. In the case of multiple, diffuse microfistulas segmental localization often is not possible, and the presence of the lesion may only be apparent after careful comparison with properly calibrated plethysmographic tracings recorded at equivalent levels on the contralateral extremity.

Arterial velocity tracings or waveforms

Extremity arterial flow is normally triphasic, with the major systolic and the minor early diastolic forward components being interrupted by a period of reversed flow. The circulation in a resting extremity is normally in a high-resistance, low-flow state to such a degree that late diastolic flow is negligible. For these reasons a VWF recorded by Doppler probe over the major inflow artery to an extremity is normally triphasic and appears to "rest" on the zero velocity baseline. Occlusive arterial lesions upstream and downstream from the monitoring Doppler probe produce characteristic abnormalities that are well known, but the changes produced by distally located AV fistulas are equally striking. Rittenhouse et al.[16] have shown that changes in peripheral arterial resistance in an otherwise normal arterial tree modify the VWF in a predictable way. Decreased peripheral resistance eliminates reversed flow and increases forward flow, particularly in diastole. As a result, end-diastolic velocity and therefore the entire VWF are elevated above the zero baseline in direct proportion to the decrease in peripheral resistance. Increases in the magnitude and steepness of the upslope of the systolic peak, as well as irregularities produced by turbulence, are also observed when peripheral resistance is significantly decreased, but these changes are not as striking or as quantifiable as the elevation in the level of end-diastolic velocity.

Hyperemia associated with exercise, the relief of ischemia, artificial warming, vasodilator drugs, inflammation, and sympathectomy all produce changes in the VWF similar to those observed with AV fistulas. However, in the usual clinical situations where the diagnosis of AV fistula is being considered, these other causes of hyperemia are unlikely and easily ruled out. Increased velocity occurs in the jet stream of a high-grade arterial stenosis, and velocity tracings recorded distal to such a lesion also are raised above the zero baseline. However, this characteristically *widens* the systolic peak and produces more irregularities, particularly on the systolic downslope. Furthermore, stenotic lesions capable of producing such waveform abnormalities also should produce *decreases* in systolic pressure distally and thus a telltale SLP gradient.

Comparison of methods

The diagnostic sensitivity of these three tests is the reverse order of their presentation, the most reliable being the VWF. However, as with other noninvasive diagnostic test situations, accuracy improves when they are considered in combination. Although we have not yet missed diagnosing an AV fistula with these screening tests, the experience of my colleagues and I is still relatively limited (37 congenital cases). We suspect that microfistulas producing small degrees of AV shunting relative to total limb blood flow (for example, 3% to 7%) might not be detected by these tests.

These screening tests have their greatest clinical application in the evaluation of patients with congenital AV fistulas, particularly (1) in determining whether or not a birthmark or hemangioma is associated with an AV fistula, (2) in ruling out AV fistulas as a cause of varicose veins of atypical distribution or early onset, and (3) in screening patients with unequal limb length to rule out the possibility of an underlying AV fistula.[18] Patients with such clinical problems are likely to be children in whom the advantages of avoiding arteriography are even greater. Also, in approximately 40% of congenital AV malformations the AV fistulas themselves cannot be visualized angiographically,[21] and diagnosis depends on indirect evidence, such as early venous filling, increase in the size or number of branches of arteries in the region, or rapid clearance of contrast material. In the study by Szilagyi et al.[21] almost 30% of the arteriograms were "normal." These tests do not eliminate the need for arteriography but limit its application to essentially therapeutic indications. Because acquired AV fistulas secondary to trauma are usually more readily diagnosed on the basis of physical examination, and because arteriography is not only definitive but necessary, the advantages of screening tests are not as great in this setting. However, the tests may be helpful in differentiating false aneurysm from AV fistula as the cause of pulsation or bruit discovered following extremity trauma.

ESTIMATING EXTREMITY AV SHUNT FLOW BY THE LABELED MICROSPHERE METHOD

The percentage of total extremity flow that passes through AV communications may be estimated by comparing the relative levels of pulmonary radioactivity following first an arterial and then a peripheral venous injection of radionuclide-labeled human albumin microspheres.[17,18] This study may be used to confirm or refute the diagnosis of extremity AV fistula if the results of the noninvasive screening tests are equivocal. It also provides a quantitative estimate of AV shunt flow, which may assist in determining the prognosis and in gauging the need for and effectiveness of therapeutic interventions.

Method

A detailed account of the preparation of the microspheres and the methodology employed in establishing and standardizing this test has been published.[8] However, the test has been simplified by the widespread and ready availability of labeled microspheres and gamma cameras. In practive a suspension of ^{99m}Tc-labeled 35 μ human albumin microspheres* is injected into the major inflow artery of the involved extremity, while the lungs are monitored by a gamma camera. The radioactivity incident to the arterial injection of microspheres is compared to that following a subsequent peripheral intravenous injection, 100% of which should be trapped by the lungs. To ensure similar counting efficiencies, the venous injectate usually contains less radioactivity than the arterial injectate (roughly one fourth to one third). The relative radioactivity of the injectates is determined by counting the syringes before and after injection. Therefore it is important that there be no extravasation at the time of injection. The percentage of extremity flow passing through AV shunts is then estimated by multiplying the ratio of pulmonary activity following the arterial injection to that following the venous injection by the ratio of the respective injectates themselves and then multiplying this product by 100. For example, if the ratio of pulmonary radioactivity incident to venous injection is 2.5 times that following arterial injection, even though the venous injectate was only one-fourth as great, the estimate of AV shunt is

$$\frac{1}{2.5} \times \frac{1}{4} \times \frac{100}{1} = 10\%$$

*3M, St. Paul, Minn.

Normally the level of AV shunting in an extremity of an unanesthetized patient is less than 3%.[17] At the time of this study a perfusion scan of the leg should also be obtained, since the distribution of the arterial injectate may not only indicate the location of a fistula but the degree to which it is "stealing" from the distal vascular bed.

Because the labeled microsphere method of studying AV fistulas supplies more objective and quantitative information than the noninvasive screening tests, it possesses a number of different clinical applications. By estimating the relative magnitude of the AV fistula, the test provides a more precise gauge of its hemodynamic significance and therefore should allow closer prediction of the likelihood of such complications as limb overgrowth, ulceration and secondary skin changes, distal arterial insufficiency secondary to the "steal" phenomenon, and systemic hemodynamic effects such as forward heart failure. Serial estimates of AV shunting may indicate whether or not to expect a stable or progressive natural course and may help to determine the need for therapeutic intervention, in the form of ablative surgery or palliative embolism, as well as gauge the effectiveness of these efforts. The test can be performed in conjunction with angiography, not only to avoid an additional arterial puncture but also to provide more precise localization, either by multiple injections from different angiographic catheter tip locations or from the same location using sphygmomanometer cuffs at different levels, temporarily inflated above systolic pressure. This test can be performed during angiographic or direct surgical attempts at fistula control to provide a more objective therapeutic end point. However, it should be remembered that both general and regional anesthetics increase shunting through naturally occurring AV communications, and this must be controlled either by an additional postinduction baseline determination or by a comparative study of the uninvolved extremity.

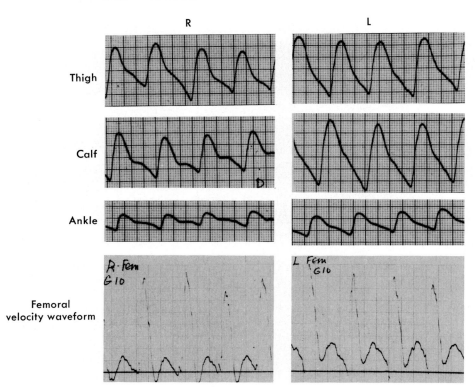

Fig. 65-1. PVRs and *(bottom)* femoral artery VWFs of young girl (S.D.) with 12% shunting through multiple congenital AV fistulas of left leg. (From Rutherford, R.B., Fleming, P.W., and McLeod, F.D.: Vascular diagnostic methods for evaluating patients with arteriovenous fistulas. In Diethrich, E.B., editor: Noninvasive cardiovascular diagnosis: current concepts, Baltimore, 1978, University Park Press.)

The varied clinical applications of both the non-invasive test and the labeled microsphere study are illustrated by the following brief case presentations.

1. S.D. (UH No. 596-978). A 10-year-old girl with hemangiomas of the left leg since birth was referred by an orthopedist for evaluation of the possibility that congenital AV fistulas might be producing progressive inequality in leg length (3 cm) and girth (2 cm), even though previous arteriography had been unable to detect them. The left extremity was somewhat warmer than the right, but there were no bruits, varicose veins, or cutaneous stigmata of chronic venous hypertension. Systolic SLPs were 10 mm Hg higher on the left at the calf but equal at other levels. However, the PVRs on the left were clearly greater

at all levels, and the femoral artery VWF on the left showed an absence of end-systolic reversal and increased diastolic velocity (Fig. 65-1). Shunt quantitation by the labeled microsphere method estimated 12% of the femoral flow passed through AV communication(s).

Comment: The diagnosis of congenital AV fistulas as the cause of unequal limb growth was easily established by relatively simple methods in spite of a "negative" arteriogram.

2. R.R. (UH No. 628-314). A 16-year-old boy with bilateral varicose veins of progressing severity since their appearance at age 2 was referred after high ligation and stripping of the left greater saphenous system caused increased discomfort and swelling with an early recurrence of the varicosities. Arteriography, performed before the surgery, "ruled out" the presence of AV fistulas. On ex-

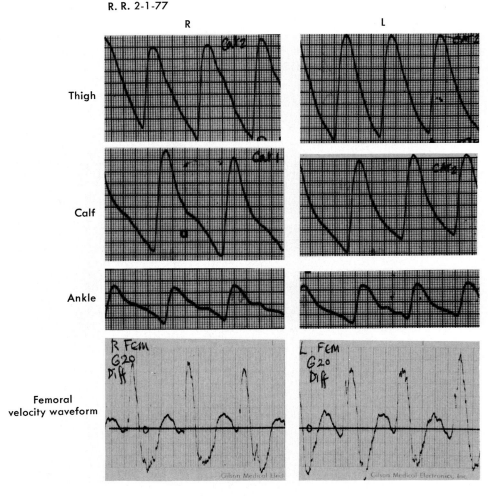

Fig. 65-2. PVRs and VWFs of 16-year-old boy (R.R.) with extensive, early-onset varicosities and cutaneous capillary hemangiomas who did not have associated AV fistulas (AV shunt, 2.1%). (From Rutherford, R.B., Fleming, P.W., and McLeod, F.D.: Vascular diagnostic methods for evaluating patients with arteriovenous fistulas. In Diethrich, E.B., editor: Noninvasive cardiovascular diagnosis: current concepts, Baltimore, 1978, University Park Press.)

amination there were extensive bilateral varicosities as well as purplish port-wine stains over both extremities. Both lower extremities seemed disproportionately large for the patient's size (height 5 feet 9 inches, shoe size 12). The diagnosis of bilateral congenital AV fistulas seemed likely in spite of the arteriogram. Systolic SLPs were equal bilaterally, as were the PVRs, although the dimensions of the latter at the thigh and calf level seemed greater than normal. However, there was no increase in diastolic velocity in either femoral artery. In fact there was an increased end-systolic reversal (Fig. 65-2). Measurement of shunt flow in the left extremity by the labeled microsphere method estimated it to be only 2.1%. Subsequent venous Doppler study demonstrated severe reflux at the femoropopliteal level bilaterally.

Comment: The clinical suspicion of AV fistula was so great that the lack of increased diastolic velocity was "ignored" and an AV shunt study obtained. Only after this confirmed the absence of significant AV shunt flow was a venous Doppler study performed to demonstrate the existence of extensive deep venous valvular insufficiency.

3. M.B. (UH No. 614-761). This 50-year-old man had a huge congenital AV malformation of the right lower extremity, causing gigantic limb overgrowth, venous "stasis" pigmentation and brawny edema with periodic ulceration. Five years earlier at another institution a surgical attack on the fistulas was abandoned after 70 units of blood had been transfused. Transaxillary angiography was performed with injection of both contrast material and labeled microspheres at several locations. The latter indicated 50% AV shunting of right common iliac flow, 65% shunting of right common femoral flow, but *no* shunting of superficial femoral flow, indicating the AV malformation was essentially limited to the distribution of the deep femoral artery. An arteriogram obtained at the same time demonstrated a major macrofistula at this location (Fig. 65-3).

Comment: The microsphere study indicated a more localized and therefore more treatable fistula than expected from physical examination and even arteriography.

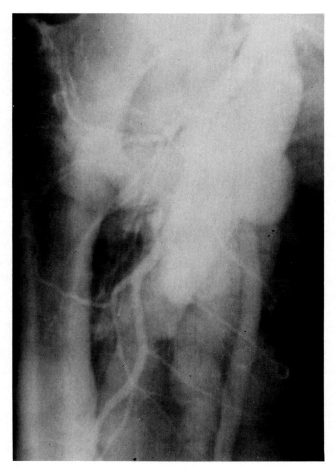

Fig. 65-3. Huge AV malformation arising near femoral artery bifurcation. AV shunting above this level was 65% but negligible more distally in the superficial femoral artery.

ULTRASONIC IMAGING

Simply placing a Doppler probe over the fistula might record characteristic changes in the velocity signals that could be diagnostic, but this is a hit-or-miss process that is not likely to succeed without definitive means of locating the fistula *and* the position of the ultrasound beam. Pulsed Doppler imaging has been used to identify AV fistulas[3] but generally is not a practical tool for this purpose. Color-coded images showing rate of flow, direction of flow, and turbulence might seem to offer advantages, but these advantages usually can be realized only in accessible, localized fistulas in which the orientation of the afferent and efferent vessel is conveniently in one plane facing the probe. Obviously the configuration of the fistulous connection and associated aneurysmal development might further complicate imaging efforts.

B-Mode scans also might visualize conveniently located fistulas, but only Duplex scanners, with the source of Doppler velocity signals accurately displayed by transducer locators, have the capability of determining the direction and velocity of flow in the vessels leading to and from the fistula.

APPLICATION OF NONINVASIVE TESTS TO THE MANAGEMENT OF PATIENTS WITH ANGIOACCESS AV FISTULAS
Preoperative monitoring

Most patients undergoing angioaccess surgery receive frequent intravenous infusions, some of which result in venous thrombosis, which may in turn dictate the placement of an AV fistula. In fact one of the accepted indications for these operations is the decreasing availability of patent peripheral veins. Therefore preoperative venous evaluation is important. This may, and in certain cases should be accomplished by venography, but a complete study of all the veins of one or more prospective extremities is impractical in most cases. On the other hand a carefully performed venous Doppler survey—"listening" over the course of the major superficial and deep veins of each extremity and observing whether the sounds are present or absent, continuous or phasic—and augmentation by compression distal to the monitoring point—constitutes a practical and inexpensive means of obtaining much of the desired information. Venography thus can be saved for the more complicated minority of cases.

Uremic, diabetic, and arteriosclerotic patients, and particularly patients with previous failed at-tempts at creation of AV fistulas, may have peripheral arterial occlusive lesions that will influence not only the choice of the "donor" artery but also the likelihood of fistula success. As with venous evaluation, the thoughtful use of noninvasive methods can reduce the need for angiography and aid in its interpretation.

The preoperative evaluation of the arterial system of an extremity that may serve as a potential site for an AV fistula or shunt should include SLPs and PVRs extended distally to include representative digits. PVRs provide important baseline information for postoperative monitoring. In addition, if consideration is being given to using either of the arteries lying parallel in the forearm or leg, for example, the radial or ulnar differential compression maneuvers should also be performed. These are analogous to the Allen patency test as applied to the ulnar and radial arteries but are more informative when carried out using a Doppler probe. Arterial velocity signals are monitored over these arteries using a directional Doppler system and a strip chart recorder, noting first if flow is normally triphasic and antegrade. If so, compression of the companion artery should result in an augmented signal. If not, there is probably an occlusive lesion in that vessel or the intervening collateral vessels. If on the other hand the artery being monitored shows retrograde flow diminished by compression of its companion vessel, it must be proximally occluded. Table 65-1 outlines all the alternative findings in performing collateral compression testing. If only one of these vessels is patent, normal SLPs and PVRs may be found. However, if one creates an AV fistula using this lone artery, the likelihood of a distal "steal" phenomenon developing is great, as is the likelihood of severe ischemia or gangrene should the fistula undergo thrombosis.

The same test can be applied to the lower extremity arteries, monitoring over the posterior tibial and dorsalis pedis arteries while compressing the companion vessel proximally. This approach has been shown by Rittenhouse and Brockenbrough[15] to predict the patency of each of the tibial arteries, even beyond a proximal occlusion.

Finally, even if these studies are normal, it is wise to do a stress test, monitoring the response of arm or ankle pressure to induced reactive hyperemia. Fee and Golding[5] have reported a case in which a femoral artery–saphenous vein fistula was created proximal to an unrecognized superficial

Table 65-1. Testing of parallel arteries with directional Doppler system and collateral compression

Condition	Direction	Form	Collateral compression
Both patent	Forward	Triphasic	Augmentation
Occluded proximally	Reversed	Triphasic	Diminution
Occluded distally	Forward	Triphasic	No response
Occluded collaterally	Forward	Triphasic	No response
Both occluded	Forward	Monophasic	No response
Common inflow occluded	Forward	Monophasic	Augmentation

femoral artery stenosis, causing distal ischemia and requiring reoperation.

Perioperative monitoring

The extremity should be studied noninvasively immediately after the creation of an AV fistula or shunt. In fact, if there is suspicion of a technical mishap, a sterilized Doppler probe can be used intraoperatively. Otherwise digital systolic pressures and plethysmography should be monitored at the end of the operation to rule out the possibility of an unrecognized complication. In addition, the point of maximum thrill or bruit should be localized and marked so it may be readily monitored during the ensuing days, when regional swelling, hematoma formation, or the need for a bulky dressing may prevent the thrill from being readily palpated. Alternatively the VWF proximal to the fistula may be recorded. If there is further doubt, a labeled microsphere study may be performed by injecting into the artery proximal to the fistula, settling any question of fistula patency.

Postoperative monitoring

As soon as the wounds have healed sufficiently and before beginning to use the fistula or shunt for dialysis, the preoperative studies should be completely repeated. The level of elevation of the Dopppler velocity tracing over the proximal artery may serve as an index of fistula flow, and the monitoring of digital pressures and plethysmographic tracings allows detection of thromboembolic complications or distal steal phenomena. Monitoring at regular intervals or at the time of development of any pain, color, or temperature changes is recommended.

In this regard it is important to recognize what changes can normally be expected after creation of AV fistulas, as nicely documented by Brenner et al.[4] Fig. 65-4 shows the characteristic change in digital pulse tracing and pressure beyond a radial artery–cephalic vein fistula. There is an *increase* in the amplitude of the plethysmographic tracing, but a *decrease* in the systolic pressure. However, Brenner showed that every patient with a radial artery–cephalic vein fistula had a drop in digital perfusion pressure, but there was rarely a further drop at the time of dialysis, even though many of the patients complained of discomfort, which was suspected to be ischemic in origin.

After a proximally placed brachial artery–axillary vein interposition AV shunt (Fig. 65-5), digital pressures dropped to an even greater extent. The plethysmographic tracings became almost flat, but with time, pulsatile flow and then pressures were restored by compensatory collateral development. In spite of this greater initial drop in digital pressure, again there was little further drop during dialysis. Thus the pressure and plethysmographic changes monitored distal to these AV fistulas are greatest in the immediate postoperative period and vary in degree with the size and location of the fistula. However, these decreases in distal perfusion improve with time and the development of collateral circulation and usually do not become much worse during dialysis.

The preceding statements apply to uncomplicated angioaccess fistulas but have even greater application in identifying postoperative complications of AV fistulas. Obviously thrombosis of the fistula itself or one of its limbs can be detected readily, particularly if postoperative baseline studies are available for comparison. This complication and either distal arterial steal or venous hypertension may all produce pain, color, or temperature changes in the hands and fingers and must be differentiated from each other. For such an evaluation, digital pressures and plethysmography should be performed at rest and then with occlusive compression of the fistula, each of its limbs, and the companion artery, as recommended by Sumner.[20]

Table 65-2 summarizes the findings in a case of radial artery–cephalic vein fistula that was stealing flow from the distal radial artery. The key obser-

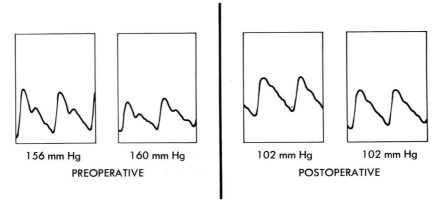

Fig. 65-4. PVRs from digits before and after creation of radial artery–cephalic vein fistula. (From Brener, B.J., Brief, D.K., and Parsonnet, A.V.: The effect of vascular access procedure on digital hemodynamics. In Diethrich, E.B., editor: Noninvasive cardiovascular diagnosis: current concepts, Baltimore, 1978, University Park Press.)

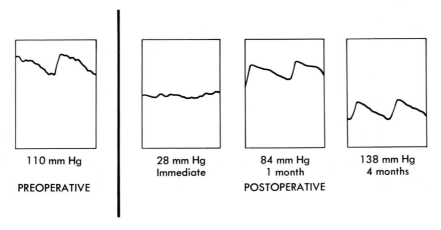

Fig. 65-5. PVRs before and after brachial artery–axillary vein graft. Plethysmographic changes are similar to digital pressure changes following insertion of prosthetic grafts. (From Brener, B.J., Brief, D.K., and Parsonnet, A.V.: The effect of vascular access procedure on digital hemodynamics. In Diethrich, E.B., editor: Noninvasive cardiovascular diagnosis: current concepts, Baltimore, 1978, University Park Press.)

Table 65-2. Radial steal—effect of ligating distal radial artery on blood pressure in the index finger ipsilateral to a radial artery–cephalic vein fistula

Blood pressure	Before ligation (mm Hg)	After ligation (mm Hg)
Brachial	100	100
Index finger		
Fistula open	32	80
Fistula occluded	68	92
Distal artery occluded	60	—
Ulnar artery occluded	0	0

From Sumner, D.S.: Diagnostic evaluation of arteriovenous fistulas. In Rutherford, R.B., editor: Vascular surgery, ed. 2, Philadelphia, 1984, W.B. Saunders Co.

Table 65-3. Distal venous hypertension—effect of ligating distal vein on blood pressure in the index finger ipsilateral to a radial artery–cephalic vein fistula

Blood pressure	Before ligation (mm Hg)	After ligation (mm Hg)
Brachial	156	160
Index finger		
Fistula open	100	110
Fistula occluded	160	186
Distal artery occluded	140	178
Proximal vein occluded	110	140
Distal vein occluded	152	110

From Sumner, D.S.: Diagnostic evaluation of arteriovenous fistulas. In Rutherford, R.B., editor: Vascular surgery, ed. 2, Philadelphia, 1984, W.B. Saunders Co.

vations are that digital pressure is greatly reduced and is improved significantly by occlusion of either the fistula itself or the radial artery distally, whereas it decreases further with occlusion of the companion artery. This interpretation was corroborated by the effects of ligation of the radial artery distal to the fistula. Thus noninvasive study not only established the diagnosis but ensured that it could be treated by distal arterial ligation without the need to interrupt the fistula.

The findings in a case of distal venous hypertension are recorded in Table 65-3. The increases in digital pressure associated with compression of the fistula and the distal radial artery indicated a distal steal phenomenon, but the resting digital pressure was not low enough to produce ischemic pain. However, the restoration of digital pressure to normal by compression of the distal vein indicated that this was the major venous outflow and was causing painful venous congestion in the hand and, as is commonly the case, in the carpal tunnel. After ligation of the distal vein, venous outflow was primarily through the proximal vein, so that its compression now raised digital pressure.

TRANSCUTANEOUS DOPPLER MEASUREMENT OF FISTULA FLOW

Ideally one would prefer to be able to monitor fistula *flow* during the postoperative period because it correlates well with fistula performance and certain flow-related complications. For example, if fistula flow is under 300 ml/min, it is probably not adequate for perfusion; if it is initially less than 150 ml/min or has been higher but is steadily drop-

ping, the fistula will inevitably undergo thrombosis. At the other end of the scale, when fistula flow increases, particularly when greater than 800 ml/min, the likelihood of distal steal is high; when fistula flow is greater than 1000 ml/min, the risk of cardiac embarrassment becomes significant, particularly in older patients.

The principle of measuring flow transcutaneously with Doppler scan is based on the equation

$$\overline{V} = \frac{\Delta f \times c}{2f(\cos\theta)}$$

where

$\overline{V}$ = Mean velocity
f = Frequency of incident sound beam
c = Velocity of sound in tissue (1.56×10^5)
θ = Angle of incident sound beam

Flow (Q) can then be calculated as the product of $\overline{V}$ and A, the cross-sectional area. The two essential components are the angle of the probe to the artery and its area. If the vessel is concentric, close, and parallel to the skin, one can establish the probe angle with reasonable accuracy and use the diameter from a power scan to estimate area. An alternative approach to quantitating velocity using a precalibrated Doppler probe is discussed in Chapter 53.

In practice a pulsed Doppler probe is scanned across the artery, giving a velocity profile that can be integrated to produce the mean velocity.[18] The same sweep can give both a depth scan and a power scan, and the arterial diameter can be determined by subtending vertical angles from the edge of the velocity profile to the depth scan. The mean ve-

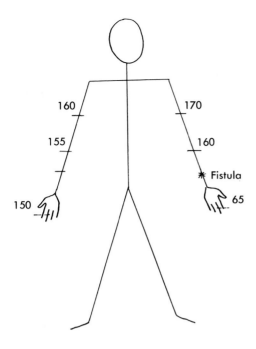

Fig. 65-6. Systolic SLPs of patient J.M. Decreased digital pressures on left indicate forearm fistula is stealing significantly from distal circulation. (From Rutherford, R.B., Fleming, P.W., and McLeod, R.D.: Vascular diagnostic methods for evaluating patients with arteriovenous fistulas. In Diethrich, E.B., editor: Noninvasive cardiovascular diagnosis: current concepts, Baltimore, 1978, University Park Press.)

locity recording is produced by using a filter to time-average the velocity profile signal. A frequency-to-voltage converter allows a direct calibrated reading of Δf, and because the other factors of the Doppler equation are constant, mean velocity can be read directly. However, it cannot be applied directly to the fistula because the probe angle cannot be established with certainty and the rapid, turbulent flow produces errors in estimating $\overline{V}$. Instead, flow over the major arterial inflow to the extremity is measured and compared with that of the contralateral normal vessel at the same level, with the difference assumed to represent fistula flow. The following case illustrates an application of this approach.

4. J.M. (UH No. 698-057), A 63-year-old woman with uremia had been on hemodialysis three times a week for more than a year using a surgically created AV fistula in the left forearm. Recently she complained of numbness and cramping of the left hand, palpitations, and fatigue. In addition to the obvious signs of a surgically created AV fistula in the left forearm, physical examination revealed a tachycardia, a soft systolic "flow" murmur, and borderline cardiomegaly without overt signs of congestive heart failure. SLPs were increased proximal to the fistula in the left arm, but digital systolic pressure was reduced to 65 mm Hg on the left, as compared to 150 mm Hg on the right (Fig. 65-6). PVRs were greatly increased proximal to the fistula but were reduced distally only at the level of the distal phalanges. Brachial VWF was normal on the right, but on the left showed greatly

increased diastolic flow (Fig. 65-7). On pulsed Doppler scan the diameter and the flow of the right brachial artery were estimated to be 7.3 mm and 212 ml/min, respectively. However, on the left the diameter was 8.7 mm with a flow of 1248 ml/min (Fig. 65-8).

Comment: The high fistula flow (>1000 ml/min) and decreased perfusion distal to the fistula were considered sufficient to explain all the patient's symptoms, and surgical reconstruction of the fistula, rather than simple banding of the proximal artery, was undertaken.

Obviously such an approach will not accurately estimate flow in an eccentrically narrowed arteriosclerotic vessel whose anatomic course in relation to the skin surface is not determinable.

The same approach to measuring AV fistula flow just described should be more readily applied using the newer prototypes of Duplex scanner now being introduced, if appropriate software modifications are made and an appropriate probe is selected for the depth of the artery. Cross-sectional areas of normal arteries should be rather easily obtained. However, the main source of error will continue to be the angle of incidence of the ultrasound beam, since being a few degrees off greatly affects the estimate of flow.

SUMMARY

Existing noninvasive diagnostic methods, although developed primarily for the detection of arterial and venous occlusive lesions, have prac-

J. M.   2-16-77

R   L

Brachial
pulse volume
recording

Forearm
pulse volume
recording

Proximal third
digit

Distal third
digit

Brachial
velocity waveform

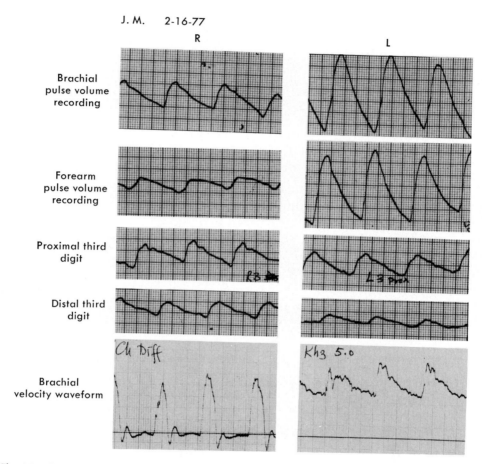

Fig. 65-7. PVRs and brachial VWFs of patient J.M. show pulse volume contours increased above and decreased below left forearm fistula, causing increased elevation of diastolic velocity in left brachial artery. (From Rutherford, R.B., Fleming, P.W., and McLeod, F.D.: Vascular diagnostic methods for evaluating patients with arteriovenous fistulas. In Diethrich, E.B., editor: Noninvasive cardiovascular diagnosis: current concepts, Baltimore, 1978, University Park Press.)

J. M.   2-16-77

R   L

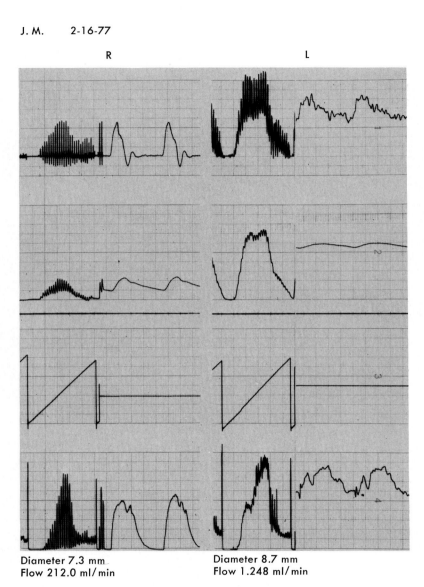

Diameter 7.3 mm
Flow 212.0 ml/min

Diameter 8.7 mm
Flow 1.248 ml/min

Fig. 65-8. Pulsed Doppler flowmeter recordings on brachial arteries of patient J.M. showing greatly increased velocity and flow caused by left forearm fistula. (From Rutherford, R.B., Fleming, P.W., and McLeod, F.D.: Vascular diagnostic methods for evaluating patients with arteriovenous fistulas. In Dietrich, E.B., editor: Noninvasive cardiovascular diagnosis: current concepts, Baltimore, 1978, University Park Press.)

tical value in the evaluation and management of AV fistulas, particularly the congenital and angioaccess types. Measurements of relative and absolute fistula flow using radionuclides and advanced Doppler instrumentation add an imporatnt quantitative dimension and, with further technical refinement, should establish their place in clinical practice.

REFERENCES

1. Anderson, C.B., et al.: Local blood flow characteristics of arteriovenous fistulas in the forearm for dialysis, Surg. Gynecol. Obstet. 144:531, 1977.
2. Barnes, R.W.: Non-invasive assessment of arteriovenous fistula, Angiology 29:691, 1978.
3. Blumoff, R.L., and Kupper, C.: Ultrasonic arteriography of femoral arteriovenous fistulae, Bruit 5:39, 1981.
4. Brener, B.J., Brief, D.K., and Parsonnet, A.V.: The effect of vascular access procedure on digital hemodynamics. In Diethrich, E.B., editor: Noninvasive cardiovascular diagnosis: current concepts, Baltimore, 1978, University Park Press.
5. Fee, H.J., and Golding, A.L.: Lower extremity ischemia after femoral arteriovenous bovine shunts, Ann. Surg. 183:42, 1976.
6. Frohlich, E.D., DeWolfe, V.G., and Vugrincic, C.F.: Unusual arteriovenous communications: arteriographic and hemodynamic studies, Cleve. Clin. Q. 38:153, 1971.
7. Gosling, R.G., and King, D.H.: Audio signals in arteriovenous bruits: use in flow monitoring and possible relevance to clotting. J. Appl. Physiol. 27:106, 1969.
8. Heitz, S.E., et al.: Value of arterial pressure measurements in the proximal and distal part of the thigh in arterial occlusive disease, Surg. Gynecol. Obstet. 146:337, 1978.
9. Holman, E., editor: Abnormal arteriovenous communications, peripheral and intra-cardiac acquired and congenital, ed. 2, Springfield, Ill., 1968, Charles C Thomas, Publisher.
10. Ingebritsen, R., and Husom, O.: Local blood pressure in congenital arteriovenous fistulae, Acta Med. Scand. 163:169, 1959.
11. Johnson, G., Jr., and Blythe, W.B.: Hemodynamic effects of arteriovenous shunts used for hemodialysis, Ann. Surg. 171:715, 1970.
12. Lichti, E.L., and Erickson, T.G.: Traumatic arteriovenous fistula: clinical evaluation and intraoperative monitoring with the Doppler ultrasonic flowmeter, Am. J. Surg. 127:333, 1974.
13. Pisko-Dubienski, Z.A., et al.: Identification and successful treatment of congenital microfistulas with the aid of directional Doppler, Surgery 78:564, 1975.
14. Rhodes, B.A., et al.: Arteriovenous shunt measurements in extremities, J. Nucl. Med. 13:357, 1972.
15. Rittenhouse, E.A., and Brockenbrough, E.C.: A method for assessing the circulation distal to a femoral artery obstruction, Surg. Gynecol. Obstet. 129:538, 1969.
16. Rittenhouse, E., et al.: Directional arterial flow velocity: a sensitive index of changes in peripheral vascular resistance. Surgery 79:350, 1976.
17. Rutherford, R.B.: Clinical applications of a method of quantitating arteriovenous shunting in extremities. In Rutherford, R.B., editor: Vascular surgery, Philadelphia, 1977, W.B. Saunders Co.
18. Rutherford, R.B., Fleming, P.W., and McLeod, R.D.: Vascular diagnostic methods for evaluating patients with arteriovenous fistulas. In Diethrich, E.B., editor: Noninvasive cardiovascular diagnosis: current concepts, Baltimore, 1978, University Park Press.
19. Strandness, D.E., Jr., Gibbons, G.E., and Bell, J.W.: Mercury strain gauge plethysmography, Arch. Surg. 85:215, 1962.
20. Sumner, D.S.: Diagnostic evaluation of arteriovenous fistulas. In Rutherford, R.B., editor: Vascular surgery, ed. 2, Philadelphia, 1984, W.B. Saunders Co.
21. Szilagyi, D.E., et al.: Congenital arteriovenous anomalies of the limbs, Arch. Surg. 111:423, 1976.
22. Yao. S.T., et al.: Limb blood flow in congenital arteriovenous fistula, Surgery 73:80, 1973.

CHAPTER 66

Noninvasive detection and evaluation of renovascular disease

ROBERT W. BARNES and C. SCOTT NORRIS

Between 20 and 30 million persons in the United States have hypertension. Of these, an estimated 5% to 10% have a correctable form of hypertension, the most common being renal artery stenosis. Unfortunately there are no reliable techniques to identify patients with renovascular hypertension. Although a number of clinical findings may suggest the diagnosis, renal arteriography remains the diagnostic standard to document this disorder. Most radiologic or hematologic screening techniques for renovascular hypertension are both insensitive and nonspecific, with no study being more than 85% accurate in detecting or excluding the diagnosis.

During the past 10 years there has been increasing emphasis on Doppler velocity signal analysis to detect arterial stenotic lesions, particularly in the extracranial carotid circulation. The present state of the art suggests that such velocity disturbances can identify advanced arterial stenosis (greater than 50%) with an accuracy exceeding 95%.[1] In addition, the systolic and diastolic flow characteristics identified within the Doppler signal are indicative of the peripheral vascular resistance.[4] During the past year we used the real-time echo Doppler (Duplex) scanner to study patients for possible renal artery stenoses.[3] The purpose of this chapter is to review our preliminary experimental and clinical studies, which suggest that Duplex scanning may be useful to screen patients for renovascular hypertension.

METHODS
Instrumentation

Initial canine studies were carried out using both continuous-wave (CW) 10 MHz and pulsed 5 MHz Doppler ultrasound to evaluate renal artery flow velocity. In studies of graded renal artery stenosis a CW Doppler detector was positioned distal to a Cushing neurosurgical screw clamp. Renal artery blood flow was determined with a Narco electromagnetic flowmeter with a probe placed on the left renal vein. In studies of parenchymal renal vascular resistance a pulsed 5 MHz Doppler ultrasonic flow probe was placed on the renal artery, and the renal blood flow recorded with an electromagnetic flow probe on the renal vein. In graded renal stenosis experiments the differential pressure from the aorta to the distal renal artery was measured with a differential pressure transducer (Hokanson, Inc.). In studies of renovascular parenchymal resistance the differential pressure from the renal artery to the renal vein also was measured with the Hokanson differential pressure transducer.

In clinical studies of patients with suspected renal artery stenosis an ultrasonic echo–Doppler Duplex scanner was employed with a real-time B-mode imaging transducer operating at 3 MHz and a pulsed Doppler transducer operating at 5 MHz.* Angiographic studies were carried out using conventional arterial contrast arteriography, usually performed with the transfemoral Seldinger technique.

EXPERIMENTAL PROTOCOL

Ten mongrel dogs weighing between 15 and 20 kg were anesthetized with sodium thiamylal (2 to 4 mg/kg/hr) and maintained on a volume respirator.† The abdominal aorta, inferior vena cava, and renal arteries and veins were isolated through a

---

*Mark V scanner, Advanced Technology Laboratories, Bellevue, Wash.
†Harvard 607.

midline abdominal incision. Pressures in the abdominal aorta and inferior vena cava were monitored with polyvinyl catheters introduced via one femoral artery and vein. The distal renal artery pressure was measured through a cannula introduced into a branch of the left renal artery in the hilum of the kidney. An electromagnetic flow probe of appropriate size was placed on the left renal vein. A neurosurgical Cushing screw clamp was placed on the proximal left renal artery. A CW 10 MHz Doppler probe was placed at a 45° angle on the left renal artery distal to the screw clamp. The probe position was maintained with a special probe holder, and acoustic coupling was accomplished with acoustic gel. Renal artery blood flow velocities were processed on a real-time fast-Fourier transform sound spectrum analyzer with integrated microprocessor.* All pressure and flow variables were recorded with a Racal FM recorder.† Aortic and distal renal artery pressures, renal venous blood flow, and renal artery CW Doppler recordings were obtained at rest and then with graded renal artery stenosis induced by the neurosurgical screw clamp.

Experimental studies of Doppler velocity correlates of parenchymal renovascular resistance were carried out during sequential injections of Sephadex gel microspheres (40 to 120 μm‡ into the aortic catheter after clamping the infrarenal aorta. Renal arteriovenous, (AV) pressure gradients, blood flow, and renal artery velocity patterns were recorded after each injection of microspheres.

Patient studies

Clinical studies of renal artery stenosis and renal parenchymal vascular resistance were carried out noninvasively using the Mark V Duplex scanner. The patients fasted overnight and were examined in the noninvasive vascular laboratory in the supine position. Acoustic gel was liberally applied over the epigastrium, and the abdominal aorta was visualized initially in longitudinal section using a 3 or 5 MHz scan head. Aortic flow velocity was recorded with the pulsed Doppler transducer; the normal aortic blood flow velocity has a characteristic low flow during diastole. Next the left renal vein was imaged and evaluated by Doppler ultrasound as it crossed anteriorly to the aorta. The cyclic flow velocity in the renal vein on respiration

was noted. Then the superior mesenteric artery was located and visualized superiorly and anteriorly to the left renal vein. The velocity characteristics in this vessel included marked pulsatility with a prominent systolic component and multiphasic low-diastolic flow velocity signals. Finally each renal artery was evaluated both visually, with the echo real-time image, and with the pulsed Doppler sound beam. The renal artery flow velocity characteristically had a higher frequency during systole and diastole than other visceral vessels. The Doppler frequency signals were displayed on a real-time sound spectrum analyzer* and the signals were stored on a magnetic disk for off-line microcomputer processing.†

Renal artery Duplex scanning was carried out on 21 normal individuals with no history of hypertension or atherosclerotic cardiovascular disease. Scans were performed on 43 patients undergoing arteriography for symptomatic aortoiliac or femoropopliteal arterial occlusive disease. Duplex scans of the renal arteries were done on 56 patients selected at random from the Medical Hypertensive Clinic.

Data analyses

Experimental studies of graded renal artery stenosis permitted correlation of renal artery flow velocity alterations with stenosis, which was graded by the degree of systolic pressure gradient from the aorta to the distal renal artery. Renal artery flow velocity abnormalities were also correlated with the percentage of reduction in renal blood flow. Using the real-time sound spectrum analyzer, microprocessing of the digitized Doppler spectra permitted assessment of three variables: (1) peak frequency, (2) mode frequency, and (3) the systolic window, which is a ratio of that portion of the "clear window" beneath the peak systolic waveform to the entire frequency envelope for 100 msec from onset of peak systole. The peak and the mode frequencies were referenced to those from the velocity recordings of the abdominal aorta to permit a dimensionless ratio.

For experiments assessing renovascular parenchymal resistance, the renal artery velocity disturbances were correlated with progressive changes in renovascular resistance, as calculated from differences in renal AV pressure divided by renal

*Angioscan II, Unigon Industries, Mt. Vernon, N.Y.
†Racal Recorders, Inc., Rockville, M.D.
‡Sigma Chemical Co., St. Louis.

*Meda Sonics, Inc., Mountain View, Calif.
†Oasis, Advanced Technology Laboratories, Bellevue, Wash.

blood flow. The renal artery velocity waveform was displayed on a real-time sound spectrum analyzer, and the ratio of the peak frequency at end diastole to the peak frequency in systole was expressed as a ratio (the so-called Pourcelot index).

Clinical studies of renal artery stenosis involved identification of renal artery flow velocity disturbances similar to those previously described for carotid artery stenoses. The normal renal artery was characterized by a smooth, pulsatile waveform, with most of the amplitude of the Doppler signal following the upper border of the envelope of the beat signal. There was prominent flow in systole and diastole. Distal to a renal artery stenosis the flow velocity was disturbed with an increase in peak frequency, spectral broadening with loss of the normally clear window beneath the systolic waveform, and continued flow disturbance throughout diastole. With advanced renal artery stenosis there was loss of the normal pulsatile signal.

In patients with increased parenchymal renovascular resistance the diastolic flow velocity was reduced, and the ratio of end-diastolic to peak systolic frequency likewise was reduced. These abnormalities in renal artery flow velocity were compared independently to arteriograms evaluated for renal artery patency, with significant stenoses classified as having greater than a 60% diameter reduction in the renal artery orifice.

RESULTS
Experimental studies

With graded renal artery stenosis in the dog there was a progressive increase in peak frequency of the renal artery Doppler velocity waveform. Significant changes in peak Doppler frequency occurred before reduction in renal artery blood flow. Detectable changes in renal artery velocity were recorded with systolic pressure gradients of 25 mm Hg or greater (Fig. 66-1).

In experimental studies of increased parenchymal renovascular resistance there was progressive diminution in renal artery diastolic blood flow velocity,[2] as shown in Fig. 66-2.

Clinical studies

Renal artery flow velocity was detectable in 94% of the patients studied. The most common reasons for nonvisualization or inability to evaluate renal artery flow signals were obesity, recent ingestion of food or fluid, previous upper abdominal surgery, or aneurysmal disease of the aorta.

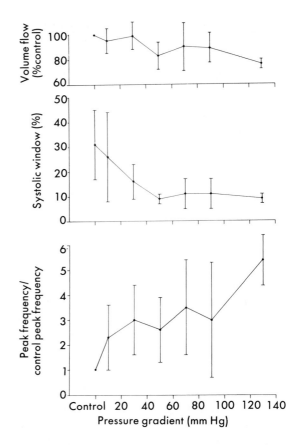

Fig. 66-1. Relationship of Doppler peak frequency and systolic window to renal bloodflow during progressive renal artery stenosis, as monitored by renal artery pressure gradients in 48 separate determinations in 10 dogs.

Patients with renal artery flow disturbance typically demonstrated increased systolic frequency and spectral broadening, as shown in Fig. 66-3. These abnormalities were present in all but 2 of the 12 patients with documented renal artery stenosis of greater that 60% diameter reduction (sensitivity of 83%). Conversely, of 76 renal arteries that were normal or had less than 60% stenosis, the renal artery Doppler spectrum was normal in 74 (specificity of 97%).

Patients with hypertension characteristically had a diastolic/systolic peak ratio significantly lower than that of normal subjects (Fig. 66-4). Patients with peripheral vascular disease who underwent arteriography characteristically had a diastolic/systolic peak frequency ratio between normal individuals and hypertensive patients.

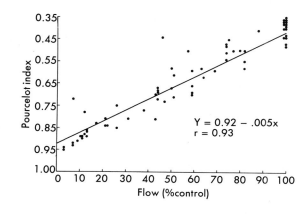

Fig. 66-2. Correlation of ratio of Doppler end-diastolic frequency to peak systolic frequency (Pourcelot index) to renal blood decrement during progressive embolization of the renal microcirculation with Sephadex gel microspheres.

$$Y = 0.92 - .005x$$
$$r = 0.93$$

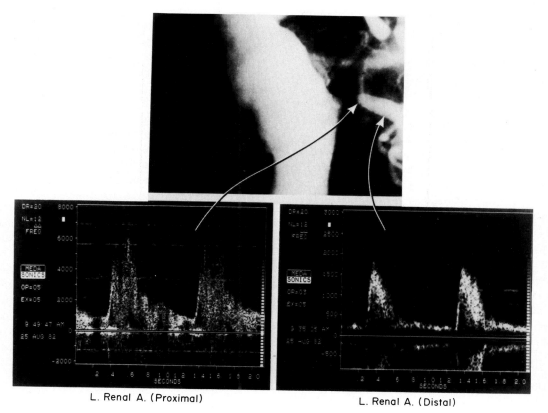

L. Renal A. (Proximal)   L. Renal A. (Distal)

Fig. 66-3. Duplex pulsed Doppler spectra from proximal *(lower left)* and distal *(lower right)* left renal artery in patient with angiographic evidence of severe renal artery stenosis *(top).*

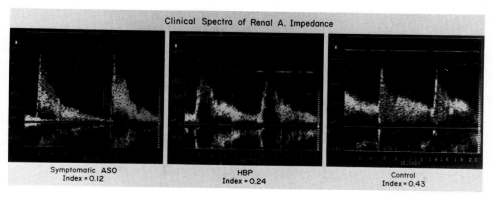

Clinical Spectra of Renal A. Impedance

Symptomatic ASO   HBP   Control
Index = 0.12   Index = 0.24   Index = 0.43

Fig. 66-4. Duplex pulsed Doppler spectra from renal artery of patients with peripheral arterial occlusive disease *(left)* and hypertension *(middle),* as contrasted with normal subject *(right).*

DISCUSSION AND CLINICAL APPLICATION

Renovascular hypertension characteristically occurs in younger patients, particularly those with recent onset of severe hypertension that may be difficult to control with oral medications. However, these clinical signs are not unique identifiers of patients with correctable renovascular disease. Many young patients fail to have renal artery stenosis documented by invasive studies and, conversely, older patients may develop renovascular hypertension. Also, some patients may progressively lose functional renal mass even though hypertension is controlled with medication. Thus the physician needs to be aware of the possibility of correctable renovascular stenosis.

The current experimental and clinical studies suggest that Doppler ultrasonic evaluation of renal artery velocity disturbances may be useful not only to detect the presence of renal artery stenosis but also to evaluate the presence of increased parenchymal renovascular resistance. The experimental studies indicate that a correlation exists between renal artery velocity disturbances and graded renal artery stenosis, as manifested by the renal artery pressure gradient. Such velocity alterations occur before a significant reduction in total renal blood flow develops. There is also a good correlation between the relationships of diastolic and systolic flow velocity and the intrarenal peripheral vascular resistance.

The clinical studies with the Duplex scanner suggest that this technique permits visualization of the renal arteries with the real-time echo scanner, as well as evaluation of renal artery flow velocity with pulsed Doppler ultrasound. The renal artery flow characteristics are similar to those of the internal carotid artery, with prominent flow throughout systole and into diastole. In renal artery stenosis characteristic changes in peak systolic frequency occur, as well as spectral broadening associated with turbulent blood flow. In addition, these clinical studies have documented characteristic diastolic flow velocity reduction in individuals with anticipated increased parenchymal renovascular resistance associated with hypertension. These findings are similar to those in the experimental models of increased renal or peripheral vascular resistance.

There are certain limitations to using Duplex scanning of renovascular disease, including obesity, previous surgery, recent ingestion of food or fluid, and aneurysmal disease. Future refinement in instrument design features possibly may improve its ability to assess renal artery flow velocity.

If future investigations further validate this technique, noninvasive Duplex scanning of renal artery flow characteristics in patients with possible renovascular hypertension may have widespread clinical application. Specifically this noninvasive technique may be refined to permit screening of hypertensive patients who may harbor renal artery lesions. The documentation of renal artery stenosis may permit more selective use of renal arteriography. Also, this technique may permit identification of those patients with increased parenchymal renovascular resistance who, despite having renal artery stenosis, may not benefit from surgical intervention. Finally the technique may permit longitudinal assessment of the natural history of medical vs. radiologic or surgical intervention for renal artery stenosis. For example, patients with documented renal artery stenosis but satisfactory control of blood pressure with medication may be followed with serial noninvasive studies. If progressive renal artery stenosis develops, possibly resulting in thrombosis and loss of renal function, surgical or radiologic intervention might be considered. Another application may be the noninvasive screening of patients who manifest progressive renal failure, with or without associated hypertension. Patients with renal flow velocity disturbances might be considered for angiography and possible radiologic or surgical intervention to preserve or improve renal function.

REFERENCES

1. Blackshear, W.M., et al.: Detection of carotid occlusive disease by ultrasonic imaging and pulsed Doppler spectrum analysis, Surgery 86:698, 1979.
2. Norris, C.S., and Barnes, R.W.: Renal artery flow velocity analysis: a sensitive measure of experimental and clinical renovascular resistance, J. Surg. Res. 36:230, 1984.
3. Norris, C.S., et al.: Noninvasive evaluation of renal artery stenosis and renovascular resistance: experimental and clinical studies, J. Vasc. Surg. 1:192, 1984.
4. Rittenhouse, E.A., et al.: Directional arterial flow velocity: a sensitive index of changes in peripheral vascular resistance, Surgery 79:350, 1976.

CHAPTER 67

Vasculogenic impotence

LUIS A. QUERAL and JAMES S.T. YAO

Awareness of male sexual dysfunction has become more prevalent in our society. However, the etiology of impotence is both multifactorial and complex. Normal penile erections are the net result of properly functioning psychologic, endocrine, neurologic, and vascular systems; impotence can occur when any of these systems malfunctions. Of all tests available for the evaluation of impotence, measurement of penile blood flow and pressure offers the most definitive technique to determine a vasculogenic cause of sexual dysfunction. This chapter discusses the vasculogenic factors responsible for impotence and methods for their detection.

An insufficient arterial blood supply to the penis results either in inability to obtain or incapacity to maintain an erection. Thus patients with vasculogenic impotence complain of weak and short-lived erections. This functional ischemia can result from an obstruction at the aortic bifurcation, an internal iliac artery occlusion, or an obliterative process of the distal branches of the internal pudendal artery.

The blood supply of the penis is derived from the paired internal pudendal arteries, which branch to become the dorsal penile, deep (corporal), and urethral arteries (Fig. 67-1). The deep corporal artery supplies blood for the erection to the corpora cavernosa. This deep artery is more laterally placed than the dorsal penile artery and is best suited for Doppler ultrasound detection. The urethral artery is the terminal branch of the perineal artery, which is another branch of the pudendal artery. Thus the entire penile blood supply is derived from the internal iliac artery.

There are various methods of measuring penile blood flow, either by pulse waveform recording or by measurement of systolic pressure; Table 67-1 summarizes the reported techniques. Of the various approaches reported, the Doppler ultrasound method appears to be the most straightforward and easiest to use and also is ideal for both office and bedside examination.

PENILE SYSTOLIC PRESSURE MEASUREMENT

Penile systolic blood pressure is measured by placing a 2.5 cm pneumatic cuff around the base of the penis and connecting the cuff to a sphygmomanometer. A 10 kHz ultrasound Doppler probe then is used to monitor flow by placing it over the deep penile artery, which is the main blood supply to the corpora cavernosa. The deep penile artery is situated laterally along the shaft on each side of the penis (Fig. 67-1). The systolic pressure is determined by inflating the cuff and then noting the return of the flow signal during deflation. In general, measurements are made on both the right and the left sides; testing is done with the patient in a supine position (Fig. 67-2). The penile systolic pressure is then divided by the brachial systolic pressure to compute the *penile-brachial index (PBI)*. In normal males the penile pressure is close to the brachial pressure, and therefore the PBI is approximately 1.0.

A PBI of 0.6 or less is compatible with vasculogenic impotence. This value has been arrived at independently by Kempczinski,[18] Engel et al.,[8] and Queral et al.[24] Although a male with normal sexual function rarely has a PBI in the 0.6 range, the converse is not true. A normal or near-normal PBI can exist in patients complaining of impotence, when this is caused by any of a variety of nonvasculogenic causes. In general a PBI greater than 0.75 is considered normal, and a PBI of 0.6 to 0.7 is compatible with, but not diagnostic of, vasculogenic impotence.

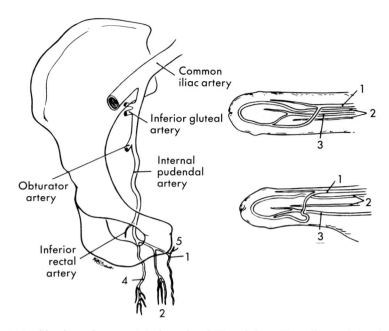

Fig. 67-1. Major blood supply to penis is from dorsal *(1)* and deep *(2)* penile arteries and the urethal artery *(3)*. These arteries are branches of internal pudendal artery, which is large branch of internal iliac artery. *(4)*, perineal artery; *(5)*, inferior hemorrhoidal artery. (From Queral, L.A., et al.: Sexual function and aortic surgery. In Bergan, J.J., and Yao, J.S.T., editors.: Surgery of the aorta and its body branches, New York, 1979, Grune & Stratton, Inc.)

Table 67-1. Techniques of measuring penile blood flow and pressure

Author	Technique	Parameters
Britt et al.[4]	Strain-gauge plethysmography	Pulse waveform
Canning et al.[5]	Impedance plethysmography	Pulse waveform
Carter (Ch. 51)	Doppler ultrasound	Systolic pressure
Engel et al.[8]	Doppler ultrasound	Systolic pressure
Gaskell[10]	Spectroscopy	Systolic pressure
Kempczinski[18]	Doppler ultrasound and pulse volume recorder	Systolic pressure and volume pulse waveform
Macvar et al.[19]	Doppler ultrasound	Flow waveform
Queral et al.[25]	Doppler ultrasound	Systolic pressure

In addition to the resting measurement, penile pressure may be recorded after leg exercise. This test, termed the *pelvic steal test*, is done in the supine position by having the patient flex and extend the legs at the knee and hip for 3 to 5 minutes.[22] A decrease of 0.15 or more in the PBI with exercise is considered abnormal.[13]

PULSE VOLUME WAVEFORMS

Pulse volume waveforms of the penis can be recorded by a pulse volume recorder[7,18] or by a digital plethysmograph.[27] The pulse volume wave-

form is then graded as good, fair, or poor. A "good" waveform contains a brisk upstroke, a sharp systolic peak, and a slower downstroke. A "fair" pulse volume waveform is of significantly lower amplitude, with more delay of the upstroke and rounding of the peak. A "poor" tracing has a marked decrease in amplitude and extreme flattening of the waveform. A comparison of simultaneously recorded digital pulses is necessary to help interpret the pulse volume waveforms.

Instead of visual inspection of the waveforms, Stauffer and DePalma[27] have suggested quantita-

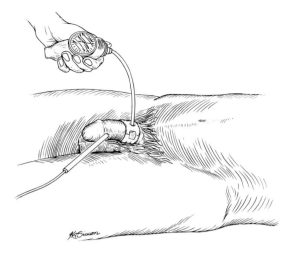

Fig. 67-2. Method of recording penile systolic pressure using Doppler ultrasound technique. (From Queral, L.A., et al.: Surgery 86:799, 1979.

tive analysis by calculating the amplitudes as well as the systolic upstroke. Their criteria for an abnormal penile pulse volume recording are (1) an amplitude less than 5 mm and (2) a systolic upstroke time longer than 0.20 seconds. Abnormal upstroke (rest time), that is, prolonged duration of upstroke, appears to correlate most reliably with presence or absence of erectile function.

As with penile pressure measurement, the penile pulse volume waveform can be recorded at rest and after postischemic reactive hyperemia.[18] The postischemic hyperemia is produced by inflating the pneumatic cuff to a pressure 50 mm Hg above the brachial systolic pressure for 5 minutes. The cuff is then deflated, and a repeat pulse volume waveform is immediately obtained. An increase in amplitude of more than 10% is considered a positive response to ischemia.

CLINICAL APPLICATIONS

The main use of penile blood flow and pressure measurement is to assess pelvic hemodynamics (1) in arterial occlusive disease, (2) in a multidisciplinary approach to impotence, and (3) after aortic surgery and renal transplantation.

Arterial occlusive disease

Leriche's syndrome (aortoiliac artery stenosis). In 1940 René Leriche described a syndrome associated with impotence and caused by thrombotic obliteration of the terminal aorta. He recognized that the condition was not rare and that the patients were young adults, mostly men. These patients complained of inability to maintain a stable erection and extreme fatigue in both lower extremities. Leriche described the findings of global atrophy of the muscles of the limbs and absence of ischemic trophic changes of the skin and nails of the feet. A decade later surgeons directed their efforts toward correcting the vascular supply to the lower extremities, without consideration of restorating blood flow to the genitalia. As techniques of aortic reconstruction became standardized, surgions became aware of persisting sexual dysfunction after aortic surgery or occurring again after aortoiliac reconstruction. Now surgeons have become interested in preventing postoperative sexual dysfunction and in attempting preoperatively to plan arterial reconstructions that will increase the blood supply to the genitalia. Thus it is important for the surgeon to monitor closely the recording of penile pressure before and after reconstructive surgery. As noted, an abnormal PBI, 0.6 or less, is compatible with vasculogenic impotence.

Pelvic steal phenomena. In addition to occlusive disease of the hypogastric artery, shunting of blood away from the pelvic region also has been related to impotence. In patients with unilateral external iliac artery occlusion and contralateral internal iliac artery stenosis, the ipsilateral internal iliac artery may act as the main blood supply to the lower limb. Queral et al.[25] have identified five patients with these anatomic findings and vasculogenic impotence. The findings have been termed the *femoral steal syndrome* because the lower extremity is taking blood that oterwise would eventually supply the pelvis and penis. Other types of steal phenomena have been described by Barker[1] and Michal et al.[20,21] The pelvic steal test or postischemic hyperemia test helps to establish the diagnosis in these patients.

Microangiopathy. Microangiopathy is a frequent

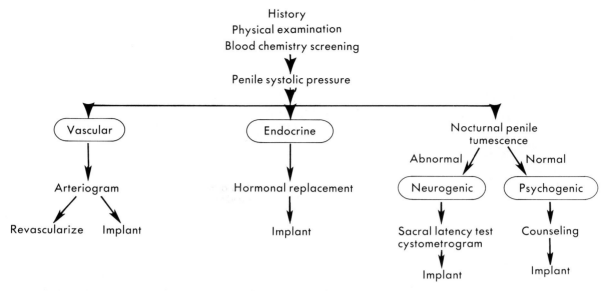

Fig. 67-3. Systematic clinical approach for evaluation of sexually impotent patient. (From Billet, A., Dagher, F.J., and Queral, L.A.: Surgery 91:108, 1982.)

complication of diabetes mellitus. Along with neuropathy, it causes impotence in approximately one fourth of all diabetic males under age 40. Those patients with juvenile onset of the disease have an even higher incidence of sexual malfunction. Obliteration of the distal branches of the internal pudendal arteries causes functional ischemia of the penis, that is vasculogenic impotence. The problem can be identified by measuring penile flow by any of the techniques listed in Table 67-1.

Radiation injury. Pelvic nerves and blood vessels can also be injured by radiation therapy, according to Swanson.[28] In a study of 23 patients who received radiation therapy for prostatic cancer, 15 experienced changes in erectile potency following radiotherapy.[14] Vascular disease was identified in all patients by a significantly decreased PBI. In 2 of these 15 patients arteriography revealed bilateral occlusive disease in the distal internal pudendal and penile arteries overlying the pelvic radiation field. These findings led Goldstein et al.[14] to conclude that vasculogenic impotence is the most consistent organic erectile abnormality in radiation-associated impotence.

Multidisciplinary approach to impotence

Recording of the penile pulse and pressure should be an integral part of the evaluation of impotence. Impotence, when presented as the patient's sole concern, requires a multidisciplinary

approach to determine its etiology.[22,26] It is also important to recognize that the presence of vasculogenic impotence, as defined by an abnormal PBI, does not rule out coexisting emotional difficulties. Therefore the approach should involve psychologic testing, a urologic examination, and a vascular evaluation.

Although nonvasculogenic causes of impotence are beyond the scope of this chapter, it is worth emphasizing the value of nocturnal penile tumescence (NPT).[17] Patients with a normal PBI can be referred to a urologist for further evaluation. Those potentially impotent patients with normal blood levels of testosterone are placed in the sleeping laboratory, and their penile tumescence is recorded during the REM phase of sleep. Those who experience erections during sleep are psychologically impaired, whereas the remainder are likely to have a neurogenic etiology for their impotence.

Fig. 67-3 illustrates an algorithmic approach using penile pressure measurement in clinical evaluation of impotence.

Assessment of pelvic hemodynamics after surgery

Aortoiliac reconstruction. Aortic surgery can adversely affect sexual function by either neurogenic or vasculogenic mechanism. Excessive dissection, with destruction of the sympathetic neural pathways located immediately adjacent to the aortic

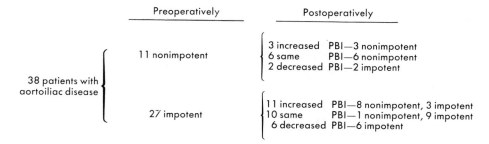

Fig. 67-4. Flow chart illustrating that, after vascular arterial reconstruction, an increase or no change in penile-brachial index (PBI) is desirable, but a decrease in PBI is associated with postoperative impotence. (From Queral, L.A., et al.: Surgery 86:799, 1979.)

bifurcation (hypogastric plexus), results in ejaculatory disturbances. Such destruction of sympathetic fibers can be readily avoided by limiting aortic dissection to the area above the origin of the inferior mesenteric artery.

The effect of surgery on pelvic hemodynamics may be assessed by recording the penile pressure before and after surgery. Changes noted in the PBI can be correlated with alterations in sexual function. The results of a study by Queral et al.[24] are summarized in Fig. 67-4. The most significant findings include (1) surgical intervention can affect the PBI; (2) an increase in PBI often can restore or improve sexual function; and (3) a decrease in PBI is detrimental to erectile capability and results in impotence. More importantly six patients who had end-to-end aortobifemoral grafts and concurrent external iliac disease experienced a significant decrease in penile pressure.[20] As a result, all became impotent after surgery. The decrease in PBI was caused by severe external iliac artery disease, which prevented retrograde flow to the internal iliac vessels. If an end-to-side anastomosis had been constructed in these patients to preserve prograde flow, a decrease in the PBI might have been avoided. Thus, maintaining penile perfusion, as emphasized by Flanigan et al.,[9] should be considered when aortic surgery is contemplated, and recording the penile pressure helps to evaluate the effect of surgery on pelvic hemodynamics.

The salient features of the effects of aortic surgery on pelvic hemodynamics are highlighted in the following two cases.

1. A 56-year-old patient had disabling bilateral buttock and lower extremity claudication and also complained of weak and short-lived erections. On physical examination femoral pulses were absent, and the PBI was 0.62. Arteriography revealed total obstruction of the aortic bi-

furcation, with reconstitution of the iliac and femoral vessels distally (Fig. 67-5, *A*). The patient underwent an aortobifemoral bypass graft (Fig. 67-5, *B*), and both his claudication and his impotence were relieved.

Comment: The aortobifemoral bypass reestablished pelvic and lower extremity blood flow. The PBI increased to 0.9 postoperatively as a result of retrograde flow up the patent external iliac arteries.

2. A 56-year-old patient complained of disabling right thigh and buttock claudication. Arteriography demonstrated aortoiliac occlusion, with extensive stenosis of both external iliac arteries (Fig. 67-6, *A*). He complained of rather soft erections but was otherwise able to function sexually. The PBI before surgery was 0.80. An aortobifemoral Dacron graft with proximal aortic transection and end-to-end anastomosis was performed. A marked increase of ankle pressure was noted, and the patient's claudication disappeared. However, repeated postoperative penile pressure measurements documented a PBI of 0.56, and the patient became impotent.

Comment: The marked decrease of penile pressure after aortoiliac reconstruction was probably related to the proximal end-to-end anastomosis. Because the aorta was transected, flow to the hypogastric arteries became dependent on retrograde flow through the external iliac arteries, which were too narrow to allow retrograde perfusion to the internal iliac vessels (Fig. 67-6, *B*). This produced a marked decrease in penile pressure, which probably was responsible for the patient's postoperative impotence.

Femorofemoral reconstruction. Both pelvic steal and femoral steal syndromes can be corrected by either aortofemoral or femorofemoral bypass grafting. The second alternative offers no chance of nerve injury, which can cause sexual dysfunction. The use of the penile pressure measurement provides an objective means to assess the result of the procedure. In five patients with the femoral steal syndrome, Queral et al.[25] have shown an improvement in PBI (0.62 to 0.86) in those patients who regained sexual capacity after femorofemoral bypass.

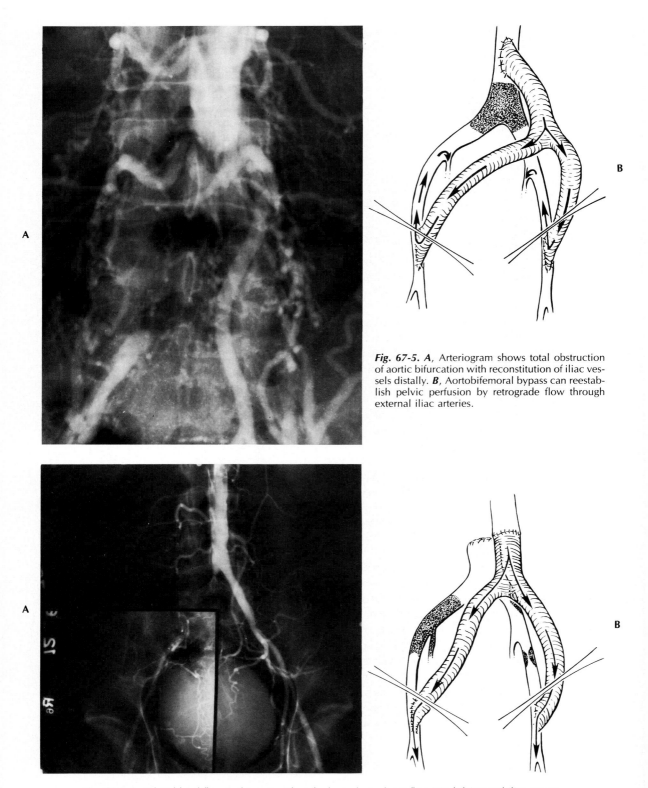

Fig. 67-5. *A*, Arteriogram shows total obstruction of aortic bifurcation with reconstitution of iliac vessels distally. ***B***, Aortobifemoral bypass can reestablish pelvic perfusion by retrograde flow through external iliac arteries.

Fig. 67-6. *A*, Pelvic blood flow in this patient largely depends on direct flow into left internal iliac artery. ***B***, End-to-end aortic grafting adversely affected pelvic hemodynamics, since retrograde flow through diseased left external iliac artery was compromised.

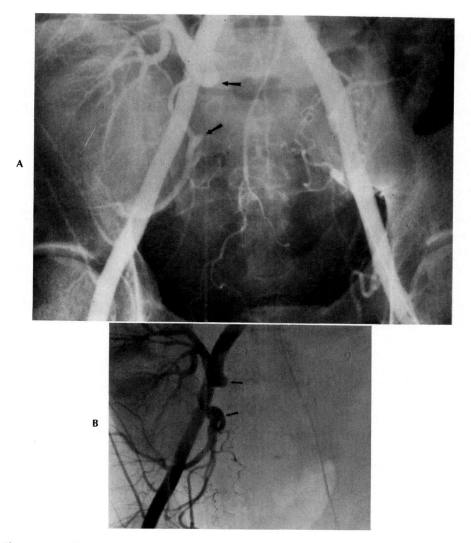

Fig. 67-7. A, Bilateral renal transplantation using internal iliac arteries *(arrows)* made this patient vasculogenically impotent. ***B***, Bypass to distal *(R)* internal iliac artery *(arrows)* restored normal pelvic flow, and sexual capacity was improved.

Renal transplantation. Recently Billet et al.[2] encountered a patient with a complaint of erectile dysfunction who had undergone ligation of both internal iliac arteries after bilateral renal transplantation. The diagnosis of vasculogenic impotence was made by the noninvasive measurement of the penile arterial systolic blood pressure (PBI of 0.64) and confirmed by pelvic arteriography (Fig. 67-7). Correction of the patient's impotence was accomplished by restoration of penile blood flow via a saphenous vein bypass between the external iliac and the internal iliac arteries. A PBI of 1.0 was obtained postoperatively, and a repeat angiogram showed a patent graft. On follow-up visits the patient stated that he had resumed normal erectile activity.

Billet et al.[2,3] reviewed sexual function and internal iliac artery patency in 24 patients who had received at least two renal transplants, one in each iliac fossa. The pelvic hemodynamics of each patient were assessed with a PBI. Sexual dysfunction, as determined by questionnaires and personal interviews, was 46% (11 of 24) in these patients with two transplants, as compared to only 21% (5 of

24) after a single transplant. None of the 11 impotent patients had bilateral internal iliac artery occlusion, and 4 of these 9 had a PBI less than 0.7. One of the 4 patients regained full sexual function after a revascularization procedure, confirming that his impotence was caused by a vascular problem. The results of the study illustrated that vascular insufficiency was present in at least 4 of the 11 impotent patients and may have been avoided by sparing at least one of the internal iliac arteries during the renal transplantation procedures.

Sexual impairment also has been noted after surgical ligation of both internal iliac arteries was performed to arrest hemorrhage in patients with pelvic trauma or to treat priapism.[11,16] Measurement of penile blood pressure allows an accurate assessment of pelvic hemodynamics in these patients.

SUMMARY

Penile blood pressure measurements and PBI are now standard in most vascular laboratories. The simplicity of the technique allows use in the physician's office. The PBI serves as the first step in identification of patients with vasculogenic impotence. Although a PBI of 0.6 or less is diagnostic of vasculogenic impotence, this number must be interpreted carefully because of the multiple factors involved in the etiology of sexual dysfunction. For vascular surgeons the PBI is useful to correlate with arteriographic findings for planning the proper procedure to preserve the blood supply to the pelvic region. More importantly recording penile pressure after surgery helps to determine the effect of aortic surgery or renal transplantation on pelvic hemodynamics.

In patients who sole complaint is impotence, a multidisciplinary evaluation approach is necessary. In these patients an abnormal penile pressure index must be correlated with other tests. If indicated, arteriography should be performed to verify an abnormal pressure index. Routine arteriography is helpful to visualize the major arteries, such as the hypogastric and internal pudendal arteries. However, for a detailed examination of the penile vasculature, selective arteriograms of the internal iliac or internal pudenal artery, performed under general or epidural anesthesia, are necessary to provide satisfactory visualization of the deep penile or deep corporal artery.[12,15] The impotent diabetic patient may have normal penile pressure, and diabetic neuropathy may be responsible for failure of erection. Conversely, a low pressure index may be recorded

in patients who are potent. As Gaylis[11] noted, penile erection is a dynamic state. Therefore recording the penile pressure at rest may not truly reflect penile status during coitus. It must be emphasized that a multidisciplinary approach is essential for evaluation of impotence, and an abnormal PBI does not confirm that ischemia is the responsible factor.

REFERENCES

1. Barker, W.F., and Garpar, N.R.: Peripheral arterial disease. In Major problems in clinical surgery, ed. 3, Philadelphia, 1981, W.B. Saunders Co.
2. Billet, A., Dagher, F.J., and Queral, L.A.: Surgical correction of vasculogenic impotence in a patient after bilateral renal transplantation, Surgery 91:108, 1982.
3. Billet, A., et al.: The effects of bilateral renal transplantation on pelvic hemodynamics and sexual function, Surgery 95:415, 1984.
4. Britt, D.B., Kemmerer, W.T., and Robinson, J.R.: Penile flow determination by mercury strain-gauge plethysmography, Invest. Urol. 8:673, 1970.
5. Canning, J.R., et al.: Genital vascular insufficiency and potency, Surg. Forum 14:298, 1963.
6. Reference deleted in proofs.
7. DePalma, R.G., Kedia, K., and Persky, L.: Vascular operations for preservation of sexual function. In Bergan, J.J., and Yao, J.S.T., editors: Surgery of the aorta and its body branches, New York, 1979, Grune & Stratton, Inc.
8. Engel, G., Burnham, S., and Carter, M.F.: Penile blood pressure in the evaluation of erectile impotence, Fertil. Steril. 30:687, 1978.
9. Flanigan, D.P., et al.: Elimination of iatrogenic impotence and improvement of sexual function after aortoiliac revascularization, Arch. Surg. 117:544, 1982.
10. Gaskell, P.: The importance of penile blood pressure in cases of impotence, Can. Med. Assoc. J. 105:1047, 1971.
11. Gaylis, H.: Penile pressure in the evaluation of impotence in aorto-iliac disease, Surgery 89:277, 1981.
12. Genestie, J.F., and Romieu, A.: Radiologic exploration of impotence, The Hague, 1978, Martinus Nijhoff Medical Division.
13. Goldstein, I., et al.: Vasculogenic impotence: role of the pelvic steal test, J. Urol. 128:300, 1982.
14. Goldstein, I., et al.: Radiation-associated impotence: a clinical study of its mechanism, JAMA 251:903, 1984.
15. Gray, R.R., et al.: Investigation of impotence by internal pudendal angiography: experience with 73 cases, Radiology 144:773, 1982.
16. Hinman, F.H.: Priapism: reasons for failure of therapy, J. Urol. 83:420, 1960.
17. Karacan, I.A.: Clinical value of nocturnal erection in the prognosis and diagnosis of impotence, Med. Aspects Hum. Sexual. 4:27, 1970.
18. Kempczinski, R.F.: Role of the vascular diagnostic laboratory in the evaluation of male impotence, Am. J. Surg. 138:278, 1979.
19. Macvar, T., Baron, T., and Clark, S.S.: Assessment of potency with the Doppler flowmeter, Urology 2:396, 1973.
20. Michal, V., Kramvar, R., and Bartak, V.: Femoropudendal bypass in the treatment of sexual impotence, J. Cardiovasc. Surg. 15:356, 1974.
21. Michal, V., Kramar, F., and Pospichal, J.: External iliac steal syndrome, J. Cardiovasc. Surg. 19:355, 1978.
22. Nath, R.L., et al.: The multidisciplinary approach to vasculogenic impotence, Surgery 89:124, 1981.

23. Pierce, G.E., et al.: Evaluation of end-to-side *v* end-to-end proximal anastomosis in aortobifemoral bypass, Arch. Surg. 117:1580, 1982.
24. Queral, L.A., et al.: Pelvic hemodynamics after aortoiliac reconstruction, Surgery 86:799, 1979.
25. Queral, L.A., et al.: Femoral steal syndrome: a report of five cases, Surg. Forum 32:344, 1981.
26. Schoenberg, H.W., Zarins, C.K., and Segraves, R.T.: Analysis of 122 unselected impotent men subjected to multidisciplinary evaluation, J. Urol. 127:445, 1982.
27. Stauffer, D., and DePalma, R.G.: A comparison of penile-brachial index (PBI) and penile pulse volume recordings for diagnosis of vasculogenic impotence, Bruit 7:29, 1983.
28. Swanson, D.A.: Cancer of the bladder and prostate: the impact of therapy on sexual function. In Von Leschenback, A.C., and Rodriguez, D.B., editors: Sexual rehabilitation of the urologic cancer patient, Boston, 1981, G.K. Hall & Co.

CHAPTER 68

Noninvasive evaluation of the cutaneous circulation

ARNOST FRONEK

Despite the skin's accessibility, there is no ideal method that permits a quantitative evaluation of skin perfusion. The only exception is the determination of digital (or toe) blood flow, which can be measured by venous occlusive plethysmography (Chapter 73). Since skin blood flow is the most essential component of digital blood flow, digital blood flow can be equated with skin blood flow. The need to determine skin perfusion at other sites, however, poses serious difficulties, especially if a quantitative evaluation is desired.

There are several indications for the determination of skin perfusion: (1) to determine optimal amputation level, (2) to evaluate vasospastic conditions, (3) to evaluate vasoactive or rheologic drugs that may have an effect on skin circulation, and (4) to predict the effectiveness of sympathectomy. Methods that can be considered in this category include the following:

1. Skin thermometry
2. Thermal conductance
3. Thermal clearance
4. Transcutaneous partial tension of oxygen (PO_2)
5. Laser Doppler flux
6. Skin arterial blood pressure
7. Epicutaneous ^{133}Xe clearance
8. Venous occlusion plethysmography
9. Photoplethysmography

Venous occlusion plethysmography and photoplethysmography are not discussed in this chapter because they are covered elsewhere in this text. In this chapter only general aspects of skin temperature measurements are discussed, since a detailed evaluation also is discussed in Chapter 75.

SKIN THERMOMETRY

Skin temperature is one of the best-known indices of skin perfusion, However, its value is limited when it is compared to superior techniques. These limitations are based on physical as well as physiologic considerations.

Skin temperature is determined by many factors, which include room temperature, humidity, circulation of the air, state of metabolic and nervous activity, vasomotor and audiomotor activity, previous exposure to nicotine, and type of food ingested. It is difficult to keep all these factors constant, especially during routine diagnostic examination conditions. On the other hand temperature differences between various sites of the body are more meaningful because the results are somewhat normalized. However, this does not prevent misinterpretations, since some vascular regions are under different vasomotor control than others, such as toes or fingers and thigh or arm. Also, absolute temperature measurements are much less useful than relative temperature measurements (topographic gradients) and dynamic skin temperature tests (temporal gradients).

An example of the limited diagnostic value of absolute temperature measurements is the finding of a highly nonlinear correlation between blood flow and skin temperature.[29] Relatively small increases in blood flow, starting with low skin temperature, result in significant increases in skin temperature, whereas a similar increase in blood flow corresponds to a minute temperature increase once the 28° C threshold is reached.

Skin thermometry can be subdivided into contact thermometry, using a thermocouple, thermistor, or liquid crystals; and noncontact thermometry (infrared thermography), using imaging and nonimaging techniques.

Contact thermometry

Thermocouples. Widely used in the past, thermocouples are being employed slightly more today after having been displaced by the more sensitive thermistors. If two different metals are joined, such as copper and constantan, a temperature-dependent potential develops.[19,37] For instance, the combination of copper and constantan has a thermoelectric sensitivity of 40 μV for each degree Celsius. This relatively small voltage compelled earlier investigators to use high-sensitivity galvanometers, which were impractical in daily laboratory routine. Low-sensitivity but more rugged recording devices required high-gain direct current (DC) amplification, which was not a simple task before the advent of operational amplifiers.

Thermistors. The electric resistance of some metals, especially alloys, exhibits considerable temperature dependence. Alloys with a high temperature coefficient of resistivity are selected as the base material for thermistors. In contrast to most metals, such as platinum, which have a positive thermal coefficient, thermistors are composed of different metallic oxides, which have a negative thermal coefficient—with increasing temperature, the resistance decreases.

Thermocouples vs. thermistors. Thermocouples usually require DC amplification when used with simple and rugged recording or monitoring devices. The availability of low-drift, high-gain, semiconductor amplifier systems has triggered a renewed interest in these instruments. Their advantage is linearity and sturdiness of the probe.

The thermistors usually need very little if any amplification because of their high thermal coefficient. Although the temperature/resistance relationship is exponential, this is usually not a serious problem. First, the range of biologic application is almost linear; second, if an extended range is needed for higher laboratory versatility, linearization can be achieved electronically.

No distinct advantages can be seen between thermocouples and thermistors for skin temperature measurement, and a choice may be made strictly on a technical basis.

Liquid crystals. Liquid crystals represent an inexpensive but far less sensitive alternative to infrared thermography. These substances behave mechanically similar to liquids but display the optical properties of crystals.[31] By mixing cholesteric substances in different proportions, specific temperature-color relationships can be produced.[93] The cholesteric liquid can be applied to the skin as a spray or as a reusable tape.[71] This method has the potential for inexpensive skin temperature scanning; the changing color combinations, as a function of changing temperature, can be photographed. The liquid crystal method has not yet found wide application in vascular diagnosis, although some early reports confirm ease of application and reliability.[35,36,71]

Infrared thermography

The skin constantly emits a certain amount of infrared energy, and interestingly its optical properties vary significantly with the wavelength.[38,107,112] To visible light, human skin is partially reflective and partially transparent. This also applies somewhat to the near infrared spectrum. However, in the far infrared region (around 10 μ) the skin behaves almost as a perfect absorber, and it is a perfect emitter of infrared energy. Thermographic instruments usually consist of an optical system, infrared detector, processing system, and display.[80] The radiation emitted by the skin is picked up by a temperature scanning and detecting system, which is synchronized with the display; this results in a picture of the scanned temperatures. The usual thermal sensitivity is around 0.1° C, with a frame time of about 2 seconds (time required to take one picture).

Some instruments include color coding as a function of temperature, whereas others use different grades of black and white. A display of the isotherm, the line connecting the same temperature points, is a useful recent improvement.

Diagnostic value. Despite the sophisticated electronics and the elegant application of complex physical principles, the same limitations described for the contact skin temperature methods apply to infrared thermography, with some exceptions. It offers a quick overview of the temperature points in the examined area more rapidly than temperature mapping, especially when using the isotherm display. Although skin temperatures can be determined quickly, the cost-effectiveness of the test remains questionable because of the limited value of skin temperature in the diagnosis of vascular disease.

THERMAL CONDUCTANCE
Principle

It can be shown mathematically that if a heat source is surrounded by an infinite mass of material, under steady-state conditions, heat production is equal to heat loss[12]:

$$J^2 \times R = 4 \times \pi \times r \times k \times \Delta t$$

where

J = Electric current of the heating system
R = Electric resistance of the heating system
r = Radius of the sphere
k = Thermal conductivity of the surrounding material
Δt = Temperature elevation of the sphere

From this it follows that thermal conductance (k) is derived as follows:

$$k = \frac{J^2 R}{4\pi r \Delta t}$$

Thermal conductance depends on the thermal conductivity of the underlying tissue and on the flow rate of blood. Provided that the first factor can be subtracted, k is proportional to blood flow rate.

Early studies

Practically all flow determination methods using thermal conductivity are based on Gibbs'[39] description of a "blood-flow recorder" using a heated thermocouple. This instrument was originally designed to measure blood flow in vessels and served as a basis for future modifications of this approach.[10,11,45,50,51]

The application of Gibbs' principle to noninvasively measure skin blood flow was first suggested by Burton[10] but was developed and analyzed by Hensel et al.[49,50,51] and Golenhofen et al.[41,42] Theoretical analysis combined with model experiments are described by Vendrik and Vos.[106] Harding et al.[47] pursued the idea of maintaining a constant temperature difference by using a servocontrol system, which compensates for the loss of heat caused by changes in blood flow rate. The changes in power are then related to flow fluctuations. This system is currently used in some commercially available transcutaneous Po$_2$ meters, which use the heating coil to obtain information about relative flow changes. A detailed technical description of this principle is given by McCaffrey and McCook.[74]

Renewed interest in this type of noninvasive skin blood flow measurement was recently initiated by Holti et al. in attempting to evaluate patients with Raynaud's disease as well as new vasoactive drugs.[40,54-56] The design is essentially based on a report by Van de Staak et al.,[105] in which the

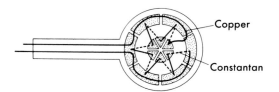

Fig. 68-1. Thermal conductance probe with copper and constantan junctions. (From Holti, G., and Mitchell, K.W.: Clin. Exp. Dermatol. 3:189, 1978.)

temperature difference is measured between a heated copper disk at the center of the probe and an unheated, concentric copper annulus at its periphery. Both temperature-sensing elements are in direct contact with the skin (Fig. 68-1). When a temperature equilibrium is established, a temperature difference of about 2° C is maintained. Changes in blood flow produce temperature changes in the tenths of 1° C. When blood flow decreases, less heat is removed from the center plate, which leads to an increased temperature difference, and vice versa. A similar system was described by Challoner[13] and also was tested with a model flow system. Recently Brown et al.,[9] using a system described by Holti and Mitchell,[56] subjected the method to a theoretical analysis and concluded that constant thermal flux caused by thermal conductivity was equal to 38 mW, whereas that caused by blood flow was only about 7 mW. This explains the requirements for high electronic stability of the system and for consideration of special precautions, such as not placing the probe in the vicinity of large vessels in order to accurately measure the small changes in temperature resulting from changes in cutaneous blood flow.

THERMAL CLEARANCE

All the previously described methods that measure thermal conductance are expressed in cal $\times$ cm^{-1} $\times$ sec^{-1} $\times$ °C^{-1}. Because of complex factors influencing the final reading, besides the desired flow-related thermal conductance, the measurements cannot be expressed in absolute values. Betz and Apfel[5] attempted to quantify these measurements and to express the results in absolute values by introducing the concept of "thermal clearance," similar to the clearance technique using radioisotope tracers.[5,76-78] In principle a certain amount of heat is injected into the tissue for a short time (slug heating), and the temperature "disappearance" curve is recorded. A normalization with

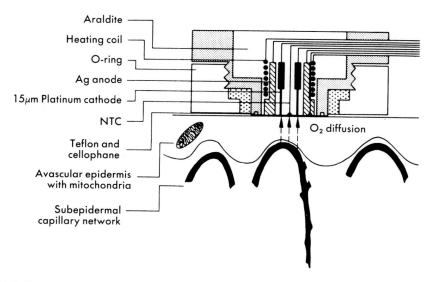

Araldite
Heating coil
O-ring
Ag anode
15μm Platinum cathode
NTC
Teflon and cellophane
Avascular epidermis with mitochondria
Subepidermal capillary network

O_2 diffusion

Fig. 68-2. Transcutaneous P_{O_2} electrode with heating coil (From Huch, A., and Huch, R.: Technical, physiological and clinical aspects of transcutaneous P_{O_2} measurements. In Taylor, D.E.M., and Whamond, J., editors: Non-invasive clinical measurements, Baltimore, 1977, University Park Press. By permission of Pitman Publishing, Ltd.)

thermal clearance under zero flow rate conditions is required. Under these conditions the temperature field (U_{slug}) of the perfused and unperfused tissue is related as follows:

$$\frac{U_{slug\,\phi}}{U_{slug\,o}} = e^{-\frac{\phi \times t}{\lambda}}$$

where ϕ is blood flow and λ is the partition coefficient for heat; indices ϕ and o correspond to perfused and unperfused tissue, respectively. A similar approach was described by Baptista[2] and included skin flow applications. Unfortunately his technique yields only a "peripheral blood circulatory index," and no absolute skin blood flow values are available.

All heat conductance techniques have one disadvantage in common: they do not offer absolute flow rate values. On the other hand, if relative flow change information is sufficient for a given project, thermal conductance is a suitable flow-related index that can be monitored with relatively inexpensive instrumentation.

On the other hand thermal clearance may supply quantitative flow information. It does not require expensive equipment but has not yet been developed for clinical application. Some doubts exist about whether the resolution will be good enough for such a relatively low-perfusion vascular bed as the skin. Further experimental information is needed.

TRANSCUTANEOUS P_{O_2} DETERMINATION
Principle

A modified Clark-type platinum oxygen electrode is used to monitor P_{O_2} from the surface of the skin during heat-induced local vasodilation.

Physiologic and physicochemical notes

The first impetus for transcutaneous P_{O_2} (tcP_{O_2}) monitoring can be traced back to a report in which an electrolytic solution at 45° C equilibrated with the arterial P_{O_2} after a finger was immersed for a sufficient time.[4] Although Evans and Naylor[27] found that the P_{O_2} on the surface of the skin was close to zero, this value could be increased up to 30 mm Hg by vasodilation. The finding that drug-induced vasodilation increases transcutaneously monitored P_{O_2}[59] led to the development of a combined electrode probe incorporating a heater system.[62,65] This represented the single most decisive improvement toward further acceptance of the method. A similar system using a heated cathode was described by Eberhard et al.[23] Standardized vasodilation is important because beyond 43° C skin temperature, the ratio of tcP_{O_2} to arterial P_{O_2} remains constant and is close to 1.[60]

The electrode design is based on the original Clark oxygen electrode,[17] using three 15 μ platinum cathodes surrounded by a common silver ring anode (Fig. 68-2). The temperature of the heating coil adjacent to the anode is controlled by a servosystem sensed by a thermistor constantly monitoring the actual skin temperature. Theoretically, this closed-loop heater control system should be capable of monitoring relative skin perfusion changes (see previous discussion on thermal conductance), but currently available systems do not reflect these changes adequately,[26,115] despite initially encouraging reports.[62,64,95] The probe designed primarily for $tcPO_2$ monitoring obviously does not fulfill the requirements for measuring exact heat consumption, as documented by a number of authors.[7,9,49,104] The electrolytic solution covering the electrodes is retained by a thin Teflon membrane. The 95% response time of this system is about 10 seconds, whereas another system[23] requires about 50 seconds because of a thicker membrane, which on the other hand reduces the oxygen consumption of the electrodes.

Using the polarographic principle, it can be shown that the resulting current (J) is determined by the following[89]:

$$J = \frac{n \times F \times A \times P_m}{V_T \times a} \, PO_2$$

where

n = Equivalents/mole
F = Faraday's constant
A = Cathode area
a = Membrane thickness
P_m = Membrane permeability
V_T = Correction for temperature

Clinical application

In view of the thin skin of newborn babies, they were obvious candidates for $tcPO_2$ monitoring and comparisons with direct PO_2 determinations.[57,59,63,66] An updated review of the application of $tcPO_2$ measurements in obstetrics and neonatology was published by Huch et al.[61] in 1979, with encouraging results, although some limitations must be recognized. First, the specific effect of some anesthetics must be considered.[43,44,94] These effects can be reduced significantly with proper design of the electrode, reducing membrane permeability and changing polarization voltage to -600 mV.[22] Unfortunately results are less reliable in cases of increased sympathetic tone and with decreased body temperature.[30]

Determination of $tcPO_2$ was successfully applied in plastic surgery to evaluate skin oxygen supply.[68]

Tønnesen[103] reported very low $tcPO_2$ values (close to zero) in patients with severe arterial oc-

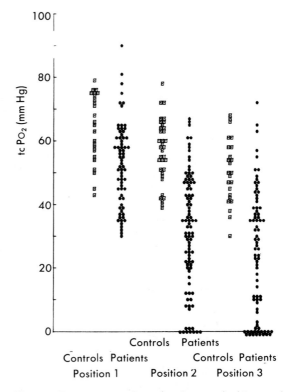

Fig. 68-3. Transcutaneous PO_2 values in control subjects and patients with peripheral arterial occlusive disease. Position 1, Chest; position 2, below knee; position 3, dorsum of foot. (From Franzeck, U.K., et al.: Surgery 91:156, 1982.)

clusive disease. The severity of ischemic disease as well as changes in leg position were well correlated with ^{99m}Tc clearance. A more systematic study, in which $tcPO_2$ values were correlated with limb position in normal control subjects, concluded that the $tcPO_2$ values varied with changes of arteriovenous pressure differences, mainly changes in hydrostatic pressure, but suddenly dropped to zero at a certain perfusion level.[113] This phenomenon, also described by Tønnesen,[103] can be explained in several ways, but one of the most plausible explanations may be that this may occur at a moment of a zero, or negative, balance between oxygen supply and oxygen consumption by the tissue and the electrodes.

Matsen et al.[73] presented $tcPO_2$ values from 13 normal subjects and nine patients with peripheral arterial disease. The $tcPO_2$ values were lower in the patient group at the below-knee (BK) and foot level. The authors concluded that all patients with a $tcPO_2$ below 20 mm Hg required some surgical

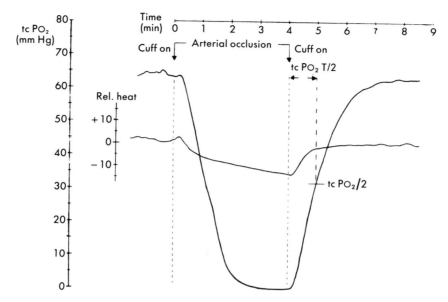

Fig. 68-4. Postocclusive reactive hyperemia response in control subject. (From Franzeck, U.K., et al.: Surgery 91:156, 1982.)

procedure (vascular reconstruction, amputation), reflecting the extreme severity of the disease.

Franzeck et al.[34] compared the tcPO$_2$ in a normal control group (24 subjects) to that of 69 patients with various degrees of arterial occlusive disease. The mean BK values in the control group were 56.8 ± 9.9 mm Hg (standard deviation), whereas the average value in the patient group was significantly lower, 31.7 ± 18.1 mm Hg (Fig. 68-3). In view of the relatively wide scatter, however, an attempt was made to investigate the effect of post-occlusive reactive hyperemia (PORH) on the tcPO$_2$ response. Fig. 68-4 illustrates the typical time course of the PORH response in a normal control subject. The tcPO$_2$ value drops to zero within 3 minutes, and reperfusion is very rapid. The half-time of the response, the time it takes until 50% of the initial tcPO$_2$ is reached, was 60.4 ± 15.2 seconds. The average halftime in the patient group was 130.6 ± 69.2 seconds. A representative tracing is shown in Fig. 68-5, in which one can see not only that the slope of the reperfusion part of the curve is shallower, but also that there is a considerable delay between cuff pressure release and the inflection point of the reperfusion curve. This delay seems to indicate severely compromised skin perfusion, since either it takes so long for the oxygen molecules to reach the surface of the skin or the amount of oxygen supplied is so small that it does not adequately cover the low oxygen requirements of the tissue and the electrode. It is possible that both factors are responsible.

In summary, although the tcPO$_2$ level is related to skin blood flow, this relationship is complex and cannot be used directly to measure skin blood flow, at least at present. On the other hand it is a very sensitive indicator of oxygen availability in the skin.

It therefore seemed appropriate for Franzeck et al.[32-34] to investigate the usefulness of the tcPO$_2$ determination as a predictor of amputation stump healing. Patients were divided into three categories: (A, successful amputation; B, prolonged healing; and C, failure). As seen in Fig. 68-6, the mean tcPO$_2$ value in 26 patients in group A was 36.5 ± 17.5 mm Hg, whereas in six patients with a failed amputation (group C) values were between 0 and 3 mm Hg. Additional experience with this method revealed some false positives and false negatives and led the investigators to increase the sensitivity and specificity of the test by adding the tcPO$_2$ response to 100% O$_2$ inhalation for 10 minutes to the initial resting tcPO$_2$ determination. Fig. 68-7 illustrates the increase in tcPO$_2$ value in normal control subjects and in different groups of patients. Although there is a striking difference in all categories, there was a false positive and a false negative in groups A and C, respectively.

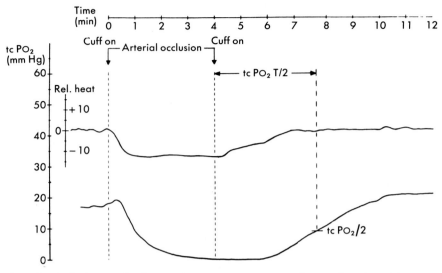

Fig. 68-5. Postocclusive reactive hyperemia response in patient with arterial occlusive disease. (From Franzeck, U.K., et al.: Surgery 91:156, 1982.)

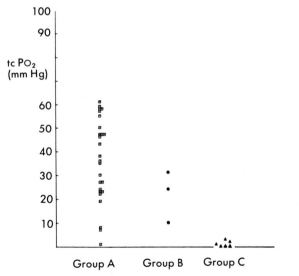

Fig. 68-6. Transcutaneous Po_2 values in patients with excellent amputation stump healing (group A), delayed healing (group B), and failure of healing (group C). (From Franzeck, U.K., et al.: Surgery 91:156, 1982.)

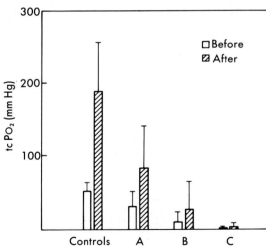

Fig. 68-7. Response to 100% O_2 breathing in control subjects and groups A, B, and C from Fig. 68-6. (From Franzeck, U.K., et al.: Surgery 91:156, 1982.)

White et al.[109] analyzed the predictive value of tcPo$_2$ in the success of spontaneous wound healing and amputation stump healing in 25 patients. They concluded that tcPo$_2$ values below 40 mm Hg predicted a poor chance of ulcer or stump healing. A postoperative improvement of tcPo$_2$ level correlated well with the long-term effectiveness of vascular bypass procedures.

Recently Hauser and Shoemaker[48] reported an interesting drop in their regional perfusion index (RPI) (tcPo$_2$ of the extremity divided by tcPo$_2$ of the chest), after standardized exercise in patients with intermittent claudication. No significant reduction was observed in asymptomatic patients, despite objective evidence of arterial occlusive disease. In a related study, using an implanted Silastic tubing permeable to oxygen, Jussila and Niinikoski[67] observed a drop in Po$_2$ in the perfused fluid after mild exercise (tiptoeing), whereas no drop was evident after successful arterial reconstruction. With more general applications in mind Chang et al.[15] used this invasive, implanted Silastic tubing technique to evaluate the optimal conditions for postoperative wound healing. Conclusions from both invasive studies are relevant to the future application of tcPo$_2$ monitoring.

Evaluation

To place the potential value of tcPo$_2$ monitoring in proper perspective, it is necessary to consider all factors that may influence the recorded tcPo$_2$ level. These include factors related to (1) morphology, especially of the skin; (2) physiology; and (3) methodology.

Morphologic factors include the diffusing capacity of the skin, thickness of various skin layers, and histologic structure of the cutaneous vasculature. The last factor may be age-dependent, which may explain why decreased tcPo$_2$ values have been observed in the chest region of older patients.[34,43]

Physiologic factors include cardiac output; degree of sympathetic stimulation, which may be a main source of discrepancies between arterial and transcutaneous Po$_2$; state of arteriovenous shunts; and oxygen consumption of the epidermis.

Methodologic factors include the effect of increased local temperature on skin blood flow and on the hemoglobin-binding curve, oxygen consumption by the electrode, and the effect of membrane quality and thickness.

Finally the observed tcPo$_2$ value is the end result of all these factors, although the most decisive one

influencing the final balance is local oxygen availability, which is ultimately a function of blood flow. Therefore we can expect that tcPo$_2$ will become a useful technique to evaluate both oxygen availability and skin viability.

LASER DOPPLER FLUX MEASUREMENT
Relationship of skin histology to cutaneous blood flow determination

To evaluate the possibilities and limitations of laser Doppler perfusion (LDP) monitoring, some basic histologic principles relating to the skin must be considered. Despite the great variability of the skin structure resulting from topographic differences (finger, forearm, foot), there is a general pattern. The epidermis is completely devoid of vascularization; it is usually a 40 to 50 μm keratin layer, which may reach a thickness up to 400 μm in the fingertips.[110] The microvascular structure starts with the feeding arterioles, which end up in a hairpinlike system of capillaries rising from the papillae of the corium to return to the subpapillary venous plexus. In contrast to the vertical takeoff of the capillaries, the larger vessels in the lower dermis run parallel to the skin surface.[46,90,96] In some sites, especially those involved in thermoregulation, arteriovenous anastomoses ($\sim$40 μm in diameter) are present and effectively shunt the capillary system if the anastomoses are dilated.

Physical principles

In contrast to the insonation of an exactly defined vessel cross-section with Doppler ultrasound, the detection of the Doppler shift signal from the cutaneous microcirculation is far more complex. First, because of the microscopic dimensions of the capillaries, relatively low-frequency ultrasonic energy cannot be used. Second, the energy beam that impinges on the microcirculatory system does not face a uniform, geometrically well-defined vasculature but rather a network of vessels crisscrossing the measurement sample site.

The selection of a very narrow monochromatic light source (laser) helped limit the difficulties posed by the complexities of skin microvasculature. However, even the application of a single, narrow-frequency light source did not solve other inherent difficulties. The incident light source reaches the capillaries and red blood cells (RBCs) at a variety of different angles because of the random orientation of the capillary loops. In addition, significant scattering occurs before the beam reaches the capillary. All this is repeated by the reflected beam on its path back to the pickup system. The incident light usually penetrates to a depth of 1.5 mm, but the actual depth of penetration is a function of technical parameters, such as power density of the source and aperture, as well as of anatomic variables, such as skin pigmentation, thickness of the epidermis, and topographic differences. However, the recorded Doppler-shifted signal corresponds to an average velocity obtained under an average angle. To complicate the matter, the resulting signal, at least in the available systems, also depends on the number of RBCs in the sample volume because of the type of signal processing currently used. The resulting signal therefore is a product of the number of RBCs moving in the sample volume and the mean velocity of the moving RBCs. Because it is neither velocity nor flow, the term *blood cell flux* has been suggested:[83,84,98]

$$\text{Flux} = \text{Red cell volume fraction} \times \text{Velocity}$$

Historical notes

In 1964 Cummins et al.[20] suggested that by applying a highly coherent monochromatic light source (laser) previously developed by Schawlow and Townes,[92] even the movement of macromolecules could be detected if a proper heterodyning technique (mixing of two close frequencies and using their difference) was used. Yeh and Cummins[114] documented that with this approach even very low flow velocities could be detected ($\sim$0.07 mm/sec). Riva et al.[86] applied this principle to the determination of retinal blood flow in the rabbit. In model experiments with glass capillaries they found a remarkable difference in the recorded frequency spectrum: a flat plateau with a sharp falloff point when using polystyrene spheres, whereas the falloff frequency was less exactly defined when using RBCs as reflecting particles, probably because of additional light scattering caused by the different RBC geometry. In subsequent studies Tanaka et al.[100,101] reported additional improvement in the signal-to-noise ratio using autocorrelation with retinal vessel application. Laser Doppler velocimetry was then directly applied in experimental microcirculatory research by Einav et al.[24,25] and Mishina et al.[75] by bringing the laser beam to the examined microvessels through a special microscope system. Le-Cong and Zweifach[70] applied the advantages of the coherent, monochromatic light source to measure not only velocities

but also microvascular dimensions. Their system, however, used the interference measurement rather than the Doppler shift signal.

Noninvasive application to monitor blood flow was first demonstrated by Stern,[97] who used a spectrum analyzer to process the Doppler-shifted signals from the fingertip. In a subsequent comprehensive theoretical and experimental analysis Stern et al.[98] obtained a good correlation with ^{133}Xe washout studies in normal subjects subjected to ultraviolet-induced local hyperemia. In all these studies root-mean-square (RMS) bandwidth of the Doppler signal was found to correlate with actual flow measurements:

$$F = \int_0^\infty \omega^2 P(\omega) d\omega$$

where F indicates the Doppler ''flow parameters'' and $P(\omega)$ denotes the power spectrum of the Doppler signal.

The advantage of this type of signal processing is its relative simplicity, although the amount of reflected energy also influences the resulting signal. Replacement of the photomultiplier type by a photodiode facilitated the more widespread use of the system because of its portability.[108] A similar system was later described by Nilsson et al.,[81-84] who improved the signal-to-noise ratio by using a differential optical system, feeding a split fiberoptic output into two identical photodiode systems (Fig. 68-8). This helps reduce the signals originating from stationary reflection sites, whereas the Doppler-shifted signals are amplified because their uniqueness precludes cancellation of the signal in the differential amplifier. Signal processing is performed in a similar way, using the RMS detection and subtracting the noise-generated signals[83]:

$$\text{RMS (blood flow)} = \sqrt{\text{RMS}^2_{(total)} - \text{RMS}^2_{noise}}$$

A more comprehensive theoretical analysis of the optimal signal processing was published by Bonner et al.[6,7] and Nilsson et al.[83]

The advantage of autocorrelation was recently emphasized by Cochrane et al.[18] in an experimental and theoretical study. Investigators using the laser Doppler system in retinal artery velocimetry reported acceptable results with simpler signal processing using a logarithmic correlation of the power output vs. frequency output.[8,86,88]

Clinical application

Although the resulting signal is a product of velocity and RBC volume, which makes it difficult

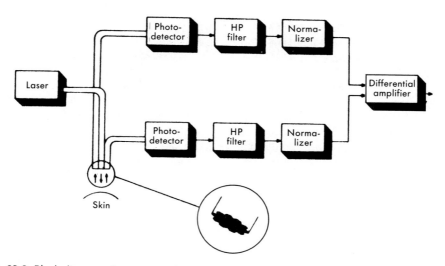

Fig. 68-8. Block diagram of compensated Laser Doppler Fluxmeter. (From Nilsson, G.E., Tenland, T., and Oberg, P.A.: Evaluation of a laser Doppler flowmeter for measurement of tissue blood flow, IEEE Trans. Biomed. Eng. 27:597, 1980. © 1980 IEEE.)

to calibrate or even to compare with existing techniques, the ease, convenience, and noninvasiveness of this method already have resulted in many studies using this technique as a prime tool to evaluate various aspects of skin perfusion.

Powers and Frayer[85] reported an application in plastic surgery, although there is no systematic study correlating output with flap viability. Holloway[52] found a significant increase in blood flow induced by needle trauma, whereas the increase caused by histamine was lower than that induced by needle trauma. These changes were significantly smaller if vasodilation (local heating) preceded the intervention. Salerud et al.[91] systematically investigated the spontaneous rhythmic microcirculatory variations previously described both in animals[14] and clinical studies.[28] Although the coefficient of variation was low in model experiments, the spatial differences in the forearm and temporal variations from day to day were significant.[102] A preliminary study by Low et al.[72] has indicated the usefulness of using laser Doppler flux metering in combination with standardized tests (inspiratory gasp, Valsalva's maneuver, cold stimulus) to separate disorders of the autonomic nervous system.

Evaluation

The advantages of laser Doppler flux metering include its noninvasive application, continuous readout, and ease of operation. The main disadvantage is the absence of calibration and inability to express results in units generally used in fluid mechanics, such as velocity or flow rate. Although the flux, RBC volume fraction multiplied by velocity, is of interest if overall questions of perfusion are investigated, an output related only to velocity or flow would be preferable. This question may be solved with appropriate signal processing.

SKIN ARTERIAL PRESSURE

In contrast to the generally accepted and highly informative arterial segmental pressure, which reflects the pressure in large arteries of the extremities, the application of skin blood pressure is still in its infancy, despite the clinical importance of skin perfusion pressure in determining skin viability, as in amputation level assessment and objective evaluation of patients with Raynaud's syndrome.

In 1967 Dahn et al.[21] used the effect of counterpressure on radioisotope clearance from the skin. The pressure at which the clearance stopped was considered the skin perfusion pressure. Besides it not being noninvasive, requiring the injection of a radioactive substance such as ^{133}Xe, this method was time-consuming and cumbersome. Lassen and Holstein[69] established the clinical value of the counterpressure technique—monitoring the effect of the increasing cuff pressure on some index of skin circulation underneath the cuff—and concluded that a skin perfusion pressure of 20 mm Hg or less predicts very poor healing for an amputation stump.

Chawatzas and Jamieson[16] described a very simple but subjective technique to estimate skin perfusion pressure: observing the blanching and reddening of the skin through a transparent sphygmomanometric cuff. Nielsen et al.[79] described an objective and simple technique to determine "systolic skin pressure" (SSP). Beneath a standard inflation cuff a flat photoelectric probe is placed in direct contact with the skin and records the reflected light from the skin. The skin becomes pale at suprasystolic pressures; during release of the cuff pressure reddening of the skin results in a change in the recorded signal. The authors used the DC mode of operation so that a change in baseline might be considered the moment of blood return to the cutaneous vascular system, the SSP. In a group of normal control subjects the SSP thus obtained was close to the diastolic pressure measured in the arm by auscultation: diastolic arm pressure, 78.2 mm Hg; SSP, 85.8 mm Hg. In a group of hypertensive patients, however, the difference between SSP and diastolic arm pressure was more pronounced: diastolic arm pressure, 106.3 mm Hg, SSP, 129.9 mm Hg. Holstein et al.[53] compared SSP in 13 normal subjects with intraarterial blood pressure obtained from the posterior tibial artery using an ultralow-compliance transducer.[3] Again the SSP was only slightly higher, 84.3 mm Hg, when compared to the direct diastolic pressure of 72 mm Hg.

We can expect this method to become an important examination technique in establishing the optimal level for dysvascular amputation.

CONCLUSIONS

Despite the number of methods available and the accessibility of the skin, there is no single technique that completely fulfills the basic requirements for evaluating skin perfusion: to determine accurately the state of skin perfusion both quantitatively and noninvasively. Of the methods described, the last three appear to have the potential to be more widely used under clinical conditions. Each reflects a different aspect of skin perfusion: transcutaneous Po_2 determination reflects oxygen availability on the surface of the skin; laser Doppler velocity metering output is a function of red blood cell velocity; and skin systolic pressure relates to the diastolic blood pressure in the large arteries. Further clinical experience will help in identifying which of these techniques is most helpful in evaluating the hemodynamics of the cutaneous circulation.

REFERENCES

1. Aschoff, J., and Wever R.: Die Anisotropic der Haut für den Wärmetr ansport, Pflügers Arch. 269:130, 1959.
2. Baptista, A.M.: A simple thermal method for the study of the peripheral blood circulation and applications, Microvasc. Res. 2:123, 1970.
3. Barras, J.-P.: Direct measurement of blood pressure by transcutaneous micropuncture of peripheral arteries—use of a new developed isovolumetric manometer, Scand. J. Clin. Lab. Invest. 128 (Suppl):153, 1973.
4. Baumberger, J.P., and Goodfriend, R.B.: Determination of arterial oxygen tension in man by equilibrium through intact skin, Feb. Proc. 10:10, 1951.
5. Betz, E., and Apfel, H.: Wärmeleitmessung und Wärmeclearance mit Thermoelementen und Thermistoren. In Hild, R., and Spann, G., editors: Therapiekontrolle in der Angiologie, Baden-Baden, West Germany, 1979, G. Witzstrock Publishers.
6. Bonner R., and Nossal, R.: Model for laser Doppler measurements of blood flow in tissue, Appl. Optics 20:2097, 1981.
7. Bonner, R.F., et al.: Laser-Doppler continuous real-time monitor of pulsatile and mean blood flow in tissue microcirculation. In: Chen, S.H., Chu, B., and Nossal, R., editors: Scattering techniques applied to supramolecular and nonequilibrium systems, NATO ASI series B, 73:685, New York, 1981, Plenum Press.
8. Brein, K.R., and Riva, Ch.E.: Laser Doppler velocimetry measurement of pulsatile blood flow in capillary tubes, Microvasc. Res. 24:114, 1982.
9. Brown, B.H., et al.: A critique of the use of a thermal clearance probe for the measurement of skin blood flow, Clin. Phys. Physiol. Meas. 1:237, 1980.
10. Burton, A.C.: The direct measurement of thermal conductance of the skin as an index of peripheral blood flow, Am. J. Physiol. 129:326, 1940.
11. Burton, A.C., and Edholm, O.G.: Man in a cold environment. London, 1955, S. Arnold Publishers.
12. Carslaw, H.S.: The mathematical theory of the conduction of heat in solids, London, 1921, Macmillan Publishers.
13. Challoner, A.V.J.: Accurate measurement of skin blood flow by a thermal conductance method, Med. Biol. Eng. 13:196, 1975.
14. Chambers, R., and Zweifach, B.W.: The topography and function of the mesenteric circulation, Am. J. Anat. 75:173, 1944.
15. Chang, N., et al.: Direct measurement of wound and tissue O_2 tension in post operative patients, Ann. Surg. 197:470, 1983.
16. Chawatzas, D., and Jamieson, C.: A simple method for approximate measurement of skin blood pressure, Lancet 1:711, 1974.
17. Clark, L.C., Jr.: Monitor and control of blood and tissue oxygen tensions, Trans. Am. Soc. Artif. Intern. Organs 2:41, 1956.
18. Cochrane, T., Earnshaw, J.C., and Love, A.H.G.: Laser Doppler measurement of blood velocity in microvessels, Med. Biol. Eng. Comput. 19:589, 1981.
19. Cromwell, F.J., Weibell, F.Y., and Pfeiffer, E.A.: Biomedical instrumentation and measurements, ed. 2, Englewood Cliffs, N.J., 1980, Prentice-Hall, Inc.
20. Cummins, H.Z., Knable, N., and Yeh, Y.: Observation of diffusion broadening of Rayleigh scattered light, Phys. Rev. Lett. 12:150, 1964.
21. Dahn, I., Lassen, N.A., and Westling, H.: Blood flow in human muscles during external pressure or venous stasis, Clin. Sci. 32:467, 1967.

22. Eberhard, P., and Mindt, N.: Interference of anesthetic gases at skin surface sensors for oxygen and carbon dioxide, Crit. Care Med. 9:717, 1981.
23. Eberhard, P., Hammacher, K., and Mindt, W.: Methode zur kutanen Messung des Sauerstoffpartialdruckes, Biomed. Tech. 18:212, 1973.
24. Einav, S., et al.: Measurements of velocity profiles of red blood cells in the microcirculation by laser Doppler anemometry (LDA), Biorheology 12:207, 1975.
25. Einav, S., et al.: Measurement of blood flow in vivo by laser Doppler anemometry through a microscope, Biorheology 12:203, 1975.
26. Enkema, L., Jr., et al.: Laser Doppler velocimetry vs. heater power as indicators of skin perfusion during transcutaneous O_2 monitoring, Clin. Chem. 27:391, 1981.
27. Evans, N.T.S., and Naylor, P.F.D.: The systemic oxygen supply to the surface of human skin, Respir. Physiol. 3:21, 1967.
28. Fagrell, B., Fronek, A., and Intaglietta, M.: A microscope-television system for studying flow velocity in human skin capillaries, Am. J. Physiol. 233:H318, 1977.
29. Felder, D., et al.: Relationship in the toe of skin surface temperature to mean blood flow measured with a plethysmograph, Clin. Sci. 13:251, 1954.
30. Fenner, A., et al.: Transcutaneous determination of arterial oxygen tension, Pediatrics 55:224, 1975.
31. Ferguson, J.L.: Liquid crystals, Sci. Am. 211:77, 1964.
32. Franzeck, U.K., et al.: Transcutaneous pO_2 measurements in health and peripheral arterial occlusive disease, Bibl. Anat. 20:688, 1981.
33. Franzeck, U.K., et al.: Transkutane pO_2—Messungen bei der peripheren arteriellen Verschlusskrankheit, Mikrocirculation und Arterielle Verschlusskrankheiten, München, 1981, Karger, Basel.
34. Franzeck, U.K., et al.: Transcutaneous pO_2 measurements in health and peripheral arterial occlusive disease, Surgery 91:156-163, 1982.
35. Gautherie, M.: Application des cristaux liquides cholestériques á la thermographie cutanée, J. Physique 30:(suppl):11-12, 1969.
36. Gautherie, M., Quenneville, Y., and Gros, Ch.: Thermographie cholestérique, Pathol. Biol. 22:553, 1974.
37. Geddes, L.A., and Baker, L.E.: Principles of applied biomedical instrumentation, ed. 2, New York, John Wiley & Sons, Inc.
38. Gershon-Cohen, J., Haberman-Brueschke, J.D., and Brueschke, E.E.: Medical thermography, Radiol. Clin. 3:403, 1965.
39. Gibbs, F.A.: A thermoelectric bloodflow recorder in the form of a needle, Proc. Soc. Exp. Biol. N.Y. 31:141, 1933.
40. Gillon, R., Holti, G., and Mitchell, K.M.: Measurement of nutrient skin bloodflow using the thermal clearance rate and cinerecordings of stereoscopic capillary microscopy, Biorheology 13:262, 1976.
41. Golenhofen, K.: Blood flow of muscle and skin studied by the local heat clearance technique, Scand. J. Clin. Lab. Invest. 19(Suppl. 99):79, 1967.
42. Golenhofen, K., Hensel, H., and Hildebrandt, G.: Durchblutungsmessung mit Wärmeleitelementen, Stuttgart, 1963, G. Thieme.
43. Gøthgen, I., and Jacobsen, E.: Transcutaneous oxygen tension measurement. I. Age variation and reproducibility, Acta Anaesthesiol. Scand. (Suppl.)67:66, 1978.
44. Gøthgen, I., and Jacobsen, E.: Transcutaneous oxygen tension measurement. II. The influence of halothane and hypotension, Acta Anaesthesiol. Scand. (Suppl.)67:71, 1978.
45. Grayson, J.: Internal calorimetry in the determinations of thermal conductivity and bloodflow, J. Physiol. 118:54, 1952.
46. Greenfield, A.D.M.: The circulation through the skin. In: II. Circulation, Hamilton, W.F., editor: Handbook of physiology. 1963, Washington, D.C., American Physiology Society.
47. Harding, D.C., Rushmer, and Baker, D.W.: Thermal transcutaneous flowmeter, Med. Biol. Eng. 5:623, 1967.
48. Hauser, C.J., and Shoemaker, W.C.: Use of a transcutaneous pO_2 regional perfusion index to quantify tissue perfusion in peripheral vascular disease, Ann. Surg. 197:337, 1983.
49. Hensel, H.: Messkopf fur Durchblutungsregistrierung an Oberflächen. Pflügers Arch. 268:604, 1959.
50. Hensel, H., and Bender, F.: Fortlaufende Bestimmung der Hautdurchblutung am Menschen mit einem elektrischen Wärmeleitmesser, Pflügers Arch. 263:603, 1956.
51. Hensel, H., Ruef, J., and Golenhofen, K.: Fortlaufende Registrierung der Muskeldurchblutung am Henschen mit der Calorimetersonde, Pflügers Arch. 259:267, 1954.
52. Holloway, G.A.: Cutaneous blood flow responses to injection trauma measured by laser Doppler velocimetry, J. Invest. Dermatol. 74:1, 1980.
53. Holstein, P., Nielsen, P.E., and Barras, J.P.: Blood flow cessation at external pressure in the skin of normal human limbs (photoelectric recordings compared to isotope washout and to local intra-arterial blood pressure), Microvasc. Res. 17:71, 1979.
54. Holti, G.: The copper-tellurite-copper thermocouple adapted as skin thermometer, Clin. Sci. 14:137, 1955.
55. Holti, G.: The assessment of the nutrient skin bloodflow with special reference to measurement of the thermal clearance rate, Biorheology 11:208, 1974.
56. Holti, G., and Mitchell, K.W.: Estimation of the nutrient skin bloodflow using a segmental thermal clearance probe, Clin. Exp. Dermatol. 3:189, 1978.
57. Huch, R., and Huch, A.: Transcutaneous Überwachung des arteriellen pO_2 in der Anesthesie. Einsatzfähikeit der Methode am Beispiel von Kurznarkosen, Anaesthetist 23:181, 1974.
58. Huch, A., Huch, R., and Lübbers, D.W.: Quantitative polarographische Sauerstoffdruckmessung auf der Kopfhaut des Neugeborenen, Arch. Gynakol. 207:443, 1969.
59. Huch, R., Huch, A., and Lübbers, D.W.: Transcutaneous measurement of blood PO_2 (t_2PO_2)—method and application in perinatal medicine, J. Perinat. Med. 1:183, 1973.
60. Huch, A., Huch, R., and Lucey, Y.F.: Continuous transcutaneous blood gas monitoring, First Int. Symp. Birth Defects Orig. Art. Series 15:1, 1979.
61. Huch, R., Huch, A., and Rolfe, P.: Transcutaneous measurement of pO_2 using electrochemical analysis. In Rolfe, P., editor: Non-invasive physiological measurements. Vol. 1, London, 1979, Academic Press.
62. Huch, R., Lübbers, D.W., and Huch, A.: Quantitative continuous measurement of partial oxygen pressure on the skin of adults and new-born babies, Pflügers Arch, 337:185, 1972.
63. Huch, R., Lübbers, D.W., and Huch, A.: Reliability of transcutaneous monitoring of arterial PO_2 in new-born infants, Arch. Dis. Child. 49:213, 1974.
64. Huch, A., Lübbers, D.W., and Huch, R.: Der periphere Perfusionsdruck: eine neue, nicht-invasive Messgrösse zur Kreislanfüberwachung von Patienten, Anaesthesist 24:39, 1975.
65. Huch, A., et al.: Eine schnelle, beheizte Pt-Oberflächenelektrode zur kontinuierlichen Überwachung des PO_2

beim Menschen, Stuttgart, 1972. Vortrag Medizin-Technik.

66. Huch, A., et al.: Continuous transcutaneous oxygen tension measured with a heated electrode, Scand. J. Clin. Lab. Invest. 31:269, 1973.

67. Jussila, E.J., and Niinikoski, J.: Effect of vascular reconstructions on tissue gas tensions in calf muscles of patients with occlusive arterial disease, Ann. Chir. Gynaecol. 70: 56, 1981.

68. Knote, G., and Bohmert, H.: Determination of the viability of skin regions in danger of necrosis by means of transcutaneous polarographic measurement of oxygen pressure, Fortschr. Med. 95:640, 1977.

69. Lassen, N.A., and Holstein, P.: Use of radioisotopes in assessment of distal blood flow and distal blood pressure in arterial insufficiency, Surg. Clin. North Am. 54:39, 1974.

70. Le-Cong, P., and Zweifach, B.W.: In vivo and in vitro velocity measurements in microvasculature with a laser, Microvasc. Res. 17:131, 1979.

71. Lee, B.Y., Trainor, F.S., and Madden, J.L.: Liquid crystal tape: its use in the evaluation of vascular diseases, Arch. Phys. Med. Rehab. 54:96, 1973.

72. Low, P.A., et al.: Evaluation of skin vasomotor reflexes by using laser Doppler velocimetry, Mayo Clin. Proc. 58:592, 1983.

73. Matsen, F.A., III., et al.: Transcutaneous oxygen tension measurement in peripheral vascular disease, Surg. Gynecol. Obstet. 150:525, 1980.

74. McCaffrey, T.V., and McCook, R.D.: A thermal method for determination of tissue blood flow, J. Appl. Physiol. 39:170, 1975.

75. Mishina, H., Koyama, T., and Asakura, T.: Velocity measurements of blood flow in the capillary and vein using a laser Doppler microscope, Appl. Optics 14:2326, 1975.

76. Müller-Schauenburg, W.: Über einen Ansatz fur Trennung von Wärmeleitung und Wärmeabtransport durch des Blut—ein neues Verfahren zur quantitativen Messung der Lokalen Gewebsdurchblutung, Thesis, University of Tübingen, 1972.

77. Müller-Schauenburg, W., and Betz, E.: Gas and heat clearance comparison and use of heat-transport for quantitative local blood flow measurements. In: Brock, M., et al., editors: Cerebral blood flow, New York, 1969, Springer-Verlag.

78. Müller-Schauenburg, W., et al.: Quantitative measurement of local blood flow with heat clearance, Basic Res. Cardiol. 70:547, 1975.

79. Nielsen, P.E., Poulsen, H.L., and Gyntelberg, F.: Arterial blood pressure in the skin measured by a photoelectric probe and external counterpressure, Vasa 2:65, 1973.

80. Nilsson, K.: Evaluation of infra-red thermography in experimental biology and medicine, Adv. Microcirc. 3:67, 1970.

81. Nilsson, G.E., Tenland, T., and Oberg, P.A.: Continuous measurement of capillary blood flow by light beating spectroscopy, Proceedings of the Conference on Transducers and Measurements, Madrid, Oct. 10-14, 1978.

82. Nilsson, G.E., Tenland, T., and Oberg, P.A.: Laser Doppler flowmetry—a non-invasive method for microvascular studies, Thirteenth Annual International Conference on Medicine and Bioengineering, Jerusalem, Aug. 19-24, 1979.

83. Nilsson, G.E., Tenland, T., and Oberg, P.A.: A new instrument for continuous measurement of tissue blood flow by light beating spectroscopy, IEEE Trans. BioMed. Eng. 27:12, 1980.

84. Nilsson, G.E., Tenland, T., and Oberg, P.A.: Evaluation of a laser Doppler flowmeter for measurement of tissue blood flow, IEEE Trans. BioMed. Eng. 27:597, 1980.

85. Powers, E.W., III, and Frayer, W.W.: Laser Doppler measurement of blood flow in the microcirculation, Plast. Reconstr. Surg. 61:250, 1978.

86. Riva, Ch.E., Grunwald, J.E., and Sinclair, S.H.: Laser Doppler measurement of relative blood velocity in the human optic nerve head, Invest. Ophthalmol. Vis. Sci. 22:241, 1982.

87. Riva, C., Ross, B., and Benedek, G.B.: Laser Doppler measurements of blood flow in capillary tubes and retinal arteries, Invest. Ophthalmol. Vis. Sci. 11:936, 1972.

88. Riva, C.E., et al.: Bi-directional LDV system for absolute measurement of blood speed in retinal vessels, Appl. Optics 18:2301, 1979.

89. Rolfe, P.: Arterial oxygen measurement in the newborn with intra-vascular transducers, IEE Med. Electr. Monogr. 18-22, London, 1976, Peter Perigrinus Ltd.

90. Ryan, J.J.: Structure and shape of blood vessels of the skin. In: Jarrett A., editor: The physiology and pathophysiology of the skin. Vol. 2, London, 1973, Academic Press.

91. Salerud, E.G., et al.: Rhythmical variations in human skin blood flow, Int. J. Microcirc. Clin. Exp. 2:91, 1983.

92. Schawlow, A.L., and Townes, C.H.: Infrared and optic lasers, Physiol. Rev. 112:1940, 1958.

93. Selawry, A.S., Selawry, H.S., and Holland, J.F.: Use of liquid cholesteric crystals for thermographic measurement of skin temperature in man, Mol. Cryst. 1:495, 1966.

94. Severinghaus, J.W., et al.: Oxygen electrode errors due to polarographic reduction of halothane, J. Appl. Physiol. 31:640, 1971.

95. Severinghaus, J.W., et al.: Workshop on methodological aspects of transcutaneous blood gas analysis, Acta Anaesthesiol. Scand. 68:1, 1978.

96. Sparks, H.V.: Skin and muscle. In Johnson, P.C., editor: Peripheral circulation, New York, 1978, John Wiley & Sons, Inc.

97. Stern, M.D.: In vivo evaluation of microcirculation by coherent light scattering, Nature 524:56, 1975.

98. Stern, M.D., et al.: Continuous measurement of tissue blood flow by laser Doppler spectroscopy, Am. J. Physiol. 232(4):H441, 1977.

99. Strandness, E.D., Jr., and Summer, D.S.: Hemodynamics for surgeons, New York, 1975, Grune & Stratton, Inc.

100. Tanaka, T., and Benedek, G.B.: Measurement of the velocity of blood flow (in vivo) using a fiber optic catheter and optical mixing spectroscopy, Appl. Optics 14:180, 1975.

101. Tanaka, T., Riva, C., and Ben-Sira, I.: Blood velocity measurements in human retinal vessels, Science 186:830, 1974.

102. Tenland, T., et al.: Spatial and temporal variations in human skin blood flow, Int. J. Microcirc. Clin. Exp. 2:81, 1983.

103. Tønnesen, K.H.: Transcutaneous oxygen tension in imminent foot gangrene, Acta Anaesthesiol. Scand. 68:107, 1978.

104. Tremper, K., and Huxtable, R.F.: Dermal heat transport analysis for transcutaneous O_2 measurement, Acta Anaesthesiol. Scand. 68:48, 1978.

105. Van de Staak, W.J.B.M., Brakkee, A.J.M., and De Rijke-Herweijer, H.E.: Measurements of the thermal conductivity of the skin as an indication of skin bloodflow, J. Invest. Dermatol. 51:149, 1968.

106. Vendrik, A.J.H., and Vos, J.J.: A method for the measurement of the thermal conductivity of human skin, J. Appl. Physiol. 11:211, 1957.

107. Wallace, J.D., and Cade, C.M: Clinical thermography, Cleveland, 1975, CRC Press.
108. Watkins, D.W., and Holloway, G.A., Jr.: An instrument to measure cutaneous blood flow using the Doppler shift of laser light, IEEE Trans. BioMed. Eng. 25:28, 1978.
109. White, R.A., et al.: Noninvasive evaluation of peripheral vascular disease using transcutaneous oxygen tension, Am. J. Surg. 144:68, 1982.
110. Whitton, J.T., and Everall, J.D.: The thickness of the epidermis, Br. J. Dermatol. 89:467, 1973.
111. Winsor, T.: Vascular aspects of thermography. J. Cardiovasc. Surg. 12:379, 1971.
112. Winsor, T., and Bendezer, J.: Thermography and the peripheral circulation, Ann. N.Y. Acad. Sci. 121:135, 1964.
113. Wyss, C.R., et al.: Dependence of transcutaneous oxygen tension on local arteriovenous pressure gradient in normal subjects, Clin. Sci. 60:499, 1981.
114. Yeh, Y., and Cummins, H.Z.: Localized fluid flow measurements with an He-Ne laser spectrometer, Appl. Physiol. Lett. 4:176, 1964.
115. Zick, G.L., Holloway, G.A., Jr., and Piraino, D.W.: Simultaneous measurement of tcPO$_2$ and capillary blood flow, Proceedings of the International Conference of Vital Parameter Determination during Extracorporeal Circulation, Nijmegan, The Netherlands, 1980.

CHAPTER 69

Controversies in the noninvasive study of peripheral arterial disease

THE EDITORS

Evaluation of peripheral arterial occlusive disease, with a careful history, physical examination, and angiography, has long been the basis of diagnosis and management. The noninvasive laboratory is an increasingly important asset in such situations, particularly since most patients are seen first by physicians who do not specialize in peripheral vascular disease. The laboratory provides an objective source of information both to help arrive at the correct diagnosis and to assess the degree of functional disability. In addition, distinguishing pseudoclaudication caused by neurospinal disorders from true arterial occlusive disease and recognizing the importance of peripheral arterial disease when combined with peripheral venous disease are readily accomplished on the basis of such laboratory data. The objective information obtained regarding the degree of functional activity then can be compared to similar data, following medical and surgical therapy, and can guide the physician's management over a long-term course.

STANDARD EXAMINATION

Through the past decade criteria for an adequate peripheral arterial examination have evolved, including tests with the patient both at rest and under stress. The mainstay of all examinations is an evaluation of peripheral pressures at rest. Earlier suggestions that the ankle blood pressure or the ankle-to-arm pressure index was an adequate measurement of peripheral arterial disease have now been replaced by a clear understanding that full segmental leg pressures are necessary. This is true because of the artifactually elevated ankle blood pressure seen in patients with rigid arteries, particularly in diabetes mellitus, and also because the ankle blood pressure alone fails to indicate the an-

atomic level of significant disease. A complete peripheral arterial examination therefore should include measurements of blood pressure at the thigh, calf, ankle, foot, and toe. In addition to artifactually elevated ankle pressure measurements, the examiner must be aware of the falsely depressed upper thigh and above-knee pressure measurements that may be observed in the presence of one or more distal occlusive lesions and that may be minimized by using more proximal sites for sensing than the toe or ankle. Toe pressure is particularly important not only as an index of significant small arterial disease in the foot, but also as a correcting factor for patients in whom ankle pressure is falsely elevated because of noncompliant arteries.

Some form of stress or exercise testing should then be used to supplement the resting pressure measurements. Such tests are appropriate because the stressed state significantly increases the sensitivity of all tests and their ability to detect and measure the functional impairment frequently associated with exercise. Three forms of stress tests are currently available: (1) the postexercise ankle blood pressure test, (2) the postocclusive reactive hyperemia test, and (3) the toe pulse reappearance time. The first two are probably equivalent in providing useful information, and at least one should be performed as a routine part of every peripheral arterial evaluation. The toe pulse reappearance time, on the other hand, is a good index of overall perfusion and collateral circulation.

CONTROVERSIAL AREAS
Pulse volume recorder

Pulse volume recorder (PVR) measurements are accurate indicators of the presence, degree, and location of peripheral arterial occlusive disease

(Chapters 17 and 54). However, they are generally used in conjunction with segmental pressure tests and other examinations. No studies have clearly identified PVR measurements as superior to segmental pressure measurements. Also, it is not clear whether PVR findings add significant data to those available from segmental pressure measurements. In the two situations when lower extremity pressure measurements are frequently artifactual—falsely depressed thigh measurement in the presence of distal occlusive lesions and falsely elevated ankle measurement in the presence of noncompliant vessels—the PVR would be expected to provide more authentic information. Since PVR measurements are based on the change in segmental volume measurements with arterial flow during each pulse, it seems likely that the PVR data would be more reliable than segmental pressure measurements under these circumstances. O'Donnell has presented data suggesting that the FP omega, which depends on the difference between PVR measurements at the thigh and calf levels, is a good indicator of leg resistance and perhaps better than segmental blood pressures. However, since convincing evidence of this has not been presented, PVR data must be considered important supplementary information to pressure measurements but without additional significance.

Quantitative Doppler velocity data

Although qualitative Doppler velocity information has been used enthusiastically by experienced investigators for many years, such data were originally difficult to quantify; comparisons from laboratory to laboratory or from time to time in the same patient were unreliable. Quantifying this information had been undertaken by a number of investigators and is discussed in detail in Chapters 3, 7, and 53. Such studies provide further support for the thesis that quantitative Doppler velocity information may permit making certain diagnoses that would not be possible from pressure and stress data alone. This is particularly true when both proximal and distal arterial occlusive disease exists, and the importance of each segment is uncertain.

Clearly, quantitative Doppler velocity measurements have not obtained widespread clinical usefulness. Among the reasons for this are a number of unresolved questions with the technique:

1. Which vessels should be studied for the most efficient and most valuable data; should popliteal and ankle vessels be analyzed?

2. Can probe-angle problems be resolved by positioning the probe to obtain the strongest Doppler signal? Will Duplex scanning devices resolve this problem of probe angle, since such systems are now commonly available for cerebrovascular studies?

3. Which of the many indices derived from Doppler velocity data are most valuable, particularly with regard to the complexity of obtaining or processing the data? Is probe calibration essential? Does the pulsatility index of Gosling provide as much useful information as the more quantitative curve analyses described by Johnston and Fronek?

4. Is special signal processing and analysis equipment helpful? Will spectral analysis using Duplex techniques enhance the diagnostic value of information obtained in the femoral area and make past problems with the zero crossing meter obsolete? How much more useful is this newer equipment in obtaining clinically worthwhile information?

5. Would Doppler velocity data obtained during or after stress of exercise be even more valuable than data obtained at rest?

6. How valuable is Doppler velocity data, of any degree of sophistication, in helping resolve the importance of the aortoiliac segment in patients with multilevel occlusive disease?

Since the Doppler velocity meter represents one of the original devices for the noninvasive study of vascular disease, it is particularly frustrating that the current role of such instruments in peripheral arterial occlusive disease cannot be placed in better perspective. However, this quandary is also an index of relative progress in other areas of instrumentation and testing during the past decade.

Evaluation of coexisting aortoiliac stenosis in multilevel occlusive disease

The detection and quantitation of peripheral arterial occlusive disease in a single anatomic location can now be performed noninvasively with precision. However, the problem of determining the significance of each segment in the face of multi-segmental disease remains difficult. Various approaches to this problem have been proposed and tested and are discussed in Chapters 50, 51, 53, 54, 56, and 59. From the point of view of the clinician, however, it is clear that no method has achieved widespread clinical usefulness, probably because no currently available method has provided satisfactory information. Therefore it seems likely that a technique involving more than one measurement will be necessary to achieve a high degree of sensitivity in evaluating the proximal aortoiliac segment in patients with combined levels of disease.

The crux of this evaluation must be pressure and velocity measurements in the common femoral artery, with the possible addition of spectral analysis and visualization of the aortoiliofemoral area with echography. In addition, a measurement of distal disease or resistance may have to be included in the index. Rather than the angiogram, direct invasive measurements such as the aortofemoral pressure gradient with and without papaverine, obtained preoperatively or intraoperatively, must remain the standard evaluation of proximal segment stenosis to which all noninvasive methods will have to be compared. The current status of this controversy is reviewed in Chapter 59, with a summary of the several promising approaches reported in the last several years.

Intraoperative monitoring

A number of techniques have been proposed for use during peripheral arterial reconstructive procedures to assess the adequacy of the reconstruction. These include distal pressure measurements at the ankle or toe, pulse volume recordings of the distal lower extremity, and other indices of flow or pressure. Earlier data, particularly from Barnes' group, suggested that these techniques were consistently valuable, not only for the demonstration of immediate operative adequacy, but also for predicting the long-term success of revascularization. Newer information suggests that this is not quite the case.

The development of signs of excellent distal flow are certainly consistent with a complete or adequate arterial reconstructive procedure and generally indicate a good prognosis. In addition, however, there are a number of patients in whom the intraoperative measurements are less than perfect, despite all operative maneuvers to improve them. Some of these patients have severe peripheral vasoconstriction as a result of cold temperature, vascular trauma, circulating catecholamines, the effects of anesthetic agents, and so forth. The well-known clinical syndrome of returning peripheral pulses, adequate circulation, and a good long-term outlook the following day has now been verified

by noninvasive measurements as well (Chapter 59).

Thus the use of intraoperative monitoring methods certainly can be encouraged, and when these demonstrate positive effects of arterial reconstruction, the additional assurance offered to the surgical team is important. However, when they fail to indicate a good result, and all measures to explore a cause for failure, including intraoperative angiography, have been exhausted, the surgeon must still consider the alternative possibilities just detailed, since a number of these patients will display perfectly acceptable results hours later. A combination of other or better measurements, perhaps associated with some pharmacologic manipulation, may be necessary to provide us with more staisfactory and secure methods of intraoperative monitoring than are currently available.

Postoperative screening

A variety of reports have emphasized the development of postoperative stenoses in relation to peripheral arterial reconstructive procedures that may be detected in a subclinical stage by the routine use of peripheral vascular laboratory monitoring. The early detection of such lesions permits their treatment, frequently by transluminal angioplasty techniques, before complete occlusion, which frequently dictates operative reconstruction and perhaps another graft. It therefore has become routine in most institutions to evaluate postoperative patients with at least an ankle blood pressure measurement. However, it appears justified to use an entire noninvasive test battery under such circumstances, rather than the single distal ankle pressure measurement, for the same reasons that a complete segmental pressure profile and stress test are appropriate in the initial clinical evaluation. Despite the known daily variations in such segmental pressure profile measurements, the pressure data, particularly when accompanied by a stress or exercise procedure, should point to earlier indications of developing or evolving stenoses and may permit separation of technical, surgically associated complications from progression of distal disease. Since the latter condition is less likely to be amenable to reconstructive surgery, the distinction is real and clinically important. A number of reports, particularly those of Berkowitz and his associates (Chapter 61), have demonstrated the usefulness of such frequent and routine postoperative checks and the ability of transluminal angioplastic procedures to successfully deal with most of these problems.

Nevertheless, the use of postoperative screening methodology has not become routine in many clinical centers. It is hoped that further evidence of the need for such regimens eventually will lead to their routine application.

SUMMARY

Noninvasive vascular laboratory measurements of peripheral arterial disease are the most quantitative and best standardized of any area of general clinical application. Use of the vascular laboratory in the initial clinical assessment of such patients raises the level of diagnostic accuracy to an expert standard. Therefore these measurements are now widespread and routine, and data collection and reporting are approaching universal usefulness. Several areas of controversy remain, however, and include (1) the need for complete segmental pressure measurements, including toe pressure measurements, as a routine; (2) the role and appropriate technique of peripheral Doppler velocity measurements; (3) techniques for separately evaluating the magnitude and functional importance of proximal aortoiliac segment disease compared with femoropopliteal and distal lower extremity lesions; and (4) the use of appropriate noninvasive techniques in the operating room and for postoperative screening purposes. Although individual investigators have achieved significant and clinically useful approaches to each of these problems, they have not yet met with widespread acceptance by the profession in general. The importance of universal standardization of measurements, both in the laboratory and in the operating room, coupled with an accepted classification of patient disease, will become increasingly obvious with time. Only such universally used approaches will allow a meaningful comparison of data between laboratories and institutions, as well as comparisons of the benefits of varying therapeutic interventions.

CHAPTER 70

The clinical spectrum of venous disease

ROBERT W. BARNES

There are six clinical syndromes of venous disease that must be recognized and accurately diagnosed by the clinician: (1) acute deep vein thrombosis, (2) recurrent deep vein thrombosis, (3) superficial thrombophlebitis, (4) varicose veins, (5) postthrombotic (postphlebitic) syndrome, and (6) pulmonary embolism. The fallibility of the clinical diagnosis of deep vein thrombosis is becoming increasingly recognized.[3] During the past 10 years several objective noninvasive diagnostic techniques have been developed to increase the accuracy of the clinical diagnosis of venous thromboembolism. It is the purpose of this chapter to review these six clinical syndromes of venous disease to permit more appropriate selection of diagnostic techniques and specific therapy of patients with suspected venous disease.

ACUTE DEEP VEIN THROMBOSIS

Acute deep vein thrombosis refers to the thrombotic occlusion of one or more veins of the deep venous system. Thrombosis most commonly occurs in the deep veins of the lower extremities, particularly the muscular veins of the calf and more proximal veins, including the popliteal, superficial femoral, and ileofemoral venous segments. Deep vein thrombosis also may involve the major veins of the upper extremity as well as the superior or inferior vena cava. Isolated venous thrombosis of the pelvic (internal iliac) veins may occur but is uncommon in the absence of pelvic inflammatory or malignant disease. The term *acute deep vein thrombosis* is currently preferred, and the previous terms *thrombophlebitis* or *phlebothrombosis* are misnomers.

Risk factors

A number of risk factors have been recognized as predisposing patients to acute deep vein thrombosis. These include prolonged bed rest, trauma, recent surgery, malignancy, severe medical illness such as chronic congestive heart failure, obesity, pregnancy, oral contraceptive use, systemic infection, varicose veins, and advancing age. Unfortunately many of these are based on previous clinical or epidemiologic studies that did not employ objective diagnosis for the documentation of venous thrombosis.

During the past decade the use of the radioactive fibrinogen uptake test has permitted more objective assessment of the incidence of deep vein thrombosis in patients screened in prospective clinical trials. However, this diagnostic test is exceedingly sensitive to minute venous thrombi, particularly in the calf, and the incidence of venous thrombosis in various prospective trials may be greater than the true incidence of major deep vein thrombosis in these reported series. Nevertheless, this diagnostic modality has greatly advanced our understanding of the potential risk of deep vein thrombosis in patients with various categories of illness. The technique has also provided objective data about the efficacy of various prophylactic measures to reduce the incidence of deep vein thrombosis.

Pathophysiology

Acute deep vein thrombosis usually begins by platelet and fibrin deposits accumulating behind venous valve cusps, which are inherent sites of venous stasis. Extension of the thrombus may result in a long, free-floating clot that may fragment and embolize to the pulmonary circulation. Alternatively the thrombus may result in progressive obstruction of venous outflow and symptoms and signs of venous thrombosis of the affected extremity. However, considerable thrombus may occur in the deep venous system without clinical manifestations because of the capacitance of the venous system and its propensity to form collateral circulation around the obstructing lesion. Eventual thrombus development results in fibrous obliteration of the venous lumen, although some degree of fibrinolysis occurs spontaneously in the deep veins. However, the extent of thrombolysis is seldom as complete as occurs in the pulmonary circulation. Organization of deep vein thrombi usually destroys the deep venous valves, which subsequently results in the postthrombotic (postphlebitic) sequelae. Such venous valvular incompetence may result in significant hypertension with ambulation, reversal of blood flow through incompetent communicating (perforating) venous valves, and collateral circulation via the superficial veins that may become varicose (secondary varicose veins).

Clinical manifestations

As many as 50% of patients with documented deep vein thrombosis may be asymptomatic and have few if any clinical signs of deep venous obstruction. The most common symptom is pain in the affected portion of the extremity. Associated tenderness includes that induced by passive dorsiflexion of the foot (*Homans' sign*), but this manifestation is exceedingly nonspecific for venous thrombosis. Edema of the affected extremity is frequently present but difficult to quantify and often absent in patients for whom bed rest has been prescribed or those with good collateral circulation. Also, edema is a nonspecific sign that accompanies many other clinical conditions in the absence of venous thrombosis. Inflammation, if marked, is unusual; fever, if other than low grade, is also uncommon in isolated deep vein thrombosis. The two most pathognomonic signs of major deep vein thrombosis are cyanosis of the extremity and prominence of the superficial veins. Venous hypertension in the affected extremity may be suspected if the superficial veins remain distended in the raised extremity when compared to the opposite limb.

Differential diagnosis

Symptoms and signs of deep vein thrombosis may be mimicked by a number of other clinical conditions, which may be categorized in three broad categories. Conditions that lead to pain include ruptured popliteal (Baker's) cyst, subfascial hematoma, ruptured plantaris muscle, nerve entrapment, and myalgia or myositis. Conditions that mimic deep vein thrombosis by causing edema of the extremity include congestive heart failure; lymphedema; extrinsic venous compression by trauma, hematoma, or malignancy; and prolonged dependency of the extremity, as in patients with paralysis, ischemic rest pain, and so on. Conditions that result in leg inflammation include lymphangitis, cellulitis, or subcutaneous fat necrosis. Many of these clinical conditions are common and emphasize the need for objective diagnosis before completing a course of therapy in a patient with suspected deep vein thrombosis.[15]

Diagnostic techniques

Contrast phlebography (venography) remains the diagnostic standard for the documentation of acute deep vein thrombosis. However, the expense, discomfort, and small but definite risk associated with this procedure have led to the proliferation of a number of noninvasive diagnostic techniques, which are discussed in subsequent chapters. With a complete laboratory any of the noninvasive techniques mentioned in this book will provide the clinician with greater diagnostic accuracy in detecting deep vein thrombosis than will the clinical examination alone. The methods most appropriate for initial screening include Doppler ultrasound, venous outflow plethysmography, phleborheography, or radioisotope venography. Radioactive fibrinogen leg scanning may be used to complement other diagnostic techniques but is not practical for the initial diagnosis because of the time and expense associated with the procedure. The intelligent application of objective diagnostic techniques before completing a course of therapy for patients with suspected deep vein thrombosis cannot be overemphasized.[29]

Complications

The two major sequelae of deep vein thrombosis are pulmonary embolism and the postthrombotic (postphlebitic) syndrome. These conditions are discussed later in this chapter.

Therapy

Acute deep vein thrombosis is usually treated with intravenous heparin anticoagulation, followed by a course of secondary prophylaxis with oral anticoagulants (warfarin). Most physicians currently use continuous intravenous heparin to reduce the risk of bleeding associated with intermittent bolus doses. After an initial bolus of approximately 5000 units intravenously, continuous infusion of 1000 to 2000 units/hr is begun to maintain the partial thromboplastin time at approximately twice the control value. After 7 to 10 days of heparin therapy the patient is maintained on oral warfarin in doses sufficient to prolong the prothrombin time at 1.5 to 2 times the control value. However, recent studies suggest that secondary prophylaxis with lower doses of warfarin may be as successful as the more traditional doses, with reduced risk of hemorrhagic complications.[19]

Thrombolytic therapy for deep vein thrombosis has been employed in a few investigative studies that have documented its efficacy in clearance of deep vein thrombosis in certain cases of disease of recent onset (less than 5 days' duration). Unfortunately many patients with deep vein thrombosis have predisposing factors that preclude the use of thrombolytic therapy. In addition, venous valvular dysfunction and postphlebitic syndrome may result despite the use of thrombolytic therapy.

Prognosis

Untreated deep vein thrombosis may be associated with pulmonary embolism in approximately 25% of patients. Heparin therapy reduces this risk approximately fivefold, but it does not prevent the development of the postthrombotic syndrome, which develops in the majority of patients if followed for a sufficient period. These sequelae can be minimized with appropriate elastic support, as mentioned later in this chapter.

RECURRENT DEEP VEIN THROMBOSIS

Recurrent deep vein thrombosis refers to the development of recurrent active thrombosis after a prior episode of acute deep vein thrombosis. Because the symptoms of recurrent deep vein thrombosis often mimic those of postthrombotic syndrome, the true incidence of this problem has probably been overemphasized in previous studies that did not employ objective diagnostic techniques to document the presence of recurrent active disease.[26]

Risk factors

The risk factors for patients with recurrent deep vein thrombosis are similar to those mentioned for acute deep vein thrombosis. The patients at greater risk are those with continuing predisposing factors such as malignancy or serious medical illness (congestive heart failure).

Clinical manifestations

The clinical manifestations also are similar to those listed for acute deep vein thrombosis: leg pain, tenderness, inflammation, swelling, cyanosis, and prominent superficial veins. Unfortunately many of these symptoms also resemble those of the chronic postthrombotic (venous stasis) syndrome. Thus the physician seeing the patient with suspected recurrent deep vein thrombosis must answer the following two questions: (1) Does the patient have venous disease? (2) If so, are the recurrent symptoms caused by active thrombosis or chronic postthrombotic (inactive) disease?

Differential diagnosis

The differential diagnosis of recurrent deep vein thrombosis is again similar to that of acute deep vein thrombosis. Any condition mimicking deep vein thrombosis (''pseudophlebitis'') may result in recurrent symptoms and thus mimic recurrent deep vein thrombosis. If a patient has venous disease, the chronic mechanical sequelae, persistent venous obstruction and/or venous valvular incompetence, may result in recurrent symptoms on a mechanical basis, the so-called postthrombotic or chronic venous stasis syndrome. These symptoms often are clinically confused with recurrent active venous thrombosis but do not require anticoagulants for their treatment.

Diagnostic techniques

The initial diagnostic screening of a patient with recurrent deep vein thrombosis may be carried out using any of the techniques employed for the detection of acute deep vein thrombosis. Doppler ultrasound, venous outflow plethysmography, phleborheography, or radioisotope venography may be used. I prefer Doppler ultrasound because this technique evaluates both venous outflow obstruction and venous valvular incompetence. If the deep veins are patent and competent, the clinician may assume that the patient has some condition mimicking venous thrombosis. If the deep veins are patent but the venous valves are incompetent, the patient may be assumed to have the postthrombotic (venous stasis) syndrome. Such patients do not require anticoagulant therapy but may be treated with bed rest, leg elevation, and elastic support for their postthrombotic symptoms. If deep venous obstruction is documented, the clinician must then define whether or not the obstruction is caused by recurrent (active) thrombosis.

The test most suited for this objective is the radioactive fibrinogen leg scan.[18,19] This test should be initiated before prescribing anticoagulant therapy, since such treatment may prevent further thrombosis and render the test negative despite the presence of recent recurrent active thrombosis. If the physician is concerned about withholding therapy during the fibrinogen uptake test, heparin may be instituted, but this may reduce the chance of demonstrating some recurrent active thrombosis. If the fibrinogen leg scan is normal, the patient may be assumed to have postthrombotic chronic venous occlusive disease. Such patients are best treated for the chronic venous insufficiency, and they do not require repeated anticoagulation. If the radioactive fibrinogen leg scan is positive, the patient may be assumed to have recurrent active venous thrombosis and appropriately treated with anticoagulants. If the fibrinogen leg scan is unavailable, I recommend contrast venography to evaluate the venous system for the presence of recent active thrombi (filling defects outlined by contrast material). If these are present, the patient is treated for recurrent active venous thrombosis. If the venogram shows only chronic obliterative venous disease with recanalization or collateral veins, I treat the patient for postthrombotic syndrome and do not use anticoagulants.

Therapy

Patients with documented recurrent active venous thrombosis usually receive anticoagulants, with a course of heparin therapy followed by secondary prophylaxis with oral anticoagulants (warfarin). Patients who develop true recurrent active venous thrombosis despite anticoagulant therapy require special diagnostic investigation for some predisposing factor leading to thrombosis, such as a hematologic abnormality (antithrombin III deficiency, platelet function abnormality). Some patients are best treated with antiplatelet therapy if an abnormality of platelet function can be documented. Rarely patients may require both oral anticoagulation and concomitant antiplatelet therapy for control of recurrent venous thrombosis, al-

though such combined therapy carries an increased risk of hemorrhagic complications.

Prognosis

Patients who do not receive secondary prophylaxis are at increased risk of developing recurrent active venous thrombosis during the first 3 months after the initial episode of thrombosis. For this reason secondary prophylaxis has been traditionally employed, with oral anticoagulants (warfarin) administered for up to 6 months or 1 year after thrombosis. However, a random clinical trial comparing oral anticoagulation therapy for 6 weeks vs. 6 months suggested no difference in the incidence of clinical recurrent venous thrombosis in either method.[26] Recent prospective clinical trials using objective diagnostic techniques to document the incidence of recurrent venous thrombosis suggest that patients treated with warfarin therapy in either traditional or low doses have an incidence of recurrent deep vein thrombosis of approximately 2%, with the low-dose regimen being associated with a significant reduction in hemorrhagic complications.[19] Low-dose subcutaneous heparin prophlaxis is associated with a higher incidence (22%) of recurrent deep vein thrombosis.[18]

SUPERFICIAL THROMBOPHLEBITIS

Superficial thrombophlebitis refers to thrombosis of the superficial veins, usually the greater or lesser saphenous veins or their branches in the lower extremities. Whereas thrombophlebitis is no longer the preferred term for deep vein thrombosis, superficial thrombophlebitis correctly describes the clinical characteristics of thrombosis of the superficial venous system. The clinical and pathologic manifestations are more inflammatory in character than with deep vein thrombosis. Similarly, superficial thrombophlebitis responds better to antiinflammatory than to anticoagulant treatment.

Risk factors

Superficial thrombophlebitis most commonly results from intravenous infusions, with the second most common predisposing factor being varicose veins. The condition may result from trauma, although this may result in subcutaneous hematomas that may be confused with superficial thrombophlebitis. A migratory superficial thrombophlebitis in the absence of other obvious predisposing factors should always suggest the possibility of severe underlying systemic disease, such as collagen disease or an occult malignancy, including carcinoma of the pancreas, lung, or prostate *(Trousseau's sign)*.

Clinical manifestations

Superficial thrombophlebitis is characterized by intense pain, redness, inflammation, swelling, and induration along the course of one or more superficial veins. There may be plainly visible varicose veins that predispose to this condition. A palpable cord typifies this disease, whereas usually cords are not expected in deep vein thrombosis. Superficial thrombophlebitis is usually a much more painful condition than deep vein thrombosis because of the proximity of cutaneous sensory nerves to the inflammatory process. A low-grade fever may be present, but a higher temperature should suggest the diagnosis of lymphangitis or cellulitis.

Differential diagnosis

The principal conditions that may be confused with superficial thrombophlebitis are lymphangitis and cellulitis. Lymphangitis, usually resulting from streptococcal infection, is associated with an initial high fever (up to 105° F), shaking chills, and vomiting followed by the development of a spreading painful, tender inflammation along the course of the lymphatics, usually on the lower extremity. There is often a portal of entry on the foot, such as a puncture wound, dermatophytosis (athlete's foot), and so on. Patients with lymphedema, either congenital or acquired, are also predisposed to lymphangitis. These conditions usually respond rapidly to antibiotic therapy, particularly intravenous penicillin.

Diagnostic techniques

The most useful diagnostic method to differentiate superficial thrombophlebitis from lymphangitis or cellulitis is a Doppler ultrasonic venous examination. This test can differentiate flow in the superficial and deep veins. If prominent flow is present in the inflamed area, lymphangitis or cellulitis is implied, with hyperemic flow resulting from the inflammation. If flow is absent in the affected superficial vein, superficial thrombophlebitis is inferred. There may be prominent arterial velocity signals as a result of the inflammation. The Doppler examination also may identify associated or causative underlying deep vein thrombosis, which may alter the therapy.[4] Contrast venography also may be used to establish the diag-

nosis of superficial thrombophlebitis, but the contrast medium may cause significant pain in this already painful condition. Other types of noninvasive or minimally invasive techniques, such as radioactive fibrinogen leg scanning, are either insensitive or nonspecific in superficial thrombophlebitis.

Complications

The principal complication of superficial thrombophlebitis is extension of the process into the deep veins, with resulting deep vein thrombosis. This complication usually develops only if the superficial thrombophlebitis is in proximity to the saphenofemoral or saphenopopliteal junction. A less common complication is the development of infection or septic thrombophlebitis, which most often is a consequence of prolonged intravenous infusion.

Therapy

Most cases of superficial thrombophlebitis respond well to antiinflammatory therapy, particularly with the use of nonsteroidal agents. A number of investigators[14,20,23] have recommended ligation and stripping of the venous system affected by superficial thrombophlebitis. Currently this treatment is most appropriate for patients with recurrent superficial thrombophlebitis and varicose veins or patients in whom the process ascends near the saphenofemoral junction, with resultant risk of deep vein thrombosis. If the latter condition is documented by Doppler ultrasound or contrast venography, anticoagulants are the treatment of choice. If septic superficial thrombophlebitis develops, incision and drainage, particularly with excision of the entire venous segment, may be necessary to control the septic process.

Prognosis

Most patients with superficial thrombophlebitis have a relatively benign course. However, superficial thrombophlebitis, particularly if migratory, may reflect a serious underlying disorder such as collagen disease or malignancy. A more serious prognosis is associated with these conditions.

VARICOSE VEINS

Varicose veins refer to dilated, elongated, and tortuous superficial veins, usually of the greater or lesser saphenous veins and their tributaries in the lower extremity.

Etiology

Varicose veins are classified as primary or secondary.[24] *Primary* varicose veins refer to isolated varicosities of the superficial venous system with normal deep and communicating veins. This disorder is usually inherited and the result of weakness of the wall constituents of the vein or absence of the deep venous valves, particularly in the iliac venous system.[24] *Secondary* varicose veins refer to varicosities in patients with underlying deep and communicating venous disease, usually the result of prior deep vein thrombosis. There may or may not be associated deep venous obstruction. Secondary varicose veins usually develop as a result of collateral circulation around the previous venous thrombosis. They also may be the result of arteriovenous fistula, either congenital or acquired. Deep venous hypoplasia or aplasia in the *Klippel-Trenaunay syndrome* results in the triad of varicose veins, port-wine stain or other congenital hemangioma, and limb overgrowth or hypertrophy.

Pathophysiology

In the normal venous system the standing superficial venous pressure at the ankle is equal to the hydrostatic pressure of the blood extending from right atrium. This pressure is usually about 120 cm saline or 100 mm Hg. With ambulation the superficial venous pressure drops to 20 to 30 cm saline *(ambulatory venous hypotension)* as blood flows from the superficial to the deep veins through the communicating veins, a result of contraction of the calf muscles (calf musculovenous pump). In patients with primary varicose veins the standing venous pressure is similar to that of normal individuals. The ambulatory venous pressure is usually 40 to 60 cm saline, with somewhat higher pressure caused by retrograde flow in the saphenous vein during the swing phase of ambulation, as blood flows retrograde from the deep veins down the incompetent venous system and then back into the deep veins through the communicating veins of the lower leg (circus motion of blood flow). In patients with secondary varicose veins the standing venous pressure also is similar to that of normal persons. However, the ambulatory venous pressure is significantly higher *(ambulatory venous hypertension)*, a result of retrograde flow of blood from deep to superficial veins through incompetent communicating (perforating) veins. In addition, the ambulatory venous hypertension may be aggravated by associated deep vein obstruction related to prior venous thrombosis. The ambulatory venous hypertension may lead to hypertension of the capillary circulation in the lower extremity, with resulting transudation and edema, rupture of the small capillaries or venules, leading to superficial hemorrhage in the microcirculation, and consequent hemosiderin deposits, accounting for the brownish pigmentation associated with chronic venous stasis disease. The capillary venous hypertension also may explain the cause of stasis ulceration in patients with secondary varicose veins and the postthrombotic syndrome.

Clinical manifestations

The most common clinical manifestation of varicose veins is the cosmetic disturbance associated with the prominent varices. Pain may occur as a result of distention of the sensitive vein walls. However, the pain in primary varicose veins is usually mild and readily controlled with adequate elastic support stocking. More severe leg pain associated with edema and stasis dermatitis or ulceration implies secondary varicose veins. The term *varicose ulcer* is a misnomer, since primary varicosities do not result in venous stasis disease.

Differential diagnosis

The differentiation of primary from secondary varicose veins is of clinical importance because of the difference in prognosis. Primary varicose veins are suggested by a family history of varicosities in the absence of postthrombotic sequelae of chronic venous stasis dermatitis, ulceration, or significant leg edema. Secondary varicose veins are typified by a past history of deep vein thrombosis and associated postthrombotic sequelae such as significant leg edema, hyperpigmentation, stasis dermatitis, and ulceration. Rarer causes of secondary varicose veins include arteriovenous fistula, either congential or acquired, with associated bruit or cutaneous stigmata of arterial venous malformations. The triad of varicose veins, limb hypertrophy, and cutaneous hemangioma is characteristic of the Klippel-Trenaunay syndrome.

Diagnostic techniques

Primary and secondary varicose veins may be differentiated by clinical bedside tests as well as noninvasive or invasive procedures. The classic procedure for competence of the deep and communicating veins is *Trendelenburg's test*. In this test the patient's extremity is elevated to empty the varices, and a latex tourniquet is applied on the proximal thigh to prevent reflux in the superficial veins as the patient assumes a standing position. If the veins remain decompressed and fill slowly from distally up the extremity, the superficial and communicating veins are assumed to be competent. Release of the tourniquet should result in rapid refilling of the varicose veins from above then downward in patients with primary varices. If rapid filling of the varicose veins occurs despite the proximal tourniquet, incompetence of deep and communicating veins is inferred. To assess the level of incompetence of communicating veins, the test may be repeated with reapplication of the tourniquet at progressively more distal levels down the leg until the venous reflux is prevented at the site immediately below the incompetent communicating vein.

A second clinical test of the patency of the deep venous system is *Perthes' test*. A latex tourniquet is applied to the proximal thigh to obstruct the superficial veins. The patient then ambulates about the room while the physician observes the superficial venous pattern. Patients with primary varicose veins may decompress the varicosities somewhat as blood is drained from the superficial to the competent deep veins and reflux is prevented by the superficial tourniquet. In patients with secondary varicose veins with patent but incompetent deep and communicating veins, the varices do not change significantly in caliber but do not distend or become painful with the application of the tourniquet. In patients with secondary varicose veins associated with deep venous obstruction, there may be increase in size of the varicosities after application of the tourniquet, and the patient may develop a sensation of congestion and pain in the extremity. In such instances the varicose veins may be serving as a collateral for venous outflow, and their stripping may be associated with an increase in symptoms postoperatively. Similarly, in patients with Klippel-Trenaunay syndrome, with deep venous hypoplasia and prominent superficial veins, the varicosities may distend with application of a superficial tourniquet. Such patients may suffer significant impairment if the varicose veins are surgically removed.

Noninvasive diagnostic techniques may be used to evaluate patients with primary or secondary varicose veins. The simplest method is Doppler ultrasound to document the incompetence of the superficial veins and the status of the communicating

and deep venous system.[2] In patients with primary varicose veins the deep and communicating veins should be patent and competent. Patients with secondary veins may manifest deep and communicating venous incompetence as well as variable degrees of deep venous obstruction. The patency and competence of deep and communicating veins may also be established by plethysmography. Venous outflow plethysmography will document venous outflow obstruction. Venous reflux plethysmography using strain-gauge[5] or photoplethysmographic[25] techniques permits quantification of the degree of deep and communicating venous reflux. Contrast phlebography permits documentation of the status of the deep and communicating veins. In primary varicose veins there is no venous reflux through incompetent deep and communicating veins. In secondary varicose veins there may be variable degrees of deep venous obstruction, radiologic abnormalities of venous valve structure and function, and documentation of incompetence of deep and communicating veins. Venous reflux may be established by descending venography from injections in the femoral vein.

Complications

The most common complication associated with varicose veins is stasis dermatitis or ulceration associated with secondary varicosities. Varicose veins may predispose patients to superficial thrombophlebitis. This complication often recurs in the same area, as the superficial thrombus recanalizes and then rethromboses.

Hemorrhage from varicose veins, particularly superficial (dermal) varices or venules near the ankle, may be prefuse if the patient remains upright and ambulatory. The hemorrhage may occur spontaneously at night and may be life-threatening.[13] Hemorrhage, when recognized, should be treated with immediate leg elevation and direct compression. This complication is an absolute indication for local surgical excision or sclerotherapy. Pulmonary embolism is a rare complication of superficial thrombophlebitis associated with varicose veins. More commonly it is a result of associated deep vein thrombosis in patients with secondary varicose veins.

Therapy

The three principal methods of treating varicose veins are the use of elastic support stockings, surgical ligation and stripping, and compression sclerotherapy. For most patients therapeutic elastic support stockings suffice to control the venous distention and the majority of symptoms. Patients with secondary varicose veins require a more heavy elastic support than do patients with the primary form. Patients who do not receive adequate relief of pain or edema with support stockings rarely benefit from surgical excision alone. Patients with secondary varicose veins and underlying deep venous disease likewise rarely are helped by isolated stripping of the superficial vein.

Surgical ligation and stripping is the most common method of treating varicose veins.[12,22] It is the treatment of choice for prominent, long saphenous varicose veins.[17] The indications for stripping include control of the cosmetic problem, relief of pain, recurrent superficial thrombophlebitis, and hemorrhage. Stripping is contraindicated in patients with extensive deep vein obstruction or the Klippel-Trenaunay syndrome. The control of an arteriovenous fistula, if etiologic, is important in addition to stripping of varicose veins.

Compression sclerotherapy is useful to eradicate small varicosities of branch veins as well as localized incompetent superficial veins associated with secondary varicose veins.[17] Either sodium tetradecylsulfate or sodium morrhuate may be injected by a small-gauge needle into the emptied varix at ''points of control'' (near underlying communicating veins), followed by firm elastic bandaging to achieve a fibrous obliteration of the veins by apposition of the walls of the collapsed vein.[17] Injection sclerotherapy carries a small risk of ulceration, deep vein thrombosis, and serious allergic systemic reaction. The technique is not widely employed in the United States.

Prognosis

Varicose veins are usually a benign disorder, particularly the primary variety. The prognosis of patients with secondary varicose veins is the same as that for the underlying chronic venous disorder. Patients with varicose veins should be informed that the varices usually do not require surgical therapy unless the specific complications just mentioned develop. Patients with chronic leg pain who undergo stripping in the absence of obvious prominent varicose veins are rendered a disservice.

POSTTHROMBOTIC SYNDROME

The postthrombotic syndrome is often termed *postphlebitic syndrome* or *chronic venous stasis*

disease. This disorder includes the constellation of sequelae that may result from deep vein thrombosis, including chronic leg pain, swelling, hyperpigmentation, stasis dermatitis, and venous stasis ulceration.

Etiology

The postthrombotic syndrome is usually the result of prior deep vein thrombosis, which may or may not have been clinically recognized.[8,9,16,21] This syndrome may also develop in patients with secondary varicose veins as a result of arteriovenous fistula.

Pathophysiology

The pathophysiology of the postthrombotic syndrome is similar to that described for patients with secondary varicose veins.[21] The clinical syndromes usually reflect the presence or absence of deep vein obstruction, deep vein valvular insufficiency (incompetence), or a combination of the two. Patients with predominant deep vein obstruction develop symptoms of recurrent leg pain with prolonged ambulation, so-called venous claudication. Patients with dominant deep and communicating venous incompetence develop symptoms of leg edema, hyperpigmentation, stasis dermatitis, and ulceration.

Clinical manifestations

Postthrombotic syndrome usually becomes manifest as progressive leg pain, swelling, hyperpigmentation, and stasis dermatitis, with or without associated venous stasis ulceration.[11,30] The hyperpigmentation is brownish in color and usually localized to the area around the medial maleous. The hyperpigmentation may extend circumferentially around the lower leg. Dermatitis with drying and scaling of the skin may simulate eczema. Stasis ulceration usually occurs in the same area as the hyperpigmentation; when cleaned, the ulcer shows a good granulating base. There may be associated varicose veins (secondary varices).

Patients with dominant deep venous obstruction manifest progressive leg pain, heaviness, and an aching or ''bursting'' sensation with prolonged walking. This venous claudication may be accompanied by edema. There may or may not be associated signs of venous stasis disease at the ankle.

Differential diagnosis

Patients with chronic venous stasis disease may be confused with those suffering from recurrent venous thrombosis. A differential diagnosis has been discussed previously. Lymphangitis and cellulitis may mimic the inflammation associated with superficial ulceration in the postthrombotic syndrome. Contact dermatitis may result in local cutaneous changes similar to those of stasis dermatitis. Other types of ulceration that may be confused with the postthrombotic syndrome include ulcers resulting from trauma or chronic arterial ischemia, hypertensive ulcers, or ulcers associated with arthritis. The chronic edema of lymphedema or congestive heart failure must be differentiated from that caused by postthrombotic chronic venous insufficiency.

Patients with venous claudication must be differentiated from those with chronic arterial occlusive disease. Likewise patients with neuromusculoskeletal conditions (pseudoclaudication) are frequently thought to have arterial or venous desease. However, the pain and disability associated with neurospinal or musculoskeletal syndromes is often inconsistent and not reproducible, as is the case in patients with vascular disorders.

Diagnostic techniques

Patients with postthrombotic syndrome are usually diagnosed from a bedside clinical examination. However, the relative magnitude of deep venous obstruction and incompetence of the deep communicating veins may be both qualitatively and quantitatively defined by noninvasive techniques. Doppler ultrasound permits rapid assessment of obstruction and incompetence of the deep, superficial, and communicating veins. Venous outflow plethysmography permits quantification of obstruction to deep venous return. Venous reflux may be quantified using strain-gauge[5] and photoplethysmographic[1,7,25] techniques. Contrast phlebography may be performed to identify deep venous obstruction and valvular incompetence.

Complications

The most common complication of postthrombotic syndrome is venous stasis ulceration. Pulmonary embolism may result from recurrent deep vein thrombosis.

Therapy

Most patients with postthrombotic syndrome may be treated adequately with elastic support stockings of therapeutic weight as well as frequent leg elevation. The stockings should be appropri-

ately fitted and provide a counterpressure of 30 to 50 mm Hg at the level of the ankle. For most patients stockings fitted below the knee are sufficient to control chronic venous stasis disease. Patients should be advised to use the stockings at all times when out of bed.

Patients with active ulceration and associated infection may require hospitalization with bed rest, leg elevation, and antibiotic therapy. However, most patients with venous stasis ulcers may be treated on an ambulatory basis using a medicated bandage (Unna boot). Once the ulcer heals, the patient should use elastic support stockings to prevent the recurrence of ulceration. In selected patients with recurrent ulceration, despite medical management, surgical intervention may be necessary. Procedures commonly recommended include excision and skin grafting, ligation of communicating veins, and stripping of secondary varicose veins. Recently a number of venous reconstructive procedures have been used on an investigational basis. These include femoral venous valvuloplasty, transposition or transplantation of vein segments carrying competent venous valves, and venous bypass procedures around obstructions of the saphenous or iliac veins. However, surgical therapy does not cure postthrombotic syndrome, and lifelong use of elastic support stockings cannot be overemphasized.

PULMONARY EMBOLISM

Pulmonary embolism refers to the embolic obstruction of the pulmonary artery and its branches by thrombi, usually from the deep venous system of the lower extremities.

Risk factors

Patients at risk of developing pulmonary embolism are similar to those at risk for deep vein thrombosis.[10] Although patients usually develop pulmonary emboli from venous thrombosis in the lower extremities, the subclavian or axillary veins rarely may cause pulmonary emboli. The use of chronic venous infusions through subclavian catheters or the use of permanent pacemakers with indwelling transvenous wires may also cause pulmonary emboli.

Pathophysiology

Patients with pulmonary embolism have a clinical spectrum of manifestations based on the magnitude of the pulmonary arterial obstruction. Patients with class 1 pulmonary embolism are asymptomatic and have normal arterial blood gas levels and normal pulmonary and systemic hemodynamics. These patients have less than 20% of the total pulmonary arteries obstructed by thrombi. Class 2 patients manifest anxiety, hyperventilation, and tachycardia and have an arterial partial tension of oxygen (PO_2) less than 80 torr, a carbon dioxide partial pressure (PCO_2) less than 35 torr, and occlusion of 20% to 30% of the pulmonary vasculature. Class 3 patients manifest dyspnea, collapse, an arterial PO_2 less than 65 torr, a PCO_2 less than 30 torr, an elevated central venous pressure, and mean pulmonary artery pressure greater than 20 mm Hg, with 30% to 50% occlusion of the pulmonary vasculature. Class 4 patients are in shock with dyspnea, arterial PO_2 less than 50 torr, PCO_2 less than 30 torr, an elevated central venous pressure, mean pulmonary artery pressure greater than 20 mm Hg, a systolic blood pressure less than 100 mm Hg, and a greater than 50% occlusion of the pulmonary vasculature. Class 5 patients represent those with chronic pulmonary hypertension associated with recurrent pulmonary emboli. They manifest dyspnea, syncope, arterial PO_2 less than 50 torr, PCO_2 less than 30 to 40 torr, a mean pulmonary artery pressure greater than 40 mm Hg, a low cardiac output, and greater than 50% occlusion of the pulmonary vasculature.

Clinical manifestations

The most common clinical manifestations of pulmonary emboli are chest pain that may be pleuritic, hemoptysis, dyspnea, tachypnea, syncope, weakness, or a feeling of impending doom.[28] Shock is present in massive pulmonary embolism. Fever is usually low grade. Unfortunately the clinical manifestations are nonspecific and often are attributed to pulmonary embolism when another disorder may be present.[27]

Differential diagnosis

Many conditions mimic pulmonary embolism, including myocardial infarction, pulmonary edema, pneumonia, atelectasis, pneumothorax, sepsis, aspiration, pericarditis, and reflux esophagitis.

Diagnostic techniques

The clinical diagnosis should prompt an objective workup for pulmonary embolism. Unfortunately the accuracy of the clinical diagnosis seldom exceeds 50%. Arterial blood gas levels are non-

specific and are of greatest value if the arterial PO_2 is normal. Hypoxia correlates with the magnitude of the embolus but is very nonspecific. There is usually associated hypocapnea, a result of the tachypnea associated with the hypoxia. There may be hypercapnea if a large embolus increases the functional dead space. The electrocardiogram is nonspecific and insensitive. Commonly associated abnormalities include a right axis deviation, an $S^1Q^3T^3$ pattern, and T wave inversion, especially in right precordial leads.

Perfusion and ventilation lung scans are the most commonly employed objective techniques to detect pulmonary emboli. Unfortunately these studies are quite nonspecific and are frequently abnormal in a number of other pulmonary conditions. Perfusion lung scans should be obtained by the technique that permits a radionuclide venogram to document a possible source of pulmonary emboli from deep vein thrombosis in the major veins of the lower extremity. A perfusion lung scan of lobar extent or greater along with a normal ventilation lung scan is of high diagnostic probability for pulmonary embolus. Unfortunately most perfusion defects are of lesser magnitude and carry lower degrees of probability of association with pulmonary emboli.

Noninvasive diagnostic techniques to screen for deep vein thrombosis are important adjuncts to increase the accuracy of the clinical diagnosis.[6] If deep vein thrombosis is documented by noninvasive screening techniques, the patient logically may be treated for pulmonary embolism. However, the deep veins are normal in approximately two thirds of individuals with suspected clinical pulmonary embolism. Such patients deserve pulmonary angiography to clarify the diagnosis unless the perfusion and ventilation lung scans indicate a high probability for an embolism.

Complications

Approximately 40% of the patients with pulmonary embolism die of the disorder. In the majority of these cases death is the result of an unrecognized diagnosis, although some patients die immediately before therapy can be instituted. Patients surviving acute pulmonary embolism may develop recurrent emboli and the syndrome of chronic pulmonary hypertension.

Therapy

Pulmonary embolism may be treated by medical or surgical techniques. The most common treatment is anticoagulation with intravenous heparin followed by subsequent secondary prophylaxis with oral anticoagulants (warfarin). Fibrinolytic therapy with streptokinase or urokinase has been shown to improve the resolution of pulmonary emboli, which may be important in patients with massive embolism associated with shock. However, the overall survival rate for patients treated with fibrinolytic therapy is not significantly different from those treated with heparin alone. The incidence of late sequelae of pulmonary embolism associated with resting or ambulatory pulmonary hypertension may be reduced with fibrinolytic therapy.

Patients who cannot be treated with anticoagulants or who develop complications while on anticoagulant therapy are candidates for interruption of the vena cava, preferably with a filter device (Greenfield) that will not result in phlebothrombosis. Pulmonary embolectomy may be done for patients with massive pulmonary embolism who are in persistent shock. The embolectomy may be performed with a catheter technique (Greenfield) or by open pulmonary embolectomy on cardiopulmonary bypass.

Prognosis

Approximately 10% of patients with massive pulmonary embolism suffer death within 1 hour of the event. Such patients cannot usually be treated and represent a principal reason for the increasing use of prophylaxis of venous thrombosis in high-risk patients. Of those who survive the initial episode of pulmonary embolism, the diagnosis is not recognized in approximately 70% of patients. Of these, about 30% will die. Of the 30% who are diagnosed with proper therapy instituted, approximately 90% survive; 10% succumb despite anticoagulant therapy. Often death is the result of a severe underlying disorder such as cardiopulmonary disease or other systemic disease, predisposing to venous thrombosis and pulmonary embolism.

SUMMARY

The clinician must recognize the importance of the various venous syndromes, including acute and recurrent deep vein thrombosis, superficial thrombophlebitis, varicose veins, postthrombotic syndrome, and pulmonary embolism. Unfortunately the clinical diagnosis is frequently erroneous, and objective diagnostic techniques must be employed to establish the diagnosis so that proper therapy

may be instituted. Fortunately the noninvasive diagnostic techniques described in this text permit rapid and safe screening of patients with suspected venous disease. Although therapy may be instituted when the diagnosis is suspected, no patient should complete therapy for venous thrombosis or pulmonary embolism without objective proof of the diagnosis. If this approach is adopted, at least 50% of patients with suspected venous disease who have an erroneous clinical diagnosis may be spared the risk and expense of unnecessary treatment.

REFERENCES

1. Abramowitz, H.G., et al.: The use of photoplethysmography in the assessment of venous insufficiency: a comparison to venous pressure measurements, Surgery 86:434, 1979.
2. Barnes, R.W., Ross, E.A., and Strandness, D.E., Jr: Differentiation of primary from secondary varicose veins by Doppler ultrasound and strain gauge plethysmography, Surg. Gynecol. Obstet. 141:207, 1975
3. Barnes, R.W., Wu, K.K., and Hoak, J.C.: Fallibility of the clinical diagnosis of venous thrombosis, JAMA, 234:605, 1975.
4. Barnes, R.W., Wu, K.K., and Hoak, J.C.: Differentiation of superficial thrombophlebitis from lymphangitis by Doppler ultrasound, Surg. Gynecol. Obstet. 143:23, 1976.
5. Barnes, R.W., et al.: Noninvasive quantitation of venous hemodynamics in the postphlebitic syndrome, Arch. Surg. 107:807, 1973.
6. Barnes, R.W., et al.: Venous thrombosis in suspected pulmonary embolism: incidence detectable by Doppler ultrasound, Thromb. Haemost. 36:150, 1976.
7. Barnes, R.W., et al.: Photoplethysmographic assessment of altered cutaneous circulation in the post-phlebitic syndrome, Proc. Assoc. Adv. Med. Instrum. 13:25, 1978.
8. Browse, N.L., and Burnand, K.G.: The cause of venous ulceration, Lancet, 2:243, 1982.
9. Browse, N.L., Clemenson, G., and Thomas, M.L.: Is the postphlebitic leg always postphlebitic? Relation between phlebographic appearances of deep-vein thrombosis and late sequelae, Br. Med. J. 281:1, 1980.
10. Coon, W.W., and Coller, F.A.: Clinicopathologic correlation in thromboembolism, Surg. Gynecol. Obstet. 109:259, 1959.
11. Cranley, J.J., Krause, R.J., and Strasser, E.S.: Chronic venous insufficiency of the lower extremity, Surgery 49:48, 1961
12. Dale, W.A.: Ligation, stripping, and excision of varicose vein, Surg. Tech. 67:389, 1970.
13. Evans, G.A., et al.: Spontaneous fatal haemorrhage caused by varicose veins, Lancet, 1973, p. 1359.
14. Hafner, C.D., et al.: A method of managing superficial thrombophlebitis, Surgery 55:201, 1964.
15. Hirsh, J.: Venous thromboembolism: diagnosis, treatment, prevention, Hosp. Pract. 10:53, 1975.
16. Hoare, M.C. et al.: The role of primary varicose veins in venous ulceration, Surgery 92:450, 1982.
17. Hobbs, J.T.: Surgery and sclerotherapy in the treatment of varicose veins, Arch. Surg. 109:793, 1974.
18. Hull, R., et al.: Warfarin sodium versus low-dose heparin in the long-term treatment of venous thrombosis, 301:855, 1979.

19. Hull, R., et al.: Different intensities of oral anticoagulant therapy in the treatment of proximal-vein thrombosis, N. Eng. J. Med. 307:1676, 1982.
20. Husni, E.A., and Williams, W.A.: Superficial thrombophlebitis of lower limbs, Surgery 91:70, 1982.
21. Linton, R.R.: The post-thrombotic ulceration of the lower extremity: its etiology and surgical treatment, Ann. Surg. 128:415, 1953.
22. Lofgren, E.P.: Present-day indications for surgical treatment of varicose veins, Mayo Clin. Proc. 41:515, 1966.
23. Lofgren, E.P., and Lofgren, K.A.: The surgical treatment of superficial thrombophlebitis, Surgery 90:49, 1981.
24. Lofgren, K.A.: Varicose veins: their symptoms, complications, and management, Postgrad. Med. 65:131, 1979.
25. Norris, C.S., Beyrau, A., and Barnes, R.W.: Quantitative photoplesthysmography in chronic venous insufficiency: a new method of noninvasive estimation of ambulatory venous pressure, Surgery 94:758, 1983.
26. O'Sullivan, E.F.: Duration of anticoagulant therapy in venous thrombo-embolism, Med. J. Aust. 2:1104, 1972.
27. Robin, E.D.: Overdiagnosis and overtreatment of pulmonary embolism: the emperor may have no clothes, Ann. Intern. Med. 87:775, 1977.
28. Sasahara, A.A., et al.: Pulmonary thromboembolism: diagnosis and treatment, Clin. Cardiol. 249:2945, 1983.
29. Strandness, D.E., Jr., Ward, K., and Krugmire, R., Jr.: The present status of acute deep venous thrombosis, Surg. Gynecol. Obstet. 145:433, 1977.
30. Thiele, B.L.: Evaluation of ulceration of the lower extremities, Vasc. Diagn. Ther. 1:33, 1980.

CHAPTER 71

Doppler ultrasonic diagnosis of venous disease

ROBERT W. BARNES

Doppler ultrasound is potentially the simplest and most rapid method to noninvasively evaluate venous disease. In experienced hands the technique is as accurate as any other noninvasive method to detect deep vein thrombosis. However, the technique demands considerable experience and attention to technical details, and these factors have limited the widespread application of this diagnostic modality. Development of a programmed audiovisual instructional series may help to facilitate the clinical use of Doppler ultrasound in venous disease.[4] However, there is no substitution for frequent clinical use of this instrument to achieve maximal accuracy in detection of venous disease. In this chapter the technique of the Doppler venous examination is reviewed, and the application of this instrument in acute and chronic venous disease and prospective screening of high-risk patients is reported.

TECHNIQUE
Instrument

I employ a portable hand-held Doppler ultrasonic detector with a transmission frequency of 5 MHz.* This unit can be readily carried in the pocket for bedside examinations. The transmission frequency is ideal for detection of venous velocity signals from the deep veins of the thigh. Flow direction–sensing capability is not necessary for conventional venous examinations.

Velocity signal

Arterial signal. Arterial blood flow velocity signals must be differentiated from venous velocity signals. The normal arterial signal (Fig. 71-1, *A*)

☐ NIH Grant, Diagnostic Techniques in Venous Thromboembolism, IROIHL 22852-02.
*Model BF4A, MedaSonics, Inc., Mountain View, Calif.

is multiphasic with a prominent systolic component and one or more diastolic sounds. Distal to an arterial obstruction, the arterial velocity signal is damped and monophasic with loss of the discrete diastolic sounds (Fig. 71-1, *B*). Arterial signals are pulsatile with each heartbeat and are not significantly influenced by limb compression maneuvers.

Venous signal. Venous velocity signals normally vary with respiration and are not pulsatile with each heartbeat. They are also significantly influenced by limb compression maneuvers. The venous velocity signal is usually of lower pitch as compared with the arterial signal, and it sounds somewhat similar to the noise of a windstorm.

There are five qualities of the venous velocity signal that must be assessed at each site of venous examination. *Spontaneity* of the signal can be elicited in all the major deep veins with the exception of the distal (posterior tibial) or superficial (saphenous) veins in vasoconstricted extremities. In the latter locations flow can be elicited by distal compression of the limb. *Phasicity* refers to the waxing and waning of the velocity signal with respiration (Fig. 71-1, *C*). In the lower extremity venous velocity is diminished or totally interrupted during inspiration when the diaphragm descends and intraabdominal pressure rises. Flow velocity is maximal during expiration. In the presence of proximal venous obstruction, distal venous flow velocity becomes more continuous and less affected by respiration (Fig. 71-1, *D*). *Augmentation* of the velocity signal can be achieved by distal limb compression or release of proximal limb compression (Fig. 71-1, *C*). In the presence of deep vein thrombosis such velocity attenuation is diminished or absent (Fig. 71-1, *D*). *Competence* of the venous valves normally prevents a flow velocity signal during proximal limb compression

(Fig. 71-1, *E*). In the presence of varicose veins or valvular destruction secondary to previous deep vein thrombosis, a reflux flow signal (Fig. 71-1, *F*) during proximal limb compression will document venous incompetence. Normally leg venous velocity signals are *nonpulsatile*, that is, they are affected by respiration and not the cardiac cycle (Fig. 71-1, *G*). With elevated systemic venous pressure, as in congestive heart failure, the lower extremity venous velocity signals may be pulsatile with each heartbeat and may be difficult to distinguish from arterial signals (Fig. 71-1, *H*). However, the influence of limb compression maneuvers or a Valsalva maneuver will alter pulsatile venous signals, in contrast with the arterial signal.

Patient position

The patient is normally examined in the supine position with the head of the bed elevated to permit pooling of blood in the leg veins. Footwear and stockings should be removed. The legs should rest in a comfortable position with the hips slightly externally rotated and the knees slightly flexed. For examination of the popliteal veins, the patient should assume the prone position with the feet elevated on a pillow.

Examination sequence

Posterior tibial vein. Initial assessment of the posterior tibial venous flow signal behind the medial malleolus permits indirect assessment of the status

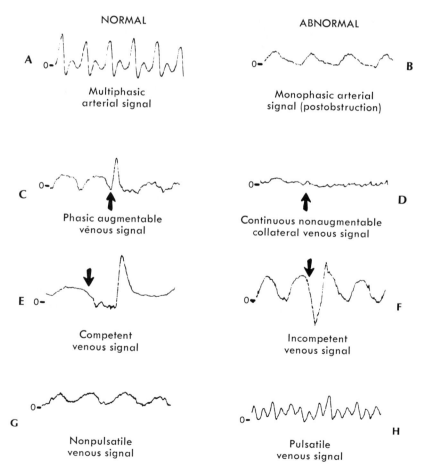

Fig. 71-1. Normal and abnormal Doppler velocity signals in peripheral arteries and veins. Upward arrows indicate distal level compression; downward arrows indicate proximal level compression. (From Barnes, R.W.: Doppler ultrasonic examination of venous disease. In Strandness, D.E., Jr., editor: Clinical handbook of ultrasonics in medicine, New York, 1978, John Wiley & Sons, Inc.)

of the calf veins. With a generous amount of acoustic gel on the Doppler probe, the posterior tibial arterial signal is initially identified, and a search is made for the low-pitched phasic venous signal. If the feet are cool and vasoconstricted, manual compression may be required to elicit the posterior tibial venous signal. The calf is then manually compressed and released to assess deep venous competence and the patency of the calf veins. Normally there should be no signal during calf compression and a prominent augmentation of venous flow on release of the calf. The amount of flow augmentation with this maneuver will be influenced by the degree of peripheral vasoconstriction but should be symmetric in the two limbs. Reduction in posterior tibial venous velocity augmentation in response to release of calf compression is the best indicator of major calf vein thrombosis.

Common femoral vein. Initially the common femoral pulse is palpated and a flow velocity signal elecited from this vessel. The common femoral vein lies medial to the artery, and the flow velocity signal is then obtained from this vessel. The influence of calf and thigh compression and a Valsalva maneuver (or abdominal compression) is noted.

Superficial femoral vein. The superficial femoral vein in the proximal third of the thigh is assessed next. The femoral artery overlies the vein, and the velocity signals normally cannot be separated. The influence of respiration and distal and proximal limb compression maneuvers is noted.

Popliteal vein. With the patient prone, the popliteal artery signal is located, and the adjacent popliteal venous signal is elicited. The effect of respiration and proximal and distal limb compression maneuvers is noted.

Other veins. In the upper extremity the brachial, axillary, and subclavian veins may be assessed. The venous signal normally is adjacent to the corresponding arterial signals. In the upper extremity the venous velocity may be more pulsatile, since the effect of right-sided heart contractions is more readily transmitted to the venous system of the arms. The internal jugular veins may be assessed adjacent to the common carotid artery signal in the neck. The high flow velocity in the internal jugular vein results in a more continuous high-pitched velocity signal.

It is important to realize that the venous evaluation in the extremities is an accurate indicator of the patency of the major intraabdominal and intrathoracic venous trunks. Thus the character of the common femoral venous velocity signal is an accurate guide to the status of the iliac veins and the inferior vena cava.

Examination of the superficial veins, particularly the greater saphenous vein, is useful not only in screening for superficial thrombophlebitis and varicose veins but also to help confirm the diagnosis of deep venous obstruction. With the latter the flow in the saphenous system may be increased compared to flow in the opposite extremity.

APPLICATION AND RESULTS
Acute deep vein thrombosis

The accuracy of the Doppler venous examination was compared with contrast phlebograms obtained in a consecutive series of 122 patients evaluated for suspected deep vein thrombosis.[4] The results of each technique were independently assessed by experienced observers who were unaware of the results of the other study. The Doppler findings agreed with the phlebographic diagnosis in 115 instances, for an overall accuracy of 94%. The Doppler findings were normal in 66 of the 70 limbs with normal phlebograms (94% specificity) and were abnormal in 49 of 52 limbs with phlebographic abnormalities (94% sensitivity). All diagnostic errors were in cases of suspected or proved calf venous disease. There were no errors in assessment of venous disease above the level of the knee. Although many noninvasive techniques are not sensitive to calf vein thrombosis, the complete Doppler venous examination can fairly reliably detect major calf vein thrombosis.[8] There was diagnostic concurrence of the Doppler and phlebographic evaluations in 46 of 55 limbs (84%) evaluated for suspected calf vein thrombosis in which disease, if proved by phlebography, was limited to the calf. The Doppler examination was abnormal in 17 of the 18 limbs with phlebographic abnormalities (94% sensitivity). The Doppler examination was normal in 29 of 37 limbs with normal phlebographic findings (78% specificity). The false-positive diagnoses were usually the result of other conditions, such as subfascial hematoma or cellulitis, which resulted in abnormalities of venous flow in the leg. Similar results have been reported by Sumner and Lambeth.[16]

The impact of Doppler screening for suspected venous disease is reflected in my initial 2-year experience in the Venous Thrombosis Laboratory at the University of Iowa.[5] Of 527 patients referred with a clinical diagnosis of leg vein thrombosis, the Doppler examination was abnormal in only 194 (37%) of the cases. In the remainder of patients some other condition was usually found that could explain the leg manifestations, such as postphlebitic stasis syndrome, symptomatic varicose veins, congestive heart failure leading to leg edema, leg trauma, occult malignancy resulting in venous or lymphatic obstruction, lymphangitis or cellulitis, and arthritis (ruptured Baker's cyst). Subclinical congestive heart failure was a frequent cause of leg edema and was evidenced by pulsatile deep venous velocity signals in the legs. The value of objective screening of patients with suspected deep vein thrombosis was particularly evident in women taking oral contraceptives, in whom only 16% proved to have abnormalities by Doppler ultrasound.[7]

My current practice is to rely on a complete Doppler examination in a patient with suspected acute deep vein thrombosis. An unequivocally normal Doppler examination leads one to consider some other diagnosis for the leg complaints. An unequivocally abnormal Doppler examination in a symptomatic extremity is justification for anticoagulant treatment for leg vein thrombosis. An equivocal Doppler examination is clarified with a contrast phlebogram.

Recurrent deep vein thrombosis

The patient with a history of deep vein thrombosis and recurrent symptoms in the leg presents a diagnostic dilemma. The leg complaints may be on the basis of postphlebitic stasis sequelae caused by residual venous obstruction or damaged deep venous valves. However, recurrent active venous thrombosis must be ruled out. Most physicians would treat such patients with anticoagulation. However, in a study of 211 patients with clinically suspected recurrent deep vein thrombosis, Doppler abnormalities were detected in only 130 individuals (62%). The remaining patients were believed to have had a previously erroneous diagnosis of venous thrombosis. The presence of Doppler abnormalities does not prove activity of venous disease, since such flow velocity alterations may persist for a considerable length of time following prior deep vein thrombosis. Such patients deserve evaluation with tests such as the [^{125}I]fibrinogen uptake test to establish the activity of the venous disease.[17] In a study of 33 patients with Doppler abnormalities and symptoms of recurrent venous thrombosis an [^{125}I]fibrinogen uptake test was positive in only 6 (18%) of these patients. The remaining patients

who were considered to have the postphlebitic syndrome were relieved by leg rest, elevation, and elastic support. I believe that the majority of patients with symptoms of recurrent disease probably do not have an active thrombotic process but are merely suffering the mechanical consequences of previous deep venous obstruction and valvular incompetence.

Postphlebitic syndrome

Doppler ultrasound is a useful method to document venous valvular incompetence in the deep, communicating, and superficial veins of patients with clinical signs of postphlebitic stasis disease. It is important to realize that incompetent deep venous flow signals may not be elicited at the ankle of such patients. Distal venous valves may remain competent if the thrombotic process does not extend to the level of the ankle. The posterior tibial vein is evaluated further up the leg, and incompetent perforators are localized by the examination technique of Folse and Alexander.[12] Such localization of incompetent perforators may permit more conservative venous ligation procedures in the treatment of postphlebitic stasis desease.

Superficial thrombophlebitis

Inflammation on the surface of the leg is often considered to be superficial thrombophlebitis. However, other conditions such as lymphangitis or cellulitis may be confused with this condition. The superficial lymphatics parallel the saphenous venous system, and inflammation of either vascular channel may mimic that of the other. In the absence of obviously thrombosed superficial varicose veins, a Doppler venous examination is a useful way to document the status of the saphenous veins.[6] In the presence of superficial thrombophlebitis, venous velocity signals cannot be elicited in the saphenous vein, although prominent arterial signals may be present in the inflammatory condition. In the presence of lymphangitis the saphenous venous velocity signal will be high-pitched and continous, reflecting the increased flow in the veins in the inflammatory state. The Doppler detector is also useful to assess the deep veins in patients with proved superficial thrombophlebitis.

Varicose veins

Varicose veins may be primary, with the abnormalities limited to the superficial (saphenous) venous system. Secondary varicose veins are the result of underlying deep vein abnormalities, usually prior venous thrombosis. It is important to distinguish between primary and secondary varicose veins, since the natural history of the two disorders may differ. The Doppler venous examination permits rapid assessment of the status of the deep veins.[3] In primary varicose veins the superficial veins are incompetent, but the deep venous system should be normal. In secondary varicose veins the superficial venous incompetence is accompanied by varying degrees of obstruction and definite incompetence of the deep venous system. Incompetent perforators are a hallmark of secondary varicose veins.

Pulmonary embolism

I have employed a screening Doppler examination in all patients with suspected pulmonary emboli. Although perfusion lung scanning is a useful guide in ruling out pulmonary emboli in patients with a normal scan, an abnormal lung scan is nonspecific and is not proof of a pulmonary embolus. If patients have a source of venous thrombosis in the lower extremities proved by Doppler examination, then the clinical diagnosis of pulmonary embolus is fairly certain. However, of 168 patients screened with a clinical diagnosis of pulmonary embolism, only 48 (28%) had venous abnormalities by Doppler examination.[9] In patients with a normal Doppler examination a diagnosis of pulmonary embolism is questionable unless the perfusion lung scan is of lobar extent or greater and the chest film is normal, or unless there is a documented mismatch between ventilation and perfusion lung scanning.[13] In other situations I would recommend pulmonary arteriography to confirm the diagnosis.

Prospective surveillance studies

Although Doppler ultrasound has been used extensively to document the presence or absence of venous disease in symptomatic patients, the technique is also useful to prospectively screen high-risk patients for the development of venous thrombosis.[1] Although there have been increasing numbers of reports suggesting the use of routine prophylactic measures such as low-dose subcutaneous heparin in such patients, a useful alternative is to prospectively screen patients by Doppler examination and treat those who develop the disease. In my experience the incidence of major deep vein thrombosis is low enough to justify such prospective surveillance, as opposed to routine anticoagulant prophylaxis in high-risk patients.

Total hip replacement. Preoperative and serial postoperative Doppler examinations were performed on 101 patients who underwent 114 total hip replacements.[11] These patients were not given routine anticoagulant prophylaxis, and patients with prior venous disease were not excluded from the study. All patients received vigorous postoperative physical therapy and were usually walking with partial weight bearing on the operated extremity within 4 or 5 days of operation. Below-knee elastic support stockings were routinely employed. There were only four instances of leg vein thrombosis detectable by Doppler ultrasound and confirmed by phlebography. In two of these, the thrombosis developed following the patient's discharge from the hospital. One additional patient had a major pulmonary embolus with no identifiable source of thrombosis by Doppler or phlebographic examination. There were no deaths from pulmonary emboli in the study. In a subsequent randomized clincial trial of the efficacy of antiembolism stockings in patients undergoing total hip replacement, Doppler ultrasound established a significant incidence (50%) of major leg vein thrombosis in patients not wearing stockings.[10] No major thrombi were detected in those wearing stockings.

Gastric bypass for morbid obesity. A prospective Doppler screening study was carried out in 58 patients undergoing gastric bypass for morbid obesity.[14] Prophylactic anticoagulants were not employed. Postoperatively only one patient had a calf vein thrombosis by Doppler examination, and this patient suffered a small pulmonary embolus. The remaining patients showed no clinical or Doppler evidence of venous thromboembolic disease.

Major leg amputation. A prospective Doppler surveillance examination was carried out on 35 patients who underwent a total of 42 below-knee amputations for advanced leg ischemia not amenable to vascular reconstruction.[2] The patients were not treated with prophylactic anticoagulants. Postoperatively no patient developed abnormalities by Doppler venous examination. One patient developed a small pulmonary embolus following discharge from the hospital after a fall on the amputation stump. The remaining patients had no clinical evidence of venous thromboembolic disease.

Abdominal surgery. A prospective study was undertaken to assess the incidence of deep vein thrombosis in patients undergoing major abdominal surgery. The patients were randomized into three groups, including a control group, a group with elastic stockings, and a group with elevation of the foot of the hospital bed. None of the 63 patients developed venous thrombosis by Doppler examination, and there was no evidence of clinical pulmonary embolism. These patients did not receive prophylactic anticoagulation. Sigel et al.[15] have used prospective Doppler surveillance of more than 2800 patients undergoing general surgery, and the risk of development of major leg vein thrombosis in the postoperative period is less than 2%. These statistics support the clinical merits of prospective screening with a simple noninvasive technique as an alternative to routine prophylaxis of high-risk patients.

SUMMARY

In experienced hands the Doppler velocity detector is the most simple, rapid, versatile, and accurate technique to evaluate venous disease. However, the technique demands considerable familiarity and attention to detail to achieve maximal accuracy. Nevertheless, this modality can be employed by a technologist. The technique depends on sound pattern recognition of phasic venous velocity signals and the response of such flow velocity to limb compression maneuvers. The routine examination includes assessment of the posterior tibial, common femoral, superficial femoral, and popliteal veins in the lower extremity. Indirect information is gained about the status of the calf veins and the intraabdominal (iliac and inferior vena cava) venous systems. Deep veins in the upper extremity and neck also may be examined. This technique is useful to evaluate patients with acute deep vein thrombosis, recurrent venous thrombosis, the postphlebitic syndrome, superficial thrombophlebitis, varicose veins, and pulmonary embolism. In addition, the simplicity, portability, and rapidity of the technique make Doppler ultrasound a useful method to prospectively screen larger numbers of patients who are at high risk of developing deep vein thrombosis.

REFERENCES

1. Barnes, R.W.: Prospective screening for deep vein thrombosis in high-risk patients, Am. J. Surg. 134:187, 1977.
2. Barnes, R.W., and Slaymaker, E.E.: Postoperative deep vein thrombosis in the lower extremity amputee: a prospective study with Doppler ultrasound, Ann. Surg. 183:429, 1976.
3. Barnes, R.W., Ross, E.A., and Strandness, D.E., Jr.: Differentiation of primary from secondary varicose veins by Doppler ultrasound and strain gauge plethysmography, Surg. Gynecol. Obstet. 141:207, 1975.
4. Barnes, R.W., Russell, H.E., and Wilson, M.R.: Doppler ultrasonic evaluation of venous disease: a programmed audiovisual instruction, ed. 2, Iowa City, 1975, University of Iowa Press.
5. Barnes, R.W., Wu, K.K., and Hoak, J.C.: The fallibility of the clinical diagnosis of venous thrombosis, J.A.M.A. 234:605, 1975.
6. Barnes, R.W., Wu, K.K., and Hoak, J.C.: Differentiation of superficial thrombophlebitis from lymphangitis by Doppler ultrasound, Surg. Gynecol. Obstet. 143:23, 1976.
7. Barnes, R.W., Krapf, T., and Hoak, J.C.: Erroneous clinical diagnosis of leg vein thrombosis in women on oval contraceptives, Surg. Gynecol. Obstet. 51:556, 1978.
8. Barnes, R.W., et al.: Accuracy by Doppler ultrasound in clinically suspected calf vein thrombosis, Surg. Gynecol. Obstet. 143:425, 1976.
9. Barnes, R.W., et al.: Venous thrombosis in suspected pulmonary embolism: incidence detectable by Doppler ultrasound, Thromb. Diath. Haemorrh. 36:150, 1976.
10. Barnes, R.W., et al.: Efficiency of graded-compression anti-embolism stockings in patients undergoing total hip replacement, Clin. Orthop. 132:61, 1978.
11. Convery, F.R., et al.: Prophylaxis against thromboembolic disease. I. Case against drug prophylaxis of thromboembolism in total hip replacement. In Harris, W., editor: The hip: proceedings of the Second Open Scientific Meeting of the Hip Society, St. Louis, 1974, The C.V. Mosby Co.
12. Folse, R., and Alexander, R.H.: Directional flow detection for localizing venous valvular incompetency, Surgery 67:114, 1970.
13. McNeil, B.J., Holman, B.L., and Adelstein, S.J.: The scintigraphic definition of pulmonary embolism, J.A.M.A. 227:753, 1974.
14. Printen, K.J., Miller, E.V., and Barnes, R.W.: Venous thromboembolism in the morbidly obese, Surg. Gynecol. Obstet. 147:63, 1978.
15. Sigel, B., Ipsen, J., and Felix, W.R., Jr.: The epidemiology of lower extremity deep venous thrombosis in surgical patients, Ann. Surg. 179:278, 1974.
16. Sumner, D.S., and Lambeth, A.: Reliability of Doppler ultrasound in the diagnosis of acute venous thrombosis both above and below the knee, Am. J. Surg. 138:205, 1979.
17. Wu, K.K., Hoak, J.C., and Barnes, R.W.: A prospective comparison of four methods for the diagnisis of deep vein thrombosis, Thromb. Diath. Haemorrh. 32:260, 1974.

CHAPTER 72

Diagnosis of deep vein thrombosis by phleborheography

JOHN J. CRANLEY

In collaboration with Larry D. Flanagan, M.D., and Eugene D. Sullivan, M.D.*

Phleborheography is a plethysmographic technique originally introduced for the noninvasive diagnosis of deep vein thrombosis of the lower extremities.[5-14] Phleborheography is defined as the tracing of flowing currents within veins. Our original concepts of the nature of deep vein thrombosis and phleborheographic instrumentation have been confirmed, modified, and broadened in the 12 years since the modality was introduced. Our understanding of venous blood flow was altered by the realization that blood flow may be substantially arrested by the extended knee, the flexed thigh, the gravid uterus, bulky movable tumors, and the position of the extremities and torso. From the beginning we recognized that the method could not detect clots outside the mainstream, for example, in the saphenous veins, the soleal veins, the deep femoral artery, and the hypogastric veins. This limitation did not prove to be the anticipated drawback, because there is evidence that thrombi in the soleal or tibial veins frequently do not become major thrombi and that most lethal emboli are large or the type that would occlude an entire segment of the femoral vein or the iliac system. Furthermore, it is probable that most small emboli are lysed in the lung without clinical sequelae.

The original phleborheograph was designed for the detection of deep vein thrombosis of the lower extremity and was a simplified version of the standard research polygraph. Now many of the features of the standard polygraph have been incorporated into the equipment, making it virtually a minipolygraph and giving it application beyond the de-

*Good Samaritan Hospital, Cincinnati, Ohio.

tection of obstruction in the deep veins of the extremities. The current model is useful not only in the analysis of venous physiology, but also for studying other physiologic variables. This model may be used as a recorder for analysis of arterial pulse waves in the extremities and in the rectum for assessing the colonic circulation. In addition, it can be used with other input signals, such as the photoelectric cell, various strain gauges, the Doppler ultrasound flow detector, and the electrocardiograph. Although it is not the universal diagnostic machine, the phleborheograph is the mainstay of noninvasive diagnosis of deep vein thrombosis in our hospital (over 27,000 extremities tested) and in many other institutions. Acute mainstream thrombi from the popliteal vein to the vena cava have been diagnosed, and the decision to hospitalize for treatment has been influenced by the results of this test.

PRINCIPLES

Reduction of respiratory waves in deep venous thrombosis. Normal breathing produces a rhythmic increase and decrease in the volume of the lower extremity, which is transmitted to the phleborheograph and recorded as an oscillation on the tracing synchronous with the wave produced by a recording cuff placed around the chest. Called respiratory waves, these oscillations are present in all normal extremities. Acute deep vein thrombosis obliterates or significantly reduces the size of the respiratory waves. With the development of collateral circulation, waves that have been absent usually reappear, and those that have been smaller become larger. The change is noticeable in approximately 2 weeks. However, although they are now present or have become larger, they may differ from normal waves in that they are relatively small and may be more rounded in configuration. In a patient with femoroiliac thrombophlebitis, respiratory waves may be visible in tracings from the leg if the veins of the leg are patent, despite the absence of waves in the thigh, probably because the respiratory influence travels down the limb through the collateral veins. Of special interest is the fact that respiratory waves in the lower extremity are usually larger in amplitude when the patient lies on his left side than those obtained when he is supine. This is thought to be a result of moving the weight of the intraabdominal viscera from the inferior vena cava and the iliac veins. Occasionally, however, the respiratory waves are larger when the patient lies on his right rather than on his left side. There is no explanation for this phenomenon.

Interference with blood outflow from the extremity. Deep vein thrombosis interferes with the normal outflow of blood from the extremity in response to rhythmic compression. Similar to active muscle contraction on walking, intermittent compression of the extremity propels blood proximally. A recording cuff proximal to the site of compression detects the momentary damming up of blood when venous thrombosis or extraluminal compression blocks its exit. Indicative of the blockage, a rise in baseline of the volume recorder takes place. However, whenever compression is applied to the normal extremity when no impediment to venous outflow is present, the baseline remains level. This penomenon localizes the site of thrombosis. If the thigh tracing shows a stepwise rise while the calf is being compressed, the level of obstruction to the deep veins is located above the thigh cuff. Rarely, external compression may be to blame; generally, intraluminal thrombosis is present.

Similarly, if there is obstruction at or above the recording cuffs, compression of the foot causes a rise in baseline of phleborheographic tracings from the leg, which is unequivocal evidence of venous obstruction.

Compression of the calf. Compression of the calf has two effects: blood is propelled up the unobstructed extremity, and blood is siphoned out of the normal foot. When the calf is compressed, a recording cuff on the foot shows a fall in baseline. Absent or less than normal foot emptying in the

presence of a rise in baseline and absent respiratory waves are indicative of acute deep vein thrombosis. More conducive to artifacts than other maneuvers, this procedure nevertheless permits detection of a normal tracing at a glance.

TECHNIQUE

The patient lies quietly in bed with the lower extremities approximately 10 degrees below heart level. The first four cuffs of the phleborheograph are for recording only. Cuff 1 is placed around the thorax, cuff 2 to the midthigh, cuffs 3, 4, and 5 to the upper calf in close approximation to each other, and cuff 6 on the foot. Cuffs 5 and 6 are used to both record transmitted impulses and apply compression (Fig. 72-1). There are three operational modes, run A, run B_1, and run B_2. In run A all cuffs on the thigh and leg record the response to compression of the foot by applying pressure to the foot cuff. In run B_1, pressure is applied to the midcalf (cuff 5). All other cuffs record the response, including the cuff on the foot (cuff 6), which records changes in pedal volume. In run B_2, cuff 5 is moved to ankle level and used to apply compression. The remaining cuffs are used for recording.

Run A: foot compression

In run A the recording cuffs are automatically inflated to 10 mm Hg pressure. The chart speed is 2.5 mm/sec. Calibration is performed by adjusting the amplification so that the 0.2 ml volume calibrator causes a 2 cm pen deflection. Respiratory waves are observed first. Following this, the compress control is operated, and three short bursts of 100 mm Hg pressure are delivered to the foot cuff (cuff 6), 0.5 second in duration and at 0.5-second intervals. About 40% of the pressure is expended in inflating the cuff so that actually only about 60 mm Hg pressure is exerted on the foot.

Although the recording pen may move erratically with application of pressure, in a normal extremity the baseline remains level (Fig. 72-2). If there is interference with the outflow of blood from the extremity, the baseline rises with each successive compression as the extremity swells. Time is allowed for venous refilling of the lower leg to occur before the next compression. This usually requires 20 seconds. This maneuver is repeated at least three times, but if there is any interference with the tracing, pressure may be applied as often as necessary.

If the respiratory waves appear to be smaller than

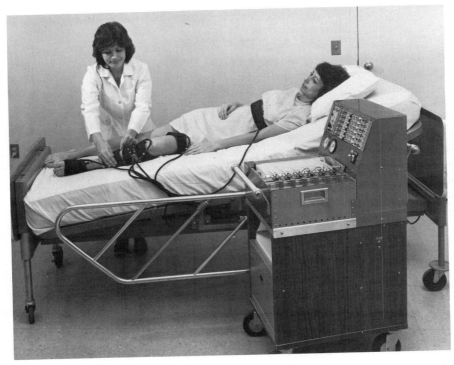

Fig. 72-1. In preparation for phleborheography of lower extremities, patient lies quietly with legs below heart level and six cuffs applied.

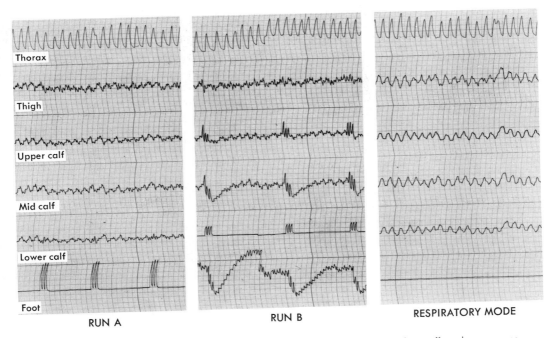

Thorax

Thigh

Upper calf

Mid calf

Lower calf

Foot

RUN A   RUN B   RESPIRATORY MODE

Fig. 72-2. Normal tracing. There are good respiratory waves throughout *run A* (foot cuff used as compression cuff) and *run B* (lower calf cuff used as compression cuff). Note absence of baseline shift when either foot or lower calf is compressed. Note also good foot emptying in *run B*. *Respiratory mode* shows good respiratory waves after arterial pulses have been filtered.

usual, the patient is turned on the left side with both knees slightly flexed, and the right leg lying behind the left. This maneuver increases the size of the respiratory waves; however, in a patient with acute deep vein thrombosis, changing the position usually does not restore the obliterated waves. If the baseline continues to show a rise with each compression or if the respiratory waves remain smaller than usual, minor positional changes may be tried in an attempt to minimize the effect of compressions on the respiratory waves. Prone or near-prone positions should not be used, since, for reasons that are unclear, these positions tend to produce a normal tracing in the presence of deep vein obstruction.

Run B₁: calf compression

In run B₁ the recording cuff on the lower part of the calf becomes a compression cuff (cuff 5), and the cuff on the foot (cuff 6) is converted to a recording cuff. In this run, operating the compress control automatically causes a 50 mm Hg pressure to compress the cuff on the calf three times, similar to compression of the foot in run A. Again, about 40% of this pressure is expended in inflating the cuff, so that actually only about 30 mm Hg pressure is exerted on the calf.

Emptying of the foot is observed. This decrease in volume of the foot is demonstrated in the tracing (cuff 6) by a fall in baseline. This test is repeated at least three times. Time must be allowed for the pen to return to its baseline before the next application of pressure. In a fully normal extremity, the pen baseline falls at least 3 cm, corresponding to a 0.3 ml volume change under the cuff, the dimensions of which are 9 x 17 cm. Return to baseline is gradual rather than abrupt.

As the lower part of the calf is compressed, the recording from the midcalf normally falls somewhat, mimicking the fall in baseline of the foot. This is thought to be an artifact caused by the proximity of cuffs 4 and 5. Meanwhile, the baseline of the tracing from the upper part of the calf and lower part of the thigh remains level. However, if any obstruction to the deep venous system exists above the recording cuff, a rise in the baseline occurs that is progressive with each compression. In extensive thrombophlebitis this may be a sharp, abrupt rise; on the other hand, a stepwise rise of greater than 1 mm is significant (Fig. 72-3).

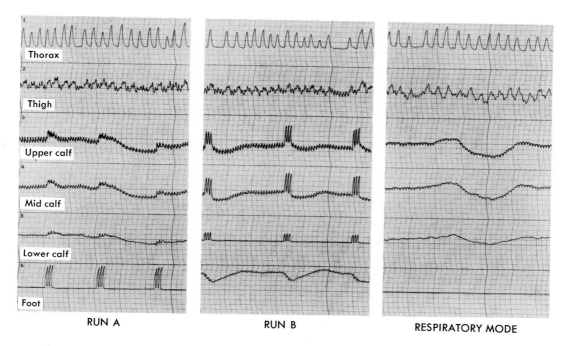

Fig. 72-3. Acute poplitical thrombosis. Note normal respiratory waves and absence of any baseline rise in thigh; however, there is obliteration of respiratory waves in calf as well as baseline elevation secondary to foot *(run A)* and calf *(run B)* compression, indicating deep venous obstruction. Note total absence of respiratory waves distal to the thigh on *respiratory mode* trace, indicating deep venous obstruction at popliteal level.

Run B_2: ankle compression

In Run B_2, the midcalf cuff (cuff 5) is moved to the ankle level and is used to deliver compressions. Cuffs 1 through 4 and cuff 6 are used for recording as in run B_1. Compressions are identical to those used in run B_1 with regard to timing, duration, and pressure.

Once again, emptying of the foot is observed as in run B_1. Unlike run B_1, however, the midcalf recording does not usually fall. The baseline of this recording cuff and the others remains level. If there is obstruction to venous outflow, a rise in baseline occurs. In addition, foot emptying may be reduced or absent.

Interpretation

Interpretation of the tracing is based on the physiologic principles previously described. Strict adherence to criteria based on over 27,000 phlebo-rheograms (PRG) and 748 phlebographic correlations is required.

In tracings of the lower extremities, it is necessary to obtain nine normal compressions, three in run A, three in run B_1, and three in run B_2. Each set of three must be obtained without changing the position of the patient; however, sets need not be consecutive. Positions used for runs A, B_1, and B_2 may differ. Only three normal compressions are required in the upper extremity, all obtained in the same position.

The characteristics of a normal compression have been precisely outlined.[5] They include the following: (1) normal respiratory wave amplitude with the amplitude averaging 50% or more of the amplitude of waves in the opposite extremity, (2) no absolute baseline rise, and (3) no dynamic baseline rise with compression. The absolute baseline is a plot of points connecting the minimum volume of each respiratory wave. The dynamic baseline is a plot of points representing the normal volume of the extremity expected at any point in the respiratory cycle. A rise greater than 1 mm in either the absolute or dynamic baseline is considered significant. Fig. 72-4 portrays tracings that illustrate abnormalities in these parameters.

Baseline elevation and respiratory waves are considered major criteria and must be normal as defined for a compression to be considered normal. The minor criteria of pulsatility and foot emptying are less important. Pulsatility refers to the amplitude of the superimposed arterial waves that are seen in the respiratory waves of every tracing.

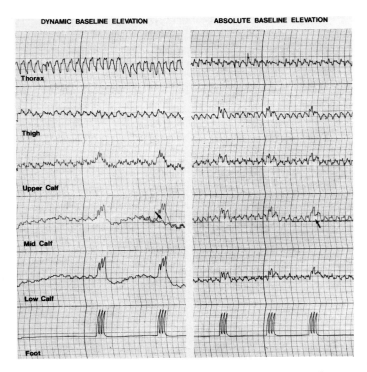

Fig. 72-4. Abnormality of dynamic baseline rise and absolute baseline rise.

When compared to the opposite leg, increased pulsatility suggests deep vein obstruction (usually acute) or the presence of a popliteal arterial aneurysm. Bilateral increased pulsatility may be seen in patients with congestive heart failure and tricuspid insufficiency. Foot emptying has been previously described. It should be noted that abnormal foot emptying or increased pulsatility are merely suggestive and not diagnostic of deep vein obstruction. Their major usefulness is to clarify an equivocal tracing.

Further consideration of a particular tracing may allow a diagnosis of acute versus chronic or complete versus partial obstruction. For example, a persistent baseline rise (dynamic or absolute) coupled with absent respiratory waves suggests acute complete obstruction. Baseline rise with near-normal respiratory waves suggests partial acute abstruction or complete obstruction with recanalization or collateralization [chronic vs. early acute (Fig. 72-5). The level of obstruction can frequently be ascertained by careful scrutiny of the changes occurring in each cuff with compression.

Serial tracings show the gradual transition from acute occlusion to the development of the chronic state or to dissolution of the thrombi. Caution and clinical judgment must be used in diagnosing the chronic process. For example, a tracing will show obstruction and large respiratory waves, indicating excellent collateral circulation, the day after ligation of the femoral vein (not for venous thrombosis). Thus the test reflects the actual state, that is, obstruction and good collateral circulation, although it is obviously not long-term. Another pitfall is a thrombus that partially but not wholly occludes a small segment of a vein, such as the popliteal or femoral, and that may cause the test to show a rise in baseline with normal respiratory waves. Instead of being a chronic occlusion, this is an early acute lesion. When the test is repeated in a day or two, respiratory waves may be absent. In other words, the partially occluding thrombus has now propagated.

UPPER EXTREMITY TECHNIQUE

Certain modifications are necessary for the upper extremity technique. Recording cuffs are placed around the thorax, upper arm, and upper and mid-

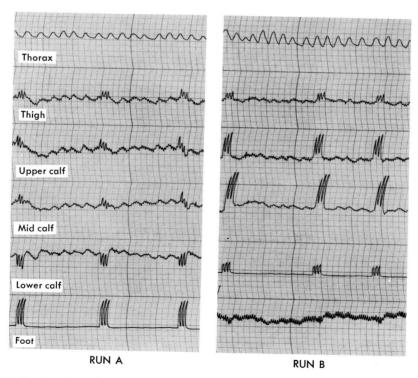

RUN A   RUN B

Fig. 72-5. Baseline rise with near normal respiratory waves suggests partial acute obstruction with recanalization or collateralization (chronic vs. early acute).

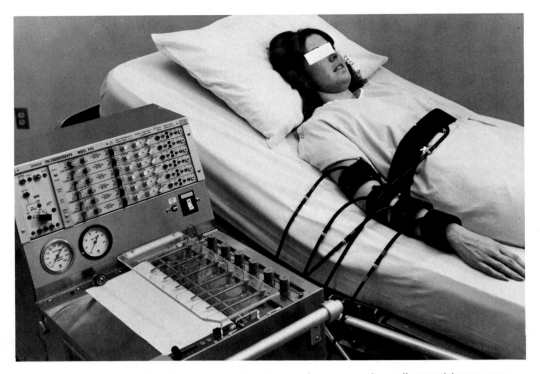

Fig. 72-6. Modified technique for upper extremity diagnosis showing recording cuffs around thorax, upper arm, and middle and lower forearm with compression cuff on wrist.

dle forearm, along with a compression cuff on the wrist (Fig. 72-6). The mode selector is turned to run B and the wrist cuff is rapidly inflated to 50 mm Hg, producing compressions that pump the blood proximally. The proximal arm cuffs record any changes in volume that occur at rest or with these volume challenges. In the upper extremity, respiratory waves can persist despite complete venous occlusion, probably because of rich venous collaterals around the shoulder. Therefore a diagnosis of upper extremity deep vein occlusion is usually based on the presence or absence of baseline rise alone.[15] However, we have seen two tracings interpreted as normal that exhibited a 50% decrease in respiratory wave amplitude compared to the opposite side and that had no baseline rise yet were shown by phlebography to contain a clot in the deep vein system.

RESULTS

Results are shown in Table 72-1. In analyzing the efficacy of the method, a subgroup of 748 lower extremities with phlebographic confirmation was studied. An equivocal tracing is usually resolved by repeating the tracing in 24 hours. At times, vein imaging using the B-mode scanner, a technique presently undergoing evaluation in our laboratory, has allowed us to confirm or refute the phleborheographic study immediately. Errors in interpretation have been determined by a review of the tracing after a phlebogram has been obtained. The technical errors have been almost completely eliminated. The percentage of inherent false negatives has remained at approximately 5% throughout the 12-year period of the instrument's availability. These false negatives have usually consisted of small clots below the knee. In a group of 60 patients with clots limited to the infrapopliteal area, 15 (25%) false negative tests have occurred.

False positives are more difficult to explain; thus studying these patients has augmented our knowledge of venous physiology. Results of upper extremity studies are shown in Table 72-2.

Venous compression

Extrinsic compression of a vein causes obstruction to the flow of venous blood, indicated by a rise in baseline. Our experience includes 10 patients with venous compression without deep vein thrombosis. Inclusion of these cases as errors is

Table 72-1. Phlebographic-phleborheographic correlations: 748 lower extremities

False negatives	
Equivocal	2/290 (0.7%)
Interpretive error	7/290 (2.4%)
True miss	15/290 (5.2%)
TOTAL	24/290 (8.3%)
False positives	
Equivocal	3/458 (0.7%)
Technical error	5/458 (1.1%)
Interpretive error	4/458 (0.9%)
True miss	11/458 (2.4%)
TOTAL	23/458 (5%)

Table 72-2. Phlebographic-phleborheographic correlations: 25 upper extremities

False negatives	
Equivocal	0/10
Interpretive error	0/10
True miss	2/10 (20%)
TOTAL	2/10 (20%)
False positives	
Equivocal	0/15
Technical error	0/15
Interpretive error	0/15
True miss	1/15 (7%)
TOTAL	1/15 (7%)

debatable, inasmuch as the test did detect the true state of affairs, namely, obstruction of venous blood flow.

In addition to the previously mentioned physiologic obstruction of venous blood flow, we re-encountered false positive tracings in several young, nervous, otherwise healthy individuals. Almost invariably, the false positive tracing becomes normal on administration of a sedative or on repeat testing. Recently, we have seen two phlebograms of young patients with a positive PRG that showed quite obvious narrowing of the femoral vein in the thigh, causing what appeared to be a significant constriction of the lumen (Fig. 72-7). We cannot explain this phenomenon at this time, but it reemphasizes the accuracy of the PRG with normal respiratory waves, indicating obstruction to the flow of blood. It also stresses the difficulty of judging whether this is or is not a false positive tracing.

Results of other investigators

Published reports of other investigations are shown in Table 72-3. At first glance Bynum et al.[2] appear to be reporting a negative experience. However, analysis of their data[8] shows that in 6 (54%) of the 11 extremities with clots below the knee, the thrombi were in the veins of the soleus-gastrocnemius muscles. In only 1 of these 6 "errors" was the clot in a named vein below the knee, which is an actual false negative test. In earlier publications we emphasized that phleborheography cannot detect clots not in the mainstream, thus excluding thrombi in veins of the soleus muscle and in the deep femoral, the hypogastric, and the saphenous veins. Therefore we have adjusted Bynum et al.'s data in the totals.

Of the four false negative tests in the femoropopliteal system, three occurred in patients with duplications of the popliteal vein. We also have observed this, most often in patients with chronic venous disease. Interestingly, in one of Bynum et al.'s three patients who had thrombosis in one of the duplicated veins, the test was positive. The fourth patient in their series with thrombi in the venous mainstream not detected by the test had Cheyne-Stokes respiration. This is a recognized source of error, a fact stressed in our training program and in earlier publications. Usually if respiratory waves are present at the time the patient is actually breathing, the major venous trunks are probably not completely occluded.

DISCUSSION

Phleborheography is noninvasive, is painless, and involves physiologic principles. Most patients can be examined in 30 to 45 minutes, although acutely ill, disabled, or less cooperative patients may require longer studies. Interpretation must be learned by each physician, and the principles previously outlined must be applied.

Nonocclusive thrombi

A thrombus that is attached to a vein wall but does not actually, or at least nearly, obstruct the flow of blood is not detected by phleborheography. As the clot occludes more and more venous flow, there may be a slight rise in baseline, but respiratory waves are still present. When the clot progresses to occlude the vein, the respiratory waves disappear. It is our impression that a thrombus attached to the vein wall over which blood continues to flow will usually lyse.

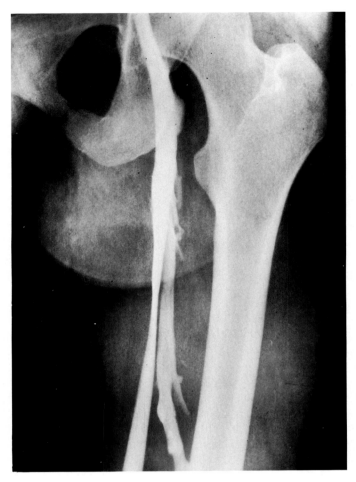

Fig. 72-7. Phlebogram showing significant narrowing of lumen of femoral vein in thigh of young patient with positive PRG with normal respiratory waves. PRG accurately showed obstruction to blood flow.

Acute and chronic deep vein thrombosis

An area of acute deep vein thrombosis may develop in an extremity with the postphlebitic syndrome. This new episode, superimposed on chronic disease, in the early stage poses some difficulties in diagnosis. In the postphlebitic limb the respiratory waves are so large that even when reduced in size as a result of obstruction by fresh thrombus they still may appear to be within normal limits. An exacerbation of existing symptoms or the onset of new ones in such a chronically insufficient limb may be indicative of acute thrombosis, and the physician should follow the patient's clinical course.

CHRONIC OCCLUSION OF MAJOR VEINS

A negative tracing in a patient with an acute obstruction of the popliteal or femoral vein has not been encountered; however, tracings on limbs with chronic occlusion of these vessels have been negative at times. Chronicity can be detected radiologically by the presence of a large number of collateral veins around the obstruction, by clot retraction, by irregularity (tree-barking) of the walls of the veins, or occasionally by clinical history.

PULMONARY EMBOLISM FOLLOWING A NEGATIVE PRG

Four instances have been observed of a pulmonary embolism following a negative PRG. Three other instances have been reported to us. In three of our patients, the embolism was fatal. The critical factor common to all seven instances is the time interval between the negative PRG and lodgment of the pulmonary embolus. In all but two patients it was between 8 and 12 days; in the re-

Table 72-3. Phlebographic-phleborheographic correlations of the lower extremities

Investigator	No. of extremities	False negatives	Sensitivity	False positives	Specificity	Overall accuracy
Sull (Nov. 1978)[17]	24	1/10 (10%)	9/10 (90%)	0/14 (0%)	14/14 (100%)	23/24 (96%)
Collins et al. (Jan. 1979)[4]	64	0/41 (0%)	41/41 (100%)	3/23 (13%)	19/23 (83%)	61/64 (95%)
Bynum et al. (Aug. 1978)[2]	59	11/35 (31%)	24/35 (69%)	0/24 (0%)	24/24 (100%)	35/59 (59%)*
Data adjusted (see text)	59	4/28 (14%)	24/28 (86%)	0/24 (0%)	24/24 (100%)	48/59 (81%)
Elliott et al. (April 1980)[15]	216	6/41 (15%)	35/41 (85%)	24/175 (14%)	151/175 (86%)	192/216 (89%)
Stallworth et al. (June 1981)[16]	39	1/13 (8%)	12/13 (92%)	1/24 (4.6%)	23/24 (96%)	35/39 (89.7%)
Classen et al. (June 1982)[3]	90	4/24 (17%)	20/24 (83%)	2/66 (3%)	64/66 (97%)	84/90 (93%)
Cranley et al. (Oct. 1983)	748	24/290 (8.3%)	266/290 (92%)	23/458 (5.1%)	435/458 (93%)	701/748 (94%)
TOTALS	1,240	40/447 (9%)	407/447 (91%)	53/784 (6.6%)	730/784 (93%)	1144/1240 (92%)

*Data include thrombi not detectable by this technique.

maining two patients, 6 days. It is believed that deep vein thrombosis may propagate at a rapid rate, so that a clot in the veins of the soleus muscle or in one of the named veins of the leg may progress to the popliteal vein and then propagate to the femoral vein in 2 or 3 days.

In our experience, there is a 25% false negative rate in PRGs performed on patients with clots limited to the veins below the knee. Usually such thrombi are small and probably do not propagate, but the potential exists that they may progress to the popliteal vein and then become lethal. Accordingly, we have adopted a policy of deferring our diagnosis whenever the PRG is normal in a patient with a tender calf, preferring to obtain repeat tests at 2-day intervals until the clinical symptoms clear or the test becomes positive, indicating that propagation to the popliteal area has taken place. In this event, treatment for deep vein thrombosis is initiated.

A small occlusive acute clot, which is a potential source of later pulmonary embolism, may be interpreted as a "chronic occlusion." The terms *acute* and *chronic* are clinical judgments, made by the clinician. The PRG is merely capable of recording presence or absence of obstruction and either large or small respiratory waves. Usually, an obstruction with the absence of collateral circulation means an acute obstruction, and the presence of large respiratory waves means a chronic obstruc-

tion. However, as we have pointed out, the day after the femoral vein has been ligated (not for venous thrombosis), a PRG tracing on that patient will indicate obstruction with normal respiratory waves. This could be interpreted as "chronic occlusion," if the clinical history were not known. Similarly, a small clot occluding a very short segment of the femoral or iliac vein might be interpreted as chronic occlusion, with the tracing showing a rising baseline combined with large respiratory waves. For this reason, tracings are now reported as either normal or abnormal. If they are abnormal because of a rise in baseline and the absence of respiratory waves, the tracing is interpreted as typical of acute deep vein thrombosis. If there is a rise in baseline and if normal appearing or larger than normal respiratory waves are seen, it is interpreted as abnormal, consistent with early acute or chronic disease. If the symptoms are acute, the patient should be followed with repeat tests at 2- to 3-day intervals.

Finally, retrospective analysis has convinced us that some patients had the pulmonary embolus before the PRG was obtained. If a large clot breaks off totally, leaving an empty vein behind, then the PRG would be normal. This problem has not been solved. However, proved clots in the lung may occur in the patient whose phlebogram shows a patent venous tree from ankles to the vena cava.

SOURCES OF ERROR IN INTERPRETATION

We now believe that most false positive tests are a result of temporary physiologic obstruction of the venous tree. Many normal patients have a segment of their tracing that appears to be positive; then simply by flexing the knee, straightening the thigh, or shifting the patient from one side to the other, the tracing becomes totally normal. At first it was difficult for us to believe this could be true, but the frequency of such occurrences plus the occasional patient in whom it was possible to document these facts has convinced us that it is a physiologic phenomenon.

Other difficulties in the statistical analysis of the accuracy of these tests stem from the fact that phlebography, the diagnostic standard, is frequently incomplete or subject to error. The possibility of obtaining 100 consecutive excellent phlebograms is virtually impossible. Yet this is a requirement if it is to be used as a standard. The most common deficiency is that the pelvic veins are not visualized. Classen et al.[3] reported 2 false positive tracings in the same patient. Visualization of the iliac veins was not obtained and possible filling defects were noted. Bi-plane films are at times essential for accurate interpretation, since the presence or absence of clots in the veins below the knee is frequently subject to contrary interpretations by different radiologists.

Skill and experience in reading the PRG tracings are of importance. In our laboratory, nine first-year Vascular Fellows successively interpreted the tests since the PRG was originated; most of their errors occurred during the early months of the academic year.

EQUIPMENT

Calibration of the phleborheograph is performed by removing precisely 0.2 cc of air from each cuff. Thus the actual size of the respiratory waves can be compared from day to day in the same patient or from patient to patient. Since it is basically an amplifier and direct-writing recorder that uses a low-pressure transducer, the equipment is highly versatile. For extended uses of the phleborheograph refer to Chapter 16.

The single greatest problem in the development of this system is that the technique is new and must be learned. Interpretation of the tracing is not always easy. In most instances, however, a physician can learn to interpret the tracings accurately in approximately 5 days of study. The test is technician sensitive, and thus the technician must be highly trained, which usually requires 3 weeks. The technician learns to recognize abnormal patterns and then maneuvers the patient to various positions to see if the tracing reverts to normal. If it does, it is considered to be normal. On the other hand, if the tracing is positive, it is impossible to make it become normal by any maneuvering of the patient's position. The most common artifact encountered is compression of the popliteal vein by the extended knee, as previously discussed. Similarly, flexing the thigh in some patients may obstruct the femoral vein in the inguinal area. In young athletic adults, compression of the veins by muscle mass may result in a false positive tracing. Many times, no explanation can be found for compression of the veins in a particular position. When the test appears to be positive, the technician turns the patient first on his left side; if the test remains abnormal, the patient is turned on his right side. Occasionally, a positive PRG then becomes normal. The reason for this phenomenon is not known, but we believe that the transmission is an accurate reflection of the physiologic status of the venous tree at the moment of recording and that the PRG is revealing some previously unrecognized physiologic state. The technician must be aware of these hemodynamic vagaries.

Phleborheography has provided physicians with a highly practical, useful modality for detecting deep vein thrombosis, which has great value in the clinical setting. A negative PRG in a patient with a hugely swollen lower extremity indicates that the swelling is not caused by deep vein thrombosis. We know of no exception to this. The patient with a positive PRG with or without clinical symptoms is admitted to the hospital for anticoagulant therapy. The patient with calf tenderness whose PRG is negative is instructed to return for a repeat test in 2 or 3 days if the clinical symptoms persist.

Phleborheography's rate of successful detection is keyed to certain limitations of physiologic transmission of hydraulic impulses. While not perfect, it is more accurate in diagnosing deep vein thrombosis than any noninvasive method with which we have had experience and is the most useful of all the tests employed in our laboratory.

REFERENCES

1. Arkoff, R.S., Gilfillan, R.S., and Burhenne, H.J.: A simple method for lower extremity phlebography: pseudo-obstruction of the popliteal vein, Radiology 90:66, 1968.
2. Bynum, L.J., et al.: Noninvasive diagnosis of deep venous thrombosis by phleborheography, Ann. Intern. Med. 89:162, 1978.
3. Classen, J.N., Richardson, J.R., and Koontz, C.: A three-year experience with phleborheography, Ann. Surg. 195:800, 1982.
4. Collins, G.J., et al.: Phleborheographic diagnosis of venous obstruction, Ann. Surg. 189:25, 1979.
5. Comerota, A.J., et al.: Phleborheography: results of a ten-year experience, Surgery 91:573, 1982.
6. Cranley, J.J.: Phleborheography, R.I. Med. J. 58:111, 1975.
7. Cranley, J.J.: Vascular surgery, vol. 2, Peripheral venous diseases, Hagerstown, Md., 1975, Harper & Row.
8. Cranley, J.J.: Phleborheography for thrombosis (letter to editor), Ann. Intern. Med. 89:1006, 1978.
9. Cranley, J.J.: Phleborheography. In Kempczinski, R.F., and Yao, J.S.T., editors: Practical noninvasive vascular diagnosis, Chicago, 1982, Year Book Medical Publishers, Inc.
10. Cranley, J.J., Canos, A.J., and Mahalingam, K.: Noninvasive diagnosis and prophylaxis of deep venous thrombosis. In Madden, J.L., and Hume, M., editors: Venous thromboembolism: prevention and treatment, New York, 1976, Appleton-Century-Crofts.
11. Cranley, J.J., Canos, A.J., and Mahalingam, K.: Diagnosis of deep venous thrombosis by phleborheography. In Gross, W., et al. editors: Symposium on venous problems in honour of Geza de Takats, Chicago, 1977, Year Book Medical Publishers, Inc.
12. Cranley, J.J., Canos, A.J., and Sull, W.J.: Diagnosis of deep venous thrombosis: fallibility of clinical symptoms and signs, Arch. Surg. 111:34, 1976.
13. Cranley, J.J., et al.: A plethysmographic technique for the diagnosis of deep venous thrombosis of the lower extremities, Surg. Gynecol. Obstet. 136:385, 1973.
14. Cranley, J.J., et al.: Phleborheographic technique for diagnosing deep venous thrombosis of the lower extremities, Surg. Gynecol. Obstet. 141:331, 1975.
15. Elliott, J.P., et al.: Phleborheography: a correlative study with venography, Henry Ford Hosp. Med. J. 28:189, 1980.
16. Stallworth, J.M., Plonk, G.W., Jr., and Horne, J.B.: Negative phleborheography: clinical follow-up in 593 patients, Arch. Surg. 116:795, 1981.
17. Sull, W.J.: Diagnosis of thrombophlebitis in the lower extremity, Mo. Med. 75:552, 1978.
18. Sullivan, E.D., Reece, C.I., and Cranley, J.J.: Phleborheography of the upper extremity, Arch. Surg. 118:1134, 1983.
19. Winsor, T., and Hyman, C.: Objective venous studies (insufficiency, obstruction and inflammation), J. Cardiovasc. Surg. 2:146, 1961.

CHAPTER 73

Strain-gauge plethysmography

DAVID S. SUMNER

Acute deep vein thrombosis and venous valvular imcompetence can be diagnosed by plethysmographic methods. Any of the various types of plethysmographs are suitable for this purpose, including the impedance, air-filled, water-filled, and strain-gauge varieties, and all yield essentially the same information. This chapter deals only with the strain-gauge plethysmograph, since the other modalities are discussed elsewhere in this book. The strain-gauge plethysmograph has some advantages when compared to the other methods: it is far less cumbersome than the water-filled type but approaches it in accuracy, and although it may be more difficult to use than the air-filled or impedance plethysmograph, it is more sensitive, more easily calibrated, and probably more reliable.

Basically, the tests include (1) measurement of calf volume expansion in response to a standardized venous congesting pressure, (2) measurement of the rate at which blood flows out of the leg after the congesting pressure has been released, (3) measurement of the rate and volume of venous reflux flow in response to sudden inflation of a thigh cuff, and (4) measurement of the rate of calf volume expansion after the venous blood has been displaced by exercise. The first two tests are used to detect deep vein thrombosis and the second two are designed to evaluate venous valvular incompetence.

CALF VOLUME EXPANSION AND VENOUS OUTFLOW

Calf volume expansion and venous outflow tests are performed with the patient in a supine position. To minimize the volume of blood in the calf and to avoid obstructing the veins in the popliteal fossa, the leg is elevated well above the level of the left atrium, and the knee is slightly flexed. In practice, this position can be achieved by placing a low pillow beneath the thigh and by supporting the foot on a foam block or pillow 20 to 30 cm high. A pneumatic cuff is applied to the thigh above the knee (Fig. 73-1). To obtain optimum venous occlusion at low pressures, the bladder of this cuff should encircle the limb completely and its width should be at least 1.2 times the diameter of the limb. A contoured cuff measuring 22 × 71 cm fulfills these requirements in most cases. In addition, the tubes leading to the cuff must have a large diameter (⅜″ ID) to permit rapid inflation and deflation.

Although a large reservoir of air can be used for accurate inflation and the cuff evacuated directly to the atmosphere, it is much easier to employ one of the solenoid-controlled inflation-deflation devices that are commercially available. These instruments, which can be set to deliver a given pressure almost instantly, are pressurized by a compressed air source or a pump. It is merely necessary to throw a switch to inflate the cuff and reverse the switch to deflate it.

Changes in calf volume are measured with a mercury-in-Silastic strain gauge wrapped around the calf at its widest point. The length of the unstretched gauge should be about 90% of the circumference of the limb. When stretched to completely encircle the calf, the gauge should exert enough tension to secure good contact with the skin but should not compress the underlying veins. Depending on the type of gauge selected, it can be applied as a single or double strand. Although it is possible to use gauges that are so long that they exceed the circumference, it may be necessary to apply correction factors to obtain valid results in such cases.[19a] Electrically calibrated plethysmo-graphs[13] are now commercially available, and they greatly simplify the calculations and procedure by avoiding the need to quantify the stretch mechanically (see Chapter 13).

Procedure

When the pneumatic cuff around the thigh is inflated to a pressure exceeding that in the under-lying vein (50 mm Hg), the calf begins to expand, at first rapidly and then more slowly, as the capacitance vessels are filled. After approximately 2 minutes a new equilibrium is attained with venous outflow again equaling the arterial inflow. At this point the venous pressure distal to the cuff equals that in the cuff (Fig. 73-2). Because of the increased capillary pressure, fluid will continue to be lost into the interstitial spaces, resulting in a slow increase in calf volume. Also there may be some continued stretch relaxation of the venous walls. Therefore a stable volume is never really reached.[22]

Calf volume expansion (sometimes called venous volume, maximal incremental venous volume, or venous capacitance) is measured by comparing the rise of the curve from the baseline with a standard stretch of the gauge (as described in Chapter 15) or against an electrical standard that indicates a 1% rise in volume (Fig. 73-3). With the electrically calibrated device, calculations are simple (div = division).

$$\frac{\text{Div rise}}{\text{Div}/1\% \text{ vol change}} = \% \text{ Vol increase} \qquad (1)$$

The results are expressed as percent volume increase or as ml/100 ml of calf volume.

After a relatively stable calf volume has been achieved in response to the 50 mm Hg congesting pressure, the cuff is suddenly deflated.[4,9,11] The rate at which the calf volume decreases can be obtained by drawing a tangent to the initial part of the down-slope. This gives the maximum venous outflow (MVO).[4] Another method, which gives lower values but equally consistent results, is to measure the extent of the volume decrease after an arbitrary period of 2 seconds following cuff deflation.[7]

As shown in Fig. 73-3, MVO can be calculated as follows, provided an electrical calibration is available:

$$\text{MVO (ml/100 ml/min)} = \qquad (2)$$
$$\frac{\text{Slope (div/min)}}{\text{Calibration (div}/1\% \text{ vol change)}}$$

The 2-second venous outflow is calculated from the following:

$$\text{2-second venous outflow (ml/100 ml/min)} = \qquad (3)$$
$$\frac{\text{Div fall} \times 30}{\text{Div}/1\% \text{ vol change}}$$

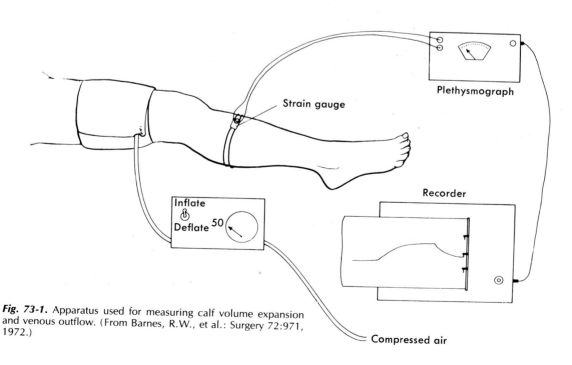

Fig. 73-1. Apparatus used for measuring calf volume expansion and venous outflow. (From Barnes, R.W., et al.: Surgery 72:971, 1972.)

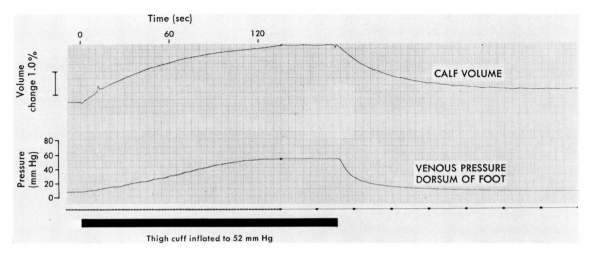

Fig. 73-2. Response of calf volume and venous pressure to inflation of pneumatic cuff placed around thigh. Although venous pressure rises to equal pressure in thigh cuff in about 2 minutes, calf volume continues to increase, albeit at a much reduced rate. (From Strandness, D.E., Jr., and Summer, D.S.: Hemodynamics for surgeons, New York, 1975, Grune & Stratton, Inc.)

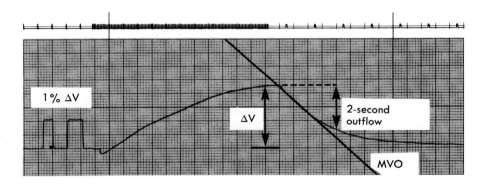

Fig. 73-3. Recording of calf volume expansion (ΔV), slope of MVO, and 2-second outflow. Paper speed in seconds is indicated at top of tracing. A 1% volume change (electrical calibration) equals 10.5 divisions. Calf volume expansion: 23 div/10.5 = 2.2 ml/100 ml; MVO: 564 div/min/10.5 = 54 ml/100 ml/min; 2-second outflow: (16 div × 30)/10.5 = 46 ml/100 ml/min.

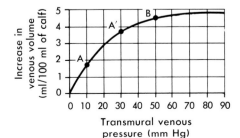

Fig. 73-4. Relationship between venous volume and transmural venous pressure. **A** indicates venous pressure and corresponding venous volume in limb of normal supine subject, **A'** indicates venous pressure and volume in limb with acute phlebitis, and **B** indicates venous pressure and volume in normal or phlebitic limb after thigh cuff has been inflated to 50 mm Hg. Note that venous wall becomes less compliant at higher pressures.

If electrical calibration is not available, the circumference of the calf must be measured and the slope compared to a standard deflection produced by a known stretch of the gauge (Chapter 15).

Calf volume expansion: interpretation of data. Normal values for calf volume expansion vary with the congesting pressure and with the time allowed before the measurement is made (usually 2 or 3 minutes from the time of cuff inflation). At a congesting pressure of 50 mm Hg, the calf volume increase approximates 2% to 3% in normal limbs.[5] In limbs with acute phlebitis, expansion of the calf is limited, usually being less than 2%.[11] The reduced expansion is probably related to the following two factors: (1) fewer veins are available for inflation, since some are occupied by thrombi, and (2) increased venous pressure distal to a proximal obstructing thrombus will have already resulted in partial venous distention. Little further expansion is possible, because the veins are already in the stiff portion of the venous compliance curve (Fig. 73-4).[22]

There are several potential sources of error in the measurement of calf expansion. First, the veins of the calf even in the normal extremity may not be completely empty before inflating the cuff. Elevation of the leg will help obviate this problem. Second, repeat determinations of calf expansion may result in stretching the veins, thereby reducing their tone and causing an increased expansion at the same congesting pressure.[14]

As shown in Table 73-1, most investigators have found statistically significant differences between the mean values for calf volume expansion obtained from normal limbs and those obtained from limbs with acute phlebitis. The differences were also sometimes significant in postphlebitic limbs but not in every study. Limbs with varicose veins appeared to have the largest venous volume. In view of the many factors influencing the extent of calf volume expansion, it is not surprising that there is considerable overlap between the values obtained from normal limbs and those obtained from limbs with venous thrombosis (Fig. 73-5). This same overlap has been observed in similar studies performed with the impedance plethysmograph (see Chapter 74).

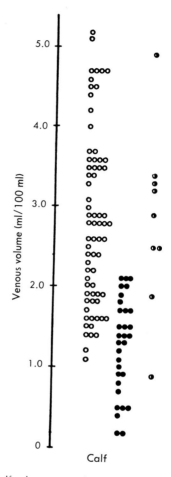

Fig. 73-5. Calf volume expansion in response to congesting pressure of 50 mm Hg. Open circles indicate normal legs; closed circles, limbs with acute phlebitis; and half-closed circles, postphlebitic limbs. (Modified from Hallböök, T., and Göthlin, J.: Acta Chir. Scand. 137:37, 1971.)

Table 73-1. Calf volume expansion (ml/100 ml of calf)*

Investigator	Cuff pressure	Normal	Limbs with varicose veins	Limbs with acute phlebitis	Postphlebitic limbs
Dahn and Eiriksson (1968)[9]	50	3.5 ± 0.6	5.1 ± 1.5†	2.4 ± 0.7†	2.7 ± 0.9†
Hallböök and Göthlin (1971)[11]	50	2.9 ± 1.1	—	1.3 ± 0.6†	2.8 ± 1.1
Sakaguchi et al. (1972)[20]	80	2.1 ± 0.6	2.4 ± 1.0	1.1 ± 0.6†	1.5 ± 0.6†
Barnes et al. (1973)[5]	50	2.1 ± 0.5	—	—	1.9 ± 0.7
Thulesius et al. (1978)[23]	60	2.7 ± 0.6	4.9 ± 1.2†	1.7 ± 0.8†	—

*Mean ± standard deviation.
†Statistically significant compared with normal values.

Table 73-2. Maximum venous outflow (ml/100 ml/min)*

Investigator	Cuff pressure	Normal	Limbs with varicose veins	Limbs with acute phlebitis	Postphlebitic limbs
Dahn and Eiriksson (1968)[9]	50	82 ± 24	168 ± 48†	16	58
Hallböök and Göthlin (1971)[11]	50	78 ± 22	—	23 ± 8†	64 ± 21
Sakaguchi et al. (1972)[20]	80	87 ± 14	110 ± 46†	32 ± 17†	55 ± 44†
Barnes et al. (1972, 1973)[4,5]	50	41 ± 11	—	12 ± 8†	34 ± 15†
Thulesius et al. (1978)[23]	60	58 ± 18	96 ± 23†	17 ± 9†	—

*Mean ± standard deviation.
†Statistically significant compared with normal values.

For these reasons, calf volume expansion has not proved to be sufficiently reliable as a diagnostic method when used alone.

Venous outflow: interpretation of data. The rate of venous outflow (Q) is directly proportional to the pressure gradient propelling blood from the calf veins (P_{cv}) to the inferior vena cava (P_{ivc}) and inversely proportional to the resistance of the venous channels lying between (R).

$$Q = \frac{P_{cv} - P_{ivc}}{R} \qquad (4)$$

Because the cuff provides a consistent congesting pressure of 50 mm Hg and because the central venous pressure is quite low, the rate of venous outflow would be expected to be decreased in the presence of acute venous thrombosis. That this is indeed the case is shown by the mean values in Table 73-2. As Barnes et al.[4] have observed, there is a good but not complete separation between normal and abnormal studies (Fig 73-6). If an outflow of 20 ml/100 ml/min is taken as the dividing line between normal and abnormal, the test is 91% sensitive for identifying limbs with acute venous thrombosis and 88% specific for identifying limbs without venous thrombosis. Using the 2-second outflow method, Barnes et al.[7] found mean values of 45 ± 18 ml/100 ml/min in normal volunteers, with a range of 20 to 91 ml/100 ml/min. Mean outflows for limbs with acute venous thrombosis were as follows: iliofemoral, 13 ± 7 ml/100 ml/min; femoropopliteal, 11 ± 4 ml/100 ml/min; and calf vein, 20 ± 16 ml/100 ml/min. When 20 ml/100 ml/min was used as the dividing line, the sensitivity of the 2-second method was 90% for thrombi detected above the knee and 66% for thrombi isolated to veins below the knee. The specificity for excluding venous thrombosis was 81% at all levels. In their study, 13 of the 16 false negative errors were in limbs with calf vein thrombi.

The venous outflow method is subject to a number of errors.[12] Acute venous thrombosis cannot be distinguished from other causes of increased venous resistance. These include the following: severe residual obstruction in the postphlebitic extremity and extrinsic pressure from tumors, hematomas, and Baker's cysts. Also, false negative studies may result when the thrombus in nonocclusive and does not seriously interfere with venous outflow. Distal thrombi in the lower leg often fall into this category.

Zetterquist et al.[24] have called attention to a biphasic pattern of the venous outflow curve that appears to occur in limbs with thrombi isolated to the iliac level when the calf and thigh veins are completely patent. In these limbs, the initial outflow slope may be quite steep (giving a normal MVO), but the second phase of the outflow slope suddenly becomes much slower. The breaking point between the two slopes always begins within 1.5 seconds of the time of cuff deflation. If the initial slope were taken as representative of the outflow, the study would be falsely interpreted as being negative when, in fact, there would be a thrombus lying in the iliac system. Use of the 2-second outflow method might avoid some of these errors.

The explanation offered for the biphasic curves is as follows: first, the inflated thigh cuff serves to empty the normal thigh veins; then when the cuff pressure is released, the blood trapped in the calf flows rapidly out to fill the space in the thigh, thus accounting for the initial rapid phase of venous emptying. Once the thigh veins are filled, the proximal obstruction in the pelvic veins impedes the further outflow of blood, producing the second more gradual slope. Similar curves have been observed in patients with increased central venous pressure caused by right ventricular heart failure. The examiner should be aware of these pitfalls when obtaining a biphasic outflow curve.

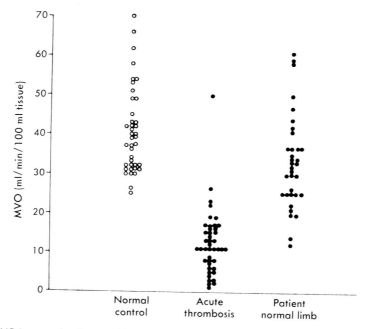

Fig. 73-6. MVO in normal patients and in patients with acute deep vein thrombosis. (From Barnes, R.W., et al.: Surgery 72:971, 1972.

RELATIONSHIP BETWEEN VENOUS OUTFLOW AND CALF VOLUME EXPANSION

Many investigators have noted a direct relationship between the rate of venous outflow and the magnitude of calf volume expansion (Fig. 73-7).[8,8a,18,19,23] In particular, those using impedance methods have combined these studies to enhance the overall accuracy of the technique, either by calculating venous outflow/venous expansion ratios or by plotting the outflow versus the calf volume expansion on a graph. A discriminate analysis line that slopes upward from left to right on a graph with venous outflow on the ordinate and venous expansion on the abscissa serves to separate normal values, which lie above the line, from abnormal values, which lie below the line (see Chapter 74).[17]

Inspection of the tracing in Fig. 73-3 reveals that the venous outflow curve is not straight but decreases in slope as the calf volume decreases.[22] Several factors are responsible for this. First, the pressure driving blood out of the leg (P_{cv}) falls rapidly following cuff deflation (equation 4). The rate at which the pressure declines is proportional to the decrease in volume of blood within the veins, which in turn depends on the resistance to venous outflow (R) and to the elasticity of the venous wall (E). If E is assumed to be the ratio of the venous transmural pressure (P) to the venous volume (V),

then the rate of venous outflow at any time after cuff release (Q_t), is as follows:

$$Q_t = \frac{E}{R} \times V_o \times e^{-(E/R)t} \tag{5}$$

where

$\quad E \quad = P/V$
$\quad V_o \quad = $ Maximum extent of calf expansion
$\quad R \quad = $ Venous resistance
$\quad t \quad = $ Time in seconds after cuff release

At the point of cuff release, when t equals zero, equation 5 reduces to the following:

$$Q_o = MVO = \frac{E}{R} \times V_o = \frac{Po}{R} \tag{6}$$

which is the same as equation 4 and is the expression for the MVO.

It can be seen from this expression that MVO increases as the stiffness of the veins (E) and the calf volume expansion (V_o) increase. Therefore, MVO is not totally dependent on venous resistance, which is the factor that we are endeavoring to measure. In fact, equation 6 can be rearranged as follows to justify the use of venous outflow/venous expansion ratios or graphic methods for assessing venous resistance:

$$R = E \times \frac{V_o}{Q_o} \tag{7}$$

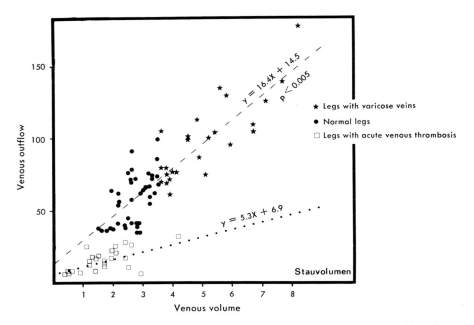

Fig. 73-7. Relationship between maximum venous outflow and venous volume in normal legs, legs with varicose veins, and legs with acute venous thrombosis. (From Thulesius, O., et al.: Diagnostik bei akuter Venethrombose der unteren Extremitäten. In Kriessman, A., and Bollinger, A., editors: Ultraschall-Doppler-Diagnostik in der Angiologie, Stuttgart, 1978, Georg Thieme Verlag.)

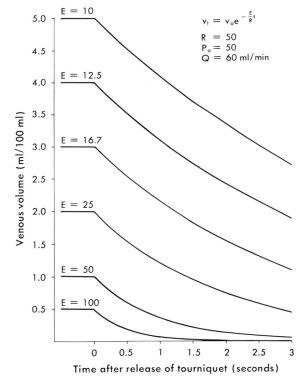

Fig. 73-8. Theoretic venous outflow curves based on equation 5. In all curves, congesting (cuff) pressure *(PO)* is 50 mm Hg; outflow resistance *(R)* is 50 mm Hg/ml⁻¹/min. Elastic modulus *(E)* is the ratio of venous transmural pressure to venous volume. Q, Flow. (From Strandness, D.E., Jr., and Summer, D.S.: Hemodynamics for surgeons, New York, 1975, Grune & Stratton, Inc.)

In other words, given a certain venous expansion (V_0), the greater the venous outflow (Q_0), the less the resistance (R) and the less likely is the limb to be the site of venous thrombosis (Fig. 73-7). Less evident is the fact that given a certain venous outflow (Q_0), the greater the venous expansion (V_0), the more likely is the limb to harbor a significant venous clot (Fig. 73-7).

Equation 6 also accounts for the different slopes of the regression lines applied to normal limbs and to those with major venous thrombosis.[18,23] Since the ratio E/R represents the slope of the line, the greater the resistance (R), the lower the slope. Thus points describing limbs with venous thrombosis have a lower slope than the line that fits the values for normal limbs (see Figs. 74-1, 74-2, and 73-7).

The second factor that complicates the interpretation of the venous outflow curve is the venous elasticity (E), which is the reciprocal of the venous compliance. Venous elasticity varies, not only from limb to limb, but also throughout the course of the venous decompression that follows release of the thigh cuff. As shown in Fig. 73-4, E is high at higher pressures where the venous wall is quite stiff but becomes low at low pressure ranges where the wall is compliant. In Fig. 73-8, a family of curves are plotted, based on equation 5, in which the congesting (cuff) pressure, the MVO, and the venous resistance (R) all remain constant. Various values of E give correspondingly different values of venous expansion. Although an accurately drawn tangent to the initial part of each curve would give identical MVOs of 60 ml/min, the 2- or 3-second outflows would differ greatly. Thus it is possible to have the same venous resistance and yet measure widely varying venous outflows. Again, from this graph one can observe the correlation of venous expansion with the 2- or 3-second venous outflow.

Clearly, the 2- or 3-second venous outflows and even the MVO are complex functions that do not solely reflect changes in venous resistance. While the discrimination of venous outflow studies used alone has been good, accuracy should be improved by incorporating volume expansion into the final analysis.[8a]

Tripolitis et al. have noted that patients undergoing operations consistently show a distinct decline in venous outflow postoperatively after a few days of bed rest.[23a] Since there has been no evidence of venous thrombosis in these patients, it is likely that the changes in venous outflow are not caused by an increase in venous resistance but rather reflect a change in venous elasticity. Again this is an argument for considering both venous volume and venous outflow when assessing the patient for deep vein thrombosis.

VENOUS REFLUX FLOW

Barnes et al.[6] have used the mercury strain gauge to measure the severity of venous valvular incompetence. The patient is positioned with legs in a horizontal position, supported only enough to prevent the calf from coming into contact with the examination table. Elevation is not desirable because it is necessary to have a supply of blood in the venous reservoirs of the leg. The apparatus is similar to that used for venous outflow studies with the exception that a narrow (arterial occlusion) cuff is placed around the thigh above the wider venous occlusion cuff (Fig. 73-9). The study is designed to measure the rate at which blood refluxes down the leg from the thigh to the calf when the venous occlusion cuff is rapidly inflated, the normal cephalad egress of blood being prevented by the arterial occlusion cuff. In addition, the total volume of the refluxed blood can be determined at any specified time after cuff inflation.

The technique is as follows: the proximal thigh cuff is inflated well above the systemic arterial pressure (250 to 300 mm Hg), and with all flow to and from the leg cut off, the distal thigh cuff (venous occlusion cuff) is suddenly inflated to 50 mm Hg. This forces the underlying blood to be displaced distally toward the calf. As shown in Fig. 73-10, the maximum venous reflux flow is quite low in subjects with normal valves but is appreciable in patients with valvular incompetence. The initial slope of the curve can be measured or the rise after a 2-second interval can be recorded. Calculations are the same as those for venous outflow (see equations 2 and 3).

In normal limbs the mean value of the maximum venous reflux flow is 3 ± 1 ml/100 ml/min, whereas that in postphlebitic limbs is several times greater, 13 ± 7 ml/100 ml/min. For normal limbs, the upper limit appears to be 6 ml/100 ml/min.[6]

The venous reflux test can be modified to differentiate primary from secondary varicose veins. A Penrose drain is applied to the calf just below the knee but well above the strain gauge. The tension on the drain should be sufficient to collapse the superficial varicosities but should not interfere with flow in the deep veins. By measuring the

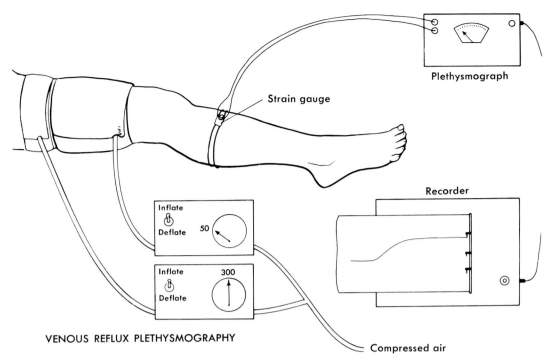

Fig. 73-9. Apparatus used for measuring venous reflux outflow. (From Barnes, R.W., et al.: Surg. Gynecol. Obstet. **136**:769, 1973.)

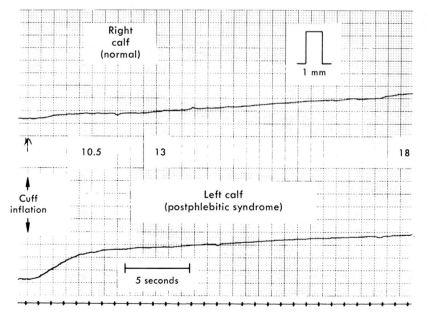

Fig. 73-10. Maximum venous reflux flow in limb with venous imcompetence (lower tracing) compared with that in normal limb (upper tracing) of same patient. (From Barnes, R.W., et al.: Surg. Gynecol. Obstet. 136:769, 1973.)

reflux flow with and without superficial venous compression, one can determine whether the venous valvular incompetence is isolated to the superficial system or whether the valves are incompetent in both the superficial and deep systems. As shown in Fig. 73-11, Barnes et al.[3] found that the maximal venous reflux flow in normal limbs (3 ± 2 ml/100 ml/min) was significantly less than that in limbs with primary (9 ± 6 ml/100 ml/min) or secondary (13 ± 7 ml/100 ml/min) varicose veins. Application of a Penrose drain tourniquet had little or no effect on the venous reflux flow in normal limbs but reduced the venous reflux flow in limbs with primary varicosities to normal levels (2 ± 1 ml/100 ml/min). However, in limbs with secondary varicose veins, the tourniquet had no consistent effect, and the maximal venous reflux flow remained high (11 ± 5 ml/100 ml/min).[3]

Venous reflux following exercise

To distinguish between primary and secondary varicose veins, Holm et al.[15,16] measure the rate at which blood returns to the calf veins after they have been emptied by exercise. A mercury strain gauge is placed around the calf at the position of maximum girth. During the test the patient stands, leaning against a wall for support; the calf veins are emptied by having the patient raise the heel three to five times. The time required for the leg volume to return to its original value is recorded.

In normal limbs, the venous return time averaged 22 ± 7 seconds. It was much more rapid in limbs with primary and secondary varicose veins, averaging 7 ± 3 seconds and 7 ± 2 seconds, respectively.[15]

After exercise in the upright position, the veins of the calf are normally refilled slowly by the arterial inflow. When the venous valves are incompetent, blood in the proximal veins rushes rapidly down the limb to fill the calf veins that have been emptied by exercise. Holm[15] observed that compression of the saphenous vein in patients with primary varicose veins restored the venous return time to within the normal range (18 ± 8 seconds). However, compression of the saphenous vein did not prevent the reflux of blood in those legs with deep venous incompetence, the average refilling time remaining quite short (7 ± 2 seconds).

Fernandes e Fernandes et al.[10] at St. Mary's Hospital in London perform a similar test for venous valvular incompetence. In their studies patients stand and raise themselves on their toes one time

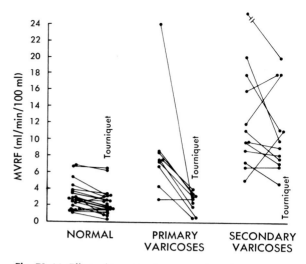

Fig. 73-11. Effect of tourniquet compression of superficial veins on maximum venous reflux flow (MVRF) in normal limbs, in limbs with primary varicose veins, and in postphlebitic limbs with secondary varicose veins. (From Barnes, R.W., Ross, E.A., and Strandness, D.E., Jr.: Surg. Gynecol. Obstet. 141:207, 1975.)

per second for a period of 20 seconds. The decrease in calf volume and the time required for the calf volume to return to preexercise levels are recorded. The test is repeated with a pneumatic tourniquet (2.5 cm wide) placed below the knee, inflated to 100 mm Hg.

The mean decrease in calf volume was 2.2 ± 0.5 ml/100 ml in normal limbs, 1.3 ± 0.3 ml/100 ml in limbs with superficial venous incompetence, 0.6 ± 0.1 ml/100 ml in limbs with deep venous incompetence, and 0.06 ± 0.5 ml/100 ml in limbs with deep venous incompetence and occlusion. A small increase in calf volume (0.4 ml/100 ml) was noted in two of the six limbs in the latter group. Application of the tourniquet had no effect on the volume change in normal limbs or in limbs with deep venous incompetence but did result in a decrease in calf volume in limbs with superficial venous incompetence.

Mean refilling times after exercise were approximately 14 seconds in normal legs, 5 seconds in legs with superficial venous incompetence, 3 seconds in legs with deep venous incompetence, and 1 second in legs with deep venous incompetence and occlusion. The tourniquet lengthened the refilling time only in those limbs with isolated superficial venous incompetence. Because the standard deviations were large, the refilling time did

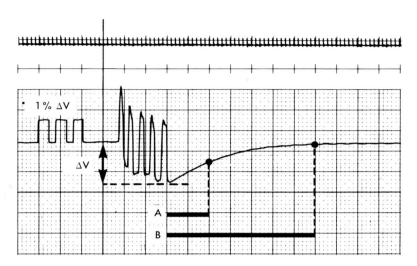

Fig. 73-12. Decrease in calf volume with exercise and recovery time. Patient is sitting with feet touching floor; five plantar flexions are performed. Volume change (ΔV) was −2 ml/100 ml. Recovery half time (**A**) was 10 seconds, and total recovery time (**B**) was 35 seconds.

not prove to be reliable as a means of distinguishing between the groups.

Because of the difficulty some patients experience in performing these tests while standing, Barnes[1] conducts similar studies with the patient sitting. With knees flexed to 90 degrees and feet on the floor, the patient performs five plantar flexions of the ankle, one per second. The decrease in calf volume, as measured by a strain gauge, was similar in normal limbs and in limbs with chronic venous insufficiency (0.95 ± 0.41 ml/100 ml and 0.90 ± 0.63 ml/100, respectively). Because it is sometimes difficult to recognize the precise point at which the calf volume returns to the baseline or levels off at a new baseline, Barnes uses a recovery half time (Fig. 73-12), defined as the time required for the calf to regain half the volume it lost during exercise. In his experience, the recovery half time was 3.4 ± 1.4 seconds in normal legs and 1.3 ± 1.0 seconds in postphlebitic limbs.

One of the problems with all the exercise tests is the development of hyperemia.[21a] The resulting increase in arterial inflow can shorten the time required for the calf to return to its original volume following exercise, and it can also lessen the magnitude of the calf volume decrease. In fact, I have observed that the volume of the normal calf muscle will decrease initially with exercise, but after a variable period of vigorous exercise, the volume will begin to rise, despite the fact that the content of venous blood has been reduced.[22] This may reflect a shortening of the muscle fibers, an increase in intracellular volume, or an increase in interstitial fluid.

Because of these concerns, Sakaguchi et al.[20,21] and more recently Barnes[2] have used mechanical compression to empty the calf muscles of venous blood. With the patient sitting, the calf muscle is squeezed manually three to five times. The decrease in calf volume was 1.4 ± 0.3 ml/100 ml in normal limbs, 1.4 ± 0.9 ml/100 ml in limbs with varicose veins, and 0.5 ± 0.3 ml/100 ml in postphlebitic limbs.[20] The rate of venous return was measured from the initial slope of the curve after cessation of the squeezing maneuvers minus the rate of arterial inflow as determined by venous occlusion plethysmography (see Chapters 13 and 15). In normal limbs, the calf filled slowly at 0.2 ± 0.8 ml/100 ml/min; but in limbs with varicose veins the refilling was much more rapid (10.2 ± 5.1 ml/100 ml/min). Postphlebitic limbs refilled at a rate of 2.2 ± 1.8 ml/100 ml/min.[20] Because the feet have little muscle mass, Schanzer et al. obviate the effect of exercise-induced hyperemia by placing the strain gauge around the foot rather than the calf.[21a]

At present this whole field is in a state of flux; new tests are constantly being introduced and old tests reevaluated. Standard values have not been established. For these reasons, readers who choose to employ any of these methods for studying venous incompetence are encouraged to modify the tests to meet their needs and to establish normal values for their own laboratory.

SUMMARY

In the United States impedance plethysmography has been more popular than strain-gauge plethysmography for the diagnosis of deep venous disease. In part the preference for impedance plethysmography may be attributed to certain apparent deficits of the strain-gauge method. Mercury strain gauges are extremely sensitive, making them responsive to the slightest movement. Unless the patient is quiet and cooperative, the tracings are apt to be erratic. In addition, it is necessary to have a battery of gauges of various lengths to fit the calves of different individuals. Furthermore, the gauges are difficult to calibrate when the mechanical method is used. Not only must the gauge be stretched precisely with a micrometer-controlled device, but also the girth of the calf must be measured accurately. Finally, the gauges are delicate and have a tendency to deteriorate because of oxidation of the mercury column.

Newer developments have overcome many of these problems. Electrical calibration, which is available on several plethysmographs, is rapid and accurate and simplifies calculations.[13] Some instruments permit volume changes to be read directly from panel meters, thus avoiding the necessity for making strip chart recordings.[7] Backing the gauges with Velcro has greatly simplified their application to the calf. Because of the way in which these new gauges contact the skin, the same gauge may be used for a variety of different calf sizes without appreciably affecting the accuracy of measurement. The substitution of an indium-gallium alloy for mercury promises to greatly extend the shelf life of the gauges.

Coupled with the obvious advantages of strain-gauge plethysmography (high sensitivity, linearity, and accuracy), these new developments should increase the use of the strain gauge in the study of venous disease. Although other simpler techniques, such as Doppler venous surveys, are equally versatile for diagnosing venous obstruction and incompetence, they do not permit the degree of obstruction or incompetence to be quantified. The ability to define numerically the extent of the functional deficit should prove valuable to the clinical investigator who wishes to document the natural history of venous disease or to the surgeon who wants to study the effect of therapeutic intervention on venous physiology.

REFERENCES

1. Barnes, R.W.: Strain gauge plethysmography (abstract), Symposium on Noninvasive Diagnostic Techniques in Vascular Disease, San Diego, 1979, p. 51.
2. Barnes, R.W.: Personal communication.
3. Barnes, R.W., Ross, E.A., and Strandness, D.E., Jr.: Differentiation of primary from secondary varicose veins by Doppler ultrasound and strain gauge plethysmography, Surg. Gynecol. Obstet. 141:207, 1975.
4. Barnes, R.W., et al.: Noninvasive quantitation of maximum venous outflow in acute thrombophlebitis, Surgery 72:971, 1972.
5. Barnes, R.W., et al.: Noninvasive quantitation of venous hemodynamics in postphlebitic syndrome, Arch. Surg. 107:807, 1973.
6. Barnes, R.W., et al.: Noninvasive quantitation of venous reflux in the postphlebitic syndrome, Surg. Gynecol. Obstet. 136:769, 1973.
7. Barnes, R.W., et al.: Detection of deep vein thrombosis with an automatic electrically calibrated strain gauge plethysmograph, Surgery 82:219, 1977.
8. Bygdeman, S., Aschberg, S., and Hindmarsh, T.: Venous plethysmography in the diagnosis of chronic venous insufficiency, Acta Chir. Scand. 137:423, 1971.
8a. Cramer, M., Beach, K.W., and Strandness, D.E., Jr.: The detection of proximal deep venous thrombosis by strain gauge plethysmography through the use of an outflow/capacitance discriminant line, Bruit 7:17, 1983.
9. Dahn, I., and Eiriksson, E.: Plethysmographic diagnosis of deep venous thrombosis of the leg, Acta Chir. Scand. Suppl. 398:33, 1968.
10. Fernandes e Fernandes, J.F., et al.: Ambulatory calf volume plethysmography in the assessment of venous insufficiency, Br. J. Surg. 66:327, 1979.
11. Hallböök, T., and Göthlin, J.: Strain-gauge plethysmography and phlebography in diagnosis of deep venous thrombosis, Acta Chir. Scand. 137:37, 1971.
12. Hallböök, T., and Ling, L.: Pitfalls in plethysmographic diagnosis of acute deep venous thrombosis, J. Cardiovasc. Surg. 14:427, 1973.
13. Hokanson, D.E., Sumner, D.S., and Strandness, D.E., Jr.: An electrically calibrated plethysmograph for direct measurement of limb blood flow, IEEE Trans. Biomed. Eng. 22(1):25, 1975.
14. Hollenberg, N.K., and Boreus, L.O.: The influence of rate of filling on apparent venous distensibility in man, Can. J. Physiol. Pharmacol. 50:310, 1972.
15. Holm, J.S.: A simple plethysmographic method for differentiating primary from secondary varicose veins, Surg. Gynecol. Obstet. 143:609, 1976.
16. Holm, J., et al.: Elective surgery for varicose veins: a simple method for evaluation of the patients, J. Cardiovasc. Surg. 15:565, 1974.
17. Hull, R., et al.: Impedance plethysmography using the occlusive cuff technique in the diagnosis of venous thrombosis, Circulation 53:696, 1976.
18. Hull, R., et al.: Impedance plethysmography: the relationship between venous filling and sensitivity and specificity for proximal vein thrombosis, Circulation 58:898, 1978.
19. Johnston, K.W., and Kakkar, V.V.: Plethysmographic diagnosis of deep vein thrombosis, Surg. Gynecol. Obstet. 138:41, 1974.
19a. Knox, R., et al.: Pitfalls of venous occlusion plethysmography, Angiology 33:268, 1982.
20. Sakaguchi, S., Ishitobi, K., and Kameda, T.: Functional segmental plethysmography with mercury strain gauge, Angiology 23:127, 1972.

21. Sakaguchi, S., et al.: Functional segmental plethysmography: a new venous function test, J. Cardiovasc. Surg. 9:87, 1968.

21a. Schanzer, H., et al.: Noninvasive evaluation of chronic venous insufficiency. Use of foot mercury strain-gauge plethysmography, Arch. Surg. 119:1013, 1984.

22. Strandness, D.E., Jr., and Sumner, D.S.: Hemodynamics for surgeons, New York, 1975, Grune & Stratton, Inc.

23. Thulesius, O., et al.: Diagnostik bei akuter Venethrombose der unteren Extremitäten. In Kriessman, A., and Bollinger, A., editors: Ultraschall-Doppler-Diagnostik in der Angiologie, Stuttgart, 1978, Georg Thieme Verlag.

23a. Tripolitis, A.J., et al.: Venous capacitance and outflow in the postoperative patient, Ann. Surg. 190:634, 1979.

24. Zetterquist, S., Ericsson, K., and Volpe, V.: The clinical significance of biphasic venous emptying curves from the lower limb in venous occlusion plethysmography, Scand. J. Clin. Lab. Invest. 35:497, 1975.

CHAPTER 74

The diagnosis of venous thrombosis by impedance plethysmography

H. BROWNELL WHEELER and FREDERICK A. ANDERSON, Jr.

Impedance plethysmography (IPG) is a widely employed noninvasive method for the diagnosis of deep vein thrombosis (DVT). The method is based on measurement of the changes in blood volume produced by temporary venous obstruction. Venous thrombosis alters this response dramatically. This chapter describes the background of the method and recent developments in its use.

When IPG was first introduced for the diagnosis of DVT, temporary venous occlusion was produced by deep inspiration or a Valsalva maneuver. Good results with this technique were obtained by several investigators,* but others reported less accurate results.[10,31] The necessity for the patient to increase intraabdominal pressure sufficiently to obstruct venous return proved to be a major limitation in both the accuracy and the usefulness of the method. Some patients were too sick or uncooperative to be tested. In evaluating the result obtained, the observer always had to take into account the response of the patient. The reliability of the test depended in large part on the experience, knowledge, and patience of the examiner.

To produce consistent results that could be reproduced by the average hospital technician, an objective and standardized method of producing temporary venous occlusion was necessary. An 8-inch pneumatic cuff was developed for this purpose. The details of the testing procedure, the instrumentation, and the method of interpretation were all made simple and objective. Minimal patient cooperation was required, and the possibility of operator error was greatly reduced. This revised occlusive cuff technique of IPG has now been stud-

ied in many laboratories* and has proven much more satisfactory than the original respiratory test.

RATIONALE

The rationale for measuring blood volume changes indirectly through changes in electrical resistance is based on Ohm's law (Voltage = Current × Resistance). Blood is a good conductor of electricity. The more blood present in the body segment being studied, the lower is the resistance to passage of an electrical current. Measurement of the resistance (or impedance) to passage of a weak, high-frequency current through the lower leg provides a convenient and safe way to measure changes in venous blood volume. The theoretic basis and experiemntal verification of IPG are explained in more detail in Chapter 15.

The physiologic basis for IPG is simple and straightforward. In normal individuals, temporary venous obstruction with continuing arterial inflow results in a marked increase in venous volume, followed by a rapid venous outflow when the obstruction is released. If thrombi are present in the major veins draining the lower leg, the venous outflow rate is diminished, often dramatically so. The initial volume increase is usually reduced as well. The outflow depends to some extent on the amount of blood dammed up following venous obstruction, and so results are more accurately evaluated when the venous outflow is expressed as a function of the venous volume increase (Figs. 74-1 and 74-2).

IPG may be thought of as a "stress test" of the venous system, which is challenged to carry away a large volume of blood within a short period of

*References 26, 27, 30, 35, 38, 39.

*References 7, 9, 12-24, 28, 29, 32-34, 36, 37, 40-42.

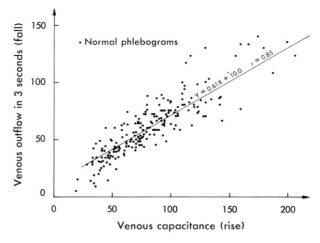

Fig. 74-1. In patients with normal venograms, occlusive IPG shows progressive increase in venous outflow as venous capacitance improves.

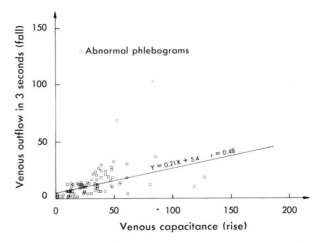

Fig. 74-2. In patients whose venograms show thrombosis in major veins. IPG indicates venous outflow is low. As venous capacitance increases, venous outflow does not increase proportionally, as occurs in normal patients.

time. Normally, the large-caliber veins of the leg can carry large quantities of blood rapidly and with minimal fluid resistance. The normal venous system is able to respond to an increasing volume challenge with a proportionately greater outflow rate. The amount of blood dammed up behind the thigh occlusion cuff will determine the venous outflow in the first few seconds after release of the cuff. However, when thrombosis is present in any of the major veins draining the lower leg, there is a marked reduction in the maximum rate of venous outflow, irrespective of the amount of blood dammed up behind the thigh occlusion cuff. An obstructed venous system will respond with an out-

flow rate proportional to the degree of obstruction but largely independent of the magnitude of the venous volume challenge (Fig. 74-3).

METHOD

The IPG test is carried out with the subject in the supine position. The leg is elevated sufficiently to facilitate venous drainage. The calf should be slightly above heart level. Usually this is best accomplished by placing the leg on a pillow and elevating the foot of the bed about 20 degrees. It is important that the patient is comfortable and that the leg muscles are relaxed.

A pneumatic cuff with a rigid backing is placed

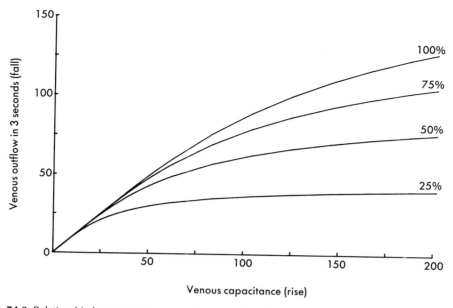

Fig. 74-3. Relationship between venous capacitance and outflow with varying degrees of venous outflow obstruction.[2]

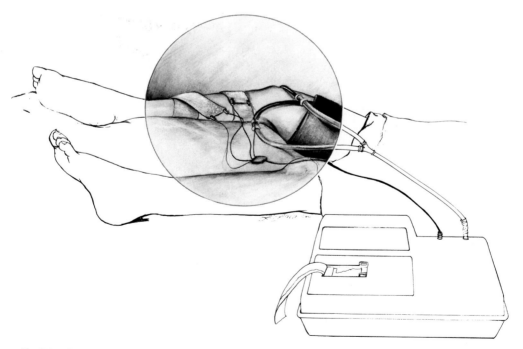

Fig. 74-4. Position for IPG. Leg is slightly elevated. Electrode bands encircle calf, and pneumatic cuff is wrapped around thigh. Electrodes and cuff are connected to IPG.

around the thigh. The cuff should not be applied tightly, or it may inadvertently act as a venous tourniquet. Circumferential electrodes are then placed around the calf (Fig. 74-4).

The electrodes are connected to an IPG (current frequency, 22 kHz; current strength, 1 mA). The pneumatic cuff is connected to an air pressure system that allows rapid deflation. The pneumatic cuff is then inflated to 70 cm H_2O pressure (about 50 mm Hg)—above venous pressure but well under arterial pressure. This pressure is maintained until the tracing "levels off," which usually occurs within 1 to 2 minutes. There is no need to time venous occlusion precisely. The thigh cuff pressure should be maintained until venous volume has

reached maximum, as shown by the tracing reaching a plateau (Fig. 74-5). This may occur in anywhere from 15 seconds to 3 minutes or more, depending on the arterial inflow, the degree of venous obstruction, and the baseline venous pressure.

It should be emphasized that the key to obtaining accurate results is maximum filling of the venous system. Prolonging the occlusion time has been well demonstrated to improve venous filling.[19] Other methods of improving venous filling include increasing the occlusion pressure, repetitive testing at the same pressure, active or passive movement of the calf muscles, use of locally applied heat, and use of vasodilating drugs. Repetitive testing and prolonged occlusion times are now standard

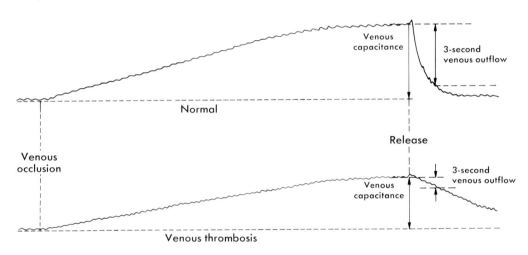

Fig. 74-5. Interpretation is based on measurement of (1) increase in blood volume that follows inflation of pneumatic cuff (venous capacitance) and (2) decrease in blood volume that follows release of cuff pressure (3-second venous outflow).

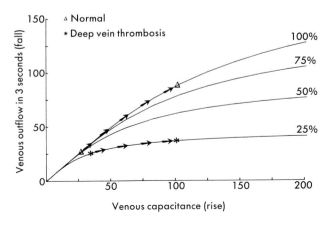

Fig. 74-6. Test points that are equivocal on initial testing are often clearly resolved by test repetition, prolonged occlusion, or other maneuvers that improve venous filling.[2]

methods of increasing venous filling. Borderline tests have then usually resolved into clearly normal or abnormal findings (Fig. 74-6).

After the tracing has leveled off and it is clear that maximum venous filling has been obtained, cuff pressure is then rapidly released. The cuff must deflate promptly, since any mechanical delay in deflation might simulate a decrease in venous outflow caused by venous thrombosis.

The increase in venous volume following inflation of the cuff and the decrease in venous volume during the first 3 seconds following release of the cuff are measured from the strip-chart recording (Fig. 74-5). These two variables, termed venous capacitance and venous outflow, are then plotted as functions of each other on a scoring graph. The method of analysis is described later. Whenever a clearly normal result is obtained, we believe the test can be terminated. However, if the result is equivocal or abnormal, we feel the test should be repeated until either a normal result has been obtained or until the examiner is sure that optimal venous filling has been obtained and that there is no technical cause for the poor tracing, such as calf muscle tension or a tourniquet effect from tight clothing, bandages, or the thigh cuff.[3] This usually requires multiple test repetitions. Others have advocated always repeating the test five times, with occlusion times of 2 minutes' duration for two of the five tests.[17-19]

FACTORS AFFECTING THE IPG RESPONSE

Although abnormal tests are nearly always the result of DVT, it is important to realize that several pathophysiologic conditions may influence the exact results obtained. In a normal subject there is a marked increase in venous volume following temporary venous obstruction. However, the rate of this increase may vary considerably, even in the same individual. The initial rate of venous pooling is a reflection of peripheral blood flow. It is influenced by cardiac output, the patency of the major arteries, the degree of peripheral vasoconstriction, and the initial venous pressure. Many pathophysiologic conditions affect one or another of these variables. Important clinical considerations are myocardial function, chronic obstructive pulmonary disease, hypovolemia, occlusive arterial disease, and peripheral vasoconstriction. Even healthy individuals exhibit peripheral vasospasm caused by apprehension, pain, or cold.

Often an improved venous capacitance is ob-

served with test repetition, particularly when the venous tourniquet is maintained in place until the tracing reaches a plateau. This probably represents the effect of compliance changes in the vein wall.

Extravascular compression

Infrequently, venous outflow may be obstructed by extravascular compression of major veins. This has been observed with cancer of the pelvis, hematomas, Baker's cysts, and other extrinsic masses that compress the venous system. Extravascular compression can also be produced by tight bandages or clothing.

A subtle but more common cause of extravascular compression is calf muscle tension. Radiologists have long been familiar with the squeezing of the calf veins that can be produced by muscle contraction during venography. For this reason, it is important to be sure that the calf muscles are relaxed during IPG.

The possibility of extravascular compression of major veins is usually apparent from a careful history or physical examination. It has rarely been a problem in the interpretation IPG results, with the exception of calf muscle tension, which may be transient and therefore difficult to recognize.

Decreased peripheral blood flow

Whenever there is impairment of arterial inflow, the early phase of the venous capacitance curve is reduced. This reduction in venous capacitance causes a corresponding reduction in the venous outflow. Reduced venous capacitance has often been observed in hypovolemic states, myocardial infarction, or congestive heart failure. It may also result from reduced arterial inflow caused by occlusive arterial disease or peripheral vasoconstriction. However, the outflow response will often be normal if the period of venous obstruction is prolonged, allowing a larger venous volume to dam up slowly behind the tourniquet.

Increased vasoconstriction may change the compliance of the venous system, as well as reduce peripheral blood flow, resulting in a diminished volume response to a given occlusion pressure. Increased vasomotor tone is often observed in patients who are apprehensive, cold, in pain, or suffering from hypovolemia or low cardiac output. With correction of the underlying cause of venoconstriction, the plethysmographic response usually reverts to normal. Dramatic improvement in venous capacitance is often seen after reactive hy-

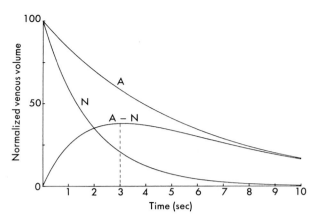

Fig. 74-7. IPG interpretation using the discriminant line as developed by Hull et al.[17]

peremia, application of local heat, peripheral vasodilator administration, or sympathetic blockade.

Interpretation of tests is often facilitated by a knowledge of concurrent physiologic conditions that may influence peripheral hemodynamics.

INTERPRETATION OF RESULTS

Venous occlusion plethysmography (VOP) has been performed for the detection of DVT using a variety of plethysmographic instruments, many of which are described elsewhere in this book. The tracings obtained are qualitatively similar to the IPG curves of Fig. 74-5. From inspection of VOP curves, it is obvious that the most dramatic difference between normal limbs and those with DVT is found in the venous outflow portion of the tracing. Most investigators have based interpretation of VOP results on some measure of venous outflow. A variety of criteria have been used, which makes it difficult to compare results between publications, even when the same instrument and test procedure have been employed (see Table 80-7).

Common indices of venous outflow used to interpret VOP tracings include the maximum venous outflow (MVO) slope and measurements of the venous outflow in a fixed time interval following the release of occlusion pressure. Based on an empiric analysis of VOP data, we found that the venous outflow volume in 3 seconds (VO_3) discriminates between normal limbs and those with DVT better than MVO or venous outflow volume at other time intervals.[4] Recently this empiric analysis has been verified experimentally.[2] Calculation of the difference in venous outflow volume versus time for an average normal and abnormal VOP curve dem-

onstrates that the maximum difference occurs 3 seconds after cuff release (Fig. 74-7). This provides objective evidence that 3 seconds is the optimal time at which to measure venous outflow differences for the detection of DVT.[2]

Accuracy of IPG results is further improved by expressing the 3-second venous outflow as a function of the amount of venous filling. IPG results are conveniently displayed on a graph in which venous filling is plotted against 3-second outflow.

There is surprisingly good separation of patients with normal venograms from those with recent thrombosis, as shown in Figs. 74-1 and 74-2. In earlier publications,[40,41] interpretation of results was based on where a given test fell in relation to overall zones of normal and abnormal, as defined by previous experience. With this method, an overall accuracy of 96% was obtained in differentiating normal patients from those with recent thrombosis of major veins.

Most commonly, interpretation has been based on a discriminate analysis line developed at McMaster University Medical Center (Fig. 74-8). This diagonal line slopes upward from left to right on a graph of venous capacitance versus venous outflow. Points that fall above the line are reported as normal. Points that fall below the line are considered abnormal. This simple classification of results provided 97% specificity and 93% sensitivity in prospective screening of mainly asymptomatic patients[17] and 95% specificity and 98% sensitivity for symptomatic patients.[18]

Both these methods of interpretation provide excellent results but suffer from being too simplistic. The results are "black or white" and do not give

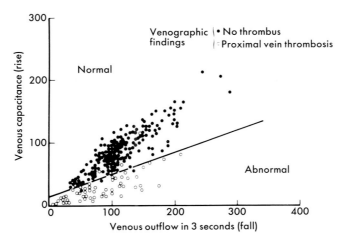

Fig. 74-8. Maximum difference between average normal *(N)* and abnormal *(A)* IPG outflow curves occurs at point approximately 3 seconds from release of venous occlusion.[2]

the full spectrum of information available from the tracings. Common sense dictates that points close to the dividing line between normal and abnormal should be considered less reliable than those some distance away. Treatment based on borderline tests may be less valid than treatment based on tests that fall clearly in the normal or abnormal zones. The possibility of inadvertent mismanagement of patients is therefore increased by these methods of data reporting.

What is the ideal way to express the results of an IPG tracing? It seems obvious that the reporting method should be simple and easy for a clinician to understand. The report should give some indication of the reliability of the result. We believe these objectives are best accomplished by reporting the IPG test in the same way that other laboratory tests are reported—by expressing the results as a number with a defined range of normal. An individual test result can then be weighed by the clinician in relation to where the specific value falls with respect to the range of normal.

We now express IPG results as a percentage of predicted normal, much as some tests of cardiac or pulmonary function are currently reported. In this method of interpretation, normality relates to the anticipated lumen diameter of the proximal veins. The percentage of predicted lumen diameter is referred to as the *venous diameter index* (VDI). A normal individual is expected to have a VDI of 75% or greater. Patients with DVT usually have a VDI of 0% to 40%. This method of interpretation is based on firm theoretic grounds and convincing

experimental data.[2,5] Equally important, it is easily understood by clinicians.

The rationale rests on actual measurements of venous diameter carried out in 100 normal extremities (using ultrasonic imaging) and in 33 limbs with DVT (using venograms). The results of VOP tracings in all limbs were correlated with the minimum venous diameter measured in the proximal veins. For a given degree of venous outflow obstruction, the time constant of venous outflow (τ) was found to vary with the amount of venous filling (VC). In mathematical terms, $\tau/VC = $ constant.* For convenience, we refer to τ/VC as F. In any given patient, the F value is constant, regardless of the degree of venous filling and reflects the degree of venous outflow obstruction. In addition to studies in patients and normal volunteers, this observation has also been confirmed in a laboratory model of the venous system of the leg under widely varying conditions.[2,5]

In 100 normal legs, the mean F value was 0.63 ± 0.16. An F value of 0.63 was therefore taken as 100% of predicted venous diameter. An inverse relationship was found between VDI and F. Thus VDI = 63/F. VDI in the 100 normal limbs varied from 63% to 188%, whereas the 33 limbs with DVT varied from 1% to 38%.

Precise calculation of VDI from F values is facilitated by a computer. However, it is also possible simply to plot VO_3 and VC on a routine scoring

*The potential value of this ratio in interpretation of VOP tracings was first suggested by Frank Ingle, Ph.D.

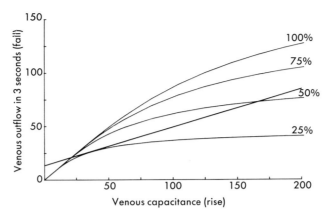

Fig. 74-9. Discriminant line divides normal and abnormal limbs at about 50% of normal venous outflow capacity.

graph to which curves approximating VDI values of 100%, 75%, 50%, and 25% have been added (Fig. 74-9). The approximate VDI can then be estimated from the graph.

CLINICAL USES OF IPG
Evaluation of symptomatic patients

In our experience, the commonest use for IPG has been to evaluate a patient with the clinical suspicion of DVT. Patients often complain of minor signs or symptoms suggesting the possibility of DVT. Many times the clinical suspicion is so slight that the physician hesitates to order a venogram with its attendant discomfort, inconvenience, and expense. However, physicians are also well aware that patients can harbor life-threatening thrombi in the deep veins, even though they may have minimal signs or symptoms. Therefore clinicians need a simple, readily available noninvasive test that answers the question "What is this patient's present risk of significant thromboembolism?" With a clearly normal IPG test, the clinician can be 99% confident that the patient does not have sufficient venous thrombosis to pose the threat of major pulmonary embolism (Chapter 80).

Even when the clinical diagnosis of DVT has been made on an apparently firm basis, IPG is useful in confirming the diagnosis. In the past, such patients have often been subjected to prolonged anticoagulant treatment on the strength of the clinical diagnosis alone. Many studies have now demonstrated the fallibility of the clinical diagnosis of DVT,[6,8,11,25] even when the signs and symptoms appear to be typical. Before treating a patient on clinical grounds alone, the diagnosis of DVT must

be confirmed with some objective diagnostic method before instituting treatment.

Screening of asymptomatic patients

The value of IPG for screening patients at risk depends on the expected incidence of DVT. When low-dose heparin or other prophylactic measures are employed, the occurrence of DVT is so infrequent in some patient groups that routine screening may not be justified. However, in patients in whom such prophylaxis is contraindicated or in patients who are at unusually high risk from DVT, IPG is a useful screening technique (Fig. 74-10). This method has been advocated for the screening of patients undergoing total hip replacement.[16,22-24] The ability of the method to detect thrombi in the groin and pelvis is particularly important in this group of patients.

Some investigators have questioned the use of IPG for screening asymptomatic patients because of its admittedly low sensitivity in the diagnosis of calf vein thrombi. Since the calf contains many veins in parallel, there is usually no detectable impairment in venous outflow until several veins are involved. However, the likelihood of major pulmonary embolism is extremely low in patients with normal impedance tests.

We observed no fatal pulmonary emboli in 1074 patients with normal IPG tests. In only 1% of these patients was there even a suspicion of nonfatal pulmonary embolism.[42] A similar low incidence of thromboembolic complications has been reported in patients with normal noninvasive tests of other types (Chapter 80).

It should be emphasized that a normal IPG test

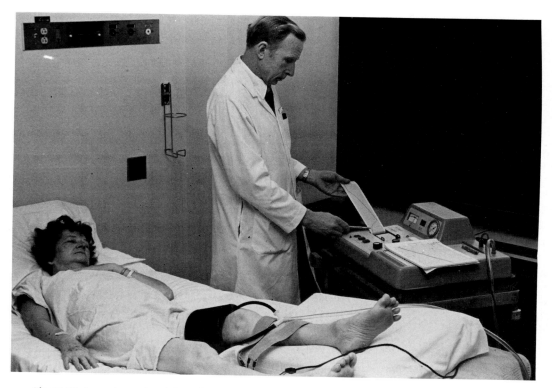

Fig. 74-10. Screening patient 4 days after aortofemoral reconstruction. Normal tracing excludes thrombosis in major veins with 99% certainty.

does *not* guarantee that the patient may not develop major venous thrombosis at a later date. When patients have continuing risk factors, we recommend repeat testing every 48 hours for as long as the patient remains at high risk.

Evaluation of suspected pulmonary embolism

IPG is also useful in the evaluation of suspected pulmonary embolism, since practically all pulmonary emboli are associated with thrombosis of the leg veins. The finding of a normal IPG test in a patient suspected of pulmonary embolism casts serious doubt on this diagnosis.[29]

Long-term management of DVT

Recent thrombosis in the popliteal, femoral, or iliac veins typically results in a marked delay in venous outflow following release of the thigh cuff. There is usually an impairment of venous capacitance as well. However, as days go by, venous capacitance improves and often returns to normal. The venous outflow rate improves more gradually but may also return to normal as collateral pathways develop. (It is sometimes useful in patients with abnormal venous outflow and a history of old DVT to place the leg slightly dependent and look for respiratory venous excursions. Such respiratory excursions are typically seen in old DVT but have not been observed in fresh venous thrombosis.) If recanalization of the vein occurs as a result of lysis, the IPG test reverts to normal. Sequential IPG results thus give the clinician an objective assessment of the extent of venous outflow obstruction. Sometimes significant outflow obstruction persists in patients who no longer have any clinical signs or symptoms to suggest DVT. Such patients should continue on anticoagulant therapy, even though they may appear to have recovered completely by clinical criteria.

Impedance phlebography has been used in this fashion to help determine the appropriate duration of anticoagulant treatment. Although most patients with proved thrombosis are maintained on oral anticoagulants for 6 months, some patients are difficult to manage on an outpatient basis. Continued anticoagulant therapy poses a risk. Under these circumstances we are willing to discontinue anticoagulant therapy if the IPG test has reverted to normal.

When the IPG test continues to show significant venous outflow obstruction, the risk of recurrent thrombophlebitis seems much higher. Since venous stasis is well recognized as one of the major factors predisposing to recurrence, we are reluctant to discontinue anticoagulation therapy for such patients. To date, recurrent thrombophlebitis has not occurred in our experience in patients with normal IPG tests in whom anticoagulant medication was discontinued.

In the future, IPG may be used to evaluate other pathophysiologic states in which peripheral hemodynamics are altered. The striking influence of peripheral vasoconstriction and reduced blood flow on the venous capacitance gives promise of clinical usefulness when these parameters have been more fully studied.

COST-BENEFIT ANALYSIS OF IPG

In proposing any new medical test, the proponent must be sensitive to the cost of the procedure and its potential effect on the already overwhelming cost of medical care. The public and third-party payers rightfully wish to know that new technology and new test procedures will not add further to this cost burden without corresponding benefits. Fortunately, with respect to IPG, the case for cost-benefit seems as compelling as the case for medical benefit (Chapter 80).[1,14,20,43]

The cost of IPG in most hospitals is roughly equivalent to that of an electrocardiogram, usually $25 to $50. This is a relatively low charge in view of the large saving possible by elimination of unnecessary or delayed treatment. From studies concerning the accuracy of the clinical diagnosis of venous thrombosis,[6,8,25] the likelihood of preventing unnecessary treatment appears to be 40% or more. Saving an unnecessary hospitalization for treatment of DVT results in considerable cost saving, as well as elimination of the risks of anticoagulant treatment and time lost from work.

According to *Professional Activity Study* data, the average length of stay for treatment of DVT is 12.6 days. Eliminating the cost of such hospitalization even occasionally would justify a great many test procedures. (Venography could be employed for the same purpose but is significantly more expensive, as well as being invasive.)

IPG often results in a firm diagnosis of venous

thrombosis earlier in the patient's hospital course than might otherwise have been the case. The duration of treatment seems likely to be shorter and the medical complications less serious than if the diagnosis and treatment were delayed. Cost savings should be significant although hard to document.

The low cost of IPG, coupled with the frequent errors in clinical diagnosis (both false positive and false negative), makes a strong circumstantial case for the cost effectiveness of this new diagnostic procedure. Recent papers have stressed the favorable cost-benefit ratio of IPG.[14,20]

SUMMARY

The accuracy of IPG is now thoroughly documented in the literature with an aggregate 93% sensitivity and 94% specificity in all reported series (2561 venograms) (see Table 80-6). The accuracy is even higher in symptomatic patients. It is widely employed in major medical centers and community hospitals. It is a simple, safe procedure that keeps the patient free from discomfort or inconvenience and provides immediate and reliable results at the bedside or in the clinic. It is particularly useful for outpatient evaluation, which saves many unnecessary hospital admissions and proves to be highly cost-effective.

The principal liability of the method has been false positive or equivocal results in patients with pathophysiologic conditions other than DVT that also affect the peripheral circulation. Severe peripheral vasoconstriction, congestive heart failure, hypotension, and severe pulmonary disease may all give abnormal tests as a result of reduced compliance of the venous system. The incidence of false positive tests in such patients is markedly reduced by multiple repetitions of the test procedure or by prolonging the duration of cuff occlusion.

Quantitative methods for interpretation of IPG results have recently been developed. Reporting test results quantitatively with an established range of normal for reference makes IPG results more understandable to clinicians and promises to further increase the usefulness of this common diagnostic test.

REFERENCES

1. Ahola, S.J., et al.: Effects of physician education on the evaluation of deep venous thrombosis in a small community hospital, Conn. Med. 47:392, 1983.
2. Anderson, F.A., Jr.: Quantification of the degree of venous outflow obstruction from venous occlusion plethysmography, doctoral dissertation, Worcester, Mass., 1984, Worcester Polytechnic Institute.

3. Anderson, F.A., Jr., and Cardullo, P.C.: Problems com monly encountered in IPG testing and their solution, Brui 4:21, 1980.

4. Anderson, F.A., Jr., and Wheeler, H.B.: Venous occlusioi plethysmography for the detection of venous thrombosis Med. Instrum. 13:350, 1979.

5. Anderson, F.A., Jr., et al.: Non-invasive quantification o the degree of venous outflow obstruction in the extremitie: by means of venous occlusion plethysmography. In Bartel D.L., editor: 1983 Advances in bioengineering, New York 1983, American Society of Mechanical Engineers.

6. Browse, N.: Deep vein thrombosis—diagnosis, Br. Med J. 4:676, 1969.

7. Clarke-Pearson, D.L., and Creasman, W.T.: Diagnosis c deep venous thrombosis in obstetrics and gynecology b impedance phlebography, Obstet. Gynecol. 58:52, 1981

8. Coon, W.W., and Coller, F.A.: Clinicopathologic corre lation in thromboembolism, Surg. Gynecol. Obstet 109:259, 1959.

9. Cooperman, M., et al.: Detection of deep venous throm bosis by impedance plethysmography, Am. J. Surg 137:252, 1979.

10. Dmochowski, J.R., Adams, D.F., and Couch, N.P Impedance measurement in the diagnosis of deep venou thrombosis, Arch. Surg. 104:170, 1972.

11. Flanc, C., Kakkar, V.V., and Clarke, M.B.: The detection of venous thrombosis of the legs using ^{125}I-labelled fibrinogen, Br. J. Surg. 55:742, 1968.

12. Flanigan, D.P., et al.: Vascular-laboratory diagnosis of clinically suspected acute deep-vein thrombosis, Lancet 2:331, 1978.

13. Foti, M.E., and Gurewich, V.: Fibrin degradation products and impedance plethysmography: measurements in the diagnosis of acute deep vein thrombosis, Arch. Intern. Med. 140:903, 1980.

14. Gross, W.S., and Burney, R.E.: Therapeutic and economic implications of emergency department evaluation for venous thrombosis, J. Am. Coll. Emer. Physicians 8:110, 1979.

15. Gross, W.S., et al.: Role of the vascular laboratory in the diagnosis of venous thrombosis. In Bergan, J.J., and Yao, J.S.T., editors: Venous problems, Chicago, 1978, Year Book Medical Publishers, Inc.

16. Harris, W.H., et al.: Cuff-impedance phlebography and ^{125}I-fibrinogen scanning versus roentgenographic phlebography for diagnosis of thrombophlebitis following hip surgery, J. Bone Joint Surg. 58A:939, 1976.

17. Hull, R., et al.: Impedance plethysmography using the occlusive cuff technique in the diagnosis of venous thrombosis, Circulation 53:696, 1976.

18. Hull, R., et al.: Combined use of leg scanning and impedance plethysmography in suspected venous thrombosis. An alternative to venography, N. Engl. J. Med. 296:1497, 1977.

19. Hull, R., et al.: Impedance plethysmography: the relationship between venous filling and sensitivity and specificity for proximal vein thrombosis, Circulation 58:898, 1978.

20. Hull, R., et al.: Cost effectiveness of clinical diagnosis, venography and noninvasive testing in patients with symptomatic deep-vein thrombosis, N. Engl. J. Med. 304:1561, 1981.

21. Hull, R., et al.: Replacement of venography in suspected venous thrombosis by impedance plethysmography and ^{125}I-fibrinogen leg scanning: a less invasive approach, Ann. Intern. Med. 94:12, 1981.

22. Hume, M., et al.: Extent of leg vein thrombosis determined by impedance and ^{125}I-fibrinogen, Am. J. Surg. 129:455, 1975.

23. Hume, M., et al.: Venous thrombosis after total hip replacement. Combined monitoring as a guide for prophylaxis and treatment, J. Bone Joint Surg. 58A:933, 1976.

24. Johnston, K.W., and Kakkar, V.V.: Plethysmographic diagnosis of deep vein thrombosis, Surg. Gynecol. Obstet. 139:41, 1974.

25. McLachlin, J., Richard, T., and Paterson, J.C.: An evaluation of clinical signs in the diagnosis of deep venous thrombosis, Arch. Surg. 85:738, 1962.

26. Mullick, S.C., Wheeler, H.B., and Songster, G.F.: Diagnosis of deep vein thrombosis by measurement of electrical impedance, Am. J. Surg. 119:417, 1970.

27. Nadeau, J.E., et al.: Impedance phlebography: accuracy of diagnosis in deep vein thrombosis, Can. J. Surg. 18:219, 1975.

28. Richards, K.L., et al.: Noninvasive diagnosis of deep venous thrombosis, Arch. Intern. Med. 136:1091, 1976.

29. Sasahara, A.A.: Current problems in pulmonary embolism: introduction, Prog. Cardiovasc. Dis. 17:161, 1974.

30. Seeber, J.J.: Impedance plethysmography: a useful method in the diagnosis of deep vein thrombophlebitis in the lower extremity, Arch. Phys. Med. Rehabil. 55:170, 1974.

31. Steer, M.L., et al.: Limitations of impedance phlebography for diagnosis of venous thrombosis, Arch. Surg. 106:44, 1973.

32. Taylor, D.W., et al.: Simplification of the sequential impedance plethysmograph technique without loss of accuracy, Thromb. Res. 17:561, 1980.

33. Toy, P.C.T.Y., and Schrier, S.L.: Occlusive impedance plethysmography, West. J. Med. 90:89, 1978.

34. Wheeler, H.B., and Anderson, F.A., Jr.: Impedance plethysmography. In Yao, S.J.T., and Kempcninski, R.F., editors: Manual for the vascular diagnostic laboratory, Chicago, Year Book Medical Publishers, Inc. (In press.)

35. Wheeler, H.B., and Mullick, S.C.: Detection of venous obstruction in the leg by measurement of electrical impedance, Ann. N.Y. Acad. Sci. 170:804, 1970.

36. Wheeler, H.B., and Patwardhan, N.A.: Evaluation of venous thrombosis by impedance plethysmography. In Madden, J.L., and Hume, M., editors: Venous thromboembolism: prevention and treatment. New York, 1976, Appleton Century-Crofts.

37. Wheeler, H.B., Patwardhan, N.A., and Anderson, F.A., Jr.: The place of occlusive impedance plethysmography in the diagnosis of venous thrombosis. In Bergan, J.J., and Yao, J.S.T., editors: Venous problems, Chicago, 1978, Year Book Medical Publishers, Inc.

38. Wheeler, H.B., et al.: Diagnosis of occult deep vein thrombosis by a noninvasive bedside technique, Surgery 70:20, 1971.

39. Wheeler, H.B., et al.: Impedance phlebography: technique, interpretation and results, Arch. Surg. 104:164, 1972.

40. Wheeler, H.B., et al.: Bedside screening for venous thrombosis using occlusive impedance phlebography, Angiology 26:199, 1975.

41. Wheeler, H.B., et al.: Occlusive impedance phlebography: a diagnostic procedure for venous thrombosis and pulmonary embolism, Prog. Cardiovasc. Dis. 17:199, 1974.

42. Wheeler, H.B., et al.: Suspected deep vein thrombosis: management by impedance plethysmography, Arch. Surg. 117:1206, 1982.

CHAPTER 75

Thermography in the diagnosis of deep vein thrombosis

ANDREW N. NICOLAIDES

The development of thermographic tests for the diagnosis of acute deep vein thrombosis (DVT) is based on the observation that the palpated skin temperature of a limb with thrombosis is often higher than that of the normal opposite limb. This temperature difference is more obvious after exposing the limbs to room temperature because of delayed cooling of the affected limb.[11] Delayed cooling was found in only 25% of limbs with DVT in one study using palpation,[5] but because of the inability of the human hand to detect a temperature difference of less than 2° C,[4] this phenomenon was investigated by Cooke and Pilcher in the early 1970s using an infrared scanning system.[6,7] By the late 1970s a diagnostic technique had become well established as a useful screening method.[4,5]

INFRARED IMAGING METHOD

The technique of examination is as follows: The limbs and lower abdomen are exposed for 10 minutes in a room with an ambient temperature of 20° C or less. Great care is taken to avoid drafts. The patient is in a supine position with the legs elevated 10 to 20 degrees with a 45-degree external rotation to prevent venous pooling. Both drafts and venous pooling interfere with the thermographic patterns by producing artifacts. Infrared images of both calves and both thighs are obtained using a thermographic scanning camera and display unit. These are recorded on Polaroid film. A temperature difference calibration scale is displayed at the lower part of the screen. Temperature differences of less than 0.2° C can be recorded.[5]

The thermogram of the normal calf and thigh shows an overall even distribution of temperature that is the same on both sides, with a slightly cooler skin overlying the tibia and patella (Fig. 75-1). In the presence of calf vein thrombosis, a diffuse area of increased temperature over most or all of the calf from ankle to knee is produced, obliterating the cooler subcutaneous border of the tibia (Fig. 75-2). Partial or complete obliteration of the cool area over the patella is good evidence of calf thrombosis extending into the thigh. The temperature difference between the two limbs is usually greater than 1.2° C, although in some patients with small thrombi it is between 0.5° and 1.2° C. Thrombi in the veins proximal to the calf, including iliac thrombosis, produce an increase in the temperature of the medial aspect of the thigh.

Several other conditions such as trauma, infection, arthritis, ruptured Baker's cyst, and superficial thrombophlebitis increase the skin temperature. Although these conditions produce characteristic patterns, their presence when DVT is suspected makes an interpretation of thermograms difficult. Therefore a different diagnostic method should be used when one or more of these conditions exist. Also, patients with arterial occlusive disease should be excluded to avoid an erroneously false positive thermographic appearance in the normal warmer limb.

A number of studies of patients presenting symptoms suggesting DVT have compared the results of thermography with venography (Table 75-1). In all of these studies, patients with obvious causes of increased skin temperature other than DVT were excluded so that the false positive rate would be kept to a minimum. The false negative rate was usually the result of small calf thrombi that, in some cases, were more than 2 weeks old.[5] The results indicate that thermography is a sensitive noninva-

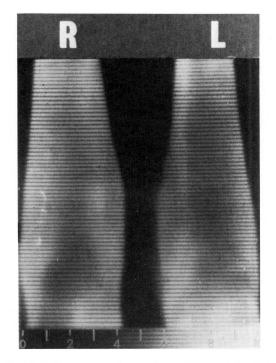

Fig. 75-1. Thermogram of normal legs. Skin overlying tibia and patella is cooler. (Courtesy Dr E. Cooke.)

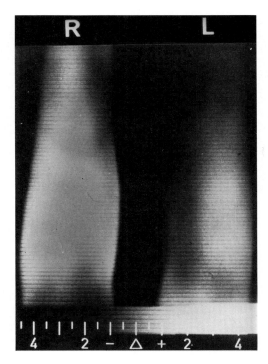

Fig. 75-2. Thermogram of patient with calf vein thrombosis. Left calf is warmer than right, with loss of pretibial cool area. (Courtesy Dr E. Cooke.)

Table 75-1. Comparison of thermography and venography in patients with suspected DVT

References	No. of patients	Incidence of DVT on venography (%)	False positive rate of thermography (%)	False negative rate of thermography (%)
Cooke and Pilcher[7]	164	46	7	8
Leiviskä and Perttala[9]	50	66	8	0
Bergqvist et al.[1]	118	72	8	2
Byström et al.[2]	51	51	0	6
Richie et al.[12]	100	34	9	18

sive method for detecting DVT. However, because of its poor specificity it is only useful as a screening test. Its value is in the fact that if the test is negative, other noninvasive or venographic investigations become unnecessary. However, if thermography is positive, the presence of thrombosis should be confirmed by another test before therapy is commenced.

"DEVE THERM" METHOD

Despite the information just presented, thermography is not widely used because the equipment is expensive and often must be placed in a draft-free constant temperature room with a supply of liquid nitrogen to cool the infrared detector. Because of this, an attempt has been made to develop a simpler, less expensive, mobile instrument using a radiation thermometer rather than a thermographic imaging system.[8,10] Such an instrument has been designed not only to be mobile, but also to produce temperature profiles of the legs, allowing direct numerical analysis of such profiles rather than the interpretation of thermographic picture patterns.

The equipment is now computerized and commercially available (DeVe Therm, Ekoscann AB, Gothenburg, Sweden). An infrared radiation trans-

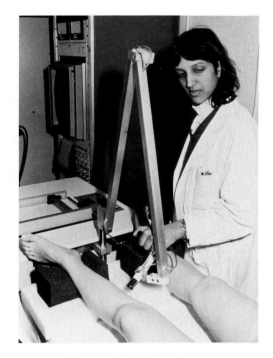

Fig. 75-3. DeVe Therm in use.

Table 75-2. Results of clinical study
by Jacobsson et al.*[8]

	Leg temperature profile		
	Positive	**Negative**	**Total**
DVT on venography	123 (95%)	7	130
No DVT on venography	38	32 (47%)	70

*Sensitivity 95%, specificity 47%.

ducer is attached to a manually directed scanning arm (Fig. 75-3) that allows the transducer to be moved along the anteromedial side of the leg from ankle to groin approximately 5 cm away from the skin surface. Potentiometers in the arm allow the sensing of position along the leg so that simultaneous recording of the temperature and position is possible on an x-y recorder. The temperature profile of one leg is subtracted from that of the other, and the temperature difference is plotted automatically. The leg is subdivided into four segments, and the mean temperature of each segment is calculated and plotted (Fig. 75-4). A difference great-

er than 0.7° C between two mean segmental temperatures is abnormal and suggests DVT in the warmer leg. A difference of less than 0.7° C is normal and indicates the absence of thrombosis. The examination is performed with the patient in a supine position after exposing the bare legs to a room temperature of 20° to 22° C for 15 minutes, with the heels supported 20 cm above the head. The calibration procedure and actual recording take less than 5 minutes.

Jacobsson et al.[8] studied a series of 200 patients, who were admitted to the hospital because of clinically suspected acute DVT, using both the DeVe Therm method and subsequent venography. The results of this study are shown in Table 75-2. Thrombosis was confined to the calf, with or without extension into the popliteal vein, in 37 limbs; it extended into more proximal veins in 86 limbs. The seven false negative tests were three iliac, two femoral, one popliteal, and one calf thrombosis. Venous occlusion plethysmography was performed on all the patients of this study and improved the sensitivity from 95% to 98%. However, as one could have predicted, the specificity was low: 47%.

My team at St Mary's Hospital, London, has been using the DeVe Therm method for several months in all patients with clinically suspected DVT. In addition to temperature profiles, patients have been investigated either by venography or a combination of impedance plethysmography, Doppler ultrasound, and [125I] fibrinogen test. To date, 50 patients have been studied. A negative thermographic examination was found in 20. In all these 20 patients the venogram or the combination of other tests just mentioned was normal.

The results of the thermographic leg temperature profiles using the DeVe Therm method indicate a sensitivity which corresponds to that of conventional thermography using an infrared imaging system. However, the equipment is more mobile, less expensive, and easy to use because of the incorporated microprocessor, which provides automatic calculation and plotting of the results, making the interpretation easier and avoiding the risk of subjective bias. This test will markedly reduce the need for further tests or venography if the result is negative, saving time and expense for many patients. It holds the promise of an excellent screening test for patients with suspected acute DVT and will likely become more widely used than the conventional thermographic imaging technique.

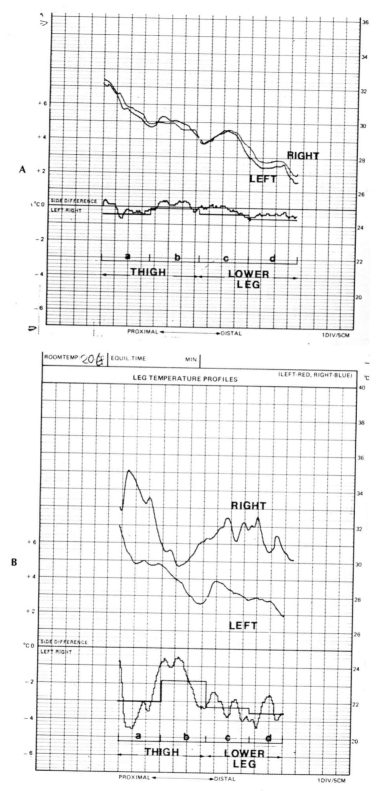

Fig. 75-4. A, Normal leg temperature profiles. Mean temperature difference between two legs is less than 0.7° C in all four segments (*a* to *d*). B, Abnormal leg temperature profiles in patient with right iliofemoral thrombosis. Right leg is warmer than left, with mean temperature difference in excess of 0.7° C in all four segments (*a* to *d*).

REFERENCES

1. Bergqvist, D., Efsing, H.O., and Hallböök, T.: Thermography. A noninvasive method for diagnosis of deep venous thrombosis, Arch. Surg. 112:600, 1977.
2. Byström, L.G., et al.: The value of thermography and the determination of fibrin-fibrinogen degradation products in the diagnosis of deep venous thrombosis, Acta Med. Scand. 202:319, 1977.
3. Cooke, E.D.: Letter: Doppler ultrasound in diagnosis of deep vein thrombosis, Br. Med. J. 1:1075, 1976.
4. Cooke, E.D.: The fundamentals of thermographic diagnosis of deep vein thrombosis, Acta Thermographica Suppl. 1, p. 1, 1978.
5. Cooke, E.D.: Thermography. In Nicolaides, A.N., and Yao, J.S.T., editors: The investigation of vascular disorders, Edinburgh, 1981, Churchill Livingstone, Inc.
6. Cooke, E.D., and Pilcher, M.F.: Thermography in diagnosis of deep venous thrombosis, Br. Med. J., 2:523, 1973.
7. Cooke, E.D., and Pilcher, M.F.: Deep vein thrombosis: preclinical diagnosis by thermography, Br. J. Surg., 61:971, 1974.
8. Jacobsson, H., et al.: Standardised leg temperature profiles in the diagnosis of acute deep venous thrombosis, Vasc. Diagn. Ther. 3:55, 1983.
9. Leiviskä, T., and Perttala, Y.: Thermography in diagnosing deep venous thrombosis of the lower limb, Radiol. Clin. (Basel) 44:417, 1975.
10. Nilsson, E., Sunden, P., and Zetterquist, S.: Leg temperature profiles with a simplified thermographic technique in the diagnosis of acute venous thrombosis, Scand. J. Clin. Lab. Invest. 39:171, 1979.
11. Pilcher, R.: Postoperative thrombosis and embolism; mortality and morbidity, Lancet 2:629, 1939.
12. Richie, W.G.M., Soulen, R.L., and Lapayowker, M.S.: Thermographic diagnosis of deep venous thrombosis, Invest. Radiol. 12:404, 1977.

CHAPTER 76

[^{125}I]fibrinogen leg scanning

RUSSELL D. HULL and JACK HIRSH

BACKGROUND AND PRINCIPLES OF USE

The diagnosis of venous thrombosis by radio-iodine-labeled fibrinogen scanning depends on incorporation of circulating labeled fibrinogen into a developing or existing thrombus; this fibrinogen is then detected by measuring the increase of overlying surface radioactivity with an isotope detector. The feasibility of this technique was demonstrated in animals and in man[5] in the early 1960s; the method has been extensively evaluated over the last decade.[17]

The equipment used initially for external scanning was cumbersome, but in the last few years portable, convenient, and sensitive equipment has become available so that the test can be performed at the patient's bedside in approximately 15 minutes. Fibrinogen leg scanning is a sensitive method for detecting calf vein thrombosis and is relatively sensitive to thrombi in the midthigh and lower thigh, but its accuracy is limited in the upper thigh, and it is totally insensitive to thrombi in the pelvis.[2,12] The insensitivity to thrombi in the pelvic veins occurs because [^{125}I]fibrinogen is a relatively low-energy gamma emitter, and its unreliability in the upper thigh is caused by high background counts as a result of radioactive urine in the bladder and circulating [^{125}I]fibrinogen in large veins and arteries.

DOSAGE, SIDE EFFECTS, AND PRECAUTIONS

The use of radioactive fibrinogen carries a theoretic risk of transmission of serum hepatitis, but this risk has been eliminated for practical purposes by preparing fibrinogen from a small number of carefully selected donors who have not transmitted hepatitis during years of frequent blood donation and who are free of hepatitis-associated antigen.

^{125}I crosses the placenta, and a small amount enters the fetal circulation.[13] The radioactivity also appears in the breast milk of lactating women.[13] For these reasons, [^{125}I]fibrinogen scanning is contraindicated during pregnancy and lactation and should not be used in young patients unless very definite indications exist, because radioiodine accumulates in the thyroid gland.

Following the injection of 100 μCi of [^{125}I]fibrinogen, approximately 200 mrem is delivered to the blood, 20 mrem to tissues, and 5 mrem to the kidneys.[13] This is less than the acceptable annual total absorbed radiation dose (500 mrad/year) recommended for the general population by the British National Council for Radiation Protection.[13]

SCANNING TECHNIQUE

Patients are scanned via a lightly shielded isotope detector probe with their legs elevated 15 degrees above horizontal to minimize venous pooling in the calf veins. Readings are taken over both legs and recorded as a percentage of the surface radioactivity measured over the heart. The surface radioactivity is measured over the femoral vein at 7 to 8 cm intervals starting just below the inguinal ligament and then at similar intervals over the medial and posterior aspects of the popliteal region and calf. The criteria for a positive leg scan have been established by a number of researchers. Venous thrombosis is suspected if there is an increase in the radioactive reading of more than 20% at any point compared with readings over adjacent points of the same leg, over the same point on a previous day, and at the corresponding point on the opposite leg. Venous thrombosis is diagnosed if the scan remains abnormal for more than 24 hours after repeated examination. The technique is simple and rapid so that up to 15 to 20 patients may be screened each day by one technician. Scanning time is limited by in vivo survival of fibrinogen so that after a single injection of 100 μCi, counting is possible for about 7 days. The thyroid gland is blocked by a daily 100 mg dose of potassium iodide given orally for 14 days to prevent excessive uptake of radioiodine. If the patient is still at risk for developing venous thrombosis after 7 days, the injection can be repeated at intervals to extend the scanning time for the high-risk period.

USES AND LIMITATIONS OF [125I]FIBRINOGEN LEG SCANNING

[125I]fibrinogen leg scanning has been a valuable research tool that has provided important information about the natural history, epidemiology, pathogenesis, and methods of prophylaxis of venous thrombosis. Leg scanning is also a useful clinical tool that can aid the clinician in the practical management of patients with venous thrombosis. It is important to recognize, however, that leg scanning has certain limitations. Its major limitations are its inability to detect the presence of venous thrombi above the inguinal ligament[3,12] and its relative unreliability for detecting thrombi in the upper thigh.[3,12] High levels of surface radioactivity in the absence of venous thrombosis are seen in patients with superficial thrombophlebitis, hematoma, cellulitis, cutaneous vasculitis, and arthritis. High counts are also seen over surgical wounds in the legs, an important limitation in patients having leg or hip surgery. Finally, if used diagnostically in patients with clinically suspected venous thrombosis, the leg scan result may not become positive for hours and sometimes even for days after injection of the isotope.

The practical indications for using [125I]fibrinogen leg scanning are as follows:

1. Screening certain high-risk patient groups in whom prophylaxis is either contraindicated or ineffective
2. As an adjunct to impedance plethysmography or Doppler ultrasound in the diagnosis of clinically suspected venous thrombosis
3. As a diagnostic test in patients with clinically suspected acute recurrent venous thrombosis
4. Screening patients who develop calf vein thrombosis when there are relative or absolute contraindications to anticoagulant therapy

Screening high-risk patients

Although screening high-risk patients by [125I]fibrinogen leg scanning to detect and treat thrombi early in their development is one approach for preventing major venous thromboembolism, it is expensive and relatively inefficient.[9] Primary prophylaxis with small doses of heparin, intermittent calf compression, or in certain circumstances, dextran or oral anticoagulant prophylaxis is much more cost-effective and is the preferred approach in most patient groups.[9]

The cost-effectiveness of primary prophylaxis versus secondary prevention by screening is illustrated by the findings of our recent cost-effectiveness analysis in high-risk general surgical patients.[9] The findings by cost-effectiveness analysis[9] are summarized in Table 76-1. Primary prophylaxis is clearly preferred to screening. Leg scanning is the most expensive of the alternative approaches and necessitates full-dose anticoagulant treatment of large numbers of patients with subclinical venous thrombi. It should therefore be reserved for patients in whom primary prophylaxis is either contraindicated or unavailable. Leg scanning may occasionally be used in addition to primary prophylaxis in the extremely high-risk patients, for example, those with a recent history of venous thrombosis who require surgery.

A number of researchers have compared results of expectant scanning and venography in general surgical and medical patients and have reported an accuracy for leg scanning of 90%.* As mentioned earlier, leg scanning has special limitations when used to screen patients for thrombosis after leg surgery.[4] This is because extravascular isotope accumulation in the hematoma and the healing wound invariably leads to scanning abnormalities at the site of surgery, so that thrombi near the wound cannot be detected. This is a major limitation in patients having hip surgery, since up to 20% of all thrombi (in about 10% of all patients) are isolated in the femoral vein close to the surgical wound.[4]

Harris et al.[4] reported on the accuracy of [125I]fibrinogen leg scanning in 83 patients who underwent leg scanning following elective hip surgery. All patients had venograms performed regardless of the result of the leg scan, so that leg scanning was compared with venography in 142 limbs. The leg scan was positive in 85% of patients

*References 1, 3, 5, 12, 15, 16.

Table 76-1. Total cost per 1000 patients of alternative approaches for the prevention of fatal pulmonary embolism in high-risk general surgical patients (1982)

Strategy	Cost ($)
SUBCUTANEOUS ADMINISTRATION OF HEPARIN IN LOW DOSES	
Administration for 7 days in 1000 patients	20,000
Ascending venography in 10 patients	880
Lung scanning in 10 patients	1170
Treatment of venous thromboembolism in 8 patients	17,672
TOTAL	39,722
INTERMITTENT PNEUMATIC COMPRESSION OF THE LEGS	
Use for 7 days in 1000 patients	33,000
Venography in 10 patients	880
Lung scanning in 10 patients	1170
Treatment of venous thromboembolism in 8 patients	17,672
TOTAL	52,722
INTRAVENOUS ADMINISTRATION OF DEXTRAN	
Administration for 4 days to 1000 patients	103,000
Venography in 20 patients	1760
Lung scanning in 10 patients	1170
Treatment of venous thromboembolism in 13 patients	28,717
TOTAL	134,647
LEG SCANNING WITH [^{125}I]FIBRINOGEN	
Scanning for 7 days in 1000 patients	85,000
Venography in 135 patients	11,880
Lung scanning in 15 patients	1755
Treatment of venous thromboembolism in 114 patients	251,826
TOTAL	350,461
TRADITIONAL (NO PROGRAM) APPROACH	
Venography in 40 patients	3520
Lung scanning in 30 patients	3510
Treatment of venous thromboembolism in 33 patients	72,897
TOTAL	79,927

who had thrombi located venographically outside the area of surgery. However, since a large number of thrombi were isolated to the femoral vein close to the site of surgery, the overall accuracy was only 50%.

We have evaluated the positive predictive value of [^{125}I]fibrinogen leg scanning for the detection of venous thrombosis in high-risk patients.[7] Leg scanning was performed in 630 patients who had gen-

eral surgical procedures and 385 patients who had hip surgery. Venography was performed if the leg scan was positive, and the positive predictive value was determined. Positive predictive value was 79% for general surgical patients and 86% for hip surgery patients. The patients were also screened with impedance plethysmosgraphy (IPG) to determine the value of adding this screening test to [^{125}I]fibrinogen leg scanning in high-risk patients.[7] The addition of the IPG to leg scanning in general surgical patients identified only one additional patient with proximal vein thrombosis (0.2%), whereas in hip surgery patients the addition of IPG identified 25 additional patients with proximal vein thombosis (6%). Thus the addition of IPG to leg scanning was not useful among general surgical patients as a screening test but was of substantial clinical value in hip surgery patients.

The results of this study were consistent with previous findings, which suggested that the majority of venous thrombi that occur in general surgical patients arise in the calf and so can be detected by leg scanning, while a considerable number of thrombi in hip surgery patients arise in the femoral vein and may occur as isolated events.

Natural history of the positive leg scan in asymptomatic patients. We have found that approximately 50% of patients who develop thrombi detected by [^{125}I]fibrinogen leg scanning postoperatively also develop new asymptomatic abnormalities in the lung scan (ventilation-perfusion mismatch), which have a high probability for pulmonary emboli, indicating that approximately 50% of leg scan–detected thrombi embolize. If the thrombi are confined to the calf, the emboli are small and rarely clinically significant. However, if the calf vein thrombi are large or if the patient has a compromised cardiac or respiratory system, even emboli that arise from a calf vein thrombus could be clinically dangerous.

Untreated, approximately 20% of silent calf vein thrombi in bedridden patients extend into the popliteal or more proximal veins. When this occurs, it is associated with a much higher risk of clinically significant thromboemboli, and, in the one small study[14] in which the silent proximal vein thrombi detected by leg scanning remained untreated, the frequency of symptomatic pulmonary emboli was reported to be approximately 50%. Most thrombi that form in surgical patients undergoing general abdominal surgical procedures or that occur in medical patients arise in the calf veins,[7] and when proximal vein thrombosis occurs, it is almost always associated with calf vein thrombosis. The site of origin of venous thrombi is different in patients who have hip and pelvic surgery.[7] In these patients, isolated proximal vein thrombosis occurs more frequently, and it is possible that in some cases of calf and proximal vein thrombosis, the proximal vein thrombi precede calf vein thrombi by a number of days and therefore may not be detected by leg scanning until distal extension to the calf occurs.

Clinical management of the positive leg scan in asymptomatic patients. The approach to the patient who develops a positive leg scan is controversial. We manage patients with a positive leg scan by performing venography and base our therapeutic decisions on the results of venography. There are two major reasons for this approach. First, between 10% and 20% of patients with positive leg scans do not have venous thrombosis by venography and these patients do not require treatment with anticoagulants. Second, the size of the venous thrombus may not be accurately reflected by the extent of positivity of the leg scan. Thus scanning may only be positive in the calf in patients who have thrombosis in the calf and in the proximal femoral or iliofemoral segment.

If contraindications to anticoagulants do not exist and the venogram confirms the presence of venous thrombosis, patients are treated with anticoagulants to prevent extension of venous thrombosis. If contraindications to anticoagulant therapy exist and the thrombus is relatively small and confined to calf veins, the patients can be followed by leg scanning and impedance plethysmography, since extension does not occur in about 80% of these patients. If the contraindication to anticoagulant therapy is transient (for example, present only in the early postoperative period), treatment with anticoagulants can be started when the contraindication is no longer present. However, if the contraindication to anticoagulants is permanent (for example, as in patients with subarachnoid hemorrhage or recent neurosurgery), then leg scanning can be continued for a prolonged period if the thrombus remains confined to the calf. If anticoagulant therapy is contraindicated and the venogram shows a large calf vein thrombus or proximal vein thrombus or if the thrombus extends, then treatment by a venous interruption procedure should be considered.

Adjunct to impedance plethysmography in the diagnosis of clinically suspected venous thrombosis

Leg scanning should never be used as the only diagnostic test in patients with clinically suspected venous thrombosis. This is because it fails to detect approximately 30% of thrombi in these patients (many of which are in the femoral or iliac veins) and because there may be a delay of hours or even days before a sufficient amount of fibrinogen accumulates in the thrombus to make the test positive. The [^{125}I]fibrinogen leg scanning test is most useful for the diagnosis of clinically suspected venous thrombosis when it is used to complement IPG.[6,8] In the majority of patients with acute venous thrombosis, the leg scan becomes positive within 24 hours of injection with [^{125}I]fibrinogen, but in some patients with symptomatic acute venous thrombosis, it may take 48 or even 72 hours for enough radioactivity to accumulate in the thrombus to allow a positive diagnosis to be made.

We have evaluated the combined use of [^{125}I]fibrinogen leg scanning and IPG in patients with clinically suspected venous thrombosis.[6] In this study patients were injected with [^{125}I]fibrinogen and had IPG performed on the day of referral. Patients then had leg scanning and IPG performed daily for the next 3 days. All patients underwent bilateral ascending venography, which was scheduled to be performed on the third day if the tests were negative or earlier if either of the tests became positive. Either leg scanning or IPG was positive in 81 of 86 patients with positive venograms (sensitivity 94%), and both tests were negative in 104 of 114 patients who had negative venograms (specificity 91%). These two tests detected all 60 patients with proximal vein thrombosis and 21 of 26 patients with calf vein thrombosis. Twenty-one of the 26 patients with calf vein thrombosis had symptoms for less than a week, and leg scanning was positive in 20 of these. The results of this study have now been confirmed in a second study of an additional 300 patients.[8]

The combined approach of IPG and leg scanning provides an alternative to venography in patients with clinically suspected deep vein thrombosis,[6,8] and it is safe to withhold anticoagulant therapy in patients who remain negative by this approach.[8]

It should be noted, however, that the use of serial IPG alone has now replaced this combined approach in patients with their first episode of venous thromboembolism.[10] Leg scanning combined with IPG remains a useful approach in selected patients with suspected acute recurrent venous thrombosis.[11] The approach of serial IPG alone for the diagnosis of suspected venous thrombosis in patients with their first episode of venous thromboembolism, and the use of leg scanning in the diagnosis of suspected acute recurrent venous thrombosis, are outlined in detail in Chapter 78.

Management of the positive [¹²⁵I]fibrinogen leg scan in patients with clinically suspected venous thrombosis. [¹²⁵I]fibrinogen is only injected into patients with clinically suspected venous thrombosis if the IPG is negative. In our experience, 10% to 15% of patients with clinically suspected venous thrombosis had a negative IPG and a positive leg scan. If cellulitis, previous knee surgery or trauma, arthritis of the knee, superficial phlebitis, or muscle injury can be excluded, then a diagnosis of deep vein thrombosis can be made with over 95% confidence. It would therefore be reasonable to base treatment on the leg scan result. If, however, the patient has clinical features that are recognized to cause a false positive leg scan, then the result of this test should be confirmed by venography before initiating anticoagulant therapy.

Diagnostic test in patients with clinically suspected acute recurrent venous thrombosis

When patients report symptoms of pain, tenderness, or swelling in a leg that has been the site of previous venous thrombosis, it may be difficult to distinguish between acute recurrent venous thrombosis and a nonthrombotic complication of chronic venous insufficiency. The clinical features may be localized to either the calf or the thigh and may appear either as an acute exacerbation on a background of long-standing less severe pain or swelling or they may occur as repeated subacute exacerbations on a background of long-standing chronic venous insufficiency. The latter is much more frequently caused by a nonthrombotic complication of the postphlebitic syndrome and usually does not require further investigation, whereas the former may or may not result from acute venous thrombosis complicating venous insufficiency.

The approach to these patients depends on the nature of their clinical presentation, on their symptoms and signs, and on whether or not there is

documented evidence of previous venous thrombosis. Venography alone is of limited diagnostic value in these patients unless the results can be compared with a previous venogram and unless a new filling defect is demonstrated. IPG may be falsely positive because of persistent venous outflow obstruction resulting from a previous episode of venous thrombosis or falsely negative because of large collateral channels that have developed consequent to the first episode. Leg scanning is useful for detecting active calf and distal thigh vein thrombi, but is relatively insensitive in the upper thigh and cannot detect external and common iliac vein thrombi. In combination, however, the approach of IPG and leg scanning plus venography has high clinical utility in the diagnosis of patients with clinically suspected acute recurrent deep vein thrombosis.[11] We have recently completed a cohort analytic study[11] incorporating long-term follow-up of 270 patients with symptoms and signs of acute recurrent deep vein thrombosis who were evaluated by combined IPG and leg scanning plus venography. The results of this study are presented in detail in Chapter 78 and provide the basis for our recommended practical approach to the diagnosis of clinically suspected acute recurrent deep vein thrombosis.

Screening patients who develop calf vein thrombosis where there are relative or absolute contrainidications to anticoagulant therapy

In addition to the use of leg scanning as a screening test in high-risk patients, a further indication for leg scanning arises in the patient who has leg pain in the early postoperative period. If venography confirms the presence of a small calf vein thrombus and anticoagulant therapy is contraindicated, then [¹²⁵I]fibrinogen can be injected and the patient followed by leg scanning and impedance plethysmography for 10 to 14 days. If extension does not occur, anticoagulant therapy can be delayed until the risk of postoperative hemorrhage has been considerably diminished.

REFERENCES

1. Becker, J.: The diagnosis of venous thrombosis in the legs using I-labelled fibrinogen. An experimental and clinical study, Acta Chir. Scand. 138:667, 1972.
2. Browse, N.L.: The ¹²⁵I-fibrinogen uptake test, Arch. Surg. 104:160, 1971.

3. Gallus, A.S., and Hirsh, J.: ^{125}I-fibrinogen leg scanning. In Fratatoni, J., and Wessler, S., editors: Prophylactic therapy for deep venous thrombosis and pulmonary embolism, DHEW Publication No. (NIH) 76-866, Washington D.C., 1975, U.S. Government Printing Office.

4. Harris, W.H., et al.: Comparison of ^{125}I-fibrinogen count scanning with phlebography for detection of venous thrombi after elective hip surgery, N. Engl. J. Med. 292:665, 1975.

5. Hobbs, J.T., and Davies, J.W.L.: Detection of venous thrombosis with ^{131}I-labelled fibrinogen in the rabbit, Lancet 2:134, 1960.

6. Hull, R., et al.: Combined use of leg scanning and impedance plethysmography in suspected venous thrombosis: an alternative to venography, N. Engl. J. Med. 296:1497, 1977.

7. Hull, R., et al.: The value of adding impedance plethysmography to ^{125}I-fibrinogen leg scanning for the detection of deep vein thrombosis in high risk surgical patients: a comparative study between patients undergoing general surgery and hip surgery, Thromb. Res. 15:227, 1979.

8. Hull, R., et al.: Replacement of venography in suspected venous thrombosis by impedance plethysmography and ^{125}I-fibrinogen leg scanning: a less invasive alternative, Ann. Intern. Med. 94:12, 1981.

9. Hull, R., et al.: Cost effectiveness of primary and secondary prevention of fatal pulmonary embolism in high-risk surgical patients, Can. Med. Assoc. J. 127:990, 1982.

10. Hull, R., et al.: A randomized trial of diagnostic strategies for symptomatic deep vein thrombosis, Thromb. Haemost. 50:160a, 1983.

11. Hull, R., et al.: The diagnosis of acute, recurrent deep-vein thrombosis: A diagnostic challenge, Circulation 67:901, 1983.

12. Kakkar, V.V.: The diagnosis of deep-vein thrombosis using the ^{125}I-fibrinogen test, Arch. Surg. 104:152, 1972.

13. Kakkar, V.V.: Fibrinogen uptake test for detection of deep vein thrombosis. A review of current practice, Semin. Nucl. Med. 7:229, 1977.

14. Kakkar, V.V., et al.: Natural history of postoperative deep vein thrombosis, Lancet 2:230, 1969.

15. Lambie, J.M., et al.: Diagnostic accuracy in venous thrombosis, Br. Med. J. 2:142, 1970.

16. Milne, R.M., et al.: Postoperative deep venous thrombosis: a comparison of diagnostic techniques, Lancet 2:445, 1971.

17. Palko, P.D., Nanson, E.M., and Fedoruk, S.O.: The early detection of deep venous thrombosis using ^{131}I-tagged human fibrinogen, Can. J. Surg. 7:215, 1964.

CHAPTER 77

The [^{99m}Tc]plasmin test

ANDREW N. NICOLAIDES and CARL-GUSTAV OLSSON

The [^{99m}Tc]plasmin test is a recently developed diagnostic test that can be used routinely in patients with symptoms and signs suggesting deep vein thrombosis.[1-5] It has been developed to overcome certain defects of the [^{125}I]fibrinogen test.

The [^{125}I]fibrinogen test (Chapter 76) is based on the observation that [^{125}I]fibrinogen injected into the circulation is incorporated into a developing thrombus as [^{125}I]fibrin, enabling the thrombus to be detected by an external scintillation counter. The [^{125}I]fibrinogen test proved a powerful research tool and provided information about the incidence of deep vein thrombosis in various groups of patients, the site of origin and the natural history of thrombi, and the efficacy of various methods of prevention. It can be used also in patients with symptoms and signs of deep vein thrombosis. Unfortunately, the diagnosis cannot be established until at least 24 to 48 hours from the time of injection of [^{125}I]fibrinogen. This is such a major drawback that the test has not been used in many such patients. In addition, it has the theoretic, although in practice very small, risk of hepatitis. The [^{99m}Tc]plasmin test has overcome these defects.

Early attempts to detect thrombi by labeling plasmin (a mixture of plasminogen and streptokinase) with ^{131}I failed.[6] This is because human plasmin is quickly bound to inhibitors in plasma, especially antiplasmin and α_2-macroglobulin, before it can attach itself to a thrombus.[5] However, porcine plasmin is not neutralized in the blood and has a high affinity for thrombi. It can be labeled with ^{99m}Tc, remaining stable for at least 29 hours.[7] It accumulates in thrombi to such an extent that the thrombi can be detected with an external scintillation apparatus.[1-5]

A lyophilized kit containing porcine plasmin (lysine-free lysofibrin, Novo Industri A/S, Copenhagen, Denmark) is now commercially available. The labeling procedure is simple[1-5] and the [^{99m}Tc]plasmin (500 μCi) is injected intravenously. The radioactivity in the legs is measured 5 and 30 minutes after the intravenous injection, over points marked at 6 to 7 cm on the thigh and calf (five thigh and six calf patients). Each leg point is measured for the same time, usually 10 seconds. Counts between 2000 and 5000 are obtained at each leg point.

The range of normal activity ratio in the plasmin test has been defined as

$$0.475 < \frac{C_R}{C_R + C_L} < 0.525 \tag{1}$$

where C_R are the counts at a measuring point on the right leg and C_L are the counts at the symmetric point on the left leg. Thus a quotient equal to or larger than 0.525 is regarded as a right-sided predominance, and a quotient equal to or less than 0.475 is regarded as a left-sided predominance. For simplicity the result is expressed in *quotient units* as follows:

$$\frac{100 \times C_R}{C_R + C_L} - 50 \tag{2}$$

where $\geq$ = indicates a right-sided and ≥ 3 a left-sided predominance. The criterion of a positive test is the presence of predominance in three adjacent measuring points on the suspected leg.

Another criterion is also used for a predominance at *one point* in one leg. In this case a quotient larger than 0.625 indicates a right-sided thrombus and a quotient less than 0.365 indicates a left-sided thrombus (in quotient units more than 13 or less than −13, respectively).

Consequently, the plasmin test indicates a pathologic condition when a predominance meets the

Table 77-1. Results of [^{99m}Tc] plasmin test compared with venography

No. of patients	Sensitivity (%)	Specificity (%)	References
93	94	48	Olsson, 1979
105	100	51	Edenbrandt et al., 1982
110	91	33	Adolfsson et al., 1982

one-point or the three-point criterion in at least one of the measuring sequences (at 5 and 30 minutes). Attempts at defining criteria for the diagnosis of bilateral thrombi with symmetric extension have failed.

In a series of 93 patients (95 legs) who had clinically suspected deep vein thrombosis, the [^{99m}Tc]plasmin test, the [^{125}I]fibrinogen test, and venography were performed.[4] The sensitivity and specificity of the [^{99m}Tc]plasmin and [^{125}I]fibrinogen tests were 94% and 97%, respectively. Unfortunately, both tests had a very poor specificity (false positives: 48%). Similar results have been reported by subsequent studies[1,3] (Table 77-1). The low false negative rate, the rapid results (within 1 hour), and the low radiation dose without the need to block the thyroid gland mean that the [^{99m}Tc]plasmin is a good screening test. If the result is negative, further investigation is unnecessary and the patient is saved from venography. Another advantage is the lack of danger of hepatitis because pigs cannot be infected by human hepatitis virus.

REFERENCES

1. Adolfsson, L., Nordenfelt, I., Olsson, H., and Torstensson, I.: Diagnosis of deep vein thrombosis with ^{99m}Tc plasmin, Acta Med. Scand. 211:365, 1982.
2. Deacon, J.M., Ell, P.J., Anderson, P., and Khan, O.: Technetium ^{99m}-plasmin: a new test for the detection of deep vein thrombosis. Br. J. Radiol. 53:673, 1980.
3. Edenbrandt, C., Nilsson, J., and Ohlin, P.: Diagnosis of deep venous thrombosis by phlebography and ^{99m}Tc-plasmin, Acta Med. Scand. 53:59, 1982.
4. Olsson, C.: On the diagnosis of deep vein thrombosis. Dissertation submitted to the Department of Clinical Physiology, University of Lund, Lund, Sweden, 1979.
5. Olsson, C.: ^{99m}Tc-plasmin: development and current status. In Nicolaides, A.N., and Yao, J.S.T., editors: The investigation of vascular disorders, Edinburgh, 1980, Churchill Livingstone.
6. Ouchi, H., and Warren, R.: Detection of intravascular thrombi by means of ^{131}I-labelled plasmin, Surgery 51:42, 1962.
7. Persson, R.B.R., and Darte, L.: ^{99m}Tc-plasmin. Int. J. Appl. Radiat. Isot. 28:97, 1977.

CHAPTER 78

Comparative value of tests for the diagnosis of venous thrombosis

RUSSELL D. HULL and JACK HIRSH

It is now widely accepted that the clinical diagnosis of venous thrombosis is inaccurate because of the low sensitivity and specificity of clinical findings.[16,17,42,48,51] The low sensitivity occurs because many potentially dangerous venous thrombi are nonobstructive and not associated with vessel wall inflammation or inflammation of the surrounding perivascular tissues and consequently have no detectable clinical manifestations. Clinical diagnosis is nonspecific because none of the symptoms or signs of venous thrombosis are unique to this condition and all can be caused by nonthrombotic disorders. The exception is the patient with phlegmasia cerulea dolens, in whom the diagnosis of massive iliofemoral thrombosis is clinically obvious and usually requires no further investigation. This syndrome constitutes less than 1% of patients who have clinically suspected venous thrombosis. In the vast majority of patients the symptoms and signs are less overt, and in more than 50% of these patients the clinical suspicion is not confirmed by objective tests.[16,17,42] It should be emphasized that patients with relatively minor symptoms and signs may have extensive venous thrombi, whereas patients with marked symptoms and signs suggesting deep vein thrombosis frequently have no objective evidence of venous thrombosis. Because of its nonspecificity, clinical diagnosis can no longer be used to make management decisions in patients who are suspected to have venous thrombosis.

The potential disadvantages of investigating all patients with clinically suspected venous thrombosis are the expense of investigation, the inconvenience to the patient, and the possible morbidity caused by the test. All of these potential disadvantages are outweighed by the advantages of investigating all patients. Thus the cost of investigation is substantially less than the cost of unnecessary hospital admission or prolongation of hospital stay and of unnecessary anticoagulant therapy in patients who have an incorrect diagnosis made.[29] The inconvenience of investigation is also minimal compared to the inconvenience of unnecessary hospitalization and treatment. Although there is some morbidity associated with venography,[6] there is virtually none associated with the noninvasive tests that can be used as an alternative to venography in the majority of patients with clinically suspected venous thrombosis. Furthermore, even the morbidity from venography is much less than the morbidity associated with anticoagulant therapy.

VENOGRAPHY

Venography is now generally accepted as the standard objective method for the diagnosis of venous thrombosis.[45,54] Although this method of investigation has been used for more than 30 years,[4] its widespread application has been delayed because the fallibility of clinical diagnosis has only been accepted in recent years.

Venography is not readily repeatable and therefore is not a suitable screening test for subclinical venous thrombosis. A number of methods for performing venography have been described.[45,54] With good technique, ascending venography outlines the deep venous system of the legs including the external and common iliac veins in most patients. However, common femoral or iliac venography may be needed if the external and common iliac veins are not properly visualized by the ascending technique or if the inferior vena cava needs to be outlined.

Ascending venography. The aim of ascending venography is to inject radiopaque contrast medium into a dorsal foot vein so that the deep venous system of the leg is clearly outlined. A number of techniques have been described for performing venograms, and in all techniques the underlying principle is to clearly opacify the deep veins of the leg.[45,54] The quality of venography can be maximized and the frequency of artifacts caused by nonfilling of venous segments reduced by injecting a large volume of dye and paying careful attention to technical detail. Filling of the calf veins is improved if the patient is examined while the table is tilted to 40 degrees from horizontal and if weight bearing on the leg being examined is avoided. The use of fluoroscopic monitoring during injection makes it possible to identify suspicious areas, which can then be examined more closely, and therefore reduces the risk of confusing a flow defect with a filling defect. These flow defects are produced when opacified blood in the major venous channel is mixed with nonopacified blood flowing in from a tributary. Such an artifact can often be distinguished from an intraluminal defect by performing a Valsalva maneuver while the dye is being injected under fluoroscopy.

The use of an ankle tourniquet to promote filling of the deep venous system by obstructing the superficial veins is controversial. Some authorities believe that it may prevent adequate filling of the deep veins and that it is unnecessary when a tilt table is used. However, in some patients with extensive superficial vein varicosities, the overlap produced by these superficial veins may obscure the deep veins; in these patients an ankle tourniquet may occasionally be helpful. The deep femoral vein and the internal iliac veins are usually not adequately visualized by ascending venography even when a Valsalva maneuver is performed.

Iliac venography. Visualization of the external and common iliac veins and the inferior vena cava can be achieved by injecting contrast medium directly into the common femoral vein,[46] by intraosseous injection,[46] or by retrograde injection through a catheter passed via the right atrium and inferior vena cava.[12] The simplest of these techniques is femoral vein puncture. This is usually performed by entering the femoral vein on the nonaffected side and by passing a catheter into the common iliac vein of the affected side using a Seldinger technique. The intraosseous technique is very painful, requires a general anesthetic, and has been reported to produce fatal fat embolism.[46] Retrograde catheterization is more complex than femoral vein puncture, but allows the internal iliac system to be examined and may be combined with pulmonary angiography.

In practice, ascending venography with careful attention to technique provides adequate visualization of the deep veins of the calf, the popliteal vein, and the femoral vein, as well as the external and common iliac veins. Occasionally a direct puncture of the femoral vein is required to clarify the nature of a suspicious defect in the common femoral or iliac veins.

Normal anatomy of the venous system

Accurate interpretation of venography requires a knowledge of the normal anatomy of the venous system and its variations. The venous system in the leg consists of three pairs of deep calf veins, the posterior tibial, the peroneal, and the anterior tibial veins, plus the soleal and gastrocnemius plexus of veins, and the superficial venous system. The soleal plexus drains into the posterior tibial vein, the gastrocnemius plexus drains into the peroneal popliteal veins, and the three pairs of deep calf veins converge to form the popliteal vein. The popliteal vein becomes the superficial femoral vein at the junction of the proximal part of the popliteal fossa and the adductor canal in the thigh. The superficial femoral vein is joined by the deep femoral vein in the upper thigh to form the common femoral vein, which becomes the external iliac vein at the level of the inguinal ligament. The external iliac vein is joined by the internal iliac vein in the pelvis to form the common iliac vein, and the common iliac veins converge to form the inferior vena cava. The superficial venous system consists of two major veins, the long and short saphenous veins, which drain into the common femoral and popliteal veins, respectively. The superficial system is connected with the deep venous system by communicating veins, which contain valves that direct flow from the superficial into the deep system. Several variations of the deep venous system are recognized, the most common being accessory popliteal veins, bifid superficial femoral veins, and an abnormally high or low origin of the popliteal vein.

Criteria for the diagnosis of venous thrombosis

A number of venographic appearances have been defined as criteria for the diagnosis of acute deep vein thrombosis.[45,54] The most reliable criterion is the presence of an intraluminal filling defect that is constant in all films and is seen in a number of projections. Other, less reliable criteria include (1) nonfilling of a segment of the deep venous system with abrupt termination of the column of contrast medium at a constant site below the segment and reappearance of the contrast medium at a constant site above the segment and (2) nonfilling of the deep venous system above the knee despite adequate venographic technique. The likelihood that these appearances are a result of venous thrombosis is increased if the abnormality is associated with the presence of abnormal collateral vessels. The presence of a constant filling defect is usually considered to represent an acute venous thrombosis, whereas the other two abnormalities or variations thereof may be caused by old venous thrombi and may be simulated by artifacts caused by incomplete mixing of contrast medium with blood, external compression of a vein, or injecting the contrast medium too far proximally in the foot.

Pitfalls of venography

Venography is a difficult technique to perform well and requires considerable experience to execute and interpret accurately. Unless care is taken to inject the dye into a dorsal foot vein distally, there may be nonfilling of calf veins, which may be incorrectly interpreted as either being caused by a thrombus (because the vein is not filled) or as normal because a filling defect is not seen. The common femoral, external iliac, and common iliac veins may not be adequately filled by ascending venography. However, frequently an incorrect diagnosis occurs because an attempt is made to interpret the results of an inadequate venogram. Once again there are two common errors; the first is to fail to detect even a large nonobstructive thrombus in the common femoral region because flow into the external iliac or common iliac vein appears to be adequate, although filling of the common femoral vein is suboptimal. The second is to incorrectly diagnose venous thrombosis because of a streaming effect in the common femoral or iliac veins caused by inadequate opacification. Misinterpreting an inadequate venogram (usually in the direction of a false positive diagnosis of venous thrombosis) is becoming an important problem, since the use of venography is increasing in centers without a special interest or expertise in this technique. It can be avoided if radiologists and clini-

cians are sensitive to the pitfalls of venography and are prepared to either repeat the venogram when the result of the test is inadequate or to base the diagnosis on the results of noninvasive tests.

Side effects of venography

Venography is an invasive procedure that may produce pain in the foot while the dye is being injected or pain in the calf 1 or 2 days after injection.[6] The radiopaque contrast medium has been shown to damage endothelial cells, and both the early pain and the delayed pain associated with injection of contrast medium are probably related to direct damage of the venous endothelium.[6]

This may result in superficial phlebitis and even in deep vein thrombosis in a small percentage of patients who have normal venograms. In our experience, 3% to 4% of patients who have negative venograms develop a positive fibrinogen leg scan after venography and about 1% to 2% develop clinically significant venous thrombosis. Others have reported a higher frequency of postphlebographic positive fibrinogen leg scan results,[1] but these differences could be a result of differences in venographic technique or in the patient population under study. It is possible, for example, that the frequency of postvenographic positive leg scan results is higher in patients who remain immobilized after venography because the thrombogenic effects of venous damage produced by the radiopaque contrast medium are combined with venous stasis.

Other less common complications of venography include hypersensitivity reactions to the radiopaque dye and local skin and tissue necrosis caused by extravasation of dye at the site of injection.[6] Many of these side effects of venography can be avoided by careful attention to detail. Care should be taken to ensure that the needle through which the dye is injected is firmly implanted in the vein and that the dye is not injected under pressure. Local pain can be reduced if lidocaine is mixed with the radiopaque material, and postvenographic phlebitis can be reduced if the leg is elevated after venography and the dye washed out with an infusion of 150 to 250 ml of normal or heparinized saline solution. The latter complications can also be reduced if isotonic radiopaque material is used. Unfortunately, however, the only preparation currently available is very expensive. Patients with a history of hypersensitivity to radiopaque dye should not have venography performed.

NONINVASIVE TESTS FOR THE DIAGNOSIS OF VENOUS THROMBOSIS

A number of noninvasive or less invasive techniques for the diagnosis of venous thrombosis have recently been developed. Of these, three have been most carefully evaluated: [^{125}I]fibrinogen leg scanning,[14,43] impedance plethysmography,[23,38,39,59,60] and Doppler ultrasonography.[13,22,54,56] Details of the methodology of these techniques are presented elsewhere in this volume. Each of these three tests has different applications depending on whether the patient has clinically suspected venous thrombosis or is being screened because of a high risk of developing venous thrombosis. A number of other diagnostic techniques, including other forms of plethysmography,[3] thermography,[10] and various isotopic methods,[20,37] have been evaluated to a limited extent. Sensitive blood tests that detect intravascular fibrin formation and lysis are currently also undergoing clinical evaluation and may be of clinical value.

[^{125}I] fibrinogen leg scanning

Principles. The diagnosis of venous thrombosis by radioiodine-labeled fibrinogen scanning depends on incorporation of circulating labeled fibrinogen into the thrombus, which is then detected by measuring the increase of overlying surface radioactivity with an isotope detector. The feasibility of this technique was demonstrated in animals[21] and in humans[52] in the early 1960s, but the method has been extensively evaluated only recently. The equipment used initially for external scanning was cumbersome, but in the last few years portable, convenient, and accurate equipment has become available so that the test can be performed at the patient's bedside.

Fibrinogen scanning can be used expectantly for screening medical and surgical patients who are at high risk of developing venous thrombosis. It can also be used to complement impedance plethysmography to confirm or exclude the diagnosis of clinically suspected venous thrombosis.

Fibrinogen leg scanning detects over 90% of acute calf vein thrombi,[14,18,41,43] but only between 60% and 80% of proximal vein thrombi, depending on their location. Leg scanning is relatively insensitive in the upper thigh and is insensitive to venous thrombi in the pelvis.[18,40]

Potential limitations of the [^{125}I]fibrinogen test. The test is insensitive to thrombi in the pelvic veins[18,41] because ^{125}I is a relatively low-energy gamma emitter and is unreliable in the upper thigh because of the proximity to the bladder, which frequently contains radioactive urine, and the presence of large veins and arteries, which produce an increase in the background count. [^{125}I]fibrinogen scanning is contraindicated during pregnancy and lactation and should not be used in young patients unless very definite indications exist.

Causes of discrepancy between results of leg scanning and venography. A leg scan abnormality in the presence of a normal venogram may be a result of hematoma, inflammation, uptake into a surgical wound, or nonvisualization of thrombus by the venogram. A false negative scan may occur in patients with an old venous thrombus that is no longer taking up fibrinogen, when a thrombus forms at a time when most radioactive fibrinogen has been cleared from the circulation, when the thrombus is too small to be detected by leg scanning, or when the thrombus is isolated in a common femoral or iliac vein.

Impedance plethysmography

Principles. Plethysmography is a noninvasive method that detects volume changes in the leg. Several plethysmographic techniques, including impedance plethysmography (IPG),[23,39,60] strain-gauge plethysmography,[3] and air cuff plethysmography,[11] have been used, but IPG has been most thoroughly evaluated.

IPG is sensitive and specific for thrombosis of the popliteal, femoral, or iliac veins (proximal veins) but is relatively insensitive to calf vein thrombosis. The principle of the method is based on the observation that blood volume changes in the calf, produced by maximum respiratory effort or by inflation or deflation of a pneumatic thigh cuff, result in changes in electrical resistance (impedance). These changes are reduced in patients with thrombosis of the popliteal or more proximal veins. The original method,[59] which used maximum respiratory effort, had shortcomings because sick patients were frequently unable to cooperate sufficiently for the test to be reliable. The test was therefore modified by using a pneumatic cuff to temporarily occlude the venous outflow (occlusive IPG).[60] This modified test is sensitive and specific for proximal vein thrombosis.[23,60]

Occlusive cuff IPG is performed with the patient in the supine position and with the lower limb elevated 25 to 30 degrees, the knee flexed 10 to 20 degrees, and the ankle 8 to 15 cm higher than the knee. A pneumatic cuff 15 cm in width is applied to the midthigh and inflated to 45 cm H_2O, thereby occluding venous return. After a predetermined period of time, the cuff is rapidly deflated, and the changes in electrical resistance (impedance) resulting from alterations in blood volume distal to the cuff are detected by circumferential calf electrodes and recorded on an electrocardiogram paper strip. The changes in impedance during cuff inflation and deflation are measured, and both the total rise during cuff inflation and the fall occurring in the first 3 seconds of deflation are plotted on a two-way IPG graph. The graph includes a "discriminant line," which was developed by a discriminant function analysis to provide optimal separation of the IPG results in normal and abnormal[23] legs for proximal vein thrombosis (Fig. 78-1).

The accuracy of IPG is critically dependent on the degree of venous filling during cuff occlusion.[25] The occlusive cuff test, as originally performed, used a 45-second occlusion time. However, it was noted that venous filling was frequently suboptimal after only 45 seconds of cuff occlusion and that, when this occurred, the accuracy of the test was compromised. Venous filling was improved by pro-

longing the period of cuff occlusion from 45 seconds to 2 minutes and by introducing repeated sequential testing. Prolonging the occlusion time to 120 seconds ensured that maximum venous filling occurred in each patient for any single test, and repeated sequential testing produced an increase in venous capacity by promoting stress relaxation of the vessel wall. These maneuvers increase both venous filling and the sensitivity and specificity of the test. It was noted that if venous filling increased there was a corresponding increase in venous emptying in normal legs but not in legs with proximal vein thrombosis, so that the regression lines relating venous filling and emptying (Fig. 78-2) in normal and abnormal legs diverged significantly ($p < .001$). Thus increased venous filling increased the separation between normal and abnormal IPG results and enhanced the accuracy of the test.

When sequential tests are performed, four patterns of IPG response are observed (Fig. 78-3). In 76% of legs that are normal by venography, the initial test in the sequence falls above the discriminant line, as do all subsequent tests. However, in 20% of legs normal by venography, the initial 45-

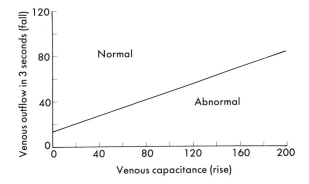

Fig. 78-1. IPG scoring graph with discriminant line. Numbers on horizontal and vertical axes refer to impedance units.

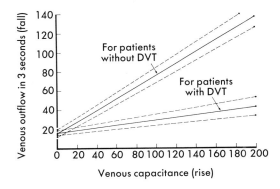

Fig. 78-2. Relationship between venous filling (IPG rise) and venous emptying (IPG fall) in patients with and without proximal deep vein thrombosis (DVT). As venous filling improves, regression lines expressing relationship between venous filling and emptying diverge and are significantly different for patients with and without proximal vein thrombosis ($p < .001$). Broken lines indicate 95% confidence limits. (From Hull, R., et al.: Circulation 58:898, 1978. By permission of the American Heart Association, Inc.)

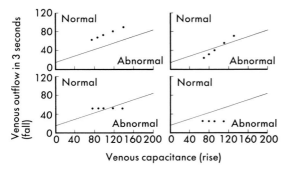

Fig. 78-3. Four patterns of IPG response observed in patients with and without proximal DVT using occlusive-cuff IPG technique with sequential testing and prolonged cuff occlusion. In 76% of legs normal by venography, initial tests fall above discriminant line, as do all subsequent tests *(a)*. In 20% of legs normal by venography, initial tests fall below discriminant line *(b)*, but subsequent tests, including test with highest rise and greatest fall, land in normal zone above line. In 10% of legs with proximal DVT, initial tests fall above line *(c)*. However, subsequent tests, including test with highest rise and greatest fall, lie below line in abnormal zone. This pattern of improved venous filling without corresponding improvement in venous emptying is commonly seen in patients with obstructive proximal venous thrombosis, resulting in fixed venous outflow. In 82% of legs with proximal DVT, initial tests and all subsequent tests fall below discriminant line *(d)*.

second test falls below the discriminant line, but when venous filling is improved by prolonging the cuff occlusion time and by performing sequential tests, the subsequent test results fall above the discriminant line. In 82% of legs that show proximal vein thrombosis by venography, the initial test and all subsequent tests fall below the discriminant line. However, in 10% the initial tests fall above the discriminant line, but as venous filling improves, it is not accompanied by corresponding improvement in venous emptying, and the tests fall below the discriminant line. This latter pattern is sometimes seen in patients with nonobstructive proximal vein thrombi. In a prospective study of 324 patients, it was found that termination of the IPG evaluation after a single 45-second occlusion time was associated with a deterioration of specificity of 20% and sensitivity of 10%. Because sequential testing is time consuming, we performed an additional study to determine whether the sequential approach could be simplified without loss of accuracy. On analysis of patients who had an abnormal IPG result and proximal vein thrombosis by venography, a "normal zone" was identified above a "stop line" parallel to the discriminant line, which allowed the multiple test sequence to be

terminated early without loss of accuracy when any test in the sequence fell above this line (Fig. 78-4). Using this approach, the IPG test sequence could have been terminated without loss of accuracy in 44% of normal patients after one test, in 59% after two tests, or in 80% after three tests.

Unrecognized contraction of leg muscles in either nervous patients or after surgery, particularly in patients with postoperative pain, is a recognized cause of false positive IPG results. The inexperienced technician and, on occasion, the experienced technician may have difficulty in distinguishing an abnormal IPG result caused by venous thrombosis from that caused by isometric muscle contraction. Since isometric muscle contraction can be measured directly by electromyography, we investigated the potential clinical value of using electromyography to detect leg muscle contraction that interferes with the IPG result.[7] It was found that voluntarily induced leg muscle contraction that altered the IPG tracing for venous filling or emptying could always be detected when the electrodes were placed both laterally and medially over the distal thigh and when a ground electrode was placed over the patella. This approach detected a threshold of isometric muscle contraction below which false positive IPG results did not occur and above which there was a very high frequency of false positive IPG results (Fig. 78-5). The attachment of the electromyograph device to the IPG machine proved to be clinically feasible, and the additional time taken to apply the skin electrodes to perform the measurements was less than 5 minutes.

Causes of discrepancy between IPG and venography. IPG only detects thrombi that produce obstruction to venous outflow. Therefore the test will not detect most calf vein thrombi, since they do not obstruct the main outflow tract, and it may not detect small nonocclusive proximal vein thrombi. The test may also be negative when proximal vein thrombosis is associated with well-developed collateral vessels.

IPG does not distinguish between thrombotic and nonthrombotic obstruction to venous outflow. Thus false positive results may be obtained if (1) a patient is positioned incorrectly or inadequately relaxed, because these positions result in constriction of veins by contracting leg muscles; (2) the vein is compressed by an extravascular mass; or (3) venous outflow is impaired by raised central venous pressure. Reduced arterial inflow to the limb caused by severe obstructive arterial disease can

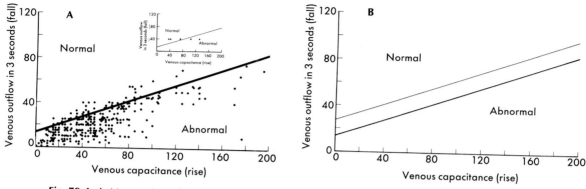

Fig. 78-4. *A,* Many points of tests early in IPG sequence of patients with proximal vein thrombosis fall above discriminant line. *B,* Second line (stop line) was drawn above and parallel to discriminant line so that it enclosed these points. Validity of this stop line was then confirmed prospectively.

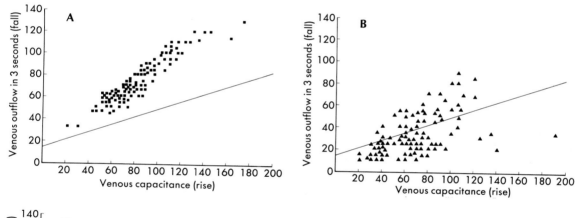

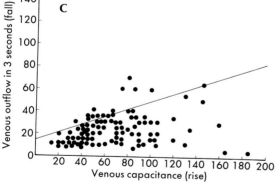

Fig. 78-5. Effects of three different levels of muscle contraction on IPG result in 100 legs with normal baseline IPG results. Test results above discriminant line are in normal zone, whereas those below line are in abnormal zone. *A,* Electromyographic readings between 0 and 25 units (mild leg muscle tension)—all IPG results are in the normal zone. *B,* Electromyographic readings between 25 and 50 units (moderate leg muscle tension)—65% of IPG results are in abnormal zone. *C,* Electromyographic readings above 50 units (severe leg muscle tension)—89% of IPG results are in abnormal zone. (From Biland, L., et al.: Thromb. Res. 14:811, 1979.)

also lead to reduced outflow and thus produce a false positive result.

Doppler ultrasonography

Principle. The Doppler ultrasound flowmeter examination is a noninvasive method that has been evaluated as a diagnostic test in patients with clinically suspected deep vein thrombosis.[55-57] In expert hands, Doppler ultrasound is a sensitive method for detecting proximal vein thrombosis but is less sensitive to calf vein thrombosis.

Positive Doppler examination. The Doppler flowmeter is highly sensitive to occluding thrombi in the popliteal and more proximal veins, but less sensitive to calf vein thrombi and nonocclusive proximal thrombi. Obstruction to venous outflow may result in loss of "phasicity" of the venous signal and may produce a continuous venous signal because of loss of the normal respiratory fluctuation. In addition, augmentation of the venous signal that normally occurs as a result of compression of the limb distal to the probe or to release of compression proximal to the probe may be diminished, may be high pitched and of short duration, or may be absent.

Causes of discrepancy between Doppler ultrasound and venography. The Doppler flowmeter method has many of the limitations of IPG. Thus it is relatively insensitive to calf vein thrombosis and may fail to detect small, partly occluding proximal vein thrombi. The technique is simple and rapid, but interpretation of results is much more dependent on the experience of the examiner than is IPG. False positive results may be obtained if the underlying vein is obstructed by compressing it with the transducer or if compression over the femoral vein or calf is carried out when the limb is drained of blood. False positive results may also be produced by incorrectly positioning the patient, since this leads to an absence or a decrease of the augmentation sound.

Other noninvasive techniques for the diagnosis of venous thrombosis

A number of other diagnostic techniques have been less intensively evaluated for the diagnosis of venous thrombosis, including phleborrheography (aircuff plethysmography),[11] strain-gauge plethysmography,[3] thermography,[10] radioisotope venography,[20,37] and blood tests that reflect intravascular fibrin formation and fibrin proteolysis. Initial stud-

ies with phleborrheography and strain-gauge plethysmography suggest that both techniques are sensitive to proximal vein thrombosis. Phleborrheography has the disadvantage that its interpretation is subjective. Promising initial results have been reported with thermography, but further studies are required before its value and limitations can be adequately assessed. Radioisotope venography is also a promising approach, but like thermography, this technique requires more adequate evaluation before its role as a practical test for the diagnosis of venous thrombosis can be determined. Sensitive and specific tests for intravascular fibrin formation and fibrin proteolysis have now been developed, but are not yet available for routine use because they are technically difficult to perform. These tests, which include the radioimmunoassay of fibrinopeptide A[61] and fragment E[62] of fibrin, are sensitive to acute venous thrombosis, but because of their very nature are nonspecific.

APPLICATION OF NONINVASIVE TESTS FOR THE DIAGNOSIS OF CLINICALLY SUSPECTED VENOUS THROMBOSIS

The objective noninvasive diagnostic tests that have been adequately evaluated in patients with clinically suspected venous thrombosis are [^{125}I]fibrinogen leg scanning, IPG, and Doppler ultrasonography. None of these tests used alone is as accurate as venography for the diagnosis of clinically suspected venous thrombosis. When used in appropriate combinations, however, these tests can replace venography in the majority of patients who have symptoms or signs suggestive of venous thrombosis. Venography may still be required when the patient has a clinical condition known to produce a false positive result with one of the noninvasive tests (for example, arterial insufficiency or congestive cardiac failure, which are known to produce false positive results with IPG, or trauma to the leg, which may produce a false positive result with [^{125}I]fibrinogen leg scanning).

[^{125}I] fibrinogen leg scanning

[^{125}I]fibrinogen leg scanning defects calf vein thrombi and thrombi in the distal half of the thigh that are actively accreting fibrin at the time of injection of ^{125}I-labeled fibrinogen. False positive results occur if scanning is performed over a hematoma, over an area of inflammation, or where there is extensive edema, but in the absence of these conditions, leg scanning is both sensitive and specific for acute calf and lower thigh vein thrombosis.

[^{125}I]fibrinogen leg scanning should never be used as the only diagnostic test in patients with clinically suspected venous thrombosis because it fails to detect many high proximal vein thrombi and because there may be a delay of hours or even days before sufficient amounts of fibrinogen accumulate in the thrombus to make the test positive. For practical purposes, these problems are overcome when [^{125}I]fibrinogen leg scanning is used to complement IPG in patients with clinically suspected venous thrombosis.[24]

IPG

A number of studies have evaluated IPG in patients with clinically suspected venous thromboembolism.[24,25,39,60] Wheeler et al.[60] compared results of IPG with venography in 168 legs. IPG was normal in 106 of 108 legs that were normal by venography and abnormal in 40 of 41 legs with venographically demonstrated recent thrombi of the popliteal, femoral, or iliac veins (proximal vein thrombosis). There were 19 calf vein thrombi detected by venography, and IPG identified only three. Johnston and Kakkar,[38] using a similar technique, detected all 20 proximal vein thrombi with IPG, which was normal in 40 of 44 legs without thrombosis and abnormal in only 5 of 15 legs with calf vein thrombi.

In a study we performed on 346 patients with suspected venous thrombosis, the IPG result was abnormal in 124 of 133 limbs that showed proximal vein thrombosis (sensitivity of 93%). Seventy-three of 88 limbs with calf vein thrombosis had a normal IPG result. An abnormal IPG result was found in the absence of thrombosis in 11 of 397 legs, the majority of which had clearly recognizable clinical conditions known to produce false positive results. Thus in patients with clinically suspected venous thrombosis, a positive IPG result can be used to make therapeutic decisions in the absence of clinical conditions known to produce false positive results (for example, congestive cardiac failure, severe peripheral vascular disease, or local leg muscle tension). A normal result essentially excludes a diagnosis of proximal vein thrombosis, but does not exclude a diagnosis of calf vein thrombosis or of a small nonocclusive proximal vein thrombus. As collateral vessels develop or as partial recanalization of the vessel occurs, the IPG may become normal.

Doppler ultrasonography

There have been several carefully performed studies comparing the results of the Doppler flowmeter examination with venography in patients with clinically suspected venous thrombosis. The results of these studies show that this technique is sensitive to proximal vein thrombosis but less sensitive to calf vein thrombosis.[55-57]

This test has both advantages and disadvantages over IPG. Its advantages are that it can be performed more conveniently and rapidly than IPG and is less expensive. The disadvantages of Doppler ultrasound are that its interpretation is subjective and it requires considerable skill and experience to perform reliably and to interpret accurately. This is its major limitation; however, in skilled hands it is almost as sensitive to symptomatic proximal vein thrombosis as is IPG and it is more sensitive to symptomatic calf vein thrombosis, detecting approximately 50% of such patients.

Doppler ultrasound is more reliable than IPG for detecting proximal vein thrombosis in patients with raised central venous pressure or arterial insufficiency and has the advantage that it can be used in patients who have their leg in plaster or who are in traction.

Tests that measure fibrin formation or its lysis in plasma or serum

The presence of intravascular fibrin can be detected by measuring fibrinopeptide A in the plasma or fibrin degradation products in the serum. The fibrinopeptide A assay is only positive if the test is performed while the thrombus is being laid down, whereas tests for fibrin degradation products may remain positive for days after the thrombotic process has been arrested. The standard tests for fibrin degradation products, such as the latex agglutination test, tagged red cell hemagglutination inhibition assay, and staphylococcal clumping, are not sufficiently sensitive to be of clinical value in patients with acute venous thrombosis. However, a recently developed radioimmunoassay for fragment E is sufficiently sensitive to be useful for excluding a diagnosis of acute venous thrombosis. Since both the fibrinopeptide A assay and the radioimmunoassay for fibrin degradation products detect intravascular fibrin formation, they are not specific for the diagnosis of acute venous thrombosis. Either of these tests has the potential to be used in combination with some of the other noninvasive diagnostic tests, but the real value has not yet been determined. The major drawbacks of these tests at present is that they are technically difficult, are not readily available, and take a number of hours to perform. However, if they were simplified, they would provide a valuable addition to the objective diagnosis of venous thrombosis.

PRACTICAL APPROACH TO THE DIAGNOSIS OF VENOUS THROMBOSIS USING NONINVASIVE TESTS IN PATIENTS WITH CLINICALLY SUSPECTED VENOUS THROMBOSIS

The noninvasive tests can be used singly or in combination to either confirm or exclude a clinical suspicion of venous thrombosis. IPG or Doppler ultrasound, when used alone, provides a sensitive approach for detecting proximal vein thrombi. However, both IPG and Doppler ultrasound are insensitive to calf vein thrombi. If the result of the IPG or Doppler ultrasound (performed with the probe placed over the femoral vein) is positive for proximal vein thrombosis in the absence of conditions known to produce false positive results, a diagnosis of venous thrombosis can be confidently made and the patient treated appropriately. If, however, the result of the Doppler ultrasound is only positive with the probe placed over the posterior tibial vein, confirmation should be obtained by venography, since the test is relatively nonspecific at this examination site.[63] If the results of these tests are negative, the clinician is faced with a number of alternatives. These alternatives are (1) to repeat the tests (IPG or Doppler) at intervals to detect extending calf vein thrombi, (2) to perform venography, or (3) to perform [125I]fibrinogen leg scanning.

IPG and [125I]fibrinogen leg scanning. As discussed earlier, IPG has the potential limitation of being insensitive to calf vein thrombosis. We therefore evaluated the combined use of IPG and [125I]fibrinogen leg scanning in 200 patients with clinically suspected venous thrombosis.[24] The investigation went as follows:

On the day of referral each patient was injected with [125I]fibrinogen, and leg scanning was carried out daily for the next 3 days. IPG was performed on the day of referral and then daily for the next 3 days. All patients underwent bilateral ascending

venography, which was scheduled to be performed on the third day if the tests were negative or earlier if either of the tests became positive. Either IPG or leg scanning was positive in 81 of 86 patients with positive venograms (sensitivity 94%), and both tests were negative in 104 of 114 patients who had negative venograms (specificity 91%). These two tests detected all 60 patients with proximal vein thrombosis, 21 of 26 patients with calf vein thrombosis, and 20 of 21 patients with calf vein thrombosis who had symptoms for less than 1 week. The findings of this initial study have been confirmed by a more recent study of 274 additional symptomatic patients.[30] Either IPG or leg scanning was positive in 103 of 114 patients with positive venograms (sensitivity 90%), and both tests were negative in 152 of 160 patients who had negative venograms (specificity 93%).[30]

This approach detected all 78 patients with proximal vein thrombosis, 25 of 36 patients with calf vein thrombosis, and 16 of 17 patients with calf vein thrombosis who had symptoms for less than 1 week.[30]

These results, therefore, confirm the finding of the initial study and indicate that the combined use of IPG and leg scanning provides an important alternative to venography in patients with clinically suspected acute deep vein thrombosis. On the basis of these two studies in patients with clinically suspected venous thrombosis, IPG should be performed first, and if this is positive in the the the absence of any of the clinical conditions known to produce false positive results, the diagnosis of venous thrombosis can be accepted. If it is negative, the patient should be injected with [125I]fibrinogen and scanned for 3 days. If the result of the leg scan becomes positive in the absence of clinical circumstances known to produce a false positive result (for example, hematoma or ruptured Baker's cyst), a diagnosis of venous thrombosis can be made.

It should be noted, however, that use of serial IPG alone has now replaced this combined approach in patients with their first episode of venous thromboembolism.[33] Leg scanning combined with IPG remains a useful approach in selected patients with suspected acute recurrent venous thrombosis.[34]

Repeated examination with IPG or Doppler ultrasound. Our current practical approach to the diagnosis of clinically suspected venous thrombosis favors the use of IPG over Doppler ultrasonography as the main test for this disorder. This is because

IPG is precise and objective, whereas the interpretation of Doppler ultrasonography is subjective and requires considerable skill and experience to perform reliably. Most importantly, however, the use of serial IPG alone has been evaluated recently in a prospective study[33] in which the safety of withholding anticoagulant therapy in patients with negative results after repeated IPG evaluation has been documented by careful long-term follow-up. To date the effectiveness and safety of using Doppler ultrasonography alone have not been formally evaluated.

The rationale of repeated IPG evaluation is based on the premise (now confirmed by observation[33]) that calf vein thrombi are only clinically important when they extend into the proximal veins, at which point detection with IPG is possible. Therefore by performing repeated examinations with IPG in patients with clinically suspected venous thrombosis, it is possible to identify patients with extending calf vein thrombosis who can be treated appropriately. Since extension occurs only in a minority of patients with calf vein thrombosis (approximately 20%), by detecting only those patients with extending calf vein thrombosis, treatment is confined to those patients who will best benefit. An alternative approach is to detect and treat all calf vein thrombi by adding leg scanning in the diagnostic approach, but this may do more harm than good because the potential benefit of anticoagulant therapy may be outweighed by the risk of bleeding.

We have recently completed a randomized clinical trial comparing combined IPG and [^{125}I]fibrinogen leg scanning with serial IPG alone for the diagnosis of clinically suspected venous thrombosis.[33] The results of this study indicate that IPG performed on the day of referral and, if negative, repeated the following day, again on the fifth to seventh day, on the tenth day, and on day 14, is as effective as the combined approach of IPG and leg scanning in the diagnosis of clinically suspected venous thrombosis. Furthermore, the clinical outcomes observed on long-term follow-up indicate that it is safe to withhold anticoagulant therapy in patients who remain negative by serial IPG for 14 days.[33]

A diagnostic algorithm for the noninvasive diagnosis of clinically suspected venous thrombosis is shown in Fig. 78-6. IPG is performed immediately on referral; if it is positive in the absence of clinical conditions that are known to produce falsely positive results, the diagnosis of venous throm-

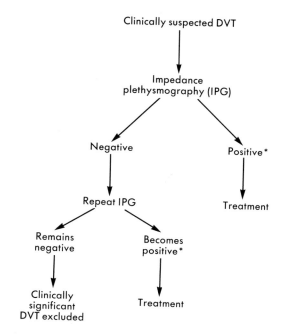

Fig. 78-6. Practical noninvasive approach for diagnosis of clinically suspected DVT using serial IPG. *Indicates absence of conditions known to produce false positive IPG result (for example, congestive cardiac failure).

bosis is established and the patient is treated accordingly. If the result of the initial IPG evaluation is negative, anticoagulant therapy is withheld, and the IPG is repeated the following day, again at the fifth to seventh days, the tenth day, and day 14. If the IPG becomes positive during this time, a diagnosis of venous thrombosis is made and anticoagulant therapy is commenced. A positive IPG in the presence of conditions known to produce a false positive result (for example, congestive cardiac failure) should be confirmed by venography.

If noninvasive tests for the diagnosis of venous thrombosis are not available, then a clinical suspicion of venous thrombosis should be objectively confirmed or excluded by performing ascending venography.

DIFFERENTIAL DIAGNOSIS IN PATIENTS WITH SUSPECTED DEEP VEIN THROMBOSIS

The differential diagnosis in patients who have clinically suspected venous thrombosis includes muscle strain (usually associated with unaccustomed exercise), direct twisting injury to the leg, vasomotor changes in a paralyzed leg, venous reflux, lymphangitis, lymphatic obstruction, muscle tear, Baker's cyst, cellulitis, internal derangement of the knee, hematoma, heart failure, and the post-phlebitic syndrome.[28] It is frequently not possible to establish an alternate diagnosis at the time of referral, but without objective testing it is not possible to rule out venous thrombosis.[28] It is often possible, however, to determine the cause of symptoms by careful follow-up once the diagnosis of venous thrombosis has been ruled out.[28] In some patients the cause of pain, tenderness, and swelling remains uncertain even after careful follow-up and is presumably a result of inflammation of other soft tissues of the leg.[28]

DIAGNOSIS OF ACUTE RECURRENT VENOUS THROMBOSIS

When patients report symptoms of pain, tenderness, or swelling in the leg that has been the site of proven or suspected previous venous thrombosis, it may be difficult to distinguish between acute recurrent thrombosis and the nonthrombotic complication of chronic venous insufficiency.

The patient with clinically suspected recurrent deep vein thrombosis presents a diagnostic challenge for the clinician because the clinical diagnosis of recurrent deep vein thrombosis is highly nonspecific, and because each of the objective diagnostic tests for deep vein thrombosis has potential limitations in this context. Recurrent leg symptoms following deep vein thrombosis may be caused by acute recurrent deep vein thrombosis, the postphlebitic syndrome, or a variety of non-thrombotic disorders. Differentiation between these three causes for recurrent leg symptoms is important because anticoagulant therapy is not required in patients with either the postphlebitic syndrome or a nonthrombotic cause for leg symptoms.

Venography alone has the limitation that the diagnostic hallmark, a constant intraluminal filling defect, may be masked because of obliteration and recanalization leading to impaired visualization. Consequently, the venographic findings may be inconclusive in patients with previous disease. IPG may be falsely positive because of persistent venous outflow obstruction resulting from a previous episode of venous thrombosis, or falsely negative because of large collateral channels that have developed consequent to the first episode. Leg scanning with [125I]fibrinogen is useful for detecting active calf and distal thigh vein thrombi, but is relatively insensitive in the upper thigh and cannot detect external and common iliac vein thrombi.

Evaluation of objective testing for suspected recurrent deep vein thrombosis

We have recently completed a cohort analytic study[34] incorporating long-term follow-up of 270 patients with symptoms and signs of acute recurrent deep vein thrombosis who were evaluated by combined IPG and [125I]fibrinogen leg scanning plus venography. The results of this study are of considerable clinical relevance because, for the first time, the clinician is provided with a practical approach to the patient with clinically suspected recurrent deep vein thrombosis.

Conventional methods could not be used to assess the accuracy of this diagnostic approach in this condition because of the lack of an acceptable reference standard for the diagnosis of acute recurrent venous thrombosis. In our study this problem was overcome by establishing a priori diagnostic criteria for the presence or absence of acute recurrence and then testing their validity by recording outcome on long-term follow-up. At the onset of the study, we decided to withhold anticoagulant therapy in patients with negative results by IPG and leg scanning, irrespective of the severity or extent of the clinical findings.

The diagnostic approach that we evaluated is outlined in Fig. 78-7. IPG was performed immediately on referral; if the results were negative, the patient was injected with [125I]fibrinogen and leg scanning was performed 1 and 3 days later, at which time the IPG was also repeated. Anticoagulant therapy was withheld in all patients whose results remained negative by noninvasive testing. If the initial IPG was positive, venography was performed. Anticoagulant therapy was begun in all patients with positive results by IPG in whom venography detected a constant intraluminal filling defect. If a constant intraluminal filling defect was not detected by venography, the patient was injected with [125I]fibrinogen and leg scanning was performed 1 and 3 days later. Anticoagulant therapy was begun if the [125I]fibrinogen leg scan result was positive. All patients were then followed up long-term at 3 months and 12 months.

One hundred and eighty-one of 270 patients (67%) had negative IPG and leg scan results (Fig. 78-7); 89 patients had positive IPG and leg scan results.[34] Anticoagulant therapy was withheld in all 181 patients with negative noninvasive testing results. On long-term follow-up, none of the 181 patients died from pulmonary emoblism and only 3 patients (1.7%) returned with objectively documented recurrent venous thromboembolism. In

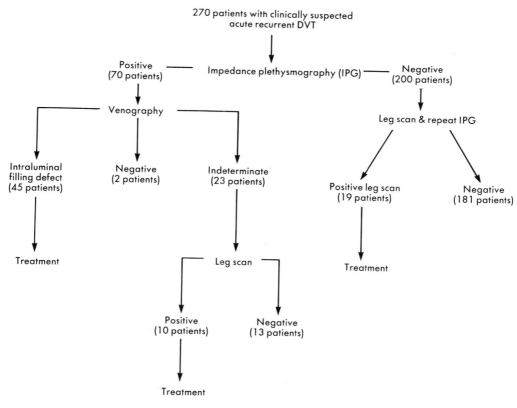

Fig. 78-7. Diagnostic process and outcome on entry in 270 patients with clinically suspected acute recurrent DVT.

contrast, 18 of 89 patients (20%) with positive IPG or leg scan results had new episodes of objectively documented venous thromboembolism, including 4 deaths (4.5%) from massive pulmonary embolism (p < .001). The results on long-term follow-up indicate that a combined approach of noninvasive testing and venography can be used to separate patients with clinically suspected recurrent deep vein thrombosis into two groups: a negative cohort in whom it is safe to withhold anticoagulant therapy and a positive cohort who require anticoagulant therapy.[57]

Clinical utility. Our diagnostic approach has high clinical utility, as definitive management was established in 95% of the 270 patients.[34] Of the 270 patients, 67% (181 patients) were spared the need for anticoagulant therapy. A definitive indication for anticoagulant therapy was established in 28% (76 patients) on the basis of positive results by IPG, leg scanning, or venography. In the remaining 5% (13 patients) with a positive IPG, an indeterminate venogram result, and a negative leg scan, acute recurrent venous thromboembolism could not be confidently ruled out. It can be argued that these patients should be treated because leg scanning is insensitive in the upper thigh and cannot detect external and common iliac vein thrombi. Given the infrequency of this combination of test results, it would be prudent to err on the side of treating these patients rather than to risk death from massive pulmonary embolism.

Differential diagnosis. In patients with recurrent leg symptoms in whom the diagnosis of acute recurrent deep vein thrombosis has been ruled out by objective testing, the differential diagnosis includes the postphlebitic syndrome and a variety of nonthrombotic causes. The presence of the postphlebitic syndrome is suggested by the presence of venous insufficiency. Incompetence of the valves of the deep veins resulting in venous insufficiency can be demonstrated by Doppler ultrasonography or by a variety of plethysmographic techniques. Nonthrombotic causes for leg symptoms should be considered when both recurrent deep vein thrombosis and the postphlebitic syndrome have been ruled out. The nonthrombotic causes for recurrent leg symptoms are essentially the same as those which are considered in patients with a first episode of clinically suspected deep vein thrombosis. In many patients, however, in whom both acute recurrence and the postphlebitic syndrome have been ruled out, a cause for leg symptoms is not identified. In these patients a diagnosis of thromboneurosis should be considered.

Thromboneurosis is a common but poorly recognized clinical syndrome that may simulate acute recurrent venous thrombosis. It occurs most frequently in patients with a morbid fear of the complications of venous thromboembolism. Thromboneurosis may occur both in patients with a previous episode of venous thrombosis documented by objective testing and in patients who were originally misdiagnosed with false positive results.

The clinical presentation of thromboneurosis includes leg pain and tenderness, and, in its most severe form, the patient may be totally incapacitated by the fear of recurrent venous thromboembolism, limb loss, and even death.

Patients with thromboneurosis frequently have a history of multiple hospital admissions for the treatment of ''recurrent venous thrombosis.'' Because of the recurrent nature of the episodes, many patients are maintained on long-term anticoagulant therapy, and some have had vena caval interruption performed. It should be emphasized that thromboneurosis is often iatrogenic in origin, and the patient's fear of recurrence is reinforced by admission to the hospital and treatment on clinical suspicion alone. Thromboneurosis can be prevented by ensuring that a clinical suspicion of acute venous thrombosis is always confirmed or excluded by objective testing.

PRACTICAL APPROACH TO THE DIAGNOSIS OF ACUTE RECURRENT VENOUS THROMBOSIS

A diagnosis of acute recurrent venous thrombosis can be made by IPG if it can be demonstrated that the test result was negative before presentation and is positive at the time of presentation. The presence of a previously normal IPG result greatly simplifies the practical diagnostic approach in patients with clinically suspected acute recurrent deep vein thrombosis.

Recurrent venous thromboembolism on adequate anticoagulant therapy is rare (less than

2%),[27,31,32] and the majority of patients who have a recurrence do so after a discontinuation of 3 months of anticoagulant therapy. In our experience 60% of patients with their first episode of extensive proximal deep vein thrombosis have a normal IPG result at the time of discontinuation of anticoagulant therapy at 3 months.[36] For this reason, we perform a baseline IPG evaluation at the time of discontinuation of long-term anticoagulant therapy in all patients with deep vein thrombosis.

Diagnostic approach in patients with a previously normal IPG result

The diagnostic algorithm for the diagnosis of clinically suspected recurrent deep vein thrombosis in patients with a previously normal IPG is shown in Fig. 78-8. We perform IPG immediately on referral and, if results are negative, anticoagulant therapy is withheld. [125I]fibrinogen leg scanning is performed daily for 72 hours, together with IPG. If the results of both IPG and leg scanning remain negative, the diagnosis of acute recurrence is excluded and the need for anticoagulant therapy avoided.

If the result of either IPG or leg scanning is positive in the absence of conditions known to produce false positive test results, a diagnosis of acute recurrent venous thrombosis is established and the patient is treated accordingly. A positive leg scan result in the presence of conditions known to produce a false positive scan (for example, hematoma) should be confirmed by venography. Venography should also be performed in patients with a concurrent condition that is known to produce a false positive IPG result (for example, congestive cardiac failure).

Diagnostic approach in patients with a previously abnormal or unknown IPG result

The diagnostic algorithm for suspected recurrent venous thrombosis in patients with a previously abnormal or unknown IPG result is shown in Figs. 78-8 and 78-9. If on referral the result of IPG is positive, then venography should be performed (Fig. 78-8) because the abnormal IPG does not distinguish between acute recurrent deep vein thrombosis and chronic venous outflow obstruction. If the venogram demonstrates a new constant intraluminal filling defect at a site not involved on the previous venogram, the diagnosis of acute recurrent deep vein thrombosis is established (Fig. 78-9). If the findings of venography are unchanged

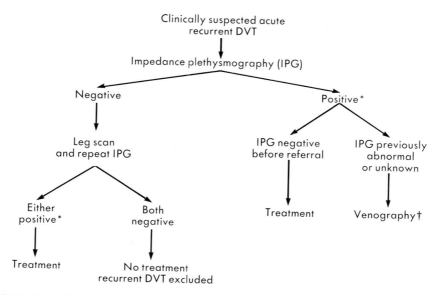

Fig. 78-8. Practical diagnostic approach in patients with clinically suspected acute recurrent DVT. *Indicates absence of conditions known to produce false positive test result. †Indicates management of results by venography shown in Fig. 78-9.

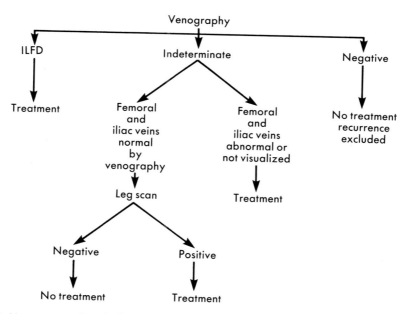

Fig. 78-9. Management of results by venography in patients with clinically suspected acute recurrent DVT. *ILFD,* Intraluminal filling defect.

or indeterminate but the common femoral and iliac veins are well visualized and normal, the patient should be injected with [^{125}I]fibrinogen and leg scanning should be performed for 72 hours. If the results of leg scanning remain negative, acute recurrent venous thrombosis can be excluded and anticoagulant therapy withheld (Fig. 78-9).

Patients with a positive IPG result, indeterminate findings by venography that include the common femoral or iliac veins (but in whom no new intraluminal filling defects can be seen), and a negative leg scan result present a diagnostic dilemma. In these patients, acute recurrence cannot be confidently excluded, and given the infrequency of this combination of test results, we prefer to err on the side of treatment rather than risk death from massive pulmonary embolism (Fig. 78-9).

The management of negative test results in patients in whom the previous IPG result was abnormal or unknown is the same as outlined for patients with a previously negative IPG (Fig. 78-8).

THE USE OF NONINVASIVE TESTS FOR SCREENING HIGH-RISK PATIENTS
[^{125}I] fibrinogen leg scanning

A number of researchers* have compared results of expectant scanning and venography in general surgical and medical patients and have reported agreement between the results of these two techniques in about 90% of the cases. Leg scanning has major limitations when used to screen patients for thrombosis after leg surgery. This is because extravascular isotope accumulation in the hematoma and the healing wound invariably leads to scan abnormalities at the site of surgery, so that thrombi near the wound cannot be detected. This is an important limitation, since up to 20% of all thrombi (in about 10% of all patients) develop as isolated thrombi in the femoral vein close to the surgical wound.

Harris et al.[18] reported on the accuracy of [^{125}I]fibrinogen leg scanning in 83 patients who underwent elective hip surgery and who had been scanned postoperatively. All patients had venograms performed regardless of the result of the leg scan, so that leg scanning was compared with venography in 142 limbs. The leg scan was positive in 86% of all thrombi that were located venographically outside the area of surgery. However, since a large number of thrombi were isolated to the

*References, 2, 5, 9, 15, 40, 44, 49, 50, 53, 58.

femoral vein close to the site of surgery, the overall accuracy was only 50%.

IPG

IPG fails to detect over 90% of asymptomatic calf vein thrombi and may not detect the occasional large nonocclusive asymptomatic proximal vein thrombi. Experience with IPG using the occlusive cuff technique as a screening test for venous thrombosis has been limited to two reports in patients undergoing elective hip surgery. In one[35] IPG detected 17 of 22 proximal thrombi, and in the other[19] it detected 7 of 10 proximal thrombi. These findings suggest that IPG, although less sensitive to proximal deep vein thrombosis when used as a screening test, is of clinical value in patients with relatively high rates of proximal vein thrombosis. Such patient groups include patients undergoing elective hip surgery, those having emergency hip surgery, and those suffering spinal cord injury.

IPG is most useful as a screening test when it is combined with [^{125}I]fibrinogen leg scanning; this is described in detail later.

Doppler ultrasonography

Doppler ultrasonography has not been adequately evaluated as a screening test. Furthermore, its application for this use is potentially limited by the need for this test to be performed by a highly experienced evaluator.

IPG and [^{125}I] fibrinogen leg scanning

We have tested the clinical value of adding IPG to [^{125}I]fibrinogen leg scanning in 630 patients who had general surgical procedures and 385 patients who had hip surgery.[26] Patients were screened with both tests, and venography was performed if either test was positive to determine the following:

1. The frequency with which proximal vein thrombosis confirmed by venography was detected by the IPG but not by leg scanning
2. The positive predictive value of these tests used either alone or in combination

Either the IPG or leg scan result was abnormal in 67 of 630 general surgical patients (11%) and in 158 of 385 hip surgery patients (41%). The positive predictive value of the tests in general surgical and hip surgery patients was 79% and 86%, respectively, for leg scanning alone, 33% and 90% for IPG alone, and 87% and 95% when both the leg scan and IPG were positive. The addition of IPG to leg scanning in general surgical patients identified only 1 additional patient with proximal vein thrombosis (0.2%), whereas in hip surgery patients the addition of IPG identified 25 additional patients with proximal vein thrombosis (6%). Thus the addition of IPG to leg scanning was not useful among general surgical patients as a screening test but was of substantial clinical value in hip surgery patients.

The results of this study were consistent with previous findings which suggested that the majority of venous thrombi occurring in general surgical patients arise in the calf and so can be detected by leg scanning, whereas a considerable number of thrombi in hip surgery patients arise in the femoral vein and may occur as isolated events. The findings also demonstrated that the likelihood that a patient would have venous thrombosis confirmed by venography if both the IPG and leg scan result were abnormal was 87% in general surgical patients and 95% in hip surgery patients. The positive predictive value of an abnormal leg scan alone was 79% in patients who had general surgery and 86% in patients who had hip surgery, whereas the positive predictive value of an abnormal IPG result alone was only 33% in patients who had general surgery and 90% in patients who had hip surgery. The poor positive predictive value of an abnormal IPG result in the presence of a normal leg scan result in general surgical patients is likely to be related to the low prevalence of proximal vein thrombosis undetected by leg scan in this group, since prevalence is an important variable that influences the positive predictive value.

REFERENCES

1. Albrechtsson, V., and Olsson, C.B.: Thrombotic side effects of lower limb phlebography, Lancet 1:723, 1976.
2. Atkins, P., and Hawkins, L.A.: Detection of venous thrombosis in the legs, Lancet 2:1217, 1965.
3. Barnes, R.W., et al.: Noninvasive quantitation of maximum venous outflow in acute thrombophlebitis, Surgery 72:971, 1972.
4. Bauer, G.: A venographic study of thromboembolic problems, Acta Chir. Scand. 84(suppl. 161):1, 1940.
5. Becker, J.: The diagnosis of venous thrombosis in the legs using I-labelled fibrinogen. An experimental and clinical study, Acta Chir. Scand. 138:667, 1972.
6. Bettman, M.A., and Paulin, S.: Leg phlebography: the incidence, nature and modification of undesirable side effects, Radiology 122:101, 1977.
7. Biland, L., et al.: The use of electromyography to detect muscle contraction responsible for falsely positive impedance plethysmographic results, Thromb. Res. 14:811, 1979.
8. Browse, N.L.: The ^{125}I-fibrinogen uptake test, Arch. Surg. 104:160, 1972.
9. Browse, N.L., et al.: Diagnosis of established deep vein thrombosis with the ^{125}I-fibrinogen uptake test, Br. Med. J. 4:325, 1971.
10. Cooke, E.D., and Pilcher, M.F.: Deep vein thrombosis: a preclinical diagnosis by thermography, Br. J. Surg. 61:971, 1974.
11. Cranley, J.J., et al.: A plethysmographic technique for the diagnosis of deep venous thrombosis of the lower extremities, Surg. Gynecol. Obstet. 136:385, 1973.
12. Dow, J.D.: Retrograde phlebography in major pulmonary embolism, Lancet 2:407, 1973.
13. Evans, D.S.: The early diagnosis of thromboembolism by ultrasound, Ann. R. Coll. Surg. Engl. 49:225, 1971.
14. Flanc, C., Kakkar, V.V., and Clarke, M.B.: The detection of venous thrombosis of the legs using ^{125}I-labelled fibrinogen, Br. J. Surg. 55:742, 1968.
15. Gallus, A.S., and Hirsh J.: ^{125}I-labelled fibrinogen leg scanning. In Frantantoni, J., and Wessler, S., editors: Prophylactic therapy for deep venous thrombosis and pulmonary embolism, DHEW Publication no. (NIH) 76-866, Washington, D.C., 1975, U.S. Government Printing Office.
16. Gallus, A.S., et al.: Diagnosis of venous thromboembolism, Semin. Thromb. Hemost. 2:203, 1976.
17. Haeger, K.: Problems of acute deep venous thrombosis. I. The interpretation of signs and symptoms, Angiology 20:219, 1969.
18. Harris, W.H., et al.: Comparison of ^{125}I-fibrinogen count scanning with phlebography for detection of venous thrombi after elective hip surgery, N. Engl. J. Med. 292:665, 1975.
19. Harris, W.H., et al.: Cuff-impedance phlebography and ^{125}I-fibrinogen scanning versus roentgenographic phlebography for diagnosis of thrombophlebitis following hip surgery, J. Bone Joint Surg. 58A:939, 1976.
20. Highman, J.H., O'Sullivan, E., and Thomas, E.: Isotope venography, Br. J. Surg. 60:52, 1973.
21. Hobbs, J.T., and Davies, J.W.L.: Detection of venous thrombosis with ^{131}I-labelled fibrinogen in the rabbit, Lancet 2: 134, 1960.
22. Holmes, M.C.G.: Deep venous thrombosis of the lower limbs diagnosed by ultrasound, Med. J. Aust. 1:427, 1973.
23. Hull, R., et al.: Impedance plethysmography using the occlusive cuff technique in the diagnosis of venous thrombosis, Circulation 53:696, 1976.
24. Hull, R., et al.: Combined use of leg scanning and impedance plethysmography in suspected venous thrombosis: an alternative to venography, N. Engl. J. Med. 296:1497, 1977.
25. Hull, R., et al.: Impedance plethysmography: the relationship between venous filling and sensitivity and specificity for proximal vein thrombosis, Circulation 58:898, 1978.
26. Hull, R., et al.: The value of adding impedance plethysmography to ^{125}I-fibrinogen leg scanning for the detection of deep vein thrombosis in high-risk surgical patients: a comparative study between patients undergoing genral surgery and hip surgery, Thromb. Res. 15:227, 1979.
27. Hull, R., et al.: Warfarin sodium versus low-dose heparin in the long-term treatment of venous thrombosis, N. Engl. J. Med. 301:855, 1979.
28. Hull, R., et al.: Clinical validity of a negative venogram in patients with clinically suspected venous thrombosis, Circulation 64(3):622, 1981.
29. Hull, R., et al.: Cost effectiveness of clinical diagnosis, venography, and noninvasive testing in patients with symptomatic deep-vein thrombosis, N. Engl. J. Med. 304:1561, 1981.
30. Hull, R., et al.: Replacement of venography in suspected venous thrombosis by impedance plethysmography and ^{125}I-fibrinogen leg scanning: a less invasive approach, Ann. Intern. Med. 94:12, 1981.

31. Hull, R., et al.: Adjusted subcutaneous heparin versus warfarin sodium in the long-term treatment of venous thrombosis, N. Engl. J. Med. 306:189, 1982.

32. Hull, R., et al.: Different intensities of oral anticoagulant therapy in the treatment of proximal vein thrombosis, N. Engl. J. Med. 307:1676, 1982.

33. Hull, R., et al.: A randomized trial of diagnostic strategies for symptomatic deep vein thrombosis, Thromb. Haemost. 50:160a, 1983.

34. Hull, R., et al.: The diagnosis of acute, recurrent, deep vein thrombosis: a diagnostic challenge, Circulation 67(4):901, 1983.

35. Hume, M., et al.: Extent of leg vein thrombosis determined by impedance and ^{125}I-fibrinogen, Am. J. Surg. 129:455, 1975.

36. Jay, R., et al.: Outcome of abnormal impedance plethysmography results in patients with proximal vein thrombosis: frequency of return to normal, Thromb. Haemost. 50:152a, 1983.

37. Johnson, W.C., et al.: Technetium 99^m isotope venography, Am. J. Surg. 127:424, 1974.

38. Johnston, K.W., and Kakkar, V.V.: Plethysmographic diagnosis of deep-vein thrombosis, Surg. Gynecol. Obstet. 139:41, 1974.

39. Johnston, K.W., et al.: A simple method for detecting deep vein thrombosis. An improved electrical impedance technique, Am. J. Surg. 127:349, 1974.

40. Kakkar, V.V.: The diagnosis of deep vein thrombosis using the ^{125}I-fibrinogen test, Arch. Surg. 104:152, 1972.

41. Kakkar, V.V.: Fibrinogen uptake test for detection of deep vein thrombosis. A review of current practice, Semin. Nucl. Med. 7:229, 1977.

42. Kakkar, V.V., et al.: Natural history of postoperative deep vein thrombosis, Lancet 2:230, 1969.

43. Kakkar, V.V., et al.: ^{125}I-labelled fibrinogen test adapted for routine screening for deep vein thrombosis, Lancet 1:540, 1972.

44. Lambie, J.M., et al.: Diagnostic accuracy in venous thrombosis, Br. Med. J. 2:142, 1970.

45. Lea Thomas, M.: Phlebography, Arch. Surg. 104:145, 1972.

46. Lea Thomas, M., and Fletcher, E.W.L.: The techniques of pelvic phlebography, Clin. Radiol. 18:399, 1967.

47. Lea Thomas, M., and Tighe, J.R.: Death from fat embolism as a complication of intraosseous phlebography, Lancet 2:1415, 1973.

48. McLachlin, J., Richard, T., and Paterson, J.D.: An evaluation of clinical signs in the diagnosis of venous thrombosis, Arch. Surg. 85:738, 1962

49. Milne, R.M., et al.: Postoperative deep venous thrombosis: a comparison of diagnostic techniques, Lancet 2:445, 1971.

50. Negus, D., et al.: ^{125}I-labelled fibrinogen in the diagnosis of deep vein thrombosis and its correlation with phlebography, Br. J. Surg. 55:835, 1968.

51. Nicolaides, A.N., et al.: The origin of deep vein thrombosis: a venographic study, Br. J. Radiol. 44:653, 1971.

52. Palko, P.D., Nanson, E.M., and Fedoruk, S.P.: The early detection of deep venous thrombosis using I^{131}-tagged human fibrinogen, Can. J. Surg. 7:215, 1964.

53. Partsch, H., Lofferer, O., and Mostbeck, A.: Diagnosis of established deep vein thrombosis in the leg using ^{131}-I fibrinogen, Angiology 25:719, 1974.

54. Rabinov, K., and Paulin, S.: Roentgen diagnosis of venous thrombosis in the leg, Arch. Surg. 104:134, 1972.

55. Sigel, B., et al.: Diagnosis of lower limb venous thrombosis by Doppler ultrasound technique, Arch. Surg. 104:174, 1972.

56. Strandness, D.E.: Postoperative deep venous thrombosis: comparison of diagnostic techniques, Lancet 2:763, 1971.

57. Strandness, D.E., and Sumner, D.S.: ULtrasonic velocity detector in the diagnosis of thrombophlebitis, Arch. Surg. 104:180, 1972.

58. Tsapogas, M.J., et al.: Postoperative venous thrombosis and the effectiveness of prophylactic measures, Arch. Surg. 103:561, 1971.

59. Wheeler, H.B., et al.: Impedance phlebography. Technique, interpretation and results, Arch. Surg. 104:164, 1972.

60. Wheeler, H.B., et al.: Bedside screening for venous thrombosis using occlusive impedance phlebography, Angiology 26:199, 1975.

61. Yudelman, I.M., et al.: Plasma fibrinopeptide A levels in symptomatic venous thromboembolism, Blood 51:1189, 1978.

62. Zielinsky, A., et al.: Evaluation of radioimmunoassay for fragment E in the diagnosis of venous thrombosis, Thromb. Haemost. 42:28, 1979.

63. Zielinsky, A., et al.: Doppler ultrasonography in patients with clinically suspected deep-vein thrombosis: improved sensitivity by inclusion of the posterior tibial vein examination site, Thromb. Haemost. 50:153a, 1983.

CHAPTER 79

Algorithms for diagnosis and therapy of venous thromboembolism

ROBERT W. BARNES

The hazards of pulmonary embolism and the morbidity of the postthrombotic syndrome make the early diagnosis and treatment of venous thromboembolic disease of great clinical importance. The fallibility of the clinical diagnosis of deep vein thrombosis[1] or pulmonary embolism has prompted physicians to recognize the importance of objective techniques to confirm the clinical diagnosis. Although contrast phlebography and pulmonary arteriography remain the standards for diagnosis of venous thromboembolic disease, the time, discomfort, risk, and expense of these procedures prevent their routine application for screening and follow-up procedures. To overcome the fallibility of clinical diagnosis, many noninvasive screening techniques have been developed to improve the accuracy of diagnosis of venous disease. Objective verification of deep vein thrombosis (DVT) or pulmonary embolism is necessary to avoid the time, expense, and risk of anticoagulation or surgical treatment of clinical conditions mimicking venous thromboembolism. In general, the various noninvasive diagnostic techniques may provide similar information with equivalent accuracy. This is particularly true of Doppler ultrasound, plethysmography, or radionuclide phlebography, all of which can provide accurate assessment of venous disease in the major veins above the level of the knee. [^{125}I]fibrinogen-uptake testing has a more limited role in the evaluation of clinically suspected venous disease. The test is particularly useful to determine the activity of recurrent DVT and to identify isolated calf vein thrombosis when the other noninvasive diagnostic techniques are normal. However, the method is not recommended as the sole means

of evaluating patients with suspected major leg vein thrombosis.

The increasing complexity of diagnostic and therapeutic decisions in medical practice has led to the use of algorithms, or decision trees, to guide the workup and management of certain disease states.[2] Even though many algorithms are rather complex and are structured according to the principles of computer decision analysis, modifications of this technique can be developed to provide logic pathways suitable for the practicing clinician. I have developed a series of diagnostic and therapeutic algorithms to assist clincians in the management of various venous disorders. The purpose of this chapter will be to review the application of these algorithms for the workup and treatment of patients with acute DVT, recurrent venous thrombosis, postthrombotic syndrome, varicose veins, superficial thrombophlebitis, and pulmonary embolism.

ACUTE DEEP VEIN THROMBOSIS

The diagnostic algorithm for evaluating the patient with clinically suspected DVT is shown in Fig. 79-1. After starting heparin therapy, the patient is screened by a noninvasive technique that is sensitive to disease in the major deep veins. In my experience Doppler ultrasound is the most reliable technique, but any technique of plethysmography or radionuclide phlebography may be used for screening. If the noninvasive diagnostic test is abnormal, the clinician should next ascertain whether an antecedent problem exists, such as limb trauma or arthritis, that may mimic DVT and result in abnormalities of diagnostic screening tests. If

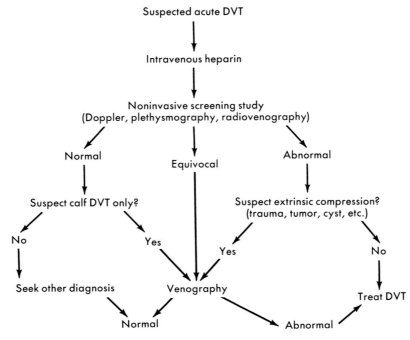

Fig. 79-1. Algorithm for diagnosis of patients with suspected acute DVT.

no antecedent factors are present, the physician can logically treat the patient for DVT. If, however, another coexistent problem exists that may make the results of noninvasive screening ambiguous, a contrast phlebogram should be obtained and the patient managed according to the result of that definitive diagnostic test. If the noninvasive screening evaluation is normal, the clinician should ascertain whether the patient's manifestations are limited to the calf. If so, most noninvasive tests are not sensitive to isolated calf vein thrombosis. In my experience a normal Doppler study is usually sensitive to any significant calf venous disease. However, to rule out calf vein thrombosis, a contrast phlebogram should be obtained and the patient treated according to the results of that study. If, however, the patient has more extensive symptoms or signs of leg vein thrombosis, a normal noninvasive screening test is sufficient evidence to rule out major leg vein thrombosis, and other diagnoses should be considered.

RECURRENT DEEP VEIN THROMBOSIS

The patient with a history of prior DVT and recurrent symptoms presents a diagnostic dilemma. Although the patient is usually treated for recurrent

venous thrombosis, many patients develop symptoms such as leg pain, edema, or inflammation on the basis of postthrombotic sequelae caused by venous abnormalities resulting from old venous thrombosis. A diagnostic algorithm to evaluate such patients is shown in Fig. 79-2. The physician plans the workup to answer the following questions:

1. Is there evidence that the patient has or has had venous disease?
2. Are the current symptoms the result of recurrent active venous thrombosis?

To answer the first question the patient can be screened with any of the noninvasive diagnostic tests that are sensitive to major deep vein obstruction and valvular incompetence, such as Doppler ultrasound or plethysmography. If the results of such tests are entirely normal, it is unlikely that the patient has or has had DVT. A venogram may be performed to establish the diagnosis. If the noninvasive screening study shows patent deep veins with valvular incompetence, the patient may be treated for postthrombotic syndrome. If the noninvasive study shows deep vein obstruction, the physician must clarify whether or not this obstruction represents new active thrombosis or residual

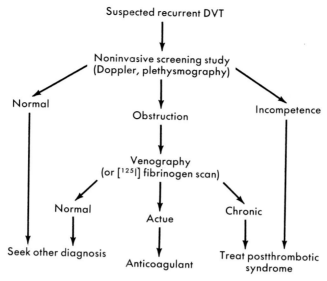

Fig. 79-2. Algorithm for diagnosis of patients with suspected recurrent DVT.

chronic inactive disease. A venogram may be performed that may show fresh thrombus outlined by contrast material, which requires anticoagulation. If chronic obstruction is seen, the patient may be treated for postthrombotic syndrome. If a [125I]fibrinogen leg scan is available, this test is specific for activity of venous thrombosis. This test may be substituted for a venogram and the patient treated for recurrent active venous thrombosis if the test is positive. If the test is negative, particularly if the patient has not received heparin therapy, the patient may be treated for postthrombotic syndrome.

POSTTHROMBOTIC SYNDROME

Patients with postthrombotic sequelae usually manifest signs of chronic venous stasis disease, such as hyperpigmentation, eczema, edema, and possible ulceration, partucularly in the skin adjacent to the medial malleolus. However, some patients with chronic leg swelling and skin changes may have these abnormalities on the basis of some other condition, such as contact dermatitis or chronic congestive heart failure.

A diagnostic algorithm for the evaluation of patients with suspected postthrombotic syndrome is shown in Fig. 79-3. The patient is evaluated by noninvasive screening studies that are sensitive to deep vein obstruction or valvular incompetence, such as Doppler ultrasound, strain-gauge plethysmography, or photoplethysmography. If these stud-

ies are normal, it is unlikely that the patient has postthrombotic disease and another diagnosis should be sought. If the noninvasive studies show deep vein obstruction, the physician should determine whether or not the patient has sufficiently disabling venous claudication to warrant surgical intervention, such as bypass of the femoral or iliac veins. Such bypass procedures are rarely necessary. If the venous symptoms are not disabling, elastic support stockings should be recommended. If the noninvasive studies show patent but incompetent deep venous valves, the therapy is dictated by the presence or absence of chronic venous stasis ulceration. If the leg is not ulcerated, elastic support therapy is prescribed. If an ulcer is present and infected, the patient should be hospitalized for local wound care and antibiotic therapy. Once the ulcer is not infected and demonstrates clean granulation tissue, further healing of the ulcer may occur with ambulatory therapy using a medicated bandage (Unna boot). Once the ulcer heals, elastic support therapy is prescribed. If the ulcer fails to heal despite such medical management, operative intervention may be necessary, including excision of chronic ulcers, split skin grafting, ligation of incompetent communicating (perforating) veins, or the investigational procedures of venous valve repair or transposition. Such surgical intervention is uncommonly necessary if diligent medical management of chronic venous disease is carried out.

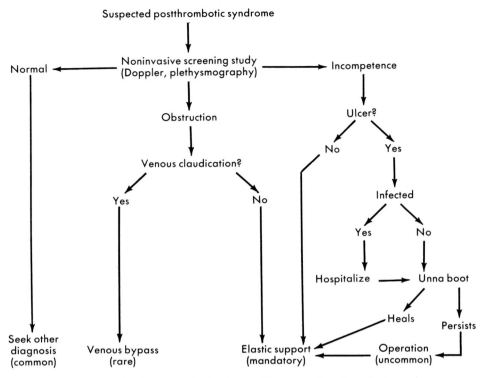

Fig. 79-3. Algorithm for diagnosis of patients with suspected postthrombotic syndrome.

VARICOSE VEINS

Varicose veins may represent a primary abnormality of dilation and valvular incompetence limited to the superficial (saphenous) veins. However, some patients with varicose veins have predisposing deep vein abnormalities, with obstruction or incompetence usually secondary to previous deep vein thrombosis. The clinician must distinguish between primary and secondary varicose veins because the therapy and prognosis of these two conditions are different. A clinical diagnosis of secondary varicose veins should be suspected if the patient manifests evidence of chronic venous stasis disease, such as marked swelling, hyperpigmentation, eczema, or stasis ulceration. However, some patients with secondary varicose veins do not have these cutaneous stigmata of the underlying abnormalities of the deep and communicating (perforating) veins. Such patients should be elevated for the integrity of the deep venous system, and a diagnostic algorithm for this workup is shown in Fig. 79-4. Noninvasive screening studies such as Doppler ultrasound, strain-gauge plethysmography or

photoplethysmography may be used to evaluate the deep, communicating, and superficial veins. If the deep veins are normal the patient is assumed to have primary varicose veins. Such patients usually require no operative intervention unless significant cosmetic problems exist or the patient develops such complications as superficial thrombophlebitis or bleeding from the varices. In such instances the patient may have surgical ligation and stripping of the varicosities and, in select patients, compression sclerotherapy may be employed. If the patients have noninvasive evidence of deep or communicating (perforating) venous abnormalities, a diagnosis of secondary varicose veins should be entertained. Surgical removal of secondary varicose veins does not usually relieve the patient's symptoms, which are primarily an expression of the associated deep or communicating venous disease. These patients must be managed similarly to patients with postthrombotic syndrome, with diligent use of elastic support therapy and medical or surgical treatment of any associated venous stasis ulceration.

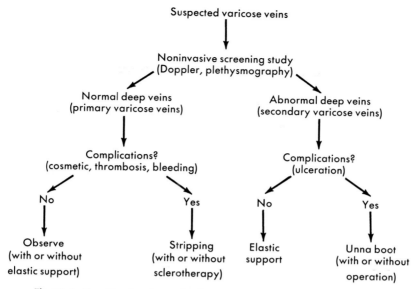

Fig. 79-4. Algorithm for diagnosis of patients with suspected varicose veins.

SUPERFICIAL THROMBOPHLEBITIS

Although patients with acute inflammation of the leg are often treated for superficial thrombophlebitis, other problems such as cellulitis or lymphangitis may mimic acute superficial venous thrombosis. A clinical diagnosis can be readily made if the inflammatory streak involves an indurated segment of a predisposing varicose vein. In the absence of such varicosities the diagnosis cannot be made with certainty. A diagnostic algorithm for the use of Doppler ultrasound in screening patients for suspected superficial thrombophlebitis is shown in Fig. 79-5. The Doppler detector is the only noninvasive technique that is uniquely suited to evaluation of the superficial venous system. In the absence of predisposing varicose veins a Doppler examination should be carried out to determine the patency of the venous system in the area of inflammation. If the Doppler examination is normal, the patient should be treated for cellulitis or lymphangitis. If the Doppler examination is abnormal or if there is an obviously thrombosed varicose vein, the next point to be clarified is whether the involvement extends toward the saphenofemoral junction. If not, distal superficial thrombophlebitis can be readily treated by local heat, antiinflammatory agents and support therapy, inasmuch as anticoagulation is not known to alter the natural history of the disease. If the process extends near the sa-

phenofemoral junction, noninvasive screening or venography of the deep veins should be carried out. If DVT is present, the patient should be treated with anticoagulants. If, however, the deep veins are patent, consideration should be given to ligation of the saphenofemoral junction to prevent extension of the process into the deep venous system.

PULMONARY EMBOLISM

Most patients with suspected pulmonary embolism are treated on the basis of the results of perfusion lung scanning. However, the fallibility of perfusion scans has been documented by several studies that have shown that the test is nonspecific and less than 50% accurate unless a perfusion defect of lobar extent or greater is present in association with a normal chest roentgenogram. Many reports have demonstrated that the specificity of pulmonary scanning is increased if both perfusion and ventilation scanning are performed to detect ventilation-perfusion mismatch associated with pulmonary embolism. In the absence of ventilation scanning capability, pulmonary arteriography may be indicated in patients with diagnostic ambiguity. A diagnostic algorithm for evaluating patients with suspected pulmonary embolism is shown in Fig. 79-6. The patient is started on intravenous heparin unless this is absolutely contraindicated. If the patient has suffered a massive embolism with symp-

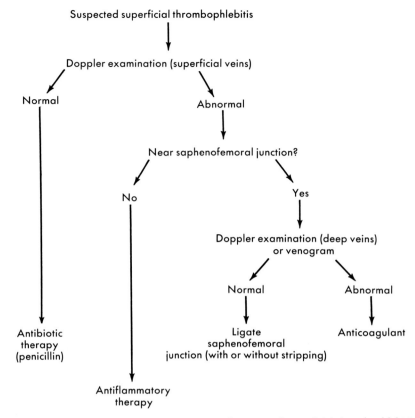

Fig. 79-5. Algorithm for diagnosis of patients with suspected superficial thrombophlebitis.

toms such as persistent shock or syncope, I prefer to proceed with pulmonary arteriography and not subject such gravely ill patients to lung scanning. These patients may require surgical intervention, such as pulmonary embolectomy or insertion of an inferior vena cava filter, and a pulmonary arteriogram should be performed before such invasive therapy. If the patient has not suffered massive embolism, a perfusion and ventilation lung scan should be obtained. These studies are of greatest diagnostic value when they are normal because a normal lung scan virtually excludes a pulmonary embolus; therefore another diagnosis should be sought. If the perfusion and ventilation scans are abnormal, a noninvasive venous examination is helpful to identify a source for the pulmonary embolus. If the noninvasive studies are abnormal, the patient may be treated for pulmonary embolism. If the noninvasive studies are normal, a pulmonary arteriogram should be considered because, in my experience, such patients have no evidence of pulmonary embolism in at least 50% of the cases. I

do not feel that the statistics of "probability" of lung scan abnormalities are sufficiently accurate to warrant therapy in an individual patient. Using this algorithmic approach, I have ruled out pulmonary embolism in 50% of the patients who otherwise would have been treated for the condition based on abnormalities of perfusion lung scanning alone.

PROSPECTIVE SURVEILLANCE OF VENOUS THROMBOSIS

The previous applications of noninvasive techniques for studying venous thrombosis have been directed to establishing a diagnosis in a patient with clinical symptoms or signs of venous disease. However, more than half of all patients with venous thrombosis are asymptomatic and are overlooked by conventional clinical techniques. During the past decade a number of prospective surveillance studies have been carried out to identify the incidence of DVT in patients at risk of developing the disease. Most of these reports have involved the use of the $[^{125}I]$fibrinogen-uptake test, with most

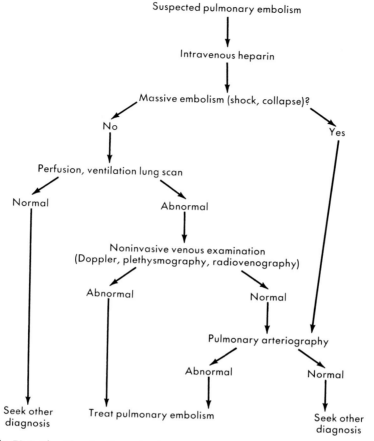

Fig. 79-6. Algorithm for diagnosis of patients with suspected pulmonary embolism.

studies being carried out in the United Kingdom and Canada. The extreme sensitivity of this diagnostic technique has resulted in the detection of a relatively high incidence of venous thrombosis in high-risk patients such as those undergoing general surgical procedures or orthopedic operations. On the basis of such studies the use of prophylactic anticoagulation, particularly with low-dose subcutaneous heparin, has been recommended and found to be efficacious in many prospective randomized studies. However, the incidence of abnormal [125I]fibrinogen-uptake tests in such patients far exceeds the frequency of clinically significant disease. It is recognized that as many as 80% of patients with an abnormal [125I]fibrinogen-uptake test have disease localized to the muscular veins of the calf, which spontaneously resolves during the course of observation. Prospective studies of DVT in general surgical patients using Doppler ultrasound reveal an incidence of DVT following

operation in less than 2% of patients during the first postoperative week. Because of the relatively low incidence of clinically significant venous thrombosis, many surgeons are reluctant to routinely administer prophylactic anticoagulants with the small but definite morbidity associated with this form of treatment.

An alternative approach to the management of venous thrombosis in high-risk patients is to perform routine prospective screening studies with noninvasive techniques. Although in many patient groups the yield of positive studies will be very low, some high-risk patients such as those undergoing orthopedic procedures or operative treatment of malignancy may be routinely screened, followed by treatment of patients with detected disease. The diagnostic modality used will depend on the experience of the examiner and the number of the patients to be screened. Doppler ultrasound is particularly useful to screen large numbers of patients since this method requires only portable instrumentation and little patient preparation. Plethysmography or [^{125}I]fibrinogen-uptake testing can also be used but requires more time, equipment, and patient preparation. Although a number of pilot prospective screening studies have been performed, it remains to be shown whether such studies are warranted as an alternative to routine anticoagulant therapy in high-risk patients.

SUMMARY

Various noninvasive diagnostic techniques are available to the clinician who must evaluate and treat patients with suspected venous thrombosis. The need for such techniques is an outgrowth of the recognized fallibility of the clinical diagnosis of venous thrombosis and the time, discomfort, expense, and potential risks of contrast phlebography. Doppler ultrasound, plethysmography, and radionuclide phlebography are particularly suited to screen patients with suspected major DVT of veins at or above the level of the knee. The [^{125}I]fibrinogen-uptake test is best suited to estab-

lishing the activity of venous thrombosis in patients with recurrent disease and to detect active isolated calf vein thrombosis. The use of these techniques for evaluation of patients with acute DVT, recurrent DVT, postthrombotic syndrome, varicose veins, superficial thrombophlebitis, and pulmonary embolism is demonstrated by means of diagnostic algorithms. Noninvasive techniques may also be useful for prospective surveillance of patients at risk of developing DVT and to identify and treat that small number of patients who develop clinically significant disease. Such prospective screening may serve as an alternative to routine prophylactic anticoagulation therapy of patients at risk of developing DVT.

REFERENCES

1. Barnes, R.W., Wu, K.K., and Hoak, J.C.: The fallibility of the clinical diagnosis of venous thrombosis, J.A.M.A. 234:605, 1975.
2. Ellis, B.W.: Use of logic-based flow patterns in the investigation and management of surgical disorders, Br. J. Surg. 62:800, 1975.

CHAPTER 80

Can noninvasive tests be used as the basis for treatment of deep vein thrombosis?

H. BROWNELL WHEELER and FREDERICK A. ANDERSON, Jr.

Because the clinical diagnosis of deep vein thrombosis (DVT) is known to be unreliable, confirmatory diagnostic tests are necessary before treatment. Some investigators have stated that venography should be obtained on every patient before treatment, but there are important practical limitations to this policy. Simpler and less expensive noninvasive tests are now available for the diagnosis of DVT, but there is controversy as to whether or not these tests are a sufficiently reliable basis for treatment. This chapter addresses that controversy.

Venography has now become the standard for diagnostic tests for DVT. It is interesting to remember that not very many years ago, venography was widely considered to be unreliable, and even dangerous. With advances in technique and extensive clinical experience, venography has now come to be regarded as highly accurate and relatively safe. Even so, a 10% error rate has been reported when the same venograms are reviewed by independent and equally experienced observers.[83] It is available in most major medical centers but not in many community hospitals across the country. Even if available in these hospitals, the accuracy and safety of this procedure cannot be assumed to be as good as have been reported by major medical centers.

Venography requires transportation of patients, sometimes critically ill, to the radiology department. Patients frequently experience pain at the injection site and occasionally complain of nausea, faintness, and other systemic side effects caused by the large amount of contrast material that must be injected. Although the occurrence of clinically apparent DVT as a result of venography is relatively rare in patients with normal venograms there is a disturbingly high incidence of [^{125}I]fibrinogen "hot spots" and frequent superficial thrombophlebitis at the injection site, clearly indicating that the contrast material is irritating to the intima and potentially thrombogenic. After injection of contrast material into an obstructed deep venous system, it seems likely that thrombosis may sometimes propagate distally. Another limitation of venography is the need for a skilled radiologist and sophisticated x-ray equipment, inevitably entailing considerable expense. Finally, because of the many reasons listed, venography is not a procedure that is easily and frequently repeatable.

These limitations in venography have led to widespread efforts to develop noninvasive tests of comparable accuracy. In the last several years, many noninvasive tests have been proposed for the diagnosis of DVT. A few of these procedures have now progressed from research status to widespread clinical use. Recent experience in community hospitals as well as in research laboratories has clarified the overall place of these tests in patient management. This discussion will consider whether we have reached the time when noninvasive tests can be used as the primary basis for diagnosis and treatment of DVT without the necessity for venography.

METHODS

Of the many noninvasive tests proposed for DVT in recent years, only a few have gained broad acceptance. These include radioisotope scanning, Doppler blood flow evaluation, thermography, and plethysmography. Other diagnostic tests also show promise and may eventually become better established. Such tests include examination of the pe-

Table 80-1. [^{125}I]fibrinogen—correlation with 718 venograms (expectant studies)

Investigator	Year	Correlation with normal venograms (specificity)	Correlation with recent DVT (sensitivity)	Location of thrombi
Negus et al.[72]	1968	60% (3/5)	100% (24/24)	Below-knee
Lambie et al.[60]	1970	90% (18/20)	90% (38/42)	Mainly below-knee
Milne et al.[68]	1971	71% (12/17)	100% (18/18)	Below-knee
Tsapogas et al.[98]	1971	100% (178/178)	92% (11/12)	Below-knee
Kakkar[57]	1972	93% (50/54)	94% (32/34)	Mainly below-knee
Becker[6]	1972	100% (74/74)	88% (15/17)	Below-knee
Walsh et al.[100]	1974	80% (12/15)	100% (50/50)	Below-knee
Hirsh and Hull[42]	1978	—	69% (37/54)	Proximal to knee
Hirsh and Hull[42]	1978	—	92% (96/104)	Below-knee
TOTALS		96% (347/363)	90% (321/355)	

OVERALL ACCURACY = 93% (668/718)

Table 80-2. [^{125}I]fibrinogen—correlation with 654 venograms in symptomatic limbs

Investigator	Year	Correlation with normal venograms (specificity)	Correlation with recent DVT (sensitivity)
Browse et al.[14]	1971	91% (91/100)	78% (66/85)
Kakkar[57]	1972	54% (15/28)	85% (63/74)
Browse[12]	1972	85% (104/123)	64% (46/72)
Walker[99]	1972	85% (46/54)	19% (22/118)
TOTALS		84% (256/305)	56% (197/349)

OVERALL ACCURACY = 69% (453/654)

Table 80-3. [^{125}I]fibrinogen—correlation with 467 venograms in hip surgery

Investigator	Year	Correlation with normal venograms (sensitivity)	Correlation with recent DVT (specificity)
Pinto[77]	1970	60% (3/5)	100% (20/20)
Field et al.[32]	1972	78% (25/32)	94% (29/31)
Harris et al.[39]	1975	86% (25/29)	49% (25/51)
Gallus and Hirsch[35]	1975	83% (24/29)	93% (38/41)
Hirsch and Hull[42]	1978	—	64% (53/83)
Sautter et al.[84]	1979	70% (67/96)	58% (29/50)
TOTALS		75% (144/191)	70% (194/276)

OVERALL ACCURACY = 72% (338/467)

ripheral blood for breakdown products of the thrombus, especially fibrin split products, and ultrasonic imaging. This chapter will deal primarily with those tests that are generally available and widely employed. A more detailed description of each of these techniques will be found elsewhere in this book.

Of the radioisotopic methods, the most popular and most extensively employed is ^{125}I-labeled fibrinogen. This tracer is incorporated into a developing thrombus, causing a local hot spot that can be detected by external scintillation counting. Use of radiolabeled fibrinogen was first described by Hobbs and Davis,[43] subsequently popularized by Kakkar et al.[56-58] and has now been studied by many investigators all over the world (Tables 80-1 to 80-3). It is the most sensitive of all noninvasive diagnostic procedures for early DVT and the only one that will reliably detect small calf vein thrombi (Table 80-1). It has been invaluable in defining the prevalence and natural history of DVT as well as in identifying risk factors and evaluating methods of prophylaxis. It is best employed for prospective screening, where the tracer can be administered to

Table 80-4. Doppler ultrasound—correlation with 2060 venograms

Investigator	Year	Correlation with normal venograms (specificity)	Correlation with recent proximal DVT (sensitivity)	Patient group
Evans[31]	1970	100% (110/110)	95% (57/60)	50% asymptomatic
Milne et al.[68]	1971	41% (7/17)	No venographically demonstrated proximal DVT	Asymptomatic
Sigel et al.[88]	1972	92% (150/165)	84% (46/55)	Symptomatic
Strandness and Sumner[91]	1972	83% (10/12)	100% (38/38)	Symptomatic
Holmes[45]	1973	94% (51/54)	100% (17/17)	Symptomatic
Johnson[55]	1974	94% (15/16)	40% (4/10)	Mainly symptomatic
Yao et al.[111]	1974	87% (27/31)	82% (104/127)	Symptomatic
Bolton and Hoffman[10]	1975	82% (32/39)	93% (13/14)	Symptomatic
Meadway et al.[67]	1975	72% (55/76)	91% (86/94)	Symptomatic
Richards et al.[79]	1976	88% (79/90)	73% (27/37)	Symptomatic
Flanigan et al.[33]	1978	96% (94/98)	65% (35/54)	Symptomatic
Nicholas et al.[73]	1977	70% (21/30)	89% (17/19)	Mainly symptomatic
Dosick and Blakemore[30]	1978	93% (100/108)	96% (50/52)	Symptomatic
Maryniak and Nicholson[65]	1979	90% (26/29)	100% (11/11)	Symptomatic
Sumner and Lambeth[94]	1979	90% (35/39)	94% (34/36)	Mainly symptomatic
Holden et al.[44]	1981	91% (87/96)	73% (22/30)	Mainly symptomatic
Hanel et al.[38]	1981	91% (118/130)	92% (49/53)	69% symptomatic
Schroeder and Dunn[85]	1982	73% (36/49)	70% (19/27)	Mainly symptomatic
Bounameaux et al.[11]	1982	62% (20/33)	83% (33/40)	Mainly symptomatic
Bendick et al.[7]	1983	90% (85/94)	73% (22/30)	Symptomatic
TOTALS		88% (1,158/1,316)	84% (627/744)	

OVERALL ACCURACY = 87% (1,785/2,060)

the patient before the period of risk. For example, it is well suited for preoperative administration to patients scheduled to undergo surgery that is known to be associated with a high risk of post-operative DVT. On the other hand, for evaluation of patients clinically suspected of DVT, the [^{125}I]fibrinogen method is less accurate (Table 80-2). A delay of 48 hours before the test can be assumed to be negative is a serious disadvantage. False negative tests have been reported to be more frequent in patients undergoing anticoagulant therapy. False positive tests may be caused by an inflammatory or infectious process in the leg. Perhaps the most serious drawback to the use of the [^{125}I]fibrinogen test is the high background radiation from the trunk that renders the test unreliable in detection of clots that originate in the groin or pelvis. Although isolated proximal thrombi are uncommon in the absence of more distal disease, they are nevertheless worrisome because of their high potential for major pulmonary embolism. For these reasons, as well as the expense of the commercially available [^{125}I]fibrinogen preparations, this method is less useful in routine clinical practice than for prospective studies. Its clinical application has been chiefly in combination with plethysmography or a Doppler system.

At about the same time that the [^{125}I]fibrinogen

technique was introduced, *ultrasonic blood flow detectors* based on the Doppler principle became available and were employed for the diagnosis of DVT by Sigel et al.,[87] Strandness and Sumner,[91] Yao et al.,[110] and many others. This method had great initial appeal because the equipment was relatively inexpensive, and the results of the test were immediately available. Although inaccurate in the detection of calf DVT, excellent sensitivity and specificity for iliac and femoral thrombosis were reported by several investigators (Table 80-4). Interpretation was subjective, based on the flow sounds heard over the venous system in response to various maneuvers designed to stimulate or impede venous flow. A number of examiners were unable to repeat the excellent results of the originators of the method, and the technique earned a possibly undeserved reputation for poor reliability. Barnes et al.[3] refined the technique and its interpretation and also developed a training program for those interested in its use. Through careful training and experience, users of the Doppler method can achieve excellent results in the detection of proximal thrombi. However, the interpretation, which remains subjective in nature, is highly dependent on the skill and experience of the examiner. Several months of supervised patient testing may be necessary before a new vascular technician is able to perform the Doppler venous test with an accuracy comparable to that reported in Table 80-4.

The Doppler method has the great advantage of using equipment that is inexpensive and portable. Even if its accuracy is somewhat less than competing methods, it may prove to be the only technique possible for laboratories with serious budgetary limitations. Also, Doppler testing may be a useful adjunct to plethysmography, particularly in patients with severe congestive heart failure (CHF), chronic obstructive pulmonary disease (COPD), or vasospasm.

The use of plethysmography for the diagnosis of DVT was given its original impetus in this country by early reports of *impedance plethysmography (IPG)*. Used to monitor changes in venous blood volume, the original IPG technique relied on measurement of respiration-induced changes in venous volume. Excellent results were obtained by several investigators*; but as in the case of Doppler examination, other investigators had less satisfactory results.[29,90]

Subsequently, using a six-channel pneumatic plethysmograph, Cranley[24-27] also studied respiration-induced changes in venous volume and added observation of volume changes proximal and distal to an inflated pneumatic cuff. This technique, known as *phleborheography (PRG)*, was more complex than the original IPG technique but also provided the examiner with more information and a slightly greater accuracy (Table 80-5).

In the meantime the inconsistencies originally encountered with the IPG technique had been identified as the result of variable patient effort in respiratory maneuvers and the necessity for the examiner to evaluate the patient effort subjectively in

*References 70, 71, 86, 103, 105, 106.

considering the results obtained. Accordingly, a more dependable method of producing venous outflow obstruction was developed to make the method simpler to perform and more objective to interpret. A 20 cm pneumatic cuff, placed around the thigh and inflated to slightly above venous pressure but well below arterial pressure, satisfied this need quite well. Following release of the occlusion cuff, the venous outflow rate was shown to be markedly impaired by DVT. The venous outflow in the first few seconds after release of the thigh occlusion cuff also increased with the amount of blood dammed up behind the cuff in normal subjects, but not in those with venous thrombosis.[104,107,108] Measurements of venous filling (after cuff occlusion) and venous emptying (after cuff release) provided a simple and objective basis for diagnosis of DVT. This "occlusive" IPG method has now been widely employed and had proved highly satisfactory in community hospitals, as well as medical centers (Table 80-6).

Several other plethysmographic techniques based on venous occlusion and measurement of venous outflow after release of the occlusion have now been described (Table 80-7). In general the results have been good to excellent, corroborating the underlying premise of this method of diagnosis. However, none of these venous occlusion techniques have been as thoroughly evaluated to date as either IPG or PRG.

Thermography was first evaluated as a method for the noninvasive diagnosis of DVT in 1973 by Cooke and Pilcher.[20] A highly sensitive instrument must be used for temperature measurement, since the typical change in the surface temperature of the leg as a result of acute DVT is only 1° C. Most investigators use an infrared camera to produce thermographic images on a television monitor. Unfortunately, this equipment is fragile, expensive,

Table 80-5. Phleborheography—correlation with 886 venograms

Investigator	Year	Correlation with normal venograms (specificity)	Correlation with recent proximal DVT (sensitivity)
Collins et al.[18]	1979	87% (20/23)	100% (41/41)
Nolan et al.[75]	1982	100% (21/21)	87% (13/15)
Comerota et al.[19]	1982	95% (418/441)	96% (247/256)
Classen et al.[17]	1982	87% (20/23)	97% (64/66)
TOTALS		94% (479/508)	97% (365/378)
OVERALL ACCURACY = 95% (844/886)			

Table 80-6. Occlusive impedance plethysmography—correlations with 2561 venograms

Investigator	Year	Correlation with normal venograms (specificity)	Correlation with recent proximal DVT (sensitivity)	Patient group
Hume et al.[53]	1975	100% (10/10)	77% (17/22)	Prospective hip surgery
Harris et al.[40]	1976	92% (55/60)	70% (7/10)	Prospective hip surgery
Todd et al.[96]	1976	100% (11/11)	100% (11/11)	Spinal cord injury
Hull et al.[46]	1976	97% (386/397)	93% (124/133)	24% asymptomatic
Hull et al.[47]	1977	95% (108/114)	98% (59/60)	Symptomatic
Toy and Schrier[97]	1978	100% (9/9)	94% (15/16)	Symptomatic
Flanigan et al.[33]	1978	95% (93/98)	96% (52/54)	Symptomatic
Hull et al.[48]	1978	96% (304/317)	92% (155/169)	40% Asymptomatic
Gross and Burney[36]	1979	94% (32/34)	100% (9/9)	Symptomatic (emergency room)
Cooperman et al.[22]	1979	96% (72/75)	87% (20/23)	Symptomatic
Wheeler and Anderson	—	92% (191/208)	98% (88/90)	Mainly symptomatic
Liapis et al.[63]	1980	90% (219/243)	91% (43/47)	Symptomatic
Foti and Gurewich[34]	1980	79% (19/24)	90% (19/21)	Symptomatic
Hull et al.[51]	1981	98% (157/160)	95% (74/78)	Symptomatic
Harris et al.[41]	1981	88% (36/41)	100% (2/2)	Hip surgery (DVT/pulmonary emboli history)
Clarke-Pearson and Creasman[16]	1981	40% (2/5)	100% (10/10)	Symptomatic pregnant
TOTALS		94% (1,704/1,806)	93% (705/755)	

OVERALL ACCURACY = 94% (2,409/2,561)

Table 80-7. Review of various nonstandard methods based on venous occlusion plethysmography

Investigator	Year	Method of interpretation	Correlation with normal venograms (specificity)	Correlation with recent proximal DVT (sensitivity)
WATER-FILLED PLETHYSMOGRAPHY				
Dahn and Eiriksson[28]	1968	VC* vs. MVO†	100% (2/2)	100% (6/6)
STRAIN-GAUGE PLETHYSMOGRAPHY				
Barnes et al.[4]	1972	MVO = 25%/min	82% (28/34)	95% (41/43)
Hallböök and Ling[37]	1974	MVO = 35%/min	100% (70/70)	100% (31/31)
Barnes et al.[5]	1977	MVO = 20%/min	No venograms	90% (28/31)
Boccalon et al.[9]	1981	VC vs. MVO	96% (27/28)	100% (26/26)
Bounameaux et al.[11]	1982	VO_3 = 1.0%	63% (21/33)	95% (35/37)
Cramer et al.[23]	1983	VC vs. $VO_{0.5-2}$	92% (11/12)	100% (12/12)
IMPEDANCE PLETHYSMOGRAPHY				
Johnston and Kakkar[56]	1974	VO_2/VC = 0.70	92% (35/38)	100% (13/13)
Yao et al.[111]	1974	MVO = 1.0%/sec	81% (22/27)	91% (84/92)
Richards et al.[79]	1976	VC vs. VO_3	87% (78/90)	83% (30/36)
Moser et al.[69]	1977	VO_{10} = 0.2%	100% (19/19)	100% (14/14)
Salles-Cunha et al.[81]	1978	VC, τ, Doppler	74% (54/73)	94% (49/52)
Lepore et al.[62]	1978	VO_2/VC = 0.65	86% (71/83)	92% (48/52)
Young et al.[112]	1978	VC vs. MVO	100% (7/7)	60% (12/20)
O'Donnell et al.[76]	1983	VC vs. VO_3	93% (53/57)	100% (23/23)
PNEUMATIC PLETHYSMOGRAPHY				
Nicholas et al.[73]	1977	VO_2/VC = 0.50	78% (36/46)	91% (21/23)
Hanel et al.[38]	1981	VC vs. MVO	62% (81/130)	77% (41/53)
Holden et al.[44]	1981	VO_2/VC = 0.70	96% (60/63)	38% (6/16)
Sufian et al.[92]	1981	VC, MVO, Doppler	98% (40/41)	83% (20/24)
McBride et al.[66]	1981	VC, MVO, MVO/VC	73% (?)	83% (?)
Schroeder and Dunn[85]	1982	VC, MVO, Doppler	84% (21/25)	66% (21/32)

*Venous capacitance.

†Maximum rate of venous outflow.

‡Venous outflow volume in n seconds following release of venous occlusion pressure.

Table 80-8. Thermography—correlation with 1164 venograms in symptomatic limbs

Investigator	Year	Correlation with normal venograms (specificity)	Correlation with recent proximal DVT (sensitivity)
Cooke and Pilcher[21]	1974	100% (49/49)	96% (51/53)
Leiviskä and Perttala[61]	1975	100% (17/17)	89% (34/38)
Bergqvist et al.[8]	1977	69% (22/32)	97% (75/77)
Bystrom et al.[15]	1977	88% (22/25)	100% (26/26)
Nilsson et al.[74]	1979	50% (7/14)	95% (35/37)
Watz and Bygdeman[101]	1979	77% (27/35)	95% (19/20)
Ritchie et al.[80]	1979	81% (113/139)	74% (53/72)
Aronen et al.[1]	1981	81% (81/100)	93% (38/41)
Lockner et al.[64]	1981	49% (31/63)	99% (95/96)
Pochaczevsky et al.[78]	1982	83% (15/18)	100% (12/12)
Jacobsson et al.[54]	1983	47% (33/70)	95% (123/130)
TOTALS		74% (417/562)	93% (561/602)

OVERALL ACCURACY = 84% (978/1,164)

and somewhat cumbersome. Recently techniques using liquid crystal thermography[78] or a portable noncontact infrared radiation transducer[54,74] have been reported. These techniques are less expensive and more portable than an infrared camera. To obtain valid data, thermography must be performed after exposing the lower half of the body to room air for at least 15 minutes. This allows the skin temperature to achieve thermal equilibrium. As presented in Table 80-8, the sensitivity reported for thermography has been quite good; however, the specificity has not been as good. This is not surprising, since numerous conditions unrelated to DVT might raise the skin temperature of the legs. It is reasonable to combine thermography with other noninvasive methods that have demonstrated a high specificity to avoid false positive results.[54]

Recently there has been considerable interest in using ultrasonic imaging devices for diagnosing DVT. When combined with pulsed Doppler technology (Duplex scanning), the conventional Doppler accuracy should improve and localize the thrombus. Disadvantages include the high cost of equipment, the need for an expert technician, and the inability to do tests at the bedside.[95]

Selection of a noninvasive test for the management of DVT is now generally considered to be a choice made from Doppler ultrasound or one of the plethysmographic techniques, usually IPG or PRG. With additional documentation, thermography, strain-gauge plethysmography (SPG), and ultrasonic imaging may also prove reliable for this purpose. Since these methods have different strengths and weaknesses, some laboratories consider the methods complementary and employ more than one method of noninvasive evaluation.

CLINICAL EXPERIENCE

Extensive and favorable clinical experience has been reported using noninvasive tests for the management of suspected DVT (Fig. 80-1). In hospitals with established reliability in noninvasive evaluation of DVT, it is safe and cost-effective to stop a diagnostic workup when normal results on DVT testing are obtained. In our experience, no fatal pulmonary emboli were observed in 1074 patients with bilaterally normal IPG tests. In only 1% of these patients was there a suspicion of nonfatal pulmonary emboli.[109] Similarly in 593 patients with negative PRG tests, Stallworth et al.[89] found a 0.7% incidence of thromboembolic complications. Only one pulmonary embolism was reported in an aggregate of 1351 patients with negative [^{125}I]fibrinogen leg scans.[13] An extremely low incidence of thromboembolic complications has also been reported in patients with normal Doppler examinations[2] or thermography.[54] Thus the risk of *not* treating patients with normal results of noninvasive tests appears to be appreciably less than the complications of anticoagulant treatment, perhaps less than the risk of venography. In addition, the cost savings are considerable.[50]

Relying on abnormal results of noninvasive tests as an indication to start treatment for DVT is associated with more risk. False positive results can be obtained with all noninvasive techniques, and anticoagulant treatment has an incidence of major complications variously reported from 1% to

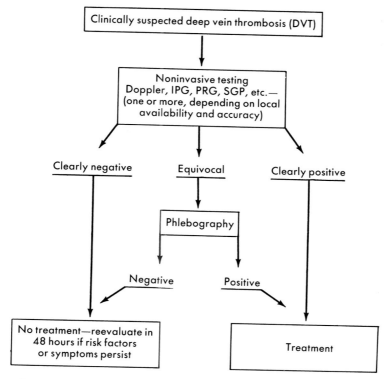

Fig. 80-1. Diagnostic approach for management of clinically suspected DVT.

20%.[82] It is a matter of clinical judgment and local laboratory accuracy as to whether or not venography should be obtained before starting anticoagulant treatment. It is our policy to rely on noninvasive test results when there is no clinical reason to suspect a false positive examination.

Use of noninvasive tests has been particularly beneficial in the emergency room and outpatient clinics when ruling out the need for venography or hospitalization. Over 90% of these patients do not have DVT; 323 patients were evaluated by IPG and 302 proved normal.[109] Some of these patients were admitted to the hospital for other reasons, but 284 were discharged with no further study or treatment. There were no pulmonary emboli, and only 1 patient (0.3%) developed DVT on further follow-up. By comparison, of 160 patients with negative venograms, 2 patients (1.25%) developed DVT on follow-up, perhaps as a result of the venography.[49]

DISCUSSION

As in the use of diagnostic tests for other disease states, the intelligent application of diagnostic tests for DVT requires an understanding of both the disease process and the test employed. There is no test that is universally applicable to all patients. To rely on noninvasive tests as the basis for treatment in a particular patient, one must take into account certain underlying principles that will be considered in the following discussion.

Natural history of DVT

There is a widespread spectrum of severity in DVT that ranges from clinically insignificant to life-threatening. The minor forms of DVT are extremely prevalent in patients who are bedridden for any great length of time. The more serious stages of the disease are fortunately much less common. The overwhelming majority of pulmonary emboli originate in the iliac or femoral veins, but a samll number do originate in the hypogastric veins or the heart. Detection of DVT in these latter locations remains an unsolved problem. In selecting which noninvasive test (or combination of tests) to use, clinicians must determine the relative importance to be attached to the detection of thrombi in different anatomic areas. It is important to remember that no test, including venography, can detect all thrombi capable of causing pulmonary emboli.

The relative importance of detecting calf vein

thrombosis, or the lack thereof, has been the source of considerable confusion. The widespread prevalence of calf vein thrombi disclosed by [^{125}I]fibrinogen studies at first amazed many clinicians. They simply could not understand the disparity between the very large number of patients with DVT documented by this extremely sensitive technique and the very small number of patients who exhibited any clinical ill effects of the disease. The implicit assumption of most physicians had been that whenever DVT existed, at whatever stage, it posed a potentially serious threat to the patient and required aggressive treatment. DVT, like pregnancy or cancer, was simplistically regarded as an all-or-nothing phenomenon. The patient either had DVT or did not, and if DVT was present, treatment was mandatory. However, with the high sensitivity of the [^{125}I]fibrinogen technique and the ability to diagnose small calf thrombi, physicians were confronted with the decision of whether or not to treat the earliest stages of the disease, which proved to be much more frequent and much more benign than had previously been suspected. The surgeon, for example, was suddenly faced with the prospect of having to prescribe anticoagulants for up to 30% of all postoperative patients over the age of 40. The risk of serious bleeding complications from such treatment is sufficiently great that such a course seemed unthinkable to most surgeons—or at least seemed riskier than leaving the patients untreated, just as they had always been left untreated before use of [^{125}I]fibrinogen testing. Dilemmas such as this raised obvious questions about the treatment of DVT. Do the earliest stages of DVT need to be treated at all? Is there not a group of patients with such minimal disease that the risk of treatment outweighs the risk of nontreatment? If so, is it really of any practical importance to detect these early stages of the disease?

There is still disagreement on these questions. However, certain facts have become well established. Thrombosis confined solely to the calf veins is extremely common in hospitalized patients. The overwhelming majority of such patients never have any untoward clinical sequelae, even if untreated. The risk of pulmonary embolism from DVT confined to one or two calf veins alone is less than the risk of anticoagulant treatment. A few calf thrombi—perhaps 20% at most—will propagate to the popliteal vein if untreated.[59] In the small percentage of patients in whom thrombus propagates

into the popliteal vein, the risk of pulmonary embolism is substantially increased. Accurate detection of popliteal vein thrombosis is an important prerequisite of any noninvasive test for DVT.

Lethal pulmonary emboli are usually very large thrombi, essentially "casts" of the iliac or femoral veins. Any noninvasive test that serves as a basis for treatment of DVT must be extremely reliable in the detection of these large thrombi in major veins.

Patients with acute DVT, reflected by signs and symptoms in the leg, usually have extensive disease. Swelling does not occur until major venous obstruction exists and is not caused by isolated calf vein thrombosis. Symptomatic patients are easily evaluated by plethysmographic or Doppler methods.

For several years our policy has been merely to observe patients with small calf thrombi who do not have major continuing risk factors but to treat those patients who either have extensive calf DVT or who have less severe calf DVT but also have major continuing risk factors, particularly prolonged bed rest. No adverse clinical consequences have led us to question this approach. However, it should be emphasized that all patients with calf vein thrombosis or with major risk factors leaving them vulnerable to DVT have been placed on continuing surveillance with noninvasive tests or given prophylactic treatment for as long as they remain at risk. If major risk factors are expected to persist indefinitely, long-term anticoagulation therapy has often been instituted.

Finally, when managing patients on the basis of noninvasive tests, it is important to understand that venous thrombosis is a dynamic disease that can change appreciably from day to day, resulting both from lysis of existing thrombus and from development of further thrombosis.[52] Such changes can occur within a few hours, but the time span is usually a few days. In choosing a suitable diagnostic test to assess the extent of venous thrombosis, it is therefore important that the test be easily repeatable.

Patient considerations

The selection of a diagnostic test may be precluded by individual considerations. Some patients are simply too sick or too difficult to transport for venography. A few patients may not be suitable for noninvasive tests because of bandages, plaster casts, extreme local discomfort, or poor cooperation. Infection or inflammation can lead to false positive [^{125}I]fibrinogen tests. Previous DVT may render the interpretation of abnormal plethysmographic or Doppler findings questionable. Severe peripheral vasoconstriction, low cardiac output, or shock may make it difficult to obtain adequate venous filling for venous occlusion plethysmography. In short, there is no diagnostic procedure that is unfailingly applicable to all patients, but this does not diminish the fact that noninvasive tests are extremely useful when appropriately applied and interpreted.

In selecting a diagnostic test, it is important to distinguish between patient groups. A test that is extremely useful in one patient group may be of less benefit in another. Patients with symptoms caused by DVT almost invariably have involvement of the popliteal, femoral, or iliac veins, or extensive calf vein disease. Often symptoms suspected to be caused by DVT are the result of other conditions, and the venous system is completely normal. Such patients are accurately assessed by plethysmographic methods, or by Doppler studies in the hands of an experienced observer. The results are immediately available, unlike the results of [^{125}I]fibrinogen testing. Plethysmographic or Doppler tests are ideal for patients who initially have signs or symptoms suggesting DVT.

If one wishes to detect asymptomatic calf vein thrombi, or the presence of fresh thrombosis in patients who have persistent venous outflow obstruction from old DVT, [^{125}I]fibrinogen testing is the most reliable noninvasive method at the present time. In patients with old DVT, the demonstration of venous obstruction by plethysmography or Doppler examination may not differentiate between recent and old thrombosis; [^{125}I]fibrinogen tests can detect fresh thrombosis in these patients more reliably. On the other hand, in patients following hip reconstruction, where potentially lethal thrombi may originate in the groin region, [^{125}I]fibrinogen testing alone is inadequate.

In summary, the physician must distinguish between patient groups to select the appropriate noninvasive test. For calf vein thrombosis studied prospectively, [^{125}I]fibrinogen testing is clearly the procedure of choice. For symptomatic patients with suspected DVT, particularly when an immediate answer is necessary, plethysmographic or Doppler examination is preferable. Individual considera-

tions may influence the applicability of a particular test procedure for a specific patient.

Selection of diagnostic tests

The prime consideration in selecting any diagnostic test is its sensitivity and specificity for a given patient group. Other factors that must be considered include the convenience and acceptability of the test procedure to the patient, as well as the ability to obtain repeat examinations for as long as the patient remains at risk. Immediate availability of results is sometimes important clinically and may lead physicians to favor procedures in which results are immediately available, such as plethysmographic or Doppler examination, rather than procedures in which the results are delayed, such as the [^{125}I]fibrinogen-uptake test. The expense of the various noninvasive procedures may also be considered but is usually not a major determinant of which tests are employed, since none of the noninvasive tests is expensive by comparison with the economic and medical importance of the information obtained. None of the noninvasive tests are recognized to involve risk for the patient, and potential complications of the procedure are not a factor in test selection.

In selecting a diagnostic test, the physician must first know its sensitivity and specificity for the patient group in question. Generalizations about overall accuracy, involving all stages of the disease and all types of patients, are meaningless with respect to the usefulness of a test in a specific patient. A test that has little use in one patient group may be the procedure of choice in another. The fact that [^{125}I]fibrinogen testing is inaccurate in the diagnosis of thrombi originating in the groin or pelvis, which are particularly important in patients undergoing total hip replacement, does not invalidate its usefulness in detecting more distal thrombi in patients undergoing abdominal or thoracic surgery. The fact that plethysomographic methods are inaccurate for isolated calf vein thrombosis does not invalidate their usefulness in the evaluation of patients who initially have signs and symptoms suggesting DVT, since symptomatic patients almost invariably have either a normal venous system or else have iliac, femoral, or popliteal thrombosis in which plethysmography is extremely reliable.

How accurate must a test be to be relied on clinically? Realistically, one must admit that a perfect test will never exist. Even venography is not perfect and is relied on as the final yardstick partly because it gives a satisfying anatomic picture of the extent of disease and partly because there is nothing known to be more reliable with which to compare it. Venography has its own errors, particularly with thrombi in the iliac veins. These errors are not infrequent in the hands of inexperienced radiologists. Sometimes thrombi in the iliac veins have been overlooked by conventional ascending venography and have then been demonstrated by noninvasive tests and subsequently confirmed by percutaneous femoral venography.

Medical practice will always be an imprecise science. The physician must decide for each individual patient whether or not a given degree of diagnostic accuracy is an adequate basis for treatment. For example, let us consider a patient known to be at high risk for DVT, who initially has unilateral leg swelling and tenderness and in whom the IPG is markedly abnormal in the affected extremity. In symptomatic patients, the accuracy of this noninvasive test alone is 95% to 100%. The typical clinical background and the physical findings add impressive corroboration. To subject such a patient to the discomfort, risk, and expense of venography is not only unnecessary but also wasteful and even unkind.

On the other hand, a bilaterally abnormal IPG in an asymptomatic patient with CHF may be a false positive result.[46,48] Without any corroborating clinical findings, the physician should have venographic confirmation of the diagnosis before treatment. If this same patient is recovering from a severe myocardial infarction and is hemodynamically unstable, the physician might hesitate to order venography and rely instead on the noninvasive procedure, particularly if the abnormal test result was unilateral. As in much of medical practice, clinical judgment is essential.

Consideration must be given to individual circumstances in arriving at a decision to base treatment on a diagnosis of DVT made by noninvasive tests with a given degree of accuracy. The risks of both treating the patient and of failing to treat the patient must be taken into account, as well as the risks of any further diagnostic procedures that might be available.

In considering how high a degree of diagnostic accuracy is necessary for treatment of DVT, one must consider the consequences of an inaccurate diagnosis. From a clinical point of view, failure to detect isolated calf vein thrombi appears to be rel-

atively inconsequential, provided the patient continues under surveillance for the duration of the period of risk. On the other hand, failure to detect large clots in the femoral or iliac vein is potentially life-threatening, not to mention the greater likelihood of a postphlebitic syndrome caused by delay in treatment. In selecting a diagnostic test, it is critical that the procedure be highly accurate in detecting main vessel thrombi of sufficient size to pose a threat of significant pulmonary embolism; but it is of much less importance whether the procedure can detect small calf thrombi, which pose little threat to the patient.

Individual hospital considerations

All the theoretic considerations discussed may be of less practical importance than local considerations in selecting a diagnostic test for DVT. All tests are not equally available, and their accuracy may vary considerably in different settings. No matter how advisable venography may be in the teaching hospital setting, a community hospital may simply not have the procedure available. Even if the local radiologist is willing to undertake venography, the accuracy and the potential risk to the patient may be quite different from that in a major medical center.

Similarly, noninvasive tests that give excellent results in the hands of research investigators may be much less reliable in the hands of a relatively inexperienced technician in a community hospital. In deciding whether or not a patient can be treated on the basis of noninvasive test results, it is important to assess the sensitivity and the specificity *locally* rather than from the literature. Tests that are relatively simple and objective may be preferable to those that are more complicated to perfrom or more subjective in their interpretation, requiring a greater degree of training and experience.

Comment

The decision as to when a diagnosis is sufficiently well established to undertake treatment is ultimately a matter of clinical judgment, based on all available clinical and laboratory information and with each patient considered as an individual problem. There is a small but inevitable element of uncertainty in the diagnosis of many diseases just as there is with DVT. It is true that if venograms are done on every patient, an absolute diagnosis can be established in many. On the other hand, an element of uncertainty will remain in some patients despite venography. Furthermore, even if the venogram is apparently negative, who can say that DVT will not be present 72 hours later, possibly even as a result of the venogram?

Now that noninvasive tests are consistently achieving overall diagnostic correlations with venography as high as 95% and even higher in certain patient groups, it becomes reasonable to use such tests as the primary basis for treatment. For a patient with a typical clinical picture of DVT and an abnormal noninvasive test that is at least 95% accurate for DVT, it seems to be poor medical practice to subject the patient to the risk, discomfort, and expense of venography.

The choice as to which noninvasive test to employ may be dictated by practical circumstances in each individual hospital. The least expensive equipment may not be the most reliable, but it may be all that is possible for small institutions or private offices. The most complicated procedure may provide the most overall information but may also require a sophisticated examiner with considerable training and experience in order to be reliable. In developing a noninvasive testing program each hospital should assess its own resources, and particularly its technical personnel, in relation to the demands made on them by the test procedure.

Several noninvasive tests have now stood the test of time, and others may establish themselves in the future. [125I]fibrinogen testing has been widely studied and is clearly the most sensitive test for the diagnosis of calf vein thrombosis. For more proximal lesions, which may well be of much greater importance clinically, Doppler ultrasound is adequate in the hands of skilled examiners, although its subjective nature leads to unacceptable results in the hands of those less experienced in its use. PRG gives excellent results in the hands of those with adequate training in its use. IPG has been used by many investigators and has proved consistently reliable for recent major DVT. It is a simpler and more objective test than PRG or Doppler. Other types of venous outflow plethysmography have been less thoroughly studied to date but have also shown generally good to excellent results. Thermography has shown excellent sensitivity, although its specificity has not been as good. In combination with plethysmography or a Doppler examination, thermography should become an acceptable method for the detection of DVT. Any of these techniques or various combinations of them can reasonably form the basis for a noninvasive

testing program, provided accuracy locally can be made comparable to the results reported in the literature. This is possible with all the above techniques but is easier with some than others.

Imaging techniques, whether based on ultrasound or radioisotopes, appear promising, although less well studied than the methods previously mentioned. They are probably an acceptable alternative, although more expensive and less convenient for the patient than the simpler bedside techniques.

No single test is ideal under all circumstances for every type of patient. In using noninvasive tests, one must be aware of those patient groups in which a particular test may have limitations or inaccuracies. The physician must be aware of the major risk factors that lead to the development of DVT and be able to identify those patients at high risk. He must understand the broad spectrum of the disease, realizing that small clots originating in the calf veins are very common but relatively innocuous and probably less dangerous to the patient than prolonged anticoagulation therapy. He must also realize that although clots originating in the groin or pelvis are relatively uncommon, they are potentially lethal. Finally, he must consider all aspects of the patient's medical condition and interpret the test result in the context of all the information available.

SUMMARY

The competent physician who understands the pathophysiology of DVT should be able to manage the great majority of patients suspected of having this disease on the basis of noninvasive tests, reserving venography for particularly complex or controversial circumstances.

REFERENCES

1. Aronen, H.J., et al.: Thermography in deep venous thrombosis of the leg, AJR 137:1179, 1981.
2. Baker, W.H., and Hayes, A.C.: The normal Doppler venous examination, Angiology 34:283, 1983.
3. Barnes, R.W., Russell, H.E., and Wilson, M.F.: Doppler ultrasonic evaluation of venous disease, a programmed audiovisual instruction, ed. 2, Iowa City, Iowa, 1975, University of Iowa.
4. Barnes, R.W., et al.: Noninvasive quantitation of maximum venous outflow in acute thrombophlebitis, Surgery 72:971, 1972.
5. Barnes, R.W., et al.: Detection of deep vein thrombosis with an automatic electrically calibrated strain gauge plethysmograph, Surgery 82:219, 1077.
6. Becker, J.: The diagnosis of venous thrombosis in the legs using I-labelled fibrinogen: an experimental and clinical study, Acta Chir. Scand. 138:667, 1972.
7. Bendick, P.J., et al.: Pitfalls of the Doppler examination for venous thrombosis, Am. Surg. 49:320, 1983.

8. Bergqvist, D., et al.: Thermography: a noninvasive method for diagnosis of deep venous thrombosis, Arch. Surg. 112:600, 1977.

9. Boccalon, H., et al.: Venous plethysmography applied in pathologic conditions, Angiology 32:822, 1981.

10. Bolton, J.P., and Hoffman, V.J.: Incidence of early postoperative iliofemoral thrombosis, Br. Med. J. 1:247, 1975.

11. Bounameaux, H., Krähenbühl, B., and Vukanovic, S.: Diagnosis of deep vein thrombosis by combination of Doppler ultrasound flow examination and strain gauge plethysmography: an alternative to venography only in particular conditions despite improved accuracy of the Doppler method, Thromb. Haemost. 47:141, 1982.

12. Browse, N.L.: The ^{125}I fibrinogen uptake test, Arch. Sug. 104:160, 1972.

13. Browse, N.L., and Thomas, M.L.: Source of nonlethal pulmonary emboli, Lancet 1(7845):258, 1974.

14. Browse, N.L., et al.: Diagnosis of established deep vein thrombosis with the 125 I-fibrinogen uptake test, Br. Med. J. 4:325, 1971.

15. Byström, L.G., et al.: The value of thermography and the determination of fibrin-fibrinogen degradation products in the diagnosis of deep vein thrombosis, Acta Med. Scand. 202:319, 1977.

16. Clarke-Pearson, D.L., and Creasman, W.T.: Diagnosis of deep venous thrombosis in obstetrics and gynecology by impedance phlebography, Obstet. Gynecol. 58:52, 1981.

17. Classen, J.N., Richardson, J.B., and Koontz, C.: A three-year experience with phleborheography: a noninvasive technique for the diagnosis of deep venous thrombosis, Ann. Surg. 195:800, 1982.

18. Collins, G.J., Jr., et al.: Phleborheographic diagnosis of venous obstruction, Ann. Surg. 189:25, 1979.

19. Comerota, A.J., et al.: Phleborheography—results of a ten-year experience, Surgery 91:573, 1982.

20. Cooke, E.D., and Pilcher, M.F.: Thermography in diagnosis of deep venous thrombosis, Br. Med. J. 2:523, 1973.

21. Cooke, E.D., and Pilcher, M.F.: Deep vein thrombosis: preclinical diagnosis by thermography, Br. J. Surg. 61:971, 1974.

22. Cooperman, M., et al.: Detection of deep venous thrombosis by impedance plethysmography, Am. J. Surg. 137:252, 1979.

23. Cramer, M., Beach, K.W., and Strandness, D.E., Jr.: The detection of proximal deep vein thrombosis by strain gauge plethysmography through the use of an outflow/capacitance discriminant line, Bruit 7:17, 1983.

24. Cranley, J.J., Canos, A.J., and Mahalingam, K.: Noninvasive diagnosis and prophylaxis of deep venous thrombosis of the lower extremity. In Madden, J.L., and Hume, M., editors: Venous thromboembolism: prevention and treatment, New York, 1976, Appleton-Century-Crofts.

25. Cranley, J.J., Canos, A.J., and Mahalingam, K.: Diagnosis of deep venous thrombosis by phleborheography. In Bergan, J.J., and Yao, J.S.T., editors: Venous problems, Chicago, 1978, Year Book Medical Publishers, Inc.

26. Cranley, J.J., et al.: A plethysmographic technique for the diagnosis of deep venous thrombosis of the lower extremities, Surg. Gynecol. Obstet. 136:385, 1973.

27. Cranley, J.J., et al.: Phleborheographic technique for diagnosing deep venous thrombosis of the lower extremities, Surg. Gynecol. Obstet. 141:331, 1975.

28. Dahn, I., and Eiriksson, E.: Plethysmographic diagnosis of deep venous thrombosis of the leg, Acta Chir. Scand. (Suppl.)398:33, 1968.

29. Dmochowski, J.R., Adams, D.F., and Couch, N.P.: Impedance measurement in the diagnosis of deep venous thrombosis, Arch. Surg. 104:170, 1972.

30. Dosick, S.M., and Blakemore, W.S.: The role of Doppler ultrasound in acute deep vein thrombosis, Am. J. Surg. 136:265, 1978.

31. Evans, D.S.: The early diagnosis of deep-vein thrombosis by ultrasound, Br. J. Surg. 57:726, 1970.

32. Field, E.S.: Deep vein thrombosis in patients with fractures of the femoral neck, Br. J. Surg. 59:377, 1972.

33. Flanigan, D.P., et al.:Vascular-laboratory diagnosis of clinically suspected acute deep vein thrombosis, Lancet 2(8085):331, 1978.

34. Foti, M.E., and Gurewich, V.: Fibrin degradation products and impedance plethysmography: measurements in the diagnosis of acute deep vein theombosis, Arch. Intern. Med. 140:903, 1980.

35. Gallus, A.S., and Hirsh, J.: ^{125}I-Fibrinogen scanning. In Mobin-Uddin, K., editor: Pulmonary thromboembolism, Springfield, Ill., 1975, Charles C Thomas, Publisher.

36. Gross, W.S., and Burney, R.E.: Therapeutic and economic implications of emergency department evaluation for venous thrombosis, J. Am. Coll. Emer. Physicians 8:110, 1979.

37. Hallböök, T., and Ling, L.: Plethysmography in the diagnosis of acute deep vein thrombosis, Vasa 3:263, 1974.

38. Hanel, K.C., et al.: The role of two noninvasive tests in deep venous thrombosis, Ann. Surg. 194:725, 1981.

39. Harris, W.H., et al.: Comparison of ^{125}I fibrinogen count scanning with phlebography for detection of venous thrombi after elective hip surgery, N. Engl. J. Med. 292:665, 1975.

40. Harris, W.H., et al.: Cuff-impedance phlebography and ^{125}I fibrinogen scanning versus roentgenographic phlebography for diagnosis of thrombophlebitis following hip surgery, J. Bone Joint Surg. 58A:939, 1976.

41. Harris, W.H., et al.: The accuracy of the *in vivo* diagnosis of deep vein thrombosis in patients with prior venous thromboembolic disease or severe varicose veins, Thromb. Res. 21:137, 1981.

42. Hirsh, J., and Hull, R.D.: Comparative value of tests for the diagnosis of venous thrombosis. In Bernstein, E.F., editor: Noninvasive diagnostic techniques in vascular disease, St. Louis, 1978, C.V. Mosby Co.

43. Hobbs, J.T., and Davies, J.W.L.: Detection of venous thrombosis with 131 I-labeled fibrinogen in the rabbit, Lancet 2(7142):134, 1960.

44. Holden, R.W., et al.: Efficacy of noninvasive modalities for diagnosis of thrombophlebitis, Diagn. Radiol. 141:63, 1981.

45. Holmes, M.C.G.: Deep venous thrombosis of the lower limbs diagnosed by ultrasound, Med. J. Aust. 1:427, 1973.

46. Hull, R., et al.: Impedance plethysmography using the occlusive cuff technique in the diagnosis of venous thrombosis, Circulation 53:696, 1976.

47. Hull, R., et al.: Combined use of leg scanning and impedance plethysmography in suspected venous thrombosis. An alternative to therapy, N. Engl. J. Med. 296:1497, 1977.

48. Hull, R., et al.: Impedance plethysmography: the relationship between venous filling and sensitivity and specificity for proximal vein thrombosis, Circulation 58:898, 1978.

49. Hull, R., et al.: Clinical validity of a negative venogram in patients with clinically suspected venous thrombosis, Circulation 64:622, 1981.

50. Hull, R. et al.: Cost effectiveness of clinical diagnosis, venography, and noninvasive testing in patients with symptomatic deep-vein thrombosis, N. Engl. J. Med. 304:1461, 1981.

51. Hull, R., et al.: Replacement of venography in suspected venous thrombosis by impedance plethysmography and ^{125}I-fibrinogen leg scanning: a less invasive approach, Ann. Intern. Med. 94:12, 1981

52. Hume, M.: Postoperative venous thrombosis—the dynamics of propagation, resolution and embolism. In Bergan, J.J., and Yao, J.S.T., editors: Venous problems, Chicago, 1978, Year Book Medical Publishers, Inc.

53. Hume, M., et al.: Extent of leg vein thrombosis determined by impedance and ^{125}I-fibrinogen, Am. J. Surg. 129:455, 1975.

54. Jacobsson, H., et al.: Standardized leg temperature profiles in the diagnosis of acute deep venous thrombosis, Vasc. Diagn. Ther. 55, May/June 1983.

55. Johnson, W.C.: Evaluation of newer techniques for the diagnosis of venous thrombosis, J. Surg. Res. 16:473, 1974.

56. Johnston, K.W., and Kakkar, V.V.: Plethysmographic diagnosis of deep vein thrombosis, Surg. Gynecol. Obstet. 139:41, 1974.

57. Kakkar, V.V.: The diagnosis of deep vein thrombosis using the ^{125}I-fibrinogen test, Arch. Surg. 104:152, 1972.

58. Kakkar, V.V.: Fibrinogen uptake test for detection of deep vein thrombosis—a review of clincial practice, Semin. Nucl. Med. 7:229, 1977.

59. Kakkar, V.V., et al.: Natural history of postoperative deep vein thrombosis, Lancet 2:230, 1969.

60. Lambie, J.M., et al.: Diagnostic accuracy in venous thrombosis, Br. Med. J. 2:142, 1970.

61. Leiviskä, T., and Perttala, Y.: Thermography in diagnosing deep venous thrombosis of the lower limb, Radiologia Clin. 44:417, 1975.

62. Lepore, T.J., et al.: Screening for lower extremity deep venous thrombosis. An improved plethysmographic and Doppler approach, Am. J. Surg. 135:529, 1978.

63. Liapis, C.D., et al.: Value of impedance plethysmography in suspected venous disease of the lower extremity, Angiology 31:522, 1980.

64. Lockner, D., et al.: Thermography in the diagnosis of DVT, Thromb. Haemost. 46:652, 1981.

65. Maryniak, O., and Nicholson, C.G.: Doppler ultrasonography for detection of deep vein thrombosis in lower extremities, Arch. Phys. Med. Rehabil. 60:277, 1979.

66. McBride, K.J., et al.: Venous volume displacement plethysmography: its diagnostic value in deep venous thrombosis as determined by receiver operator characteristic curves, Bulletin of Texas Heart Institute 8:499, 1981.

67. Meadway, J., et al.: Value of Doppler ultrasound in diagnosis of clinically suspected deep venous thrombosis, Br. Med. J. 4:552, 1975.

68. Milne, R.M., et al.: Postoperative deep venous thrombosis: a comparison of diagnostic techniques, Lancet 2:445, 1971.

69. Moser, K.M., Brach, B.B., and Dolan, G.F.: Clinically suspected deep venous thrombosis of the lower extremities: a comparison of venography, impedance plethysmography, and radiolabeled fibrinogen, JAMA 237:2195, 1977.

70. Mullick, S.C., Wheeler, H.B., and Songster, G.F.: Diagnosis of deep venous thrombosis by measurement of electrical impedance, Am. J. Surg. 119:417, 1970.

71. Nadeau, J.E., et al.: Impedance phlebography: accuracy of diagnosis in deep vein thrombosis, Can. J. Surg. 18:219, 1975.

72. Negus, D., et al.: ^{125}I-labelled fibrinogen in the diagnosis of deep vein thrombosis and its correlation with phlebography, Br. J. Surg. 55:835, 1968.

73. Nicholas, G.G., et al.: Clinical vascular laboratory diagnosis of deep venous thrombosis, Ann. Surg. 186:213, 1977.

74. Nilsson, E., Sundén, P., and Zetterquist, S.: Leg temperature profiles with a simplified thermographic technique in the diagnosis of acute venous thrombosis, Scand. J. Clin. Lab. Invest. 39:171, 1979.

75. Nolan, T.R., et al.: Diagnostic accuracy of phleborheography in deep venous thrombosis, Am. Surg. 48:77, 1982.

76. O'Donnell, J.A., et al.: Impedance plethysmography: noninvasive diagnosis of deep venous thrombosis and arterial insufficiency, Am. Surg. 49:26, 1983.

77. Pinto, D.J.: Controlled trial of an anticoagulant (warfarin sodium) in the prevention of venous thrombosis following hip surgery, Br. J. Surg. 57:349, 1970.

78. Pochaczevsky, R., et al.: Liquid crystal contact thermography of deep venous thrombosis, AJR 138:717, 1982.

79. Richards, K.L., et al.: Noninvasive diagnosis of deep venous thrombosis, Arch. Intern. Med. 136:1091, 1976.

80. Ritchie, W.G., et al.: Thermographic diagnosis of deep venous thrombosis, Radiology 131:341, 1979.

81. Salles-Cunha, S.X., Bernhard, V.M., and Imray, T.J.: Reliability of Doppler and impedance techniques for the diagnosis of thrombophlebitis, Med. Instrum. 12:117, 1978.

82. Salzman, E.W., and Davies, G.C.: Prophylaxis of venous thromboembolism: analysis of cost effectiveness, Ann. Surg. 191:207, 1980.

83. Sauerbrei, E., et al.: Observer variation in lower limb venography, J. Can. Assoc. Radiol. 31:28, 1981.

84. Sautter, R.D., et al.: The limited utility of fibrinogen I-125 leg scanning, Arch. Intern. Med. 139:148, 1979.

85. Schroeder, P.J., and Dunn, E.: Mechanical plethysmography and Doppler ultrasound, Arch. Surg. 117:301, 1982.

86. Seeber, J.J.: Impedance plethysmography: a useful method in the diagnosis of deep vein thrombophlebitis in the lower extremity, Arch. Phys. Med. Rehabil. 55:170, 1974.

87. Sigel, B., et al.: A Doppler ultrasound method for diagnosing lower extremity venous disease, Surg. Gynecol. Obstet. 127:339, 1968.

88. Sigel, B., et al.: Diagnosis of lower limb venous thrombosis by Doppler ultrasound technique, Arch. Surg. 104:174, 1972.

89. Stallworth, J.M., et al.: Negative phleborheography, Arch. Surg. 116:175, 1981.

90. Steer, M.L., et al.: Limitations of impedance phlebography for diagnosis of venous thrombosis, Arch. Surg. 106:44, 1973.

91. Strandness, D.E., Jr., and Sumner, D.S.: Ultrasonic velocity detector in the diagnosis of thrombophlebitis, Arch. Surg. 104:180, 1972.

92. Sufian, S.: Noninvasive vascular laboratory diagnosis of deep venous thrombosis, Am. Surg. 47:254, 1981.

93. Sumner, D.S.: The approach to diagnosis and monitoring of venous disease. In Rutherford, R.B., editor: Vascular surgery, Philadelphia, 1977, W.B. Saunders Co.

94. Sumner, D.S., and Lambeth, A.: Reliability of Doppler ultrasound in the diagnosis of acute venous thrombosis both above and below the knee, Am. J. Surg. 138:205, 1979.

95. Talbot, S.R.: Use of real-time imaging in identifying deep venous obstruction: a preliminary report, Bruit 6:41, 1982.

96. Todd, J.W., et al.: Deep venous thrombosis in acute spinal cord injury: a comparison of ^{125}I fibrinogen leg scanning and venography, Paraplegia 14:50, 1976.

97. Toy, P.T.C.Y., and Schrier, S.L.: Occlusive impedance plethysmography. A noninvasive method of diagnosis of deep vein thrombosis, West. J. Med. 129:89, 1978.

98. Tsapogas, M.J., et al.: Postoperative venous thrombosis and the effectiveness of prophylactic measures, Arch. Surg. 103:561, 1971.

99. Walker, M.G.: The natural history of venous thromboembolism, Br. J. Surg. 59:753, 1972.

100. Walsh, J.J., Bonnar, J., and Wright, F.W.: A study of pulmonary embolism and deep leg vein thrombosis after major gynaecological surgery using labelled fibrinogenphlebography and lung scanning, J. Obstet. Gynaecol. Br. Commonw. 81:311, 1974.

101. Watz, R., et al.: Noninvasive diagnosis of acute deep vein thrombosis, Acta Med. Scand. 206:463, 1979.

102. Wheeler, H.B.: Plethysmographic diagnosis of deep venous thrombosis. In Rutherford, R.B., editor: Vascular surgery, ed. 2, Philadelphia, 1984, W.B. Saunders Co.

103. Wheeler, H.B., and Mullick, S.C.: Detection of venous obstruction in the leg by measurement of electrical impedance, Ann. N.Y. Acad. Sci. 170:804, 1970.

104. Wheeler, H.B., Patwardhan, N.A., and Anderson, F.A., Jr.: The place of occlusive impedance plethysmography in the diagnosis of venous thrombosis. In Bergan, J.J., and Yao, J.S.T., editors: Venous problems, Chicago, 1978, Year Book Medical Publishers, Inc.

105. Wheeler, H.B., et al.: Diagnosis of occult deep vein thrombosis by a noninvasive bedside technique, Surgery 70:20, 1971.

106. Wheeler, H.B., et al.: Impedance phlebography: technique, interpretation and results, Arch. Surg. 104:164, 1972.

107. Wheeler, H.B., et al.: Occlusive impedance phlebography: a diagnostic procedure for venous thrombosis and pulmonary embolism, Prog. Cardiovasc. Dis. 17:199, 1974.

108. Wheeler, H.B., et al.: Bedside screening for venous thrombosis using occlusive impedance phlebography, Angiology 26:199, 1975.

109. Wheeler, H.B., et al.: Suspected deep vein thrombosis: management by impedance plethysmography, Arch. Surg. 117:1206, 1982.

110. Yao, J.S.T., Gourmos, C., and Hobbs, J.T.: Detection of proximal vein thrombosis by Doppler ultrasound flow-detection method, Lancet 1(7740):1, 1972.

111. Yao, J.S.T., Henkin, R.E., and Bergan, J.J.: Venous thromboembolic disease: evaluation of new methodology in treatment, Arch. Surg. 109:664, 1974.

112. Young, A.E., et al.: Impedance plethysmography: its limitations as a substitute for phlebography, Cardiovasc. Rad. 1:233, 1978.

CHAPTER 81

Cost-effectiveness of noninvasive diagnosis of deep vein thrombosis in symptomatic patients

RUSSELL D. HULL, GARY E. RASKOB, and JACK HIRSH

This cost-effectiveness analysis is based to a large extent on data derived from approximately 500 patients with clinically suspected deep vein thrombosis (DVT) studied at McMaster University between 1975 and 1979.[8] All of these patients were carefully assessed clinically by a limited number of competent physicians according to a standard protocol by impedance plethysmography, [^{125}I]fibrinogen leg scanning, and venography.[8]

Cost-effectiveness analysis is an economic tool that when applied to health care evaluation allows ranking of alternative approaches to the same health problem to determine which is "best."[17] The best approach in economic terms can be defined as the approach that (1) accomplishes the desired health effect at minimum cost (cost minimization), (2) produces maximum health benefit for a given cost, or (3) carries the maximum effectiveness/cost ratio.

The application of cost-effectiveness analysis to the diagnosis of DVT is readily accomplished using cost minimization.[8] This cost-effectiveness technique makes it possible to rank the diagnostic approaches from "worst" to "best," with the best approach defined as that which accomplishes the desired health effect at minimum cost.

Effectiveness (health benefit) may be defined in this context as the number or proportion of patients with DVT correctly identified by objective testing. The reasons for correctly identifying DVT are (1) to treat patients with DVT in an attempt to prevent fatal pulmonary embolism and (2) to obviate the need for treatment and hospital admission for patients with clinically suspected DVT in whom the diagnosis is not confirmed by objective tests. It is generally accepted that proximal vein thrombosis is much more likely to lead to fatal pulmonary embolism[14,15] than is calf vein thrombosis and that the incidence of fatal pulmonary embolism can be markedly reduced if DVT is treated with heparin. Prevention of fatal pulmonary embolism is therefore used as a major parameter for assessing effectiveness. A second important complication of DVT is postphlebitic syndrome. However, no reliable information is available on the prevalence of postphlebitic syndrome in treated versus untreated DVT. This important complication therefore is not considered further in the cost-effectiveness analysis.

The parameters considered in the cost are the intrinsic costs of the tests, the cost of hospitalization, and the cost of treatment, which are the major costs for which hard data are available.[8] Other costs include the cost of treating side effects of the diagnostic procedure and of patient treatment (bleeding).[8] These costs are relatively minor and are not considered in the cost analysis, although they would detract from the effectiveness of any approach with which they were associated. The costs used in this analysis are based on mean conservative figures derived from a number of regions in North America; they are based on 1980 U.S. dollars and have been adjusted to reflect 1984 costs by applying an inflation index of 25% for the period 1980 to 1984.

The parameters considered in determining effectiveness are the proportion of patients with proximal vein thrombosis and with calf vein thrombosis correctly identified and the number of patients in whom fatal pulmonary embolism will be prevented by correct identification and treatment of DVT. Hard facts are provided for the proportion of patients with DVT correctly identified by testing, but the proportion of deaths averted by correct identification and treatment of DVT is based in part on hard data and in part on extrapolation from information obtained from (1) the frequency of fatal pulmonary embolism in patients with untreated DVT reported by Zilliacus[18] in the 1940s before anticoagulant therapy was available, (2) more recent studies by Barrit and Jordan[1] and by Kakkar et al.,[14] and (3) a number of recent reports in the literature[2,16] and our own experience[4] regarding the effectiveness of heparin therapy for the treatment of objectively documented DVT. In the report by Zilliacus, between 11% and 22% of patients with clinically diagnosed DVT died from major pulmonary embolism. This estimate of mortality for untreated DVT is supported by the findings of more recent studies that show that (1) 50% of patients with proximal vein thrombosis develop clinical pulmonary embolism, (2) 25% of patients with untreated pulmonary embolism develop a fatal pulmonary embolic event,[1] and (3) more than 50% of patients suffering a fatal pulmonary embolic event do so without premonitory pulmonary embolic episodes.[3] By extrapolation, these later findings support the more conservative estimate of an 11% fatality rate from pulmonary embolism in patients with untreated clinically suspected DVT.

Heparin therapy followed by orally administered anticoagulant therapy is effective in averting death from pulmonary embolism.[1-4,6,10-12,16] Commencement of anticoagulant therapy at the time of diagnosis of DVT is clearly preferable to treating the complicating pulmonary embolic events, as half of the fatal pulmonary embolic events would not be averted by the latter approach.

Approaches to the diagnosis of DVT in symptomatic patients include clinical diagnosis, venography, and one or more noninvasive approaches. The best evaluated of the noninvasive approaches are impedance plethysmography (IPG), Doppler ultrasonography, and [125I]fibrinogen leg scanning.[4]

The data that provided the basis for this cost-effectiveness analysis were derived from a study of approximately 500 patients referred to the Hamilton Regional Thromboembolism Programme with a first episode of clinically suspected DVT.[8] All were assessed clinically and were then investigated by venography, IPG, and, if the IPG was negative, leg scanning, which was carried out for 72 hours. Adequate venograms were obtained in 478 of these patients[8] (Fig. 81-1).

Treatment with heparin for 10 to 14 days plus orally administered anticoagulants for 3 months was given to patients in whom a positive diagnosis of acute DVT was made. None of the patients in

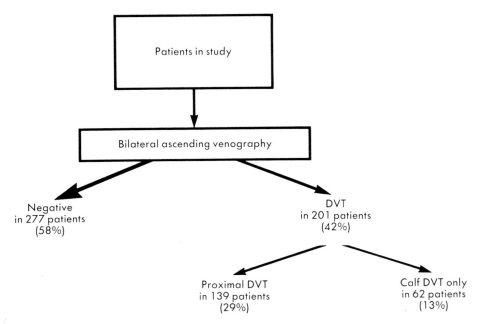

Fig. 81-1. Data that provided basis for this cost-effectiveness analysis were derived from study of 478 patients with first episodes of clinically suspected deep vein thrombosis, all of whom underwent bilateral ascending venography and noninvasive testing.

this study died from pulmonary embolism, and there were no fatal bleeding episodes in patients receiving anticoagulant therapy.[8]

Because all patients with negative IPG results underwent leg scanning, the effectiveness of serial IPG evaluations (used alone) could not be directly measured from this study.[4] We have recently completed a randomized clinical trial comparing combined IPG and [^{125}I]fibrinogen leg scanning with serial IPG alone for the diagnosis of clinically suspected venous thrombosis.[13] The results of this randomized trial provide relevant new data enabling the cost-effectiveness of serial IPG alone to be accurately evaluated (p. 824). Doppler ultrasonography was not formally evaluated in the study and therefore is not discussed here, but the cost-effectiveness of Doppler ultrasound can be approximated by interchanging the anticipated results obtained by Doppler ultrasound with those obtained by IPG. It should be noted, however, that the safety of withholding anticoagulant therapy on the basis of Doppler ultrasonography has not been formally evaluated.[4]

The simplified economic analysis of the results are displayed in two ways: (1) as though the patient had no co-morbid condition requiring in-hospital care and (2) as though the patient had co-morbid conditions requiring hospital care.

COST-EFFECTIVENESS OF DIAGNOSTIC APPROACHES FOR DVT IN PATIENTS WITHOUT CO-MORBID CONDITIONS REQUIRING HOSPITAL ADMISSION
Clinical diagnosis

Of the 478 patients with clinically suspected DVT the diagnosis was not confirmed by venography in 277 (58%). This figure for false positive results is remarkably similar to that obtained in a number of other studies evaluating the specificity of clinical diagnosis.[5] Thus, if admission to the hospital and treatment were based on clinical diagnosis, over 50% of patients would have been inappropriately admitted to the hospital and exposed to the hazards of short- and long-term anticoagulant therapy and the psychologic effects of an incorrect diagnosis of DVT.

An alternative approach to treatment in all patients with clinically suspected DVT would be to attempt to subselect for treatment those patients with severe symptoms. However, further analysis of the symptoms and signs leading to a clinical diagnosis of DVT revealed that no clinical findings

alone or in combination had sufficiently high predictive power to appreciably lessen this false positive rate. Furthermore, many patients with extensive proximal vein thrombosis did not have florid symptoms or signs of DVT, and many with "severe" clinical features did not have DVT. Thus selection of patients on clinical grounds would both expose patients without DVT to inappropriate admission to the hospital and treatment and would result in failure to treat a large proportion of patients with extensive DVT.

It is evident that selection of patients for anticoagulant therapy on clinical grounds exposes untreated patients to the risk of massive or fatal pulmonary embolism. It follows, therefore, that if clinical diagnosis is not corroborated by objective tests, all patients with clinically suspected DVT would have to receive treatment to reduce pulmonary embolic deaths to a minimum.

The most important complication (side effect) of anticoagulant therapy is major bleeding. In our experience this occurs in approximately 7% of patients receiving anticoagulant therapy. This is an undesirable and needless risk in patients who are subsequently shown not to have DVT on objective testing. Because the cost of this complication is relatively low compared with other costs and because death caused by bleeding is extremely infrequent (none of the patients receiving anticoagulant therapy in our study died from bleeding), neither the cost nor the effect of this side effect is formally evaluated in this analysis.[8]

It can be estimated from the information given previously that the mortality from pulmonary embolism or bleeding will be less than 1% in patients with treated DVT. The cost and effectiveness of clinical diagnosis are shown in Table 81-1.

The analysis is based on cost of the test, cost of hospitalization, and cost of treatment. The total cost of clinical diagnosis in 478 patients at $3063 per patient was $1,464,114. Thus the cost of clinical diagnosis for a yield of 201 patients with DVT correctly diagnosed and treated was $1,464,114, or $7284 per patient.

The total cost of clinical diagnosis for a yield of 53 deaths from pulmonary embolism averted was $1,464,114; therefore the cost for each death from pulmonary embolism averted was $27,625. Thus the cost-effectiveness of clinical diagnosis of DVT was $7284 per patient with DVT correctly identified and treated and $27,625 for each pulmonary embolic death averted.

Table 81-1. Cost-effectiveness of clinical diagnosis alone

Cost		Effectiveness*
Intrinsic technical cost	$0	Correctly identified DVT in 201 patients
Cost of hospital room at $250/day for 10 days	$2500	Averted 53 deaths from pulmonary embolism by giving treatment to all 478 patients with a clinical diagnosis of DVT
Cost of therapy and laboratory testing and monitoring (inpatient and outpatient)	$563	
Total cost per patient	$3063	
Total cost for 478 patients	$1,464,114	
COST-EFFECTIVENESS OF DESIRED HEALTH EFFECT		
Cost for each correct diagnosis of DVT	$7284	
Cost for each death from pulmonary embolism averted	$27,625	

*Desired health effect in 478 patients with clinical diagnosis of DVT.

Table 81-2. Cost-effectiveness of ascending venography as an outpatient diagnostic approach

Cost		Effectiveness*
Intrinsic cost of venography at $438/patient for 478 patients	$209,364	Correctly identified DVT in 201 patients
Cost of hospital room at $250/day for 10 days per patient for 201 patients with DVT	$502,500	Averted 53 deaths from pulmonary embolism by treating DVT in all 201 patients
Cost of therapy, laboratory tests, and monitoring at $563/patient for 201 patients with DVT	$113,163	
Total cost for 478 patients	$825,297	
COST-EFFECTIVENESS OF DESIRED HEALTH EFFECT		
Cost for each correct diagnosis of DVT	$4106	
Cost for each death from pulmonary embolism averted	$15,572	

*Desired health effect in 478 patients with clinical diagnosis of DVT.

Venography

Venography is accepted as the diagnostic reference standard for venous thrombosis against which noninvasive tests are measured. However, venography has disadvantages in that it is invasive, is associated with patient morbidity, and may not be readily available on an outpatient basis and so requires admission to the hospital. The cost will be considered on the basis of outpatient diagnosis and inpatient diagnosis.

Venography as an outpatient diagnostic approach. The cost and effectiveness of venography used as an outpatient diagnostic approach are shown in Table 81-2. Venography yielded negative results in 277 of 478 patients; thus the major cost incurred in this group was the cost of venography. The diagnosis of DVT was established in 201 patients (Fig. 81-1); thus the major costs incurred by these patients included not only the cost of venography but also of inpatient care and treatment. There were no deaths from pulmonary embolism (or bleeding).

As shown in Table 81-2, the total cost of this diagnostic approach in 478 patients was $825,297. Thus the cost of using outpatient venography as a diagnostic approach for a yield of 201 patients with DVT correctly diagnosed and treated was $825,297. Therefore the cost for each patient with DVT correctly diagnosed and treated was $4106.

The total cost of using outpatient venography as a diagnostic approach with a yield of 53 deaths from pulmonary embolism averted was $825,297. Therefore the cost for each death from pulmonary embolism averted was $15,572.

Venography as an elective inpatient diagnostic approach. Lack of availability of immediate outpatient venography may require that symptomatic pa-

Table 81-3. Cost-effectiveness of ascending venography applied as an inpatient elective diagnostic approach

Cost		Effectiveness*
Intrinsic cost of venography at $438/patient for 478 patients	$209,364	Correctly identified DVT in 201 patients
Cost of hospital room at $250/day for 10 days per patient for 201 patients with DVT	$502,500	Averted 53 deaths from pulmonary embolism by treating DVT in all 201 patients
Cost of therapy, laboratory tests, and monitoring at $563/patient for 201 patients with DVT	$113,163	
Cost of 3 days of in-hospital care and treatment with negative results at $938/patient for 277 patients	$259,826	
Total cost for 478 patients	$1,085,123	
COST-EFFECTIVENESS OF DESIRED HEALTH EFFECT		
Cost for each correct diagnosis of DVT	$5399	
Cost for each death from pulmonary embolism averted	$20,474	

*Desired health effect in 478 patients with clinical diagnosis of DVT.

tients be admitted to the hospital for elective venography. In our experience patients with clinically suspected DVT subsequently shown by elective venography not to have DVT had an average hospital stay of 3 days. If all 478 symptomatic patients were admitted to the hospital for elective venography, 277 patients (Fig. 81-1) would have been admitted to the hospital unnecessarily, incurring the costs of anticoagulant therapy and hospitalization for 3 days. The cost and effectiveness of this diagnostic approach are shown in Table 81-3.

The total cost of this diagnostic approach in 478 patients was $1,085,123. Thus the cost of using inpatient venography as a diagnostic approach for a yield of 201 patients with DVT correctly diagnosed and treated was $1,085,123. Therefore the cost for each patient with DVT correctly diagnosed and treated was $5399.

The total cost of using inpatient venography as a diagnostic approach for a yield of 53 deaths from pulmonary embolism averted was $1,085,123. Therefore the cost for each death from pulmonary embolism averted was $20,474.

Combined occlusive cuff impedance plethysmography–[125I]fibrinogen leg scanning: an alternative to venography

Combined IPG and [125I]fibrinogen leg scanning as a diagnostic approach for DVT is described in Chapter 78. The high sensitivity and specificity of combined IPG and leg scanning provide the clinician with a noninvasive alternative to venography that is versatile and can be performed at the pa-

tient's bedside or in the outpatient clinic or emergency room.[5,9]

The two tests combined detected DVT in 184 (92%) of 201 patients, proximal vein thrombosis in 138 of 139 (sensitivity 99%), and calf vein thrombosis in 46 of 62 (sensitivity 74%). The majority of calf thrombi not detected were in patients with long-standing symptoms, and their clinical significance is uncertain. Because they were inactive by the [125I]fibrinogen uptake test, we considered that these thrombi would be unlikely to extend proximally and to lead to clinically significant pulmonary embolism. We therefore elected not to give these patients anticoagulant therapy, and none developed pulmonary embolism at early or long-term follow-up. Of the 31 patients with acute symptoms resulting from calf DVT, leg scanning detected calf DVT in 29 (sensitivity 94%). These active calf thrombi are more likely to extend into the proximal veins if untreated, placing the patient at risk for massive pulmonary embolism. The combined approach yielded negative results in 256 of the 277 patients without venous thrombosis (specificity 92%) and was falsely positive in 21 patients (8%). All patients with proximal vein thrombosis or active calf vein thrombosis were given anticoagulant therapy. There were no deaths from pulmonary embolism or bleeding.[8] The cost and effectiveness of combined IPG and leg scanning are shown in Table 81-4.

The cost of this diagnostic approach in 478 patients was $720,647. Thus the cost of combined IPG and leg scanning as a diagnostic approach for

Table 81-4. Cost-effectiveness of combined IPG and [^{125}I]fibrinogen leg scanning

Cost		Effectiveness*
Intrinsic cost of IPG at $44/patient for 478 patients	$21,032	Correctly identified DVT in 184 patients
Intrinsic cost of leg scanning at $150/patient for 478 patients	$71,700	Averted 53 deaths from pulmonary embolism by treating DVT in all 184 patients
Cost of hospital room at $250/day for 10 days/patient for 205 patients	$512,500	
Cost of therapy, laboratory tests, and monitoring at $563/patient for 205 patients	$115,415	
Total cost for 478 patients	$720,647	
COST-EFFECTIVENESS OF DESIRED HEALTH EFFECT		
Cost for each correct diagnosis of DVT	$3917	
Cost for each death from pulmonary embolism averted	$13,597	

*Desired health effect in 478 patients with clinical diagnosis of DVT.

a yield of 184 patients with DVT correctly diagnosed and treated was $720,647. Therefore the cost for each of the patients with correctly diagnosed and treated DVT was $3917.

The total cost of combined IPG and leg scanning as a diagnostic approach for a total of 53 deaths from pulmonary embolism averted was $720,647. Therefore the cost for each death from pulmonary embolism averted was $13,597.

Serial occlusive cuff impedance plethysmography alone

IPG using the occlusive cuff technique is sensitive and specific for proximal vein thrombosis but is insensitive to calf thrombi. IPG is an objective diagnostic method that can be carried out in the outpatient clinic, ward, or emergency room.

IPG detected proximal vein thrombosis in 132 (95%) of 139 patients and calf DVT in 10 (16%) of 62. Thus a correct diagnosis was made in 142 (71%) of 201 patients with DVT. The IPG was falsely positive in 5 patients.

We have recently completed a randomized clinical trial[13] comparing serial IPG alone with a reference standard, combined IPG plus [^{125}I]fibrinogen leg scanning, which is essentially as accurate as venography. IPG was performed serially to detect both proximal vein thrombosis and extending calf DVT. The important practical finding of our randomized trial is the observation that it is safe to withhold anticoagulant therapy in patients with clinically suspected venous thrombosis if the results by serial IPG remain negative.[13] On referral, results were initially negative by IPG in 634 pa-

tients. Anticoagulant therapy was withheld in all 634 patients, who were then randomized to receive noninvasive testing with serial IPG alone or with combined IPG and leg scanning. During the initial diagnostic assessment none of the 634 patients in whom anticoagulant therapy was withheld on the basis of negative IPG results on referral died from pulmonary embolism. One of the 634 patients suffered a submassive pulmonary embolism; this patient had been ramdomized to combined testing with IPG plus leg scanning. Thus the frequency of pulmonary embolism in patients with negative IPG results at the time of referral in our study was 1 in 634 patients (0.16%; 95% confidence limits, −0.15% to 0.47%).

Anticoagulant therapy was withheld in all patients in whom results of serial noninvasive testing remained negative, and was commenced in those patients in whom results became positive. All patients were followed up at 3 months and 1 year. At 1-year follow-up none of the 634 patients had died from pulmonary embolism. Six of 311 patients randomized to receive noninvasive testing with serial IPG alone returned with objectively documented venous thromboembolism, a frequency of 1.9% (95% confidence limits, 0.4% to 3.4%). Seven of 323 patients randomized to receive combined IPG plus leg scanning returned with objectively documented venous thromboembolism, a frequency of 2.2% (95% confidence limits, 0.6% to 3.8%). Because the observed difference between the two comparative diagnostic groups was 0.36%, which favors IPG alone, it is unlikely ($p < .05$) that a true difference in favor of serial IPG alone would

Table 81-5. Cost-effectiveness of serial IPG alone using the occlusive cuff technique

Cost		Effectiveness*
Intrinsic cost of IPG at $44/patient for 478 patients	$21,032	Correctly identified DVT in 142 patients
Cost of hospital room at $250/day for 10 days per patient for 147 patients with positive IPG results	$367,500	Averted 53 deaths from pulmonary embolism by treating DVT in 142 patients†
Cost of therapy, laboratory tests, and monitoring at $563/patient for 147 patients	$82,761	
Total cost for 478 patients	$471,293	
COST-EFFECTIVENESS OF DESIRED HEALTH EFFECT		
Cost for each correct diagnosis of DVT	$3319	
Cost for each death from pulmonary embolism averted	$8892	

*Desired health effect in 478 patients with clinical diagnosis of DVT.
†Calf DVT not detected in 52 patients and therefore not treated (see text).

be higher than 2.4%, and the difference could be as much at 2.1% in favor of the combined approach. These findings indicate that IPG performed on the day of referral and, if negative, repeated the following day, again on day 5 to 7, day 10, and on day 14, is as effective as the combined approach for the diagnosis of clinically suspected venous thrombosis.[13]

We have previously demonstrated that the combined approach of IPG plus leg scanning is essentially as accurate and safe as venography.[5,7,9] These observations, when taken together with the findings of our randomized trial, indicate that serial IPG alone is as effective as venography. The outcomes of long-term follow-up indicate that it is safe to withhold anticoagulant therapy in symptomatic patients in whom results are negative by repeat evaluation with IPG. Thus the use of serial IPG alone is as effective as venography for the diagnosis of venous thrombosis and for averting death from pulmonary embolism in patients with clinically suspected DVT. The cost and effectiveness of serial occlusive cuff IPG used alone are shown in Table 81-5.

The total cost of this diagnostic approach in 478 patients was $471,293. Thus the cost of IPG used alone as a diagnostic approach for a yield of 142 patients with DVT correctly diagnosed and treated was $471,293. Therefore the cost for each patient with DVT correctly identified and treated was $3319.

The total cost of using serial IPG alone as a diagnostic approach for a yield of 53 deaths from pulmonary embolism averted was $471,293. Therefore the cost for each death from pulmonary embolism averted was $8892.

Comparison of diagnostic approaches by cost-effectiveness analysis

The cost-effectiveness of each diagnostic approach is summarized in Table 81-6. The "worst" approach is clearly clinical diagnosis and the "best" the approach of IPG alone performed serially.

COST-EFFECTIVENESS OF DIAGNOSTIC APPROACHES FOR DVT IN PATIENTS WITH CO-MORBID CONDITIONS REQUIRING HOSPITAL ADMISSION

The assumption has been made in this economic analysis that the reason for admitting or keeping the patient in the hospital is the diagnosis of DVT. Clearly a proportion of patients will have co-morbid conditions that may have been the primary reason for hospital admission or that may require continuing in-hospital care and treatment irrespective of the complication of DVT. It is inappropriate to charge the cost of the hosptial room against the diagnostic approach in these patients.

Table 81-7 summarizes the cost-effectiveness of the diagnostic approaches, excluding the cost of the hospital room. It is evident that the noninvasive tests are slightly less expensive than venography. The most cost-effective of the alternative approaches is the approach of serial IPG alone.

Relative cost-effectiveness

The relative cost-effectiveness of the diagnostic approaches in patients without co-morbid conditions requiring hospitalization is shown in Table 81-8. The net savings of each of the diagnostic approaches in comparison with clinical diagnosis is substantial for each of the objective approaches.

Table 81-6. Cost-effectiveness of diagnostic approaches for DVT

Diagnostic approach	Total cost for each patient with DVT correctly diagnosed ($)	Total cost for each death from pulmonary embolism averted ($)	Comment
Clinical diagnosis	7284	27,625	All patients with clinically suspected DVT admitted to hospital and treated
Venography			
Outpatient	4106	15,572	Patients with findings positive for DVT admitted to hospital and treated
Inpatient	5399	20,474	All patients admitted to hospital and given treatment initially, but patients with findings negative for DVT subsequently discharged at a mean time of 72 hours
Combined IPG and leg scanning	3917	13,597	Patients with findings positive for DVT admitted to hospital and given treatment
IPG alone performed serially	3319	8892	Patients with findings positive for DVT admitted to hospital and given treatment

Table 81-7. Cost-effectiveness of diagnostic approaches for DVT excluding the cost of the hospital room in patients with other conditions requiring hospitalization

Diagnostic approach	Total cost for each patient with DVT correctly diagnosed ($)	Total cost for each death from pulmonary embolism averted ($)
Clinical diagnosis	1339	5078
Immediate venography	1606	6091
Combined IPG and leg scanning	1131	3297
IPG alone	731	1958

Table 81-8. Relative cost-effectiveness of objective diagnostic approaches for DVT

Objective diagnostic approach and its cost for each correct diagnosis of DVT ($)		Net savings* for each correct diagnosis of DVT using objective diagnosis ($)
Venography		
Outpatient	4106	3178
Inpatient	5399	1885
Combined IPG and leg scanning	3917	3367
IPG alone	3319	3965

*Compared with clinical diagnosis at a cost of $7284 for each correct diagnosis.

The greatest net savings is achieved with IPG alone, followed by the combination of IPG with leg scanning.

Similarly, the net savings of objective diagnosis can be calculated in patients with the clinical diagnosis of DVT who are in the hospital or admitted to the hospital for co-morbid conditions. The least expensive approach is IPG alone, followed by IPG combined with leg scanning.

Future relevance of cost in this analysis

Although the actual cost of each component will vary according to regional differences and will change in the future, it is apparent that the proportion each parameter contributes (to the total cost) will remain linked. Thus ranking of the diagnostic approaches from worst to best as determined by cost-effectiveness analysis should continue to be relevant. Inpatient diagnosis is likely to remain a major cost; therefore emphasis should be placed on outpatient diagnosis.[8]

SUMMARY

The diagnostic approaches to DVT include clinical diagnosis, venography, and noninvasive approaches used alone or in combination. The clinical diagnosis of DVT is nonspecific and insensitive. In approximately 50% or more of patients with clinically diagnosed DVT results of objective testing are negative. Thus this approach is cost-ineffective because one of two patients with clinically diagnosed DVT is inappropriately admitted to the hospital and given anticoagulant therapy. Patients with DVT can be accurately identified by using venography or a combination of noninvasive tests.

At present venography is the standard diagnostic reference test against which the noninvasive tests are evaluated. Disadvantages of venography are that it is invasive, is associated with patient discomfort, and induces postvenography phlebitis in approximately 1% to 3% of patients.[4] In many centers venography is not readily available on an outpatient basis; consequently, patients with clinically suspected DVT are admitted to the hospital, anticoagulant therapy is begun and the diagnosis is confirmed or ruled out later by elective venography. This approach is cost-ineffective in patients subsequently found not to have DVT because they are admitted to the hospital unnecessarily and exposed to the hazards and added costs of anticoagulant therapy.[8]

In ranking the approaches discussed, it is evident that clinical diagnosis is the least cost-effective. Serial IPG alone is the most cost-effective and is as effective as the combined approach of IPG and leg scanning (and hence as effective as venography).[5,9,13] Serial IPG alone is less expensive than venography, is more versatile, and can be carried out in the outpatient clinic, ward, or emergency room. Noninvasive testing with serial IPG avoids the risk of unnecessary anticoagulant therapy in those patients subsequently shown by elective inpatient venography not to have DVT, and its ease of access obviates the need to admit the patient to the hospital and the cost of an unnecessary hospital stay.

ACKNOWLEDGMENT

We thank Greg Stoddart, Ph.D., Health Economist, McMaster University, for assistance.

REFERENCES

1. Barrit, D.W., and Jordan, S.L.: Anticoagulant drugs in the treatment of pulmonary embolism: A controlled trial, Lancet 1:1309, 1960.
2. Basu, D., Gallus, A., Hirsh, J., and Cade, J.F.: A prospective study of the value of monitoring heparin treatment with the activated partial thromboplastin time, N. Engl. J. Med. 287:324, 1972.
3. Gallus, A.S., and Hirsh, J.: Diagnosis of venous thromboembolism, Semin. Throm. Hemost. 2:203, 1976.
4. Hull, R., and Hirsh, J.: Advances and controversies in the diagnosis, prevention and treatment of venous thromboembolism, Prog. Hematol. 12:73, 1981.
5. Hull, R., et al.: Combined use of leg scanning and impedance plethysmography in suspected venous thrombosis: an alternative to venography, N. Engl. J. Med. 296:1497, 1977.
6. Hull, R., et al.: Warfarin sodium versus low-dose heparin in the long-term treatment of venous thrombosis, N. Engl. J. Med. 301:855, 1979.
7. Hull, R., et al.: Clinical validity of a negative venogram in patients with clinically suspected venous thrombosis, Circulation 64:622, 1981.
8. Hull, R., et al.: Cost effectiveness of clinical diagnosis, venography, and noninvasive testing in patients with symptomatic deep-vein thrombosis, N. Engl. J. Med. 304:1561, 1981.
9. Hull, R., et al.: Replacement of venography in suspected venous thrombosis by impedance plethysmography and ^{125}I-fibrinogen leg scanning: a less invasive approach, Ann. Intern. Med. 94:12, 1981.
10. Hull, R., et al.: Adjusted subcutaneous heparin versus warfarin sodium in the long-term treatment of venous thrombosis, N. Engl. J. Med. 306:189, 1982.
11. Hull, R., et al.: Different intensities of oral anticoagulant therapy in the treatment of proximal-vein thrombosis, N. Engl. J. Med. 307:1676, 1982.
12. Hull, R., et al.: The diagnosis of acute, recurrent, deep-vein thrombosis: a diagnostic challenge, Circulation 67:901, 1983.
13. Hull, R., et al.: A randomized trial of diagnostic strategies for symptomatic deep-vein thrombosis, Thromb. Hemost. 50:160a, 1983.
14. Kakkar, V.V., et al.: Natural history of post-operative deep-vein thrombosis, Lancet 2:230, 1969.
15. Mavor, G.E., and Galloway, J.M.D.: The iliofemoral venous segment as a source of pulmonary embolism, Lancet 1:871, 1967.
16. Salzman, E.W., Deykin, D., and Shapiro, R.M.: Management of heparin therapy, N. Engl. J. Med. 292:1046, 1975.
17. Weinstein, M.C., and Stason, W.B.: Foundations of cost-effectiveness analysis for health and medical practices, N. Engl. J. Med. 296:716, 1977.
18. Zilliacus, H.: On specific treatment of thrombosis and pulmonary embolism with anticoagulants with particular reference to the post-thrombotic sequelae. Acta Med. Scand. [Suppl.] 171:1, 1946.

CHAPTER 82

Foot volumetry

OLAV THULESIUS

Noninvasive diagnosis of chronic venous disease has been very limited compared with the multiplying techniques available for diagnosis of arterial disease. This situation is out of proportion considering the high prevalence of chronic venous insufficiency. In a population study of 4529 apparently healthy workers from Basel, Switzerland, it was concluded that 8% of those aged 25 to 54 years had significant venous disease, and if these findings were extrapolated to the whole Swiss population aged 25 to 74 years there was an estimated prevalence of 14%.[9]

Until recently, functional studies for the venous circulation have been limited to the study of venous pressure changes during exercise and Doppler ultrasonic testing of valvular function (Chapter 48). My colleagues and I[8] introduced a new method for truly noninvasive testing of venous function based on the concept that measurements of venous pressure and volume rely on similar mechanisms. Photoplethysmography as described in Chapter 70 relies on a similar principle except that quantitative evaluation only relies on recovery time, which is equivalent to refilling time, but not on actual venous volume.

During quiet standing in the upright position the hydrostatic pressure in the lower extremity venous system is a function of the vertical height of the blood column from the heart to the foot. With exercise and competent venous valves, standing venous pressure at the ankle is reduced from 90 to 20 mm Hg.[7] This reduction in peripheral venous pressure is caused by the central dislocation of blood secondary to the massaging action of the contracting calf muscles and the stretching forces of moving connective tissue (fascia) acting on compressible vessels.

Competent valves disrupt the blood column on the venous side and thereby eliminate the hydrostatic pressure in the distal vessels, leaving the hydraulic pressure transmitted from the arterial side as the main factor. This physiologic response of peripheral venous pressure in the foot to exercise has been used by many as a functional test for the quantitative evaluation of the calf muscle pump and the efficiency of the venous valves.[1]

Venous pressure measurement, however, is an invasive principle requiring puncture of a foot vein, which is uncomfortable for the patient and therefore reduces its usefulness. In addition, it is impractical at repeated intervals. Noninvasive assessment of foot volume changes with exercise are much easier to perform, and the findings correlate well with pressure measurements.[4-6]

PRINCIPLE

The foot volumeter is an open, water-filled box designed to measure the foot volume at rest and its changes with exercise. The water level, initially 14 cm from the bottom, is sensed by a critically damped photoelectric float-sensor, which operates an optical wedge, the output of which is continuously recorded on a strip-chart recorder. During exercise blood is expelled from the foot vessels, and therefore the water displacement is reduced in proportion to the volume of dislocated blood. After a series of knee bends the blood volume gradually declines until it reaches a steady state, usually after 20 knee bends in rapid succession. The initial resting volume is again reached a varying length of time after completion of the exercise test.

Refilling flow is normally exclusively from the arterial side, but in cases of venous insufficiency retrograde flow (reflux) from proximally located

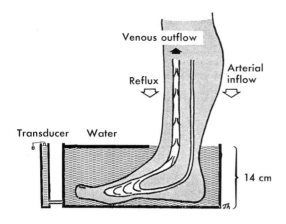

Fig. 82-1. Principle of volumetry: an open, water-filled box (plethysmograph) for continuous measurement of water level.

veins occurs (Fig. 82-1). Usually two volumeters are used, one for each foot, and a volume record is made on a two-channel recorder.

METHOD

The feet are placed in the volumeter, which is rapidly filled from a thermostated water line at a temperature of 32° C. Thereafter calibration is performed with a water-filled syringe. When a steady baseline is achieved in the standing position, a standard exercise is performed, consisting of 20 knee bends in 40 seconds, paced with a metronome. After completion of the exercise the patient stands quietly until volume restitution has been completed. To facilitate the exercise procedure the patient grips handlebars with both hands (Figs. 82-2 and 82-3). To differentiate between superficial and deep venous insufficiency repeated measurements are performed after tourniquet compression of superficial veins below the knee and just above the ankle. After completion of the exercise the water is sucked out of the volumeter and the total foot volume measured with a calibrated reservoir.

Fig. 82-4 shows a recording from a normal individual and one from a patient with varicose veins together with the different variables that can be measured from the curve; these data are also presented in Table 82-1. The most important variables are the expelled volume (EV) and the refilling flow (Q). EV is measured in absolute units (milliliters) or given in relation to foot volume. (When measured per 100 ml tissue the result is the expelled volume [EVr]).

Refilling flow is normally equal to arterial inflow, but in patients with venous insufficiency it also reflects retrograde flow through incompetent veins. The abbreviation and explanation of the different variables together with the experimental errors are given in Table 82-1. Table 82-2 presents normal values from our laboratory and from researchers from Austria and the United Kingdom. Another valuable measure is the time required to refill the initial foot volume, or the more easily determined half refilling time. The ratio of refilling flow and expelled volume (Q/EVr) combines two parameters and is the most sensitive determinant for the diagnosis of venous insufficiency.

CLINICAL APPLICATION

Foot volumetry evaluates the functional capacity of the peripheral venous system of the leg by assessing valvular function and the capacity of the calf-foot pump. A common question to be studied is the presence and extent of superficial or deep venous insufficiency. Foot volumetry is performed, and if reflux or a decreased expelled blood volume is detected, a repeat measurement is performed with tourniquet occlusion and compression, first below the knee and then just above the water level to exclude insufficient superficial veins. If volumetry is performed together with intravenous pressure measurement, it is possible to calculate the distensibility characteristics of the venous bed.[3]

Foot volumetry provides a quantitative estimation of the *degree of venous insufficiency* as shown by Norgren et al.[4] and Partsch[5] from Austria and Lawrence and Kakkar[2] from the United Kingdom. It is also possible to use volumetry for prospective studies in patients with deep venous thrombosis to determine the incidence of postthrombotic valvular insufficiency. Lawrence and Kakkar[2] showed that within 9 months of suffering a major deep venous thrombosis, half the patients already showed evidence of severe functional derangement.

DISCUSSION

Volumetry is a functional test of the venous circulation. To obtain reliable information it is necessary to adhere to a strict protocol. Among other things, it is essential to have a standardized *exercise* procedure of 20 knee bends every other second with knee flexion of 70 degrees. The bath temperature is important and should be kept between 30° and 32° C. The higher temperature of 37° C, as used by Lawrence and Kakkar,[2] increases arterial inflow

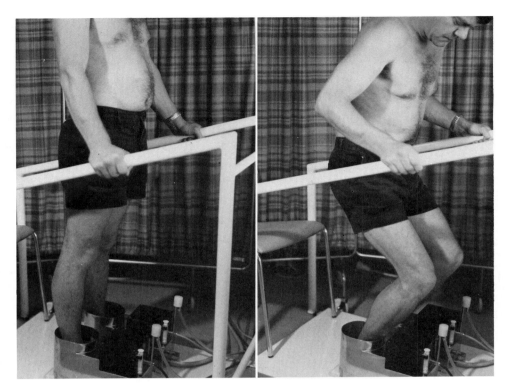

Fig. 82-2. Performance of foot volumetry with knee-bending exercise.

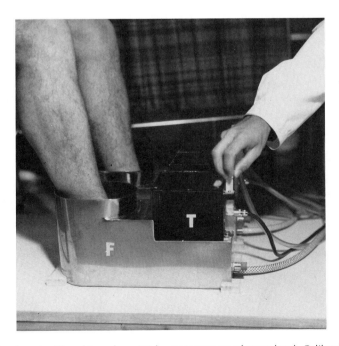

Fig. 82-3. Foot volumeter *(F)* and transducer *(T)* for measurement of water level. Calibration with syringe is shown.

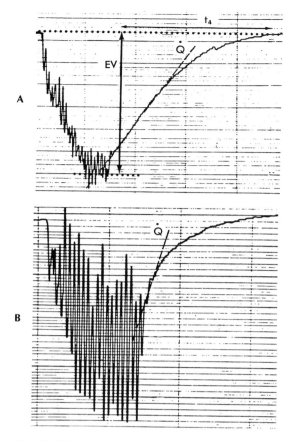

Fig. 82-4. Volumetric recordings from two patients. *A,* Normal individual. *B,* Patient with superficial venous insufficiency. *EV,* Expelled volume; *Q,* refilling flow; t_4 refilling time.

to the foot and may therefore obscure increments of flow because of reflux. The Q values of these authors are higher than ours[4] (Table 82-2). Foot volume at rest may be of importance in conjunction with evaluation of certain drug effects.[4] We found a statistical relationship between body surface area (BSA) and foot volume (V) as follows (holds if the foot is immersed to 14 cm from the sole):

$$V = 617.3 \times BSA + 44.7$$

Among the three diagnostic determinants, the flow volume factor Q/EVr is the best discriminating value when comparing control groups, patients with varicose veins, and patients with deep venous insufficiency.[4]

Table 82-1. Volumetric variables with abbreviations and error of determination according to Norgren et al.[4] (values of Partsch[5] given in parentheses)

Variable	Unit	Error (%)
Foot volume (V)	ml	1.1
Expelled volume (EV)	ml	4.3
Expelled volume per 100 ml tissue (EVr)	ml/100 ml	(9.8)
Refilling flow (Q)	ml/100 ml · min	32.3
Time factor (Q/EVr)	1/min	—
Half refilling time (t_3)	sec	16.2 (25.7)
Refilling time (t_4)	sec	—

Table 82-2. Normal values for volumetric parameters from three different studies*

Variable	Norgren et al.[4]		Partsch[5]	Lawrence and Kakkar[2]
V = 617.3 × BSA† + 44.7	—	—	1219.7 ± 163.9	—
EV	17.0 ± 7.5	8.8 ± 3.7	18.3 ± 6.8	21.2 ± 4.8
EVr	1.5 ± 0.5	0.8 ± 0.3	1.4 ± 0.4	1.9 ± 0.4
Q	2.3 ± 1.1	2.1 ± 0.7	2.2 ± 1.0	2.9
Q/EVr	1.6 ± 0.8	2.8 ± 1.2	1.5 ± 0.6	2.1 ± 0.9
t_3	25.9 ± 12.0	13.2 ± 5.0	26.4 ± 10.2	19.8 ± 8.3
t_4	101.2 ± 38.8	—	86.9 ± 34.3	—
n‡	29	17	36	14
Age (years)	31 (20 to 50)	68 (62 to 75)	35.4	Not stated

*Abbreviations and units given in Table 82-1; mean values ± 1 standard deviation, range in parentheses.
†BSA, Body surface area.
‡n, Number of observations.

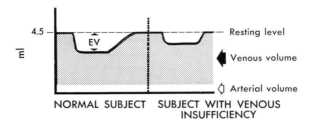

Fig. 82-5. Schematic illustration of effect of exercise on expelled volume *(EV)*.

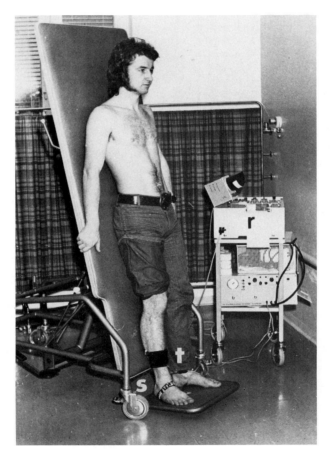

Fig. 82-6. Foot volumetry with strain-gauge band applied to top part of foot. *s,* Strain gauge; *t,* tourniquet; *r,* recorder.

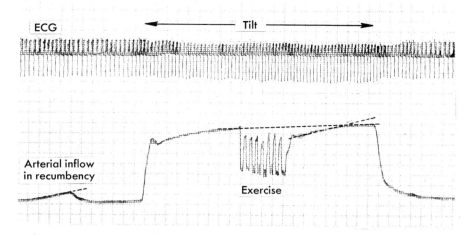

Fig. 82-7. Example of foot volumetry using strain gauge.

Exercise involving the calf-foot pump dislocates only about 30% to 40% of the total blood volume contained in the foot vessels and mainly affects the volume of the larger veins. The main volume contained in the venules and capillary bed is not affected (Fig. 82-5). Some of the dislocated foot volume presumably comes from lymphatic vessels that are slowly refilled after completion of venous filling. An indication of this comes from observations with simultaneous pressure measurements: resting venous pressure is always reached first, and thereafter foot volume is reached. This means that the full hydrostatic column is attained after filling of the large veins when slow filling is still going on, presumably in the lymphatic vessels. Total venous refilling according to pressure measurement occurred at 55% of volume restitution time in normal individuals and in patients with uncomplicated varicose veins but at 38% in patients with chronic venous insufficiency.[5] This may reflect a greater amount of tissue fluid or lymph dislocation in the latter group, and hence delayed replenishment in these cases presumably is the result of edema.

Foot volumetry can also be performed with the aid of girth-measuring strain gauges. The precalibrated strain gauge (Fig. 82-6) can be applied to the foot and measurements can be performed with the patient in the supine and vertical positions, with venous stasis at the ankle (lying), and with exercise in the standing position (Fig. 82-7). This method is easy to perform but gives less reliable results and does not provide absolute values of the expelled volume in milliliters.

REFERENCES

1. Kriessmann, A.: Periphere phlebodynomometrie, Vasa Suppl. 4:1, 1975.
2. Lawrence, D., and Kakkar, V.V.: Venous pressure measurement and foot volumetry in venous disease. In Verstraete, M., editor: Techniques in angiology, The Hague, 1979, Martinus Nijhoff, NV.
3. Norgren, L., and Thulesius, O.: Pressure-volume characteristics of foot veins in normal cases and patients with venous insufficiency. Blood Vessels 12:1, 1975.
4. Norgren, L., et al.: Foot-volumetry and simultaneous venous pressure measurements for evaluation of venous insufficiency, Vasa 3:140, 1974.
5. Partsch, H.: Simultane Venendruckmessung und Plethysmographie am Fuss. In May, R., and Kriessmann, A., editors: Periphere Venendruckmessung, Stuttgart, 1978, Georg Thieme, Verlag KG.
6. Partsch, H., and Gisel, J.: Funktionelle Indikation zur Krampfaderoperation, Wien. Klin. Wochenschr. 89:627, 1977.
7. Pollack, A.A., and Wood, E.H.: Venous pressure in saphenous vein at the ankle in man during exercise and changes in posture, J. Appl. Physiol. 1:649, 1949.
8. Thulesius, O., Norgren, L., and Gjöres, J.E.: Foot volumetry: A new method for objective assessment of edema and venous function, Vasa 2:325, 1973.
9. Widmer, L.: Peripheral venous disorders, Berne, Switzerland, 1978, Hans Huber Medical Publisher.

CHAPTER 83

Venous pressure measurements

NORMAN L. BROWSE

Although the pressure gradient between the left ventricle and the right atrium is sufficient to maintain continuous blood flow, the adoption by humans of the erect posture placed such a strain on the venous return from the lower limbs that a supplementary peripheral venous pump developed. Most chronic ''venous'' disease of the lower limb is caused by derangements of this peripheral pump.

Because the veins have functions other than simple blood conduction, for example, thermoregulation, the peripheral venous system has become a complex two-chamber system. The superficial vessels, which are concerned with temperature control, form one chamber, which is connected to the vessels within the muscle pump, the second chamber, by small valved communicating (perforating) veins.

Any test that purports to measure the function of the peripheral venous pump should be able to measure all its properties: the inflow to the pump, the pump ejection fraction, the competence of the valves between the chambers of the pump, the quantity of regurgitation through any set of incompetent valves, and the state of the outflow tract.

None of our current methods of investigation achieves this ideal, least of all the measurement of foot vein pressure. However, this is the oldest of the techniques available[3,4] and is usually used as the standard for the comparative assessment of new methods.

When the calf pump is working normally it ejects blood from within the muscles toward the heart along the deep axial veins. When the muscles relax blood flows from the superficial veins into the intramuscular veins through the communicating veins. Consequently, the pressure in the superficial veins of the leg, which are on the upstream side of the pump, reflects calf pump efficiency in much

the same way as central venous pressure reflects cardiac efficiency. But it only indicates the overall effect of the pump. It does not indicate the site or degree of any individual abnormality without the additional use of corrective tourniquets. When there are multiple pump defects the measurement of foot vein pressure, even with the use of tourniquets, rarely gives anything more than a crude evaluation of total calf pump function.

METHODS
The vein

The foot is richly endowed with subcutaneous veins. Any one may be catheterized, but the most suitable is a vein running straight down the middle of the dorsum of the foot that can be entered 2 to 5 cm (1 to 2 inches) above an interdigital cleft so that the needle or catheter can lie comfortably inside the vein without impinging on the vein wall.

The catheter

Many workers use a short butterfly-type needle. This can have two disadvantages. It is short and can slip out of the vein, and to make the venipuncture simple and less painful, many are tempted to use a very fine needle. Fine needles damp the pressure-detecting system. Although the frequency of venous pressure changes is slow compared with the frequency of the arterial pressure wave, the best traces are obtained by using a catheter of a size that does not cause damping. I prefer to use a short fine (0.5 mm internal diameter) catheter inserted through a small stab wound with the patient under local anesthesia.

Skin anesthesia

A small intradermal bleb of 2% lignocaine is sufficient to make the skin stab or venipuncture painless. The vein is marked with the patient standing, but the venipuncture is done with the patient lying down after producing venous congestion with an ankle tourniquet, because a number of patients faint if they feel pain while they are standing. It is not necessary to infiltrate deep into the skin. Anesthetic agents around the vein alter its tone.

Catheter, transducer, and recorder

It is important to use a transducer of sufficient sensitivity. The pressure may vary between 30 and 150 mm Hg, but the transducer must reliably detect changes of 2 to 5 mm Hg without excessive amplification. The frequency of the pressure waves will depend on the type and rate of exercise, but the transducer should have a greater than 95% response to changes of at least 10 Hz. The center of the transducer diaphragm should be fixed level with the tip of the intravenous catheter. The connecting catheter should be as short as possible and not allowed to bounce about.

Any form of recorder may be used. The wider the paper and the tracing, the easier it is to measure gradients. I have an intrinsic distrust of computerized systems that calculate rate of change electronically and present a number without displaying the tracing. I prefer to see the trace and decide that it is acceptable before making calculations from it.

System check

Transducer and pressure measurements have become so commonplace that many forget to check the system at regular intervals throughout a study.

1. Check that there are no air bubbles in any part of the catheter-transducer system.
2. Flush the catheter at regular intervals to prevent a blood clot from occluding its lumen. A continuous flushing system using heparinized saline solution prevents this complication.
3. Before each exercise test put a very short high-pressure flush into the system and watch the trace. It should rise and fall vertically and return immediately to the baseline. Any tailing off of the rate of fall as it approaches its original resting level indicates damping caused by problems such as a clot in the catheter, bubbles in the system, too fine a catheter, the catheter tip resting on the vein wall, or an inadequate transducer. I prefer to see a ''flush'' in published recordings of pressure traces; it indicates that the operator knows the system and recognizes the problems.
4. Ask the patient to perform a Valsalva maneuver. Foot vein pressure should rise slightly if the system is working well.

Type of exercise

The venous pump must work with the patient standing, so foot vein pressures should be measured in this position. The most common form of exercise is to have the patient raise both heels off the ground as high as possible at a regular rate, usually one/sec, in time to a metronome.

Many laboratories also assess calf pump function by foot volumetry[6]; the exercise test for this consists of repeated knee bending because the foot must remain still. It would seem sensible to use the same type of exercise for both methods, which means using knee bending for pressure studies.

The exercise should continue until a new stable pressure is reached. One of the objects of the test is to determine the maximum pressure fall obtainable. This is judged by watching the tracing.

At least 2, preferably 5, minutes' rest should be allowed between each period of exercise.

Tourniquets

The information gained from this test can be expanded by the application of tourniquets, which produce superficial vein obstruction. A tourniquet placed around the midthigh should prevent refilling down an incompetent long saphenous vein; one just below the knee should prevent refilling through both long and short saphenous veins; and one just above the ankle should stop refilling from all superficial to deep connections, that is, the long and short saphenous veins and any incompetent communicating veins.

The problem is to find a tourniquet pressure that occludes the superficial but not the deep veins. In a leg with an average layer of fat, Nicolaides and Yao[5] have shown that a narrow (2.5 cm) cuff inflated to a pressure of 120 mm Hg at the ankle or 180 mm Hg at midthigh will occlude the superficial but not the deep veins. However, this does not hold in every case. The effect of the cuff will be affected by its width, the size of the leg, the depth of the fat layer, and the anatomy of the veins. There is no 100% reliable test to confirm superficial vein occlusion. I find the Doppler flow probe useful for detecting flow beneath the cuff and a helpful guide when adjusting the pressure in the tourniquet. An alternative technique is to inflate the tourniquet slowly until the respiratory fluctuations seen in the foot vein pressure disappear and then increase the tourniquet pressure by 10 mm Hg.

NORMAL FOOT VEIN PRESSURES
Resting pressure

The pressure in the veins of the feet when the patient is standing quietly is equal to the hydrostatic pressure produced by the column of blood between the head and the foot. It is usually 80 to 90 mm Hg, varies with the height of the patient, and shows small fluctuations corresponding to respiration.

Effect of exercise

Calf pump activity expels blood through the popliteal vein toward the heart. Between contractions, when the intramuscular vein pressure is zero, blood flows in from the subcutaneous veins through the communicating veins. The superficial vein pressure falls. Normally the pressure falls by 60% to 80%, that is, from 80 to 90 mm Hg down to 20 to 30 mm Hg. When the subject stops exercising the pressure returns to the preexercise level. Three measurements can be made from the trace: rate of fall, maximum fall, and rate of recovery.

Rate of fall. The rate of fall is affected by the power of the calf pump, obstruction or reflux in the pump outflow tract, and reflux back and forth between the superficial reservoir and the pump through the communicating veins, or the saphenopopliteal junction. The rate of fall is a measure of the rate of pump emptying and is difficult to measure accurately. It is also entirely dependent on the way the patient performs the exercise. It is not usually measured, because it is unusual to see the emptying time prolonged even in the presence of severe outflow obstruction.

Maximum fall. During the reduction of calf volume the superficial venous pressure fluctuates in time to the heel raising. Once the maximum fall is reached the fluctuations become smaller and it is easy to measure their upper and lower limits and calculate the mean. The mean lowest pressure is also visible for a brief moment after cessation of exercise. The percent fall in pressure is a good indicator of the overall efficiency of the calf muscle pump and the state of the inflow and outflow tracts. It is particularly affected by incompetent communicating veins and deep vein damage.[1,7]

Rate of recovery. The rate of recovery depends on the relative proportions of normal inflow from the arterial side of the circulation and retrograde flow down the deep and superficial veins. It is usually measured by drawing and extending the slope of the first few seconds of the pressure trace, immediately after cessation of exercise, and then calculating the time taken for the pressure to return halfway to normal. All of these measurements should be repeated before and after the inflation of superficial vein–occluding tourniquets.

Normal values

Although the reduction of pressure is reproducible from laboratory to laboratory, the rates of emptying and refilling vary according to the nature of the exercise used. Each laboratory must establish its own normal values before attempting to assess patients with disordered calf pumps.

PRESSURE TRACES IN VENOUS DISEASE
Long saphenous vein incompetence

The most common abnormality of the venous system of the lower limb is simple long saphenous vein incompetence (LSI). The calf pump can usually cope with the extra load presented by reflux in this system of veins, and thus the rate and degree of foot vein pressure reduction during exercise may be normal or only just outside normal limits. The rate of refilling after exercise is increased and should be corrected by a midthigh superficial vein–occluding tourniquet. If LSI is the only abnormality, then restoration of the pressure trace to normality by a midthigh cuff confirms the diagnosis and predicts a good response to long saphenous vein ligation. Pressure traces after the operation should be restored to the normal range.

Short saphenous vein incompetence

The pressure profile of short saphenous vein incompetence (SSI) is similar to that of LSI and should be corrected by a below-knee superficial vein–occluding tourniquet. However LSI and SSI often occur simultaneously. In such cases a midthigh tourniquet will prolong the refilling time but not restore it to normal, and the below-knee tourniquet will have a greater effect. If there is no communicating vein incompetence, a below-knee tourniquet should restore the pressure profile to normal in combined LSI and SSI as well as pure SSI and pure LSI.

Communicating vein incompetence

Incompetence of the communicating veins allows blood to flow into the superficial system at a variety of points between the knee and the ankle during calf muscle exercise. Consequently, the foot vein pressure fails to fall during exercise. If no other veins are incompetent the refilling time is normal, because there is not a large volume of blood available within the deep veins to flow outward into the superficial reservoir after exercise in the way that LSI allows, unless the whole of the deep system is also incompetent. A superficial vein–occluding tourniquet at the ankle may improve the pressure drop during exercise but rarely restores it to normal, because (1) the communicating vein leak makes the whole pump inefficient, so it fails to empty the superficial veins of the foot, and (2) the tourniquet often fails to separate all the incompetent communicating veins from the foot, because although most of them are above it, there is often a communicator below the tourniquet just behind and below the malleolus. Communicating vein incompetence is mainly diagnosed by exclusion, that is, when the above- and below-knee tourniquets fail to restore the refilling rate to normal and it is known by other means (usually phlebography) that there is no deep axial vein obstruction or incompetence. The communicating vein leakage cannot be quantified by any of the superficial reservoir pressure or volume measuring techniques.

Deep axial vein obstruction

A major obstruction in the popliteal or femoral vein would be expected to slow the rate of emptying during exercise and reduce the total expelled volume. Such changes are only apparent when the obstruction is extremely severe. In most cases there is sufficient power in the pump and the collateral vessels are big enough to allow normal emptying rates. Emptying is also dependent on the speed and strength of calf muscle contraction, a factor difficult to standardize. The absence of a detectable obstruction to outflow during laboratory exercise does not mean that one does not exist during the hyperemia of prolonged normal exercise.

If all of the collateral vessels bypassing a deep block are in the subcutaneous tissues, a superficial vein–occluding tourniquet may prolong the rate of emptying. This is a rare situation, and invariably there is edema and venous claudication.

The refilling rate should be normal in pure deep vein obstruction unless there are very inadequate collateral vessels. However, in most such limbs there is secondary incompetence of the superficial varicose veins, so the rate of refilling may be increased and the application of a midthigh cuff may

prolong both emptying and refilling. Interpretation of such a pressure trace is extremely difficult.

Deep axial vein incompetence

Severe deep vein incompetence reduces pump efficiency and thus the expelled volume and the pressure fall of exercise and increases the rate of refilling. The rate of refilling will not be corrected by superficial vein–occluding cuffs wherever they are placed. However, because most of these patients have some degree of secondary superficial vein incompetence, there is usually some response to a midthigh tourniquet, which confuses the interpretation. Rapid refilling unaffected by a superficial vein–occluding cuff is one of the abnormalities best detected by foot vein pressure measurements.

ABSOLUTE VALUES

It can be seen from the preceding and the singular lack of actual pressure measurements in this chapter that more is learned from a change in pressure profile in response to maneuvers such as the application of tourniquets than can be deduced from the absolute values of the pressures or their rate of change. Each laboratory must determine its own normal range, but most investigators quickly find that the normal range is so wide and the overlap between normal and abnormal so great that the interpretation of different values between individual patients is impossible. The only reliable and reproducible measurement is the 60% to 80% fall in foot vein pressure during exercise in normal individuals. Pressure falls of less than 60% signal an abnormality, but beyond this the investigator must rely on interpretation of the changes in pressure profile caused by the inflation of pneumatic cuffs at different positions on the leg. This is not a very scientific approach and emphasizes the fact that foot vein pressure measurements, although better than many other techniques, only indicate overall calf pump efficiency and the possible presence of superficial or deep reflux. Pressure measurements cannot measure individual abnormalities in the presence of multiple abnormalities—the usual clinical situation—and therefore cannot be used to assess treatment except when only one abnormality is corrected.[2]

SUMMARY

Foot vein pressure measured during exercise, with and without the application of superficial vein–occluding tourniquets, gives a crude indication of calf pump function and may demonstrate the presence of superficial or deep vein reflux. The pressure changes do not give a precise measurement of any particular feature of calf pump function. In most cases there is more than one abnormality of the pump, often undetected by our present forms of investigation and inadequately corrected by our current methods of treatment, so it is not surprising that pressure profiles are rarely restored to normal by surgery.

REFERENCES

1. Bjordal, R.I.: Pressure patterns in the saphenous system in patients with venous leg ulcers, Acta Chir. Scand. 137:495, 1971.
2. Burnand, K.G., O'Donnell, T.F., Lea, T.M., and Browse, N.L.: The relative importance of incompetent communicating veins in the production of varicose veins and venous ulcers, Surgery 82:9, 1977.
3. McPheeters, H.O., Merkel, C.E., and Lundblad, R.A.: The mechanics of the reverse flow of blood in varicose veins as proved by blood pressure readings, Surg. Gynecol. Obstet. 55:298, 1932.
4. Moritz, F., and Tabora, D.: Uber eine Methode beim Menschen den Druck in oberflachlichen Venen exakt zu bestimmen, Deutsch. Arch. Klin. Med. 98:475, 1910.
5. Nicolaides, A., and Yao, J.S.T.: The investigation of vascular disorders, Edinburgh, 1980, Churchill Livingstone, Inc.
6. Thulesuis, O., Norgren, L., and Gjores, J.E.: Foot volumetry: a new method for objective assessment of oedema and venous function, Vasa 2:325, 1973.
7. Warren, R., White, E.A., and Belcher, C.D.: Venous pressure in the saphenous system in normal, varicose and postphlebitic extremities, Surgery 26:435, 1949.

CHAPTER 84

Noninvasive techniques in chronic venous insufficiency

ROBERT W. BARNES

Three clinical disorders constitute the syndrome of chronic venous insufficiency: varicose veins, postthrombotic syndrome, and recurrent deep vein thrombosis (DVT). Each of these disorders may present diagnostic ambiguities for the clinician. In a patient with varicose veins, the physician must determine whether the abnormalities are limited to the superficial veins (primary varicose veins) or whether the varicosities are associated with an underlying venous problem (secondary varicose veins). In a patient with chronic leg pain, swelling, and possible ulceration, the postthrombotic syndrome must be differentiated from other conditions, such as edema from congestive heart failure or lymphedema, contact dermatitis, ischemic ulceration, or ulceration from other conditions such as hypertension or vasculitis. Finally, the patient with recurrent leg pain and swelling is often treated for recurrent venous thrombosis when in actuality the patient may be suffering from chronic postthrombotic sequelae caused by mechanical dysfunction of the deep venous system. Therefore the physician should be familiar with various objective diagnostic techniques to clarify the ambiguities.

The traditional methods of evaluating patients with a suspected chronic venous insufficiency include contrast venography and ambulatory venous pressure measurements.[24,35] However, the expense and discomfort associated with these procedures have limited their application in patients with chronic venous disease. Many of the noninvasive techniques discussed in this book have been used to evaluate patients with acute DVT. However, many methods are also applicable to patients with chronic venous disease. The techniques permit evaluation of the three major pathophysiologic sequelae of venous thrombosis: venous outflow obstruction, venous valvular incompetence, and venous thrombosis. This chapter will review the principles and applications of various noninvasive techniques in the systematic evaluation of patients with suspected chronic venous insufficiency. More detailed analysis of the individual diagnostic techniques will be found in separate chapters of this book.

TESTS OF VENOUS OUTFLOW OBSTRUCTION
Qualitative techniques

Doppler ultrasound permits the most rapid, sensitive, and versatile method of evaluating obstruction of the venous system.[8] The technique has been reviewed in Chapter 73 and by others.[3,29-31] The method is subjective and requires considerable experience for maximal accuracy. However, Doppler ultrasound permits localization of venous thrombi and differentiation of disease in the deep and superficial veins.[7] It is sensitive to major venous thrombi in the calf,[9] as well as the more proximal veins of the lower and upper extremities. The technique may be used in modified form for patients in traction or plaster casts. In addition, Doppler ultrasound provides qualitative estimation of venous valvular incompetence in the deep, communicating, and superficial veins.[15] In experienced hands the method has a sensitivity of approximately 95% and a specificity of 85% for the diagnosis of venous outflow obstruction when compared to contrast venography. The lower specificity is a reflection of the functional venous flow velocity abnormalities that may be noted in patients with extrinsic venous obstruction in the absence of true venous thrombosis, such as subfascial hematomas, malignancy, or Baker's cyst.

Phleborheography (PRG) provides functional assessment of the venous system in a manner somewhat similar to that of Doppler ultrasound.[12] By means of segmental alterations in limb volumetric responses to respiration and pneumatic limb compression maneuvers, qualitative assessment of deep venous obstruction and valvular incompetence can be graphically recorded. The technique is reviewed in detail in Chapter 74. In patients with acute DVT the segmental limb volumetric responses to respiration are attenuated or absent, and significant increases in segmental limb volume result in response to distal limb compression maneuvers. In chronic venous insufficiency the residual venous outflow obstruction may be identified as segmental limb volume increases in response to distal limb compression in the face of normal volumetric fluctuations in response to respiration. Like Doppler ultrasound, PRG is sensitive to major deep venous obstruction of the calf, as well as the more proximal veins, and the technique may be also modified for use on the upper extremity. The sensitivity of the method in experienced centers approaches 95%.

Quantitative techniques

Venous outflow plethysmography refers to methods that graphically record the rates of decrease in calf circumference or volume in response to deflation of a proximal venoocclusive thigh pneumatic cuff. The principle and techniques of the method are described in Chapters 73 and 74. Several plethysmographic techniques are available, including strain-gauge,[2,5,10] impedance,[36] air,[28,37] and water transducers. The latter method is technically complex and not currently in widespread use. The most commonly used methods are strain-gauge and impedence plethysmography. The principle of venous outflow plethysmography is the same, regardless of the type of transducer used on the calf.

With the patient in the supine position, the lower extremity is elevated to empty the deep venous system. After applying the transducer to the calf and balancing and calibrating the apparatus, a pneumatic cuff on the thigh is inflated to a pressure that occludes venous return (30 to 50 mm Hg). After the calf volume stabilizes (usually in 1 or 2 minutes) the pneumatic cuff is rapidly deflated and the rate of change in calf circumference is graphically recorded. From the decrement in calf circumference or volume, the maximum venous outflow may be inferred. The rate of decrease in calf dimensions per unit time is usually related to the

incremental increase during venous occlusion and is plotted on a graph or expressed as a percentage. With the strain-gauge or water plethysmograph, maximum venous outflow may be expressed in milliliters per minute per 100 ml of calf tissue.[5] The test may be repeated with the application of superficial tourniquets to prevent venous return via the superficial system. This technique is important in patients with chronic venous insufficiency who may have much of the venous outflow of the limb occurring via the superficial veins.

Venous outflow plethysmography is useful in patients with chronic venous insufficiency for three purposes. First, the technique permits quantification of the degree of chronic venous outflow obstruction,[33] which may have implications for surgical therapy in select patients. Second, the method permits longitudinal follow-up of the degree of resolution of venous obstruction as the result of endogenous fibrinolysis, venous collateral development, or the effect of therapeutic fibrinolysis. Finally, objective documentation of increased venous outflow obstruction in the late postthrombotic period may be an indirect clue to the development of recurrent active venous thrombosis.

TESTS OF VENOUS VALVULAR INCOMPETENCE

Noninvasive diagnostic techniques permit qualitative and quantitative detection and localization of venous valvular incompetence in the deep, communicating (perforating), and superficial veins.

Deep vein incompetence

Qualitative assessment of venous valvular incompetence of the deep veins is rapidly carried out with continuous-wave (CW) Doppler ultrasound.[3,8,15,29-31,33] The technique of a venous Doppler examination is described in greater detail in Chapter 73. In principle, the Doppler velocity detector permits assessment of venous flow during manual compression of the limb proximal to the Doppler probe or during a Valsalva maneuver. Normally such maneuvers result in interruption in venous flow velocity; but in the presence of deep venous valvular incompetence, retrograde flow through incompetent venous valves will be heard with the Doppler instrument. This technique permits assessment of valvular competence in the posterior tibial (calf), popliteal, superficial femoral, and common femoral veins and, indirectly, the iliac veins. In the upper extremities, the brachial, axillary, and subclavian veins may be assessed for valvular incompetence.

PRG is an air plethysmographic technique that permits qualitative assessment of deep venous valvular incompetence.[12] This technique is described in greater detail in Chapter 72. In principle, the phleborheograph permits recording of the rate of recovery in foot or calf venous volume in response to temporary pneumatic compression of the calf or thigh proximal to the recording cuff. The normal recovery time for return of foot or calf volume to baseline is 10 seconds or greater, whereas in patients with deep venous incompetence the limb volume returns to normal within a few seconds after cessation of calf or thigh compression.

Quantitative measurement of deep venous valvular incompetence is possible with strain-gauge plethysmography.[5,10] This technique may be performed in one of two ways. With the patient supine, the strain gauge on the calf records calf volumetric changes in response to temporary pneumatic compression of the thigh distal to a proximal thigh tourniquet.[4] Normally the underlying thigh venous blood cannot be displaced distally if the venous valves are competent. In the presence of deep venous incompetence, a distal thigh cuff will permit translocation of thigh venous blood by an amount and rate proportional to the incompetence of the deep venous valves. In patients in the upright position, a strain gauge on the calf permits recording of calf volumetric changes during static calf muscle exercise[18] or during ambulation on a treadmill. Normally the calf volume decreases initially and then will increase during exercise. After cessation of exercise the calf venous volume returns to normal baseline levels in 10 seconds or more. In the presence of deep venous incompetence, the calf volume will increase rapidly within a few seconds after cessation of exercise. The maximal decrement in calf venous volume immediately after upright exercise is at least 2% of the resting calf volume. In patients with deep venous incompetence this decrement is attenuated or absent. Similar studies may be obtained with the pneumatic phethysmograph.[28,37] Water plethysmography with the so-called foot volumeter permits assessment of total foot volumetric changes in response to upright exercise.[32] This technique is reviewed in Chapter 85. With the patient in the standing position, both feet are placed in the water plethysmograph. Using a sensitive fluid-level transducer, the amount of decrement in foot volume in response to leg exercise (multiple knee-bends) may be recorded. In patients with deep venous incompetence the amount of decrease in foot volume during upright exercise and the length of time for recovery to preexercise resting volumes are decreased.

Communicating (perforating) venous incompetence

Qualitative assessment of the presence and location of incompetent communicating veins in the lower leg may be determined with Doppler ultrasound by the technique of Folse and Alexander.[15] In this technique, the patient is examined in the sitting position. A tourniquet is applied to the calf immediately below the knee to prevent reflux of blood through incompetent superficial veins. Acoustic gel is applied liberally over the skin of the medial aspect of the lower leg. Using CW (preferably bidirectional) Doppler detector, sites of reflux venous flow signals are mapped out on the lower leg during repeated compression of the calf above the tourniquet. Normally such compression maneuvers will not result in reflux flow signals in the skin of the distal leg. However, in the presence of incompetent deep and communicating (perforating) veins, short bursts of reflux venous flow velocity will be heard with the Doppler probe at the site of incompetent perforators or in superficial veins in juxtaposition to incompetent perforating veins.

Photoplethysmography (PPG) may be used to detect incompetence in communicating veins using either a qualitative[1,6,22,26] or quantitative[25] technique. In the qualitative method, the patient is examined in the sitting position (Fig. 84-1). The PPG transducer is taped with two-faced clear plastic tape to the skin on the medial aspect of each lower leg. After connecting the transducer to the amplifier and recorder, the photoplethysmograph is calibrated and balanced. The stylus of the recorder is adjusted to the upper level of the recording tracing. The patient then plantar flexes the foot five times, and the decrement in skin blood content of the lower leg is recorded with the photoplethysmograph. The recording is continued until the skin blood content returns to baseline. The test is repeated after application of a tourniquet to the calf to prevent reflux through incompetent superficial veins. The skin blood content normally requires 10 to 20 seconds

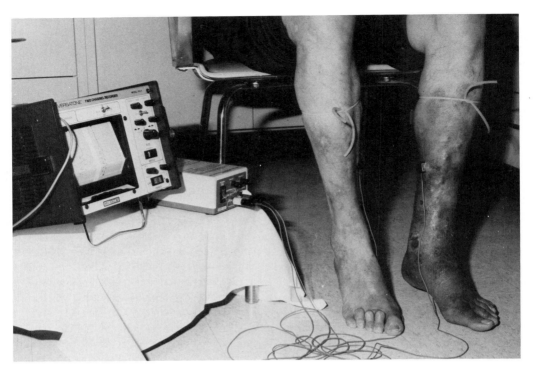

Fig. 84-1. Technique of qualitative venous reflux photoplethysmography (PPG).

or more to return to baseline levels after a brief period of upright leg exercise (Fig. 84-2). In incompetent deep and communicating (perforating) veins, the recovery time will be shortened. In addition, the amount of decrease in the skin blood content may be attenuated or absent in the presence of significant deep and communicating venous incompetence.

To quantify the skin blood content change with exercise, the photoplethysmograph may be calibrated in vivo.[25] With the patient in the supine position, the PPG transducer on each lower leg is balanced and calibrated with the tracing on the recorder set to a zero baseline. The patient then assumes the standing position and after equilibration of skin blood content by stability of the tracing, the gain of the photoplethysmograph recorder is adjusted such that the stylus position reflects the calculated hydrostatic pressure in the superficial veins, as measured by the distance from the right atrium to the site of the transducer on the lower leg (usually about 100 mm Hg or 130 cm saline). The patient again assumes the supine position and alternates this with a standing position until the zero baseline and the standing levels of skin blood

content approximate that predicted from calculation of the hydrostatic pressure. The patient then walks on a treadmill for 30 seconds and comes to a stop while standing upright. The decrement in skin blood content as recorded by the photoplethysmograph is proportional to the degree of fall in ambulatory venous pressure as measured by intravenous pressure measurement recordings. In addition to the decrement in skin blood content, the recovery time for the tracing to return to baseline is recorded. Finally, the patient again assumes the supine position to see if the zero baseline is approximated on the recording.

A less common technique to record the site of incompetent perforating veins is thermography.[11,14] Sites of increased temperature on the skin surface when the patient moves from the supine to the upright position have been correlated with sites of incompetent communicating veins. A similar technique is the detection of fluorescein,[14,23] which is injected into a superficial vein of the foot distal to a tourniquet at the ankle. These techniques have not proved to be sufficiently accurate or simple enough to warrant widespread clinical application.

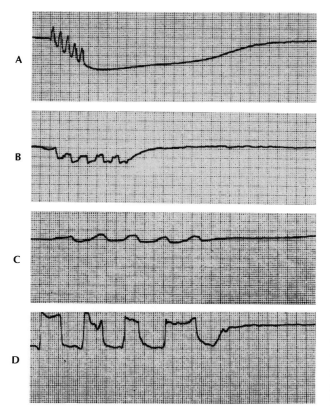

Fig. 84-2. Photoplethysmographic recordings during and after calf muscle exercise while sitting in *A*, normal subject, and in patients with chronic venous insufficiency showing *B*, decompressive, *C*, static, and *D*, congestive venous patterns.

Superficial veins

Doppler ultrasound permits qualitative assessment of primary and secondary varicose veins.[7] These two types of varicosities must be distinguished because of their different etiology, natural history, and treatment. With primary varicose veins the underlying deep venous system should be normal, and communicating (perforating) veins are also usually competent in this disorder. With the CW Doppler velocity detector, patients with primary varicose veins have incompetent venous flow in the superficial veins in response to proximal compression on the varices or a Valsalva maneuver. The deep veins should be patent and competent by Doppler venous examination. In patients with secondary varicose veins, the deep veins are always incompetent, as are the communicating veins in most instances. There may be associated venous obstruction as a result of old DVT.

Quantitative assessment of varicose veins is fea-

sible with various types of plethysmographs. The simplest technique is to quantify the recovery time of the skin blood content using a photoplethysmograph while the patient is sitting.[6,22,26] This technique is similar to that described previously for photoplethysmographic assessment of communicating venous incompetence. In primary varicose veins the recovery time will be shortened, but with application of a superficial tourniquet the skin blood content recovery time should be normalized. With secondary varicose veins the abnormally short recovery time is persistent despite the application of the superficial tourniquet. Estimation of ambulatory venous pressure using quantitative PPG also may be carried out to distinguish primary from secondary varicose veins.[25] With primary varicose veins the skin blood content should decrease in response to treadmill exercise, although this drop may not be as great as in normal individuals. However, application of a superficial tourniquet to the leg should normalize the decrement in skin blood content during walking. With secondary varicose veins the drop in skin blood content during exercise is attenuated or absent even with the application of a rubber tourniquet to the leg. Similar studies may be carried out with air[28,37] and strain-gauge[7] plethysmography, although the results may be somewhat ambiguous unless the varices are large, because superficial veins normally contribute little to the total calf circumference.

TESTS FOR ACTIVITY OF THROMBOSIS

Patients with suspected recurrent venous thrombosis must be evaluated not only for the presence of venous disease but also for the activity of the thrombotic process. Of the various techniques to document active thrombus formation, the [^{125}I]fibrinogen leg scan is the most specific. However, other techniques have been investigated, including other radionuclide techniques, thermography, and evaluation of various by-products of blood coagulation in the circulating plasma or serum. Finally, conventional contrast venography permits evaluation of recent active thrombi.

[^{125}I]fibrinogen leg scanning

The radioactive fibrinogen-uptake test[17] is described more completely in Chapter 76. This test is very useful in evaluating patients with suspected recurrent active thrombosis.[16,38] Because of the time and expense associated with this procedure it should not be the first diagnostic study ordered for such patients. I recommend initial screening with other noninvasive techniques to define the presence of deep venous obstruction. If the deep veins are normal or are widely patent with only venous valvular incompetence, recurrent active thrombosis is probably not the cause of the patient's symptoms and I recommend no further evaluation. If, however, the noninvasive studies suggest deep vein obstruction, then it becomes incumbent on the physician to rule out acute DVT. The [^{125}I]fibrinogen-uptake test should be performed in such patients, but heparin therapy should probably be started first to protect the patient during the 24- to 72-hour delay. If the test is abnormal, the patient may be appropriately treated for recurrent active venous thrombosis. If, however, the test is normal, the deep venous obstruction may be assumed to be old, presumably the result of unresolved old venous thrombosis that poses no current threat of embolism to the patient. Such patients are best treated with bed rest, leg elevation, and elastic support for the chronic (postthrombotic) venous stasis syndrome.

Other techniques

Radioactive streptokinase,[20] urokinase,[27] plasmin,[13] platelets,[21] and heparin[34] have all been used to define activity of suspected recurrent DVT. Although these tests are promising, they remain investigational and have not been widely applied. Thermography has been employed to define areas of increased heat in association with active venous thrombosis.[11] However, patients with proven DVT often manifest increased heat irradiation from the leg for many weeks or months after the thrombotic process develops. The true specificity for thermography in defining recurrent active thrombosis remains to be established. Other hemologic studies,[19] such as determination of β-thromboglobulin and fibrinopeptide A[19] or other products of the coagulation process, have been used to define the presence of recurrent active venous thrombosis. The sensitivity and specificity of these tests remains to be established and most studies are investigational.

In the absence of the radioactive fibrinogen-uptake test, all patients with suspected recurrent venous thrombosis who have documented deep venous obstruction by noninvasive techniques should undergo venography.[16] Patients who show venographic abnormalities suggestive of chronic venous obstruction are treated for the postthrombotic venous stasis syndrome with leg elevation and elastic

support. Such patients have not been treated with anticoagulants, and there has been no instance of pulmonary embolism in these patients. On the other hand, if a fresh thrombus is outlined with contrast material as a persistent filling defect in the venous system, the patient is treated for recurrent venous thrombosis with anticoagulants. With this approach, the number of patients requiring anticoagulant therapy for symptoms of recurrent venous thrombosis is less than 30%.

CLINICAL APPLICATIONS

An approach to the use of various noninvasive diagnostic techniques for the evaluation of chronic venous insufficiency is illustrated by algorithms in Chapter 79. Individual clinical applications of the various diagnostic techniques listed in this chapter may be found in other chapters of the book devoted to specific diagnostic modalities. Current recommendations for the evaluation of patients with varicose veins, postthrombotic syndrome and recurrent DVT are summarized in the remainder of this chapter.

Patients with suspected or clinically evident varicose veins should be evaluated initially with the Doppler ultrasonic velocity detector.[7] Some patients with prominent superficial veins have intact venous valves and do not have reflux flow signals and thus do not truly have varicose veins. Doppler ultrasound is most helpful in distinguishing those patients with varicose veins and a normal deep venous system (primary varicose veins) from patients with evidence of deep and communicating venous incompetence with or without deep venous obstruction (secondary varicose veins). The latter patients rarely have complete relief of symptoms by varicose vein stripping and these patients are advised to use chronic elastic support therapy for their postthrombotic problem. On the other hand, patients with primary varicose veins may be counseled that their condition is not serious and that unless a serious cosmetic disorder exists or subsequent superficial complications occur (such as thrombosis or bleeding), they may be followed nonoperatively without the likelihood of significant future complications.

To quantify abnormalities in patients with varicose veins, quantitative PPG[25] is appropriate to define the presence and magnitude of ambulatory venous hypertension in patients before and after application of a superficial tourniquet to the leg. If a patient develops normal reduction in skin blood content during exercise with a tourniquet on the leg, it is likely that any symptoms caused by the varicosities will be relieved by their removal. If, however, ambulatory venous hypertension is suggested by quanitative PPG despite the application of a tourniquet, stripping of varicose veins is not recommended unless the patient realizes that any cosmetic benefit may not be accompanied by significant relief of symptoms of pain, edema, or stasis changes of the lower leg. Strain-gauge plethysmography or foot volumetry may also be used to quantify these responses to standing leg exercise before and after application of tourniquets.

Patients with postthrombotic venous stasis syndrome are initially screened with Doppler ultrasound.[3,5,8] If the superficial, communicating, and deep veins are normal, the patient should be evaluated for other conditions mimicking stasis disease, such as contact dermatitis, congestive heart failure, and vasculitis. If superficial and deep venous incompetence is documented, the symptoms and signs may be attributed to postthrombotic disease. Most patients do not have significant venous outflow obstruction. Quantification of the hemodynamic abnormalities may be carried out with strain-gauge plethysmography,[4] PPG,[6] or foot volumetry.[32] If ambulatory venous hypertension exists despite the application of tourniquets, some patients may benefit from subfascial ligation of communicating (perforating) veins. However, such surgical intervention is usually reserved for patients who have chronic ulceration that is resistant to healing with medicated bandages and other conservative therapy. Recent techniques of venous valvular reconstruction, venous transposition, or transplantation of competent valve-bearing venous segments may be evaluated using quantitative plethysmography. Although some patients have beeen shown to have striking hemodynamic improvement is not sustained over the course of time. Further investigation using objective outcome criteria will be necessary to evaluate these experimental techniques. Likewise, in patients with documented deep venous outflow obstruction, venous bypass procedures have been recommended, such as popliteal-femoral bypass using the ipsilaterial saphenous vein or femoral-femoral corssover bypass using the saphenous vein from the opposite extremity. Such procedures also may be evaluated by the objective quantitative plethysmographic techniques

listed in this chapter. To date, there has been little objective verification of the hemodynamic improvement associated with these procedures and they remain investigational. It is also unclear which, if any, noninvasive tests best correlate with postoperative clinical result.

Patients with suspected recurrent DVT should initially be evaluated by Doppler ultrasound or one of the plethysmographic techniques. If the deep veins are patent and competent by these studies, the patient should be evaluated for some other condition mimicking recurrent venous thrombosis. If the deep veins are patent but are incompetent, the patient may be assumed to have postthrombotic chronic venous insufficiency. If deep venous obstruction is present, the patient should have some additional objective evaluation of the activity of venous thrombosis. Although the radioactive fibrinogen-uptake test is ideal for this purpose,[38] contrast venography may be carried out to establish the presence or absence of fresh clot outlined by contrast material.[16]

CONCLUSIONS

This chapter has reviewed the currently available noninvasive and minimally invasive diagnostic techniques to evaluate patients for chronic venous insufficiency. The three venous syndromes of varicose veins, postthrombotic chronic venous stasis syndrome, and recurrent venous thrombosis may be evaluated by systematic use of these noninvasive techniques. Although many of these disorders may be initially assessed by simple bedside physical examination, the true status of the superficial, communicating, and deep veins can only be ascertained by more objective techniques. Using both qualitative and quantitative noninvasive techniques, the physician can establish whether or not the patients have chronic venous disease and, if so, can determine the relative contribution of venous outflow obstruction and venous valvular incompetence, which are the two major pathophysiologic sequelae of venous thrombosis. In addition, patients with suspected recurrent venous thrombosis may be evaluated for activity of venous disease using tests specific for this disorder. Only by systematic evaluation of these patients will the physician be able to properly diagnose and treat those patients who have disabling chronic venous insufficiency, while excluding from unnecessary therapy those patients who have some other disorder mimicking this condition.

REFERENCES

1. Abramowitz, H.B., et al.: The use of photoplethysmography in the assessment of venous insufficiency: a comparison to venous pressure measurements, Surgery 86:434, 1979.
2. Anastasios, J.T., et al.: The physiology of venous claudication, Am. J. Surg. 139:447, 1980.
3. Barnes, R.W.: Doppler ultrasonic examination of venous disease. In de Vlieger, M., et al. editors: Handbook of clinical ultrasound, New York, 1978, John Wiley & Sons, Inc.
4. Barnes, R.W., et al.: Noninvasive quantitation of venous reflux in the postphlebitic syndrome, Surg. Gynecol. Obstet. 136:769, 1973.
5. Barnes, R.W., et al.: Noninvasive quantitation of venous hemodynamics in the postphlebitic syndrome, Arch. Surg. 107:307, 1973.
6. Barnes, R.W., et al.: Photoplethysmographic assessment of altered cutaneous circulation in the postphlebitic syndrome, Proc. Assoc. Adv. Med. Instrum. 13:25, 1978.
7. Barnes, R.W., Ross, E.A., and Strandness, D.E.: Differentiation of primary from secondary varicose veins by Doppler ultrasound and strain gauge plethysmography, Surg. Gynecol. Obstet. 141:207, 1975.
8. Barnes, R.W., Russell, H.E., and Wilson, M.R.: Doppler ultrasonic evaluation of venous disease: a programmed audiovisual instruction, ed. 2nd, Iowa City, 1975, University of Iowa Press.
9. Barnes, R.W., et al.: Accuracy of Doppler ultrasound in clinically suspected venous thrombosis of the calf, Surg. Gynecol. Obstet. 143:425, 1976.
10. Bygdeman, S., Aschberg, S., and Hindmarsh, T.: Venous plethysmography in the diagnosis of chronic venous insufficiency, Acta Chir. Scand. 137:423, 1971.
11. Cooke, E.D., and Bowcock, S.A.: Investigation of chronic venous insufficiency by thermography, Vasc. Diagn. Ther., Oct./Nov. 1982.
12. Cranley, J.J., Grass, A.M., and Simeone, F.A.: A plethysmographic technique for the diagnosis of deep venous thrombosis of the lower extremities, Surg. Gynecol. Obstet. 136:385, 1973.
13. Deacon, J.M., et al.: Technetium 99m-plasmin: a new test for the detection of deep vein thrombosis, Br. J. Radiol. 53:673, 1980.
14. Elem, B., Shorey, B.A., and Williams, K.L.: Comparison between thermography and fluorescein test in the detection of incompetent perforating veins, Br. Med. J. 11:651, 1971.
15. Folse, R., and Alexander, R.H.: Directional flow detection for localizing venous valvular incompetency, Surgery 67:114, 1970.
16. Harris, W.H., et al.: The accuracy of the *in vivo* diagnosis of deep vein thrombosis in patients with prior venous thromboembolic disease or severe varicose veins, Thromb. Res. 21:137, 1981.
17. Hirsh, J., and Gallus, A.S.: I-labeled fibrinogen scanning, JAMA 233:970, 1975.
18. Holm, J.S.E.: A simple plethysmographic method for differentiating primary from secondary varicose veins, Surg. Gynecol. Obstet. 143:609, 1976.
19. Hulsteijn, H.V., Bertina, R., and Briet, E.: A one-year follow-up study of plasma fibrinopeptide A and beta-thromboglobulin after deep vein thrombosis and pulmonary embolism, Thromb. Res. 27:225, 1982.
20. Kempi, V., Linden, W.V.D., and Scheele, C.V.: Diagnosis of deep vein thrombosis with 99m Tc-streptokinase: a clincial comparison with phlebography, Br. Med. J. 28:748, 1974.
21. Knight, L.C., et al.: Comparison of In-111-labeled platelets and iodinated fibrinogen for the detection of deep vein thrombosis, J. Nucl. Med. 19:391, 1978.
22. Li, J.M., Anderson, F.A., and Wheeler, H.B.: Noninvasive testing for venous reflux using photoplethysmography: standardization of technique and evaluation of interpretation criteria, Bruit 7:25, 1983.
23. Lofqvist, J., et al.: Evaluation of the fluorescein test in the diagnosis of incompetent perforating veins, Vasa 12:46, 1983.
24. Nicolaides, A., et al.: The value of ambulatory venous pressure in the assessment of venous insufficiency, Vasc. Diagn. Ther., Dec./Jan. 1982.
25. Norris, C.S., Beyrau, A., and Barnes, R.W.: Quantitative photoplethysmography in chronic venous insufficiency: a new method of noninvasive estimation of ambulatory venous pressure, Surgery 94:758, 1983.
26. Pearce, W.H., et al.: Hemodynamic assessment of venous problems, Surgery 93:715, 1983.
27. Rhodes, B.A., et al.: Radioactive urokinase for blood clot scanning, J. Nucl. Med. 13:646, 1972.
28. Sakaguchi, S., et al.: Functional segmental plethysmography: a new nenous function test, J. Cardiovasc. Surg. 9:87, 1968.
29. Sigel, B., et al.: Diagnosis of lower limb venous thrombosis by Doppler ultrasound technique, Arch. Surg. 104:174, 1972.
30. Strandness, D.E., and Sumner, D.S.: Ultrasonic velocity detector in the diagnosis of thrombophlebitis, Arch. Surg. 104:180, 1972.
31. Sumner, D.S., Baker, D.W., and Strandness, D.E.: The ultrasonic velocity detector in a clinical study of venous disease. Arch. Surg. 97:75, 1968.
32. Thulesius, O., Norgren, L., and Gjores, J.E.: Foot-volumetry, a new method for objective assessment of edema and venous function, Vasa 2:325, 1973.
33. Tibbs, D.J., and Fletcher, E.W.L.: Direction of flow in superficial veins as a guide to venous disorders in lower limbs, Surgery 93:758, 1983.
34. Utne, H.E., Nielsen, S.P., and Nielsen, H.V.: A gamma camera method for the evaluation of deep-vein thrombosis in the leg, Eur. J. Nucl. Med. 6:237, 1981.
35. Warren, R., White, E.A., and Belcher, C.D.: Venous pressures in the saphenous system in normal, varicose and postphlebitis extremities. Alterations following femoral vein ligation, Surgery 26:135, 1949.
36. Wheeler, H.B., et al.: Diagnosis of occult deep vein thrombosis by a noninvasive bedside technique, Surgery 70:20, 1971.
37. Winsor, T., and Hyman, C.: Objective venous studies (insufficiency, obstruction and inflammation), J. Cardiovasc. Surg. 2:146, 1961.
38. Wu, K.K., Hoak, J.C., and Barnes, R.W.: A prospective comparison of four methods for the diagnosis of deep vein thrombosis, Thrombos. Diath. Haemorrh. 32:260, 1974.

CHAPTER 85

Role of noninvasive tests in the management of acute and chronic venous disease

THE EDITORS

The previous chapters in this section suggest that there are a number of reasons why noninvasive diagnostic techniques may play a valuable role in the diagnosis and management of patients with venous disease:

1. The clinical diagnosis of acute deep vein thrombosis (DVT) is both insensitive and nonspecific, with the bedside appraisal of the patient seldom being more than 50% accurate.
2. Several acute and chronic venous diseases require objective diagnosis for proper management, including acute DVT, recurrent DVT, superficial thrombophlebitis, postthrombotic stasis disease, primary and secondary varicose veins, and pulmonary embolism.
3. The diagnostic standards, both contrast phlebography and pulmonary arteriography, impose such significant expense, discomfort, and risk to the patients as to preclude their use for routine screening and follow-up procedures.
4. Since the validity of certain noninvasive diagnostic techniques has become established, these methods can be used to manage patients with suspected venous disease in the absence of contrast studies.
5. The use of noninvasive diagnostic techniques in venous disease is proving cost-effective.

To summarize and place in proper perspective the previous material in this section, the following discussion will identify the attributes and limitations of the various techniques based on their diagnostic principles and will review the most appropriate methods for use in the various venous disorders. The conclusion will address some principles to keep in mind when choosing one or more instruments for the laboratory.

DIAGNOSTIC PRINCIPLES

The two pathophysiologic sequelae of venous disease that result in hemodynamic abnormalities detected by noninvasive techniques are *venous obstruction* to outflow from the limb and *venous reflux* through incompetent venous valves. In venous obstruction the presence of thrombotic activity must be established, particularly in patients with suspected recurrent venous thrombosis.

Venous outflow obstruction may be assessed qualitatively by Doppler ultrasound and quantitatively by the various plethysmographic techniques, including impedance plethysmography (IPG), strain-gauge plethysmography (SPG), and phleborheography (PRG). Visualization of obstructed venous segments proximal to the knee is possible with radionuclide phlebography. Of these techniques only Doppler ultrasound and PRG are capable of detecting major calf vein thrombi. Doppler ultrasound is capable of distinguishing superficial as well as deep venous obstruction and also may be used to screen for venous thrombosis of the upper extremities. Doppler ultrasound is the only technique that allows screening of patients in traction or plaster casts or in the presence of major limb amputation. Although it is the least expensive and the most versatile technique, Doppler ultrasound suffers the limitation of being the most vulnerable to subjective misinterpretation, and considerable experience is required for maximal accuracy with this technique. The other plethysmographic techniques, although more expensive,

Table 85-1. Characteristics of noninvasive venous diagnostic techniques*

Technique	Simplicity	Portability	Versatility	Inexpense	Sensitivity Proximal	Calf	Specificity Proximal	Calf
Doppler ultrasound	±	+	+	+	+	±	+	±
IPG	+	+	0	0	+	0	+	0
SPG	+	+	+	±	+	0	+	0
PRG	±	+	+	0	+	±	+	±
PPG	+	+	+	±	0	+	0	+
Foot volumetry	+	±	0	±	0	+	0	+
[125I]fibrinogen-uptake test	±	+	0	0	±	+	±	±
Radionuclide phlebography	0	0	0	0	+	0	+	0

* +, good; ±, fair; 0, poor.

are more objective and reproducible, making them more useful for initial equipment in most laboratories.

Venous reflux in postthrombotic disease and primary or secondary varicose veins may be assessed by both Doppler ultrasound and plethysmographic techniques. Qualitative assessment of the competence of deep, communicating (perforating), and superficial veins may be carried out with nondirectional or directional Doppler equipment, with or without recordings. This technique also permits concomitant assessment of superficial and deep venous obstruction in these chronic venous disorders. Quantitative assessment of deep or superficial venous competence is feasible using SPG, photoplethysmography (PPG), or foot volumetry. The phleborheograph also has the capability of measuring altered foot venous volume responses in chronic venous insufficiency, although the technique has not been exploited in this area.

Thrombotic activity is defined only by the [125I]fibrinogen-uptake test. Although other hematologic methods, including determination of fibrin split products or fibrin monomers, have been used to identify active venous thrombosis, such methods are not in widespread use. [125I]fibrinogen leg scanning is the most sensitive technique to identify active calf vein thrombi. It is also particularly useful to define the presence or absence of true recurrent active venous thrombosis, particularly in patients with proven prior deep venous obstruction who may develop recurrent symptoms on the basis of mechanical venous obstruction rather than recurrent thrombotic activity. The technique is expensive and time-consuming and has been primarily limited to prospective investigative studies of high-risk patients. Although the method may not be

useful for routine screening for acute DVT, its selective use in patients in whom definition of thrombotic activity is important makes it an useful adjunct to other noninvasive techniques.

Table 85-1 summarizes some attributes and limitations of the various noninvasive diagnostic techniques in venous disease.

CLINICAL APPLICATION
Acute deep vein thrombosis

Patients with an initial episode of suspected acute DVT may be screened by many of the techniques that are sensitive to a major venous obstruction. These include Doppler ultrasound and the various plethysmographic techniques, including IPG, SPG, and PRG. In experienced hands such techniques are capable of detecting proximal venous thrombosis with an accuracy approaching 95%. Doppler ultrasound and PRG are also sensitive to calf vein thrombosis, although these techniques are less specific in this area. [125I]fibrinogen leg scanning is the most sensitive technique to identify isolated calf vein thrombosis. However, the technique is only accurate during the active phase of the disease, and the time and expense for the procedure preclude its use for routine diagnostic assessment of patients with suspected acute venous thrombosis. Fibrinogen leg scanning is best reserved for patients in whom other noninvasive techniques are negative and in whom isolated calf vein thrombosis is suspected. Radionuclide phlebography is sensitive to major obstructive disease of the proximal leg veins, but the technique is best suited for use in conjunction with perfusion lung scans and to document the status of the intraabdominal veins.

Patients with clinical signs and symptoms of major leg vein thrombosis in whom noninvasive tests are normal may be safely managed without anticoagulant therapy while being investigated for some other cause of the leg complaints. Patients in whom venous thrombosis is suspected and in whom a noninvasive test is unequivocally abnormal may be appropriately treated with anticoagulants for DVT. If diagnostic ambiguity is present, contrast phlebography should be carried out.

Acute superficial thrombophlebitis

Although thrombosis of a prominent varicose vein presents no diagnostic dilemma, patients with superficial inflammation in the absence of varices may have lymphangitis or cellulitis, which may be confused with superficial thrombophlebitis. To distinguish these conditions, which require different therapy, Doppler ultrasound is the most appropriate noninvasive technique to assess the patency of the superficial venous system. Although contrast phlebography may be performed, the pain and inflammation associated with this procedure may aggravate the existing leg inflammation. Doppler ultrasound is also useful to define the status of the deep veins, which may be occasionally thrombosed in the presence of superficial thrombophlebitis. In such instances anticoagulation therapy is indicated, whereas an antiinflammatory agent is usually the only medication required for superficial thrombophlebitis.

Recurrent deep vein thrombosis

The patient who has acute leg pain or swelling following a previous clinical history of leg vein thrombosis presents a diagnostic dilemma. Many patients with prior DVT have residual deep venous obstruction, as well as valvular incompetence, both of which may lead to the postthrombotic sequelae of leg pain and edema, which may be confused with recurrent active thrombosis. Some patients who have recurrent symptoms have actually never had venous disease and suffer from some other problem. To evaluate such patients, initial screening should be carried out with noninvasive techniques sensitive to major venous obstruction, such as Doppler ultrasound or some type of plethysmography. If such studies are normal, recurrent venous thrombosis is improbable and some other diagnosis should be sought. If the noninvasive studies (particularly Doppler ultrasound) reveal patent but incompetent deep veins, the patient may be treated for postthrombotic syndrome with rest, leg elevation, and elastic support. If, however, such

venous screening procedures suggest venous obstruction, the presence or absence of active thrombosis must be established. To this end, [^{125}I]fibrinogen leg scanning is most appropriate, and this study should be carried out preferably before the patient is given anticoagulants. If the test is positive, the patient should be treated for recurrent venous thrombosis. If the [^{125}I]fibrinogen-uptake test is negative, the patient should be treated for the postthrombotic syndrome with bed rest, leg elevation, and elastic support. Anticoagulants in such instances are not necessary. If fibrinogen leg scanning is not available, contrast venography may be used to differentiate active thrombosis (fresh clot outlined by contrast material) from chronic venous occlusion (obstruction with prominent collaterals, wall irregularity, and valvular change).

Postthrombotic syndrome

Patients with the postthrombotic (chronic venous stasis) syndrome usually suffer from marked deep venous incompetence and valvular insufficiency of the communicating (perforating) veins of the lower leg. In approximately 33% of patients, abnormalities of venous outflow contribute to the syndrome. Such patients are best studied by techniques that assess both venous outflow obstruction and venous reflux. Qualitative evaluation with Doppler ultrasound is the most simple and rapid method. This technique also permits mapping of the location of the incompetent communicating (perforating) veins, which may be selectively ligated through small superficial incisions. Quantification of superficial and deep venous incompetence is possible with SPG or PPG. PRG provides some measure of deep venous incompetence, but the technique has been primarily used for assessment of obstruction to venous outflow.

Varicose veins

It is important to distinguish primary varicose veins, which are an isolated superficial disorder, from secondary varicose veins associated with underlying deep venous disease. Secondary varices are usually the result of antecedent DVT. Surgical treatment of secondary varices rarely results in complete relief of symptoms because of the residual venous dysfunction of the deep and communicating (perforating) veins. Although the presence of postthrombotic stasis dermatitis or ulceration is almost always a reflection of deep venous pathology, occasionally secondary varicose veins may be

Table 85-2. Role of noninvasive techniques in the diagnosis of venous disease*

Technique	Acute DVT	Recurrent DVT	Superficial thrombophlebitis	Venous insufficiency	Pulmonary embolism
Doppler	+	±	+	+	±
IPG	+	±	0	0	±
SPG	+	±	0	+	±
PRG	+	±	0	±	±
PPG	0	0	0	+	0
Foot volumetry	0	0	0	+	0
[^{125}I]fibrinogen-uptake test	±	+	0	0	±
Radionuclide phlebography	+	±	0	0	±

* +, good; ±, equivocal; 0, poor.

present with little postthrombotic stigmata. Objective documentation of the status of the deep veins should be carried out before surgical treatment of varicose veins. Doppler ultrasound provides qualitative assessment of the presence of deep venous obstruction or incompetence. In the absence of such disorders the varices may be assumed to be primary. If deep or communicating venous abnormalities are present, surgical therapy of the secondary varicose veins should be undertaken with caution, and the patient should be warned of the possibility of recurrent varices, recurrent venous thrombosis, and possible subsequent postthrombotic leg sequelae. SPG or PPG may be used to quantify abnormalities of venous outflow and venous reflux. Longitudinal follow-up studies are useful to define the natural history of previous venous thrombosis and the development of recurrent venous thrombosis or the efficacy of medical or surgical therapy of chronic venous disease.

Pulmonary embolism

Patients with clinically suspected pulmonary embolism should be evaluated for both the presence of a source of embolus (venous thrombosis) and the existence of an embolus in the lung. Screening of the lower extremities of such patients may be carried out by Doppler ultrasound, plethysmography, or radionuclide phlebography. If venous thrombosis is present, the clinical diagnosis of pulmonary embolus is given credence. However, the majority of such patients have normal leg veins, and the diagnosis of pulmonary embolus is then in question. Although perfusion and ventilation lung scans have been the standard for diagnosis of pulmonary embolus, the nonspecificity of these techniques is becoming increasingly apparent. If a per-

fusion defect of lobar extent or greater is present in association with a normal chest x-ray film, particularly if the area is normally ventilated, the diagnosis of pulmonary embolism can be assumed, with an accuracy approaching 90%. However, perfusion defects of lesser extent, regardless of the status of the chest film, are associated with a significant incidence of false positive results when pulmonary arteriography is carried out. Unless a source of venous thrombosis is established in the extremities, such patients should probably undergo pulmonary arteriography to clarify the diagnosis.

Table 85-2 summarizes the role of the various noninvasive techniques in acute and chronic venous disease.

CHOICE OF NONINVASIVE TECHNIQUES

The selection of one or more of the available noninvasive diagnostic techniques presents a challenge to the clinician desiring to initiate a vascular laboratory. A number of factors must be considered in deciding on the most appropriate technique, including the requirements of portability, frequency of use, cost, the individual to be performing the tests, the use for diagnostic or for prospective studies, and the type of diseases to be studied. The least expensive and most portable and versatile technique is Doppler ultrasound, which is particularly useful for screening both acute and chronic venous disease. Its ability to evaluate the venous system of extremities in traction or in plaster casts makes it particularly useful for orthopedic patients. However, the subjective nature of the method and the requirement for considerable experience before maximal accuracy is achieved have detracted from its widespread use by clinicians. Most laboratories will be best served by the incorporation of a plethysmographic method to screen for venous disease. For high-volume studies, dedicated equipment such as that used in IPG provides simple and rapid screening of patients. For more versatility in the assessment of both acute and chronic venous disease, as well as peripheral arterial disease, SPG, PPG, or PRG should be considered. [^{125}I]fibrinogen leg scanning plays a complementary role in the assessment of thrombotic activity, but its expense and time-consuming characteristics will preclude its routine use except for the screening of patients with suspected recurrent venous thrombosis. Radionuclide phlebography is widely available in hospitals, but its application will probably be limited to patients who are to undergo perfusion lung scanning.

Contrast phlebography (venography) remains the diagnostic standard for venous thrombosis and is the technique by which the noninvasive methods must be validated. For many physicians, contrast phlebography will be the primary objective method to establish the diagnosis. However, the expense, discomfort, and potential morbidity associated with phlebography should prompt physicians to consider noninvasive screening for acute and chronic venous disease. Not only have the methods been validated in recent years, but there is now evidence that these techniques may prove to be the most cost-effective method of managing patients with venous disorders.

PART THREE

PRACTICAL ASPECTS

CHAPTER 86

Organization of the vascular laboratory

CYNTHIA A. KUPPER and M. LEE NIX

During the past decade, noninvasive vascular testing has spread from centers primarily involved in research and development of instrumentation to many clinically oriented laboratories. Although acceptance of this discipline is gratifying, it is also disturbing that the increase in quantity has not consistently produced an increase in quality. Unfortunately, the development of sophisticated instrumentation has not been paralleled by an equal increase in knowledge of the technology. This chapter addresses the issue of the contributions and interrelationships of the physician, technologist, and instrumentation to form the foundation of a clinical vascular laboratory.

THE PHYSICIAN

The first task in the establishment of the vascular laboratory is selection of the medical director. As in any patient-care service, the primary motivation of the physician should be to provide excellent patient care and useful diagnostic information in the evaluation of disease. Physicians should be compensated for their input, although the primary motivation should not be monetary gain; therefore it is important to select an individual who is willing to make a commitment. The physician with an interest in vascular disease has an advantage because of his knowledge of the natural history and evaluation of patients with these problems. Only recently have physicians been exposed to noninvasive vascular studies that investigate hemodynamic variables and provide complementary physiologic and anatomic information to the usual evaluation by history, physical examination, and arteriography. In-depth formal education in noninvasive techniques for physicians has been limited to postgraduate fellowships in vascular surgery and continuing education courses.

When a physician makes the decision to become director of a vascular laboratory, a major time commitment is involved. This commitment of time, support, and interest will be concentrated in the developmental phase of the laboratory, but must continue on a lesser scale after establishment of the routine procedures. If the physician is inexperienced in noninvasive testing, an even greater investment will be required, since he must first acquire an appropriate base of knowledge about the capabilities and limitations of the techniques. As this knowledge is gained, the physician will become aware of the interrelationship of physician involvement, examiner input, and test modality capabilities and limitations. This will allow the physician to select the appropriate instruments and hire staff capable of fulfilling job expectations. Because an experienced staff is usually not available, the physician must work with the inexperienced staff until an acceptable level of competence is reached. Initially it will be necessary for the physician to select the appropriate tests for each patient, interpret the results, and communicate the results to the referring physician. As director, the physician is also responsible for correlation of test results with the more traditional contrast arteriograms. This initial process of physician input and interaction with his staff is the foundation of all later laboratory activity and is important for the survival and success of the operation.

After the proficiency and competence of the laboratory are established, the physician may choose to continue his active participation by overseeing all aspects of the operation or he may choose to be involved in a less demanding role by delegating most aspects to examiners. This decision is strongly influenced by the availability of the director for decision making on a patient-to-patient basis. In addition, this delegation of responsibility may occur only if the examiners have demonstrated their ability to function independently.

In situations where the physician is interested in continuing an active, participatory role in the laboratory, he chooses a supervisory role. The active role includes selection of the appropriate procedures, overseeing the performance of the tests, interpretation of the results, and communication of the results to the referring physician. This requires a significant time commitment on a daily basis, as well as accessibility for consultations with the examiners and referring physicians.

A physician with limited time should choose a collaborative relationship with a capable examiners staff rather than a supervisory role that requires regular supervision of patient examinations. A collaborative relationship implies that the physician depends on the examiners to make decisions appropriate to each testing situation and assumes a high level of confidence in their competence. The wise physician looks beyond the initial role he must assume and seeks to hire an individual who will complement his input.

THE EXAMINER: TECHNICIAN OR TECHNOLOGIST?

When more than half a dozen noninvasive examinations a week are to be done, the physician should hire an examiner to perform the procedures. This examiner is either a technician or a technologist. A technician has acquired the technique of a specialized skill, whereas a technologist is capable of independent work and selects appropriate tests as dictated by the clinical situation.

A technician should work efficiently and accurately in the performance of objective tests according to strict procedure protocols. In the small hospital or office practice where fewer than five vascular tests are performed daily, a technician can also perform a variety of other tasks. Such an arrangement can be cost-effective provided that the physician/director assumes an active role in the decision-making process in the vascular laboratory. Problems will inevitably follow if either of two situations occurs. First, if the physician does not maintain a supervisory role, quality will suffer. Second, if the technician is expected to perform subjective testing, not only will quality suffer but the technician may also become frustrated and overwhelmed by the responsibility.

The technologist is capable of performing both objective and subjective tests and should be knowledgeable about vascular disease and test capabilities and limitations. This enables him to evaluate the noninvasive test data obtained during the course of the examination and to modify the procedure to better assess the results. This interactive process of using clinical and technical expertise allows the technologist to individualize the examination and is critical for obtaining accurate data and maximizing the amount of information in those situations when a physician supervisor is not available. The technologist is best suited to work in a large community hospital, private laboratory, or medical center where at least five procedures are performed daily. The technologist should be capable of initiating research, evaluating current technology, educating patients about vascular disease, and interpreting test results. This expanded role is essential for the individual with the broad knowledge required for this role and is important for job satisfaction. The physician-director plays a key role in promoting job satisfaction for the technologist by providing time for correlation of noninvasive test results with contrast radiographic results, encouragement for reviewing pertinent periodical information and for interfacing with other medical personnel regarding noninvasive vascular testing, and opportunity for participation in vascular conferences and rounds.

Education for technologists and technicians is in its infancy; the number of centers that offer formal education in the field of noninvasive vascular technology is currently less than five, and none are on the baccalaureate level. Education of the vascular technologist and technician relies primarily on self-initiated study and experience gained during employment. For this reason it is important that the individual hired for a technical position has a background that includes a knowledge of anatomy, physiology, medical ethics, disease processes, and biophysicical principles. An understanding of the scientific method and statistics is necessary as well, and in the clinical setting a medical background in patient care is valuable. Other desirable characteristics in a technologist are inquisitiveness, independence, and motivation. Such an individual will seek out answers to physiologic questions and monitor current state-of-the-art technology.

Once a technologist or technician has been hired he should proceed with a course of study structured by the physician. This should include a review of pertinent anatomy, physiology, and pathophysiology. Programmed texts such as the Barnes' series[1-3] afford a simplified review and information about the use of Doppler evaluation of the arterial, venous, and cerebrovascular systems. It is helpful to begin learning test procedures by examining normal volunteers. This allows the examiner to become familiar with the variations that occur among normal subjects. Establishing expertise in one area of testing before learning another promotes confidence and reduces frustration.

It is wise to establish good rapport with the radiologist, since feedback from radiologic procedures is a primary learning tool in identification of problems in technique and in defining limitations of the test method. Physicians who refer patients for invasive radiologic procedures may be approached about the possibility of performing noninvasive tests at no charge to the patient. Not only does this provide feedback regarding accuracy for the novice, but it will also help establish the accuracy of the procedure for the particular laboratory.

Once the basic principles of testing are understood, there is no substitute for working with a knowledgeable preceptor; if the director has a working knowledge of noninvasive testing, he can provide this valuable resource. Otherwise it will be necessary for the the physician and the examiner to seek assistance from an established resource.

TESTING MODALITIES

Equipment selection is a major issue in the organization of the vascular laboratory; the choice between objective and subjective test modalities should be based on the scope of clinical questions to be addressed. Objective tests are those performed according to a defined protocol and require minimal operator input. Although objective tests are restricted in the clinical information they provide, the examiner may be trained to perform these tests in a short time. The use of a stethoscope to obtain blood pressure is an example of an objective test, since the examiner can be taught the procedure quickly, and it is not necessary to understand Korotkoff's sounds or physiologic variables that affect pressure changes to obtain accurate pressure measurements. The parallel in the vascular laboratory is the measurement of segmental pressures in the limb by Doppler ultrasound.

In general, subjective testing is more versatile, addresses a broader spectrum of clinical questions,

and requires maximum operator input to obtain the largest amount of accurate information. The operator must modify the test during the procedure in accordance with knowledge of anatomy, physiology, pathophysiology, hemodynamics, and instrumentation. An example of such a test is the venous Doppler examination. The use of Doppler ultrasound to assess the deep venous system for obstruction requires the examiner to understand the deep and superficial venous systems and how they relate, the hemodynamics involved in the venous muscle pump and the effect of respiration on venous blood flow, the physical principles involved in extrinsic and intrinsic venous obstruction, Doppler ultrasound and its limitations, and the variations common to venous anatomy.

Testing modalities that involve the use of plethysmography generally are objective in nature and those using ultrasound, either Doppler or real-time imaging, are generally subjective. Occasionally an instrument can be used for either subjective or objective testing. Doppler ultrasound may be an objective instrument in blood pressure measurement, but can be subjective in analysis of arterial, venous, and carotid velocity signals. However, it must be understood that the subjective and objective methods rarely assess the exact same variables. An oculoplethysmograph may provide information about the presence of an uncompensated internal carotid lesion, but it cannot provide comprehensive information about the status of the cervical carotid bifurcation specifically. Such information must be obtained with Doppler ultrasound or real-time imaging by direct examination of the cervical carotid arteries. An oculoplethysmographic examination may be carried out with little or no understanding of the results, whereas a Doppler examination of the carotid bifurcation requires that the technologist have extensive knowledge of anatomy, physiology, and the possible variations.

Another consideration in the choice of subjective or objective test modalities is the availability of contrast arteriographic and venographic studies for validation of noninvasive test results. Without contrast verification of noninvasive examination results, the logical choices for noninvasive tests would be those that allow standardized results and little examiner input or variability. Unfortunately, standardization of test results has been slow in developing. Subjective examinations require ongoing monitoring of results and contrast radiography is currently the diagnostic standard in this assessment;

it is the only credible verification method. Correlation of these findings requires the participation of a knowledgeable physician.

Adequate numbers of examinations are required to develop proficiency with the subjective tests. A minimum of 6 to 10 studies per week is necessary to attain and maintain an appropriate level of competence with subjective testing modalities. For example, if a review of venograms with a competent interpreter is not possible or if fewer than 6 venous Doppler examinations are performed per week, then the selection of an objective technique is recommended.

Turnover in technical staff affects the selection of instrumentation. If frequent turnover is anticipated, objective testing modalities should be used. Because of the shorter learning curve involved, these skills are more easily transferred from one individual to another. Conversely, subjective testing modalities require an extended learning curve that may approach a year if the technologist is to perform comprehensive testing in the areas of cerebrovascular, arterial, and venous assessment.

INTERRELATIONSHIP OF PHYSICIAN, EXAMINER, AND TESTING MODALITIES

The organizational base for the vascular laboratory depends on the interrelationship of the physician, examiner, and the tests performed (Fig. 86-1). This interrelationship will serve effectively if it is structured according to either of the following triads (Fig. 86-2). The inner triad, which addresses a limited clinical role, has a physician in a supervisory role, a vascular technician, and objective testing modalities. The outer triad, which encompasses a more comprehensive range of clinical testing, illustrates the laboratory structured with a physician in a collaborative role, a technologist, and subjective procedures. If factors between the two triads are exchanged, the basic foundation of the laboratory will be weakened, which results in a sacrifice of quality and personnel conflicts.

In the inner triad the desired clinical information is restricted in scope (Fig. 86-2). Objective tests are performed competently by a technician under the direction of a physician supervisor. In this pattern the physician is available to interface with the referring physician and the technician on a patient-to-patient basis. Should the physician supervisor be inaccessible, the technician will function beyond his capability (Fig. 86-3) and laboratory credibility will suffer. In addition, the technician may feel frustrated and cost-effectiveness and patient safety may be jeopardized if the referring physician, unfamiliar with noninvasive testing or clinical presentation of vascular disease, requests an inappropriate examination. At best the result would be a failure to provide diagnostic information. At worst, the incorrect procedure may result in patient injury. Such a situation might occur if segmental pressures were requested for a patient with confusing clinical signs, such as limb edema and diminished pulses,

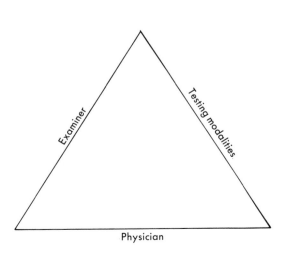

Fig. 86-1. Organizational base for vascular laboratory: physician, examiner, and testing modalities.

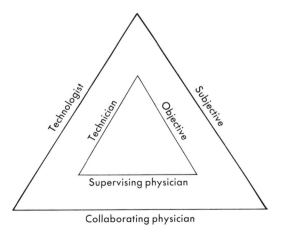

Fig. 86-2. Triads representing appropriate organization of vascular laboratory. Outer triad represents structure required to address entire scope of vascular testing. Inner triad represents structure recommended for laboratories addressing most clinical questions.

and the test resulted in dislodgement of thrombotic material from a deep vein thrombosis. Another aberration is shown in Fig. 86-4. This illustrates the situation in which subjective testing is performed by a technician who is supervised by the laboratory director. Quality cannot be maintained unless the laboratory director oversees and assumes the responsibility for each subjective testing procedure, and few physicians have the time to participate in each examination. A final variation of the inner triad is to have a technologist fill the role of a technician examiner (Fig. 86-5). Since the technologist is capable of functioning in a more independent role, it is likely that job dissatisfaction and termination of employment will occur.

If maximum efficiency and clinical information are desired, the outer triad should be selected (Fig. 86-2). Subjective techniques may be used by the technologist in collaboration with the medical director to address a broad scope of clinical questions. This outer triad functions effectively when the physician delegates responsibility to a technologist who is capable of and willing to function independently. It must be stressed that it is the responsibility of the physician to delegate responsibility only if the technologist has demonstrated an appropriate level of knowledge and expertise. The most dangerous variation of either triad is to place the technician in the position of performing subjective tests when the physician performs only

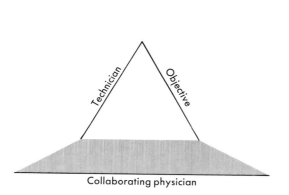

Fig. 86-3. Laboratory credibility decreases because of lack of consistent physician input.

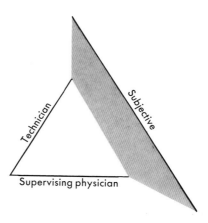

Fig. 86-4. Scope of subjective testing exceeds capability of technician.

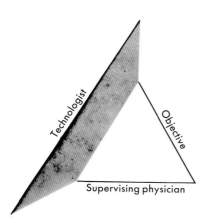

Fig. 86-5. Technologist is underused in role of technician.

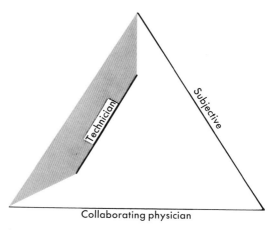

Fig. 86-6. Most dangerous variation of either triad. Technician is expected to function beyond capability.

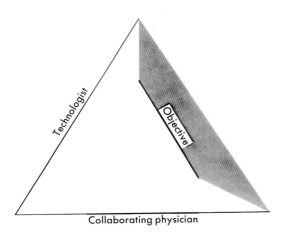

Fig. 86-7. Limited scope of testing modalities underuses capabilities of personnel.

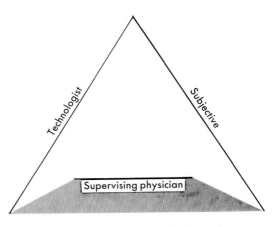

Fig. 86-8. Least dangerous variation of either triad. However, personnel conflicts are likely to occur.

a collaborative role (Fig. 86-6). Since a technician is not capable of making independent clinical decisions and the physician is not present during the examination to make these decisions, the accuracy of the results must suffer. Two other variations of the outer triad are illustrated in Figs. 86-7 and 86-8. Both of these will result in job dissatisfaction for the technologist. When objective techniques are used, the technologist will become bored (Fig. 86-7). When the physician functions as a supervisor, the technologist will be stifled (Fig. 86-8).

SUMMARY

During the initial organizational phase of the vascular laboratory it is essential to define precisely the roles of the physician and examiner in relation to the equipment chosen for the laboratory. A laboratory planned in accordance with the capability of the director and the examiner is preferred to one

that evolves around premature purchase of instruments. With proper planning, an appropriate relationship may be designed for any given laboratory situation. Attention to this relationship in the planning stage will lead to the development of a harmonious and capable vascular laboratory.

REFERENCES

1. Barnes, R.W., and Wilson, M.R.: Doppler ultrasonic evaluation of cerebrovascular disease: a programmed instruction, Iowa City, Iowa, 1975, University of Iowa Audiovisual Center.
2. Barnes, R.W., Russell, H.E., and Wilson, M.R.: Doppler ultrasonic evaluation of venous disease: a programmed audiovisual instruction, ed. 2, Iowa City, Iowa, 1975, University of Iowa Press.
3. Barnes, R.W., and Wilson, M.R.: Doppler ultrasonic evaluation of peripheral arterial disease: a programmed audiovisual instruction, Iowa City, Iowa, 1976, University of Iowa Press.

CHAPTER 87

Evaluation of noninvasive testing procedures: data analysis and interpretation

DAVID S. SUMNER

In clinical practice, many factors influence the choice of a noninvasive test, including availability of the instrument, cost, experience of the technician, convenience, personal prejudices, and accuracy. Of these, accuracy is certainly the most important. Without sufficient accuracy, the results of a test are meaningless and its performance not only constitutes a waste of time but also results in an uncompensated expense for the patient in terms of money, unwarranted concern over a falsely positive diagnosis, or neglect of a lesion that should be treated. Unlike older diagnostic modalities, noninvasive tests came along at a time when investigators were sensitive to the need for demonstrating their accuracy. To the credit of those in the field, earnest efforts have been made to employ statistical methods and to be as objective as possible. Despite these efforts, bias invariably creeps in; the multiplicity of instruments, techniques, and methods of analysis has added to the confusion.

This chapter describes some of the statistical methods used to evaluate the accuracy of noninvasive tests, describes how these methods may be used to compare the accuracy of one test with another, examines some of the subtle ways that results may be biased, discusses the advantages and disadvantages of using multiple tests, and points out how some of the statistical attributes relate to the practical application of these tests.

BASIC CONSIDERATIONS

The fact that measurements made on one group of patients differ statistically from those made on another group does not mean that these measurements are sufficiently accurate to effectively distinguish between the two groups. For example, the

average weight of 50 females on two hospital wards was significantly lower (p < .001) than that of 50 males on the same wards; yet, as shown in Fig. 87-1, the spread of the data was so great in both groups that given a certain weight it would be impossible to predict with any degree of confidence whether the individual was male or female.

To evaluate the accuracy of a diagnostic test, the results of the test must be compared with the results obtained on the same patient (or same artery or vein) with a reliable, well-established diagnostic standard (frequently referred to as a ''gold standard''). Use of a diagnostic standard is necessary since the true diagnosis is often unknown. In the simplest case, the diagnosis and the test results are considered to be either positive or negative (Table 87-1). *True negative* (TN) results are those in which both the noninvasive test and the diagnostic standard results are negative; *true positive* (TP) results are those in which both the noninvasive test and the diagnostic standard results are positive. *False negative* (FN) results are those in which the noninvasive test is negative but the definitive test is positive, indicating the presence of disease. *False positive* (FP) results are those in which the noninvasive test is positive but the diagnostic standard is negative, indicating the absence of disease.

From Table 87-1, four useful parameters describing the accuracy of the test can be derived. *Sensitivity*, which is the ability of a test to recognize the presence of disease, is calculated by dividing the number of true positive results by the total number of positive results obtained with the diagnostic standard. *Specificity*, which is the ability to recognize the absence of disease, is calculated

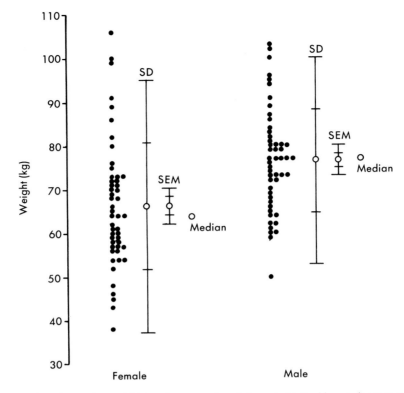

Fig. 87-1. Weights of 50 males and 50 females on two hospital wards. Vertical bars indicate two standard deviations of mean *(SD)* or two standard errors of the mean *(SEM)*. t = 3.866, df = 98, p < .001.

Table 87-1. Matrix for calculating parameters of accuracy

| Noninvasive test results | Distribution according to diagnostic standard | | Noninvasive test total |
	Negative	Positive	
Negative	TN	FN	TN + FN
Positive	FP	TP	TP + FP
TOTAL FOR DIAGNOSTIC STANDARD	TN + FP	TP + FN	

by dividing the number of true negative results by the total number of negative results obtained with the diagnostic standard.

$$\text{Sensitivity} = \frac{TP}{TP + FN} \quad (1)$$

$$\text{Specificity} = \frac{TN}{TN + FP} \quad (2)$$

Although sensitivity and specificity are the best parameters for comparing the accuracy of one test with that of another, the clinician receiving the results of a test is more concerned with predictive value. *Positive predictive value* (PPV) represents the likelihood that a positive test result actually implies the presence of disease, whereas *negative predictive value* (NPV) is the likelihood that a negative test result actually implies the absence of disease. PPV is the ratio of true positive results to the total number of positive test results, and NPV is the ratio of true negative results to the total number of negative test results.

$$\text{PPV} = \frac{TP}{TP + FP} \quad (3)$$

$$\text{NPV} = \frac{TN}{TN + FN} \quad (4)$$

Dividing the sum of the test results that agree with the diagnostic standard results by the total number of tests performed gives the *overall accuracy*.

$$\text{Accuracy} = \frac{TN + TP}{TN + FN + TP + FP} \quad (5)$$

Calculated in this way, accuracy is not very descriptive, since it does not directly reflect the values of the more critical parameters. As shown in Table 87-2, two tests with identical accuracies can have widely different sensitivities, specificities, PPVs, and NPVs. Except in the unique case when sensitivity and specificity are equal, the prevalence of the disease in the population being studied will also affect overall accuracy, despite the facts that the same test is being used and that sensitivity and specificity remain the same (Table 87-3). Overall accuracy alone, therefore, provides the reader with insufficient information to evaluate the merits of a test.

Prevalence refers to the proportion of the population being studied that actually has the disease. In retrospective studies, prevalence can be calculated by dividing the number of positive results as determined by the diagnostic standard (TP + FN) by the total number of tests performed; in actual practice, prevalence is seldom known with certainty.

$$\text{Prevalence} = \frac{\text{TP} + \text{FN}}{\text{TN} + \text{FN} + \text{TP} + \text{FP}} \qquad (6)$$

Table 87-3 illustrates how variations in prevalence can affect predictive values, even when the same test is used. In each of the three examples, sensitivity and specificity are unchanged; however, the PPV increases when prevalence is high and decreases when prevalence is low. Conversely, NPV increases when prevalence is low but decreases when prevalence is high. These relationships are shown graphically in Figs. 87-2 and 87-3.

The important relationships between sensitivity and specificity and predictive values are also illustrated in Figs. 87-2 and 87-3. Given the same specificity, an improvement in sensitivity will have little effect on the PPV (Fig. 87-2) but will have a major effect on the NPV (Fig. 87-3). On the other hand, given the same sensitivity, an improvement in specificity will have little effect on the NPV (Fig. 87-3) but will have a major effect on the PPV (Fig. 87-2). In other words, if the investigation requires a high PPV, a test with a high specificity should be selected—even at the expense of a low sensitivity. If a high NPV is desired, a test with a high sensitivity should be used. How this relates to actual clinical practice will be discussed later in this chapter.

Predictive values can be calculated for any disease prevalence if sensitivities and specificities are known. In Table 87-4, the TN, TP, FN, and FP results have been expressed in terms of prevalence, sensitivity, and specificity. This permits the following equations to be derived:

Table 87-2. Relationship of accuracy to sensitivity and specificity (different tests, same accuracy)

Noninvasive test results	Distribution according to diagnostic standard		Noninvasive test total
	Negative	Positive	
TEST A*			
Negative	84	8	92
Positive	16	92	108
TEST B†			
Negative	98	22	120
Positive	2	78	80

*Accuracy, 88%; sensitivity, 92%; specificity, 84%; PPV, 85%; NPV, 91%.
†Accuracy, 88%; sensitivity, 78%; specificity, 98%; PPV, 98%; NPV, 82%.

Table 87-3. Effect of prevalence on accuracy and predictive values (same test, three different populations)

Noninvasive test results	Distribution according to diagnostic standard		Noninvasive test total
	Negative	Positive	
POPULATION A*—50% PREVALENCE			
Negative	80	10	90
Positive	20	90	110
POPULATION B†—10% PREVALENCE			
Negative	144	2	146
Positive	36	18	54
POPULATION C‡—90% PREVALENCE			
Negative	16	18	34
Positive	4	162	166

*Accuracy, 85%; sensitivity, 90%; specificity, 80%; PPV, 82%; NPV, 89%.
†Accuracy, 81%; sensitivity, 90%; specificity, 80%; PPV, 33%; NPV, 99%.
‡Accuracy, 89%; sensitivity, 90%; specificity, 80%; PPV, 98%; NPV, 47%.

$$\text{PPV} = \frac{\text{PA}}{(1 - \text{P})(1 - \text{B}) + \text{PA}} \qquad (7)$$

$$\text{NPV} = \frac{\text{B}(1 - \text{P})}{\text{B}(1 - \text{P}) + \text{P}(1 - \text{A})} \qquad (8)$$

$$\text{ACC} = \text{B} + \text{P}(\text{A} - \text{B}) \qquad (9)$$

where P indicates prevalence; A, sensitivity; and B, specificity. P, A, and B are expressed in decimal fractions and are always less than 1. These equations prove very useful in selecting a test to fit a particular study population.

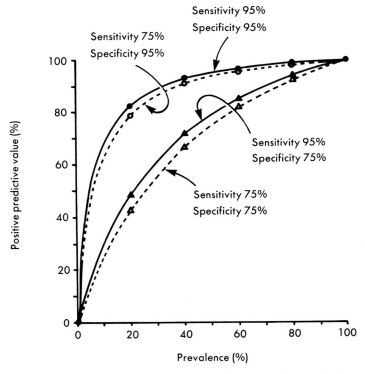

Fig. 87-2. Effect of sensitivity, specificity, and prevalence on positive predictive value.

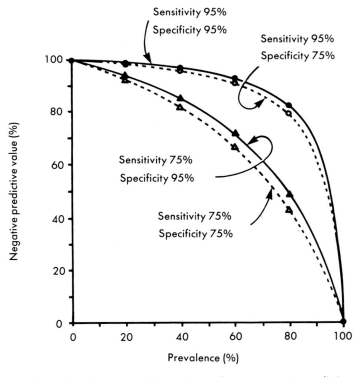

Fig. 87-3. Effect of sensitivity, specificity, and prevalence on negative predictive value.

Table 87-4. Matrix for calculating PPV and NPV from sensitivity, specificity, and prevalence

Noninvasive test results	Distribution according to diagnostic standard		Noninvasive test total
	Negative	Positive	
Negative	$B (1 - P)$	$P (1 - A)$	$B (1 - P) + P (1 - A)$
Positive	$(1 - P) (1 - B)$	PA	$(1 - P) (1 - B) + PA$
TOTAL FOR DIAGNOSTIC STANDARD	$1 - P$	P	**1**

P, Prevalence; A, sensitivity; B, specificity.

GRADATIONS OF DISEASE

In most of the conditions to which noninvasive testing is applied, there is a gradation in the severity of the disease process. Arteriosclerosis, for example, can be absent, produce nonstenotic plaques, cause varying degrees of stenosis, or result in total arterial occlusion. A noninvasive test may be called on to detect the presence or absence of any disease regardless of its severity, to distinguish between hemodynamically significant and nonhemodynamically significant stenoses, or to differentiate between stenotic and totally occluded arteries. It is necessary, therefore, to establish some guidelines to determine what magnitude of disease is to be considered negative and what, positive.

Many noninvasive tests (such as oculoplethysmography or impedance plethysmography) do not become positive unless disease of a certain severity is present. Moreover, the percentage of positive test results increases as the severity of the disease process increases. For this reason, the same test applied to the same population will usually appear to be more sensitive and less specific when the criterion for a positive result is set at a high degree of stenosis and less sensitive and more specific when the criterion is set at a lower level of stenosis. How this occurs is shown in Fig. 87-4. A hypothetical population consisting of equal numbers of arteries in each of six categories of stenosis is illustrated. To the right of the vertical line indicating the *test threshold*, the results of the noninvasive test are positive; to the left, the test results are negative. In the category of no disease (0% diameter stenosis), most of the test results are negative; in the category of total occlusion (100% diameter stenosis), most of the test results are positive. When the degree of stenosis is less severe (for example, 25% to 49% diameter stenosis), the number of positive and negative test results are

almost equal. If the criteria for a positive test were set at 50% diameter stenosis, 79% of the arteries with stenoses >50% would have positive studies and 76% of those with stenoses <50% would have negative studies. On the other hand, if the test were called on to distinguish between total occlusion and any degree of stenosis (criterion 100%), the sensitivity would rise to 91% and the specificity would fall to 56%. For detecting any stenosis, the sensitivity would drop to 60% and the specificity would increase to 91%.

It is critically important, therefore, when one compares the results of two diagnostic tests to be aware of the criteria used to distinguish between the presence and absence of disease. Medical literature contains many examples of tests that appear to be highly sensitive merely because the dividing line has been set at a high level of disease ($\geq$70% to 80%). If these same tests had been employed to differentiate between <50% diameter stenosis and >50% or between 0% stenosis and $\geq$1% stenosis, the results, in terms of sensitivity, would have been considerably less impressive.

DISTRIBUTION OF DISEASE

Because the percentage of positive test results usually increases with the severity of disease, the distribution of disease in a study population will affect the various parameters of accuracy. As shown in Table 87-5, a test will appear to be most sensitive and specific when the distribution is skewed toward the more severe and less severe ends of the disease spectrum and least sensitive and specific when the numbers are concentrated in the midportion of the spectrum. When the disease is evenly distributed between the four categories of stenosis, the parameters of accuracy lie between the two extremes. In these three examples, the parameters of accuracy vary even though the same test is used

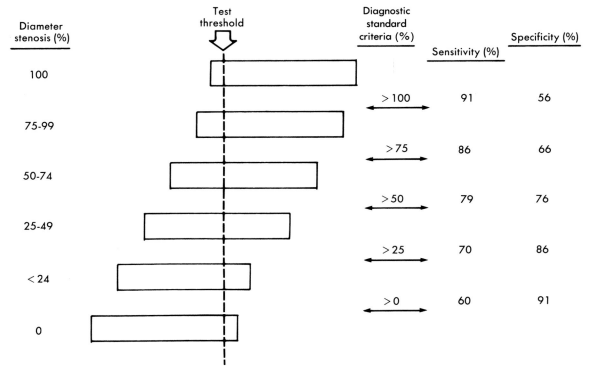

Fig. 87-4. Effect of varying positive criteria for presence of disease on sensitivity and specificity. Test threshold is fixed.

Table 87-5. Effect of disease distribution on sensitivity and specificity (same test, three different populations; dividing line between positive and negative set at 50% diameter stenosis)

Noninvasive test results	Distribution according to diagnostic standard (% Stenosis)			
	Negative		Positive	
	0-24	25-49	50-74	75-100
EVEN DISTRIBUTION*				
Negative	95	65	35	5
Positive	5	35	65	95
SKEWED TOWARD EXTREMES†				
Negative	171	13	7	9
Positive	9	7	13	171
CONCENTRATED IN MIDPORTION‡				
Negative	19	117	63	1
Positive	1	63	117	19

*Sensitivity, 80%; specificity, 80%; prevalence, 50%.
†Sensitivity, 92%; specificity, 92%; prevalence, 50%.
‡Sensitivity, 68%; specificity, 68%; prevalence, 50%.

and the apparent disease prevalence remains constant. In Table 87-5, the *percentage* of positive test results from the three populations was the same: 5% positive in the range of 0% to 24% diameter stenosis, 35% positive in the 25% to 49% disease range, 65% positive in the 50% to 74% range, and 95% positive in the 75% to 100% range.

In comparing the test results the reader should be careful to examine the distribution of disease in the study populations. One test may appear better than another merely because the study includes a large number of normal or occluded vessels.

RECEIVER OPERATING CHARACTERISTIC CURVES

In the preceding discussion, test results have been considered to be positive or negative. The results of most noninvasive tests, however, are not so easily classified. For example, carotid Doppler spectra have a wide range of peak frequencies and bandwidths, and the degree of stenosis estimated from pulsed Doppler images may vary from none

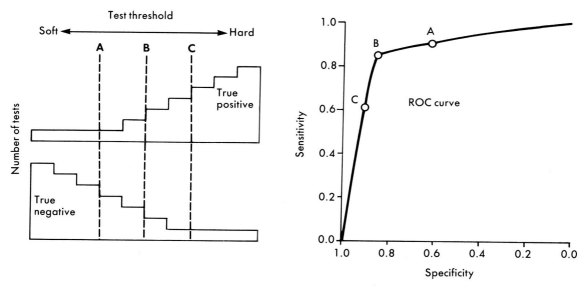

Fig. 87-5. Generation of ROC curve. With varying test threshold, sensitivity and specificity shift in opposite directions. (Reprinted from Ref. 14a, p. 177, by courtesy of Marcel Dekker, Inc.)

to total occlusion. Other examples of tests in which results vary continuously over a wide range include ankle pressure measurements, venous plethysmography, oculopneumoplethysmography (OPG-Gee), and pulse-delay oculoplethysmography (OPG-Kartchner). To apply these tests, the investigator must decide what level of ankle pressure, rate of venous outflow, intraocular/arm pressure ratio, or pulse delay to call normal and what to call abnormal. A threshold or cutoff point must be selected to divide positive from negative results.

Where this threshold is set will have a major effect on the sensitivity and specificity of the test. As shown in Fig. 87-5, if the criterion for a positive test is made very strict (hard reading, indicated by *C*), few lesions that are negative by the diagnostic standard criterion will be called positive, but many positive lesions will be missed. On the other hand, if the criterion for a positive test is made very lenient (soft reading, indicated by *A*), few lesions that are positive by the diagnostic standard criterion will be called negative, but many negative lesions will be wrongly identified as being positive. In other words, when the test reading is hard, specificity increases (few false positives), but sensitivity decreases (many false negatives); when the test reading is soft, sensitivity increases (few false negatives), but specificity decreases (many false positives).

Receiver operating characteristic (ROC) curves are constructed by plotting the sensitivity of the test vs. its specificity at various thresholds. In the example shown in Fig. 87-5, at point *A* (soft threshold) the sensitivity of the test is 92% and its specificity 62%; at point *C* (hard threshold) the sensitivity is 62% and the specificity is 92%; at point *B* (intermediate threshold) both are 85%. The best compromise would appear to be threshold *B*, but under certain circumstances the purposes of the investigator might be better served by selecting one of the other thresholds.

ROC curves can be used to compare the accuracy of tests at various thresholds. Of the three tests whose ROC curves are illustrated in Fig. 87-6, test *x* is clearly the best. A soft reading of test *y*, however, will provide sensitivities almost as good as those of test *x*, albeit at the expense of specificity. A hard reading of test *z* yields specificities comparable to test *x*, but the sensitivity is reduced. For some purposes, therefore, substitution of test *y* or *z* for test *x* might be justified, especially when *y* or *z* is less expensive, less time consuming, less technically demanding, or more readily available than test *x*.

A family of ROC curves is required to document the accuracy of any given test when different definitive criteria are used to define the presence or absence of disease. Figs. 34-4 and 40-4 illustrate

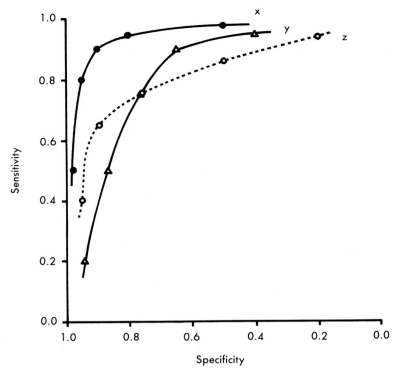

Fig. 87-6. ROC curves for three different tests, *x,y,* and *z.* Point on each curve closest to upper left-hand corner is best cutoff point in terms of making fewest mistakes (smallest number of false positive and false negative studies). Test *x* is generally more accurate than tests *y* and *z.*

this point. At all test thresholds, sensitivities improve and specificities decline as the definitive criteria for positivity shift toward more significant disease, causing the inflexion of the ROC curve to move upward and to the left. Obviously, the same definitive criterion must be in effect when the ROC curves of two tests are compared.

PRESENTATION OF DATA

Since both the distribution of disease in the study population and the degree of positivity of the test results vary, presentation of data in a 2 × 2 format often obscures differences between studies that may be critical for evaluating the accuracy of a test. Without knowledge of the distribution of disease, the three tests in Table 87-5 would have been interpreted as having widely different accuracies. Without some indication of the threshold criterion employed for the test, ROC curves cannot be constructed—again, making it difficult to compare test results. For these reasons, it is preferable to present raw data in tables with enough columns and rows to adequately display categories of increasing disease severity on one axis and categories of increas-

ing test positivity on the other (Tables 40-1 and 40-3).

In some cases there may be multiple disease categories but the test results are either positive or negative; in others, there may be several gradations of test positivity but only two categories of disease. In most cases more than two rows and columns will be required to display the data. The number of cells in such a table will be equal to the product of the number of columns and the number of rows (Fig. 87-7). In the better tests, cells corresponding to high-grade disease and normal or almost normal test results and cells corresponding to low-grade disease and markedly abnormal test results will be empty, or nearly so, whereas those in which the disease grade and the test results correlate will be relatively full. Deviations from this ideal pattern are easily perceived; their severity is immediately apparent; and the correlations most responsible for errors are readily identified.

By adjusting the line dividing positive from negative disease categories and the orthogonal line dividing positive from negative test results, the reader is able to calculate the sensitivity and specificity

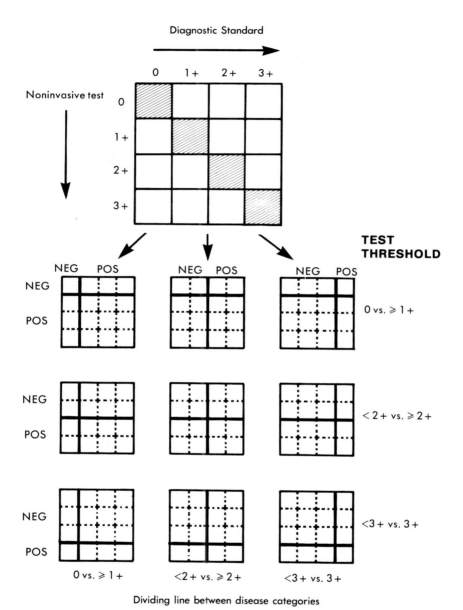

Diagnostic Standard

TEST THRESHOLD

Dividing line between disease categories

Fig. 87-7. Method for obtaining sensitivities and specificities for different levels of disease and for different test thresholds. Shaded areas in upper diagram indicate perfect correlation. Dark lines in lower diagrams indicate dividing lines between positive and negative disease levels or test thresholds.

of the test for different disease severities and the ROC curves defining the characteristics of the test for each disease category (Fig. 87-7). From a 4 × 4 matrix, nine sets of sensitivities and specificities can be calculated—the number of sets being equal to the number of columns minus one times the number of rows minus one.

When the data vary continuously, they may be presented with greater precisión in a scatter diagram, the coordinates of each point being determined by the test results on one axis and the disease severity (diagnostic standard results) on the other (Fig. 87-8). In some cases, test results vary continuously but disease severity is discontinuous; in others, the opposite occurs. Data from such studies can be presented in columns corresponding to the discontinuous parameter with the vertical position of the points in each column corresponding to the values of the continuous parameter (Fig. 87-1). Continuous data, of course, can be analyzed in the same fashion as categorized data by constructing vertical and horizontal dividing lines across the display, thus separating positive from negative disease states and positive from negative test results. Sensitivities and specificities are calculated by

counting the number of points in each of the four resulting quadrants and performing the appropriate mathematical manipulations.

κ STATISTIC

For the most part, the preceding discussions have considered only the ability of noninvasive tests to distinguish disease of lesser severity from that of greater severity. In addition, some noninvasive tests are capable of predicting the actual magnitude of the disease process within certain limits. For example, spectrum analysis, pulsed Doppler imaging, and B-mode scans can be used not only to discriminate between hemodynamically and non-hemodynamically significant disease at the carotid bifurcation but also to estimate the degree of stenosis of the internal carotid artery.

To evaluate how well the results of a noninvasive test correlate with the results of the diagnostic standard, a number of investigators have employed the κ statistic, which is a coefficient of agreement for nominal scales. With the data arranged in a matrix with n columns and n rows, there will be n cells in which there are perfect agreement. In Fig. 87-9, there are four columns, four rows, and four cells with perfect agreement (A_1, A_2, A_3, and A_4). The proportion of results that agree perfectly with

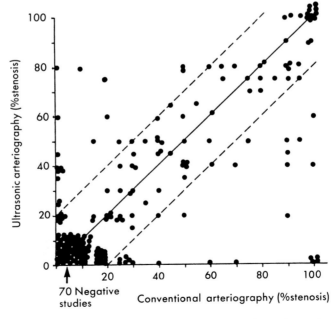

Fig. 87-8. Scatter diagram of continuously varying data comparing ultrasonic arteriography with conventional arteriography in detecting internal carotid artery stenosis in 209 vessels from 122 patients. Results of conventional arteriography are on abscissa and results of ultrasonic arteriography are on ordinate. (From Sumner, D.S., et al.: Arch. Surg. 114:1222, 1979. Copyright 1979, American Medical Association.)

the diagnostic standard (P_0) may be obtained by adding the numbers within the A cells and dividing the total by the total number of studies performed (N):

$$P_0 = \frac{\sum_1^n A}{N} \qquad (10)$$

The total number of results in each row is obtained by adding the numbers in each cell of that row. This figure is designated by M, or the "marginal" for that row. Similarly, the total number of results in each column is indicated by the marginal, M'. The proportion of agreement expected by chance (P_c) is the sum of the products of the marginals of each corresponding row and column divided by the square of the total number of studies performed.

$$P_c = \frac{\sum_1^n MM'}{N^2} \qquad (11)$$

κ is obtained from the observed proportion of agreement (P_0) and that expected by chance (P_c) by means of the following formula:

$$\kappa = \frac{P_0 - P_c}{1 - P_c} \qquad (12)$$

The standard error of κ is given by:

$$\sigma_\kappa = \left(\frac{P_0 (1 - p_0)}{N (1 - p_0)^2} \right)^{1/2} \qquad (13)$$

Table 87-6 demonstrates the use of equations 10 through 13 to calculate κ and its standard error from hypothetical data comparing a noninvasive test having four grades of positivity with a diagnostic standard having four similar grades of positivity. In this example, 84.4% of the results of the noninvasive test and the diagnostic standard agreed ($P_0 = 0.844$); but 25.4% of the studies could have agreed by chance ($P_c = 0.254$). The difference between the observed agreement and chance agreement divided by the difference between perfect agreement (1.0) and chance gives a κ value of 0.791. The standard error is 0.055; therefore the 95% confidence limits of κ are 0.791 ± 1.96 (0.055) or 0.683 to 0.899.

When the results are "perfectly" randomly distributed, P_0 and P_c are identical and κ equals 0.0, indicating the total lack of correlation (Table 87-7). Perfect correlation, on the other hand, yields a κ value of $+1.0$ (Table 87-7). Reversed correlations are also possible, in which case κ has a negative sign. A perfect negative correlation would have a κ value of -1.0. In other words, κ values may vary from -1.0 through 0.0 to $+1.0$. As κ approaches 1.0, the correlation improves between the noninvasive test and the diagnostic standard.

Even when there is an absolute lack of correlation between the noninvasive test and the diagnostic standard, it is unlikely that the results will be as perfectly distributed as they are in the upper

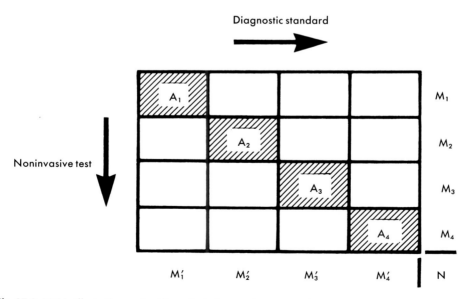

Fig. 87-9. Matrix illustrating method for calculating κ value. Areas of perfect agreement are indicated by *A*, marginal totals by *M*, and total number of studies by *N*. See text for explanation.

Table 87-6. Calculating κ value

Noninvasive test results	Distribution according to diagnostic standard				Noninvasive test totals
	9	1 +	2 +	3 +	
0	20	2	1	0	23
1 +	2	15	1	0	18
2 +	0	3	16	2	21
3 +	0	0	1	14	15
TOTAL FOR DIAGNOSTIC STANDARD	22	20	19	16	77

$$P_0 = \frac{20 + 15 + 16 + 14}{77} = 0.844.$$

$$P_c = \frac{23(22) + 18(20) + 21(19) + 15(16)}{(77)^2} = 0.254.$$

$$\kappa = \frac{0.844 - 0.254}{1 - 0.254} = 0.791.$$

$$\sigma_\kappa = \left(\frac{0.844(1 - 0.844)}{77(1 - 0.254)^2}\right)^{1/2} = 0.055.$$

Table 87-7. Properties of the κ statistic.

Noninvasive test results	Distribution according to diagnostic standard				Noninvasive test total
	0	1 +	2 +	3 +	
*PERFECT RANDOM DISTRIBUTION**					
0	16	12	8	4	40
1 +	12	9	6	3	30
2 +	8	6	4	2	20
3 +	4	3	2	1	10
PERFECT CORRELATION†					
0	40	0	0	0	40
1 +	0	30	0	0	30
2 +	0	0	20	0	20
3 +	0	0	0	10	10

$$*P_0 = \frac{16 + 9 + 4 + 1}{100} = 0.3.$$

$$P_c = \frac{(40)^2 + (30)^2 + (20)^2 + (10)^2}{(100)^2} = 0.3.$$

$$\kappa = \frac{0.3 - 0.3}{1 - 0.3} = 0.0.$$

$$†P_0 = \frac{40 + 30 + 20 + 10}{100} = 1.0.$$

$$P_c = \frac{(40)^2 + (30)^2 + (20)^2 + (10)^2}{(100)^2} = 0.3.$$

$$\kappa = \frac{1.0 - 0.3}{1 - 0.3} = 1.0.$$

Table 87-8. Effect of number of cells on κ value

Noninvasive test results	Distribution according to diagnostic standard						Noninvasive test total
	0	**1 +**	**2 +**	**3 +**	**4 +**	**5 +**	
6 × 6 MATRIX*							
0	10	5	2	1	0	0	18
1 +	5	10	5	2	1	0	23
2 +	2	5	10	5	2	1	25
3 +	1	2	5	10	5	2	25
4 +	0	1	2	5	10	5	23
5 +	0	0	1	2	5	10	18

3 × 3 MATRIX†				
	0 to 1 +	**2 + to 3 +**	**4 + to 5 +**	
0 to 1 +	30	10	1	41
2 + to 3 +	10	30	10	50
4 + to 5 +	1	10	30	41

*p_0, .455; p_c, .170; κ, 0.343; standard deviation, 0.052.
†p_0, .682; p_c, .336; κ, 0.521; standard deviation, 0.061.

part of Table 87-7. For example, the κ values of three 4 × 4 matrices in which the 16 cells were filled with random numbers from 1 to 10 were 0.106 ± 0.065, 0.074 ± 0.071, and 0.103 ± 0.061. Thus slight positive or negative correlations are likely to happen by chance. That these three κ values are not statistically significantly different from zero becomes evident when their relatively large standard errors are considered. In each case, the 95% confidence limit extends below zero.

The κ statistic can be used to compare the accuracy of one test with that of another; the test with the higher κ value would be expected to be the better predictor of disease severity. The standard errors of the tests must, of course, be considered in determining whether the differences could have occurred by chance. Another pitfall concerns the fact that κ values for the same data are increased when the data are condensed in a matrix with fewer cells (Table 87-8). Therefore when comparing tests one must be careful to make sure that the same number of cells are employed.

One further note: Pearson correlation coefficients (r) can also be applied to grouped data. Analyzed in this way, the data in Table 87-6 give an r value of 0.920, a value that is considerably higher than the κ value for this table, 0.791.

PREDICTING SEVERITY OF DISEASE

The κ statistic measures the overall correlation between the noninvasive test and the diagnostic standard results but does not tell the clinician how

reliable a report indicating a specific level of disease is likely to be. To illustrate this point, the data in each test category of Table 87-6 have been divided by appropriate row totals and are listed as percentages in Table 87-9. Although 87% of the 0 noninvasive tests had 0 disease according to the diagnostic standard, 9% had 1 + disease and 4% had 2 + disease. Similarly, 83% of the 1 +, 76% of the 2 +, and 93% of the 3 + noninvasive tests were correct. If it were assumed that all future test results from the same laboratory were likely to have a similar distribution, the clinician receiving a report of 2 + disease could predict that this patient has a 76% chance of having 2 + disease, a 14% chance of having 1 + disease, and a 10% chance of having 3 + disease. The clinician could be reasonably sure, however, that the patient had at least some disease. Likewise, a report of 0 or 1 + would virtually rule out 3 + disease, and a report of 3 + would make 0 or 1 + disease highly unlikely.

An example of this kind of analysis is given in Table 34-4, which summarizes the distribution of degree of internal carotid stenosis according to the ultrasonic arteriographic reading. Presenting the data in this way enables the clinician to determine what level of confidence to attach to any given test result.

Calculations of sensitivity and specificity by the method illustrated in Fig. 87-7 may give a distorted impression of the ability of a noninvasive test to discriminate between levels of disease. As the data in Table 87-10 show, ultrasonic arteriography (UA) has a sensitivity of 86%, a specificity of 85%, and an overall accuracy of 85% for distinguishing internal carotid artery stenoses of <25% from stenoses >25%. Yet, χ^2 analysis fails to demonstrate a statistically significant difference between the distribution of UA findings in the 1% to 24% lesions and the 25% to 49% lesions. While this may represent a type II statistical error (too few examples to reach statistical significance), it does show that the test is not very good for discriminating between these disease levels. Similarly, the test cannot re-

liably discriminate 50% to 74% lesions from 75% to 99% lesions despite a sensitivity of 69%, a specificity of 91%, and an accuracy of 88%. The test does, however, appear to be capable of discriminating between no disease and 1% to 24% stenoses, between 25% to 49% and 50% to 74% stenoses, and between 75% to 99% stenosis and total occlusion. Medical literature contains many examples in which the accuracy implied by sensitivity and specificity data misrepresents the actual capabilities of the noninvasive test.

PROSPECTIVE VS. RETROSPECTIVE

After data have been accumulated and compared with the diagnostic standard, the investigator may examine it retrospectively to determine what test threshold provides the optimum combination of sensitivity and specificity. From this retrospective examination, accuracy parameters may (and often are) reported. But when retrospectively determined test thresholds are applied prospectively to new sets of data, the investigator may be disappointed to find that sensitivities and specificities are no longer satisfactory. The data are then reexamined; a new

Table 87-9. Predictive value (%) of noninvasive test results (derived from Table 87-6)

Noninvasive test results	Distribution of noninvasive percentages according to diagnostic standard			
	0	1+	2+	3+
0	87	9	4	0
1+	11	83	6	0
2+	0	14	76	10
3+	0	0	7	93

Table 87-10. Ability of noninvasive test to discriminate between levels of disease: comparing the results of ultrasonic arteriography and conventional arteriography in 232 internal carotid arteries

Results of ultrasonic arteriography (%Stenosis)	Conventional arteriography (%Stenosis)					
	Normal	1-24	25-49	50-74	75-99	Total occlusion
Normal	92	14	4	1	0	0
1-24	12	8	7	0	0	0
25-49	10	5	10	2	1	1
50-74	0	1	3	9	9	0
75-99	2	0	1	8	9	1
Total occlusion	3	2	0	2	2	13

	0% vs. 1% to 24%	1% to 24% vs. 25% to 49%	25% to 49% vs. 50% to 74%	50% to 74% vs. 75% to 99%	75% to 99% vs. 100%
	92 14	22 11	21 3	12 10	19 2
	27 16	8 14	4 19	10 11	2 13
χ^2 (Yates)	9.5174	3.7431	20.4553	0.02221	18.3673
	p < 0.005	0.05 < p < .10	p < .0005	0.80 < p < .90	p < .0005
	0% vs. ≥1%	≤24% vs. ≥25%	≤49% vs. ≥50%	≤74% vs. ≥75%	≤99% vs. 100%
Sensitivity	83	86	91	69	87
Specificity	77	85	93	91	96
Accuracy	80	85	93	88	95

threshold is selected based on the new data; and again, sensitivities and specificities are retrospectively reported. This process, of course, ensures that the reported accuracies will always be good. It does not, however, ensure that they will be representative of the capabilities of the test.

To illustrate these points, the data in Table 87-11 were developed using a random number generator programmed to provide 80% negative test results in the 0 range, 6% in the 1+ range, 6% in the 2+ range, and 8% in the 3+ range for an infinite number of trials in which the diagnostic standard is negative. An opposite distribution is assumed for trials in which the standard is positive. Prevalence is assumed to be 50% for all trials. In trial 1, in which 50 studies were performed, it appears that the optimum threshold would be ≥3+. This would provide a sensitivity and specificity of 92%. Applying this same threshold to 50 more studies in trial 2 gives a sensitivity of only 72%. By readjusting the threshold to ≥1+, the sensitivity is again 92% and the specificity is a respectable 88%. Unfortunately if this new threshold were reapplied to the data in trial 1, the specificity would fall to 72%. When figures for 23 more trials (1150 studies) are accumulated, it becomes apparent that a ≥2+ threshold provides the best compromise between sensitivity and specificity. With the increasing number of studies, the randomly allocated data approaches the infinite distribution, confirming what is already evident—the larger the study population, the more closely the results approximate truth. Other thresholds could be selected if the investigator wished to optimize sensitivity at the expense of specificity, or vice versa.

As long as the test itself has not been changed (no new instruments, no new technicians, etc.), it is not only valid but quite important to update accuracy figures by a retrospective examination of the data; however, to minimize errors, all of the preceding test results should be included in the review, not just those resulting from the most recent trial. Armed with this information, the results of a prospective trial of 50 new studies—such as trial 2—in which sensitivities drop need not be viewed with alarm but could be recognized for what they are, merely the vagaries of chance.

The warning for the student of the medical literature is simply to view with some skepticism accuracy figures derived from retrospective reviews.

CONFIDENCE LIMITS

The previous discussion raises questions regarding the certainty that sensitivities and specificities reported from a limited sample actually represent *true values* (the values expected if the test had applied to an infinitely large population). Is test A with a reported sensitivity of 80% inferior to test B with a reported sensitivity of 90%, or could the difference be the result of chance? One way of approaching this problem is to calculate the 95% confidence limits of the sensitivity and specificity.

Although confidence limits for means are commonly reported in medical literature (that is, the mean ± the standard error of the mean), similar data for proportions seldom appear. Sensitivity and specificity are proportions, the former being the proportion of positive noninvasive tests in the sample of tests that are positive according to the di-

Table 87-11. Variations in accuracy caused by sampling (prevalence, 50%)

Noninvasive test results	Distribution according to standard, infinite trials		Distribution according to standard, trial 1		Distribution according to standard, trial 2		Distribution according to standard, trials 3-25	
	Negative	Positive	Negative	Positive	Negative	Positive	Negative	Positive
0	80%	8%	18	1	22	2	453	34
1+	6%	6%	2	0	1	3	44	33
2+	6%	6%	3	1	1	2	32	42
3+	8%	80%	2	23	1	18	46	466
Threshold	**Specificity**	**Sensitivity**	**Specificity**	**Sensitivity**	**Specificity**	**Sensitivity**	**Specificity**	**Sensitivity**
≥1+	80%	92%	72%	96%	88%	92%	79%	94%
≥2+	86%	86%	80%	96%	92%	80%	86%	88%
≥3+	92%	80%	92%	92%	96%	72%	92%	81%

Table 87-12. Binomial theorem: probability distribution of positive test results, f(x), in samples of 20 studies

Positive results (%)	No. of positive studies (x)	Test A (p = .80)		Test B (p = .90)	
		f(x)	$\Sigma_0^x f(x)$	f(x)	$\Sigma_0^x f(x)$
0	0	1×10^{-14}	0.000	1×10^{-20}	0.000
5	1	8×10^{-13}	0.000	2×10^{-18}	0.000
10	2	3×10^{-11}	0.000	2×10^{-16}	0.000
15	3	8×10^{-10}	0.000	8×10^{-15}	0.000
20	4	1×10^{-8}	0.000	3×10^{-13}	0.000
25	5	2×10^{-7}	0.000	9×10^{-12}	0.000
30	6	2×10^{-6}	0.000	2×10^{-10}	0.000
35	7	1×10^{-5}	0.000	4×10^{-9}	0.000
40	8	9×10^{-5}	0.000	5×10^{-8}	0.000
45	9	5×10^{-4}	0.000	7×10^{-7}	0.000
50	10	0.002	0.003	6×10^{-6}	0.000
55	11	0.007	0.010	5×10^{-5}	0.000
60	12	0.022	0.032	4×10^{-4}	0.000
65	13	0.055	0.087	0.002	0.002
70	14	0.109	0.196	0.009	0.011
75	15	0.175	0.370	0.032	0.043
80	16	0.218	0.589	0.090	0.133
85	17	0.205	0.794	0.190	0.323
90	18	0.137	0.931	0.285	0.608
95	19	0.058	0.988	0.270	0.878
100	20	0.012	1.000	0.122	1.000

agnostic standard and the latter being the proportion of negative tests in the sample that are negative according to the diagnostic standard.

To illustrate the vagaries of sampling, consider an infinitely large, well-defined population in which test A has a true sensitivity of 80%. Thus the probability (p) that any individual study will correctly identify the presence of disease is .80. Now suppose an investigator applies the test to a group of patients from this population in which 20 of the diagnostic standard results turn out to be positive. What is the likelihood that exactly 16 (80%) of the test results will also be positive? The answer, somewhat surprisingly, is that in only about 22% of such samples will exactly 16 studies be positive. Unfortunately, an investigator attempting to estimate the sensitivity of the test from a sample of 20 has a 78% chance of arriving at an erroneous value. In fact, in over 5% of such samples, as few as 13 or as many as 19 positive studies can be expected. In the former case the sensitivity would appear to be 65% and, in the latter case, 95%. Table 87-12 lists the probability, f(x), that a certain number of positive test results, x, will be found in samples of n = 20, when p = .80. These probabilities are derived from the binomial theorem

$$f(x) = \frac{n!}{x!(n-x)!} p^x (1-p)^{n-x} \tag{14}$$

The calculation for 16 positive studies is as follows:

$$f(16) = \frac{20!}{16!(4)!} 0.8^{16}(0.2)^4 = 0.218$$

Because of the factorials these calculations are cumbersome to do by hand but are easily accomplished with a programmable calculator, a computer, or the aid of tables.

As indicated in Table 87-12, the sum of all the probabilities $\Sigma f(x)$, from x = 0 to x = 20 is 1.0. Since only 1% of the samples would have 11 or fewer positive results ($\Sigma_0^{11} f(x) = 0.010$), it is unlikely that the investigators would conclude that the sensitivity of the test is 55% or less. Also, it is unlikely that all 20 studies would be positive (f(x) = 0.012). On the other hand, there is a 21% chance that the sample of 20 would include 18 or more positive studies ($\Sigma_{18}^{20} f(x) = 0.137 + 0.058 + 0.012$), leading to the mistaken conclusion that the sensitivity of the test is 90% or better. There is a 60% chance that the sample of 20 will produce 15 to 17 positive studies, implying a sensitivity of 75% to 85%, which is equal to or within 5% of the true sensitivity of 80%.

(To make these observations more intuitively evident, it is helpful to consider an analogous situation. Suppose that we have a sack containing 8000 red marbles and 2000 white marbles; each time a marble is removed blindly from the sack and then replaced, the probability (p) that it will be red is .8. If one removes, inspects, and replaces 20 marbles, one would not be surprised to find that the sample of 20 has not produced exactly 16 red marbles but rather, 14, 15, 17, or 18 red marbles. However, one would not expect the sample to contain all red marbles or less than 10 or 11 red marbles.)

The probability distribution, f(x), of another test (test B) with a true sensitivity of 90% (p = .90) is also shown in Table 87-12. Almost 29% of the samples of 20 studies in which the diagnostic standard is positive would be expected to yield 18 positive test results. In other words, the estimated sensitivity would be correct 29% of the time. But 13% of the samples would indicate a sensitivity of 80% or less $(\Sigma_0^{16} f(x) = .133)$. Since 21% of the samples from test A might indicate a sensitivity greater than 90%, it would be possible to conclude—given the vagaries of sampling—that test B was inferior to test A. It is interesting that the chances of obtaining exactly 17 positive test results (estimated sensitivity, 85%) are almost the same with either test.

These examples emphasize the difficulties involved in making inferences regarding the true sensitivity (or specificity) of a test from a limited number of studies. It seems obvious that inferences could be improved by increasing the sample size. If, instead of 20 marbles, 100 marbles were withdrawn from the sack, the likelihood that exactly 80% would be red is reduced from 22% to 10% but the likelihood that 75% to 85% will be red is increased from 60% to 83%. In fact, with a sample size of 100, 62% of the samples should consist of 77% to 83% red marbles. In other words, increasing the sample size reduces the likelihood that the precise sensitivity of a test would be discovered but permits a more accurate estimation of the range in which the precise sensitivity is likely to occur.

In actual practice, the true sensitivity or specificity of a test is never known. The best that the

investigator can do is to estimate the sensitivity or specificity from the proportion of successes (positive results in the case of sensitivity, negative results in the case of specificity) that are found in a sample consisting of positive or negative diagnostic standard results. The estimated probability of success is indicated by $\hat{p}$ to distinguish it from the true probability of success, p. Therefore:

$$\hat{p} = x'/n \tag{15}$$

where x' is the number of successes observed in a sample size of n (x' and n, of course, are always positive integers).

For any $\hat{p}$, 95% confidence limits can be defined. The lower limit of the true probability (p_a) is that which would be expected to yield x' or more success in only 2.5% of samples of size n; the upper limit of the true probability (p_b) is that which would be expected to yield x' or fewer successes in only 2.5% of samples of size n. Expressed mathematically, the lower limit (p_a) is that which satisfies the following equations:

$$\sum_{x'}^{n} f(x, n, p_a) = 0.025 \tag{16}$$

$$\sum_{0}^{x'-1} f(x, n, p_a) = 0.975 \tag{17}$$

and the upper limit is expressed as

$$\sum_{0}^{x'} f(x, n, p_b) = 0.025 \tag{18}$$

$$\sum_{x'+1}^{n} f(x, n, p_b) = 0.975 \tag{19}$$

Suppose an investigator analyzes data and finds that a noninvasive test is positive in 17 of 20 arteries that had positive results for carotid artery disease according to the diagnostic standard. The number of successes (x') is 17, the sample size (n) is 20, and the estimated sensitivity ($\hat{p}$) is 0.85. To determine the lower limit, p_a, the investigator applies equation 14, uses 17, 18, 19, and 20 for x, and guesses what the p_a value should be. The resulting probabilities are added, as in equation 16, and inspected to see how closely the sum approximates 0.025. If the first estimation of p_a had been .5, the resulting sum would be 0.0013 (Table 87-13). Since this value is too low, the estimated p_a

Table 87-13. Finding the 95% confidence limits for $\hat{p} = .85$ (n = 20, x' = 17)

p_a	$\Sigma_{17}^{20}f(x,\ n,\ p_a)$	p_b	$\Sigma_0^{17}f(x,\ n,\ p_b)$
.500	.0013	.950	.0755
.600	.0016	.960	.0439
.620	.0245	.967	.0269
.621	**.0250**	**.968**	**.0249**
.622	.0255	.969	.0229
.650	.0444	.975	.0130
.700	.1071	.980	.0071

must be too low. The process is then repeated, this time using a p_a of .7. This gives a sum of 0.1071, indicating that over 10% of the samples taken with a p of .7 would yield 17 or more successes. Thus p_a must lie between .5 and .7. By repeating the process, the p_a can be narrowed down to .621, a value that would yield 17 or more successes in only 2.5% of samples having an n of 20.

To determine p_b, the investigator again applies equation 14, this time using all the integers from 0 through 17 for x and totaling the resulting probabilities as in equation 18. If the first guess at a value for p_b had been .95, the sum would be too high (0.0755), indicating that almost 8% of the samples would yield 17 or fewer successes (Table 87-13). A p_b of .98 would be too high, since the percentage of samples yielding 17 or fewer successes is far less than 2.5%. By process of elimination, .968 appears to be the best approximation for p_b.

The investigator can now report that the sensitivity of this test is 85% with the 95% confidence limits being 62.1% and 96.8%. Clearly, this range would encompass the true p values of test A (.80) and test B (.90) in Table 87-12, both of which would frequently yield a $\hat{p}$ of .85. As expected, increasing the sample size narrows the confidence limits. If the sample size had been 100 and the apparent sensitivity had been 85% (x' = 85), the 95% confidence limits would be 76.5% and 91.5%.

Calculating confidence limits in this way can be extremely time consuming and cumbersome, even with the help of a programmable calculator. Computer programs, charts, and tables are, however available to simplify the task.

Returning to the original question—is test A with a reported sensitivity of 80% inferior to test B with a sensitivity of 90%? If for both tests the positive sample according to the diagnostic standard consisted of 20 arteries, the 95% confidence limits of test A would be 56.3% to 94.3% and that for test B would be 68.3% to 98.8%. Because of the considerable overlap, it is apparent that the two tests could easily be identical. It is quite possible that test B could be inferior to test A. χ^2 with Yates correction is only 0.196, indicating that differences as large as those observed have a 60% to 70% likelihood of occurring by chance. Suppose the sample for test A were increased to 75 and that for test B to 50 and that both retained the same sensitivity. The narrowed confidence limits for test A (69.2% to 98.4%) would still overlap those for test B (78.2% to 96.7%). χ^2 with Yates correction (1.550) would still be insufficient to reject the null hypothesis (.20 < p< .30). It would take sample sizes of about 120 for each of the tests to reject the null hypothesis at the 5.0% level. With these numbers the 95% confidence limits would show little overlap (A ~ 73% to 86% and B ~83% to 94%).

While the facts that confidence limits overlap and tests for significant differences between proportions (χ^2 or Fisher's exact test) fail to reject the null hypothesis at the 5.0% levels do not mean that the sensitivities (or specificities) of two tests are not really different, it is wise to consider the possibility that the differences are less than they appear to be and could have occurred by chance. The cautious investigator may wish to defer judgment on the relative merits of two tests until sufficient data have accumulated to establish with reasonable certainty that one is better than the other. Unfortunately, there is a tendency to accept data at face value, with the result that some tests are discarded prematurely and others accepted too readily. Publications of confidence limits for sensitivity and specificity would do much to dispel this source of confusion.

RELIABILITY OF THE DIAGNOSTIC STANDARD

Ideally the accuracy of a noninvasive test should be evaluated based on concrete knowledge of the presence or absence of disease or its relative severity. Since the truth is seldom known, it is usually necessary to substitute a diagnostic standard. A variety of standards have been used; some are clinical (relief of claudication), others are physiologic

Table 87-14. Demonstrating the effect of diagnostic standard errors on the apparent accuracy of a noninvasive test, given the true disease status

DIAGNOSTIC STANDARD VS. TRUE DISTRIBUTION*			
Diagnostic standard results	True distribution		Diagnostic standard total
	Negative	Positive	
Negative	285	5	290
Positive	15	95	110

NONINVASIVE TEST VS. TRUE DISTRIBUTION†			
Noninvasive test results	True distribution		Noninvasive test total
	Negative	Positive	
Negative	285	5	290
Positive	15	95	110

NONINVASIVE TEST VS. DIAGNOSTIC STANDARD‡			
Noninvasive test results	Distribution according to diagnostic standard		Noninvasive test total
	Negative	Positive	
Negative	270	20	290
Positive	20	90	110

SUMMARY			
Diagnostic standard results	Noninvasive test results	True distribution	
		Negative	Positive
Negative	Negative	270	0
Negative	Positive	15	5
Positive	Negative	15	5
Positive	Positive	0	90

*Sensitivity, 95%; specificity, 95%; PPV, 86%; NPV, 98%; accuracy, 95%.
†Sensitivity, 95%; specificity, 95%; PPV, 86%; NPV, 98%; accuracy, 95%.
‡Sensitivity, 82%; specificity, 93%; PPV, 82%; NPV, 93%; accuracy, 90%.

(invasive pressure measurements); but most are anatomic (angiography). Diagnostic standards should be selected to coincide with the objectives of the noninvasive test. For example, it would be more appropriate to compare noninvasive pressure measurements to invasive pressure measurements than to arteriography. Another guideline for selecting the diagnostic standard should be its accuracy. Unfortunately, these guidelines are frequently neglected, and the most readily available, conventionally used method for diagnosing disease is employed.

All too often, the accuracy of a diagnostic standard is unknown. Recently, there have been several reports questioning the reliability of conventional arteriography for assessing disease at the carotid bifurcation. Since most noninvasive tests designed to assess the severity of disease at the carotid bi-

furcation have been compared to arteriography, it is informative to consider what effect errors made by the diagnostic standard might have on the apparent accuracy of the noninvasive tests.

Table 87-14 illustrates a unique situation in which we are privileged to know the truth regarding the presence or absence of disease. Based on the true condition, a noninvasive test and its diagnostic standard are both quite accurate, both having sensitivities and specificities of 95%. For the most part, the results coincide; but in a few cases, they disagree. When the test is compared to the diagnostic standard rather than to the true condition, the apparent sensitivity of the test falls to 82%; the other parameters (specificity, PPV, NPV, and overall accuracy) also suffer. Thus it is possible that the true accuracy of a test may be considerably better than its apparent accuracy.

On the other hand, a noninvasive test and its diagnostic standard may be subject to the same errors, in which case the apparent accuracy of the test may exceed its true accuracy.

NONINVASIVE DIAGNOSTIC STANDARDS

In a few reports, one noninvasive test has been employed as the diagnostic standard for another. This practice is perhaps even more likely to yield distorted parameters of accuracy than the use of an independent diagnostic standard, such as conventional arteriography. The accuracy of the noninvasive test being evaluated may appear inferior to that of the test used as the diagnostic standard when, in fact, its true accuracy may be equally as good or even better. How this can happen is shown in Table 87-15. Test B, with a true sensitivity and specificity of 95% appears to have a sensitivity and specificity of only 80% when test A, with a true sensitivity and specificity of 85% serves as the definitive test. Similarly, if test B were selected as the diagnostic standard, test A would appear to have a sensitivity and specificity of 80%. Either way, the parameters of accuracy of the test being evaluated are erroneously low.

If, however, the two tests are basically similar and are likely to make the same errors, the apparent sensitivity and specificity will be deceptively high. Test C in Table 87-15 has a true sensitivity and specificity of 86%, only slightly better than test A; but because they tend to make the same mistakes, test C appears to have a sensitivity and specificity of 97% when compared with test A.

In general, therefore, it seems advisable to avoid using one noninvasive test as the standard for evaluating the accuracy of another. Data derived from studies that employ this approach must be viewed with some skepticism.

VARIABILITY OF TEST RESULTS

Like all clinical determinations, the results of noninvasive tests are subject to three main sources of variability: true biologic, temporal, and measurement error. Intersubject biologic variability includes those differences that relate to the many factors that distinguish one individual from another; temporal variability refers to biologic differences occurring within a single individual from one time to the next; and measurement errors relate to differences attributable to the instruments, test procedures, or interpretation. Since the goals of noninvasive testing are to identify the presence of disease, assess its severity, determine its location, and evaluate disease progression, the clinician must

Table 85-15. Effect of using noninvasive tests as diagnostic standards

Noninvasive test result	Distribution according to noninvasive test A*		True distribution	
	Negative	Positive	Negative	Positive
TEST B†				
Negative	80	20	95	5
Positive	20	80	5	95
TEST C‡				
Negative	97	3	86	14
Positive	3	97	14	86

SUMMARY

Tests B vs. A		True distribution		Tests C vs. A		True distribution	
		Negative	Positive			Negative	Positive
Negative	Negative	80	0	Negative	Negative	84	13
Positive	Negative	5	15	Positive	Negative	1	2
Negative	Positive	15	5	Negative	Positive	2	1
Positive	Positive	0	80	Positive	Positive	13	84

*True sensitivity, 85%; true specificity, 85%.
†Apparent sensitivity using Test A as diagnostic standard, 80%; apparent specificity, 80%; true sensitivity, 95%; true specificity, 95%.
‡Apparent sensitivity using test A as diagnostic standard, 97%; apparent specificity, 97%; true sensitivity, 86%; true specificity, 86%.

be able to distinguish pathologic changes from normal variation or measurement error. Accomplishing this requires an awareness of the extent to which the test results vary in normal subjects. Ideally, confidence limits should be established so that the likelihood that any result is abnormal (or normal) can be predicted.

Of the three sources of variability, that caused by biologic factors has been the most frequently investigated. Information is available on the range of normal values for many noninvasive tests, including ankle pressure indices, venous outflow, and ophthalmic pressures. Indeed, the calculation of sensitivity and specificity is predicated on knowledge of the spread of normal values (intersubject variability). Less attention, however, has been given to the analysis of temporal variation (intrasubject variability). For some easily repeated tests, such as the determination of ankle pressures, several measurements may be made on the same visit, and the results analyzed to give a single value. But many tests are too difficult, too time consuming, too expensive, or too uncomfortable to be repeated. In such cases, every effort should be made to perform the measurements when the patient has rested long enough to minimize the effects of previous activity or excitement. Variability between visits is usually higher than that observed during any single visit. Between-visits variability may be reduced by careful attention to decreasing the factors implicit in single-visit variability by making the measurements at the same time of day (to standardize the effects of circadian rhythms) and by striving to maintain the same laboratory conditions. Despite all efforts at standardization, there will always be some temporal variation. Unless the extent of this variation is known, the clinician may be uncertain whether a change in the results of a noninvasive test represents a worsening (or improvement) of the patient's condition or merely reflects intrasubject variability. For this reason, serial interpretation of tests that do not lend themselves readily to numerical measurement, such as B-mode scans or Doppler venous surveys, may be difficult.

Measurement errors, of course, influence apparent biologic and temporal variability. Although measurement errors cannot be eliminated, they should be sought out, their source identified, their magnitude determined, and—if possible—their cause corrected. Any of the multiple factors that interact to produce the final result of the noninvasive test may be responsible: Instruments may

be poorly designed, lack stability, or have a tendency to malfunction; technicians may be inadequately trained, careless, fatigued, or distracted; the patient's physique, mental condition, or physiologic state may preclude an adequate study. Tests that require additional interpretation are conducive to further error—the more subjective the test, the less likely that one interpreter will agree with another or even with himself if given the same data at a later date. Finally, the rationale of the test may not be based on sound physiologic principles.

Inaccuracy may represent bias, lack of precision, or both. Since the average results of an unbiased test should approach the true or correct value, bias can usually be recognized by comparing the data derived from the test with the results of a reliable diagnostic standard. The precision of noninvasive tests is less easily determined and consequently is seldom reported. A precise test yields results with little spread. Unfortunately, it may be difficult to distinguish variability resulting from lack of precision from that caused by temporal factors. Although the precision of some noninvasive tests can be evaluated by comparing the results to those obtained simultaneously with an accurate invasive test, many noninvasive tests have no readily available invasive counterpart. It is possible, however, by suitably blinding the interpreters to determine the precision with which tests are read. Recent reports concerning the interpretation of carotid arteriograms have called attention to a surprisingly high degree of interobserver and intraobserver variability. The fact that arteriography—which is ordinarily considered to be highly objective—is subject to diverse interpretations should serve as a warning to those of us who employ noninvasive tests.

The message is clear: Each laboratory should define the extent of the biologic and temporal variability of the population it serves and should determine the reliability and precision of the tests it employs. Only in this way can the significance of aberrant values be determined. Documentation of variability is particularly important when noninvasive tests are used to diagnose disease progression or to define the natural history of a disease.

MULTIPLE TESTS

To improve the accuracy of the overall result, laboratories often employ two or more noninvasive tests concurrently. The intuitive rationale for this approach is that if one test is good, two must be

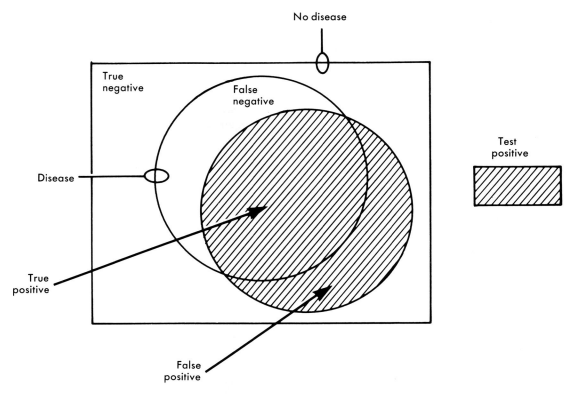

Fig. 87-10. Venn diagram depicting relationship of one test with diagnostic standard.

better, and three or more should be best. But each additional test adds to the expense and time required to complete the evaluation. Because of these factors, it is important to examine carefully the premise that a battery of tests will provide superior results.

Venn diagrams help explain the interaction of multiple noninvasive tests and the study population. In Fig. 87-10, the rectangle represents all the patients included in the study. Patients with disease are represented by the contents of the open circle. Those with no disease are represented by the space between that circle and the rectangle. Positive test results are indicated by the shaded circle and negative results by the space between the shaded circle and the rectangle. If the test were 100% sensitive and specific, the two circles would coincide. As it is, the overlapping areas represent the TP studies, the remaining crescent of the open or "disease" circle represents FN studies, and the shaded crescent outside the disease circle includes all of the FP results. Thus the shaded portion of the disease circle corresponds to the sensitivity of the test. The space within the rectangle not occupied by either of the circles represents TN studies and corresponds to the specificity of the test.

The more the shaded circle overlaps the disease circle, the greater the sensitivity and specificity become, and vice versa—the less the overlap, the poorer the sensitivity and specificity. Although the two circles in Fig. 87-10 are of equal size, they would not necessarily be so. For example, the shaded circle could be smaller or larger than the disease circle, indicating more or less positive studies than the number of patients with disease. In other words, the Venn diagram functions as a graphic representation of Table 87-1.

Consider two similar tests, subject to the same types of error, that are applied to the same population. An example would be two forms of pulse-delay oculoplethysmography, such as the OPG-Kartchner and the OPG-Zira. In Fig. 87-11 the test represented by the inner shaded circle (test A) is somewhat less sensitive but more specific than the test represented by the outer shaded circle (test B). For each battery of two tests there are four possible combinations of results: (1) both tests positive, (2) both tests negative, (3) test *A* positive, test *B* negative, and (4) test *A* negative, test *B* positive. In this particular example, however, there are no tests that fall into the A positive, B negative category. If the two tests agree, there will be no problem in

Both tests negative

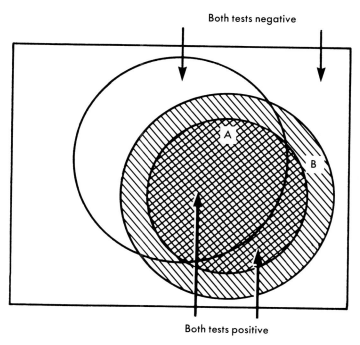

Both tests positive

Fig. 87-11. Venn diagram illustrating relationship between two dependent tests and diagnostic standard. Tests are convergent: Test *A* is more likely to be positive when test *B* is positive than when test *B* is negative.

classifying the overall result, but when *B* is positive and *A* is negative, should the overall result be called positive or negative? If we decide to accept the *B* reading, then the overall sensitivity will be greater, but the specificity will be less than if we had accepted the *A* reading. Either way, the overall result would be the same as if we had employed only one test, the test whose results we decide to accept. If, on the other hand, we decide to discard all those studies that do not coincide, a number of studies made in both the disease and no disease categories will be considered uninterpretable and will disappear from the denominator in the sensitivity and specificity calculations. This approach may or may not have a favorable effect on the overall accuracy and is always done at the cost of an increased number of uninterpretable studies. The conclusion that must be drawn from this diagram is that combining similar tests will not materially affect overall accuracy.

Fig. 87-12 shows a Venn diagram of two dissimilar, totally independent tests. An example of two such tests would be ultrasonic B-mode scanning of the carotid bifurcation and oculopneumoplethysmography. Because the rationals of these tests are different, they would not necessarily make the same errors. Although the two tests depicted in the diagram are equally sensitive and specific,

they frequently disagree. All possible combinations of results are pictured: (1) both tests positive, (2) both negative, (3) test *A* (horizontal shading) positive, test *B* (diagonal shading) negative, and (4) test *A* negative, test *B* positive. Both tests can agree and both be falsely positive, falsely negative, truly positive, or truly negative. When the tests disagree, one test will be falsely negative while the other is truly positive or one test will be falsely positive while the other is truly negative. Again when the tests agree, there will be no problem in classifying the overall result. When some of the tests disagree, three options are possible:

1. Those tests that disagree can be disregarded and only those that agree considered in formulating the overall result.
2. The overall result can be called positive if one or both tests are positive, and negative if both tests are negative.
3. The overall result can be called positive if both tests are positive, and negative if one or both tests are negative.

As Fig. 87-12 clearly shows, if option 2 is selected, the disease circle is nearly occupied by positive studies, but an increased portion of the area outside the circle (the area corresponding to no disease) is also occupied by positive studies. Thus calling the result positive when any one or both

Both tests negative

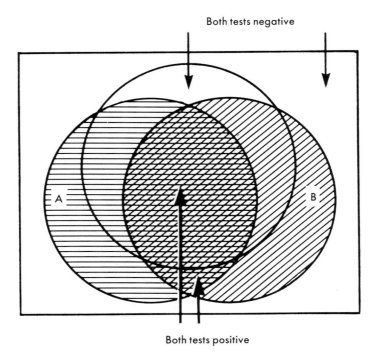

Both tests positive

Fig. 87-12. Venn diagram illustrating relationship between two independent tests and diagnostic standard. To be completely independent, positivity rate of test **A** should be same for patients with positive or negative results of test **B**.

tests are positive and negative when both are negative always increases sensitivity at the expense of specificity.

The reverse is true when option 3 is selected. In this event, only the areas where the two tests are both positive are considered positive (the crosshatched area in Fig. 87-12). Since this leaves a large portion of the disease circle unoccupied, sensitivity is always decreased. Specificity is always increased because only a small part of the area outside the circle is occupied by the intersection of positive tests.

Overall results are less easily predicted when option 1 is selected. While the elimination of tests that do not agree always increases the number of uninterpretable studies, this undesirable feature may be offset by an increased accuracy. Although the relationships are complicated, sensitivity and specificity both tend to increase when the major portion of the overlapping area of the positive circles of both tests (the crosshatched area in Fig. 87-12) lies in the disease circle with little remaining in the nondiseased area outside. Although it is possible that considering only tests that agree could decrease sensitivity and specificity compared to a single test, this seldom happens in practice.

To summarize, options rank as follows, in regard to sensitivity:
Option 2 > option 1 > option 3
Option 2 > single test > option 3
Option 1 <, =, or > single test
In regard to specificity:
Option 3 > option 1 > option 2
Option 3 > single test > option 2
Option 1 <, =, or > single test

When three or more tests are included in the battery, similar generalizations pertain. Fig. 87-13 illustrates the effects on overall sensitivity and specificity that result from the use of multiple tests. All tests are assumed to be totally independent and to have a sensitivity and specificity of 60%. If option 1 is used (all tests must agree to be considered), sensitivity and specificity both increase as more tests are added, but the percentage of tests that agree rapidly declines (Fig. 87-13, left). Although the accuracy obtained when four tests agree is much improved over that obtained with a single test, only 16% of the total studies can be used; the remaining 84% would be considered uninterpretable. Eventually accuracy for agreeing tests would approach 100%, but the percentage that agree would approach 0%.

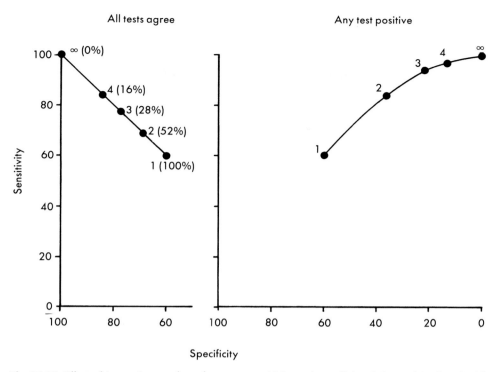

Fig. 87-13. Effect of increasing number of tests on sensitivity and specificity. *Left panel* (option 1): All tests must agree to be positive. *Right panel* (option 2): Overall result considered to be positive if one or more test results are positive. Percentages in parentheses (left panel) indicate percentage of total studies that agree.

When option 2 is used (overall result positive if one or more tests are positive, overall result negative only if all tests are negative), increasing the number of tests rapidly improves sensitivity at the expense of rapidly decreasing specificity (Fig. 87-13, right). With three or four tests the sensitivity exceeds 90%, but the 20% specificity is unacceptably low. The graph for option 3 (overall result negative if any test is negative) would be identical to that for option 2 except that the labeling of the axes would be reversed. Adding tests would increase specificity but decrease sensitivity.

As implied by the graphs in Fig. 87-13, not only are the beneficial effects of adding more tests offset by the detrimental effects, but also the incremental increase in accuracy rapidly declines (the sensitivity of four tests is little better than that of three). Thus there appears to be scant justification for using more than two, perhaps three, rarely four tests even if they are totally independent. To illustrate these points, low sensitivities and specificities were deliberately selected for calculating the data in Fig. 87-13. However, the curves would be similar,

though less exaggerated, if higher values had been employed. The *all tests agree* curve would rotate upward and the *any test positive* curve would shift to left and rotate upward. In other words, increasing the sensitivity and specificity of any or all of the tests used would further decrease the relative benefits of adding more tests.

Bayes theorem

The algorithm in Fig. 87-14 illustrates another approach to combining the results of multiple tests. Since any of the tests must be either positive or negative, the number of combinations is equal to 2^n. Thus three tests yield 8 combinations and four tests yield 16 combinations. By means of a retrospective review of accumulated data, one could determine what percentage of a given combination of test results was actually found to be associated with the presence of disease when the results were compared with a diagnostic standard. For example, the combination $A+$, $B-$, $C+$, $D+$ might have a PPV of 94%, whereas another combination, $A-$, $B+$, $C-$, $D-$, might have a PPV of only 8% (a

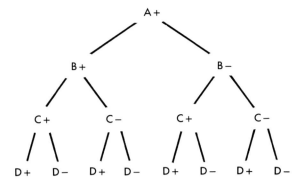

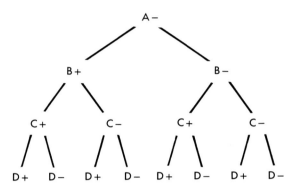

Fig. 87-14. Algorithm illustrating various possible combinations of results from four diagnostic tests.

NPV of 92%). If enough examples of each combination are available for analysis and if the data are continuously updated, this approach provides a rational method of using multiple tests to predict the likelihood of disease.

Bayes theorem provides a mathematic approach to the same problem. In the following calculations, $p(D+)$ denotes the probability that disease is present, and $p(D-)$ denotes the probability of no disease. These symbols refer to the *prior probability* in that these calculations assume knowledge of the prevalence (prior probability) of the disease in the population being studied. Symbolically, prior probability is:

$$p(D+) = \frac{TP + FN}{TN + FN + TP + FP} = \text{Prevalence} \quad (20)$$

Similarly, the prior probability of no disease is

$$p(D-) = \frac{TN + FP}{TN + FN + TP + FP} = 1 - \text{Prevalence} \quad (21)$$

In equations 22 and 23, $p(T+ \mid D+)$ and $p(T+ \mid D-)$ are the *conditional probabilities* that the test will be positive when disease is either

present or absent, respectively, and are expressed symbolically as follows:

$$p(T+ \mid D+) = \frac{TP}{TP + FN} = \text{Sensitivity} \quad (22)$$

$$p(T+ \mid D-) = \frac{FP}{TN + FP} = 1 - \text{Specificity} \quad (23)$$

Bayes theorem calculates the *posterior probability* that disease is present given a positive test result as follows:

$$p(D+ \mid T+) = \quad (24)$$

$$\frac{p(D+) \cdot p(T+ \mid D+)}{p(D+) \cdot p(T+ \mid D+) + p(D-) \cdot p(T+ \mid D-)} =$$

$$\frac{(\text{Prevalence})(\text{Sensitivity})}{(\text{Prevalence})(\text{Sensitivity}) + (1 - \text{Prevalence})(1 - \text{Specificity})} =$$

$$\frac{TP}{FP + TP} = \text{PPV}$$

Thus this formula is merely a complex method of stating the PPV. The conditional probabilities that the test will be negative $(T-)$ when disease is present or absent are expressed as follows:

$$P(T- \mid D+) = \frac{FN}{TP + FN} = 1 - \text{Sensitivity} \quad (25)$$

$$P(T- \mid D-) = \frac{TN}{Tn + FP} = \text{Specificity} \quad (26)$$

The posterior probability that disease is present given a negative test result is:

$$P(D+ \mid T-) = \quad (27)$$

$$\frac{P(D+) \cdot P(T- \mid D+)}{P(D+) \cdot P(T- \mid D+) + P(D-) \cdot P(T- \mid D-)} =$$

$$\frac{(\text{Prevalence})(1 - \text{Sensitivity})}{(\text{Prevalence})(1 - \text{Sensitivity}) + (1 - \text{Prevalence})(\text{Specificity})} =$$

$$\frac{FN}{FN + TN} = 1 - \text{NPV}$$

For any given combination of tests, some of which may be positive (subscript i) and some negative (subscript j), formulas 24 and 27 can be combined to calculate the probability of disease:

$$p(D+ \mid T_{ij}) = \quad (28)$$

$$\frac{(\text{Prevalence})(\text{Sensitivity}_i)(1 - \text{Sensitivity}_j)}{\begin{array}{c}(\text{Prevalence})(\text{Sensitivity}_i)(1 - \text{Sensitivity}_j) + \\ (1 - \text{Prevalence})(1 - \text{Specificity}_i)(\text{Specificity}_j)\end{array}}$$

Consider three tests, A with a sensitivity of 80% and a specificity of 70%, B with a sensitivity of 60% and a specificity of 90%, and C with a sensitivity of 90% and a specificity of 50%. If tests A and B were positive and test C were negative

Table 87-16. Probability of disease (prevalence 30%): random number generator vs. Bayes theorem

Test results			Random number generator				Bayes theorem
A*	B†	C‡	Disease present	Disease absent	Total	Probability of disease	Probability of disease
+	+	+	108	0	108	1.000	.982
+	+	−	44	15	59	.746	.720
+	−	+	20	12	32	.625	.771
+	−	−	9	97	106	.085	.139
−	+	+	14	12	26	.538	.600
−	+	−	9	85	94	.096	.067
−	−	+	3	37	40	.075	.086
−	−	−	3	232	235	.013	.004

*Sensitivity, 90%; specificity, 80%.
†Sensitivity, 80%; specificity, 80%.
‡Sensitivity, 70%; specificity, 80%.

and if the prevalence were 30%, the calculated disease probability would be as follows:

$$\frac{(0.3)(0.8)(0.6)(1 - 0.9)}{(0.3)(0.8)(0.6)(1 - 0.9) + (1 - 0.3)(1 - 0.7)(1 - 0.9)(0.5)} =$$

$$= 0.578$$

Table 87-16 compares the disease probabilities calculated with Bayes theorem to the disease probabilities obtained with a random number generator programmed to simulate an algorithmic analysis of the results of three totally independent tests. The sample included 700 studies, each consisting of the three tests, and, for most of the eight combinations, this sample provided numbers adequate to estimate disease probability. The fact that the results of the two approaches were quite similar supports the validity of Bayes theorem.

Aside from its labor-saving features, the primary advantage of the Bayes approach is that it allows prediction of disease probability for any combination of tests based on knowledge of sensitivity, specificity, and estimated prevalence (prior probability) even when the number of studies previously performed by the laboratory is insufficient to use the algorithmic approach. Moreover, in the event that all three tests could not be performed on a given patient, the Bayes approach would still be applicable. The disadvantage of Bayes theorem—and for that matter, any of the previously discussed schemes for using combinations of tests—is that it is valid only when the tests are totally independent. Obviously, if two tests were similar (as in Fig. 87-10), the results would be fallacious. A further disadvantage is that it presupposes a reasonably accurate estimate of disease prevalence, which varies

ies from time to time in the same laboratory and from one population to the next.

In reality most tests are not entirely independent. For example, even though the methodologies of pulse-delay oculoplethysmography and supraorbital Doppler sonography are dissimilar, both depend on the development of collaterals in response to a hemodynamically significant lesion at the carotid bifurcation. Furthermore, independence is sacrificed when the result of one test is allowed to influence the reading of another. This is especially likely to happen when both tests are interpreted by the same individual. Consequently, most combinations of tests will fall somewhere between the two extremes of providing little or no benefit (all tests measuring the same parameter, as in Fig. 87-11) and providing maximal benefit (all tests independent, as in Fig. 87-12). This generalization applies to all methods used to combine test results.

It is probable that most laboratories employing multiple-test batteries do not adhere to a strict protocol based on the number of positive or negative tests. The natural tendency of the interpreter is to weigh—either consciously or unconsciously—his perception of the relative merits of each test before arriving at a conclusion. No matter how accurate the conclusions, this approach is not particularly satisfying from a scientific viewpoint.

In summary, the use of multiple tests is not without its price. The cost for improving the accuracy of one parameter is borne by the loss of accuracy of another or by an increased incidence of uninterpretable studies. Whether the additional time and expense are justified depends on the goals of the investigator and the demonstration by objective

Table 87-17. Effect of prevalence on posterior probability of disease

Test	Sensitivity	Specificity	Prior probability of disease — Prevalence	Posterior probability of disease (Positive test)		Posterior probability of disease (Negative test)	
				PPV	PPV − Prevalence	1 − NPV	(1 − NPV) − Prevalence
A	0.70	0.90	0.05	0.27	+0.22	0.02	−0.03
			0.40	0.82	+0.42	0.18	−0.22
			0.70	0.94	+0.24	0.44	−0.26
			0.90	0.98	+0.08	0.75	−0.15
B	0.90	0.70	0.05	0.14	+0.09	0.01	−0.04
			0.40	0.67	+0.27	0.09	−0.31
			0.70	0.88	+0.18	0.25	−0.45
			0.90	0.96	+0.06	0.56	−0.34
C	0.90	0.90	0.05	0.32	+0.27	0.01	−0.04
			0.40	0.86	+0.46	0.07	−0.33
			0.70	0.96	+0.26	0.21	−0.49
			0.90	0.99	+0.09	0.50	−0.40

clinical studies that the battery of tests does in fact enhance overall accuracy. Because the point of diminishing returns is rapidly reached as new tests are added, it is usually sufficient to employ two, possibly three, but rarely four well-established, independently read tests based on different physiologic principles.

APPLICATION

In general, very sensitive tests (or batteries of tests, such as option 2) should be selected when the goal is to rule out disease. As indicated in Fig. 87-3, the influence of sensitivity on the NPV far outweighs that of specificity. On the other hand, when confirmation of the presence of disease becomes the primary goal, a very specific test (or battery of tests, such as option 3) should be employed. In other words, PPV is more dependent on specificity than it is on sensitivity (Fig. 87-2). Thus sensitive tests are used to narrow the range of diagnostic hypotheses, and specific tests are used to increase the level of diagnostic confidence when there is a strong clinical suspicion that a certain disease is present. No test can establish the presence or absence of disease with absolute certainty. The purpose of all noninvasive tests is to reduce the range of uncertainty.

As a rule, tests are most helpful when the prior (pretest) probability of disease is in the 50% range and least helpful when the likelihood of disease is either very low or very high. The figures in Table 87-17 illustrate this point. For example, suppose

test B has a sensitivity of 90% and a specificity of 70% and the prior probability of disease was considered to be very small (estimated prevalence = .05); the PPV or posterior (posttest) probability of disease given a positive test result (equation 24) would increase to .14, which represents a change of only +.09 (+9%) from the prior probability (PPV − Prevalence). Similarly, if the results of test B were negative (equation 27), the posterior probability of disease being present (1-NPV) would diminish to .01, a change of only −.04 (−4%). In other words, applying test B to a population in which the prevalence of disease is suspected to be very low would not materially affect the likelihood that the individual patient does or does not have the disease. Even if the results were positive, the odds are still 6 to 1 against him having the disease (.86:.14).

At the other extreme, applying test A with a sensitivity of 70% and a specificity of 90% to a population with a high likelihood of disease (90%) would increase the likelihood by only 8% if the test were positive and would decrease the likelihood by a modest 15% if the test were negative. Even with a negative test, the odds are still 3 to 1 that the patient has the disease (.75:.25). Consequently, one would be reluctant to discard the diagnosis based on a negative test result.

If the prior probability were 70% (which in our experience approximates the probability that a patient referred to our laboratory with a clinical diagnosis of transient ischemic attack [TIA] will have

Table 87-18. Apparent prevalence compared with true prevalence of disease

Noninvasive test results	True distribution		Noninvasive test total
	Negative	**Positive**	
Negative	855	5	860
Positive	95	45	140
TRUE TOTAL	950	50	1000

Apparent prevalence, 14%; true prevalence 5%.

a lesion in the appropriate carotid artery) and test C, with a sensitivity and specificity of 90%, were applied, the posterior probability given a positive result would rise to .96—virtually confirming the presence of disease. A negative result would lower the probability of disease significantly to .21, stimulating one to consider other diagnoses. In other words, with a negative result the odds against the patient having the disease rise from .4:1 to 3.8:1. Of course, the decision to discard a diagnosis will depend not only on the posterior probability of disease but also on one's clinical judgment regarding the potential harm that would ensue if vital treatment were withheld. Therefore if the patient had had a classic TIA, most clinicians would still pursue the diagnosis of carotid disease despite a negative test result. On the other hand, the decision to accept a positive diagnosis will depend on the potential harm that would ensue from a FP diagnosis.

Table 87-17 further confirms what has been mentioned about the relative value of sensitivity and specificity for diagnosing or ruling out disease. A positive result with a very specific test, such as test A or C, will greatly increase the posterior probability of disease in the middle ranges of prevalence; whereas a negative result with a very sensitive test, such as test B or C, will significantly reduce the likelihood that disease is present.

After the first test (or series of tests) has been performed, the clinician may then decide whether further tests are necessary. For the second test, the posterior probability following the first test now becomes the prior probability (estimated prevalence) for the second test. Remembering this fact may influence the decision to select a highly sensitive or highly specific test. The ultimate results of any series of tests follow the precepts of Bayes theorem.

Interpretation of screening tests must be done cautiously. Consider a population in which the true prevalence of disease is only 5% (Table 87-18). If, in an attempt to assess the prevalence of disease, a highly sensitive (90%) and specific (90%) test is used, the investigator may conclude that the prevalence is much higher, 14%. This, in fact, was the conclusion of a study in which noninvasive tests with this degree of accuracy were used to ascertain the prevalence of >75% stenosis of the internal carotid artery in a series of patients undergoing cardiovascular and peripheral vascular surgery. Although the use of the test does define two populations—one with a greater likelihood of having the disease than the other—any inferences regarding the true prevalence of disease are likely to be quite inaccurate.

BIBLIOGRAPHY

1. Beyer, W.H., editor: Handbook of tables for probability and statistics, ed. 2, Boca Raton, Fla., 1968, CRC Press, Inc.
2. Cohen, J.: A coefficient of agreement for nominal scales, Educ. Psychol. Measures 20:37, 1960.
3. Cohen, J.: Weighted kappa: nominal scale agreement with provision for scaled disagreement or partial credit, Psychol. Bull. 70:213, 1968.
4. Colton, T.: Statistics in medicine, Boston, 1974, Little, Brown, & Co.
5. Griner, P.F., et al.: Selection and interpretation of diagnostic tests and procedures. Principles and application, Ann. Intern. Med. 94:553, 1981.
6. Hall, G.H.: The clinical application of Bayes' theorem, Lancet 2:555, 1967.
7. Haynes, R.B.: Interpretation of diagnostic data. 2. How to do it with a simple table (part A), Can. Med. Assoc. J. 129:559, 1983.
8. Haynes, R.B.: Interpretation of diagnostic data. 3. How to do it with a simple table (part B), Can. Med. Assoc. J. 129:705, 1983.
9. Ingelfinger, J.A., et al.: Biostatistics in clinical medicine, New York, 1983, Macmillan, Inc.
10. Lusted, L.B.: Introduction to medical decision making, Springfield, Ill., 1968, Charles C Thomas, Publisher.
11. McNeil, B.J., Keeler, E., and Adelstein, S.J.: Primer on certain elements of medical decision making, N. Engl. J. Med. 293:211, 1975.
12. Metz, C.E.: Basic principles of ROC analysis, Semin. Nucl. Med. 8:283, 1978.
13. Sackett, D.L.: Interpretation of diagnostic data. 1. How to do it with pictures, Can. Med. Assoc. J. 129:429, 1983.
14. Sackett, D.L.: Interpretation of diagnostic data. 5. How to do it with simple maths, Can. Med. Assoc. J. 129:947, 1983.
14a. Sumner, D.S.: Noninvasive investigation of the arterial supply to the brain and eye. In Warlow, C., and Morris, P.J., editors: Transient ischemic attack, New York, 1982, Marcel Dekker, Inc.
15. Trout, K.S.: Interpretation of diagnostic data. 6. How to do it with more complex maths, Can. Med. Assoc. J. 129:1093, 1983.
16. Tugwell, P.X.: Interpretation of diagnostic data. 4. How to do it with a more complex table, Can. Med. Assoc. J. 129:832, 1983.
17. Vecchio, T.J.: Predictive value of a single diagnostic test in unselected populations, N. Engl. J. Med. 274:1171, 1966.

INDEX